Place-of-Service Codes for Professional Claims

Listed below are place-of-service codes and descriptions. These codes should be used on professional claims to specify the entity where service(s) were rendered. Check with individual payers (eg, Medicare, Medicaid, other private insurance) for reimbursement policies regarding these codes. If you would like to comment on a code(s) or description(s), please send your request to posinfo@cms.hhs.gov.

Place of Service Code(s)	Place of Service Name	Place of Service Description
01	Pharmacy	A facility or location where drugs and other medically related items and services are sold, dispensed, or otherwise provided directly to patients. (Effective 10/1/05)
02	Unassigned	N/A
03	School	A facility whose primary purpose is education.
04	Homeless Shelter	A facility or location whose primary purpose is to provide temporary housing to homeless individuals (eg, emergency shelters, individual or family shelters).
05	Indian Health Service Free-Standing Facility	A facility or location, owned and operated by the Indian Health Service, which provides diagnostic, therapeutic (surgical and non-surgical), and rehabilitation services to American Indians and Alaska Natives who do not require hospitalization.
06	Indian Health Service Provider-Based Facility	A facility or location, owned and operated by the Indian Health Service, which provides diagnostic, therapeutic (surgical and non-surgical), and rehabilitation services rendered by, or under the supervision of, physicians to American Indians and Alaska Natives admitted as inpatients or outpatients.
07	Tribal 638 Free-Standing Facility	A facility or location owned and operated by a federally recognized American Indian or Alaska Native tribe or tribal organization under a 638 agreement which provides diagnostic, therapeutic (surgical and non-surgical), and rehabilitation services to tribal members who do not require hospitalization.
08	Tribal 638 Provider-Based Facility	A facility or location owned and operated by a federally recognized American Indian or Alaska Native tribe or tribal organization under a 638 agreement which provides diagnostic, therapeutic (surgical and non-surgical), and rehabilitation services to tribal members admitted as inpatients or outpatients.
09	Prison/Correctional Facility	A prison, jail, reformatory, work farm, detention center, or any other similar facility maintained by either Federal, State, or local authorities for the purpose of confinement or rehabilitation of adult or juvenile criminal offenders. (Effective 7/1/06)
10	Unassigned	N/A
11	Office	Location, other than a hospital, skilled nursing facility (SNF), military treatment facility, community health center, State or local public health clinic, or intermediate care facility (ICF), where the health professional routinely provides health examinations, diagnosis, and treatment of illness or injury on an ambulatory basis.
12	Home	Location, other than a hospital or other facility, where the patient receives care in a private residence.
13	Assisted Living Facility	Congregate residential facility with self-contained living units providing assessment of each resident's needs and on-site support 24 hours a day, 7 days a week, with the capacity to deliver or arrange for services including some health care and other services. (Effective 10/1/03)
14	Group Home	A residence, with shared living areas, where clients receive supervision and other services such as social and/or behavioral services, custodial service, and minimal services (eg, medication administration). (Effective 10/1/03)
15	Mobile Unit	A facility/unit that moves from place-to-place equipped to provide preventive, screening, diagnostic, and/or treatment services.
16	Temporary Lodging	A short term accommodation such as a hotel, camp ground, hostel, cruise ship or resort where the patient receives care, and which is not identified by any other POS code. (Effective 4/1/08)
17	Walk-in Retail Health Clinic	A walk-in health clinic, other than an office, urgent care facility, pharmacy, or independent clinic, which is not described by any other Place of Service code, that is located within a retail operation and provides, on an ambulatory basis, preventive and primary care services. (Effective 5/1/10)
18	Place of Employment—Worksite	A location, not described by any other POS code, owned or operated by a public or private entity where the patient is employed, and where a health professional provides on-going or episodic occupational medical, therapeutic or rehabilitative services to the individual. (This code is available for use effective January 1, 2013 but no later than May 1, 2013.)
19	Unassigned	N/A
20	Urgent Care Facility	Location, distinct from a hospital emergency room, an office, or a clinic, whose purpose is to diagnose and treat illness or injury for unscheduled, ambulatory patients seeking immediate medical attention. (Effective 1/1/03)
21	Inpatient Hospital	A facility, other than psychiatric, which primarily provides diagnostic, therapeutic (both surgical and non-surgical), and rehabilitation services by, or under, the supervision of physicians to patients admitted for a variety of medical conditions.
22	Outpatient Hospital	A portion of a hospital which provides diagnostic, therapeutic (both surgical and non-surgical), and rehabilitation services to sick or injured persons who do not require hospitalization or institutionalization.
23	Emergency Room—Hospital	A portion of a hospital where emergency diagnosis and treatment of illness or injury is provided.
24	Ambulatory Surgical Center	A free-standing facility, other than a physician's office, where surgical and diagnostic services are provided on an ambulatory basis.
25	Birthing Center	A facility, other than a hospital's maternity facilities or a physician's office, which provides a setting for labor, delivery, and immediate postpartum care as well as immediate care of newborn infants.
26	Military Treatment Facility	A medical facility operated by one or more of the Uniformed Services. Military treatment facility (MTF) also refers to certain former U.S. Public Health Service (USPHS) facilities now designated as Uniformed Service Treatment Facilities (USTF).
27-30	Unassigned	N/A

31	Skilled Nursing Facility	A facility that primarily provides inpatient skilled nursing care and related services to patients who require medical, nursing, or rehabilitative services but does not provide the level of care or treatment available in a hospital.
32	Nursing Facility	A facility that primarily provides to residents skilled nursing care and related services for the rehabilitation of injured, disabled, or sick persons, or, on a regular basis, health-related care services above the level of custodial care to other than mentally retarded individuals.
33	Custodial Care Facility	A facility that provides room, board, and other personal assistance services, generally on a long-term basis, and which does not include a medical component.
34	Hospice	A facility, other than a patient's home, in which palliative and supportive care for terminally ill patients and their families are provided.
35-40	Unassigned	N/A
41	Ambulance—Land	A land vehicle specifically designed, equipped and staffed for lifesaving and transporting the sick or injured.
42	Ambulance—Air or Water	An air or water vehicle specifically designed, equipped, and staffed for lifesaving and transporting the sick or injured.
43-48	Unassigned	N/A
49	Independent Clinic	A location, not part of a hospital and not described by any other Place of Service code, that is organized and operated to provide preventive, diagnostic, therapeutic, rehabilitative, or palliative services to outpatients only. (Effective 10/1/03)
50	Federally Qualified Health Center	A facility located in a medically underserved area that provides Medicare beneficiaries preventive primary medical care under the general direction of a physician.
51	Inpatient Psychiatric Facility	A facility that provides inpatient psychiatric services for the diagnosis and treatment of mental illness on a 24-hour basis, by or under the supervision of a physician.
52	Psychiatric Facility—Partial Hospitalization	A facility for the diagnosis and treatment of mental illness that provides a planned therapeutic program for patients who do not require full time hospitalization, but who need broader programs than are possible from outpatient visits to a hospital-based or hospital-affiliated facility.
53	Community Mental Health Center	A facility that provides the following services: outpatient services, including specialized outpatient services for children, the elderly, individuals who are chronically ill, and residents of the CMHC's mental health services area who have been discharged from inpatient treatment at a mental health facility; 24 hour a day emergency care services; day treatment, other partial hospitalization services, or psychosocial rehabilitation services; screening for patients being considered for admission to State mental health facilities to determine the appropriateness of such admission; and consultation and education services.
54	Intermediate Care Facility/Mentally Retarded	A facility that primarily provides health-related care and services above the level of custodial care to mentally retarded individuals but does not provide the level of care or treatment available in a hospital or SNF.
55	Residential Substance Abuse Treatment Facility	A facility which provides treatment for substance (alcohol and drug) abuse to live-in residents who do not require acute medical care. Services include individual and group therapy and counseling, family counseling, laboratory tests, drugs and supplies, psychological testing, and room and board.
56	Psychiatric Residential Treatment Center	A facility or distinct part of a facility for psychiatric care which provides a total 24-hour therapeutically planned and professionally staffed group living and learning environment.
57	Non-residential Substance Abuse Treatment Facility	A location that provides treatment for substance (alcohol and drug) abuse on an ambulatory basis. Services include individual and group therapy and counseling, family counseling, laboratory tests, drugs and supplies, and psychological testing. (Effective 10/1/03)
58-59	Unassigned	N/A
60	Mass Immunization Center	A location where providers administer pneumococcal pneumonia and influenza virus vaccinations and submit these services as electronic media claims, paper claims, or using the roster billing method. This generally takes place in a mass immunization setting, such as, a public health center, pharmacy, or mall but may include a physician office setting.
61	Comprehensive Inpatient Rehabilitation Facility	A facility that provides comprehensive rehabilitation services under the supervision of a physician to inpatients with physical disabilities. Services include physical therapy, occupational therapy, speech pathology, social or psychological services, and orthotics and prosthetics services.
62	Comprehensive Outpatient Rehabilitation Facility	A facility that provides comprehensive rehabilitation services under the supervision of a physician to outpatients with physical disabilities. Services include physical therapy, occupational therapy, and speech pathology services.
63-64	Unassigned	N/A
65	End-Stage Renal Disease Treatment Facility	A facility other than a hospital, which provides dialysis treatment, maintenance, and/or training to patients or caregivers on an ambulatory or home-care basis.
66-70	Unassigned	N/A
71	Public Health Clinic	A facility maintained by either State or local health departments that provides ambulatory primary medical care under the general direction of a physician.
72	Rural Health Clinic	A certified facility which is located in a rural medically underserved area that provides ambulatory primary medical care under the general direction of a physician.
73-80	Unassigned	N/A
81	Independent Laboratory	A laboratory certified to perform diagnostic and/or clinical tests independent of an institution or a physician's office.
82-98	Unassigned	N/A
99	Other Place of Service	Other place of service not identified above.

current procedural terminology

cpt® 2016

Standard Edition

Jay T. Ahlman
Angela J. Boudreau
Judy Connelly
Rick A. Crosslin
Biljana Dimovski, MS, RHM, CDC
Martha Espronceda
Desiree D. Evans, AAS
Lauren M. Feldman

DeHandro Hayden, BS
Nadia Khalid, MJ, RHIA, RMM
Elizabeth Lumakovska, MPA, RHIT
Janette Meggs, RHIA
Marie L. Mindeman, BA, RHIT
Karen E. O'Hara, BS, CCS-P
Mary R. O'Heron, RHIA
Danielle Pavloski, BS, RHIT, CCS-P

Desiree Rozell, MPA
Nancy Spector, BSN, MSC
Lianne Stancik, RHIT
Ada Walker, CCA
Arletrice Watkins, MHA, RHIA
Rejina L. Young

AMA
AMERICAN MEDICAL
ASSOCIATION

Standard ISBN: 978-1-62202-208-3
ISSN: 0276-8283

Foreword

Current Procedural Terminology (CPT®), Fourth Edition, is a listing of descriptive terms and identifying codes for reporting medical services and procedures performed by physicians. The purpose of the terminology is to provide a uniform language that will accurately describe medical, surgical, and diagnostic services, and will thereby provide an effective means for reliable nationwide communication among physicians, patients, and third parties. *CPT 2016* is the most recent revision of a work that first appeared in 1966.

CPT descriptive terms and identifying codes currently serve a wide variety of important functions in the field of medical nomenclature. The CPT code set is useful for administrative management purposes such as claims processing and for the development of guidelines for medical care review. The uniform language is also applicable to medical education and outcomes, health services, and quality research by providing a useful basis for local, regional, and national utilization comparisons. The CPT code set is the most widely accepted nomenclature for the reporting of physician procedures and services under government and private health insurance programs. In 2000, the CPT code set was designated by the Department of Health and Human Services as the national coding standard for physician and other health care professional services and procedures under the Health Insurance Portability and Accountability Act (HIPAA). This means that for all financial and administrative health care transactions sent electronically, the CPT code set will need to be used.

The changes that appear in this revision have been prepared by the CPT Editorial Panel with the assistance of physicians representing all specialties of medicine, and with important contributions from many third-party payers and governmental agencies.

The American Medical Association trusts that this revision will continue the usefulness of its predecessors in identifying, describing, and coding medical, surgical, and diagnostic services.

Acknowledgments

Publication of the annual CPT codebook represents many challenges and opportunities. From reconciling the many differences of opinion about the best way to describe a procedure, to the last details on placement of a semicolon, many individuals and organizations devote their energies and expertise to the preparation of this revision.

The editorial staff wishes to express sincere thanks to the many national medical specialty societies, health insurance organizations and agencies, and individual physicians and other health professionals who have made contributions.

Thanks are due to Claudia Bonnell, Blue Cross and Blue Shield Association; Nelly Leon-Chisen, American Hospital Association; Sue Bowman, RHIA, American Health Information Management Association; and Raemarie Jiminez, CPC, American Academy of Professional Coders, for their invaluable assistance in enhancing the CPT code set.

AMA CPT Editorial Panel

Chair
Peter A. Hollmann, MD*

Vice-Chair
Kenneth P. Brin, MD, PhD, FACC*

Albert E. Bothe, Jr, MD, FACS
Boyd R. Buser, DO, FACOFP
Leslie F. Davidson, PhD, OTR/L
Frank J. Dubeck, Jr, MD, FACP*
Richard Duszak, Jr, MD, FACR*
David A. Ellington, MD
Edith Hambrick, MD, JD
R. Patrick Jacob, MD, FACS†
Christopher L. Jagmin, MD
Katharine Krol, MD, FSIR, FACR
Bernard A. Pfeifer, MD
Julia M. Pillsbury, DO, FAAP, FACOP
Jordan G. Pritzker, MD, MBA, FACOG†
Antonio E. Puente, PhD
Mark S. Synovec, MD*

Secretary
Marie L. Mindeman, BA, RHIT

*Member of the CPT Executive Committee
†New Panel Member
‡New Advisors

AMA CPT Advisory Committee

American Academy of Allergy, Asthma and Immunology
Donald W. Aaronson, MD, JD, MPH

American Academy of Child & Adolescent Psychiatry
Benjamin N. Shain, MD, PhD
Jason Chang, MD‡

American Academy of Dermatology
Alexander Miller, MD
Ann F. Haas, MD

American Academy of Disability Evaluating Physicians
Douglas W. Martin, MD, FAADEP, FACOEM
James B. Talmage, MD

American Academy of Family Physicians
Robert J. Carr, Jr, MD
Gretchen M. Dickson, MD, MBA

American Academy of Neurology
Marc R. Nuwer, MD, PhD, FAAN, FACP
Bruce H. Cohen, MD, FAAN

American Academy of Ophthalmology
Michael X. Repka, MD, MBA
John M. Haley, MD

American Academy of Orthopaedic Surgeons
Richard J. Friedman, MD, FACSC
M. Bradford Henley, MD, MBA

American Academy of Otolaryngic Allergy
Paul T. Fass, MD, FACS

American Academy of Otolaryngology Head and Neck Surgery
Bradley F. Marple, MD, FAAOA
Lawrence M. Simon, MD, FAAP

American Academy of Pain Medicine
Eduardo M. Fraifeld, MD

American Academy of Pediatrics
Joel F. Bradley, Jr, MD, FAAP
David M. Kanter, MD, MBA, CPC, FAAP‡

American Academy of Physical Medicine and Rehabilitation
Jeffrey S. Brault, DO
Annie D. Purcell, DO

American Academy of Sleep Medicine
Dennis Hwang, MD‡
William C. Sherrill, Jr, MD

American Association for Clinical Chemistry
William A. Clark, PhD, DABCC, FACB

American Association for Thoracic Surgery
Kirk R. Kanter, MD
Stephen J. Lahey, MD

American Association of Clinical Endocrinologists
Eric A. Orzeck, MD, FACP, FACE
William C. Biggs, MD, FACE, ECNU‡

American Association of Neurological Surgeons
Joseph S. Cheng, MD, MS, FACS, FAANS‡
Jeffrey W. Cozzens, MD, FACS‡

American Association of Neuromuscular and Electrodiagnostic Medicine
John C. Kincaid, MD‡

American Clinical Neurophysiology Society
Marc R. Nuwer, MD, PhD, FAAN, FACP
Ronald G. Emerson, MD

American College of Allergy, Asthma and Immunology
Gary N. Gross, MD

American College of Cardiology
Robert N. Piana, MD, FACC
Randall C. Thompson, MD

American College of Chest Physicians
Steve G. Peters, MD
Michael E. Nelson, MD, FCCP

American College of Emergency Physicians
Kenneth L. DeHart, MD, FACEP
Jacob Mark J. Meredith, III, MD, MMM, FACEP

American College of Gastroenterology
Christopher Y. Kim, MD, MBA, FACG, FASGE, AGAF, FACP
Daniel C. DeMarco, MD, FACG

American College of Medical Genetics and Genomics
David B. Flannery, MD

American College of Medical Quality
Joel Grossman, MD

American College of Mohs Surgery
David B. Pharis, MD, PC

American College of Nuclear Medicine
Scott C. Bartley, MD

American College of Occupational and Environmental Medicine
Lee S. Glass, MD, JD

American College of Phlebology
Bruce R. Hoyle, MD‡

American College of Physicians
Jeannine Z. Engel, MD, FACP
Tiffany R. Groover, MD, MPH‡

American College of Radiation Oncology
Andy W. Su, MD
Paul E. Wallner, DO, FACR, FAOCR, FASTRO, FACRO

American College of Radiology
Daniel Picus, MD, FACR, RCC
Timothy A. Crummy, MD, RCC

American College of Rheumatology
Gerald M. Eisenberg, MD, FACP, FACR
Robert J. Lloyd, MD, FACP, FACR

American College of Surgeons
Linda M. Barney, MD, FACS
Mark T. Savarise, MD, FACS

American Congress of Obstetricians and Gynecologists
Judith K. Volkar, MD
Mark R. Hoffman, MD‡

American Dental Association
Anthony M. Spina, DDS, MD
Joshua E. Everts, DDS, MD

American Gastroenterological Association
Joel V. Brill, MD, FACP, AGAF
Braden Kuo, MD‡

American Geriatrics Society
Robert A. Zorowitz, MD, MBA, FACP, AGSF, CMD

American Institute of Ultrasound in Medicine
Harvey L. Nisenbaum, MD

American Medical Directors Association
Dennis L. Stone, MD, MBA

American Orthopaedic Association
Blair C. Filler, MD

American Orthopaedic Foot and Ankle Society
Walter J. Pedowitz, MD
David I. Pedowitz, MD

American Osteopathic Association
Judith A. O'Connell, DO, FAAO
Brian E. Kaufman, DO

American Psychiatric Association
David K. Nace, MD
Jeremy S. Musher, MD

American Roentgen Ray Society
Mark D. Alson, MD, FACR, RCC

American Society for Aesthetic Plastic Surgery, Inc.
Paul R. Weiss, MD

American Society for Clinical Pathology
Lee H. Hilborne, MD, MPH, FASCP

American Society for Dermatologic Surgery
Murad Alam, MD
Jeremy S. Bordeaux, MD, MPH

American Society for Gastrointestinal Endoscopy
Glenn D. Littenberg, MD, MACP

American Society for Metabolic and Bariatric Surgery
Matthew L. Brengman, MD‡

American Society for Radiation Oncology
William F. Hartsell, MD

American Society for Reproductive Medicine
Beth W. Rackow, MD, FACOG‡

American Society for Surgery of the Hand
Daniel J. Nagle, MD
Leon S. Benson, MD

American Society of Anesthesiologists
Peter A. Goldzweig, DO
Kevin E. Vorenkamp, MD

American Society of Cataract and Refractive Surgery
Stephen S. Lane, MD

American Society of Clinical Oncology
Christian A. Thomas, MD

American Society of Colon and Rectal Surgeons
Stephen M. Sentovich, MD, MBA, FACS, FASCRS
William J. Harb, MD, FACS

American Society of Cytopathology
Carol A. Filomena, MD

American Society of General Surgeons
George K. Gillian, MD, FACS
Christopher C. Smith, MD

American Society of Hematology
Samuel M. Silver, MD, PhD, FACP, FAHA
Robert Weinstein, MD

American Society of Interventional Pain Physicians
Frank J.E. Falco, MD
Sachin Jha, MD, MS

American Society of Neuroradiology
Raymond K. Tu, MD, FACR
Jacqueline A. Bello, MD, FACR

American Society of Ophthalmic Plastic and Reconstructive Surgery
L. Neal Freeman, MD, MBA, CCS-P, FACS

American Society of Plastic Surgeons
Raymond V. Janevicius, MD
Deborah S. Bash, MD

American Thoracic Society
Stephen P. Hoffmann, MD

American Urological Association
Jeffrey A. Dann, MD, MBA
Ronald P. Kaufman, Jr, MD, FACS

Association of University Radiologists
Robert K. Zeman, MD, FACR

College of American Pathologists
Michael D. McEachin, MD
Ronald W. McLawhon, MD, PhD‡

Congress of Neurological Surgeons
Henry H. Woo, MD, FACS, FAANS‡

Heart Rhythm Society
Oussama M. Wazni, MD
Joseph E. Marine, MD

Infectious Disease Society of America
Steven K. Schmitt, MD
Lyssette L. Cardona, MD, MPH, MSHA

International Society for the Advancement of Spine Surgery
Morgan L. Lorio, MD, FACS‡

International Spinal Intervention Society
Scott I. Horn, DO
Claire Tibiletti, MD

National Association of Medical Examiners
John S. Denton, MD

North American Spine Society
William Mitchell, MD
David R. O'Brien, Jr, MD

Radiological Society of North America
Timothy A. Crummy, MD
Eric M. Rubin, MD‡

Renal Physicians Association
Chester A. Amedia, Jr, MD, FACP
Timothy A. Pflederer, MD

Society for Cardiovascular Angiography and Interventions
Arthur C. Lee, MD, FSCAI

Society for Investigative Dermatology
Stephen P. Stone, MD

Society for Vascular Surgery
Sean P. Roddy, MD, FACS

Society of American Gastrointestinal Endoscopic Surgeons
John S. Roth, MD, FACS
Kevin E. Wasco, MD, FACS

Society of Critical Care Medicine
George A. Sample, MD, FCCP

Society of Interventional Radiology
Timothy L. Swan, MD
Donald F. Denny, Jr, MD

Society of Nuclear Medicine and Molecular Imaging
Gary L. Dillehay, MD, FACNP, FACR

Society of Thoracic Surgeons
Francis C. Nichols, III, MD
Jeffrey P. Jacobs, MD, FACS, FACC, FCCP

The Endocrine Society
Carol H. Wysham, MD‡

The Triological Society
Richard W. Waguespack, MD, FACS

United States and Canadian Academy of Pathology
David S. Wilkinson, MD, PhD

AMA Health Care Professionals Advisory Committee (HCPAC)

Peter A. Hollmann, MD*, Co-Chair
AMA CPT Editorial Panel
Antonio E. Puente, PhD, Co-Chair
AMA CPT Editorial Panel

Academy of Nutrition and Dietetics
Keith-Thomas Ayoob, EdD, RN, FADA, CSP
Jessie M. Pavlianc, MS, RD, CSR, LD

American Academy of Audiology
Brad A. Stach, PhD
Paul M. Pessis, AuD

American Academy of Physician Assistants
Patrick J. Cafferty, MPAS, PA-C

American Association of Naturopathic Physicians
Wendell B. Milliman, ND
Eva Miller, ND

American Association for Respiratory Care
Susan Rinaldo-Gallo, MEd, RRT, FAARC

American Chiropractic Association
Leo Bronston DC, MAppSc

American Massage Therapy Association
Nancy M. Porambo, BA, MS, LMT, NCTMB
Glyn Desmond, LMP‡

American Nurses Association
Jamesetta A. Newland, PhD, RN, FNP-BC, FAANP, DPNAP
Leslie C. Verucci, RN, MSN, CNS, CRNP, APRN-BC

American Occupational Therapy Association
Mary Jo McGuire, MS, OTR/L, FAOTA
Doris J. Shriver, OTR, FAOTA, QRC, CLCP

American Optometric Association
Douglas C. Morrow, OD
Rebecca H. Wartman, OD

American Physical Therapy Association
Helene M. Fearon, PT
Kathleen M. Picard, PT

American Podiatric Medical Association
Phillip E. Ward, DPM
Ira H. Kraus, DPM

American Psychological Association
Neil H. Pliskin, PhD, ABPP-CN
Randy E. Phelps, PhD

American Speech-Language-Hearing Association
Stuart G. Trembath, MA, CCC-A

National Athletic Trainers' Association
Karen D. Fennell, MS, ATC
Clark E. Simpson, MBA, Med, ATC‡

National Association of Social Workers
Mirean F. Coleman, MSW, LICSW

National Society of Genetic Counselors
Leslie H. Cohen, MS, CGC

Pharmacy Health Information Technology Collaborative
Daniel E. Buffington, PharmD, MBA
Brian J. Isetts, PhD, BCPS, FAPhA‡

Contents

Contents

Introduction

Current Procedural Terminology (CPT®), Fourth Edition, is a set of codes, descriptions, and guidelines intended to describe procedures and services performed by physicians and other health care professionals, or entities. Each procedure or service is identified with a five-digit code. The use of CPT codes simplifies the reporting of procedures and services. In the CPT code set, the term "procedure" is used to describe services, including diagnostic tests.

Inclusion of a descriptor and its associated five-digit code number in the CPT Category I code set is based on whether the procedure or service is consistent with contemporary medical practice and is performed by many practitioners in clinical practice in multiple locations. Inclusion in the CPT code set does not represent endorsement by the American Medical Association (AMA) of any particular diagnostic or therapeutic procedure or service. Inclusion or exclusion of a procedure or service does not imply any health insurance coverage or reimbursement policy.

The CPT code set is published annually in the late summer or early fall as both electronic data files and books. The release of CPT data files on the Internet typically precedes the book by several weeks. In any case, January 1 is the effective date for use of the update of the CPT code set. The interval between the release of the update and the effective date is considered the implementation period and is intended to allow physicians and other providers, payers, and vendors to incorporate CPT changes into their systems. The exceptions to this schedule of release and effective dates are CPT Category III and vaccine product codes, which are released twice a year on January 1 or July 1 with effective dates for use six months later, and CPT Category II codes. Changes to the CPT code set are meant to be applied prospectively from the effective date.

The main body of the Category I section is listed in six sections. Each section is divided into subsections with anatomic, procedural, condition, or descriptor subheadings. The procedures and services with their identifying codes are presented in numeric order with one exception—the entire **Evaluation and Management** section (99201-99499) appears at the beginning of the listed procedures. These items are used by most physicians in reporting a significant portion of their services.

Section Numbers and Their Sequences

Evaluation and Management 99201-99499

Anesthesiology 00100-01999, 99100-99140

Surgery 10021-69990

Radiology (Including Nuclear Medicine
and Diagnostic Ultrasound) 70010-79999

Pathology and Laboratory 80047-89398

Medicine (except
Anesthesiology) 90281-99199, 99500-99607

The first and last code numbers and the subsection name of the items appear at the top margin of most pages (eg, "11010-11306 Surgery/Integumentary System"). The continuous pagination of the CPT codebook is found on the lower margin of each page along with explanation of any code symbols that are found on that page.

Instructions for Use of the CPT Codebook

Select the name of the procedure or service that accurately identifies the service performed. Do not select a CPT code that merely approximates the service provided. If no such specific code exists, then report the service using the appropriate unlisted procedure or service code. In surgery, it may be an operation; in medicine, a diagnostic or therapeutic procedure; in radiology, a radiograph. Other additional procedures performed or pertinent special services are also listed. When necessary, any modifying or extenuating circumstances are added. Any service or procedure should be adequately documented in the medical record.

It is equally important to recognize that as techniques in medicine and surgery have evolved, new types of services, including minimally invasive surgery, as well as endovascular, percutaneous, and endoscopic interventions have challenged the traditional distinction of Surgery vs Medicine. Thus, the listing of a service or procedure in a specific section of this book should not be interpreted as strictly classifying the service or procedure as "surgery" or "not surgery" for insurance or other purposes. The placement of a given service in a specific section of the book may reflect historical or other considerations (eg, placement of the percutaneous peripheral vascular endovascular interventions in the Surgery/Cardiovascular System section, while the percutaneous coronary interventions appear in the Medicine/Cardiovascular section).

When advanced practice nurses and physician assistants are working with physicians, they are considered as working in the exact same specialty and exact same subspecialties as the physician. A "physician or other qualified health care professional" is an individual who is qualified by education, training, licensure/regulation (when applicable), and facility privileging (when applicable) who performs a professional service within his/her scope of practice and independently reports that professional service. These professionals are distinct from "clinical staff." A clinical staff member is a person who works under the supervision of a physician or other qualified health care professional and who is allowed by law, regulation, and facility policy to perform or assist in the performance of a specified professional service, but who does not individually report that professional service. Other policies may also affect who may report specific services.

Throughout the CPT code set the use of terms such as "physician," "qualified health care professional," or "individual" is not intended to indicate that other entities may not report the service. In selected instances, specific instructions may define a service as limited to professionals or limited to other entities (eg, hospital or home health agency).

Instructions, typically included as parenthetical notes with selected codes, indicate that a code should not be reported with another code or codes. These instructions are intended to prevent errors of significant probability and are not all inclusive. For example, the code with such instructions may be a component of another code and therefore it would be incorrect to report both codes even when the component service is performed. These instructions are not intended as a listing of all possible code combinations that should not be reported, nor do they indicate all possible code combinations that are appropriately reported. When reporting codes for services provided, it is important to assure the accuracy and quality of coding through verification of the intent of the code by use of the related guidelines, parenthetical instructions, and coding resources, including *CPT Assistant* and other publications resulting from collaborative efforts of the American Medical Association with the medical specialty societies (ie, *Clinical Examples in Radiology*).

Format of the Terminology

The CPT code set has been developed as stand-alone descriptions of medical procedures. However, some of the procedures in the CPT codebook are not printed in their entirety but refer back to a common portion of the procedure listed in a preceding entry. This is evident when an entry is followed by one or more indentations. This is done in an effort to conserve space.

Example

25100 Arthrotomy, wrist joint; with biopsy

25105   with synovectomy

Note that the common part of code 25100 (the part before the semicolon) should also be considered part of code 25105. Therefore, the full procedure represented by code 25105 should read:

25105 Arthrotomy, wrist joint; with synovectomy

Requests to Update the CPT Nomenclature

The effectiveness of the CPT nomenclature depends on constant updating to reflect changes in medical practice. This can only be accomplished through the interest and timely suggestions of practicing physicians and other qualified health care professionals, specialty/professional societies, state medical associations, organizations, agencies, individual users of the CPT code set, and other stakeholders. Accordingly, the AMA welcomes correspondence, inquiries, and suggestions concerning CPT coding and nomenclature for old and new procedures and services, as well as any matters relating to the CPT code set.

For information on submission of an application to add, delete, or revise codes contained in the CPT code set, please see www.ama-assn.org/go/cpt-processfaq or contact:

CPT Editorial Research & Development
American Medical Association
330 North Wabash Avenue
Suite 39300
Chicago IL 60611-5885

Code change applications are available at the AMA's CPT website: www.ama-assn.org/go/cpt-application.

All proposed changes to the CPT code set will be considered by the CPT Editorial Panel, in consultation with medical specialty societies as represented by the CPT Advisory Committee, other health care professional societies as represented by the Health Care Professionals Advisory Committee (HCPAC), and other interested parties.

Application Submission Requirements

All complete CPT code change applications are reviewed and evaluated by the CPT staff, the CPT/HCPAC Advisory Committee, and the CPT Editorial Panel. Strict conformance with the following is required for review of a code change application:

- Submission of a complete application, including all necessary supporting documents
- Adherence to all posted deadlines
- Cooperation with requests from the CPT staff and/or Editorial Panel members for clarification and information; *and*
- Compliance with CPT Lobbying Policy

General Criteria for Category I and Category III Codes

All Category I or Category III code change applications must satisfy each of the following criteria:

- The proposed descriptor is unique, well-defined, and describes a procedure or service that is clearly identified and distinguished from existing procedures and services already in the CPT code set.
- The descriptor structure, guidelines, and instructions are consistent with the current CPT Editorial Panel standards for maintenance of the code set.
- The proposed descriptor for the procedure or service is neither a fragmentation of an existing procedure or service nor currently reportable as a complete service by one or more existing codes (with the exclusion of unlisted codes). However, procedures and services frequently performed together may require new or revised codes.
- The structure and content of the proposed code descriptor accurately reflects the procedure or service as typically performed. If always or frequently performed with one or more other procedures or services, the descriptor structure and content will reflect the typical combination or complete procedure or service.
- The descriptor for the procedure or service is not proposed as a means to report extraordinary circumstances related to the performance of a procedure or service already described in the CPT code set; *and*

- The procedure or service satisfies the category-specific criteria set forth below.

Category-Specific Requirements

Category I Criteria

A proposal for a new or revised Category I code must satisfy all of the following criteria:

- All devices and drugs necessary for performance of the procedure or service have received FDA clearance or approval when such is required for performance of the procedure or service.

- The procedure or service is performed by many physicians or other qualified health care professionals across the United States.

- The procedure or service is performed with frequency consistent with the intended clinical use (ie, a service for a common condition should have high volume, whereas a service commonly performed for a rare condition may have low volume).

- The procedure or service is consistent with current medical practice.

- The clinical efficacy of the procedure or service is documented in literature that meets the requirements set forth in the CPT code change application.

Category III Criteria

The following **criteria** are used by the CPT/HCPAC Advisory Committee and the CPT Editorial Panel for evaluating Category III code **applications**:

- The procedure or service is currently or recently performed in humans; **and**

At least one of the following additional criteria has been met:

- The application is supported by at least one CPT or HCPAC advisor representing practitioners who would use this procedure or service; **or**

- The actual or potential clinical efficacy of the specific procedure or service is supported by peer reviewed literature, which is available in English for examination by the CPT Editorial Panel; **or**

- There is (a) at least one Institutional Review Board– approved protocol of a study of the procedure or service being performed; (b) a description of a current and ongoing United States trial outlining the efficacy of the procedure or service; or (c) other evidence of evolving clinical utilization.

Guidelines

Specific guidelines are presented at the beginning of each of the sections. These guidelines define items that are necessary to appropriately interpret and report the procedures and services contained in that section. For example, in the **Medicine** section, specific instructions are provided for handling unlisted services or procedures, special reports, and supplies and materials provided. Guidelines also provide explanations regarding terms that apply only to a particular section. For instance, **Radiology Guidelines** provide a definition of the unique term, "radiological supervision and interpretation." While in **Anesthesia**, a discussion of reporting time is included.

▶A written report (eg, handwritten or electronic) signed by the interpreting individual should be considered an integral part of a radiologic procedure or interpretation. Please see the guidelines regarding Imaging Guidance in each individual section.◀

Add-on Codes

Some of the listed procedures are commonly carried out in addition to the primary procedure performed. These additional or supplemental procedures are designated as add-on codes with the ✚ symbol and they are listed in **Appendix D** of the CPT codebook. Add-on codes in *CPT 2016* can be readily identified by specific descriptor nomenclature that includes phrases such as "each additional" or "(List separately in addition to primary procedure)."

The add-on code concept in *CPT 2016* applies only to add-on procedures or services performed by the same physician. Add-on codes describe additional intra-service work associated with the primary procedure, eg, additional digit(s), lesion(s), neurorrhaphy(s), vertebral segment(s), tendon(s), joint(s).

Add-on codes are always performed in addition to the primary service or procedure and must never be reported as a stand-alone code. All add-on codes found in the CPT codebook are exempt from the multiple procedure concept (see the modifier 51 definition in **Appendix A**).

Modifiers

A modifier provides the means to report or indicate that a service or procedure that has been performed has been altered by some specific circumstance but not changed in its definition or code. Modifiers also enable health care professionals to effectively respond to payment policy requirements established by other entities. The judicious application of modifiers obviates the necessity for separate procedure listings that may describe the modifying circumstance. Modifiers may be used to indicate to the recipient of a report that:

- A service or procedure had both a professional and technical component.

- A service or procedure was performed by more than one physician or other health care professional and/or in more than one location.

- A service or procedure was increased or reduced.

- Only part of a service was performed.

- An adjunctive service was performed.

- A bilateral procedure was performed.

- A service or procedure was provided more than once.

- Unusual events occurred.

Example

A physician providing diagnostic or therapeutic radiology services, ultrasound, or nuclear medicine services in a hospital would add modifier 26 to report the professional component.

73090 with modifier 26 = Professional component only for an X-ray of the forearm

Example

Two surgeons may be required to manage a specific surgical problem. When two surgeons work together as primary surgeons performing distinct part(s) of a procedure, each surgeon should report his/her distinct operative work by adding modifier 62 to the procedure code and any associated code(s) for that procedure as long as both surgeons continue to work together as primary surgeons. Each surgeon should report the co-surgery once using the same procedure code. Modifier 62 would be applicable. For instance, a neurological surgeon and an otolaryngologist are working as co-surgeons in performing transphenoidal excision of a pituitary neoplasm.

The first surgeon would report:

61548 62 = Hypophysectomy or excision of pituitary tumor, transnasal or transseptal approach, nonstereotactic + two surgeons modifier

and the second surgeon would report:

61548 62 = Hypophysectomy or excision of pituitary tumor, transnasal or transseptal approach, nonstereotactic + two surgeons modifier

If additional procedure(s) (including add-on procedure[s]) are performed during the same surgical session, separate code(s) may also be reported with modifier 62 added. It should be noted that if a co-surgeon acts as an assistant in the performance of additional procedure(s) during the same surgical session, those services may be reported using separate procedure code(s) with modifier 80 or modifier 82 added, as appropriate. A complete listing of modifiers is found in **Appendix A**.

Place of Service and Facility Reporting

Some codes have specified places of service (eg, evaluation and management codes are specific to a setting). Other services and procedures may have instructions specific to the place of service (eg, therapeutic, prophylactic, and diagnostic injections and infusions). The CPT code set is designated for reporting physician and qualified health care professional services. It is also the designated code set for reporting services provided by organizations or facilities (eg, hospitals) in specific circumstances. Throughout the CPT code set, the use of terms such as "physician," "qualified health care professional," or "individual" is not intended to indicate that other entities may not report the service. In selected instances, specific instructions may define a service as limited to professionals or limited to other entities (eg, hospital or home health agency). The CPT code set uses the term "facility" to describe such providers and the term "nonfacility" to describe services settings or circumstances in which no facility reporting may occur. Services provided in the home by an agency are facility services. Services provided in the home by a physician or other qualified health care professional who is not a representative of the agency are nonfacility services.

Unlisted Procedure or Service

It is recognized that there may be services or procedures performed by physicians or other qualified health care professionals that are not found in the CPT code set. Therefore, a number of specific code numbers have been designated for reporting unlisted procedures. When an unlisted procedure number is used, the service or procedure should be described (see specific section guidelines). Each of these unlisted procedural code numbers (with the appropriate accompanying topical entry) relates to a specific section of the book and is presented in the guidelines of that section.

In some cases alternative coding and procedural nomenclature as contained in other code sets may allow appropriate reporting of a more specific code. CPT references to use an unlisted procedure code do not preclude the reporting of an appropriate code that may be found in other code sets.

Results, Testing, Interpretation, and Report

Results are the technical component of a service. Testing leads to results; results lead to interpretation. Reports are the work product of the interpretation of test results. Certain procedures or services described in CPT involve a technical component (eg, tests) which produces "results" (eg, data, images, slides). For clinical use, some of these results require interpretation. Some CPT descriptors specifically require interpretation and reporting to report that code.

Special Report

A service that is rarely provided, unusual, variable, or new may require a special report. Pertinent information should include an adequate definition or description of the nature, extent, and need for the procedure and the time, effort, and equipment necessary to provide the service.

Time

The CPT code set contains many codes with a time basis for code selection. The following standards shall apply to time measurement, unless there are code or code-range–specific instructions in guidelines, parenthetical instructions, or code descriptors to the contrary. Time is the face-to-face time with the patient. Phrases such as "interpretation and report" in the code descriptor are not intended to indicate in all cases that report writing is part of the reported time. A unit of time is attained when the mid-point is passed. For example, an hour is attained when 31 minutes have elapsed (more than midway between zero and sixty minutes). A second hour is attained when a total of 91 minutes have elapsed. When codes are ranked in sequential typical times and the actual time is between two typical times, the code with the typical time closest to the actual time is used. See also the **Evaluation and Management (E/M) Services Guidelines**. When another service is performed concurrently with a time-based service, the time associated with the concurrent service should not be included in the time used for reporting the time-based service. Some services measured in units other than days extend across calendar dates. When this occurs a continuous service does not reset and create a first hour. However, any disruption in the service does create a new initial service. For example, if intravenous hydration

(96360, 96361) is given from 11 PM to 2 AM, 96360 would be reported once and 96361 twice. For facility reporting on a single date of service or for continuous services that last beyond midnight (ie, over a range of dates), report the total units of time provided continuously.

Code Symbols

A summary listing of additions, deletions, and revisions applicable to the CPT codebook is found in **Appendix B**. New procedure numbers added to the CPT codebook are identified throughout the text with the symbol ● placed before the code number. In instances where a code revision has resulted in a substantially altered procedure descriptor, the symbol ▲ is placed before the code number. The symbols ► ◄ are used to indicate new and revised text other than the procedure descriptors. These symbols indicate CPT Editorial Panel actions. The symbol ○ is used to indicate reinstated/recycled code. The AMA reserves the right to correct typographical errors and make stylistic improvements.

CPT add-on codes are annotated by the symbol ✛ and are listed in **Appendix D**. The symbol ⊘ is used to identify codes that are exempt from the use of modifier 51 but have not been designated as CPT add-on procedures or services. A list of codes exempt from modifier 51 usage is included in **Appendix E**. The symbol ⊙ is used to identify codes that include moderate sedation (see **Appendix G**). The symbol ⁄ is used to identify codes for vaccines that are pending FDA approval (see **Appendix K**). The symbol # is used to identify codes that are listed out of numerical sequence (see **Appendix N**).

Resequenced codes that are not placed numerically are identified with the # symbol, and a reference placed numerically (ie, Code is out of numerical sequence. See…) as a navigational alert to direct the user to the location of the out-of-sequence code (see **Appendix N**). Resequencing is utilized to allow placement of related concepts in appropriate locations within the families of codes regardless of the availability of numbers for sequential numerical placement.

Alphabetical Reference Index

This codebook features an expanded alphabetical index that includes listings by procedure and anatomic site. Procedures and services commonly known by their eponyms or other designations are also included.

CPT 2016 in Electronic Formats

CPT 2016 procedure codes and descriptions are also available as data file on CD-ROM or as downloadable data file. The CPT data file is available in ASCII and EBCDIC formats and provides a convenient way to import the 2016 CPT codes and descriptions into existing documentation or into any billing and claims reporting software that accepts a text (.TXT) file format. The data file contains the complete official AMA CPT guidelines, descriptor package, and new descriptors for consumers and clinicians. For more information call 800 621-8335 or visit amastore.com.

Other AMA CPT Resources

Individual back issues of the *CPT Assistant* and *Clinical Examples in Radiology* are available for purchase by calling 800 621-8335 or at **amastore.com**.

CPT Assistant and *Clinical Examples in Radiology* are now online! Based on the best-selling hard copy newsletters, *CPT Assistant Online* and *Clinical Examples in Radiology Online* put the content medical coding professionals rely on daily in a more user-friendly format. Benefits exclusive to the online versions include:

- Monthly (*CPT Assistant*) and quarterly (*Clinical Examples in Radiology*) updates! The home screen notifies you when a new issue is available and you can review the latest issue in its entirety.

- Unlimited access to every archived issue and article dating back to when the newsletter first published.

- A historical CPT code list that references when a code was added, deleted, and/or revised since 1990.

- Simple search capabilities, including intuitive menus and a cumulative index of article titles.

- Anatomical illustrations, charts, and graphs for quick reference.

For more information call 800 621-8335.

Current and past editions of *CPT Changes: An Insider's View* can be purchased by calling the AMA's Unified Service Center at 800 621-8335 or visiting **amastore.com**.

In addition, *CPT Changes: An Insider's View* is now available online. Instantly access current CPT code changes and historical changes dating back to 2000. This invaluable online library provides you with an easy and efficient way to search every edition of *CPT Changes: An Insider's View* (from 2000 to the current year) for the official interpretation and rationale behind every code and guideline change. For more information call 800 621-8335.

Illustrated Anatomical and Procedural Review

It is essential that coders have a thorough understanding of medical terminology and anatomy to code accurately. The following section reviewing the basics of vocabulary and anatomy can be used as a quick reference to help you with your coding. It is not intended as a replacement for up-to-date medical dictionaries and anatomy texts, which are essential tools for accurate coding.

Prefixes, Suffixes, and Roots

Although medical terminology may seem complex, many medical terms can be broken into component parts, which makes them easier to understand. Many of these terms are derived from Latin or Greek words, but some include the names of physicians.

Prefixes are word parts that appear at the beginning of a word and modify its meaning; suffixes are found at the end of words. By learning what various prefixes and suffixes mean, it is possible to decipher the meaning of a word quickly. The following lists are a quick reference for some common prefixes and suffixes.

Numbers

Prefix	Meaning	Example
mono-, uni-	one	monocyte, unilateral
bi-	two	bilateral
tri-	three	triad
quadr-	four	quadriplegia
hex-, sex-	six	hexose
diplo-	double	diplopia

Surgical Procedures

Suffix	Meaning	Example
-centesis	puncture a cavity to remove fluid	amniocentesis
-ectomy	surgical removal (excision)	appendectomy
-ostomy	a new permanent opening	colostomy
-otomy	cutting into (incision)	tracheotomy
-orrhaphy	surgical repair/suture	herniorrhaphy
-opexy	surgical fixation	nephropexy
-oplasty	surgical repair	rhinoplasty
-otripsy	crushing, destroying	lithotripsy

Conditions

Prefix	Meaning	Example
ambi-	both	ambidextrous
aniso-	unequal	anisocoria
dys-	bad, painful, difficult	dysphoria
eu-	good, normal	euthanasia
hetero-	different	heterogeneous
homo-	same	homogeneous
hyper-	excessive, above	hypergastric
hypo-	deficient, below	hypogastric
iso-	equal, same	isotonic
mal-	bad, poor	malaise
megalo-	large	megalocardia

Suffix	Meaning	Example
-algia	pain	neuralgia
-asthenia	weakness	myasthenia
-emia	blood	anemia
-iasis	condition of	amebiasis
-itis	inflammation	appendicitis
-lysis	destruction, break down	hemolysis
-lytic	destroy, break down	hemolytic
-oid	like	lipoid
-oma	tumor	carcinoma
-opathy	disease of	arthropathy
-orrhagia	hemorrhage	menorrhagia
-orrhea	flow or discharge	amenorrhea
-osis	abnormal condition of	tuberculosis
-paresis	weakness	hemiparesis
-plasia	growth	hyperplasia
-plegia	paralysis	paraplegia
-pnea	breathing	apnea

Directions and Positions

Prefix	Meaning	Example
ab-	away from	abduction
ad-	toward	adduction
ecto, exo-	outside	ectopic, exocrine
endo-	within	endoscope
epi-	upon	epigastric
infra-	below, under	infrastructure
ipsi-	same	ipsilateral
meso-	middle	mesopexy
meta-	after, beyond, transformation	metastasis
peri-	surrounding	pericardium
retro-	behind, back	retroversion
trans-	across, through	transvaginal

Word	Meaning
anterior or ventral	at or near the front surface of the body
posterior or dorsal	at or near the back surface of the body
superior	above
inferior	below
lateral	side
distal	farthest from center
proximal	nearest to center
medial	middle
supine	face up or palm up
prone	face down or palm down
sagittal	vertical body plane, divides the body into equal right and left sides
transverse	horizontal body plane, divides the body into top and bottom sections
coronal	vertical body plane, divides the body into front and back sections

Additional References

For best coding results, you will need to use other reference materials in addition to your CPT® coding books. These references include medical dictionaries and anatomy books.

Medical Dictionaries

Dorland's Illustrated Medical Dictionary, 32nd ed.
Philadelphia, PA: Elsevier; 2011

Stedman's CPT® Dictionary, 2nd ed.
Chicago, IL: American Medical Association; 2009.
OP:300609

Stedman's Medical Dictionary. 28th ed.
Philadelphia, PA: Lippencott; 2005.

Anatomy References

Bernard, SP. *Netter's Atlas of Human Anatomy for CPT® Surgery*
Chicago, IL: American Medical Association; Spring, 2015.

Kirschner, CG. *Netter's Atlas of Human Anatomy for CPT® Coding*, 2nd ed.
Chicago, IL: American Medical Association; 2009.
OP:490609

Netter, FH. *Atlas of Human Anatomy*, 6th ed.
Philadelphia, PA; Elsevier; 2014
OP:936714

List of Illustrations

To further aid coders in properly assigning CPT codes, the codebook contains a number of anatomical illustrations.

Anatomical Illustrations

On the following pages (xix-xxvii), there are 31 anatomical illustrations:

Figure	Illustration Title
Figure 1A	Body Planes—3/4 View
Figure 1B	Body Aspects—Side View
Figure 1C	Body Planes—Front View
Figure 2	Structure of Skin
Figure 3	Skeletal System
Figure 4	Skull
Figure 5A	Muscular System—Front
Figure 5B	Muscular System—Back
Figure 6A	Thoracic Vertebra—Superior View
Figure 6B	Lumbar Vertebra—Superior View
Figure 6C	Lumbar Vertebrae—Lateral View
Figure 7	Bones, Muscles, and Tendons of Hand
Figure 8	Bones and Muscles of Foot
Figure 9	Paranasal Sinuses
Figure 10	Respiratory System
Figure 11	Aortic Anatomy
Figure 12	Cardiac Anatomy
Figure 13A	Circulatory System—Arteries
Figure 13B	Circulatory System—Veins
Figure 14	Brachial Artery
Figure 15	Lymphatic System
Figure 16	Digestive System
Figure 17	Urinary System
Figure 18A	Male Genital System
Figure 18B	Female Genital System
Figure 19	Nervous System
Figure 20A	Brain Anatomy
Figure 20B	Sagittal Section of Brain and Brain Stem
Figure 21	Eye Anatomy
Figure 22	Ear Anatomy
Figure 23	Endocrine System

Figure 1A
Body Planes — 3/4 View

Coronal (frontal) plane

Sagittal plane (at the body's median)

Horizontal or transverse plane

Figure 1B
Body Aspects — Side View

Superior (cranial) aspect

Posterior aspect

Anterior aspect

Dorsal surface of hand

Palmar surface of hand

Dorsal surface of foot

Plantar surface of foot

Inferior aspect

Figure 1C
Body Planes — Front View

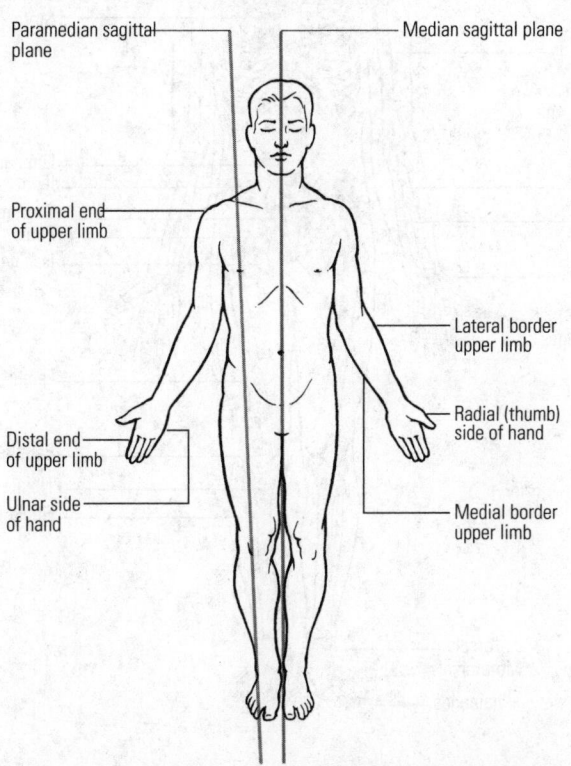

Paramedian sagittal plane

Median sagittal plane

Proximal end of upper limb

Lateral border upper limb

Radial (thumb) side of hand

Distal end of upper limb

Ulnar side of hand

Medial border upper limb

Figure 2
Structure of Skin

Hair shaft

Hair root

Epidermis

Dermis

Subcutaneous tissue

Sebaceous gland

Nerve endings

Hair bulb

Sweat gland

Cutaneous nerve

Blood vessels

Figure 3
Skeletal System

Skull

Maxilla

Mandible

Cervical vertebra

First rib

Clavicle

Scapula

Sternum

Humerus

Radius

Ulna

Carpals

Metacarpals

Phalanges

Lumbar vertebra

Ilium

Sacrum

Pubis

Ischium

Femur

Patella

Tibia

Fibula

Tarsals

Metatarsals

Phalanges

Figure 4
Skull

Parietal bone

Temporal bone

Sphenoid bone

Zygomatic bone

Maxilla

Mandible

Frontal bone

Nasal bone

Frontal bone

Nasal bone

Zygomatic bone

Maxilla bone

Mandible

Parietal bone

Occipital bone

Temporal bone

Temporomandibular joint

Figure 5A
Muscular System — Front

Sternocleidomastoid m.
Omohyoid m.
Sternohyoid m.
Trapezius m.
Deltoid m.
Pectoralis major m.
Latissimus dorsi m.
Serratas anterior m.
Oblique external m.
Rectus abdominus m.

Biceps m.
Brachialus m.
Brachioradialus m.
Pronator teres m.
Flexor carpi radialus m.
Palmaris longus m.
Flexor digitorum superficialus m.
Flexor carpi ulnaris m.

Pectineus m.
Adductor longus m.
Adductor magnus m.
Gracilis m.
Sartorius m.
Rectus femoris m.
Vastus medialis m.
Vastus lateralis m. } Quadriceps

Peroneus longus m.
Tibialis anterior m.
Gastrocnemius m.
Extensor digitorum longus m.
Soleus m.

Figure 5B
Muscular System — Back

Trapezius m.
Deltoid m.
Infraspinatus m.
Teres minor m.
Teres major m.
Triceps m.
Latissimus dorsi m.
Anconeus m.
Extensor carpi radialis longus m.
Flexor carpi ulnaris m.
Extensor carpi radialis brevis m.
Extensor digitorum m.
Extensor carpi ulnaris m.
Abductor pollicis longus m.
Extensor pollicis brevis m.

Gluteus medius m.
Gluteus maximus m.
Adductor magnus m.
Biceps femoris m.
Semitendinosus m.
Gracilis m.
Semimembranosus m.
Vastus lateralis m.
Sartorius m.

Gastrocnemius m.

Peroneus longus m.
Flexor hallicis longus m.

Figure 6A
Thoracic Vertebra — Superior View

Spinous process
Lamina
Transverse process
Spinal canal
Transverse costal facet
Pedicle
Superior articular facet
Superior costal facet
Vertebral body

Figure 6B
Lumbar Vertebra — Superior View

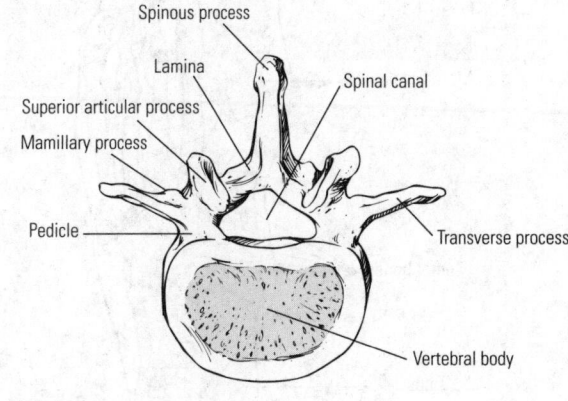

Spinous process
Lamina
Superior articular process
Mamillary process
Spinal canal
Pedicle
Transverse process
Vertebral body

Figure 6C
Lumbar Vertebrae — Lateral View

Pedicle
Superior articular process
Transverse process
Spinous process
Inferior articular process
Inferior vertebral notch
Intervertebral foramen
Superior vertebral notch

Vertebral body
L1
Intervertebral discs
L2
L3
L4
L5

Figure 7
Bones, Muscles, and Tendons of Hand

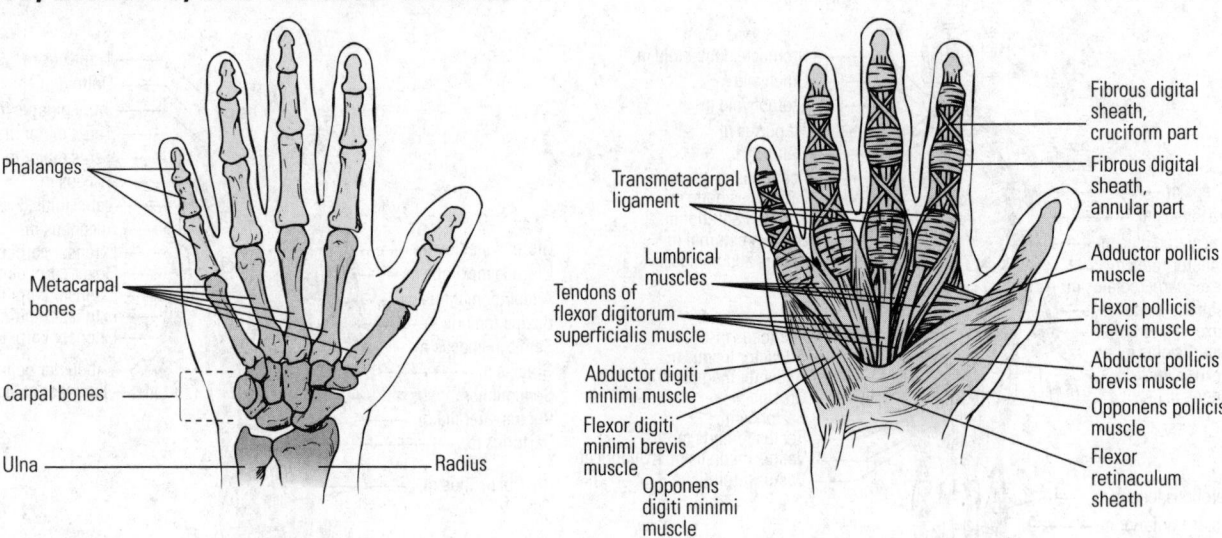

Phalanges

Metacarpal bones

Carpal bones

Ulna

Radius

Transmetacarpal ligament

Lumbrical muscles

Tendons of flexor digitorum superficialis muscle

Abductor digiti minimi muscle

Flexor digiti minimi brevis muscle

Opponens digiti minimi muscle

Fibrous digital sheath, cruciform part

Fibrous digital sheath, annular part

Adductor pollicis muscle

Flexor pollicis brevis muscle

Abductor pollicis brevis muscle

Opponens pollicis muscle

Flexor retinaculum sheath

Figure 8
Bones and Muscles of Foot

Phalanges

Metatarsal bones

Tarsal bones

Talus

Calcaneus

Tendon of flexor hallucis longus muscle

Flexor hallucis brevis muscle

Abductor hallucis muscle

Lumbrical muscles

Flexor digitorum brevis muscle

Flexor digiti minimi brevis muscle

Abductor digiti minimi muscle

Figure 9
Paranasal Sinuses

Frontal

Ethmoid

Sphenoid

Maxillary

Figure 10
Respiratory System

Nasal cavity

Nasopharynx

Oropharynx

Epiglottis

Larynx

Esophagus

Trachea

Right bronchus

Left bronchus

Right lung

Left lung

Figure 11
Aortic Anatomy

Left common carotid artery

Innominate artery

Left subclavian artery

Aortic arch

Ascending aorta

Descending thoracic aorta

Sinotubular junction

Sinus of Valsava

Root

Diaphragm

Abdominal aorta

Common iliac artery

Figure 12
Cardiac Anatomy

Superior vena cava

Aorta

Right pulmonary artery

Pulmonary artery

Pulmonary valve

Left atrium

Location of sinoatrial node

Aortic valve

Location of atrioventricular node

Mitral valve

Right atrium

Left ventricle

Tricuspid valve

Ventricular septum

Right ventricle

Descending thoracic aorta

Inferior vena cava

Figure 13A
Circulatory System—Arteries

Superficial temporal a.
Posterior auricular a.
Common carotid a.
Subclavian a.
Brachiocephalic trunk
Axillary a.
Deep brachial a.
Brachial a.
Aorta
Radial a.
Interosseous a.
Ulnar a.
Deep palmar arch
Superficial palmar arch
Descending genicular a.

External carotid a.
Internal carotid a.
Vertebral a.
Aorta and arch
Pulmonary a.
Cardiac a.
Thoracic aorta
Celiac trunk
Superior mesenteric a.
Renal a.
Gonadal a.
Inferior mesenteric a.
Common iliac a.
External iliac a.
Internal iliac a.
Deep femoral a.
Femoral a.
Popliteal a.
Anterior tibial a.
Peroneal a.
Posterior tibial a.

Figure 13B
Circulatory System—Veins

Superficial temporal v.
External jugular v.
Subclavian v.
Brachiocephalic v.
Axillary v.
Brachial v.
Cepalic v.
Basilic v.
Median cubital v.
Medial antebrachial v.
Superficial venous palmar arch
Small saphenous v.

Facial v.
Internal jugular v.
Superior vena cava
Hepatic v.
Renal v.
Gonadal v.
Inferior vena cava
Common iliac v.
Internal iliac v.
External iliac v.
Deep femoral v.
Femoral v.
Great saphenous v.
Popliteal v.
Anterior tibial v.
Posterior tibial v.
Dorsal venous arch

Figure 14
Brachial Artery

Brachiocephalic vein
Subclavian vein
Superior vena cava
Upper arm cephalic vein
Brachial artery
Brachial vein
Basilic vein
Radial artery
Lower arm cephalic vein
Ulnar artery

Figure 15
Lymphatic System

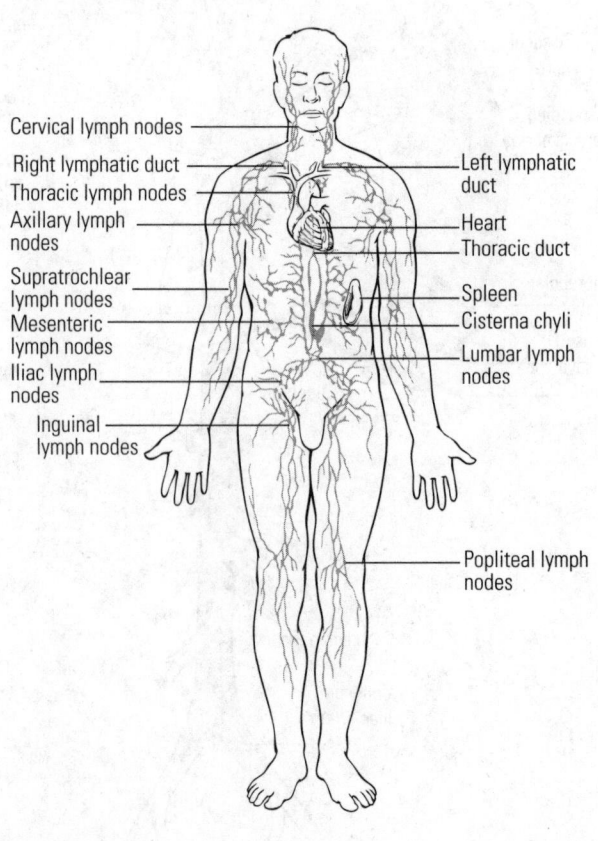

Cervical lymph nodes
Right lymphatic duct
Thoracic lymph nodes
Axillary lymph nodes
Supratrochlear lymph nodes
Mesenteric lymph nodes
Iliac lymph nodes
Inguinal lymph nodes

Left lymphatic duct
Heart
Thoracic duct
Spleen
Cisterna chyli
Lumbar lymph nodes
Popliteal lymph nodes

Figure 16
Digestive System

Oral cavity
Tongue
Oropharynx
Esophagus
Liver
Stomach
Gall bladder
Pancreas
Duodenum
Transverse colon
Ascending colon
Jejunum
Ileum
Cecum
Appendix
Sigmoid colon
Rectum
Anal canal and anus

Figure 17
Urinary System

Right kidney
Left kidney
Ureters
Urinary bladder
Urethra (empties through penis or in front of vagina)

Figure 18A
Male Genital System

Deferent duct
Urinary bladder and cavity
Seminal vesicle
Corpus cavernosa
Ejaculatory duct
Corpus spongiosum
Prostate gland
Penis
Spermatic cord and deferent duct
Glans penis
Epididymus
Prepuce
Testes
Scrotum

Figure 18B
Female Genital System

Uterine tube
Fundus of uterus
Ampulla
Infundibulum with fimbriae
Ligament of ovary
Ovary
Body of uterus and uterine cavity
Cervix and cervical canal
Vagina

Figure 19
Nervous System

- Brachial plexus
- Musculocutaneous n.
- Radial nerve
- Median nerve
- Iliohypogastric nerve
- Ilioinguinal nerve
- Deep branch of radial nerve
- Lat. femoral cutaneous nerve
- Genitofemoral nerve
- Superficial branch of radial nerve
- Obturator nerve
- Ulnar nerve
- Common peroneal nerve
- Deep peroneal nerve
- Superficial peroneal nerve

- Brain
- Cerebellum
- Spinal cord
- Intercostal nerves (with ribs)
- Subcostal nerve (12th thoracic)
- Lumbar plexus
- Sacral plexus
- Femoral nerve
- Pudendal nerve
- Sciatic nerve
- Muscular branches of femoral nerve
- Saphenous nerve
- Tibial nerve

Figure 20A
Brain Anatomy

- Longitudinal fissure
- Frontal lobes
- Parietal lobes
- Occipital lobes
- Frontal lobe
- Parietal lobe
- Occipital lobe
- Temporal lobe
- Cerebellum

Figure 20B
Sagittal Section of Brain and Brain Stem

- Cerebrum
- Corpus collosum
- Ventricles
- Thalamus
- Midbrain
- Cerebellum
- Brain stem
- Hypothalamus
- Pituitary gland
- Pons
- Medulla

Figure 21
Eye Anatomy

Figure 22
Ear Anatomy

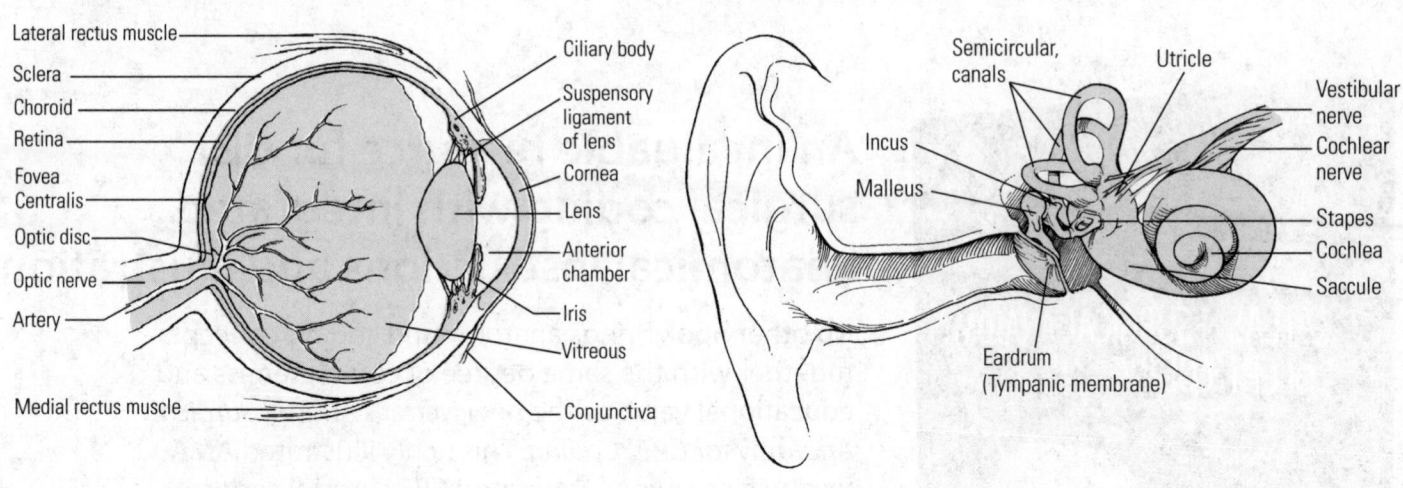

Lateral rectus muscle
Sclera
Choroid
Retina
Fovea
Centralis
Optic disc
Optic nerve
Artery
Medial rectus muscle

Ciliary body
Suspensory
ligament
of lens
Cornea
Lens
Anterior
chamber
Iris
Vitreous
Conjunctiva

Semicircular,
canals
Incus
Malleus
Utricle
Vestibular
nerve
Cochlear
nerve
Stapes
Cochlea
Saccule
Eardrum
(Tympanic membrane)

Figure 23
Endocrine System

Hypothalamus
Pineal body
Pituitary
Parathyroids
Thyroid gland
Thymus gland
Adrenal glands
Pancreas
Ovaries
Testes

Evaluation and Management (E/M) Services Guidelines

In addition to the information presented in the Introduction, several other items unique to this section are defined or identified here.

Classification of Evaluation and Management (E/M) Services

The E/M section is divided into broad categories such as office visits, hospital visits, and consultations. Most of the categories are further divided into two or more subcategories of E/M services. For example, there are two subcategories of office visits (new patient and established patient) and there are two subcategories of hospital visits (initial and subsequent). The subcategories of E/M services are further classified into levels of E/M services that are identified by specific codes. This classification is important because the nature of work varies by type of service, place of service, and the patient's status.

The basic format of the levels of E/M services is the same for most categories. First, a unique code number is listed. Second, the place and/or type of service is specified, eg, office consultation. Third, the content of the service is defined, eg, comprehensive history and comprehensive examination. (See "Levels of E/M Services," page 3, for details on the content of E/M services.) Fourth, the nature of the presenting problem(s) usually associated with a given level is described. Fifth, the time typically required to provide the service is specified. (A detailed discussion of time is provided on page 4.)

Definitions of Commonly Used Terms

Certain key words and phrases are used throughout the E/M section. The following definitions are intended to reduce the potential for differing interpretations and to increase the consistency of reporting by physicians in differing specialties. E/M services may also be reported by other qualified health care professionals who are authorized to perform such services within the scope of their practice.

New and Established Patient

Solely for the purposes of distinguishing between new and established patients, **professional services** are those face-to-face services rendered by physicians and other qualified health care professionals who may report evaluation and management services reported by a specific CPT code(s). A new patient is one who has not received any professional services from the physician/ qualified health care professional or another physician/ qualified health care professional of the **exact** same specialty **and subspecialty** who belongs to the same group practice, within the past three years.

An established patient is one who has received professional services from the physician/qualified health care professional or another physician/qualified health care professional of the **exact** same specialty **and subspecialty** who belongs to the same group practice, within the past three years. See Decision Tree.

In the instance where a physician/qualified health care professional is on call for or covering for another physician/qualified health care professional, the patient's encounter will be classified as it would have been by the physician/qualified health care professional who is not available. When advanced practice nurses and physician assistants are working with physicians they are considered as working in the exact same specialty and exact same subspecialties as the physician.

No distinction is made between new and established patients in the emergency department. E/M services in the emergency department category may be reported for any new or established patient who presents for treatment in the emergency department.

The decision tree on page 2 is provided to aid in determining whether to report the E/M service provided as a new or an established patient encounter.

Chief Complaint

A chief complaint is a concise statement describing the symptom, problem, condition, diagnosis, or other factor that is the reason for the encounter, usually stated in the patient's words.

Concurrent Care and Transfer of Care

Concurrent care is the provision of similar services (eg, hospital visits) to the same patient by more than one physician or other qualified health care professional on the same day. When concurrent care is provided, no special reporting is required. Transfer of care is the process whereby a physician or other qualified health care professional who is providing management for some or all of a patient's problems relinquishes this responsibility to another physician or other qualified health care professional who explicitly agrees to accept this responsibility and who, from the initial encounter, is not providing consultative services. The physician or other qualified health care professional transferring care is then no longer providing care for these problems though he or she may continue providing care for other conditions when appropriate. Consultation codes should not be reported by the physician or other qualified health care professional who has agreed to accept transfer of care before an initial evaluation but are appropriate to report if the decision to accept transfer of care cannot be made until after the initial consultation evaluation, regardless of site of service.

Decision Tree for New vs Established Patients

Decision Tree for New vs Established Patients

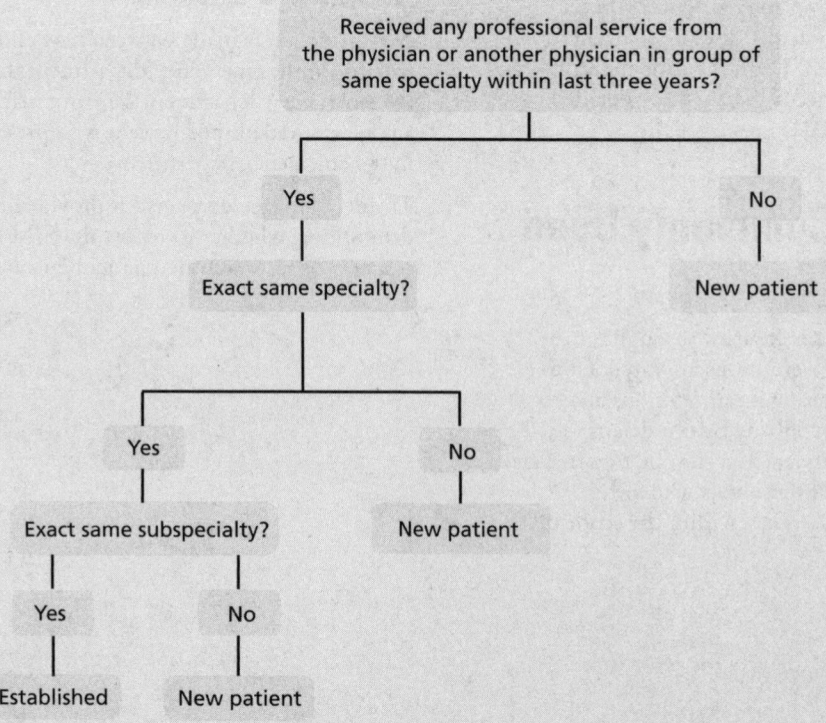

⊙=Moderate sedation   ✚=Add-on code   ✔=FDA approval pending   #=Resequenced code   ○=Recycled/reinstated code

Counseling

Counseling is a discussion with a patient and/or family concerning one or more of the following areas:

- Diagnostic results, impressions, and/or recommended diagnostic studies
- Prognosis
- Risks and benefits of management (treatment) options
- Instructions for management (treatment) and/or follow-up
- Importance of compliance with chosen management (treatment) options
- Risk factor reduction
- Patient and family education

      (For psychotherapy, see 90832-90834, 90836-90840)

Family History

A review of medical events in the patient's family that includes significant information about:

- The health status or cause of death of parents, siblings, and children
- Specific diseases related to problems identified in the Chief Complaint or History of the Present Illness, and/or System Review
- Diseases of family members that may be hereditary or place the patient at risk

History of Present Illness

A chronological description of the development of the patient's present illness from the first sign and/or symptom to the present. This includes a description of location, quality, severity, timing, context, modifying factors, and associated signs and symptoms significantly related to the presenting problem(s).

Levels of E/M Services

Within each category or subcategory of E/M service, there are three to five levels of E/M services available for reporting purposes. Levels of E/M services are **not** interchangeable among the different categories or subcategories of service. For example, the first level of E/M services in the subcategory of office visit, new patient, does not have the same definition as the first level of E/M services in the subcategory of office visit, established patient.

The levels of E/M services include examinations, evaluations, treatments, conferences with or concerning patients, preventive pediatric and adult health supervision, and similar medical services, such as the determination of the need and/or location for appropriate care. Medical screening includes the history, examination, and medical decision-making required to determine the need and/or location for appropriate care and treatment

of the patient (eg, office and other outpatient setting, emergency department, nursing facility). The levels of E/M services encompass the wide variations in skill, effort, time, responsibility, and medical knowledge required for the prevention or diagnosis and treatment of illness or injury and the promotion of optimal health. Each level of E/M services may be used by all physicians or other qualified health care professionals.

The descriptors for the levels of E/M services recognize seven components, six of which are used in defining the levels of E/M services. These components are:

- History
- Examination
- Medical decision making
- Counseling
- Coordination of care
- Nature of presenting problem
- Time

The first three of these components (history, examination, and medical decision making) are considered the **key** components in selecting a level of E/M services. (See "Determine the Extent of History Obtained," page 6.)

The next three components (counseling, coordination of care, and the nature of the presenting problem) are considered **contributory** factors in the majority of encounters. Although the first two of these contributory factors are important E/M services, it is not required that these services be provided at every patient encounter.

Coordination of care with other physicians, other health care professionals, or agencies without a patient encounter on that day is reported using the case management codes.

The final component, time, is discussed in detail on page 4.

Any specifically identifiable procedure (ie, identified with a specific CPT code) performed on or subsequent to the date of initial or subsequent E/M services should be reported separately.

The actual performance and/or interpretation of diagnostic tests/studies ordered during a patient encounter are not included in the levels of E/M services. Physician performance of diagnostic tests/studies for which specific CPT codes are available may be reported separately, in addition to the appropriate E/M code. The physician's interpretation of the results of diagnostic tests/studies (ie, professional component) with preparation of a separate distinctly identifiable signed written report may also be reported separately, using the appropriate CPT code with modifier 26 appended.

The physician or other health care professional may need to indicate that on the day a procedure or service identified by a CPT code was performed, the patient's

Evaluation/Management

condition required a significant separately identifiable E/M service above and beyond other services provided or beyond the usual preservice and postservice care associated with the procedure that was performed. The E/M service may be caused or prompted by the symptoms or condition for which the procedure and/or service was provided. This circumstance may be reported by adding modifier 25 to the appropriate level of E/M service. As such, different diagnoses are not required for reporting of the procedure and the E/M services on the same date.

Nature of Presenting Problem

A presenting problem is a disease, condition, illness, injury, symptom, sign, finding, complaint, or other reason for encounter, with or without a diagnosis being established at the time of the encounter. The E/M codes recognize five types of presenting problems that are defined as follows:

Minimal: A problem that may not require the presence of the physician or other qualified health care professional, but service is provided under the physician's or other qualified health care professional's supervision.

Self-limited or minor: A problem that runs a definite and prescribed course, is transient in nature, and is not likely to permanently alter health status OR has a good prognosis with management/compliance.

Low severity: A problem where the risk of morbidity without treatment is low; there is little to no risk of mortality without treatment; full recovery without functional impairment is expected.

Moderate severity: A problem where the risk of morbidity without treatment is moderate; there is moderate risk of mortality without treatment; uncertain prognosis OR increased probability of prolonged functional impairment.

High severity: A problem where the risk of morbidity without treatment is high to extreme; there is a moderate to high risk of mortality without treatment OR high probability of severe, prolonged functional impairment.

Past History

A review of the patient's past experiences with illnesses, injuries, and treatments that includes significant information about:

- Prior major illnesses and injuries
- Prior operations
- Prior hospitalizations
- Current medications
- Allergies (eg, drug, food)
- Age appropriate immunization status
- Age appropriate feeding/dietary status

Social History

An age appropriate review of past and current activities that includes significant information about:

- Marital status and/or living arrangements
- Current employment
- Occupational history
- Military history
- Use of drugs, alcohol, and tobacco
- Level of education
- Sexual history
- Other relevant social factors

System Review (Review of Systems)

An inventory of body systems obtained through a series of questions seeking to identify signs and/or symptoms that the patient may be experiencing or has experienced. For the purposes of the CPT codebook the following elements of a system review have been identified:

- Constitutional symptoms (fever, weight loss, etc)
- Eyes
- Ears, nose, mouth, throat
- Cardiovascular
- Respiratory
- Gastrointestinal
- Genitourinary
- Musculoskeletal
- Integumentary (skin and/or breast)
- Neurological
- Psychiatric
- Endocrine
- Hematologic/lymphatic
- Allergic/immunologic

The review of systems helps define the problem, clarify the differential diagnosis, identify needed testing, or serves as baseline data on other systems that might be affected by any possible management options.

Time

The inclusion of time in the definitions of levels of E/M services has been implicit in prior editions of the CPT codebook. The inclusion of time as an explicit factor beginning in *CPT 1992* is done to assist in selecting the most appropriate level of E/M services. It should be recognized that the specific times expressed in the visit code descriptors are averages and, therefore, represent a range of times that may be higher or lower depending on actual clinical circumstances.

Time is **not** a descriptive component for the emergency department levels of E/M services because emergency department services are typically provided on a variable intensity basis, often involving multiple encounters with several patients over an extended period of time. Therefore, it is often difficult to provide accurate estimates of the time spent face-to-face with the patient.

Studies to establish levels of E/M services employed surveys of practicing physicians to obtain data on the amount of time and work associated with typical E/M services. Since "work" is not easily quantifiable, the codes must rely on other objective, verifiable measures that correlate with physicians' estimates of their "work." It has been demonstrated that estimations of **intraservice** time (as explained on the next page), both within and across specialties, is a variable that is predictive of the "work" of E/M services. This same research has shown there is a strong relationship between intraservice time and total time for E/M services. Intraservice time, rather than total time, was chosen for inclusion with the codes because of its relative ease of measurement and because of its direct correlation with measurements of the total amount of time and work associated with typical E/M services.

Intraservice times are defined as **face-to-face** time for office and other outpatient visits and as **unit/floor** time for hospital and other inpatient visits. This distinction is necessary because most of the work of typical office visits takes place during the face-to-face time with the patient, while most of the work of typical hospital visits takes place during the time spent on the patient's floor or unit. When prolonged time occurs in either the office or the inpatient areas, the appropriate add-on code should be reported.

Face-to-face time (office and other outpatient visits and office consultations): For coding purposes, face-to-face time for these services is defined as only that time spent face-to-face with the patient and/or family. This includes the time spent performing such tasks as obtaining a history, examination, and counseling the patient.

Time is also spent doing work before or after the face-to-face time with the patient, performing such tasks as reviewing records and tests, arranging for further services, and communicating further with other professionals and the patient through written reports and telephone contact.

This **non-face-to-face** time for office services—also called pre- and postencounter time—is not included in the time component described in the E/M codes. However, the pre- and post-non-face-to-face work associated with an encounter was included in calculating the total work of typical services in physician surveys.

Thus, the face-to-face time associated with the services described by any E/M code is a valid proxy for the total work done before, during, and after the visit.

Unit/floor time (hospital observation services, inpatient hospital care, initial inpatient hospital consultations, nursing facility): For reporting purposes, intraservice time for these services is defined as unit/floor time, which includes the time present on the patient's hospital unit and at the bedside rendering services for that patient. This includes the time to establish and/or review the patient's chart, examine the patient, write notes, and communicate with other professionals and the patient's family.

In the hospital, pre- and post-time includes time spent off the patient's floor performing such tasks as reviewing pathology and radiology findings in another part of the hospital.

This pre- and postvisit time is not included in the time component described in these codes. However, the pre- and postwork performed during the time spent off the floor or unit was included in calculating the total work of typical services in physician surveys.

Thus, the unit/floor time associated with the services described by any code is a valid proxy for the total work done before, during, and after the visit.

Unlisted Service

An E/M service may be provided that is not listed in this section of the CPT codebook. When reporting such a service, the appropriate unlisted code may be used to indicate the service, identifying it by "Special Report," as discussed in the following paragraph. The "Unlisted Services" and accompanying codes for the E/M section are as follows:

99429	**Unlisted preventive** medicine service
99499	**Unlisted evaluation and management** service

Special Report

An unlisted service or one that is unusual, variable, or new may require a special report demonstrating the medical appropriateness of the service. Pertinent information should include an adequate definition or description of the nature, extent, and need for the procedure and the time, effort, and equipment necessary to provide the service. Additional items that may be included are complexity of symptoms, final diagnosis, pertinent physical findings, diagnostic and therapeutic procedures, concurrent problems, and follow-up care.

Clinical Examples

Clinical examples of the codes for E/M services are provided to assist in understanding the meaning of the descriptors and selecting the correct code. The clinical examples are listed in Appendix C. Each example was developed by the specialties shown.

The same problem, when seen by different specialties, may involve different amounts of work. Therefore, the appropriate level of encounter should be reported using the descriptors rather than the examples.

Instructions for Selecting a Level of E/M Service

Review the Reporting Instructions for the Selected Category or Subcategory

Most of the categories and many of the subcategories of service have special guidelines or instructions unique to that category or subcategory. Where these are indicated, eg, "Inpatient Hospital Care," special instructions will be presented preceding the levels of E/M services.

Review the Level of E/M Service Descriptors and Examples in the Selected Category or Subcategory

The descriptors for the levels of E/M services recognize seven components, six of which are used in defining the levels of E/M services. These components are:

- History
- Examination
- Medical decision making
- Counseling
- Coordination of care
- Nature of presenting problem
- Time

The first three of these components (ie, history, examination, and medical decision making) should be considered the **key** components in selecting the level of E/M services. An exception to this rule is in the case of visits that consist predominantly of counseling or coordination of care (see numbered paragraph 3, page 7).

The nature of the presenting problem and time are provided in some levels to assist the physician in determining the appropriate level of E/M service.

Determine the Extent of History Obtained

The extent of the history is dependent upon clinical judgment and on the nature of the presenting problem(s). The levels of E/M services recognize four types of history that are defined as follows:

Problem focused: Chief complaint; brief history of present illness or problem.

Expanded problem focused: Chief complaint; brief history of present illness; problem pertinent system review.

Detailed: Chief complaint; extended history of present illness; problem pertinent system review extended to include a review of a limited number of additional systems; **pertinent** past, family, and/or social history **directly related to the patient's problems.**

Comprehensive: Chief complaint; extended history of present illness; review of systems that is directly related to the problem(s) identified in the history of the present illness plus a review of all additional body systems; **complete** past, family, and social history.

The comprehensive history obtained as part of the preventive medicine E/M service is not problem-oriented and does not involve a chief complaint or present illness. It does, however, include a comprehensive system review and comprehensive or interval past, family, and social history as well as a comprehensive assessment/history of pertinent risk factors.

Determine the Extent of Examination Performed

The extent of the examination performed is dependent on clinical judgment and on the nature of the presenting problem(s). The levels of E/M services recognize four types of examination that are defined as follows:

Problem focused: A limited examination of the affected body area or organ system.

Expanded problem focused: A limited examination of the affected body area or organ system and other symptomatic or related organ system(s).

Detailed: An extended examination of the affected body area(s) and other symptomatic or related organ system(s).

Comprehensive: A general multisystem examination or a complete examination of a single organ system. **Note:** The comprehensive examination performed as part of the preventive medicine E/M service is multisystem, but its extent is based on age and risk factors identified.

For the purposes of these CPT definitions, the following body areas are recognized:

- Head, including the face
- Neck
- Chest, including breasts and axilla
- Abdomen
- Genitalia, groin, buttocks
- Back
- Each extremity

For the purposes of these CPT definitions, the following organ systems are recognized:

- Eyes
- Ears, nose, mouth, and throat
- Cardiovascular
- Respiratory
- Gastrointestinal
- Genitourinary
- Musculoskeletal
- Skin
- Neurologic
- Psychiatric
- Hematologic/lymphatic/immunologic

Determine the Complexity of Medical Decision Making

Medical decision making refers to the complexity of establishing a diagnosis and/or selecting a management option as measured by:

- The number of possible diagnoses and/or the number of management options that must be considered
- The amount and/or complexity of medical records, diagnostic tests, and/or other information that must be obtained, reviewed, and analyzed
- The risk of significant complications, morbidity, and/or mortality, as well as comorbidities, associated with the patient's presenting problem(s), the diagnostic procedure(s), and/or the possible management options

Four types of medical decision making are recognized: straightforward, low complexity, moderate complexity, and high complexity. To qualify for a given type of decision making, two of the three elements in Table 1 must be met or exceeded.

Comorbidities/underlying diseases, in and of themselves, are not considered in selecting a level of E/M services *unless* their presence significantly increases the complexity of the medical decision making.

Select the Appropriate Level of E/M Services Based on the Following

1. For the following categories/subcategories, **all of the key components,** ie, history, examination, and medical decision making, must meet or exceed the stated requirements to qualify for a particular level of E/M service: office, new patient; hospital observation services; initial hospital care; office consultations; initial inpatient consultations; emergency department services; initial nursing facility care; domiciliary care, new patient; and home, new patient.

2. For the following categories/subcategories, **two of the three key components** (ie, history, examination, and medical decision making) must meet or exceed the stated requirements to qualify for a particular level of E/M services: office, established patient; subsequent hospital care; subsequent nursing facility care; domiciliary care, established patient; and home, established patient.

3. When counseling and/or coordination of care dominates (more than 50%) the encounter with the patient and/or family (face-to-face time in the office or other outpatient setting or floor/unit time in the hospital or nursing facility), then **time** shall be considered the key or controlling factor to qualify for a particular level of E/M services. This includes time spent with parties who have assumed responsibility for the care of the patient or decision making whether or not they are family members (eg, foster parents, person acting in loco parentis, legal guardian). The extent of counseling and/or coordination of care must be documented in the medical record.

Table 1
Complexity of Medical Decision Making

Number of Diagnoses or Management Options	Amount and/or Complexity of Data to be Reviewed	Risk of Complications and/or Morbidity or Mortality	Type of Decision Making
minimal	minimal or none	minimal	**straightforward**
limited	limited	low	**low complexity**
multiple	moderate	moderate	**moderate complexity**
extensive	extensive	high	**high complexity**

Evaluation/Management

Evaluation and Management

Office or Other Outpatient Services

The following codes are used to report evaluation and management services provided in the office or in an outpatient or other ambulatory facility. A patient is considered an outpatient until inpatient admission to a health care facility occurs.

To report services provided to a patient who is admitted to a hospital or nursing facility in the course of an encounter in the office or other ambulatory facility, see the notes for initial hospital inpatient care (page 11) or initial nursing facility care (page 19).

For services provided in the emergency department, see 99281-99285.

For observation care, see 99217-99226.

For observation or inpatient care services (including admission and discharge services), see 99234-99236.

New Patient

99201 **Office or other outpatient visit** for the evaluation and management of a new patient, which requires these 3 key components:

- **A problem focused history;**
- **A problem focused examination;**
- **Straightforward medical decision making.**

Counseling and/or coordination of care with other physicians, other qualified health care professionals, or agencies are provided consistent with the nature of the problem(s) and the patient's and/or family's needs.

Usually, the presenting problem(s) are self limited or minor. Typically, 10 minutes are spent face-to-face with the patient and/or family.

99202 **Office or other outpatient visit** for the evaluation and management of a new patient, which requires these 3 key components:

- **An expanded problem focused history;**
- **An expanded problem focused examination;**
- **Straightforward medical decision making.**

Counseling and/or coordination of care with other physicians, other qualified health care professionals, or agencies are provided consistent with the nature of the problem(s) and the patient's and/or family's needs.

Usually, the presenting problem(s) are of low to moderate severity. Typically, 20 minutes are spent face-to-face with the patient and/or family.

99203 **Office or other outpatient visit** for the evaluation and management of a new patient, which requires these 3 key components:

- **A detailed history;**
- **A detailed examination;**
- **Medical decision making of low complexity.**

Counseling and/or coordination of care with other physicians, other qualified health care professionals, or agencies are provided consistent with the nature of the problem(s) and the patient's and/or family's needs.

Usually, the presenting problem(s) are of moderate severity. Typically, 30 minutes are spent face-to-face with the patient and/or family.

99204 **Office or other outpatient visit** for the evaluation and management of a new patient, which requires these 3 key components:

- **A comprehensive history;**
- **A comprehensive examination;**
- **Medical decision making of moderate complexity.**

Counseling and/or coordination of care with other physicians, other qualified health care professionals, or agencies are provided consistent with the nature of the problem(s) and the patient's and/or family's needs.

Usually, the presenting problem(s) are of moderate to high severity. Typically, 45 minutes are spent face-to-face with the patient and/or family.

99205 **Office or other outpatient visit** for the evaluation and management of a new patient, which requires these 3 key components:

- **A comprehensive history;**
- **A comprehensive examination;**
- **Medical decision making of high complexity.**

Counseling and/or coordination of care with other physicians, other qualified health care professionals, or agencies are provided consistent with the nature of the problem(s) and the patient's and/or family's needs.

Usually, the presenting problem(s) are of moderate to high severity. Typically, 60 minutes are spent face-to-face with the patient and/or family.

Established Patient

99211 **Office or other outpatient visit** for the evaluation and management of an established patient, that may not require the presence of a physician or other qualified health care professional. Usually, the presenting problem(s) are minimal. Typically, 5 minutes are spent performing or supervising these services.

99212   **Office or other outpatient visit** for the evaluation and management of an established patient, which requires at least 2 of these 3 key components:

- **A problem focused history;**
- **A problem focused examination;**
- **Straightforward medical decision making.**

Counseling and/or coordination of care with other physicians, other qualified health care professionals, or agencies are provided consistent with the nature of the problem(s) and the patient's and/or family's needs.

Usually, the presenting problem(s) are self limited or minor. Typically, 10 minutes are spent face-to-face with the patient and/or family.

99213   **Office or other outpatient visit** for the evaluation and management of an established patient, which requires at least 2 of these 3 key components:

- **An expanded problem focused history;**
- **An expanded problem focused examination;**
- **Medical decision making of low complexity.**

Counseling and coordination of care with other physicians, other qualified health care professionals, or agencies are provided consistent with the nature of the problem(s) and the patient's and/or family's needs.

Usually, the presenting problem(s) are of low to moderate severity. Typically, 15 minutes are spent face-to-face with the patient and/or family.

99214   **Office or other outpatient visit** for the evaluation and management of an established patient, which requires at least 2 of these 3 key components:

- **A detailed history;**
- **A detailed examination;**
- **Medical decision making of moderate complexity.**

Counseling and/or coordination of care with other physicians, other qualified health care professionals, or agencies are provided consistent with the nature of the problem(s) and the patient's and/or family's needs.

Usually, the presenting problem(s) are of moderate to high severity. Typically, 25 minutes are spent face-to-face with the patient and/or family.

99215   **Office or other outpatient visit** for the evaluation and management of an established patient, which requires at least 2 of these 3 key components:

- **A comprehensive history;**
- **A comprehensive examination;**
- **Medical decision making of high complexity.**

Counseling and/or coordination of care with other physicians, other qualified health care professionals, or agencies are provided consistent with the nature of the problem(s) and the patient's and/or family's needs.

Usually, the presenting problem(s) are of moderate to high severity. Typically, 40 minutes are spent face-to-face with the patient and/or family.

Hospital Observation Services

The following codes are used to report evaluation and management services provided to patients designated/admitted as "observation status" in a hospital. It is not necessary that the patient be located in an observation area designated by the hospital.

If such an area does exist in a hospital (as a separate unit in the hospital, in the emergency department, etc.), these codes are to be utilized if the patient is placed in such an area.

For definitions of key components and commonly used terms, please see **Evaluation and Management Services Guidelines.**

Observation Care Discharge Services

Observation care discharge of a patient from "observation status" includes final examination of the patient, discussion of the hospital stay, instructions for continuing care, and preparation of discharge records. For observation or inpatient hospital care including the admission and discharge of the patient on the same date, see codes 99234-99236 as appropriate.

99217   **Observation care discharge** day management (This code is to be utilized to report all services provided to a patient on discharge from "observation status" if the discharge is on other than the initial date of "observation status." To report services to a patient designated as "observation status" or "inpatient status" and discharged on the same date, use the codes for Observation or Inpatient Care Services [including Admission and Discharge Services, 99234-99236 as appropriate.])

Initial Observation Care

New or Established Patient

The following codes are used to report the encounter(s) by the supervising physician or other qualified health care professional with the patient when designated as "observation status." This refers to the initiation of observation status, supervision of the care plan for observation and performance of periodic reassessments. For observation encounters by other physicians, see office or other outpatient consultation codes (99241-99245) or subsequent observation care codes (99224-99226) as appropriate.

To report services provided to a patient who is admitted to the hospital after receiving hospital observation care services on the same date, see the notes for initial hospital inpatient care (page 11). For observation care services on other than the initial or discharge date, see subsequent observation services codes (99224-99226). For a patient admitted to the hospital on a date subsequent to the date of observation status, the hospital admission would be

Evaluation/Management

reported with the appropriate initial hospital care code (99221-99223). For a patient admitted and discharged from observation or inpatient status on the same date, the services should be reported with codes 99234-99236 as appropriate. Do not report observation discharge (99217) in conjunction with a hospital admission (99221-99223).

When "observation status" is initiated in the course of an encounter in another site of service (eg, hospital emergency department, office, nursing facility) all evaluation and management services provided by the supervising physician or other qualified health care professional in conjunction with initiating "observation status" are considered part of the initial observation care when performed on the same date. The observation care level of service reported by the supervising physician or other qualified health care professional should include the services related to initiating "observation status" provided in the other sites of service as well as in the observation setting.

Evaluation and management services including new or established patient office or other outpatient services (99201-99215), emergency department services (99281-99285), nursing facility services (99304-99318), domiciliary, rest home, or custodial care services (99324-99337), home services (99341-99350), and preventive medicine services (99381-99429) on the same date related to the admission to "observation status" should not be reported separately.

These codes may not be utilized for post-operative recovery if the procedure is considered part of the surgical "package." These codes apply to all evaluation and management services that are provided on the same date of initiating "observation status."

99218 Initial observation care, per day, for the evaluation and management of a patient which requires these 3 key components:

- **A detailed or comprehensive history;**
- **A detailed or comprehensive examination; and**
- **Medical decision making that is straightforward or of low complexity.**

Counseling and/or coordination of care with other physicians, other qualified health care professionals, or agencies are provided consistent with the nature of the problem(s) and the patient's and/or family's needs.

Usually, the problem(s) requiring admission to "observation status" are of low severity. Typically, 30 minutes are spent at the bedside and on the patient's hospital floor or unit.

99219 Initial observation care, per day, for the evaluation and management of a patient, which requires these 3 key components:

- **A comprehensive history;**
- **A comprehensive examination; and**
- **Medical decision making of moderate complexity.**

Counseling and/or coordination of care with other physicians, other qualified health care professionals, or agencies are provided consistent with the nature of the problem(s) and the patient's and/or family's needs.

Usually, the problem(s) requiring admission to "observation status" are of moderate severity. Typically, 50 minutes are spent at the bedside and on the patient's hospital floor or unit.

99220 Initial observation care, per day, for the evaluation and management of a patient, which requires these 3 key components:

- **A comprehensive history;**
- **A comprehensive examination; and**
- **Medical decision making of high complexity.**

Counseling and/or coordination of care with other physicians, other qualified health care professionals, or agencies are provided consistent with the nature of the problem(s) and the patient's and/or family's needs.

Usually, the problem(s) requiring admission to "observation status" are of high severity. Typically, 70 minutes are spent at the bedside and on the patient's hospital floor or unit.

Subsequent Observation Care

All levels of subsequent observation care include reviewing the medical record and reviewing the results of diagnostic studies and changes in the patient's status (ie, changes in history, physical condition, and response to management) since the last assessment.

\# **99224** Subsequent observation care, per day, for the evaluation and management of a patient, which requires at least 2 of these 3 key components:

- **Problem focused interval history;**
- **Problem focused examination;**
- **Medical decision making that is straightforward or of low complexity.**

Counseling and/or coordination of care with other physicians, other qualified health care professionals, or agencies are provided consistent with the nature of the problem(s) and the patient's and/or family's needs.

Usually, the patient is stable, recovering, or improving. Typically, 15 minutes are spent at the bedside and on the patient's hospital floor or unit.

\# **99225** Subsequent observation care, per day, for the evaluation and management of a patient, which requires at least 2 of these 3 key components:

- **An expanded problem focused interval history;**
- **An expanded problem focused examination;**
- **Medical decision making of moderate complexity.**

Counseling and/or coordination of care with other physicians, other qualified health care professionals, or agencies are provided consistent with the nature of the problem(s) and the patient's and/or family's needs.

Usually, the patient is responding inadequately to therapy or has developed a minor complication. Typically, 25 minutes are spent at the bedside and on the patient's hospital floor or unit.

 # 99226   **Subsequent observation care,** per day, for the evaluation and management of a patient, which requires at least 2 of these 3 key components:

- **A detailed interval history;**
- **A detailed examination;**
- **Medical decision making of high complexity.**

Counseling and/or coordination of care with other physicians, other qualified health care professionals, or agencies are provided consistent with the nature of the problem(s) and the patient's and/or family's needs.

Usually, the patient is unstable or has developed a significant complication or a significant new problem. Typically, 35 minutes are spent at the bedside and on the patient's hospital floor or unit.

Hospital Inpatient Services

The following codes are used to report evaluation and management services provided to hospital inpatients. Hospital inpatient services include those services provided to patients in a "partial hospital" setting. These codes are to be used to report these partial hospitalization services. See also psychiatry notes in the full text of the CPT code set.

For definitions of key components and commonly used terms, please see **Evaluation and Management Services Guidelines.** For Hospital Observation Services, see 99218-99220, 99224-99226. For a patient admitted and discharged from observation or inpatient status on the same date, the services should be reported with codes 99234-99236 as appropriate.

Initial Hospital Care

New or Established Patient

The following codes are used to report the first hospital inpatient encounter with the patient by the admitting physician.

For initial inpatient encounters by physicians other than the admitting physician, see initial inpatient consultation codes (99251-99255) or subsequent hospital care codes (99231-99233) as appropriate.

For admission services for the neonate (28 days of age or younger) requiring intensive observation, frequent interventions, and other intensive care services, see 99477.

When the patient is admitted to the hospital as an inpatient in the course of an encounter in another site of service (eg, hospital emergency department, observation status in a hospital, office, nursing facility) all evaluation and management services provided by that physician in conjunction with that admission are considered part of the initial hospital care when performed on the same date as the admission. The inpatient care level of service reported by the admitting physician should include the services related to the admission he/she provided in the other sites of service as well as in the inpatient setting.

Evaluation and management services including new or established patient office or other outpatient services (99201-99215), emergency department services (99281-99285), nursing facility services (99304-99318), domiciliary, rest home, or custodial care services (99324-99337), home services (99341-99350), and preventive medicine services (99381-99397) on the same date related to the admission to "observation status" should **not** be reported separately. For a patient admitted and discharged from observation or inpatient status on the same date, the services should be reported with codes 99234-99236 as appropriate.

99221   **Initial hospital care,** per day, for the evaluation and management of a patient, which requires these 3 key components:

- **A detailed or comprehensive history;**
- **A detailed or comprehensive examination; and**
- **Medical decision making that is straightforward or of low complexity.**

Counseling and/or coordination of care with other physicians, other qualified health care professionals, or agencies are provided consistent with the nature of the problem(s) and the patient's and/or family's needs.

Usually, the problem(s) requiring admission are of low severity. Typically, 30 minutes are spent at the bedside and on the patient's hospital floor or unit.

99222   **Initial hospital care,** per day, for the evaluation and management of a patient, which requires these 3 key components:

- **A comprehensive history;**
- **A comprehensive examination; and**
- **Medical decision making of moderate complexity.**

Counseling and/or coordination of care with other physicians, other qualified health care professionals, or agencies are provided consistent with the nature of the problem(s) and the patient's and/or family's needs.

Usually, the problem(s) requiring admission are of moderate severity. Typically, 50 minutes are spent at the bedside and on the patient's hospital floor or unit.

99223   **Initial hospital care,** per day, for the evaluation and management of a patient, which requires these 3 key components:

- **A comprehensive history;**
- **A comprehensive examination; and**
- **Medical decision making of high complexity.**

Counseling and/or coordination of care with other physicians, other qualified health care professionals, or agencies are provided consistent with the nature of the problem(s) and the patient's and/or family's needs.

Usually, the problem(s) requiring admission are of high severity. Typically, 70 minutes are spent at the bedside and on the patient's hospital floor or unit.

99224   Code is out of numerical sequence. See 99224-99226

99225   Code is out of numerical sequence. See 99224-99226

99226   Code is out of numerical sequence. See 99224-99226

Subsequent Hospital Care

All levels of subsequent hospital care include reviewing the medical record and reviewing the results of diagnostic studies and changes in the patient's status (ie, changes in history, physical condition and response to management) since the last assessment.

99231   **Subsequent hospital care,** per day, for the evaluation and management of a patient, which requires at least 2 of these 3 key components:

- **A problem focused interval history;**
- **A problem focused examination;**
- **Medical decision making that is straightforward or of low complexity.**

Counseling and/or coordination of care with other physicians, other qualified health care professionals, or agencies are provided consistent with the nature of the problem(s) and the patient's and/or family's needs.

Usually, the patient is stable, recovering or improving. Typically, 15 minutes are spent at the bedside and on the patient's hospital floor or unit.

99232   **Subsequent hospital care,** per day, for the evaluation and management of a patient, which requires at least 2 of these 3 key components:

- **An expanded problem focused interval history;**
- **An expanded problem focused examination;**
- **Medical decision making of moderate complexity.**

Counseling and/or coordination of care with other physicians, other qualified health care professionals, or agencies are provided consistent with the nature of the problem(s) and the patient's and/or family's needs.

Usually, the patient is responding inadequately to therapy or has developed a minor complication. Typically, 25 minutes are spent at the bedside and on the patient's hospital floor or unit.

99233   **Subsequent hospital care,** per day, for the evaluation and management of a patient, which requires at least 2 of these 3 key components:

- **A detailed interval history;**
- **A detailed examination;**
- **Medical decision making of high complexity.**

Counseling and/or coordination of care with other physicians, other qualified health care professionals, or agencies are provided consistent with the nature of the problem(s) and the patient's and/or family's needs.

Usually, the patient is unstable or has developed a significant complication or a significant new problem. Typically, 35 minutes are spent at the bedside and on the patient's hospital floor or unit.

Observation or Inpatient Care Services (Including Admission and Discharge Services)

The following codes are used to report observation or inpatient hospital care services provided to patients admitted and discharged on the same date of service. When a patient is admitted to the hospital from observation status on the same date, only the initial hospital care code should be reported. The initial hospital care code reported by the admitting physician or other qualified health care professional should include the services related to the observation status services he/she provided on the same date of inpatient admission.

When "observation status" is initiated in the course of an encounter in another site of service (eg, hospital emergency department, office, nursing facility) all evaluation and management services provided by the supervising physician or other qualified health care professional in conjunction with initiating "observation status" are considered part of the initial observation care when performed on the same date. The observation care level of service should include the services related to initiating "observation status" provided in the other sites of service as well as in the observation setting when provided by the same individual.

For patients admitted to observation or inpatient care and discharged on a different date, see codes 99218-99220, 99224-99226, 99217, or 99221-99223, 99238 and 99239.

99234   **Observation or inpatient hospital care,** for the evaluation and management of a patient including admission and discharge on the same date, which requires these 3 key components:

- **A detailed or comprehensive history;**
- **A detailed or comprehensive examination; and**
- **Medical decision making that is straightforward or of low complexity.**

Counseling and/or coordination of care with other physicians, other qualified health care professionals, or agencies are provided consistent with the nature of the problem(s) and the patient's and/or family's needs.

Usually the presenting problem(s) requiring admission are of low severity. Typically, 40 minutes are spent at the bedside and on the patient's hospital floor or unit.

99235 **Observation or inpatient hospital care,** for the evaluation and management of a patient including admission and discharge on the same date, which requires these 3 key components:

- **A comprehensive history;**
- **A comprehensive examination; and**
- **Medical decision making of moderate complexity.**

Counseling and/or coordination of care with other physicians, other qualified health care professionals, or agencies are provided consistent with the nature of the problem(s) and the patient's and/or family's needs.

Usually the presenting problem(s) requiring admission are of moderate severity. Typically, 50 minutes are spent at the bedside and on the patient's hospital floor or unit.

99236 **Observation or inpatient hospital care,** for the evaluation and management of a patient including admission and discharge on the same date, which requires these 3 key components:

- **A comprehensive history;**
- **A comprehensive examination; and**
- **Medical decision making of high complexity.**

Counseling and/or coordination of care with other physicians, other qualified health care professionals, or agencies are provided consistent with the nature of the problem(s) and the patient's and/or family's needs.

Usually the presenting problem(s) requiring admission are of high severity. Typically, 55 minutes are spent at the bedside and on the patient's hospital floor or unit.

Hospital Discharge Services

The hospital discharge day management codes are to be used to report the total duration of time spent by a physician for final hospital discharge of a patient. The codes include, as appropriate, final examination of the patient, discussion of the hospital stay, even if the time spent by the physician on that date is not continuous, instructions for continuing care to all relevant caregivers, and preparation of discharge records, prescriptions and referral forms. For a patient admitted and discharged from observation or inpatient status on the same date, the services should be reported with codes 99234-99236 as appropriate.

99238 **Hospital discharge day management**; 30 minutes or less

99239 more than 30 minutes

(These codes are to be utilized to report all services provided to a patient on the date of discharge, if other than the initial date of inpatient status. To report services to a patient who is admitted as an inpatient and discharged on the same date, see codes 99234-99236 for observation or inpatient hospital care including the admission and discharge of the patient on the same date. To report concurrent care services provided by an individual other than the physician or qualified health care professional performing the discharge day management service, use subsequent hospital care codes [99231-99233] on the day of discharge.)

(For Observation Care Discharge, use 99217)

(For observation or inpatient hospital care including the admission and discharge of the patient on the same date, see 99234-99236)

(For Nursing Facility Care Discharge, see 99315, 99316)

(For discharge services provided to newborns admitted and discharged on the same date, use 99463)

Consultations

A consultation is a type of evaluation and management service provided at the request of another physician or appropriate source to either recommend care for a specific condition or problem or to determine whether to accept responsibility for ongoing management of the patient's entire care or for the care of a specific condition or problem.

A physician consultant may initiate diagnostic and/or therapeutic services at the same or subsequent visit.

A "consultation" initiated by a patient and/or family, and not requested by a physician or other appropriate source (eg, physician assistant, nurse practitioner, doctor of chiropractic, physical therapist, occupational therapist, speech-language pathologist, psychologist, social worker, lawyer, or insurance company), is not reported using the consultation codes but may be reported using the office visit, home service, or domiciliary/rest home care codes as appropriate.

The written or verbal request for consult may be made by a physician or other appropriate source and documented in the patient's medical record by either the consulting or requesting physician or appropriate source. The consultant's opinion and any services that were ordered or performed must also be documented in the patient's medical record and communicated by written report to the requesting physician or other appropriate source.

If a consultation is mandated (eg, by a third-party payer) modifier 32 should also be reported.

Any specifically identifiable procedure (ie, identified with a specific CPT code) performed on or subsequent to the date of the initial consultation should be reported separately.

Evaluation/Management

If subsequent to the completion of a consultation the consultant assumes responsibility for management of a portion or all of the patient's condition(s), the appropriate **Evaluation and Management** services code for the site of service should be reported. In the hospital or nursing facility setting, the consultant should use the appropriate inpatient consultation code for the initial encounter and then subsequent hospital or nursing facility care codes. In the office setting, the consultant should use the appropriate office or other outpatient consultation codes and then the established patient office or other outpatient services codes.

To report services provided to a patient who is admitted to a hospital or nursing facility in the course of an encounter in the office or other ambulatory facility, see the notes for Initial Hospital Inpatient Care (page 11) or Initial Nursing Facility Care (page 19).

For definitions of key components and commonly used terms, please see **Evaluation and Management Services Guidelines.**

Office or Other Outpatient Consultations

New or Established Patient

The following codes are used to report consultations provided in the office or in an outpatient or other ambulatory facility, including hospital observation services, home services, domiciliary, rest home, or emergency department (see the preceding consultation definition above). Follow-up visits in the consultant's office or other outpatient facility that are initiated by the consultant or patient are reported using the appropriate codes for established patients, office visits (99211-99215), domiciliary, rest home (99334-99337), or home (99347-99350). If an additional request for an opinion or advice regarding the same or a new problem is received from another physician or other appropriate source and documented in the medical record, the office consultation codes may be used again. Services that constitute transfer of care (ie, are provided for the management of the patient's entire care or for the care of a specific condition or problem) are reported with the appropriate new or established patient codes for office or other outpatient visits, domiciliary, rest home services, or home services.

99241 **Office consultation** for a new or established patient, which requires these 3 key components:

- **A problem focused history;**
- **A problem focused examination; and**
- **Straightforward medical decision making.**

Counseling and/or coordination of care with other physicians, other qualified health care professionals, or agencies are provided consistent with the nature of the problem(s) and the patient's and/or family's needs.

Usually, the presenting problem(s) are self limited or minor. Typically, 15 minutes are spent face-to-face with the patient and/or family.

99242 **Office consultation** for a new or established patient, which requires these 3 key components:

- **An expanded problem focused history;**
- **An expanded problem focused examination; and**
- **Straightforward medical decision making.**

Counseling and/or coordination of care with other physicians, other qualified health care professionals, or agencies are provided consistent with the nature of the problem(s) and the patient's and/or family's needs.

Usually, the presenting problem(s) are of low severity. Typically, 30 minutes are spent face-to-face with the patient and/or family.

99243 **Office consultation** for a new or established patient, which requires these 3 key components:

- **A detailed history;**
- **A detailed examination; and**
- **Medical decision making of low complexity.**

Counseling and/or coordination of care with other physicians, other qualified health care professionals, or agencies are provided consistent with the nature of the problem(s) and the patient's and/or family's needs.

Usually, the presenting problem(s) are of moderate severity. Typically, 40 minutes are spent face-to-face with the patient and/or family.

99244 **Office consultation** for a new or established patient, which requires these 3 key components:

- **A comprehensive history;**
- **A comprehensive examination; and**
- **Medical decision making of moderate complexity.**

Counseling and/or coordination of care with other physicians, other qualified health care professionals, or agencies are provided consistent with the nature of the problem(s) and the patient's and/or family's needs.

Usually, the presenting problem(s) are of moderate to high severity. Typically, 60 minutes are spent face-to-face with the patient and/or family.

99245 **Office consultation** for a new or established patient, which requires these 3 key components:

- **A comprehensive history;**
- **A comprehensive examination; and**
- **Medical decision making of high complexity.**

Counseling and/or coordination of care with other physicians, other qualified health care professionals, or agencies are provided consistent with the nature of the problem(s) and the patient's and/or family's needs.

Usually, the presenting problem(s) are of moderate to high severity. Typically, 80 minutes are spent face-to-face with the patient and/or family.

Inpatient Consultations

New or Established Patient

The following codes are used to report physician or other qualified health care professional consultations provided to hospital inpatients, residents of nursing facilities, or patients in a partial hospital setting. Only one consultation should be reported by a consultant per admission. Subsequent services during the same admission are reported using subsequent hospital care codes (99231-99233) or subsequent nursing facility care codes (99307-99310), including services to complete the initial consultation, monitor progress, revise recommendations, or address a new problem. Use subsequent hospital care codes (99231-99233) or subsequent nursing facility care codes (99307-99310) to report transfer of care services (see page 5, Concurrent Care and Transfer of Care definitions).

When an inpatient consultation is performed on a date that a patient is admitted to a hospital or nursing facility, all evaluation and management services provided by the consultant related to the admission are reported with the inpatient consultation service code (99251-99255). If a patient is admitted after an outpatient consultation (office, emergency department, etc), and the patient is not seen on the unit on the date of admission, only report the outpatient consultation code (99241-99245). If the patient is seen by the consultant on the unit on the date of admission, report all evaluation and management services provided by the consultant related to the admission with either the inpatient consultation code (99251-99255) or with the initial inpatient admission service code (99221-99223). Do not report both an outpatient consultation (99241-99245) and inpatient consultation (99251-99255) for services related to the same inpatient stay. When transfer of care services are provided on a date subsequent to the outpatient consultation, use the subsequent hospital care codes (99231-99233) or subsequent nursing facility care codes (99307-99310).

99251 **Inpatient consultation** for a new or established patient, which requires these 3 key components:

- **A problem focused history;**
- **A problem focused examination; and**
- **Straightforward medical decision making.**

Counseling and/or coordination of care with other physicians, other qualified health care professionals, or agencies are provided consistent with the nature of the problem(s) and the patient's and/or family's needs.

Usually, the presenting problem(s) are self limited or minor. Typically, 20 minutes are spent at the bedside and on the patient's hospital floor or unit.

99252 **Inpatient consultation** for a new or established patient, which requires these 3 key components:

- **An expanded problem focused history;**
- **An expanded problem focused examination; and**
- **Straightforward medical decision making.**

Counseling and/or coordination of care with other physicians, other qualified health care professionals, or agencies are provided consistent with the nature of the problem(s) and the patient's and/or family's needs.

Usually, the presenting problem(s) are of low severity. Typically, 40 minutes are spent at the bedside and on the patient's hospital floor or unit.

99253 **Inpatient consultation** for a new or established patient, which requires these 3 key components:

- **A detailed history;**
- **A detailed examination; and**
- **Medical decision making of low complexity.**

Counseling and/or coordination of care with other physicians, other qualified health care professionals, or agencies are provided consistent with the nature of the problem(s) and the patient's and/or family's needs.

Usually, the presenting problem(s) are of moderate severity. Typically, 55 minutes are spent at the bedside and on the patient's hospital floor or unit.

99254 **Inpatient consultation** for a new or established patient, which requires these 3 key components:

- **A comprehensive history;**
- **A comprehensive examination; and**
- **Medical decision making of moderate complexity.**

Counseling and/or coordination of care with other physicians, other qualified health care professionals, or agencies are provided consistent with the nature of the problem(s) and the patient's and/or family's needs.

Usually, the presenting problem(s) are of moderate to high severity. Typically, 80 minutes are spent at the bedside and on the patient's hospital floor or unit.

99255 **Inpatient consultation** for a new or established patient, which requires these 3 key components:

- **A comprehensive history;**
- **A comprehensive examination; and**
- **Medical decision making of high complexity.**

Counseling and/or coordination of care with other physicians, other qualified health care professionals, or agencies are provided consistent with the nature of the problem(s) and the patient's and/or family's needs.

Usually, the presenting problem(s) are of moderate to high severity. Typically, 110 minutes are spent at the bedside and on the patient's hospital floor or unit.

Emergency Department Services

New or Established Patient

The following codes are used to report evaluation and management services provided in the emergency department. No distinction is made between new and established patients in the emergency department.

An emergency department is defined as an organized hospital-based facility for the provision of unscheduled episodic services to patients who present for immediate medical attention. The facility must be available 24 hours a day.

For critical care services provided in the emergency department, see Critical Care notes and 99291, 99292.

For evaluation and management services provided to a patient in an observation area of a hospital, see 99217-99220.

For observation or inpatient care services (including admission and discharge services), see 99234-99236.

99281　**Emergency department visit** for the evaluation and management of a patient, which requires these 3 key components:

- **A problem focused history;**
- **A problem focused examination; and**
- **Straightforward medical decision making.**

Counseling and/or coordination of care with other physicians, other qualified health care professionals, or agencies are provided consistent with the nature of the problem(s) and the patient's and/or family's needs.

Usually, the presenting problem(s) are self limited or minor.

99282　**Emergency department visit** for the evaluation and management of a patient, which requires these 3 key components:

- **An expanded problem focused history;**
- **An expanded problem focused examination; and**
- **Medical decision making of low complexity.**

Counseling and/or coordination of care with other physicians, other qualified health care professionals, or agencies are provided consistent with the nature of the problem(s) and the patient's and/or family's needs.

Usually, the presenting problem(s) are of low to moderate severity.

99283　**Emergency department visit** for the evaluation and management of a patient, which requires these 3 key components:

- **An expanded problem focused history;**
- **An expanded problem focused examination; and**
- **Medical decision making of moderate complexity.**

Counseling and/or coordination of care with other physicians, other qualified health care professionals, or agencies are provided consistent with the nature of the problem(s) and the patient's and/or family's needs.

Usually, the presenting problem(s) are of moderate severity.

99284　**Emergency department visit** for the evaluation and management of a patient, which requires these 3 key components:

- **A detailed history;**
- **A detailed examination; and**
- **Medical decision making of moderate complexity.**

Counseling and/or coordination of care with other physicians, other qualified health care professionals, or agencies are provided consistent with the nature of the problem(s) and the patient's and/or family's needs.

Usually, the presenting problem(s) are of high severity, and require urgent evaluation by the physician, or other qualified health care professionals but do not pose an immediate significant threat to life or physiologic function.

99285　**Emergency department visit** for the evaluation and management of a patient, which requires these 3 key components within the constraints imposed by the urgency of the patient's clinical condition and/or mental status:

- **A comprehensive history;**
- **A comprehensive examination; and**
- **Medical decision making of high complexity.**

Counseling and/or coordination of care with other physicians, other qualified health care professionals, or agencies are provided consistent with the nature of the problem(s) and the patient's and/or family's needs.

Usually, the presenting problem(s) are of high severity and pose an immediate significant threat to life or physiologic function.

Other Emergency Services

In directed emergency care, advanced life support, the physician or other qualified health care professional is located in a hospital emergency or critical care department, and is in two-way voice communication with ambulance or rescue personnel outside the hospital. Direction of the performance of necessary medical procedures includes but is not limited to: telemetry of cardiac rhythm; cardiac and/or pulmonary resuscitation; endotracheal or esophageal obturator airway intubation; administration of intravenous fluids and/or administration of intramuscular, intratracheal or subcutaneous drugs; and/or electrical conversion of arrhythmia.

99288　**Physician or other qualified health care professional direction of** emergency medical systems (EMS) emergency care, advanced life support

Critical Care Services

Critical care is the direct delivery by a physician(s) or other qualified health care professional of medical care for a critically ill or critically injured patient. A critical illness or injury acutely impairs one or more vital organ systems such that there is a high probability of imminent or life threatening deterioration in the patient's condition. Critical care involves high complexity decision making to assess, manipulate, and support vital system function(s) to treat single or multiple vital organ system failure and/or to prevent further life threatening deterioration of the patient's condition. Examples of vital organ system failure include, but are not limited to: central nervous system failure, circulatory failure, shock, renal, hepatic, metabolic, and/or respiratory failure. Although critical care typically requires interpretation of multiple physiologic parameters and/or application of advanced technology(s), critical care may be provided in life threatening situations when these elements are not present. Critical care may be provided on multiple days, even if no changes are made in the treatment rendered to the patient, provided that the patient's condition continues to require the level of attention described above.

Providing medical care to a critically ill, injured, or post-operative patient qualifies as a critical care service only if both the illness or injury and the treatment being provided meet the above requirements. Critical care is usually, but not always, given in a critical care area, such as the coronary care unit, intensive care unit, pediatric intensive care unit, respiratory care unit, or the emergency care facility.

Inpatient critical care services provided to infants 29 days through 71 months of age are reported with pediatric critical care codes 99471-99476. The pediatric critical care codes are reported as long as the infant/young child qualifies for critical care services during the hospital stay through 71 months of age. Inpatient critical care services provided to neonates (28 days of age or younger) are reported with the neonatal critical care codes 99468 and 99469. The neonatal critical care codes are reported as long as the neonate qualifies for critical care services during the hospital stay through the 28th postnatal day. The reporting of the pediatric and neonatal critical care services is not based on time or the type of unit (eg, pediatric or neonatal critical care unit) and it is not dependent upon the type of physician or other qualified health care professional delivering the care. To report critical care services provided in the outpatient setting (eg, emergency department or office), for neonates and pediatric patients up through 71 months of age, see the critical care codes 99291, 99292. If the same individual provides critical care services for a neonatal or pediatric patient in both the outpatient and inpatient settings on the same day, report only the appropriate neonatal or pediatric critical care code 99468-99472 for all critical care services provided on that day. Also report 99291-99292 for neonatal or pediatric critical care services provided by the individual providing critical care at one facility but transferring the patient to another facility. Critical care services provided by a second individual of a different specialty not reporting a per day neonatal or pediatric critical care code can be reported with codes 99291, 99292. For additional instructions on reporting these services, see the Neonatal and Pediatric Critical Care section and codes 99468-99476.

Services for a patient who is not critically ill but happens to be in a critical care unit are reported using other appropriate E/M codes.

Critical care and other E/M services may be provided to the same patient on the same date by the same individual.

For reporting by professionals, the following services are included in critical care when performed during the critical period by the physician(s) providing critical care: the interpretation of cardiac output measurements (93561, 93562), chest X-rays (71010, 71015, 71020), pulse oximetry (94760, 94761, 94762), blood gases, and information data stored in computers (eg, ECGs, blood pressures, hematologic data [99090]); gastric intubation (43752, 43753); temporary transcutaneous pacing (92953); ventilatory management (94002-94004, 94660, 94662); and vascular access procedures (36000, 36410, 36415, 36591, 36600). Any services performed that are not included in this listing should be reported separately. Facilities may report the above services separately.

Codes 99291, 99292 should be reported for the attendance during the transport of critically ill or critically injured patients older than 24 months of age to or from a facility or hospital. For transport services of critically ill or critically injured pediatric patients 24 months of age or younger, see 99466, 99467.

Codes 99291, 99292 are used to report the total duration of time spent in provision of critical care services to a critically ill or critically injured patient, even if the time spent providing care on that date is not continuous. For any given period of time spent providing critical care services, the individual must devote his or her full attention to the patient and, therefore, cannot provide services to any other patient during the same period of time.

Time spent with the individual patient should be recorded in the patient's record. The time that can be reported as critical care is the time spent engaged in work directly related to the individual patient's care whether that time was spent at the immediate bedside or elsewhere on the floor or unit. For example, time spent on the unit or at the nursing station on the floor reviewing test results or imaging studies, discussing the critically ill patient's care with other medical staff or documenting critical care services in the medical record would be reported as critical care, even though it does not occur at the bedside.

Also, when the patient is unable or lacks capacity to participate in discussions, time spent on the floor or unit with family members or surrogate decision makers obtaining a medical history, reviewing the patient's condition or prognosis, or discussing treatment or limitation(s) of treatment may be reported as critical care, provided that the conversation bears directly on the management of the patient.

Time spent in activities that occur outside of the unit or off the floor (eg, telephone calls whether taken at home, in the office, or elsewhere in the hospital) may not be reported as critical care since the individual is not immediately available to the patient. Time spent in activities that do not directly contribute to the treatment of the patient may not be reported as critical care, even if they are performed in the critical care unit (eg, participation in administrative meetings or telephone calls to discuss other patients). Time spent performing separately reportable procedures or services should not be included in the time reported as critical care time. No individual may report remote real-time interactive video-conferenced critical care services (0188T, 0189T) for the period in which any other physician or qualified health care professional reports codes 99291, 99292.

Code 99291 is used to report the first 30-74 minutes of critical care on a given date. It should be used only once per date even if the time spent by the individual is not continuous on that date. Critical care of less than 30 minutes total duration on a given date should be reported with the appropriate E/M code.

Code 99292 is used to report additional block(s) of time, of up to 30 minutes each beyond the first 74 minutes. (See the following table.)

The following examples illustrate the correct reporting of critical care services:

Total Duration of Critical Care Codes

less than 30 minutes	appropriate E/M codes
30-74 minutes (30 minutes - 1 hr. 14 min.)	99291 X 1
75-104 minutes (1 hr. 15 min. - 1 hr. 44 min.)	99291 X 1 AND 99292 X 1
105-134 minutes (1 hr. 45 min. - 2 hr. 14 min.)	99291 X 1 AND 99292 X 2
135-164 minutes (2 hr. 15 min. - 2 hr. 44 min.)	99291 X 1 AND 99292 X 3
165-194 minutes (2 hr. 45 min. - 3 hr. 14 min.)	99291 X 1 AND 99292 X 4
195 minutes or longer (3 hr. 15 min. - etc.)	99291 and 99292 as appropriate (see illustrated reporting examples above)

99291   **Critical care, evaluation and management** of the critically ill or critically injured patient; first 30-74 minutes

+ 99292   each additional 30 minutes (List separately in addition to code for primary service)

(Use 99292 in conjunction with 99291)

Nursing Facility Services

The following codes are used to report evaluation and management services to patients in nursing facilities (formerly called skilled nursing facilities [SNFs], intermediate care facilities [ICFs], or long-term care facilities [LTCFs]).

These codes should also be used to report evaluation and management services provided to a patient in a psychiatric residential treatment center (a facility or a distinct part of a facility for psychiatric care, which provides a 24-hour therapeutically planned and professionally staffed group living and learning environment). If procedures such as medical psychotherapy are provided in addition to evaluation and management services, these should be reported in addition to the evaluation and management services provided.

Nursing facilities that provide convalescent, rehabilitative, or long term care are required to conduct comprehensive, accurate, standardized, and reproducible assessments of each resident's functional capacity using a Resident Assessment Instrument (RAI). All RAIs include the Minimum Data Set (MDS), Resident Assessment Protocols (RAPs), and utilization guidelines. The MDS is the primary screening and assessment tool; the RAPs trigger the identification of potential problems and provide guidelines for follow-up assessments.

Physicians have a central role in assuring that all residents receive thorough assessments and that medical plans of care are instituted or revised to enhance or maintain the residents' physical and psychosocial functioning. This role includes providing input in the development of the MDS and a multi-disciplinary plan of care, as required by regulations pertaining to the care of nursing facility residents.

Two major subcategories of nursing facility services are recognized: Initial Nursing Facility Care and Subsequent Nursing Facility Care. Both subcategories apply to new or established patients.

For definitions of key components and commonly used terms, please see **Evaluation and Management Services Guidelines.**

(For care plan oversight services provided to nursing facility residents, see 99379-99380)

Initial Nursing Facility Care

New or Established Patient

When the patient is admitted to the nursing facility in the course of an encounter in another site of service (eg, hospital emergency department, office), all evaluation and management services provided by that physician in conjunction with that admission are considered part of the initial nursing facility care when performed on the same date as the admission or readmission. The nursing facility care level of service reported by the admitting physician should include the services related to the admission he/she provided in the other sites of service as well as in the nursing facility setting.

Hospital discharge or observation discharge services performed on the same date of nursing facility admission or readmission may be reported separately. For a patient discharged from inpatient status on the same date of nursing facility admission or readmission, the hospital discharge services should be reported with codes 99238, 99239 as appropriate. For a patient discharged from observation status on the same date of nursing facility admission or readmission, the observation care discharge services should be reported with code 99217. For a patient admitted and discharged from observation or inpatient status on the same date, see codes 99234-99236.

(For nursing facility care discharge, see 99315, 99316)

99304   Initial nursing facility care, per day, for the evaluation and management of a patient, which requires these 3 key components:

- **A detailed or comprehensive history;**
- **A detailed or comprehensive examination; and**
- **Medical decision making that is straightforward or of low complexity.**

Counseling and/or coordination of care with other physicians, other qualified health care professionals, or agencies are provided consistent with the nature of the problem(s) and the patient's and/or family's needs.

Usually, the problem(s) requiring admission are of low severity. Typically, 25 minutes are spent at the bedside and on the patient's facility floor or unit.

99305   Initial nursing facility care, per day, for the evaluation and management of a patient, which requires these 3 key components:

- **A comprehensive history;**
- **A comprehensive examination; and**
- **Medical decision making of moderate complexity.**

Counseling and/or coordination of care with other physicians, other qualified health care professionals, or agencies are provided consistent with the nature of the problem(s) and the patient's and/or family's needs.

Usually, the problem(s) requiring admission are of moderate severity. Typically, 35 minutes are spent at the bedside and on the patient's facility floor or unit.

99306   Initial nursing facility care, per day, for the evaluation and management of a patient, which requires these 3 key components:

- **A comprehensive history;**
- **A comprehensive examination; and**
- **Medical decision making of high complexity.**

Counseling and/or coordination of care with other physicians, other qualified health care professionals, or agencies are provided consistent with the nature of the problem(s) and the patient's and/or family's needs.

Usually, the problem(s) requiring admission are of high severity. Typically, 45 minutes are spent at the bedside and on the patient's facility floor or unit.

Subsequent Nursing Facility Care

All levels of subsequent nursing facility care include reviewing the medical record and reviewing the results of diagnostic studies and changes in the patient's status (ie, changes in history, physical condition, and response to management) since the last assessment by the physician or other qualified health are professional.

99307   Subsequent nursing facility care, per day, for the evaluation and management of a patient, which requires at least 2 of these 3 key components:

- **A problem focused interval history;**
- **A problem focused examination;**
- **Straightforward medical decision making.**

Counseling and/or coordination of care with other physicians, other qualified health care professionals, or agencies are provided consistent with the nature of the problem(s) and the patient's and/or family's needs.

Usually, the patient is stable, recovering, or improving. Typically, 10 minutes are spent at the bedside and on the patient's facility floor or unit.

99308   Subsequent nursing facility care, per day, for the evaluation and management of a patient, which requires at least 2 of these 3 key components:

- **An expanded problem focused interval history;**
- **An expanded problem focused examination;**
- **Medical decision making of low complexity.**

Counseling and/or coordination of care with other physicians, other qualified health care professionals, or agencies are provided consistent with the nature of the problem(s) and the patient's and/or family's needs.

Usually, the patient is responding inadequately to therapy or has developed a minor complication. Typically, 15 minutes are spent at the bedside and on the patient's facility floor or unit.

Evaluation/Management

99309 Subsequent nursing facility care, per day, for the evaluation and management of a patient, which requires at least 2 of these 3 key components:

- **A detailed interval history;**
- **A detailed examination;**
- **Medical decision making of moderate complexity.**

Counseling and/or coordination of care with other physicians, other qualified health care professionals, or agencies are provided consistent with the nature of the problem(s) and the patient's and/or family's needs.

Usually, the patient has developed a significant complication or a significant new problem. Typically, 25 minutes are spent at the bedside and on the patient's facility floor or unit.

99310 Subsequent nursing facility care, per day, for the evaluation and management of a patient, which requires at least 2 of these 3 key components:

- **A comprehensive interval history;**
- **A comprehensive examination;**
- **Medical decision making of high complexity.**

Counseling and/or coordination of care with other physicians, other qualified health care professionals, or agencies are provided consistent with the nature of the problem(s) and the patient's and/or family's needs.

The patient may be unstable or may have developed a significant new problem requiring immediate physician attention. Typically, 35 minutes are spent at the bedside and on the patient's facility floor or unit.

Nursing Facility Discharge Services

The nursing facility discharge day management codes are to be used to report the total duration of time spent by a physician or other qualified health care professional for the final nursing facility discharge of a patient. The codes include, as appropriate, final examination of the patient, discussion of the nursing facility stay, even if the time spent on that date is not continuous. Instructions are given for continuing care to all relevant caregivers, and preparation of discharge records, prescriptions and referral forms.

99315 Nursing facility discharge day management; 30 minutes or less

99316 more than 30 minutes

Other Nursing Facility Services

99318 Evaluation and management of a patient involving an annual nursing facility assessment, which requires these 3 key components:

- **A detailed interval history;**
- **A comprehensive examination; and**
- **Medical decision making that is of low to moderate complexity.**

Counseling and/or coordination of care with other physicians, other qualified health care professionals, or agencies are provided consistent with the nature of the problem(s) and the patient's and/or family's needs.

Usually, the patient is stable, recovering, or improving. Typically, 30 minutes are spent at the bedside and on the patient's facility floor or unit.

(Do not report 99318 on the same date of service as nursing facility services codes 99304-99316)

Domiciliary, Rest Home (eg, Boarding Home), or Custodial Care Services

The following codes are used to report evaluation and management services in a facility which provides room, board and other personal assistance services, generally on a long-term basis. They also are used to report evaluation and management services in an assisted living facility.

The facility's services do not include a medical component.

For definitions of key components and commonly used terms, please see **Evaluation and Management Services Guidelines**.

(For care plan oversight services provided to a patient in a domiciliary facility under the care of a home health agency, see 99374, 99375, and for hospice agency, see 99377, 99378. For care plan oversight provided to a patient under hospice or home health agency care, see 99339, 99340)

New Patient

99324 Domiciliary or rest home visit for the evaluation and management of a new patient, which requires these 3 key components:

- **A problem focused history;**
- **A problem focused examination; and**
- **Straightforward medical decision making.**

Counseling and/or coordination of care with other physicians, other qualified health care professionals, or agencies are provided consistent with the nature of the problem(s) and the patient's and/or family's needs.

Usually, the presenting problem(s) are of low severity. Typically, 20 minutes are spent with the patient and/or family or caregiver.

99325 Domiciliary or rest home visit for the evaluation and management of a new patient, which requires these 3 key components:

- **An expanded problem focused history;**
- **An expanded problem focused examination; and**
- **Medical decision making of low complexity.**

Counseling and/or coordination of care with other physicians, other qualified health care professionals, or agencies are provided consistent with the nature of the problem(s) and the patient's and/or family's needs.

Usually, the presenting problem(s) are of moderate severity. Typically, 30 minutes are spent with the patient and/or family or caregiver.

99326 Domiciliary or rest home visit for the evaluation and management of a new patient, which requires these 3 key components:

- **A detailed history;**
- **A detailed examination; and**
- **Medical decision making of moderate complexity.**

Counseling and/or coordination of care with other physicians, other qualified health care professionals, or agencies are provided consistent with the nature of the problem(s) and the patient's and/or family's needs.

Usually, the presenting problem(s) are of moderate to high severity. Typically, 45 minutes are spent with the patient and/or family or caregiver.

99327 Domiciliary or rest home visit for the evaluation and management of a new patient, which requires these 3 key components:

- **A comprehensive history;**
- **A comprehensive examination; and**
- **Medical decision making of moderate complexity.**

Counseling and/or coordination of care with other physicians, other qualified health care professionals, or agencies are provided consistent with the nature of the problem(s) and the patient's and/or family's needs.

Usually, the presenting problem(s) are of high severity. Typically, 60 minutes are spent with the patient and/or family or caregiver.

99328 Domiciliary or rest home visit for the evaluation and management of a new patient, which requires these 3 key components:

- **A comprehensive history;**
- **A comprehensive examination; and**
- **Medical decision making of high complexity.**

Counseling and/or coordination of care with other physicians, other qualified health care professionals, or agencies are provided consistent with the nature of the problem(s) and the patient's and/or family's needs.

Usually, the patient is unstable or has developed a significant new problem requiring immediate physician attention. Typically, 75 minutes are spent with the patient and/or family or caregiver.

Established Patient

99334 Domiciliary or rest home visit for the evaluation and management of an established patient, which requires at least 2 of these 3 key components:

- **A problem focused interval history;**
- **A problem focused examination;**
- **Straightforward medical decision making.**

Counseling and/or coordination of care with other physicians, other qualified health care professionals, or agencies are provided consistent with the nature of the problem(s) and the patient's and/or family's needs.

Usually, the presenting problem(s) are self-limited or minor. Typically, 15 minutes are spent with the patient and/or family or caregiver.

99335 Domiciliary or rest home visit for the evaluation and management of an established patient, which requires at least 2 of these 3 key components:

- **An expanded problem focused interval history;**
- **An expanded problem focused examination;**
- **Medical decision making of low complexity.**

Counseling and/or coordination of care with other physicians, other qualified health care professionals, or agencies are provided consistent with the nature of the problem(s) and the patient's and/or family's needs.

Usually, the presenting problem(s) are of low to moderate severity. Typically, 25 minutes are spent with the patient and/or family or caregiver.

99336 Domiciliary or rest home visit for the evaluation and management of an established patient, which requires at least 2 of these 3 key components:

- **A detailed interval history;**
- **A detailed examination;**
- **Medical decision making of moderate complexity.**

Counseling and/or coordination of care with other physicians, other qualified health care professionals, or agencies are provided consistent with the nature of the problem(s) and the patient's and/or family's needs.

Usually, the presenting problem(s) are of moderate to high severity. Typically, 40 minutes are spent with the patient and/or family or caregiver.

99337 Domiciliary or rest home visit for the evaluation and management of an established patient, which requires at least 2 of these 3 key components:

- **A comprehensive interval history;**
- **A comprehensive examination;**
- **Medical decision making of moderate to high complexity.**

Counseling and/or coordination of care with other physicians, other qualified health care professionals, or agencies are provided consistent with the nature of the problem(s) and the patient's and/or family's needs.

Usually, the presenting problem(s) are of moderate to high severity. The patient may be unstable or may have developed a significant new problem requiring immediate physician attention. Typically, 60 minutes are spent with the patient and/or family or caregiver.

Domiciliary, Rest Home (eg, Assisted Living Facility), or Home Care Plan Oversight Services

(For instructions on the use of 99339, 99340, see introductory notes for 99374-99380)

(For care plan oversight services for patients under the care of a home health agency, hospice, or nursing facility, see 99374-99380)

(Do not report 99339, 99340 for time reported with 98966-98969, 99441-99444)

99339 Individual physician supervision of a patient (patient not present) in home, domiciliary or rest home (eg, assisted living facility) requiring complex and multidisciplinary care modalities involving regular physician development and/or revision of care plans, review of subsequent reports of patient status, review of related laboratory and other studies, communication (including telephone calls) for purposes of assessment or care decisions with health care professional(s), family member(s), surrogate decision maker(s) (eg, legal guardian) and/or key caregiver(s) involved in patient's care, integration of new information into the medical treatment plan and/or adjustment of medical therapy, within a calendar month; 15-29 minutes

99340 30 minutes or more

(Do not report 99339, 99340 for patients under the care of a home health agency, enrolled in a hospice program, or for nursing facility residents)

(Do not report 99339, 99340 during the same month with 99487-99489)

(Do not report 99339, 99340 when performed during the service time of codes 99495 or 99496)

Home Services

The following codes are used to report evaluation and management services provided in a private residence.

For definitions of key components and commonly used terms, please see **Evaluation and Management Services Guidelines.**

(For care plan oversight services provided to a patient in the home under the care of a home health agency, see 99374, 99375, and for hospice agency, see 99377, 99378. For care plan oversight provided to a patient under hospice or home health agency care, see 99339, 99340)

New Patient

99341 **Home visit** for the evaluation and management of a new patient, which requires these 3 key components:

- **A problem focused history;**
- **A problem focused examination; and**
- **Straightforward medical decision making.**

Counseling and/or coordination of care with other physicians, other qualified health care professionals, or agencies are provided consistent with the nature of the problem(s) and the patient's and/or family's needs.

Usually, the presenting problem(s) are of low severity. Typically, 20 minutes are spent face-to-face with the patient and/or family.

99342 **Home visit** for the evaluation and management of a new patient, which requires these 3 key components:

- **An expanded problem focused history;**
- **An expanded problem focused examination; and**
- **Medical decision making of low complexity.**

Counseling and/or coordination of care with other physicians, other qualified health care professionals, or agencies are provided consistent with the nature of the problem(s) and the patient's and/or family's needs.

Usually, the presenting problem(s) are of moderate severity. Typically, 30 minutes are spent face-to-face with the patient and/or family.

99343 **Home visit** for the evaluation and management of a new patient, which requires these 3 key components:

- **A detailed history;**
- **A detailed examination; and**
- **Medical decision making of moderate complexity.**

Counseling and/or coordination of care with other physicians, other qualified health care professionals, or agencies are provided consistent with the nature of the problem(s) and the patient's and/or family's needs.

Usually, the presenting problem(s) are of moderate to high severity. Typically, 45 minutes are spent face-to-face with the patient and/or family.

99344 **Home visit** for the evaluation and management of a new patient, which requires these 3 key components:

- **A comprehensive history;**
- **A comprehensive examination; and**
- **Medical decision making of moderate complexity.**

Counseling and/or coordination of care with other physicians, other qualified health care professionals, or agencies are provided consistent with the nature of the problem(s) and the patient's and/or family's needs.

Usually, the presenting problem(s) are of high severity. Typically, 60 minutes are spent face-to-face with the patient and/or family.

99345   **Home visit** for the evaluation and management of a new patient, which requires these 3 key components:

- **A comprehensive history;**
- **A comprehensive examination; and**
- **Medical decision making of high complexity.**

Counseling and/or coordination of care with other physicians, other qualified health care professionals, or agencies are provided consistent with the nature of the problem(s) and the patient's and/or family's needs.

Usually, the patient is unstable or has developed a significant new problem requiring immediate physician attention. Typically, 75 minutes are spent face-to-face with the patient and/or family.

Established Patient

99347   **Home visit** for the evaluation and management of an established patient, which requires at least 2 of these 3 key components:

- **A problem focused interval history;**
- **A problem focused examination;**
- **Straightforward medical decision making.**

Counseling and/or coordination of care with other physicians, other qualified health care professionals, or agencies are provided consistent with the nature of the problem(s) and the patient's and/or family's needs.

Usually, the presenting problem(s) are self limited or minor. Typically, 15 minutes are spent face-to-face with the patient and/or family.

99348   **Home visit** for the evaluation and management of an established patient, which requires at least 2 of these 3 key components:

- **An expanded problem focused interval history;**
- **An expanded problem focused examination;**
- **Medical decision making of low complexity.**

Counseling and/or coordination of care with other physicians, other qualified health care professionals, or agencies are provided consistent with the nature of the problem(s) and the patient's and/or family's needs.

Usually, the presenting problem(s) are of low to moderate severity. Typically, 25 minutes are spent face-to-face with the patient and/or family.

99349   **Home visit** for the evaluation and management of an established patient, which requires at least 2 of these 3 key components:

- **A detailed interval history;**
- **A detailed examination;**
- **Medical decision making of moderate complexity.**

Counseling and/or coordination of care with other physicians, other qualified health care professionals, or agencies are provided consistent with the nature of the problem(s) and the patient's and/or family's needs.

Usually, the presenting problem(s) are moderate to high severity. Typically, 40 minutes are spent face-to-face with the patient and/or family.

99350   **Home visit** for the evaluation and management of an established patient, which requires at least 2 of these 3 key components:

- **A comprehensive interval history;**
- **A comprehensive examination;**
- **Medical decision making of moderate to high complexity.**

Counseling and/or coordination of care with other physicians, other qualified health care professionals, or agencies are provided consistent with the nature of the problem(s) and the patient's and/or family's needs.

Usually, the presenting problem(s) are of moderate to high severity. The patient may be unstable or may have developed a significant new problem requiring immediate physician attention. Typically, 60 minutes are spent face-to-face with the patient and/or family.

Prolonged Services

Prolonged Service With Direct Patient Contact

►Codes 99354-99357 are used when a physician or other qualified health care professional provides prolonged service(s) involving direct patient contact that is provided beyond the usual service in either the inpatient or outpatient setting. Direct patient contact is face to face and includes additional non-face-to-face services on the patient's floor or unit in the hospital or nursing facility during the same session. This service is reported in addition to the primary procedure (ie, the designated evaluation and management services at any level or psychotherapy, code 90837, 60 minutes with patient and/or family member) and any other services provided at the same session. Appropriate codes should be selected for supplies provided or other procedures performed in the care of the patient during this period.◄

Codes 99354-99355 are used to report the total duration of face-to-face time spent by a physician or other qualified health care professional on a given date providing prolonged service in the office or other outpatient setting, even if the time spent by the physician or other qualified health care professional on that date is not continuous. Codes 99356-99357 are used to report the total duration of time spent by a physician or other qualified health care professional at the bedside and on the patient's floor or unit in the hospital or nursing facility on a given date providing prolonged service to a patient, even if the time spent by the physician or other qualified health care professional on that date is not continuous.

►Time spent performing separately reported services other than the E/M or psychotherapy service is not counted toward the prolonged services time.◄

Code 99354 or 99356 is used to report the first hour of prolonged service on a given date, depending on the place of service.

►Either code should be used only once per date, even if the time spent by the physician or other qualified health care professional is not continuous on that date. Prolonged service of less than 30 minutes total duration on a given date is not separately reported because the work involved is included in the total work of the evaluation and management or psychotherapy codes.◄

Code 99355 or 99357 is used to report each additional 30 minutes beyond the first hour, depending on the place of service. Either code may also be used to report the final 15-30 minutes of prolonged service on a given date. Prolonged service of less than 15 minutes beyond the first hour or less than 15 minutes beyond the final 30 minutes is not reported separately.

The use of the time based add-on codes requires that the primary evaluation and management service has a typical or specified time published in the CPT codebook.

►For E/M services that require prolonged clinical staff time and may include face-to-face services by the physician or other qualified health care professional, use 99415, 99416. Do not report 99354 or 99355 with 99415 or 99416.

The following table illustrates the correct reporting of prolonged physician or other qualified health care professional service with direct patient contact in the office setting beyond the usual service time.◄

Total Duration of Prolonged Services	Code(s)
less than 30 minutes	Not reported separately
30-74 minutes (30 minutes - 1 hr. 14 min.)	99354 X 1
75-104 minutes (1 hr. 15 min. - 1 hr. 44 min.)	99354 X 1 AND 99355 X 1
105 minutes or more (1 hr. 45 min. or more)	99354 X 1 AND 99355 X 2 or more for each additional 30 minutes.

+▲ 99354 Prolonged evaluation and management or psychotherapy service(s) (beyond the typical service time of the primary procedure) in the office or other outpatient setting requiring direct patient contact beyond the usual service; first hour (List separately in addition to code for office or other outpatient **Evaluation and Management** or psychotherapy service)

(Use 99354 in conjunction with 90837, 99201-99215, 99241-99245, 99324-99337, 99341-99350)

►(Do not report 99354 in conjunction with 99415, 99416)◄

+▲ 99355 each additional 30 minutes (List separately in addition to code for prolonged service)

(Use 99355 in conjunction with 99354)

►(Do not report 99355 in conjunction with 99415, 99416)◄

+ 99356 Prolonged service in the inpatient or observation setting, requiring unit/floor time beyond the usual service; first hour (List separately in addition to code for inpatient **Evaluation and Management** service)

(Use 99356 in conjunction with 90837, 99218-99220, 99221-99223, 99224-99226, 99231-99233, 99234-99236, 99251-99255, 99304-99310)

+ 99357 each additional 30 minutes (List separately in addition to code for prolonged service)

(Use 99357 in conjunction with 99356)

Prolonged Service Without Direct Patient Contact

Codes 99358 and 99359 are used when a prolonged service is provided that is neither face-to-face time in the office or outpatient setting, nor additional unit/floor time in the hospital or nursing facility setting during the same session of an evaluation and management service and is beyond the usual physician or other qualified health care professional service time.

This service is to be reported in relation to other physician or other qualified health care professional services, including evaluation and management services at any level. This prolonged service may be reported on a different date than the primary service to which it is related. For example, extensive record review may relate to a previous evaluation and management service performed earlier and commences upon receipt of past records. However, it must relate to a service or patient where (face-to-face) patient care has occurred or will occur and relate to ongoing patient management. A typical time for the primary service need not be established within the CPT code set.

Codes 99358 and 99359 are used to report the total duration of non-face-to-face time spent by a physician or other qualified health care professional on a given date providing prolonged service, even if the time spent by the physician or other qualified health care professional on that date is not continuous. Code 99358 is used to report the first hour of prolonged service on a given date regardless of the place of service. It should be used only once per date.

Prolonged service of less than 30 minutes total duration on a given date is not separately reported.

Code 99359 is used to report each additional 30 minutes beyond the first hour regardless of the place of service. It may also be used to report the final 15 to 30 minutes of prolonged service on a given date.

Prolonged service of less than 15 minutes beyond the first hour or less than 15 minutes beyond the final 30 minutes is not reported separately.

Do not report 99358, 99359 for time spent in care plan oversight services (99339, 99340, 99374-99380), anticoagulant management (99363, 99364), medical team conferences (99366-99368), on-line medical evaluations (99444), or other non-face-to-face services that have more specific codes and no upper time limit in the CPT code set. Codes 99358, 99359 may be reported when related to other non-face-to-face services codes that have a published maximum time (eg, telephone services).

99358　**Prolonged evaluation and management service** before and/or after direct patient care; first hour

+ 99359　　　each additional 30 minutes (List separately in addition to code for prolonged service)

(Use 99359 in conjunction with 99358)

(Do not report 99358, 99359 during the same month with 99487-99489)

(Do not report 99358, 99359 when performed during the service time of codes 99495 or 99496)

►Prolonged Clinical Staff Services With Physician or Other Qualified Health Care Professional Supervision◄

►Codes 99415, 99416 are used when a prolonged evaluation and management (E/M) service is provided in the office or outpatient setting that involves prolonged clinical staff face-to-face time beyond the typical face-to-face time of the E/M service, as stated in the code description. The physician or qualified health care professional is present to provide direct supervision of the clinical staff. This service is reported in addition to the designated E/M services and any other services provided at the same session as E/M services.

Codes 99415, 99416 are used to report the total duration of face-to-face time spent by clinical staff on a given date providing prolonged service in the office or other outpatient setting, even if the time spent by the clinical staff on that date is not continuous. Time spent performing separately reported services other than the E/M service is not counted toward the prolonged services time.

Code 99415 is used to report the first hour of prolonged clinical staff service on a given date. Code 99415 should be used only once per date, even if the time spent by the clinical staff is not continuous on that date. Prolonged service of less than 45 minutes total duration on a given date is not separately reported because the clinical staff time involved is included in the E/M codes. The typical face-to-face time of the primary service is used in defining when prolonged services time begins. For example, prolonged clinical staff services for 99214 begin after 25 minutes, and 99415 is not reported until at least 70 minutes total face-to-face clinical staff time has been performed. When face-to-face time is noncontiguous, use only the face-to-face time provided to the patient by the clinical staff.

Code 99416 is used to report each additional 30 minutes of prolonged clinical staff service beyond the first hour. Code 99416 may also be used to report the final 15-30 minutes of prolonged service on a given date. Prolonged service of less than 15 minutes beyond the first hour or less than 15 minutes beyond the final 30 minutes is not reported separately.

Codes 99415, 99416 may be reported for no more than two simultaneous patients. The use of the time-based add-on codes requires that the primary E/M service has a typical or specified time published in the CPT code set.

For prolonged services by the physician or qualified health care professional, use 99354, 99355. Do not report 99415 or 99416 with 99354 or 99355.

Facilities may not report 99415, 99416.◄

#+● 99415　　Prolonged clinical staff service (the service beyond the typical service time) during an evaluation and management service in the office or outpatient setting, direct patient contact with physician supervision; first hour (List separately in addition to code for outpatient **Evaluation and Management** service)

►(Use 99415 in conjunction with 99201, 99202, 99203, 99204, 99205, 99211, 99212, 99213, 99214, 99215)◄

►(Do not report 99415 in conjunction with 99354, 99355)◄

#+● 99416　　each additional 30 minutes (List separately in addition to code for prolonged service)

►(Use 99416 in conjunction with 99415)◄

►(Do not report 99416 in conjunction with 99354, 99355)◄

▶The Total Duration of Prolonged Services Table illustrates the correct reporting of prolonged services provided by clinical staff with physician supervision in the office setting beyond the initial 45 minutes of clinical staff time:◀

▶Total Duration of Prolonged Services	Code(s)
less than 45 minutes	Not reported separately
45-74 minutes (45 minutes - 1 hr. 14 min.)	99415 X 1
75-104 minutes (1 hr. 15 min. - 1 hr. 44 min.)	99415 X 1 AND 99416 X 1
105 minutes or more (1 hr. 45 min. or more)	99415 X 1 AND 99416 X 2 or more for each additional 30 minutes.◀

Standby Services

Code 99360 is used to report physician or other qualified health care professional standby services that are requested by another individual and that involve prolonged attendance without direct (face-to-face) patient contact. Care or services may not be provided to other patients during this period. This code is not used to report time spent proctoring another individual. It is also not used if the period of standby ends with the performance of a procedure, subject to a surgical package by the individual who was on standby.

Code 99360 is used to report the total duration of time spent on a given date on standby. Standby service of less than 30 minutes total duration on a given date is not reported separately.

Second and subsequent periods of standby beyond the first 30 minutes may be reported only if a full 30 minutes of standby was provided for each unit of service reported.

99360   **Standby service,** requiring prolonged attendance, each 30 minutes (eg, operative standby, standby for frozen section, for cesarean/high risk delivery, for monitoring EEG)

        (For hospital mandated on call services, see 99026, 99027)

        (99360 may be reported in addition to 99460, 99465 as appropriate)

        (Do not report 99360 in conjunction with 99464)

Case Management Services

Case management is a process in which a physician or another qualified health care professional is responsible for direct care of a patient and, additionally, for coordinating, managing access to, initiating, and/or supervising other health care services needed by the patient.

Anticoagulant Management

Anticoagulant services are intended to describe the outpatient management of warfarin therapy, including ordering, review, and interpretation of International Normalized Ratio (INR) testing, communication with patient, and dosage adjustments as appropriate.

When reporting these services, the work of anticoagulant management may not be used as a basis for reporting an evaluation and management (E/M) service or care plan oversight time during the reporting period. Do not report these services with 98966-98969, 99441-99444 when telephone or on-line services address anticoagulation with warfarin management. If a significant, separately identifiable E/M service is performed, report the appropriate E/M service code using modifier 25.

These services are outpatient services only. When anticoagulation therapy is initiated or continued in the inpatient or observation setting, a new period begins after discharge and is reported with 99364. Do not report 99363-99364 with 99217-99239, 99291-99292, 99304-99318, 99471-99480 or other code(s) for physician review, interpretation, and patient management of home INR testing for a patient with mechanical heart valve(s).

Any period less than 60 continuous outpatient days is not reported. If less than the specified minimum number of services per period are performed, do not report the anticoagulant management services (99363-99364).

99363   Anticoagulant management for an outpatient taking warfarin, physician review and interpretation of International Normalized Ratio (INR) testing, patient instructions, dosage adjustment (as needed), and ordering of additional tests; initial 90 days of therapy (must include a minimum of 8 INR measurements)

99364   each subsequent 90 days of therapy (must include a minimum of 3 INR measurements)

        (Do not report 99363, 99364 during the same month with 99487-99489)

        (Do not report 99363, 99364 when performed during the service time of codes 99495 or 99496)

Medical Team Conferences

Medical team conferences include face-to-face participation by a minimum of three qualified health care professionals from different specialties or disciplines (each of whom provide direct care to the patient), with or without the presence of the patient, family member(s), community agencies, surrogate decision maker(s) (eg, legal guardian), and/or caregiver(s). The participants are actively involved in the development, revision, coordination, and implementation of health care services needed by the patient. Reporting participants shall have performed face-to-face evaluations or treatments of the patient, independent of any team conference, within the previous 60 days.

Physicians or other qualified health care professionals who may report evaluation and management services should report their time spent in a team conference with the patient and/or family present using evaluation and management (E/M) codes (and time as the key controlling factor for code selection when counseling and/or coordination of care dominates the service). These introductory guidelines do not apply to services reported using E/M codes (see E/M services guidelines). However, the individual must be directly involved with the patient, providing face-to-face services outside of the conference visit with other physicians, and qualified health care professionals, or agencies.

Reporting participants shall document their participation in the team conference as well as their contributed information and subsequent treatment recommendations.

No more than one individual from the same specialty may report 99366-99368 at the same encounter.

Individuals should not report 99366-99368 when their participation in the medical team conference is part of a facility or organizational service contractually provided by the organization or facility.

The team conference starts at the beginning of the review of an individual patient and ends at the conclusion of the review. Time related to record keeping and report generation is not reported. The reporting participant shall be present for all time reported. The time reported is not limited to the time that the participant is communicating to the other team members or patient and/or family. Time reported for medical team conferences may not be used in the determination of time for other services such as care plan oversight (99374-99380), home, domiciliary, or rest home care plan oversight (99339-99340), prolonged services (99354-99359), psychotherapy, or any E/M service. For team conferences where the patient is present for any part of the duration of the conference, nonphysician qualified health care professionals (eg, speech-language pathologists, physical therapists, occupational therapists, social workers, dietitians) report the team conference face-to-face code 99366.

Medical Team Conference, Direct (Face-to-Face) Contact With Patient and/or Family

99366   **Medical team conference** with interdisciplinary team of health care professionals, face-to-face with patient and/or family, 30 minutes or more, participation by nonphysician qualified health care professional

(Team conference services of less than 30 minutes duration are not reported separately)

(For team conference services by a physician with patient and/or family present, see Evaluation and Management services)

(Do not report 99366 during the same month with 99487-99489)

(Do not report 99366 when performed during the service time of codes 99495 or 99496)

Medical Team Conference, Without Direct (Face-to-Face) Contact With Patient and/or Family

99367   **Medical team conference** with interdisciplinary team of health care professionals, patient and/or family not present, 30 minutes or more; participation by physician

99368   participation by nonphysician qualified health care professional

(Team conference services of less than 30 minutes duration are not reported separately)

(Do not report 99367, 99368 during the same month with 99487-99489)

(Do not report 99367, 99368 when performed during the service time of codes 99495 or 99496)

Care Plan Oversight Services

Care plan oversight services are reported separately from codes for office/outpatient, hospital, home, nursing facility or domiciliary, or non-face-to-face services. The complexity and approximate time of the care plan oversight services provided within a 30-day period determine code selection. Only one individual may report services for a given period of time, to reflect the sole or predominant supervisory role with a particular patient. These codes should not be reported for supervision of patients in nursing facilities or under the care of home health agencies unless they require recurrent supervision of therapy.

The work involved in providing very low intensity or infrequent supervision services is included in the pre- and post-encounter work for home, office/outpatient and nursing facility or domiciliary visit codes.

(For care plan oversight services of patients in the home, domiciliary, or rest home [eg, assisted living facility], see 99339, 99340, and for hospice agency, see 99377, 99378)

(Do not report 99374-99380 for time reported with 98966-98969, 99441-99444)

(Do not report 99374-99378 during the same month with 99487-99489)

(Do not report 99374-99380 when performed during the service time of codes 99495 or 99496)

99374 **Supervision** of a patient under care of home health agency (patient not present) in home, domiciliary or equivalent environment (eg, Alzheimer's facility) requiring complex and multidisciplinary care modalities involving regular development and/or revision of care plans by that individual, review of subsequent reports of patient status, review of related laboratory and other studies, communication (including telephone calls) for purposes of assessment or care decisions with health care professional(s), family member(s), surrogate decision maker(s) (eg, legal guardian) and/or key caregiver(s) involved in patient's care, integration of new information into the medical treatment plan and/or adjustment of medical therapy, within a calendar month; 15-29 minutes

99375 30 minutes or more

99377 **Supervision** of a hospice patient (patient not present) requiring complex and multidisciplinary care modalities involving regular development and/or revision of care plans by that individual, review of subsequent reports of patient status, review of related laboratory and other studies, communication (including telephone calls) for purposes of assessment or care decisions with health care professional(s), family member(s), surrogate decision maker(s) (eg, legal guardian) and/or key caregiver(s) involved in patient's care, integration of new information into the medical treatment plan and/or adjustment of medical therapy, within a calendar month; 15-29 minutes

99378 30 minutes or more

99379 **Supervision** of a nursing facility patient (patient not present) requiring complex and multidisciplinary care modalities involving regular development and/or revision of care plans by that individual, review of subsequent reports of patient status, review of related laboratory and other studies, communication (including telephone calls) for purposes of assessment or care decisions with health care professional(s), family member(s), surrogate decision maker(s) (eg, legal guardian) and/or key caregiver(s) involved in patient's care, integration of new information into the medical treatment plan and/or adjustment of medical therapy, within a calendar month; 15-29 minutes

99380 30 minutes or more

Preventive Medicine Services

The following codes are used to report the preventive medicine evaluation and management of infants, children, adolescents, and adults.

The extent and focus of the services will largely depend on the age of the patient.

If an abnormality is encountered or a preexisting problem is addressed in the process of performing this preventive medicine evaluation and management service, and if the problem or abnormality is significant enough to require additional work to perform the key components of a problem-oriented E/M service, then the appropriate Office/Outpatient code 99201-99215 should also be

reported. Modifier 25 should be added to the Office/Outpatient code to indicate that a significant, separately identifiable evaluation and management service was provided on the same day as the preventive medicine service. The appropriate preventive medicine service is additionally reported.

An insignificant or trivial problem/abnormality that is encountered in the process of performing the preventive medicine evaluation and management service and which does not require additional work and the performance of the key components of a problem-oriented E/M service should not be reported.

The "comprehensive" nature of the Preventive Medicine Services codes 99381-99397 reflects an age and gender appropriate history/exam and is **not** synonymous with the "comprehensive" examination required in Evaluation and Management codes 99201-99350.

▶Codes 99381-99397 include counseling/anticipatory guidance/risk factor reduction interventions which are provided at the time of the initial or periodic comprehensive preventive medicine examination. (Refer to 99401, 99402, 99403, 99404, 99411, and 99412 for reporting those counseling/anticipatory guidance/risk factor reduction interventions that are provided at an encounter separate from the preventive medicine examination.)

(For behavior change intervention, see 99406, 99407, 99408, 99409)◀

Vaccine/toxoid products, immunization administrations, ancillary studies involving laboratory, radiology, other procedures, or screening tests (eg, vision, hearing, developmental) identified with a specific CPT code are reported separately. For immunization administration and vaccine risk/benefit counseling, see 90460, 90461, 90471-90474. For vaccine/toxoid products, see 90476-90749.

New Patient

99381 **Initial comprehensive preventive medicine** evaluation and management of an individual including an age and gender appropriate history, examination, counseling/anticipatory guidance/risk factor reduction interventions, and the ordering of laboratory/diagnostic procedures, new patient; infant (age younger than 1 year)

99382 early childhood (age 1 through 4 years)

99383 late childhood (age 5 through 11 years)

99384 adolescent (age 12 through 17 years)

99385 18-39 years

99386 40-64 years

99387 65 years and older

Established Patient

99391   **Periodic comprehensive preventive medicine** reevaluation and management of an individual including an age and gender appropriate history, examination, counseling/anticipatory guidance/risk factor reduction interventions, and the ordering of laboratory/diagnostic procedures, established patient; infant (age younger than 1 year)

99392   early childhood (age 1 through 4 years)

99393   late childhood (age 5 through 11 years)

99394   adolescent (age 12 through 17 years)

99395   18-39 years

99396   40-64 years

99397   65 years and older

Counseling Risk Factor Reduction and Behavior Change Intervention

New or Established Patient

▶These codes are used to report services provided face-to-face by a physician or other qualified health care professional for the purpose of promoting health and preventing illness or injury. They are distinct from evaluation and management (E/M) services that may be reported separately with modifier 25 when performed. Risk factor reduction services are used for persons without a specific illness for which the counseling might otherwise be used as part of treatment.◀

Preventive medicine counseling and risk factor reduction interventions will vary with age and should address such issues as family problems, diet and exercise, substance use, sexual practices, injury prevention, dental health, and diagnostic and laboratory test results available at the time of the encounter.

▶Behavior change interventions are for persons who have a behavior that is often considered an illness itself, such as tobacco use and addiction, substance abuse/misuse, or obesity. Behavior change services may be reported when performed as part of the treatment of condition(s) related to or potentially exacerbated by the behavior or when performed to change the harmful behavior that has not yet resulted in illness. Any E/M services reported on the same day must be distinct and reported with modifier 25, and time spent providing these services may not be used as a basis for the E/M code selection. Behavior change services involve specific validated interventions of assessing readiness for change and barriers to change, advising a change in behavior, assisting by providing specific suggested actions and motivational counseling, and arranging for services and follow-up.◀

For counseling groups of patients with symptoms or established illness, use 99078.

Health and Behavior Assessment/Intervention services (96150-96155) should not be reported on the same day as codes 99401-99412.

Preventive Medicine, Individual Counseling

99401   **Preventive medicine counseling** and/or risk factor reduction intervention(s) provided to an individual (separate procedure); approximately 15 minutes

99402   approximately 30 minutes

99403   approximately 45 minutes

99404   approximately 60 minutes

Behavior Change Interventions, Individual

99406   Smoking and tobacco use cessation counseling visit; intermediate, greater than 3 minutes up to 10 minutes

99407   intensive, greater than 10 minutes

(Do not report 99407 in conjunction with 99406)

99408   Alcohol and/or substance (other than tobacco) abuse structured screening (eg, AUDIT, DAST), and brief intervention (SBI) services; 15 to 30 minutes

(Do not report services of less than 15 minutes with 99408)

99409   greater than 30 minutes

(Do not report 99409 in conjunction with 99408)

(Do not report 99408, 99409 in conjunction with 99420)

(Use 99408, 99409 only for initial screening and brief intervention)

Preventive Medicine, Group Counseling

99411   **Preventive medicine counseling** and/or risk factor reduction intervention(s) provided to individuals in a group setting (separate procedure); approximately 30 minutes

99412   approximately 60 minutes

99415   Code is out of numerical sequence. See 99358-99416

99416   Code is out of numerical sequence. See 99358-99416

Other Preventive Medicine Services

99420   **Administration and interpretation** of health risk assessment instrument (eg, health hazard appraisal)

99429   **Unlisted preventive** medicine service

Evaluation/Management

Non-Face-to-Face Services

Telephone Services

Telephone services are non-face-to-face evaluation and management (E/M) services provided to a patient using the telephone by a physician or other qualified health care professional, who may report evaluation and management services. These codes are used to report episodes of patient care initiated by an established patient or guardian of an established patient. If the telephone service ends with a decision to see the patient within 24 hours or next available urgent visit appointment, the code is not reported; rather the encounter is considered part of the preservice work of the subsequent E/M service, procedure, and visit. Likewise if the telephone call refers to an E/M service performed and reported by that individual within the previous seven days (either requested or unsolicited patient follow-up) or within the postoperative period of the previously completed procedure, then the service(s) are considered part of that previous E/M service or procedure. (Do not report 99441-99443 if reporting 99441-99444 performed in the previous seven days.)

> (For telephone services provided by a qualified nonphysician who may not report evaluation and management services [eg, speech-language pathologists, physical therapists, occupational therapists, social workers, dietitians], see 98966-98968)

99441 Telephone evaluation and management service by a physician or other qualified health care professional who may report evaluation and management services provided to an established patient, parent, or guardian not originating from a related E/M service provided within the previous 7 days nor leading to an E/M service or procedure within the next 24 hours or soonest available appointment; 5-10 minutes of medical discussion

99442 11-20 minutes of medical discussion

99443 21-30 minutes of medical discussion

> (Do not report 99441-99443 when using 99339-99340, 99374-99380 for the same call[s])

> (Do not report 99441-99443 for anticoagulation management when reporting 99363, 99364)

> (Do not report 99441-99443 during the same month with 99487-99489)

> (Do not report 99441-99443 when performed during the service time of codes 99495 or 99496)

On-Line Medical Evaluation

An on-line electronic medical evaluation is a non-face-to-face evaluation and management (E/M) service by a physician to a patient using Internet resources in response to a patient's on-line inquiry. Reportable services involve the physician's personal timely response to the patient's inquiry and must involve permanent storage (electronic or hard copy) of the encounter. This service is reported only once for the same episode of care during a seven-day period, although multiple physicians could report their exchange with the same patient. If the on-line medical evaluation refers to an E/M service previously performed and reported by the physician within the previous seven days (either physician requested or unsolicited patient follow-up) or within the postoperative period of the previously completed procedure, then the service(s) are considered covered by the previous E/M service or procedure. A reportable service encompasses the sum of communication (eg, related telephone calls, prescription provision, laboratory orders) pertaining to the on-line patient encounter.

> (For an on-line medical evaluation provided by a qualified nonphysician health care professional, use 98969)

99444 Online evaluation and management service provided by a physician or other qualified health care professional who may report evaluation and management services provided to an established patient or guardian, not originating from a related E/M service provided within the previous 7 days, using the Internet or similar electronic communications network

> (Do not report 99444 when using 99339, 99340, 99374-99380 for the same communication[s])

> (Do not report 99444 for anticoagulation management when reporting 99363, 99364)

> (Do not report 99444 during the same month with 99487-99489)

> (Do not report 99444 when performed during the service time of codes 99495 or 99496)

Interprofessional Telephone/Internet Consultations

The consultant should use the following codes to report interprofessional telephone/Internet consultations. An interprofessional telephone/Internet consultation is an assessment and management service in which a patient's treating (eg, attending or primary) physician or other qualified health care professional requests the opinion and/or treatment advice of a physician with specific specialty expertise (the consultant) to assist the treating physician or other qualified health care professional in the diagnosis and/or management of the patient's problem without the need for the patient's face-to-face contact with the consultant.

These services are typically provided in complex and/or urgent situations where a timely face-to-face service with the consultant may not be feasible (eg, geographic distance). These codes should not be reported by a consultant who has agreed to accept transfer of care before the telephone/Internet assessment, but are appropriate to report if the decision to accept transfer of care cannot be made until after the initial interprofessional telephone/Internet consultation.

The patient for whom the interprofessional telephone/Internet consultation is requested may be either a new patient to the consultant or an established patient with a new problem or an exacerbation of an existing problem. However, the consultant should not have seen the patient in a face-to-face encounter within the last 14 days. When the telephone/Internet consultation leads to an immediate transfer of care or other face-to-face service (eg, a surgery, a hospital visit, or a scheduled office evaluation of the patient) within the next 14 days or next available appointment date of the consultant, these codes are not reported.

Review of pertinent medical records, laboratory studies, imaging studies, medication profile, pathology specimens, etc may be required and transmitted electronically by fax or by mail immediately before the telephone/Internet consultation or following the consultation.

The review of this data is included in the telephone/Internet consultation service and should not be reported separately. The majority of the service time reported (greater than 50%) must be devoted to the medical consultative verbal/Internet discussion. This service should not be reported more than once within a seven-day interval.

If more than one telephone/Internet contact(s) is required to complete the consultation request (eg, discussion of test results), the entirety of the service and the cumulative discussion and information review time should be reported with a single code.

The written or verbal request for telephone/Internet advice by the treating/requesting physician or other qualified health care professional should be documented in the patient's medical record, including the reason for the request, and concludes with a verbal opinion report and written report from the consultant to the treating/requesting physician or other qualified health care professional.

Telephone/Internet consultations of less than five minutes should not be reported. Consultant communications with the patient and/or family may be reported using 99441, 99442, 99443, 99444, 98966, 98967, 98968, 98969 and the time related to these services is not used in reporting 99446, 99447, 99448, 99449.

When the sole purpose of the telephone/Internet communication is to arrange a transfer of care or other face-to-face service, these codes are not reported.

The treating/requesting physician or other qualified health care professional may report the prolonged service codes 99354, 99355, 99356, 99357 for the time spent on the interprofessional telephone/Internet discussion with

the consultant (eg, specialist) if the time **exceeds 30 minutes** beyond the typical time of the appropriate E/M service performed and the patient is present (on-site) and accessible to the treating/requesting physician or other qualified health care professional. If the interprofessional telephone/Internet assessment and management service occurs when the patient is not present or on-site, and the discussion time **exceeds 30 minutes** beyond the typical time of the appropriate E/M service performed, then the non-face-to-face prolonged service codes 99358, 99359 may be reported by the treating/requesting physician or other qualified health care professional.

> (For telephone services provided by a physician to a patient, see 99441, 99442, 99443)
>
> (For telephone services provided by a qualified health care professional to a patient, see 98966, 98967, 98968)
>
> (For an on-line medical evaluation provided by a physician to a patient, use 99444)
>
> (For an on-line assessment and management service provided by a qualified health care professional to a patient, use 98969)

99446   Interprofessional telephone/Internet assessment and management service provided by a consultative physician including a verbal and written report to the patient's treating/requesting physician or other qualified health care professional; 5-10 minutes of medical consultative discussion and review

99447   11-20 minutes of medical consultative discussion and review

99448   21-30 minutes of medical consultative discussion and review

99449   31 minutes or more of medical consultative discussion and review

Special Evaluation and Management Services

The following codes are used to report evaluations performed to establish baseline information prior to life or disability insurance certificates being issued. This service is performed in the office or other setting, and applies to both new and established patients. When using these codes, no active management of the problem(s) is undertaken during the encounter.

If other evaluation and management services and/or procedures are performed on the same date, the appropriate E/M or procedure code(s) should be reported in addition to these codes.

Basic Life and/or Disability Evaluation Services

99450 **Basic life** and/or disability examination that includes:

- **Measurement of height, weight, and blood pressure;**
- **Completion of a medical history following a life insurance pro forma;**
- **Collection of blood sample and/or urinalysis complying with "chain of custody" protocols; and**
- **Completion of necessary documentation/ certificates.**

Work Related or Medical Disability Evaluation Services

99455 **Work related** or medical disability examination by the treating physician that includes:

- **Completion of a medical history commensurate with the patient's condition;**
- **Performance of an examination commensurate with the patient's condition;**
- **Formulation of a diagnosis, assessment of capabilities and stability, and calculation of impairment;**
- **Development of future medical treatment plan; and**
- **Completion of necessary documentation/ certificates and report.**

99456 **Work related** or medical disability examination by other than the treating physician that includes:

- **Completion of a medical history commensurate with the patient's condition;**
- **Performance of an examination commensurate with the patient's condition;**
- **Formulation of a diagnosis, assessment of capabilities and stability, and calculation of impairment;**
- **Development of future medical treatment plan; and**
- **Completion of necessary documentation/ certificates and report.**

(Do not report 99455, 99456 in conjunction with 99080 for the completion of Workman's Compensation forms)

Newborn Care Services

The following codes are used to report the services provided to newborns (birth through the first 28 days) in several different settings. Use of the normal newborn codes is limited to the initial care of the newborn in the first days after birth prior to home discharge.

Evaluation and Management (E/M) services for the newborn include maternal and/or fetal and newborn history, newborn physical examination(s), ordering of diagnostic tests and treatments, meetings with the family, and documentation in the medical record.

When delivery room attendance services (99464) or delivery room resuscitation services (99465) are required, report these in addition to normal newborn services Evaluation and Management codes.

For E/M services provided to newborns who are other than normal, see codes for hospital inpatient services (99221-99233) and neonatal intensive and critical care services (99466-99469, 99477-99480). When normal newborn services are provided by the same individual on the same date that the newborn later becomes ill and receives additional intensive or critical care services, report the appropriate E/M code with modifier 25 for these services in addition to the normal newborn code.

Procedures (eg, 54150, newborn circumcision) are not included with the normal newborn codes, and when performed, should be reported in addition to the newborn services.

When newborns are seen in follow-up after the date of discharge in the office or outpatient setting, see 99201-99215, 99381, 99391 as appropriate.

99460 Initial hospital or birthing center care, per day, for evaluation and management of normal newborn infant

99461 Initial care, per day, for evaluation and management of normal newborn infant seen in other than hospital or birthing center

99462 Subsequent hospital care, per day, for evaluation and management of normal newborn

99463 Initial hospital or birthing center care, per day, for evaluation and management of normal newborn infant admitted and discharged on the same date

(For newborn hospital discharge services provided on a date subsequent to the admission date, see 99238, 99239)

Delivery/Birthing Room Attendance and Resuscitation Services

99464 Attendance at delivery (when requested by the delivering physician or other qualified health care professional) and initial stabilization of newborn

(99464 may be reported in conjunction with 99460, 99468, 99477)

(Do not report 99464 in conjunction with 99465)

99465   Delivery/birthing room resuscitation, provision of positive pressure ventilation and/or chest compressions in the presence of acute inadequate ventilation and/or cardiac output

(99465 may be reported in conjunction with 99460, 99468, 99477)

(Do not report 99465 in conjunction with 99464)

(Procedures that are performed as a necessary part of the resuscitation [eg, intubation, vascular lines] are reported separately in addition to 99465. In order to report these procedures, they must be performed as a necessary component of the resuscitation and not as a convenience before admission to the neonatal intensive care unit)

Inpatient Neonatal Intensive Care Services and Pediatric and Neonatal Critical Care Services

Pediatric Critical Care Patient Transport

Codes 99466, 99467 are used to report the physical attendance and direct face-to-face care by a physician during the interfacility transport of a critically ill or critically injured pediatric patient 24 months of age or younger. Codes 99485, 99486 are used to report the control physician's non-face-to-face supervision of interfacility transport of a critically ill or critically injured pediatric patient 24 months of age or younger. These codes are not reported together for the same patient by the same physician. For the purpose of reporting 99466 and 99467, face-to-face care begins when the physician assumes primary responsibility of the pediatric patient at the referring facility, and ends when the receiving facility accepts responsibility for the pediatric patient's care. Only the time the physician spends in direct face-to-face contact with the patient during the transport should be reported. Pediatric patient transport services involving less than 30 minutes of face-to-face physician care should not be reported using 99466, 99467. Procedure(s) or service(s) performed by other members of the transporting team may not be reported by the supervising physician.

Codes 99485, 99486 are used to report control physician's non-face-to-face supervision of interfacility pediatric critical care transport, which includes all two-way communication between the control physician and the specialized transport team prior to transport, at the referring facility and during transport of the patient back to the receiving facility. The "control" physician is the physician directing transport services. These codes do not include pretransport communication between the control physician and the referring facility before or following

patient transport. These codes are only reported for patients 24 months of age or younger who are critically ill or critically injured. The control physician provides treatment advice to a specialized transport team who are present and delivering the hands-on patient care. The control physician does not report any services provided by the specialized transport team. The control physician's non-face-to-face time begins with the first contact by the control physician with the specialized transport team and ends when the patient's care is handed over to the receiving facility team. Refer to 99466 and 99467 for face-to-face transport care of the critically ill/injured patient. Time spent with the individual patient's transport team and reviewing data submissions should be recorded. Code 99485 is used to report the first 16-45 minutes of direction on a given date and should only be used once even if time spent by the physician is discontinuous. Do not report services of 15 minutes or less or any time when another physician is reporting 99466, 99467. Do not report 99485 or 99486 in conjunction with 99466, 99467 when performed by the same physician.

For the definition of the critically injured pediatric patient, see the **Neonatal and Pediatric Critical Care Services** section.

The non-face-to-face direction of emergency care to a patient's transporting staff by a physician located in a hospital or other facility by two-way communication is not considered direct face-to-face care and should not be reported with 99466, 99467. Physician-directed non-face-to-face emergency care through outside voice communication to transporting staff personnel is reported with 99288 or 99485, 99486 based upon the age and clinical condition of the patient.

Emergency department services (99281-99285), initial hospital care (99221-99223), critical care (99291, 99292), initial date neonatal intensive (99477) or critical care (99468) are only reported after the patient has been admitted to the emergency department, the inpatient floor, or the critical care unit of the receiving facility. If inpatient critical care services are reported in the referring facility prior to transfer to the receiving hospital, use the critical care codes (99291, 99292).

The following services are included when performed during the pediatric patient transport by the physician providing critical care and may not be reported separately: routine monitoring evaluations (eg, heart rate, respiratory rate, blood pressure, and pulse oximetry), the interpretation of cardiac output measurements (93562), chest X-rays (71010, 71015, 71020), pulse oximetry (94760, 94761, 94762), blood gases and information data stored in computers (eg, ECGs, blood pressures, hematologic data) (99090), gastric intubation (43752, 43753), temporary transcutaneous pacing (92953), ventilatory management (94002, 94003, 94660, 94662), and vascular access procedures (36000, 36400, 36405, 36406, 36415, 36591, 36600). Any services performed which are not listed above should be reported separately.

Evaluation/Management

Services provided by the specialized transport team during non-face-to-face transport supervision are not reported by the control physician.

Code 99466 is used to report the first 30 to 74 minutes of direct face-to-face time with the transport pediatric patient and should be reported only once on a given date. Code 99467 is used to report each additional 30 minutes provided on a given date. Face-to-face services of less than 30 minutes should not be reported with these codes.

Code 99485 is used to report the first 30 minutes of non-face-to-face supervision of an interfacility transport of a critically ill or critically injured pediatric patient and should be reported only once per date of service. Only the communication time spent by the supervising physician with the specialty transport team members during an interfacility transport should be reported. Code 99486 is used to report each additional 30 minutes beyond the initial 30 minutes. Non-face-to-face interfacility transport of 15 minutes or less is not reported.

> (For total body and selective head cooling of neonates, use 99184)

99466   **Critical care** face-to-face services, during an interfacility transport of critically ill or critically injured pediatric patient, 24 months of age or younger; first 30-74 minutes of hands-on care during transport

+ 99467   each additional 30 minutes (List separately in addition to code for primary service)

> (Use 99467 in conjunction with 99466)

> (Critical care of less than 30 minutes total duration should be reported with the appropriate E/M code)

 # 99485   Supervision by a control physician of interfacility transport care of the critically ill or critically injured pediatric patient, 24 months of age or younger, includes two-way communication with transport team before transport, at the referring facility and during the transport, including data interpretation and report; first 30 minutes

#+ 99486   each additional 30 minutes (List separately in addition to code for primary procedure)

> (Use 99486 in conjunction with 99485)

> (For physician direction of emergency medical systems supervision for a pediatric patient older than 24 months of age, or at any age if not critically ill or injured, use 99288)

> (Do not report 99485, 99486 with any other services reported by the control physician for the same period)

> (Do not report 99485, 99486 in conjunction with 99466, 99467 when performed by the same physician)

Inpatient Neonatal and Pediatric Critical Care

The same definitions for critical care services apply for the adult, child, and neonate.

Codes 99468, 99469 are used to report the services of directing the inpatient care of a critically ill neonate or infant 28 days of age or younger. They represent care starting with the date of admission (99468) to a critical care unit and subsequent day(s) (99469) that the neonate remains critical. These codes may be reported only by a single individual and only once per day, per patient, per hospital stay in a given facility. If readmitted to the neonatal critical care unit during the same day **or stay**, report the subsequent day(s) code 99469 for the first day of readmission to critical care, and 99469 for each day of critical care following readmission.

The initial day neonatal critical care code (99468) can be used in addition to 99464 or 99465 as appropriate, when the physician or other qualified health care professional is present for the delivery (99464) or resuscitation (99465) is required. Other procedures performed as a necessary part of the resuscitation (eg, endotracheal intubation [31500]) are also reported separately when performed as part of the pre-admission delivery room care. In order to report these procedures separately, they must be performed as a necessary component of the resuscitation and not simply as a convenience before admission to the neonatal intensive care unit.

Codes 99471-99476 are used to report direction of the inpatient care of a critically ill infant or young child from 29 days of postnatal age through less than 6 years of age. They represent care starting with the date of admission (99471, 99475) to all subsequent day(s) (99472, 99476) the infant or child remains critical. These codes may be reported only by a single individual and only once per day, per patient in a given setting. Services for the critically ill or critically injured child 6 years of age or older would be reported with the time based critical care codes (99291, 99292). Report 99471, 99475 only once per hospital stay in a given facility. If readmitted to the pediatric critical care unit during the same **day or** stay, report 99472 or 99476 for the first day of readmission to critical care and 99472 for each day of critical care following readmission.

The pediatric and neonatal critical care codes include those procedures listed for the critical care codes (99291, 99292). In addition, the following procedures are also included (and are not separately reported by professionals, but may be reported by facilities) in the pediatric and neonatal critical care service codes (99468-99472, 99475, 99476) and the intensive care services codes (99477-99480).

Any services performed that are not included in these listings may be reported separately. For initiation of selective head or total body hypothermia in the critically ill neonate, report 99184. Facilities may report the included services separately.

Invasive or non-invasive electronic monitoring of vital signs

Vascular access procedures

    Peripheral vessel catheterization (36000)

    Other arterial catheters (36140, 36620)

    Umbilical venous catheters (36510)

    Central vessel catheterization (36555)

    Vascular access procedures (36400, 36405, 36406)

    Vascular punctures (36420, 36600)

    Umbilical arterial catheters (36660)

Airway and ventilation management

    Endotracheal intubation (31500)

    Ventilatory management (94002-94004)

    Bedside pulmonary function testing (94375)

    Surfactant administration (94610)

    Continuous positive airway pressure (CPAP) (94660)

Monitoring or interpretation of blood gases or oxygen saturation (94760-94762)

Car Seat Evaluation (94780-94781)

Transfusion of blood components (36430, 36440)

Oral or nasogastric tube placement (43752)

Suprapubic bladder aspiration (51100)

Bladder catheterization (51701, 51702)

Lumbar puncture (62270)

Any services performed which are not listed above may be reported separately.

When a neonate or infant is not critically ill but requires intensive observation, frequent interventions, and other intensive care services, the Continuing Intensive Care Services codes (99477-99480) should be used to report these services.

To report critical care services provided in the outpatient setting (eg, emergency department or office) for neonates and pediatric patients of any age, see the Critical Care codes 99291, 99292. If the same individual provides critical care services for a neonatal or pediatric patient less than 6 years of age in both the outpatient and inpatient settings on the same day, report only the appropriate Neonatal or Pediatric Critical Care codes 99468-99476 for all critical care services provided on that day. Critical care services provided by a second individual of a different specialty not reporting a per-day neonatal or pediatric critical care code can be reported with 99291, 99292.

When critical care services are provided to neonates or pediatric patients less than 6 years of age at two separate institutions by an individual from a different group on the same date of service, the individual from the referring institution should report their critical care services with the time-based critical care codes (99291, 99292) and the receiving institution should report the appropriate initial day of care code 99468, 99471, 99475 for the same date of service.

Critical care services to a pediatric patient 6 years of age or older are reported with the time based critical care codes 99291, 99292.

When the critically ill neonate or pediatric patient improves and is transferred to a lower level of care to another individual in another group within the same facility, the transferring individual does not report a per day critical care service. Subsequent hospital care (99231-99233) or time-based critical care services (99291-99292) is reported, as appropriate based upon the condition of the neonate or child. The receiving individual reports subsequent intensive care (99478-99480) or subsequent hospital care (99231-99233) services, as appropriate based upon the condition of the neonate or child.

When the neonate or infant becomes critically ill on a day when initial or subsequent intensive care services (99477-99480), hospital services (99221-99233), or normal newborn services (99460, 99461, 99462) have been performed by one individual and is transferred to a critical care level of care provided by a different individual in a different group, the transferring individual reports either the time-based critical care services performed (99291, 99292) for the time spent providing critical care to the patient, the intensive care service (99477-99480), hospital care services (99221-99233), or normal newborn service (99460, 99461, 99462) performed, but only one service. The receiving individual reports initial or subsequent inpatient neonatal or pediatric critical care (99468-99476), as appropriate based upon the patient's age and whether this is the first or subsequent admission to the critical care unit for the hospital stay.

When a newborn becomes critically ill on the same day they have already received normal newborn care (99460, 99461, 99462), and the same individual or group assumes critical care, report initial critical care service (99468) with modifier 25 in addition to the normal newborn code.

When a neonate, infant, or child requires initial critical care services on the same day the patient already has received hospital care or intensive care services by the same individual or group, only the initial critical care service code (99468, 99471, 99475) is reported.

Time-based critical care services (99291, 99292) are not reportable by the same individual or different individual within the same group when neonatal or pediatric critical care services (99468-99476) are reported for the same patient on the same day.

No individual may report remote real-time videoconferenced critical care (0188T, 0189T) when neonatal or pediatric intensive or critical care services (99468-99476) are reported.

99468   **Initial inpatient neonatal critical care,** per day, for the evaluation and management of a critically ill neonate, 28 days of age or younger

99469   **Subsequent inpatient neonatal critical care,** per day, for the evaluation and management of a critically ill neonate, 28 days of age or younger

99471   **Initial inpatient pediatric critical care,** per day, for the evaluation and management of a critically ill infant or young child, 29 days through 24 months of age

99472   **Subsequent inpatient pediatric critical care,** per day, for the evaluation and management of a critically ill infant or young child, 29 days through 24 months of age

99475   **Initial inpatient pediatric critical care,** per day, for the evaluation and management of a critically ill infant or young child, 2 through 5 years of age

99476   **Subsequent inpatient pediatric critical care,** per day, for the evaluation and management of a critically ill infant or young child, 2 through 5 years of age

Initial and Continuing Intensive Care Services

Code 99477 represents the initial day of inpatient care for the child who is not critically ill but requires intensive observation, frequent interventions, and other intensive care services. Codes 99478-99480 are used to report the subsequent day services of directing the continuing intensive care of the low birth weight (LBW 1500-2500 grams) present body weight infant, very low birth weight (VLBW less than 1500 grams) present body weight infant, or normal (2501-5000 grams) present body weight newborn who does not meet the definition of critically ill but continues to require intensive observation, frequent interventions, and other intensive care services. These services are for infants and neonates who are not critically ill but continue to require intensive cardiac and respiratory monitoring, continuous and/or frequent vital sign monitoring, heat maintenance, enteral and/or parenteral nutritional adjustments, laboratory and oxygen monitoring, and constant observation by the health care team under direct supervision of the physician or other qualified health care professional. Codes 99477-99480 may be reported by a single individual and only once per day, per patient in a given facility. If readmitted to the intensive care unit during the same hospital stay, report 99478-99480 for the first day of intensive care and for each successive day that the child requires intensive care services.

These codes include the same procedures that are outlined in the **Neonatal and Pediatric Critical Care Services** section and these services should not be separately reported.

The initial day neonatal intensive care code (99477) can be used in addition to 99464 or 99465 as appropriate, when the physician or other qualified health care professional is present for the delivery (99464) or resuscitation (99465) is required. In this situation, report 99477 with modifier 25. Other procedures performed as a necessary part of the resuscitation (eg, endotracheal intubation [31500]) are also reported separately when performed as part of the pre-admission delivery room care. In order to report these procedures separately, they must be performed as a necessary component of the resuscitation and not simply as a convenience before admission to the neonatal intensive care unit.

The same procedures are included as bundled services with the neonatal intensive care codes as those listed for the neonatal (99468, 99469) and pediatric (99471-99476) critical care codes.

When the neonate or infant improves after the initial day and no longer requires intensive care services and is transferred to a lower level of care, the transferring individual does not report a per day intensive care service. Subsequent hospital care (99231-99233) or subsequent normal newborn care (99460, 99462) is reported as appropriate based upon the condition of the neonate or infant. If the transfer to a lower level of care occurs on the same day as initial intensive care services were provided by the transferring individual, 99477 may be reported.

When the neonate or infant is transferred after the initial day within the same facility to the care of another individual in a different group, both individuals report subsequent hospital care (99231-99233) services. The receiving individual reports subsequent hospital care (99231-99233) or subsequent normal newborn care (99462).

When the neonate or infant becomes critically ill on a day when initial or subsequent intensive care services (99477-99480) have been reported by one individual and is transferred to a critical care level of care provided by a different individual from a different group, the transferring individual reports either the time-based critical care services performed (99291, 99292) for the time spent providing critical care to the patient or the initial or subsequent intensive care (99477-99480) service, but not both. The receiving individual reports initial or subsequent inpatient neonatal or pediatric critical care (99468-99476) based upon the patient's age and whether this is the first or subsequent admission to critical care for the same hospital stay.

When the neonate or infant becomes critically ill on a day when initial or subsequent intensive care services (99477-99480) have been performed by the same individual or group, report only initial or subsequent inpatient neonatal or pediatric critical care (99468-99476) based upon the patient's age and whether this is the first or subsequent admission to critical care for the same hospital stay.

For the subsequent care of the sick neonate younger than 28 days of age but more than 5000 grams who does not require intensive or critical care services, use codes 99231-99233.

99477   **Initial hospital care,** per day, for the evaluation and management of the neonate, 28 days of age or younger, who requires intensive observation, frequent interventions, and other intensive care services

     (For the initiation of inpatient care of the normal newborn, use 99460)

     (For the initiation of care of the critically ill neonate, use 99468)

     (For initiation of inpatient hospital care of the ill neonate not requiring intensive observation, frequent interventions, and other intensive care services, see 99221-99223)

99478   **Subsequent intensive care,** per day, for the evaluation and management of the recovering very low birth weight infant (present body weight less than 1500 grams)

99479   **Subsequent intensive care,** per day, for the evaluation and management of the recovering low birth weight infant (present body weight of 1500-2500 grams)

99480   **Subsequent intensive care,** per day, for the evaluation and management of the recovering infant (present body weight of 2501-5000 grams)

     (99481, 99482 have been deleted. To report, use 99184)

99485   Code is out of numerical sequence. See 99466-99486

99486   Code is out of numerical sequence. See 99466-99486

Care Management Services

Care management services are management and support services provided by clinical staff, under the direction of a physician or other qualified health care professional, to a patient residing at home or in a domiciliary, rest home, or assisted living facility. Services may include establishing, implementing, revising, or monitoring the care plan, coordinating the care of other professionals and agencies, and educating the patient or caregiver about the patient's condition, care plan, and prognosis. The physician or other qualified health care professional provides or oversees the management and/or coordination of services, as needed, for all medical conditions, psychosocial needs, and activities of daily living.

A plan of care must be documented and shared with the patient and/or caregiver. A care plan is based on a physical, mental, cognitive, social, functional, and environmental assessment. It is a comprehensive plan of care for all health problems. It typically includes, but is not limited to, the following elements: problem list, expected outcome and prognosis, measurable treatment goals, symptom management, planned interventions, medication management, community/social services

ordered, how the services of agencies and specialists unconnected to the practice will be directed/coordinated, identification of the individuals responsible for each intervention, requirements for periodic review, and, when applicable, revision of the care plan.

Codes 99487, 99489, 99490 are reported only once per calendar month and may only be reported by the single physician or other qualified health care professional who assumes the care management role with a particular patient for the calendar month.

The face-to-face and non-face-to-face time spent by the clinical staff in communicating with the patient and/or family, caregivers, other professionals, and agencies; revising, documenting, and implementing the care plan; or teaching self-management is used in determining the care management clinical staff time for the month. Only the time of the clinical staff of the reporting professional is counted. Only count the time of one clinical staff member when two or more clinical staff members are meeting about the patient. **Note:** Do not count any clinical staff time on a day when the physician or qualified health care professional reports an E/M service (office or other outpatient services 99201, 99202, 99203, 99204, 99205, 99211, 99212, 99213, 99214, 99215, domiciliary, rest home services 99324, 99325, 99326, 99327, 99328, 99334, 99335, 99336, 99337, home services 99341, 99342, 99343, 99344, 99345, 99347, 99348, 99349, 99350).

Care management activities performed by clinical staff typically include:

- communication and engagement with patient, family members, guardian or caretaker, surrogate decision makers, and/or other professionals regarding aspects of care;

- communication with home health agencies and other community services utilized by the patient;

- collection of health outcomes data and registry documentation;

- patient and/or family/caregiver education to support self-management, independent living, and activities of daily living;

- assessment and support for treatment regimen adherence and medication management;

- identification of available community and health resources;

- facilitating access to care and services needed by the patient and/or family;

- management of care transitions not reported as part of transitional care management (99495, 99496);

- ongoing review of patient status, including review of laboratory and other studies not reported as part of an E/M service, noted above;

- development, communication, and maintenance of a comprehensive care plan.

The care management office/practice must have the following capabilities:

■ provide 24/7 access to physicians or other qualified health care professionals or clinical staff including providing patients/caregivers with a means to make contact with health care professionals in the practice to address urgent needs regardless of the time of day or day of week;

■ provide continuity of care with a designated member of the care team with whom the patient is able to schedule successive routine appointments;

■ provide timely access and management for follow-up after an emergency department visit or facility discharge;

■ utilize an electronic health record system so that care providers have timely access to clinical information;

■ use a standardized methodology to identify patients who require care management services;

■ have an internal care management process/function whereby a patient identified as meeting the requirements for these services starts receiving them in a timely manner;

■ use a form and format in the medical record that is standardized within the practice;

■ be able to engage and educate patients and caregivers as well as coordinate care among all service professionals, as appropriate for each patient.

E/M services may be reported separately by the same physician or other qualified health care professional during the same calendar month. Care management services include care plan oversight services (99339, 99340, 99374-99380), prolonged services without direct patient contact (99358, 99359), anticoagulant management (99363, 99364), medical team conferences (99366, 99367, 99368), education and training (98960, 98961, 98962, 99071, 99078), telephone services (99366, 99367, 99368, 99441, 99442, 99443), on-line medical evaluation (98969, 99444), preparation of special reports (99080), analysis of data (99090, 99091), transitional care management services (99495, 99496), medication therapy management services (99605, 99606, 99607) and, if performed, these services may not be reported separately during the month for which 99487, 99489, 99490 are reported. All other services may be reported. Do not report 99487, 99489, 99490 if reporting ESRD services (90951-90970) during the same month. If the care management services are performed within the postoperative period of a reported surgery, the same individual may not report 99487, 99489, 99490.

Care management may be reported in any calendar month during which the clinical staff time requirements are met. If care management resumes after a discharge during a new month, start a new period or report transitional care management services (99495, 99496) as appropriate. If discharge occurs in the same month, continue the reporting period or report Transitional Care Management Services. Do not report 99487, 99489, 99490 for any post-discharge care management services for any days within 30 days of discharge, if reporting 99495, 99496.

Chronic Care Management Services

Chronic care management services are provided when medical and/or psychosocial needs of the patient require establishing, implementing, revising, or monitoring the care plan. Patients who receive chronic care management services have two or more chronic continuous or episodic health conditions that are expected to last at least 12 months, or until the death of the patient, and that place the patient at significant risk of death, acute exacerbation/decompensation, or functional decline. Code 99490 is reported when, during the calendar month, at least 20 minutes of clinical staff time is spent in care management activities.

99490   Chronic care management services, at least 20 minutes of clinical staff time directed by a physician or other qualified health care professional, per calendar month, with the following required elements:

■ multiple (two or more) chronic conditions expected to last at least 12 months, or until the death of the patient;

■ chronic conditions place the patient at significant risk of death, acute exacerbation/decompensation, or functional decline;

■ comprehensive care plan established, implemented, revised, or monitored.

(Chronic care management services of less than 20 minutes duration, in a calendar month, are not reported separately)

Complex Chronic Care Management Services

Complex chronic care management services are provided during a calendar month that includes criteria for chronic care management services as well as establishment or substantial revision of a comprehensive care plan; medical, functional, and/or psychosocial problems requiring medical decision making of moderate or high complexity; and clinical staff care management services for at least 60 minutes, under the direction of a physician or other qualified health care professional. Physicians or other qualified health care professionals may not report complex chronic care management services if the care plan is unchanged or requires minimal change (eg, only a medication is changed or an adjustment in a treatment modality is ordered). Medical decision making as defined in the Evaluation and Management (E/M) guidelines is determined by the problems addressed by the reporting individual during the month.

Patients who require complex chronic care management services may be identified by practice-specific or other published algorithms that recognize multiple illnesses, multiple medication use, inability to perform activities of daily living, requirement for a caregiver, and/or repeat admissions or emergency department visits. Typical adult patients who receive complex chronic care management services are treated with three or more prescription medications and may be receiving other types of therapeutic interventions (eg, physical therapy, occupational therapy). Typical pediatric patients receive three or more therapeutic interventions (eg, medications, nutritional support, respiratory therapy). All patients have two or more chronic continuous or episodic health conditions that are expected to last at least 12 months, or until the death of the patient, and that place the patient at significant risk of death, acute exacerbation/decompensation, or functional decline. Typical patients have complex diseases and morbidities and, as a result, demonstrate one or more of the following:

- need for the coordination of a number of specialties and services;

- inability to perform activities of daily living and/or cognitive impairment resulting in poor adherence to the treatment plan without substantial assistance from a caregiver;

- psychiatric and other medical comorbidities (eg, dementia and chronic obstructive pulmonary disease or substance abuse and diabetes) that complicate their care; and/or

- social support requirements or difficulty with access to care.

Total Duration of Staff Care Management Services	Complex Chronic Care Management
Less than 60 minutes	Not reported separately
60 to 89 minutes (1 hour - 1 hr. 29 min.)	99487
90 - 119 minutes (1 hr. 30 min. - 1 hr. 59 min.)	99487 and 99489 X 1
120 minutes or more (2 hours or more)	99487 and 99489 X 2 and 99489 for each additional 30 minutes

99487   Complex chronic care management services, with the following required elements:

- multiple (two or more) chronic conditions expected to last at least 12 months, or until the death of the patient,

- chronic conditions place the patient at significant risk of death, acute exacerbation/decompensation, or functional decline,

- establishment or substantial revision of a comprehensive care plan,

- moderate or high complexity medical decision making;

- 60 minutes of clinical staff time directed by a physician or other qualified health care professional, per calendar month.

(Complex chronic care management services of less than 60 minutes duration, in a calendar month, are not reported separately)

(99488 has been deleted. To report one or more face-to-face visits by the physician or other qualified health care professional that are performed in the same month as 99487, use the appropriate E/M code[s])

+ 99489   each additional 30 minutes of clinical staff time directed by a physician or other qualified health care professional, per calendar month (List separately in addition to code for primary procedure)

(Report 99489 in conjunction with 99487)

(Do not report 99489 for care management services of less than 30 minutes additional to the first 60 minutes of complex chronic care management services during a calendar month)

(Do not report 99487, 99489, 99490 during the same month with 90951-90970, 98960-98962, 98966-98969, 99071, 99078, 99080, 99090, 99091, 99339, 99340, 99358, 99359, 99363, 99364, 99366-99368, 99374-99380, 99441-99444, 99495, 99496, 99605-99607)

99490   Code is out of numerical sequence. See 99487-99490

Transitional Care Management Services

Codes 99495 and 99496 are used to report transitional care management services (TCM). These services are for a new or established patient whose medical and/or psychosocial problems require moderate or high complexity medical decision making during transitions in care from an inpatient hospital setting (including acute hospital, rehabilitation hospital, long-term acute care hospital), partial hospital, observation status in a hospital, or skilled nursing facility/nursing facility to the patient's community setting (home, domiciliary, rest home, or assisted living). TCM commences upon the date of discharge and continues for the next 29 days.

TCM is comprised of one face-to-face visit within the specified timeframes, in combination with non-face-to-face services that may be performed by the physician or other qualified health care professional and/or licensed clinical staff under his/her direction.

Non-face-to-face services provided by clinical staff, under the direction of the physician or other qualified health care professional, may include:

- communication (with patient, family members, guardian or caretaker, surrogate decision makers, and/or other professionals) regarding aspects of care,

- communication with home health agencies and other community services utilized by the patient,

- patient and/or family/caretaker education to support self-management, independent living, and activities of daily living,

- assessment and support for treatment regimen adherence and medication management,

- identification of available community and health resources,

- facilitating access to care and services needed by the patient and/or family

Non-face-to-face services provided by the physician or other qualified health care provider may include:

- obtaining and reviewing the discharge information (eg, discharge summary, as available, or continuity of care documents);

- reviewing need for or follow-up on pending diagnostic tests and treatments;

- interaction with other qualified health care professionals who will assume or reassume care of the patient's system-specific problems;

- education of patient, family, guardian, and/or caregiver;

- establishment or reestablishment of referrals and arranging for needed community resources;

- assistance in scheduling any required follow-up with community providers and services.

TCM requires a face-to-face visit, initial patient contact, and medication reconciliation within specified time frames. The first face-to-face visit is part of the TCM service and not reported separately. Additional E/M services provided on subsequent dates after the first face-to-face visit may be reported separately. TCM requires an interactive contact with the patient or caregiver, as appropriate, within two business days of discharge. The contact may be direct (face-to-face), telephonic, or by electronic means. Medication reconciliation and management must occur no later than the date of the face-to-face visit.

These services address any needed coordination of care performed by multiple disciplines and community service agencies. The reporting individual provides or oversees the management and/or coordination of services, as needed, for all medical conditions, psychosocial needs and activity of daily living support by providing first contact and continuous access.

Medical decision making and the date of the first face-to-face visit are used to select and report the appropriate TCM code. For 99496, the face-to-face visit must occur within 7 calendar days of the date discharge and medical decision making must be of high complexity. For 99495, the face-to-face visit must occur within 14 calendar days of the date of discharge and medical decision making must be of at least moderate complexity.

Type of Medical Decision Making	Face-to-face visit within 7 days	Face to face visit within 8 to 14 days
Moderate Complexity	99495	99495
High Complexity	99496	99495

Medical decision making is defined by the E/M Services Guidelines. The medical decision making over the service period reported is used to define the medical decision making of TCM. Documentation includes the timing of the initial post discharge communication with the patient or caregivers, date of the face-to-face visit, and the complexity of medical decision making.

Only one individual may report these services and only once per patient within 30 days of discharge. Another TCM may not be reported by the same individual or group for any subsequent discharge(s) within the 30 days. The same individual may report hospital or observation discharge services and TCM. However, the discharge service may not constitute the required face-to-face visit. The same individual should not report TCM services provided in the postoperative period of a service that the individual reported.

A physician or other qualified health care professional who reports codes 99495, 99496 may not report care plan oversight services (99339, 99340, 99374-99380), prolonged services without direct patient contact (99358, 99359), anticoagulant management (99363, 99364), medical team conferences (99366-99368), education and training (98960-98962, 99071, 99078), telephone services (98966-98968, 99441-99443), end stage renal disease services (90951-90970), online medical evaluation services (98969, 99444), preparation of special reports (99080), analysis of data (99090, 99091), complex chronic care coordination services (99487-99489), medication therapy management services (99605-99607), during the time period covered by the transitional care management services codes.

99495 **Transitional Care Management Services** with the following required elements:

- Communication (direct contact, telephone, electronic) with the patient and/or caregiver within 2 business days of discharge

- Medical decision making of at least moderate complexity during the service period

- Face-to-face visit, within 14 calendar days of discharge

99496   **Transitional Care Management Services** with the following required elements:

- Communication (direct contact, telephone, electronic) with the patient and/or caregiver within 2 business days of discharge
- Medical decision making of high complexity during the service period
- Face-to-face visit, within 7 calendar days of discharge

(Do not report 90951-90970, 98960-98962, 98966-98969, 99071, 99078, 99080, 99090, 99091, 99339, 99340, 99358, 99359, 99363, 99364, 99366-99368, 99374-99380, 99441-99444, 99487-99489, 99605-99607 when performed during the service time of codes 99495 or 99496)

Advance Care Planning

Codes 99497, 99498 are used to report the face-to-face service between a physician or other qualified health care professional and a patient, family member, or surrogate in counseling and discussing advance directives, with or without completing relevant legal forms. An advance directive is a document appointing an agent and/or recording the wishes of a patient pertaining to his/her medical treatment at a future time should he/she lack decisional capacity at that time. Examples of written advance directives include, but are not limited to, Health Care Proxy, Durable Power of Attorney for Health Care, Living Will, and Medical Orders for Life-Sustaining Treatment (MOLST).

When using codes 99497, 99498, no active management of the problem(s) is undertaken during the time period reported.

Codes 99497, 99498 may be reported separately if these services are performed on the same day as another Evaluation and Management service (99201-99215, 99217, 99218, 99219, 99220, 99221, 99222, 99223, 99224, 99225, 99226, 99231, 99232, 99233, 99234, 99235, 99236, 99238, 99239, 99241, 99242, 99243, 99244, 99245, 99251, 99252, 99253, 99254, 99255, 99281, 99282, 99283, 99284, 99285, 99304, 99305, 99306, 99307, 99308, 99309, 99310, 99315, 99316, 99318, 99324, 99325, 99326, 99327, 99328, 99334, 99335, 99336, 99337, 99341, 99342, 99343, 99344, 99345, 99347, 99348, 99349, 99350, 99381-99397, 99495, 99496).

99497   Advance care planning including the explanation and discussion of advance directives such as standard forms (with completion of such forms, when performed), by the physician or other qualified health care professional; first 30 minutes, face-to-face with the patient, family member(s), and/or surrogate

+ 99498   each additional 30 minutes (List separately in addition to code for primary procedure)

(Use 99498 in conjunction with 99497)

(Do not report 99497 and 99498 on the same date of service as 99291, 99292, 99468, 99469, 99471, 99472, 99475, 99476, 99477, 99478, 99479, 99480)

Other Evaluation and Management Services

99499   **Unlisted evaluation and management** service

Evaluation/Management

Notes

Anesthesia Guidelines

Services involving administration of anesthesia are reported by the use of the anesthesia five-digit procedure code (00100-01999) plus modifier codes (defined under "Anesthesia Modifiers" later in these Guidelines).

The reporting of anesthesia services is appropriate by or under the responsible supervision of a physician. These services may include but are not limited to general, regional, supplementation of local anesthesia, or other supportive services in order to afford the patient the anesthesia care deemed optimal by the anesthesiologist during any procedure. These services include the usual preoperative and postoperative visits, the anesthesia care during the procedure, the administration of fluids and/or blood and the usual monitoring services (eg, ECG, temperature, blood pressure, oximetry, capnography, and mass spectrometry). Unusual forms of monitoring (eg, intra-arterial, central venous, and Swan-Ganz) are not included.

Items used by all physicians in reporting their services are presented in the **Introduction.** Some of the commonalities are repeated in this section for the convenience of those physicians referring to this section on **Anesthesia.** Other definitions and items unique to anesthesia are also listed.

To report moderate (conscious) sedation provided by a physician also performing the service for which conscious sedation is being provided, see codes 99143-99145.

For the procedures listed in Appendix G, when a second physician other than the health care professional performing the diagnostic or therapeutic services provides moderate (conscious) sedation in the facility setting (eg, hospital, outpatient hospital/ambulatory surgery center, skilled nursing facility), the second physician reports the associated moderate sedation procedure/service 99148-99150; when these services are performed by the second physician in the nonfacility setting (eg, physician office, freestanding imaging center), codes 99148-99150 would not be reported. Moderate sedation does not include minimal sedation (anxiolysis), deep sedation, or monitored anesthesia care (00100-01999).

To report regional or general anesthesia provided by a physician also performing the services for which the anesthesia is being provided, see modifier 47 in Appendix A.

Time Reporting

Time for anesthesia procedures may be reported as is customary in the local area. Anesthesia time begins when the anesthesiologist begins to prepare the patient for the induction of anesthesia in the operating room (or in an equivalent area) and ends when the anesthesiologist is no longer in personal attendance, that is, when the patient may be safely placed under postoperative supervision.

Anesthesia Services

Services rendered in the office, home, or hospital; consultation; and other medical services are listed in the **Evaluation and Management Services** section (99201-99499 series) on page 8. "Special Services and Reporting" (99000-99091 series) are listed in the **Medicine** section.

Supplied Materials

Supplies and materials provided (eg, sterile trays, drugs) over and above those usually included with the office visit or other services rendered may be listed separately. Drugs, tray supplies, and materials provided should be listed and identified with 99070 or the appropriate supply code.

Separate or Multiple Procedures

When multiple surgical procedures are performed during a single anesthetic administration, the anesthesia code representing the most complex procedure is reported. The time reported is the combined total for all procedures.

Special Report

A service that is rarely provided, unusual, variable, or new may require a special report. Pertinent information should include an adequate definition or description of the nature, extent, and need for the procedure and the time, effort, and equipment necessary to provide the service.

Anesthesia Modifiers

All anesthesia services are reported by use of the anesthesia five-digit procedure code (00100-01999) plus the addition of a physical status modifier. The use of other optional modifiers may be appropriate.

Physical Status Modifiers

Physical Status modifiers are represented by the initial letter 'P' followed by a single digit from 1 to 6 as defined in the following list:

P1: A normal healthy patient

P2: A patient with mild systemic disease

P3: A patient with severe systemic disease

P4: A patient with severe systemic disease that is a constant threat to life

P5: A moribund patient who is not expected to survive without the operation

P6: A declared brain-dead patient whose organs are being removed for donor purposes

These six levels are consistent with the American Society of Anesthesiologists (ASA) ranking of patient physical status. Physical status is included in the CPT codebook to distinguish among various levels of complexity of the anesthesia service provided.

Example: 00100-P1

Qualifying Circumstances

More than one qualifying circumstance may be selected.

Many anesthesia services are provided under particularly difficult circumstances, depending on factors such as extraordinary condition of patient, notable operative conditions, and/or unusual risk factors. This section includes a list of important qualifying circumstances that significantly affect the character of the anesthesia service provided. These procedures would not be reported alone but would be reported as additional procedure numbers qualifying an anesthesia procedure or service.

+ 99100 Anesthesia for patient of extreme age, younger than 1 year and older than 70 (List separately in addition to code for primary anesthesia procedure)

(For procedure performed on infants younger than 1 year of age at time of surgery, see 00326, 00561, 00834, 00836)

+ 99116 Anesthesia complicated by utilization of total body hypothermia (List separately in addition to code for primary anesthesia procedure)

+ 99135 Anesthesia complicated by utilization of controlled hypotension (List separately in addition to code for primary anesthesia procedure)

+ 99140 Anesthesia complicated by emergency conditions (specify) (List separately in addition to code for primary anesthesia procedure)

(An emergency is defined as existing when delay in treatment of the patient would lead to a significant increase in the threat to life or body part)

Anesthesia

Head

00100   Anesthesia for procedures on salivary glands, including biopsy

00102   Anesthesia for procedures involving plastic repair of cleft lip

00103   Anesthesia for reconstructive procedures of eyelid (eg, blepharoplasty, ptosis surgery)

00104   Anesthesia for electroconvulsive therapy

00120   Anesthesia for procedures on external, middle, and inner ear including biopsy; not otherwise specified

00124   otoscopy

00126   tympanotomy

00140   Anesthesia for procedures on eye; not otherwise specified

00142   lens surgery

00144   corneal transplant

00145   vitreoretinal surgery

00147   iridectomy

00148   ophthalmoscopy

00160   Anesthesia for procedures on nose and accessory sinuses; not otherwise specified

00162   radical surgery

00164   biopsy, soft tissue

00170   Anesthesia for intraoral procedures, including biopsy; not otherwise specified

00172   repair of cleft palate

00174   excision of retropharyngeal tumor

00176   radical surgery

00190   Anesthesia for procedures on facial bones or skull; not otherwise specified

00192   radical surgery (including prognathism)

00210   Anesthesia for intracranial procedures; not otherwise specified

00211   craniotomy or craniectomy for evacuation of hematoma

00212   subdural taps

00214   burr holes, including ventriculography

00215   cranioplasty or elevation of depressed skull fracture, extradural (simple or compound)

00216   vascular procedures

00218   procedures in sitting position

00220   cerebrospinal fluid shunting procedures

00222   electrocoagulation of intracranial nerve

Neck

00300   Anesthesia for all procedures on the integumentary system, muscles and nerves of head, neck, and posterior trunk, not otherwise specified

00320   Anesthesia for all procedures on esophagus, thyroid, larynx, trachea and lymphatic system of neck; not otherwise specified, age 1 year or older

00322   needle biopsy of thyroid

(For procedures on cervical spine and cord, see 00600, 00604, 00670)

00326   Anesthesia for all procedures on the larynx and trachea in children younger than 1 year of age

(Do not report 00326 in conjunction with 99100)

00350   Anesthesia for procedures on major vessels of neck; not otherwise specified

00352   simple ligation

(For arteriography, use 01916)

Thorax (Chest Wall and Shoulder Girdle)

00400   Anesthesia for procedures on the integumentary system on the extremities, anterior trunk and perineum; not otherwise specified

00402   reconstructive procedures on breast (eg, reduction or augmentation mammoplasty, muscle flaps)

00404   radical or modified radical procedures on breast

00406   radical or modified radical procedures on breast with internal mammary node dissection

00410   electrical conversion of arrhythmias

00450   Anesthesia for procedures on clavicle and scapula; not otherwise specified

(00452 has been deleted)

00454   biopsy of clavicle

00470   Anesthesia for partial rib resection; not otherwise specified

00472   thoracoplasty (any type)

00474   radical procedures (eg, pectus excavatum)

▲=Revised code   ●=New code   ►◄=Contains new or revised text   ⊘=Modifier 51 exempt

Intrathoracic

00500 Anesthesia for all procedures on esophagus

00520 Anesthesia for closed chest procedures; (including bronchoscopy) not otherwise specified

00522 needle biopsy of pleura

00524 pneumocentesis

00528 mediastinoscopy and diagnostic thoracoscopy not utilizing 1 lung ventilation

(For tracheobronchial reconstruction, use 00539)

00529 mediastinoscopy and diagnostic thoracoscopy utilizing 1 lung ventilation

00530 Anesthesia for permanent transvenous pacemaker insertion

00532 Anesthesia for access to central venous circulation

00534 Anesthesia for transvenous insertion or replacement of pacing cardioverter-defibrillator

(For transthoracic approach, use 00560)

00537 Anesthesia for cardiac electrophysiologic procedures including radiofrequency ablation

00539 Anesthesia for tracheobronchial reconstruction

00540 Anesthesia for thoracotomy procedures involving lungs, pleura, diaphragm, and mediastinum (including surgical thoracoscopy); not otherwise specified

00541 utilizing 1 lung ventilation

(For thoracic spine and cord anesthesia procedures via an anterior transthoracic approach, see 00625-00626)

00542 decortication

00546 pulmonary resection with thoracoplasty

00548 intrathoracic procedures on the trachea and bronchi

00550 Anesthesia for sternal debridement

00560 Anesthesia for procedures on heart, pericardial sac, and great vessels of chest; without pump oxygenator

00561 with pump oxygenator, younger than 1 year of age

(Do not report 00561 in conjunction with 99100, 99116, and 99135)

00562 with pump oxygenator, age 1 year or older, for all noncoronary bypass procedures (eg, valve procedures) or for re-operation for coronary bypass more than 1 month after original operation

00563 with pump oxygenator with hypothermic circulatory arrest

00566 Anesthesia for direct coronary artery bypass grafting; without pump oxygenator

00567 with pump oxygenator

00580 Anesthesia for heart transplant or heart/lung transplant

Spine and Spinal Cord

00600 Anesthesia for procedures on cervical spine and cord; not otherwise specified

(For percutaneous image-guided spine and spinal cord anesthesia procedures, see 01935, 01936)

00604 procedures with patient in the sitting position

00620 Anesthesia for procedures on thoracic spine and cord, not otherwise specified

(00622 has been deleted)

00625 Anesthesia for procedures on the thoracic spine and cord, via an anterior transthoracic approach; not utilizing 1 lung ventilation

00626 utilizing 1 lung ventilation

(For anesthesia for thoracotomy procedures other than spinal, see 00540-00541)

00630 Anesthesia for procedures in lumbar region; not otherwise specified

00632 lumbar sympathectomy

(00634 has been deleted)

00635 diagnostic or therapeutic lumbar puncture

00640 Anesthesia for manipulation of the spine or for closed procedures on the cervical, thoracic or lumbar spine

00670 Anesthesia for extensive spine and spinal cord procedures (eg, spinal instrumentation or vascular procedures)

Upper Abdomen

00700 Anesthesia for procedures on upper anterior abdominal wall; not otherwise specified

00702 percutaneous liver biopsy

00730 Anesthesia for procedures on upper posterior abdominal wall

00740 Anesthesia for upper gastrointestinal endoscopic procedures, endoscope introduced proximal to duodenum

00750 Anesthesia for hernia repairs in upper abdomen; not otherwise specified

00752 lumbar and ventral (incisional) hernias and/or wound dehiscence

00754 omphalocele

00756 transabdominal repair of diaphragmatic hernia

00770 Anesthesia for all procedures on major abdominal blood vessels

00790 Anesthesia for intraperitoneal procedures in upper abdomen including laparoscopy; not otherwise specified

00792 partial hepatectomy or management of liver hemorrhage (excluding liver biopsy)

⊙=Moderate sedation ✚=Add-on code ✗=FDA approval pending #=Resequenced code ○=Recycled/reinstated code

00794	pancreatectomy, partial or total (eg, Whipple procedure)
00796	liver transplant (recipient)
	(For harvesting of liver, use 01990)
00797	gastric restrictive procedure for morbid obesity

Lower Abdomen

00800	Anesthesia for procedures on lower anterior abdominal wall; not otherwise specified
00802	panniculectomy
00810	Anesthesia for lower intestinal endoscopic procedures, endoscope introduced distal to duodenum
00820	Anesthesia for procedures on lower posterior abdominal wall
00830	Anesthesia for hernia repairs in lower abdomen; not otherwise specified
00832	ventral and incisional hernias
	(For hernia repairs in the infant 1 year of age or younger, see 00834, 00836)
00834	Anesthesia for hernia repairs in the lower abdomen not otherwise specified, younger than 1 year of age
	(Do not report 00834 in conjunction with 99100)
00836	Anesthesia for hernia repairs in the lower abdomen not otherwise specified, infants younger than 37 weeks gestational age at birth and younger than 50 weeks gestational age at time of surgery
	(Do not report 00836 in conjunction with 99100)
00840	Anesthesia for intraperitoneal procedures in lower abdomen including laparoscopy; not otherwise specified
00842	amniocentesis
00844	abdominoperineal resection
00846	radical hysterectomy
00848	pelvic exenteration
00851	tubal ligation/transection
00860	Anesthesia for extraperitoneal procedures in lower abdomen, including urinary tract; not otherwise specified
00862	renal procedures, including upper one-third of ureter, or donor nephrectomy
00864	total cystectomy
00865	radical prostatectomy (suprapubic, retropubic)
00866	adrenalectomy
00868	renal transplant (recipient)
	(For donor nephrectomy, use 00862)
	(For harvesting kidney from brain-dead patient, use 01990)
00870	cystolithotomy

00872	Anesthesia for lithotripsy, extracorporeal shock wave; with water bath
00873	without water bath
00880	Anesthesia for procedures on major lower abdominal vessels; not otherwise specified
00882	inferior vena cava ligation

Perineum

(For perineal procedures on integumentary system, muscles and nerves, see 00300, 00400)

00902	Anesthesia for; anorectal procedure
00904	radical perineal procedure
00906	vulvectomy
00908	perineal prostatectomy
00910	Anesthesia for transurethral procedures (including urethrocystoscopy); not otherwise specified
00912	transurethral resection of bladder tumor(s)
00914	transurethral resection of prostate
00916	post-transurethral resection bleeding
00918	with fragmentation, manipulation and/or removal of ureteral calculus
00920	Anesthesia for procedures on male genitalia (including open urethral procedures); not otherwise specified
00921	vasectomy, unilateral or bilateral
00922	seminal vesicles
00924	undescended testis, unilateral or bilateral
00926	radical orchiectomy, inguinal
00928	radical orchiectomy, abdominal
00930	orchiopexy, unilateral or bilateral
00932	complete amputation of penis
00934	radical amputation of penis with bilateral inguinal lymphadenectomy
00936	radical amputation of penis with bilateral inguinal and iliac lymphadenectomy
00938	insertion of penile prosthesis (perineal approach)
00940	Anesthesia for vaginal procedures (including biopsy of labia, vagina, cervix or endometrium); not otherwise specified
00942	colpotomy, vaginectomy, colporrhaphy, and open urethral procedures
00944	vaginal hysterectomy
00948	cervical cerclage
00950	culdoscopy
00952	hysteroscopy and/or hysterosalpingography

Pelvis (Except Hip)

01112   Anesthesia for bone marrow aspiration and/or biopsy, anterior or posterior iliac crest

01120   Anesthesia for procedures on bony pelvis

01130   Anesthesia for body cast application or revision

01140   Anesthesia for interpelviabdominal (hindquarter) amputation

01150   Anesthesia for radical procedures for tumor of pelvis, except hindquarter amputation

01160   Anesthesia for closed procedures involving symphysis pubis or sacroiliac joint

01170   Anesthesia for open procedures involving symphysis pubis or sacroiliac joint

01173   Anesthesia for open repair of fracture disruption of pelvis or column fracture involving acetabulum

01180   Anesthesia for obturator neurectomy; extrapelvic

01190   intrapelvic

Upper Leg (Except Knee)

01200   Anesthesia for all closed procedures involving hip joint

01202   Anesthesia for arthroscopic procedures of hip joint

01210   Anesthesia for open procedures involving hip joint; not otherwise specified

01212   hip disarticulation

01214   total hip arthroplasty

01215   revision of total hip arthroplasty

01220   Anesthesia for all closed procedures involving upper two-thirds of femur

01230   Anesthesia for open procedures involving upper two-thirds of femur; not otherwise specified

01232   amputation

01234   radical resection

01250   Anesthesia for all procedures on nerves, muscles, tendons, fascia, and bursae of upper leg

01260   Anesthesia for all procedures involving veins of upper leg, including exploration

01270   Anesthesia for procedures involving arteries of upper leg, including bypass graft; not otherwise specified

01272   femoral artery ligation

01274   femoral artery embolectomy

Knee and Popliteal Area

01320   Anesthesia for all procedures on nerves, muscles, tendons, fascia, and bursae of knee and/or popliteal area

01340   Anesthesia for all closed procedures on lower one-third of femur

01360   Anesthesia for all open procedures on lower one-third of femur

01380   Anesthesia for all closed procedures on knee joint

01382   Anesthesia for diagnostic arthroscopic procedures of knee joint

01390   Anesthesia for all closed procedures on upper ends of tibia, fibula, and/or patella

01392   Anesthesia for all open procedures on upper ends of tibia, fibula, and/or patella

01400   Anesthesia for open or surgical arthroscopic procedures on knee joint; not otherwise specified

01402   total knee arthroplasty

01404   disarticulation at knee

01420   Anesthesia for all cast applications, removal, or repair involving knee joint

01430   Anesthesia for procedures on veins of knee and popliteal area; not otherwise specified

01432   arteriovenous fistula

01440   Anesthesia for procedures on arteries of knee and popliteal area; not otherwise specified

01442   popliteal thromboendarterectomy, with or without patch graft

01444   popliteal excision and graft or repair for occlusion or aneurysm

Lower Leg (Below Knee, Includes Ankle and Foot)

01462   Anesthesia for all closed procedures on lower leg, ankle, and foot

01464   Anesthesia for arthroscopic procedures of ankle and/or foot

01470   Anesthesia for procedures on nerves, muscles, tendons, and fascia of lower leg, ankle, and foot; not otherwise specified

01472   repair of ruptured Achilles tendon, with or without graft

01474   gastrocnemius recession (eg, Strayer procedure)

01480   Anesthesia for open procedures on bones of lower leg, ankle, and foot; not otherwise specified

01482   radical resection (including below knee amputation)

01484   osteotomy or osteoplasty of tibia and/or fibula

01486	total ankle replacement
01490	Anesthesia for lower leg cast application, removal, or repair
01500	Anesthesia for procedures on arteries of lower leg, including bypass graft; not otherwise specified
01502	embolectomy, direct or with catheter
01520	Anesthesia for procedures on veins of lower leg; not otherwise specified
01522	venous thrombectomy, direct or with catheter

Shoulder and Axilla

Includes humeral head and neck, sternoclavicular joint, acromioclavicular joint, and shoulder joint.

01610	Anesthesia for all procedures on nerves, muscles, tendons, fascia, and bursae of shoulder and axilla
01620	Anesthesia for all closed procedures on humeral head and neck, sternoclavicular joint, acromioclavicular joint, and shoulder joint
01622	Anesthesia for diagnostic arthroscopic procedures of shoulder joint
01630	Anesthesia for open or surgical arthroscopic procedures on humeral head and neck, sternoclavicular joint, acromioclavicular joint, and shoulder joint; not otherwise specified
01634	shoulder disarticulation
01636	interthoracoscapular (forequarter) amputation
01638	total shoulder replacement
01650	Anesthesia for procedures on arteries of shoulder and axilla; not otherwise specified
01652	axillary-brachial aneurysm
01654	bypass graft
01656	axillary-femoral bypass graft
01670	Anesthesia for all procedures on veins of shoulder and axilla
01680	Anesthesia for shoulder cast application, removal or repair; not otherwise specified
01682	shoulder spica

Upper Arm and Elbow

01710	Anesthesia for procedures on nerves, muscles, tendons, fascia, and bursae of upper arm and elbow; not otherwise specified
01712	tenotomy, elbow to shoulder, open
01714	tenoplasty, elbow to shoulder
01716	tenodesis, rupture of long tendon of biceps

01730	Anesthesia for all closed procedures on humerus and elbow
01732	Anesthesia for diagnostic arthroscopic procedures of elbow joint
01740	Anesthesia for open or surgical arthroscopic procedures of the elbow; not otherwise specified
01742	osteotomy of humerus
01744	repair of nonunion or malunion of humerus
01756	radical procedures
01758	excision of cyst or tumor of humerus
01760	total elbow replacement
01770	Anesthesia for procedures on arteries of upper arm and elbow; not otherwise specified
01772	embolectomy
01780	Anesthesia for procedures on veins of upper arm and elbow; not otherwise specified
01782	phleborrhaphy

Forearm, Wrist, and Hand

01810	Anesthesia for all procedures on nerves, muscles, tendons, fascia, and bursae of forearm, wrist, and hand
01820	Anesthesia for all closed procedures on radius, ulna, wrist, or hand bones
01829	Anesthesia for diagnostic arthroscopic procedures on the wrist
01830	Anesthesia for open or surgical arthroscopic/endoscopic procedures on distal radius, distal ulna, wrist, or hand joints; not otherwise specified
01832	total wrist replacement
01840	Anesthesia for procedures on arteries of forearm, wrist, and hand; not otherwise specified
01842	embolectomy
01844	Anesthesia for vascular shunt, or shunt revision, any type (eg, dialysis)
01850	Anesthesia for procedures on veins of forearm, wrist, and hand; not otherwise specified
01852	phleborrhaphy
01860	Anesthesia for forearm, wrist, or hand cast application, removal, or repair

Radiological Procedures

01916	Anesthesia for diagnostic arteriography/venography
	(Do not report 01916 in conjunction with therapeutic codes 01924-01926, 01930-01933)

Anesthesia

01920 Anesthesia for cardiac catheterization including coronary angiography and ventriculography (not to include Swan-Ganz catheter)

01922 Anesthesia for non-invasive imaging or radiation therapy

01924 Anesthesia for therapeutic interventional radiological procedures involving the arterial system; not otherwise specified

01925   carotid or coronary

01926   intracranial, intracardiac, or aortic

01930 Anesthesia for therapeutic interventional radiological procedures involving the venous/lymphatic system (not to include access to the central circulation); not otherwise specified

01931   intrahepatic or portal circulation (eg, transvenous intrahepatic portosystemic shunt[s] [TIPS])

01932   intrathoracic or jugular

01933   intracranial

01935 Anesthesia for percutaneous image guided procedures on the spine and spinal cord; diagnostic

01936   therapeutic

Burn Excisions or Debridement

01951 Anesthesia for second- and third-degree burn excision or debridement with or without skin grafting, any site, for total body surface area (TBSA) treated during anesthesia and surgery; less than 4% total body surface area

01952   between 4% and 9% of total body surface area

+ 01953   each additional 9% total body surface area or part thereof (List separately in addition to code for primary procedure)

(Use 01953 in conjunction with 01952)

Obstetric

01958 Anesthesia for external cephalic version procedure

01960 Anesthesia for vaginal delivery only

01961 Anesthesia for cesarean delivery only

01962 Anesthesia for urgent hysterectomy following delivery

01963 Anesthesia for cesarean hysterectomy without any labor analgesia/anesthesia care

01965 Anesthesia for incomplete or missed abortion procedures

01966 Anesthesia for induced abortion procedures

01967 Neuraxial labor analgesia/anesthesia for planned vaginal delivery (this includes any repeat subarachnoid needle placement and drug injection and/or any necessary replacement of an epidural catheter during labor)

+ 01968 Anesthesia for cesarean delivery following neuraxial labor analgesia/anesthesia (List separately in addition to code for primary procedure performed)

(Use 01968 in conjunction with 01967)

+ 01969 Anesthesia for cesarean hysterectomy following neuraxial labor analgesia/anesthesia (List separately in addition to code for primary procedure performed)

(Use 01969 in conjunction with 01967)

Other Procedures

01990 Physiological support for harvesting of organ(s) from brain-dead patient

01991 Anesthesia for diagnostic or therapeutic nerve blocks and injections (when block or injection is performed by a different physician or other qualified health care professional); other than the prone position

01992   prone position

(Do not report 01991 or 01992 in conjunction with 99143-99150)

(When regional intravenous administration of local anesthetic agent or other medication in the upper or lower extremity is used as the anesthetic for a surgical procedure, report the appropriate anesthesia code. To report a Bier block for pain management, use 64999)

(For intra-arterial or intravenous therapy for pain management, see 96373, 96374)

01996 Daily hospital management of epidural or subarachnoid continuous drug administration

(Report code 01996 for daily hospital management of continuous epidural or subarachnoid drug administration performed after insertion of an epidural or subarachnoid catheter)

01999 Unlisted anesthesia procedure(s)

Surgery Guidelines

Guidelines to direct general reporting of services are presented in the **Introduction.** Some of the commonalities are repeated here for the convenience of those referring to this section on **Surgery.** Other definitions and items unique to Surgery are also listed.

Services

Services rendered in the office, home, or hospital, consultations, and other medical services are listed in the **Evaluation and Management Services** section (99201-99499) beginning on page 8. "Special Services and Reports" (99000-99091) are listed in the **Medicine** section.

CPT Surgical Package Definition

By their very nature, the services to any patient are variable. The CPT codes that represent a readily identifiable surgical procedure thereby include, on a procedure-by-procedure basis, a variety of services. In defining the specific services "included" in a given CPT surgical code, the following services related to the surgery when furnished by the physician or other qualified health care professional who performs the surgery are included in addition to the operation per se:

- Evaluation and Management (E/M) service(s) subsequent to the decision for surgery on the day before and/or day of surgery (including history and physical)
- Local infiltration, metacarpal/metatarsal/digital block or topical anesthesia
- Immediate postoperative care, including dictating operative notes, talking with the family and other physicians or other qualified health care professionals
- Writing orders
- Evaluating the patient in the postanesthesia recovery area
- Typical postoperative follow-up care

Follow-Up Care for Diagnostic Procedures

Follow-up care for diagnostic procedures (eg, endoscopy, arthroscopy, injection procedures for radiography) includes only that care related to recovery from the diagnostic procedure itself. Care of the condition for which the diagnostic procedure was performed or of

other concomitant conditions is not included and may be listed separately.

Follow-Up Care for Therapeutic Surgical Procedures

Follow-up care for therapeutic surgical procedures includes only that care which is usually a part of the surgical service. Complications, exacerbations, recurrence, or the presence of other diseases or injuries requiring additional services should be separately reported.

Supplied Materials

Supplies and materials (eg, sterile trays/drugs), over and above those usually included with the procedure(s) rendered are reported separately. List drugs, trays, supplies, and materials provided. Identify as 99070 or specific supply code.

Reporting More Than One Procedure/Service

When more than one procedure/service is performed on the same date, same session or during a post-operative period (subject to the "surgical package" concept), several CPT modifiers may apply (see Appendix A for definition).

Separate Procedure

Some of the procedures or services listed in the CPT codebook that are commonly carried out as an integral component of a total service or procedure have been identified by the inclusion of the term "separate procedure." The codes designated as "separate procedure" should not be reported in addition to the code for the total procedure or service of which it is considered an integral component.

However, when a procedure or service that is designated as a "separate procedure" is carried out independently or considered to be unrelated or distinct from other procedures/services provided at that time, it may be reported by itself, or in addition to other procedures/services by appending modifier 59 to the specific "separate procedure" code to indicate that the procedure is not considered to be a component of another procedure, but is a distinct, independent procedure. This may represent a different session, different procedure or surgery, different site or organ system, separate incision/excision, separate lesion, or separate injury (or area of injury in extensive injuries).

Unlisted Service or Procedure

A service or procedure may be provided that is not listed in this edition of the CPT codebook. When reporting such a service, the appropriate "Unlisted Procedure" code may be used to indicate the service, identifying it by "Special Report" as discussed in the section below. The "Unlisted Procedures" and accompanying codes for **Surgery** are as follows:

15999   Unlisted procedure, excision pressure ulcer

17999   Unlisted procedure, skin, mucous membrane and subcutaneous tissue

19499   Unlisted procedure, breast

20999   Unlisted procedure, musculoskeletal system, general

21089   Unlisted maxillofacial prosthetic procedure

21299   Unlisted craniofacial and maxillofacial procedure

21499   Unlisted musculoskeletal procedure, head

21899   Unlisted procedure, neck or thorax

22899   Unlisted procedure, spine

22999   Unlisted procedure, abdomen, musculoskeletal system

23929   Unlisted procedure, shoulder

24999   Unlisted procedure, humerus or elbow

25999   Unlisted procedure, forearm or wrist

26989   Unlisted procedure, hands or fingers

27299   Unlisted procedure, pelvis or hip joint

27599   Unlisted procedure, femur or knee

27899   Unlisted procedure, leg or ankle

28899   Unlisted procedure, foot or toes

29799   Unlisted procedure, casting or strapping

29999   Unlisted procedure, arthroscopy

30999   Unlisted procedure, nose

31299   Unlisted procedure, accessory sinuses

31599   Unlisted procedure, larynx

31899   Unlisted procedure, trachea, bronchi

32999   Unlisted procedure, lungs and pleura

33999   Unlisted procedure, cardiac surgery

36299   Unlisted procedure, vascular injection

37501   Unlisted vascular endoscopy procedure

37799   Unlisted procedure, vascular surgery

38129   Unlisted laparoscopy procedure, spleen

38589   Unlisted laparoscopy procedure, lymphatic system

38999   Unlisted procedure, hemic or lymphatic system

39499   Unlisted procedure, mediastinum

39599   Unlisted procedure, diaphragm

40799   Unlisted procedure, lips

40899   Unlisted procedure, vestibule of mouth

41599   Unlisted procedure, tongue, floor of mouth

41899   Unlisted procedure, dentoalveolar structures

42299   Unlisted procedure, palate, uvula

42699   Unlisted procedure, salivary glands or ducts

42999   Unlisted procedure, pharynx, adenoids, or tonsils

43289   Unlisted laparoscopy procedure, esophagus

43499   Unlisted procedure, esophagus

43659   Unlisted laparoscopy procedure, stomach

43999   Unlisted procedure, stomach

44238   Unlisted laparoscopy procedure, intestine (except rectum)

44799   Unlisted procedure, small intestine

44899   Unlisted procedure, Meckel's diverticulum and the mesentery

44979   Unlisted laparoscopy procedure, appendix

45399   Unlisted procedure, colon

45499   Unlisted laparoscopy procedure, rectum

45999   Unlisted procedure, rectum

46999   Unlisted procedure, anus

47379   Unlisted laparoscopic procedure, liver

47399   Unlisted procedure, liver

47579   Unlisted laparoscopy procedure, biliary tract

47999   Unlisted procedure, biliary tract

48999   Unlisted procedure, pancreas

49329   Unlisted laparoscopy procedure, abdomen, peritoneum and omentum

49659   Unlisted laparoscopy procedure, hernioplasty, herniorrhaphy, herniotomy

49999   Unlisted procedure, abdomen, peritoneum and omentum

50549   Unlisted laparoscopy procedure, renal

50949   Unlisted laparoscopy procedure, ureter

51999   Unlisted laparoscopy procedure, bladder

53899   Unlisted procedure, urinary system

54699   Unlisted laparoscopy procedure, testis

55559   Unlisted laparoscopy procedure, spermatic cord

Surgery

55899	Unlisted procedure, male genital system
58578	Unlisted laparoscopy procedure, uterus
58579	Unlisted hysteroscopy procedure, uterus
58679	Unlisted laparoscopy procedure, oviduct, ovary
58999	Unlisted procedure, female genital system (nonobstetrical)
59897	Unlisted fetal invasive procedure, including ultrasound guidance, when performed
59898	Unlisted laparoscopy procedure, maternity care and delivery
59899	Unlisted procedure, maternity care and delivery
60659	Unlisted laparoscopy procedure, endocrine system
60699	Unlisted procedure, endocrine system
64999	Unlisted procedure, nervous system
66999	Unlisted procedure, anterior segment of eye
67299	Unlisted procedure, posterior segment
67399	Unlisted procedure, extraocular muscle
67599	Unlisted procedure, orbit
67999	Unlisted procedure, eyelids
68399	Unlisted procedure, conjunctiva
68899	Unlisted procedure, lacrimal system
69399	Unlisted procedure, external ear
69799	Unlisted procedure, middle ear
69949	Unlisted procedure, inner ear
69979	Unlisted procedure, temporal bone, middle fossa approach

Special Report

A service that is rarely provided, unusual, variable, or new may require a special report. Pertinent information should include an adequate definition or description of the nature, extent, and need for the procedure, and the time, effort, and equipment necessary to provide the service.

►Imaging Guidance◄

►When imaging guidance or imaging supervision and interpretation is included in a surgical procedure, guidelines for image documentation and report, included in the guidelines for Radiology (Including Nuclear Medicine and Diagnostic Ultrasound) will apply.◄

Surgical Destruction

Surgical destruction is a part of a surgical procedure and different methods of destruction are not ordinarily listed separately unless the technique substantially alters the standard management of a problem or condition. Exceptions under special circumstances are provided for by separate code numbers.

Surgery

General

(For percutaneous image-guided fluid collection drainage by catheter of soft tissue [eg, extremity, abdominal wall, neck], use 10030)

10021 Fine needle aspiration; without imaging guidance

10022 with imaging guidance

(For placement of percutaneous localization device[s] [eg, clip, metallic pellet, during breast biopsy], see 19081-19086)

(For radiological supervision and interpretation, see 76942, 77002, 77012, 77021)

(For percutaneous needle biopsy other than fine needle aspiration, see 19081-19086 for breast, 20206 for muscle, 32400 for pleura, 32405 for lung or mediastinum, 42400 for salivary gland, 47000 for liver, 48102 for pancreas, 49180 for abdominal or retroperitoneal mass, 50200 for kidney, 54500 for testis, 54800 for epididymis, 60100 for thyroid, 62267 for nucleus pulposus, intervertebral disc, or paravertebral tissue, 62269 for spinal cord)

(For evaluation of fine needle aspirate, see 88172, 88173)

Integumentary System

Skin, Subcutaneous, and Accessory Structures

Introduction and Removal

⊙ **10030** Image-guided fluid collection drainage by catheter (eg, abscess, hematoma, seroma, lymphocele, cyst), soft tissue (eg, extremity, abdominal wall, neck), percutaneous

(Report 10030 for each individual collection drained with a separate catheter)

(Do not report 10030 in conjunction with 75989, 76942, 77002, 77003, 77012, 77021)

(For image-guided fluid collection drainage, percutaneous or transvaginal/transrectal of visceral, peritoneal, or retroperitoneal collections, see 49405-49407)

▶Soft tissue-marker placement with imaging guidance is reported with 10035 and 10036. If a more specific site descriptor than soft tissue is applicable (eg, breast), use the site-specific codes for marker placement at that site. Report 10035 and 10036 only once per target, regardless of how many markers (eg, clips, wires, pellets, radioactive seeds) are used to mark that target.◀

● **10035** Placement of soft tissue localization device(s) (eg, clip, metallic pellet, wire/needle, radioactive seeds), percutaneous, including imaging guidance; first lesion

+● **10036** each additional lesion (List separately in addition to code for primary procedure)

▶(Use 10036 in conjunction with 10035)◀

▶(Do not report 10035, 10036 in conjunction with 76942, 77002, 77012, 77021)◀

▶(To report a second procedure on the same side or contralateral side, use 10036)◀

Incision and Drainage

(For excision, see 11400, et seq)

10040 Acne surgery (eg, marsupialization, opening or removal of multiple milia, comedones, cysts, pustules)

10060 Incision and drainage of abscess (eg, carbuncle, suppurative hidradenitis, cutaneous or subcutaneous abscess, cyst, furuncle, or paronychia); simple or single

10061 complicated or multiple

10080 Incision and drainage of pilonidal cyst; simple

10081 complicated

(For excision of pilonidal cyst, see 11770-11772)

10120 Incision and removal of foreign body, subcutaneous tissues; simple

10121 complicated

(To report wound exploration due to penetrating trauma without laparotomy or thoracotomy, see 20100-20103, as appropriate)

(To report debridement associated with open fracture(s) and/or dislocation(s), use 11010-11012, as appropriate)

10140 Incision and drainage of hematoma, seroma or fluid collection

(If imaging guidance is performed, see 76942, 77012, 77021)

10160 Puncture aspiration of abscess, hematoma, bulla, or cyst

(If imaging guidance is performed, see 76942, 77012, 77021)

10180 Incision and drainage, complex, postoperative wound infection

(For secondary closure of surgical wound, see 12020, 12021, 13160)

Debridement

Wound debridements (11042-11047) are reported by depth of tissue that is removed and by surface area of the wound. These services may be reported for injuries, infections, wounds and chronic ulcers. When performing debridement of a single wound, report depth using the deepest level of tissue removed. In multiple wounds, sum the surface area of those wounds that are at the same depth, but do not combine sums from different depths. For example: When bone is debrided from a 4 sq cm heel ulcer and from a 10 sq cm ischial ulcer, report the work with a single code, 11044. When subcutaneous tissue is debrided from a 16 sq cm dehisced abdominal wound and a 10 sq cm thigh wound, report the work with 11042 for the first 20 sq cm and 11045 for the second 6 sq cm. If all four wounds were debrided on the same day, use modifier 59 with either 11042, or 11044 as appropriate.

(For dermabrasions, see 15780-15783)

(For nail debridement, see 11720-11721)

(For burn(s), see 16000-16035)

(For pressure ulcers, see 15920-15999)

11000   Debridement of extensive eczematous or infected skin; up to 10% of body surface

(For abdominal wall or genitalia debridement for necrotizing soft tissue infection, see 11004-11006)

+ 11001   each additional 10% of the body surface, or part thereof (List separately in addition to code for primary procedure)

(Use 11001 in conjunction with 11000)

11004   Debridement of skin, subcutaneous tissue, muscle and fascia for necrotizing soft tissue infection; external genitalia and perineum

11005   abdominal wall, with or without fascial closure

11006   external genitalia, perineum and abdominal wall, with or without fascial closure

(If orchiectomy is performed, use 54520)

(If testicular transplantation is performed, use 54680)

+ 11008   Removal of prosthetic material or mesh, abdominal wall for infection (eg, for chronic or recurrent mesh infection or necrotizing soft tissue infection) (List separately in addition to code for primary procedure)

(Use 11008 in conjunction with 10180, 11004-11006)

(Do not report 11008 in conjunction with 11000-11001, 11010-11044)

(Report skin grafts or flaps separately when performed for closure at the same session as 11004-11008)

(When insertion of mesh is used for closure, use 49568)

11010   Debridement including removal of foreign material at the site of an open fracture and/or an open dislocation (eg, excisional debridement); skin and subcutaneous tissues

11011   skin, subcutaneous tissue, muscle fascia, and muscle

11012   skin, subcutaneous tissue, muscle fascia, muscle, and bone

(For debridement of skin, ie, epidermis and/or dermis only, see 97597, 97598)

(For active wound care management, see 97597, 97598)

(For debridement of burn wounds, see 16020-16030)

11042   Debridement, subcutaneous tissue (includes epidermis and dermis, if performed); first 20 sq cm or less

(For debridement of skin [ie, epidermis and/or dermis only], see 97597, 97598)

#+ 11045   each additional 20 sq cm, or part thereof (List separately in addition to code for primary procedure)

(Use 11045 in conjunction with 11042)

11043   Debridement, muscle and/or fascia (includes epidermis, dermis, and subcutaneous tissue, if performed); first 20 sq cm or less

#+ 11046   each additional 20 sq cm, or part thereof (List separately in addition to code for primary procedure)

(Use 11046 in conjunction with 11043)

11044   Debridement, bone (includes epidermis, dermis, subcutaneous tissue, muscle and/or fascia, if performed); first 20 sq cm or less

11045   Code is out of numerical sequence. See 11000-11047

11046   Code is out of numerical sequence. See 11000-11047

+ 11047   each additional 20 sq cm, or part thereof (List separately in addition to code for primary procedure)

(Do not report 11042-11047 in conjunction with 97597-97602 for the same wound)

(Use 11047 in conjunction with 11044)

Paring or Cutting

(To report destruction, see 17000-17004)

11055   Paring or cutting of benign hyperkeratotic lesion (eg, corn or callus); single lesion

11056   2 to 4 lesions

11057   more than 4 lesions

Biopsy

During certain surgical procedures in the integumentary system, such as excision, destruction, or shave removals, the removed tissue is often submitted for pathologic examination. The obtaining of tissue for pathology during the course of these procedures is a routine component of such procedures. This obtaining of tissue is not considered a separate biopsy procedure and is not separately reported. The use of a biopsy procedure code (eg, 11100, 11101) indicates that the procedure to obtain tissue for pathologic examination was performed

Integumentary

independently, or was unrelated or distinct from other procedures/services provided at that time. Such biopsies are not considered components of other procedures when performed on different lesions or different sites on the same date, and are to be reported separately.

(For biopsy of conjunctiva, use 68100; eyelid, use 67810)

11100 Biopsy of skin, subcutaneous tissue and/or mucous membrane (including simple closure), unless otherwise listed; single lesion

+ 11101 each separate/additional lesion (List separately in addition to code for primary procedure)

(Use 11101 in conjunction with 11100)

Removal of Skin Tags

Removal by scissoring or any sharp method, ligature strangulation, electrosurgical destruction or combination of treatment modalities, including chemical destruction or electrocauterization of wound, with or without local anesthesia.

11200 Removal of skin tags, multiple fibrocutaneous tags, any area; up to and including 15 lesions

+ 11201 each additional 10 lesions, or part thereof (List separately in addition to code for primary procedure)

(Use 11201 in conjunction with 11200)

Shaving of Epidermal or Dermal Lesions

Shaving is the sharp removal by transverse incision or horizontal slicing to remove epidermal and dermal lesions without a full-thickness dermal excision. This includes local anesthesia, chemical or electrocauterization of the wound. The wound does not require suture closure.

11300 Shaving of epidermal or dermal lesion, single lesion, trunk, arms or legs; lesion diameter 0.5 cm or less

11301 lesion diameter 0.6 to 1.0 cm

11302 lesion diameter 1.1 to 2.0 cm

11303 lesion diameter over 2.0 cm

11305 Shaving of epidermal or dermal lesion, single lesion, scalp, neck, hands, feet, genitalia; lesion diameter 0.5 cm or less

11306 lesion diameter 0.6 to 1.0 cm

11307 lesion diameter 1.1 to 2.0 cm

11308 lesion diameter over 2.0 cm

11310 Shaving of epidermal or dermal lesion, single lesion, face, ears, eyelids, nose, lips, mucous membrane; lesion diameter 0.5 cm or less

11311 lesion diameter 0.6 to 1.0 cm

11312 lesion diameter 1.1 to 2.0 cm

11313 lesion diameter over 2.0 cm

Excision—Benign Lesions

Excision (including simple closure) of benign lesions of skin (eg, neoplasm, cicatricial, fibrous, inflammatory, congenital, cystic lesions), includes local anesthesia. See appropriate size and area below. For shave removal, see 11300 et seq, and for electrosurgical and other methods see 17000 et seq.

Excision is defined as full-thickness (through the dermis) removal of a lesion, including margins, and includes simple (non-layered) closure when performed. Report separately each benign lesion excised. Code selection is determined by measuring the greatest clinical diameter of the apparent lesion plus that margin required for complete excision (lesion diameter plus the most narrow margins required equals the excised diameter). The margins refer to the most narrow margin required to adequately excise the lesion, based on individual judgment. The measurement of lesion plus margin is made prior to excision. The excised diameter is the same whether the surgical defect is repaired in a linear fashion, or reconstructed (eg, with a skin graft).

The closure of defects created by incision, excision, or trauma may require intermediate or complex closure. Repair by intermediate or complex closure should be reported separately. For excision of benign lesions requiring more than simple closure, ie, requiring intermediate or complex closure, report 11400-11446 in addition to appropriate intermediate (12031-12057) or complex closure (13100-13153) codes. For reconstructive closure, see 15002-15261, 15570-15770. For excision performed in conjunction with adjacent tissue transfer, report only the adjacent tissue transfer code (14000-14302). Excision of lesion (11400-11446) is not separately reportable with adjacent tissue transfer. See page 58 for the definition of *intermediate* or *complex* closure.

11400 Excision, benign lesion including margins, except skin tag (unless listed elsewhere), trunk, arms or legs; excised diameter 0.5 cm or less

11401 excised diameter 0.6 to 1.0 cm

11402 excised diameter 1.1 to 2.0 cm

11403 excised diameter 2.1 to 3.0 cm

11404 excised diameter 3.1 to 4.0 cm

11406 excised diameter over 4.0 cm

(For unusual or complicated excision, add modifier 22)

11420 Excision, benign lesion including margins, except skin tag (unless listed elsewhere), scalp, neck, hands, feet, genitalia; excised diameter 0.5 cm or less

11421 excised diameter 0.6 to 1.0 cm

11422 excised diameter 1.1 to 2.0 cm

11423 excised diameter 2.1 to 3.0 cm

11424 excised diameter 3.1 to 4.0 cm

11426   excised diameter over 4.0 cm

       (For unusual or complicated excision, add modifier 22)

11440   Excision, other benign lesion including margins, except skin tag (unless listed elsewhere), face, ears, eyelids, nose, lips, mucous membrane; excised diameter 0.5 cm or less

11441   excised diameter 0.6 to 1.0 cm

11442   excised diameter 1.1 to 2.0 cm

11443   excised diameter 2.1 to 3.0 cm

11444   excised diameter 3.1 to 4.0 cm

11446   excised diameter over 4.0 cm

       (For unusual or complicated excision, add modifier 22)

       (For eyelids involving more than skin, see also 67800 et seq)

11450   Excision of skin and subcutaneous tissue for hidradenitis, axillary; with simple or intermediate repair

11451   with complex repair

11462   Excision of skin and subcutaneous tissue for hidradenitis, inguinal; with simple or intermediate repair

11463   with complex repair

11470   Excision of skin and subcutaneous tissue for hidradenitis, perianal, perineal, or umbilical; with simple or intermediate repair

11471   with complex repair

       (When skin graft or flap is used for closure, use appropriate procedure code in addition)

       (For bilateral procedure, add modifier 50)

Excision—Malignant Lesions

Excision (including simple closure) of malignant lesions of skin (eg, basal cell carcinoma, squamous cell carcinoma, melanoma) includes local anesthesia. (See appropriate size and body area below.) For destruction of malignant lesions of skin, see destruction codes 17260-17286.

Excision is defined as full-thickness (through the dermis) removal of a lesion including margins, and includes simple (non-layered) closure when performed. Report separately each malignant lesion excised. Code selection is determined by measuring the greatest clinical diameter of the apparent lesion plus that margin required for complete excision (lesion diameter plus the most narrow margins required equals the excised diameter). The margins refer to the most narrow margin required to adequately excise the lesion, based on the physician's judgment. The measurement of lesion plus margin is made prior to excision. The excised diameter is the same whether the surgical defect is repaired in a linear fashion, or reconstructed (eg, with a skin graft).

The closure of defects created by incision, excision, or trauma may require intermediate or complex closure. Repair by intermediate or complex closure should be reported separately. For excision of malignant lesions requiring more than simple closure, ie, requiring intermediate or complex closure, report 11600-11646 in addition to appropriate intermediate (12031-12057) or complex closure (13100-13153) codes. For reconstructive closure, see 15002-15261, 15570-15770. For excision performed in conjunction with adjacent tissue transfer, report only the adjacent tissue transfer code (14000-14302). Excision of lesion (11600-11646) is not separately reportable with adjacent tissue transfer. See page 79 [of the professional codebook] for the definition of *intermediate* or *complex* closure.

When frozen section pathology shows the margins of excision were not adequate, an additional excision may be necessary for complete tumor removal. Use only one code to report the additional excision and re-excision(s) based on the final widest excised diameter required for complete tumor removal at the same operative session. To report a re-excision procedure performed to widen margins at a subsequent operative session, see codes 11600-11646, as appropriate. Append modifier 58 if the re-excision procedure is performed during the postoperative period of the primary excision procedure.

11600   Excision, malignant lesion including margins, trunk, arms, or legs; excised diameter 0.5 cm or less

11601   excised diameter 0.6 to 1.0 cm

11602   excised diameter 1.1 to 2.0 cm

11603   excised diameter 2.1 to 3.0 cm

11604   excised diameter 3.1 to 4.0 cm

11606   excised diameter over 4.0 cm

11620   Excision, malignant lesion including margins, scalp, neck, hands, feet, genitalia; excised diameter 0.5 cm or less

11621   excised diameter 0.6 to 1.0 cm

11622   excised diameter 1.1 to 2.0 cm

11623   excised diameter 2.1 to 3.0 cm

11624   excised diameter 3.1 to 4.0 cm

11626   excised diameter over 4.0 cm

11640   Excision, malignant lesion including margins, face, ears, eyelids, nose, lips; excised diameter 0.5 cm or less

11641   excised diameter 0.6 to 1.0 cm

11642   excised diameter 1.1 to 2.0 cm

11643   excised diameter 2.1 to 3.0 cm

11644   excised diameter 3.1 to 4.0 cm

11646   excised diameter over 4.0 cm

       (For eyelids involving more than skin, see also 67800 et seq)

Integumentary

Nails

(For drainage of paronychia or onychia, see 10060, 10061)

11719 Trimming of nondystrophic nails, any number

11720 Debridement of nail(s) by any method(s); 1 to 5

11721 6 or more

11730 Avulsion of nail plate, partial or complete, simple; single

+ 11732 each additional nail plate (List separately in addition to code for primary procedure)

(Use 11732 in conjunction with 11730)

11740 Evacuation of subungual hematoma

11750 Excision of nail and nail matrix, partial or complete (eg, ingrown or deformed nail), for permanent removal;

11752 with amputation of tuft of distal phalanx

(For skin graft, if used, use 15050)

11755 Biopsy of nail unit (eg, plate, bed, matrix, hyponychium, proximal and lateral nail folds) (separate procedure)

11760 Repair of nail bed

11762 Reconstruction of nail bed with graft

11765 Wedge excision of skin of nail fold (eg, for ingrown toenail)

Pilonidal Cyst

11770 Excision of pilonidal cyst or sinus; simple

11771 extensive

11772 complicated

(For incision of pilonidal cyst, see 10080, 10081)

Introduction

11900 Injection, intralesional; up to and including 7 lesions

11901 more than 7 lesions

(11900, 11901 are not to be used for preoperative local anesthetic injection)

(For veins, see 36470, 36471)

(For intralesional chemotherapy administration, see 96405, 96406)

11920 Tattooing, intradermal introduction of insoluble opaque pigments to correct color defects of skin, including micropigmentation; 6.0 sq cm or less

11921 6.1 to 20.0 sq cm

+ 11922 each additional 20.0 sq cm, or part thereof (List separately in addition to code for primary procedure)

(Use 11922 in conjunction with 11921)

11950 Subcutaneous injection of filling material (eg, collagen); 1 cc or less

11951 1.1 to 5.0 cc

11952 5.1 to 10.0 cc

11954 over 10.0 cc

11960 Insertion of tissue expander(s) for other than breast, including subsequent expansion

(For breast reconstruction with tissue expander(s), use 19357)

11970 Replacement of tissue expander with permanent prosthesis

11971 Removal of tissue expander(s) without insertion of prosthesis

11976 Removal, implantable contraceptive capsules

11980 Subcutaneous hormone pellet implantation (implantation of estradiol and/or testosterone pellets beneath the skin)

11981 Insertion, non-biodegradable drug delivery implant

11982 Removal, non-biodegradable drug delivery implant

11983 Removal with reinsertion, non-biodegradable drug delivery implant

Repair (Closure)

Use the codes in this section to designate wound closure utilizing sutures, staples, or tissue adhesives (eg, 2-cyanoacrylate), either singly or in combination with each other, or in combination with adhesive strips. Wound closure utilizing adhesive strips as the sole repair material should be coded using the appropriate E/M code.

Definitions

The repair of wounds may be classified as Simple, Intermediate, or Complex.

Simple repair is used when the wound is superficial; eg, involving primarily epidermis or dermis, or subcutaneous tissues without significant involvement of deeper structures, and requires simple one layer closure. This includes local anesthesia and chemical or electrocauterization of wounds not closed.

Intermediate repair includes the repair of wounds that, in addition to the above, require layered closure of one or more of the deeper layers of subcutaneous tissue and superficial (non-muscle) fascia, in addition to the skin (epidermal and dermal) closure. Single-layer closure of heavily contaminated wounds that have required extensive cleaning or removal of particulate matter also constitutes intermediate repair.

Complex repair includes the repair of wounds requiring more than layered closure, viz., scar revision, debridement (eg, traumatic lacerations or avulsions), extensive undermining, stents or retention sutures. Necessary preparation includes creation of a limited defect for repairs or the debridement of complicated lacerations or avulsions. Complex repair does not include excision of benign (11400-11446) or malignant (11600-11646) lesions, excisional preparation of a wound bed (15002-15005) or debridement of an open fracture or open dislocation.

Instructions for listing services at time of wound repair:

1. The repaired wound(s) should be measured and recorded in centimeters, whether curved, angular, or stellate.

2. When multiple wounds are repaired, add together the lengths of those in the same classification (see above) and from all anatomic sites that are grouped together into the same code descriptor. For example, add together the lengths of intermediate repairs to the trunk and extremities. Do not add lengths of repairs from different groupings of anatomic sites (eg, face and extremities). Also, do not add together lengths of different classifications (eg, intermediate and complex repairs).

When more than one classification of wounds is repaired, list the more complicated as the primary procedure and the less complicated as the secondary procedure, using modifier 59.

3. Decontamination and/or debridement: Debridement is considered a separate procedure only when gross contamination requires prolonged cleansing, when appreciable amounts of devitalized or contaminated tissue are removed, or when debridement is carried out separately without immediate primary closure.

> (For extensive debridement of soft tissue and/or bone, not associated with open fracture(s) and/or dislocation(s) resulting from penetrating and/or blunt trauma, see 11042-11047.)

> (For extensive debridement of subcutaneous tissue, muscle fascia, muscle, and/or bone associated with open fracture(s) and/or dislocation(s), see 11010-11012.)

4. Involvement of nerves, blood vessels and tendons: Report under appropriate system (Nervous, Cardiovascular, Musculoskeletal) for repair of these structures. The repair of these associated wounds is included in the primary procedure unless it qualifies as a complex repair, in which case modifier 59 applies.

Simple ligation of vessels in an open wound is considered as part of any wound closure.

Simple "exploration" of nerves, blood vessels or tendons exposed in an open wound is also considered part of the essential treatment of the wound and is not a separate procedure unless appreciable dissection is required. If the wound requires enlargement, extension of dissection (to determine penetration), debridement, removal of foreign body(s), ligation or coagulation of minor subcutaneous and/or muscular blood vessel(s) of the subcutaneous tissue, muscle fascia, and/or muscle, not requiring thoracotomy or laparotomy, use codes 20100-20103, as appropriate.

Repair—Simple

Sum of lengths of repairs for each group of anatomic sites.

12001	Simple repair of superficial wounds of scalp, neck, axillae, external genitalia, trunk and/or extremities (including hands and feet); 2.5 cm or less
12002	2.6 cm to 7.5 cm
12004	7.6 cm to 12.5 cm
12005	12.6 cm to 20.0 cm
12006	20.1 cm to 30.0 cm
12007	over 30.0 cm
12011	Simple repair of superficial wounds of face, ears, eyelids, nose, lips and/or mucous membranes; 2.5 cm or less
12013	2.6 cm to 5.0 cm
12014	5.1 cm to 7.5 cm
12015	7.6 cm to 12.5 cm
12016	12.6 cm to 20.0 cm
12017	20.1 cm to 30.0 cm
12018	over 30.0 cm
12020	Treatment of superficial wound dehiscence; simple closure
12021	with packing

(For extensive or complicated secondary wound closure, use 13160)

Repair—Intermediate

Sum of lengths of repairs for each group of anatomic sites.

12031	Repair, intermediate, wounds of scalp, axillae, trunk and/or extremities (excluding hands and feet); 2.5 cm or less
12032	2.6 cm to 7.5 cm
12034	7.6 cm to 12.5 cm
12035	12.6 cm to 20.0 cm
12036	20.1 cm to 30.0 cm
12037	over 30.0 cm
12041	Repair, intermediate, wounds of neck, hands, feet and/or external genitalia; 2.5 cm or less
12042	2.6 cm to 7.5 cm
12044	7.6 cm to 12.5 cm
12045	12.6 cm to 20.0 cm
12046	20.1 cm to 30.0 cm
12047	over 30.0 cm
12051	Repair, intermediate, wounds of face, ears, eyelids, nose, lips and/or mucous membranes; 2.5 cm or less

Integumentary

12052	2.6 cm to 5.0 cm
12053	5.1 cm to 7.5 cm
12054	7.6 cm to 12.5 cm
12055	12.6 cm to 20.0 cm
12056	20.1 cm to 30.0 cm
12057	over 30.0 cm

Repair—Complex

Reconstructive procedures, complicated wound closure.

Sum of lengths of repairs for each group of anatomic sites.

(For full thickness repair of lip or eyelid, see respective anatomical subsections)

13100 Repair, complex, trunk; 1.1 cm to 2.5 cm

(For 1.0 cm or less, see simple or intermediate repairs)

13101 2.6 cm to 7.5 cm

+ 13102 each additional 5 cm or less (List separately in addition to code for primary procedure)

(Use 13102 in conjunction with 13101)

13120 Repair, complex, scalp, arms, and/or legs; 1.1 cm to 2.5 cm

(For 1.0 cm or less, see simple or intermediate repairs)

13121 2.6 cm to 7.5 cm

+ 13122 each additional 5 cm or less (List separately in addition to code for primary procedure)

(Use 13122 in conjunction with 13121)

13131 Repair, complex, forehead, cheeks, chin, mouth, neck, axillae, genitalia, hands and/or feet; 1.1 cm to 2.5 cm

(For 1.0 cm or less, see simple or intermediate repairs)

13132 2.6 cm to 7.5 cm

+ 13133 each additional 5 cm or less (List separately in addition to code for primary procedure)

(Use 13133 in conjunction with 13132)

(13150 has been deleted)

(For 1.0 cm or less, see simple or intermediate repairs)

13151 Repair, complex, eyelids, nose, ears and/or lips; 1.1 cm to 2.5 cm

13152 2.6 cm to 7.5 cm

+ 13153 each additional 5 cm or less (List separately in addition to code for primary procedure)

(Use 13153 in conjunction with 13152)

13160 Secondary closure of surgical wound or dehiscence, extensive or complicated

(For packing or simple secondary wound closure, see 12020, 12021)

Adjacent Tissue Transfer or Rearrangement

For full thickness repair of lip or eyelid, see respective anatomical subsections.

Codes 14000-14302 are used for excision (including lesion) and/or repair by adjacent tissue transfer or rearrangement (eg, Z-plasty, W-plasty, V-Y plasty, rotation flap, random island flap, advancement flap). When applied in repairing lacerations, the procedures listed must be performed by the surgeon to accomplish the repair. They do not apply to direct closure or rearrangement of traumatic wounds incidentally resulting in these configurations. Undermining alone of adjacent tissues to achieve closure, without additional incisions, does not constitute adjacent tissue transfer, see complex repair codes 13100-13160. The excision of a benign lesion (11400-11446) or a malignant lesion (11600-11646) is not separately reportable with codes 14000-14302.

Skin graft necessary to close secondary defect is considered an additional procedure. For purposes of code selection, the term "defect" includes the primary and secondary defects. The primary defect resulting from the excision and the secondary defect resulting from flap design to perform the reconstruction are measured together to determine the code.

14000 Adjacent tissue transfer or rearrangement, trunk; defect 10 sq cm or less

14001 defect 10.1 sq cm to 30.0 sq cm

14020 Adjacent tissue transfer or rearrangement, scalp, arms and/or legs; defect 10 sq cm or less

14021 defect 10.1 sq cm to 30.0 sq cm

14040 Adjacent tissue transfer or rearrangement, forehead, cheeks, chin, mouth, neck, axillae, genitalia, hands and/or feet; defect 10 sq cm or less

14041 defect 10.1 sq cm to 30.0 sq cm

14060 Adjacent tissue transfer or rearrangement, eyelids, nose, ears and/or lips; defect 10 sq cm or less

14061 defect 10.1 sq cm to 30.0 sq cm

(For eyelid, full thickness, see 67961 et seq)

14301 Adjacent tissue transfer or rearrangement, any area; defect 30.1 sq cm to 60.0 sq cm

+ 14302 each additional 30.0 sq cm, or part thereof (List separately in addition to code for primary procedure)

(Use 14302 in conjunction with 14301)

14350 Filleted finger or toe flap, including preparation of recipient site

Skin Replacement Surgery

Skin replacement surgery consists of **surgical preparation** and topical placement of an **autograft** (including tissue cultured autograft) or **skin substitute graft** (ie, homograft, allograft, xenograft). The graft is anchored using the individual's choice of fixation. When services are performed in the office, routine dressing supplies are not reported separately.

The following definition should be applied to those codes that reference "100 sq cm or 1% of body area of infants and children" when determining the involvement of body size: The measurement of 100 sq cm is applicable to adults and children 10 years of age and older; and percentages of body surface area apply to infants and children younger than 10 years of age. The measurements apply to the size of the recipient area.

Procedures involving wrist and/or ankle are reported with codes that include arm or leg in the descriptor.

When a primary procedure requires a skin substitute or skin autograft for definitive skin closure (eg, orbitectomy, radical mastectomy, deep tumor removal), use 15100-15278 in conjunction with primary procedure.

For biological implant for soft tissue reinforcement, use 15777 in conjunction with primary procedure.

The supply of skin substitute graft(s) should be reported separately in conjunction with 15271-15278.

Definitions

Surgical preparation codes 15002-15005 for skin replacement surgery describe the initial services related to preparing a clean and viable wound surface for placement of an autograft, flap, skin substitute graft or for negative pressure wound therapy. In some cases, closure may be possible using adjacent tissue transfer (14000-14061) or complex repair (13100-13153). In all cases, appreciable nonviable tissue is removed to treat a burn, traumatic wound or a necrotizing infection. The clean wound bed may also be created by incisional release of a scar contracture resulting in a surface defect from separation of tissues. The intent is to heal the wound by primary intention, or by the use of negative pressure wound therapy. Patient conditions may require the closure or application of graft, flap, or skin substitute to be delayed, but in all cases the intent is to include these treatments or negative pressure wound therapy to heal the wound. Do not report 15002-15005 for removal of nonviable tissue/debris in a chronic wound (eg, venous or diabetic) when the wound is left to heal by secondary intention. See active wound management codes (97597, 97598) and debridement codes (11042-11047) for this service. For necrotizing soft tissue infections in specific anatomic locations, see 11004-11008.

Select the appropriate code from 15002-15005 based upon location and size of the resultant defect. For multiple wounds, sum the surface area of all wounds from all anatomic sites that are grouped together into the same code descriptor. For example, sum the surface area of all wounds on the trunk and arms. Do not sum wounds from different groupings of anatomic sites (eg, face and arms). Use 15002 or 15004, as appropriate, for excisions and incisional releases resulting in wounds up to and including 100 sq cm of surface area. Use 15003 or 15005 for each additional 100 sq cm or part thereof. For example: Surgical preparation of a 20 sq cm wound on the right hand and a 15 sq cm wound on the left hand would be reported with a single code, 15004. Surgical preparation of a 75 sq cm wound on the right thigh and a 75 sq cm wound on the left thigh would be reported with 15002 for the first 100 sq cm and 15003 for the second 50 sq cm. If all four wounds required surgical preparation on the same day, use modifier 59 with 15002, and 15004.

Autografts/tissue cultured autografts include the harvest and/or application of an autologous skin graft. Repair of donor site requiring skin graft or local flaps is reported separately. Removal of current graft and/or simple cleansing of the wound is included, when performed. Do not report 97602. Debridement is considered a separate procedure only when gross contamination requires prolonged cleansing, when appreciable amounts of devitalized or contaminated tissue are removed, or when debridement is carried out separately without immediate primary closure.

Select the appropriate code from 15040-15261 based upon type of autograft and location and size of the defect. The measurements apply to the size of the recipient area. For multiple wounds, sum the surface area of all wounds from all anatomic sites that are grouped together into the same code descriptor. For example, sum the surface area of all wounds on the trunk and arms. Do not sum wounds from different groupings of anatomic sites (eg, face and arms).

Skin substitute grafts include non-autologous human skin (dermal or epidermal, cellular and acellular) grafts (eg, homograft, allograft), non-human skin substitute grafts (ie, xenograft), and biological products that form a sheet scaffolding for skin growth. These codes are not to be reported for application of non-graft wound dressings (eg, gel, ointment, foam, liquid) or injected skin substitutes. Removal of current graft and/or simple cleansing of the wound is included, when performed. Do not report 97602. Debridement is considered a separate procedure only when gross contamination requires prolonged cleansing, when appreciable amounts of devitalized or contaminated tissue are removed, or when debridement is carried out separately without immediate primary closure.

Select the appropriate code from 15271-15278 based upon location and size of the defect. For multiple wounds, sum the surface area of all wounds from all anatomic sites that are grouped together into the same code descriptor. For example, sum the surface area of all wounds on the trunk and arms. Do not sum wounds from different groupings of anatomic sites (eg, face and arms).

Surgical Preparation

15002 Surgical preparation or creation of recipient site by excision of open wounds, burn eschar, or scar (including subcutaneous tissues), or incisional release of scar contracture, trunk, arms, legs; first 100 sq cm or 1% of body area of infants and children

(For linear scar revision, see 13100-13153)

+ 15003   each additional 100 sq cm, or part thereof, or each additional 1% of body area of infants and children (List separately in addition to code for primary procedure)

(Use 15003 in conjunction with 15002)

15004 Surgical preparation or creation of recipient site by excision of open wounds, burn eschar, or scar (including subcutaneous tissues), or incisional release of scar contracture, face, scalp, eyelids, mouth, neck, ears, orbits, genitalia, hands, feet and/or multiple digits; first 100 sq cm or 1% of body area of infants and children

+ 15005   each additional 100 sq cm, or part thereof, or each additional 1% of body area of infants and children (List separately in addition to code for primary procedure)

(Use 15005 in conjunction with 15004)

Autografts/Tissue Cultured Autograft

15040 Harvest of skin for tissue cultured skin autograft, 100 sq cm or less

15050 Pinch graft, single or multiple, to cover small ulcer, tip of digit, or other minimal open area (except on face), up to defect size 2 cm diameter

15100 Split-thickness autograft, trunk, arms, legs; first 100 sq cm or less, or 1% of body area of infants and children (except 15050)

+ 15101   each additional 100 sq cm, or each additional 1% of body area of infants and children, or part thereof (List separately in addition to code for primary procedure)

(Use 15101 in conjunction with 15100)

15110 Epidermal autograft, trunk, arms, legs; first 100 sq cm or less, or 1% of body area of infants and children

+ 15111   each additional 100 sq cm, or each additional 1% of body area of infants and children, or part thereof (List separately in addition to code for primary procedure)

(Use 15111 in conjunction with 15110)

15115 Epidermal autograft, face, scalp, eyelids, mouth, neck, ears, orbits, genitalia, hands, feet, and/or multiple digits; first 100 sq cm or less, or 1% of body area of infants and children

+ 15116   each additional 100 sq cm, or each additional 1% of body area of infants and children, or part thereof (List separately in addition to code for primary procedure)

(Use 15116 in conjunction with 15115)

15120 Split-thickness autograft, face, scalp, eyelids, mouth, neck, ears, orbits, genitalia, hands, feet, and/or multiple digits; first 100 sq cm or less, or 1% of body area of infants and children (except 15050)

+ 15121   each additional 100 sq cm, or each additional 1% of body area of infants and children, or part thereof (List separately in addition to code for primary procedure)

(Use 15121 in conjunction with 15120)

(For eyelids, see also 67961-67975)

15130 Dermal autograft, trunk, arms, legs; first 100 sq cm or less, or 1% of body area of infants and children

+ 15131   each additional 100 sq cm, or each additional 1% of body area of infants and children, or part thereof (List separately in addition to code for primary procedure)

(Use 15131 in conjunction with 15130)

15135 Dermal autograft, face, scalp, eyelids, mouth, neck, ears, orbits, genitalia, hands, feet, and/or multiple digits; first 100 sq cm or less, or 1% of body area of infants and children

+ 15136   each additional 100 sq cm, or each additional 1% of body area of infants and children, or part thereof (List separately in addition to code for primary procedure)

(Use 15136 in conjunction with 15135)

15150 Tissue cultured skin autograft, trunk, arms, legs; first 25 sq cm or less

+ 15151   additional 1 sq cm to 75 sq cm (List separately in addition to code for primary procedure)

(Do not report 15151 more than once per session)

(Use 15151 in conjunction with 15150)

+ 15152   each additional 100 sq cm, or each additional 1% of body area of infants and children, or part thereof (List separately in addition to code for primary procedure)

(Use 15152 in conjunction with 15151)

15155 Tissue cultured skin autograft, face, scalp, eyelids, mouth, neck, ears, orbits, genitalia, hands, feet, and/or multiple digits; first 25 sq cm or less

+ 15156   additional 1 sq cm to 75 sq cm (List separately in addition to code for primary procedure)

(Do not report 15156 more than once per session)

(Use 15156 in conjunction with 15155)

+ 15157   each additional 100 sq cm, or each additional 1% of body area of infants and children, or part thereof (List separately in addition to code for primary procedure)

(Use 15157 in conjunction with 15156)

15200   Full thickness graft, free, including direct closure of donor site, trunk; 20 sq cm or less

+ 15201   each additional 20 sq cm, or part thereof (List separately in addition to code for primary procedure)

(Use 15201 in conjunction with 15200)

15220   Full thickness graft, free, including direct closure of donor site, scalp, arms, and/or legs; 20 sq cm or less

+ 15221   each additional 20 sq cm, or part thereof (List separately in addition to code for primary procedure)

(Use 15221 in conjunction with 15220)

15240   Full thickness graft, free, including direct closure of donor site, forehead, cheeks, chin, mouth, neck, axillae, genitalia, hands, and/or feet; 20 sq cm or less

(For finger tip graft, use 15050)

(For repair of syndactyly, fingers, see 26560-26562)

+ 15241   each additional 20 sq cm, or part thereof (List separately in addition to code for primary procedure)

(Use 15241 in conjunction with 15240)

15260   Full thickness graft, free, including direct closure of donor site, nose, ears, eyelids, and/or lips; 20 sq cm or less

+ 15261   each additional 20 sq cm, or part thereof (List separately in addition to code for primary procedure)

(Use 15261 in conjunction with 15260)

(For eyelids, see also 67961-67975)

(Repair of donor site requiring skin graft or local flaps is considered a separate procedure)

Skin Substitute Grafts

The supply of skin substitute graft(s) should be reported separately in conjunction with 15271-15278. For biologic implant for soft tissue reinforcement, use 15777 in conjunction with code for primary procedure.

15271   Application of skin substitute graft to trunk, arms, legs, total wound surface area up to 100 sq cm; first 25 sq cm or less wound surface area

+ 15272   each additional 25 sq cm wound surface area, or part thereof (List separately in addition to code for primary procedure)

(Use 15272 in conjunction with 15271)

(For total wound surface area greater than or equal to 100 sq cm, see 15273, 15274)

(Do not report 15271, 15272 in conjunction with 15273, 15274)

15273   Application of skin substitute graft to trunk, arms, legs, total wound surface area greater than or equal to 100 sq cm; first 100 sq cm wound surface area, or 1% of body area of infants and children

+ 15274   each additional 100 sq cm wound surface area, or part thereof, or each additional 1% of body area of infants and children, or part thereof (List separately in addition to code for primary procedure)

(Use 15274 in conjunction with 15273)

(For total wound surface area up to 100 sq cm, see 15271, 15272)

15275   Application of skin substitute graft to face, scalp, eyelids, mouth, neck, ears, orbits, genitalia, hands, feet, and/or multiple digits, total wound surface area up to 100 sq cm; first 25 sq cm or less wound surface area

+ 15276   each additional 25 sq cm wound surface area, or part thereof (List separately in addition to code for primary procedure)

(Use 15276 in conjunction with 15275)

(For total wound surface area greater than or equal to 100 sq cm, see 15277, 15278)

(Do not report 15275, 15276 in conjunction with 15277, 15278)

15277   Application of skin substitute graft to face, scalp, eyelids, mouth, neck, ears, orbits, genitalia, hands, feet, and/or multiple digits, total wound surface area greater than or equal to 100 sq cm; first 100 sq cm wound surface area, or 1% of body area of infants and children

+ 15278   each additional 100 sq cm wound surface area, or part thereof, or each additional 1% of body area of infants and children, or part thereof (List separately in addition to code for primary procedure)

(Use 15278 in conjunction with 15277)

(For total wound surface area up to 100 sq cm, see 15275, 15276)

(Do not report 15271-15278 in conjunction with 97602)

Flaps (Skin and/or Deep Tissues)

The regions listed refer to the recipient area (not the donor site) when a flap is being attached in a transfer or to a final site.

The regions listed refer to a donor site when a tube is formed for later transfer or when a "delay" of flap occurs prior to the transfer. Codes 15732-15738 are described by donor site of the muscle, myocutaneous, or fasciocutaneous flap.

Codes 15570-15738 do not include extensive immobilization (eg, large plaster casts and other immobilizing devices are considered additional separate procedures).

A repair of a donor site requiring a skin graft or local flaps is considered an additional separate procedure.

> (For microvascular flaps, see 15756-15758)
>
> (For flaps without inclusion of a vascular pedicle, see 15570-15576)
>
> (For adjacent tissue transfer flaps, see 14000-14302)

15570 Formation of direct or tubed pedicle, with or without transfer; trunk

15572 scalp, arms, or legs

15574 forehead, cheeks, chin, mouth, neck, axillae, genitalia, hands or feet

15576 eyelids, nose, ears, lips, or intraoral

15600 Delay of flap or sectioning of flap (division and inset); at trunk

15610 at scalp, arms, or legs

15620 at forehead, cheeks, chin, neck, axillae, genitalia, hands, or feet

15630 at eyelids, nose, ears, or lips

15650 Transfer, intermediate, of any pedicle flap (eg, abdomen to wrist, Walking tube), any location

> (For eyelids, nose, ears, or lips, see also anatomical area)
>
> (For revision, defatting or rearranging of transferred pedicle flap or skin graft, see 13100-14302)

15731 Forehead flap with preservation of vascular pedicle (eg, axial pattern flap, paramedian forehead flap)

> (For muscle, myocutaneous, or fasciocutaneous flap of the head or neck, use 15732)

15732 Muscle, myocutaneous, or fasciocutaneous flap; head and neck (eg, temporalis, masseter muscle, sternocleidomastoid, levator scapulae)

> (For forehead flap with preservation of vascular pedicle, use 15731)

15734 trunk

15736 upper extremity

15738 lower extremity

Other Flaps and Grafts

Code 15740 describes a cutaneous flap, transposed into a nearby but not immediately adjacent defect, with a pedicle that incorporates an anatomically named axial vessel into its design. The flap is typically transferred through a tunnel underneath the skin and sutured into its new position. The donor site is closed directly.

Neurovascular pedicle procedures are reported with 15750. This code includes not only skin but also a functional motor or sensory nerve(s). The flap serves to reinnervate a damaged portion of the body dependent on touch or movement (eg, thumb).

Repair of donor site requiring skin graft or local flaps should be reported as an additional procedure.

For random island flaps, V-Y subcutaneous flaps, advancement flaps, and other flaps from adjacent areas without clearly defined anatomically named axial vessels, see 14000-14302.

15740 Flap; island pedicle requiring identification and dissection of an anatomically named axial vessel

15750 neurovascular pedicle

15756 Free muscle or myocutaneous flap with microvascular anastomosis

> (Do not report code 69990 in addition to code 15756)

15757 Free skin flap with microvascular anastomosis

> (Do not report code 69990 in addition to code 15757)

15758 Free fascial flap with microvascular anastomosis

> (Do not report code 69990 in addition to code 15758)

15760 Graft; composite (eg, full thickness of external ear or nasal ala), including primary closure, donor area

15770 derma-fat-fascia

15775 Punch graft for hair transplant; 1 to 15 punch grafts

15776 more than 15 punch grafts

> (For strip transplant, use 15220)

+ 15777 Implantation of biologic implant (eg, acellular dermal matrix) for soft tissue reinforcement (ie, breast, trunk) (List separately in addition to code for primary procedure)

> (For implantation of biologic implants for soft tissue reinforcement in tissues other than breast and trunk, use 17999)
>
> (For bilateral breast procedure, report 15777 with modifier 50)
>
> (For implantation of mesh or other prosthesis for open incisional or ventral hernia repair, use 49568 in conjunction with 49560-49566)
>
> (For insertion of mesh or other prosthesis for closure of a necrotizing soft tissue infection wound, use 49568 in conjunction with 11004-11006)
>
> (For topical application of skin substitute graft to a wound surface, see 15271-15278)
>
> (For repair of anorectal fistula with plug (eg, porcine small intestine submucosa [SIS]), use 46707)
>
> (For insertion of mesh or other prosthesis for repair of pelvic floor defect, use 57267)
>
> (The supply of biologic implant should be reported separately in conjunction with 15777)

Other Procedures

15780 Dermabrasion; total face (eg, for acne scarring, fine wrinkling, rhytids, general keratosis)

15781 segmental, face

15782 regional, other than face

15783 superficial, any site (eg, tattoo removal)

15786 Abrasion; single lesion (eg, keratosis, scar)

+ **15787** each additional 4 lesions or less (List separately in addition to code for primary procedure)

(Use 15787 in conjunction with 15786)

15788 Chemical peel, facial; epidermal

15789 dermal

15792 Chemical peel, nonfacial; epidermal

15793 dermal

15819 Cervicoplasty

15820 Blepharoplasty, lower eyelid;

15821 with extensive herniated fat pad

15822 Blepharoplasty, upper eyelid;

15823 with excessive skin weighting down lid

(For bilateral blepharoplasty, add modifier 50)

15824 Rhytidectomy; forehead

(For repair of brow ptosis, use 67900)

15825 neck with platysmal tightening (platysmal flap, P-flap)

15826 glabellar frown lines

15828 cheek, chin, and neck

15829 superficial musculoaponeurotic system (SMAS) flap

(For bilateral rhytidectomy, add modifier 50)

15830 Excision, excessive skin and subcutaneous tissue (includes lipectomy); abdomen, infraumbilical panniculectomy

(Do not report 15830 in conjunction with 12031-12037, 13100-13102, 14000, 14001, 14302)

15832 thigh

15833 leg

15834 hip

15835 buttock

15836 arm

15837 forearm or hand

15838 submental fat pad

15839 other area

(For bilateral procedure, add modifier 50)

15840 Graft for facial nerve paralysis; free fascia graft (including obtaining fascia)

(For bilateral procedure, add modifier 50)

15841 free muscle graft (including obtaining graft)

15842 free muscle flap by microsurgical technique

(Do not report code 69990 in addition to code 15842)

15845 regional muscle transfer

(For intravenous fluorescein examination of blood flow in graft or flap, use 15860)

(For nerve transfers, decompression, or repair, see 64831-64876, 64905, 64907, 69720, 69725, 69740, 69745, 69955)

+ **15847** Excision, excessive skin and subcutaneous tissue (includes lipectomy), abdomen (eg, abdominoplasty) (includes umbilical transposition and fascial plication) (List separately in addition to code for primary procedure)

(Use 15847 in conjunction with 15830)

(For abdominal wall hernia repair, see 49491-49587)

(To report other abdominoplasty, use 17999)

15850 Removal of sutures under anesthesia (other than local), same surgeon

15851 Removal of sutures under anesthesia (other than local), other surgeon

15852 Dressing change (for other than burns) under anesthesia (other than local)

15860 Intravenous injection of agent (eg, fluorescein) to test vascular flow in flap or graft

15876 Suction assisted lipectomy; head and neck

15877 trunk

15878 upper extremity

15879 lower extremity

Pressure Ulcers (Decubitus Ulcers)

15920 Excision, coccygeal pressure ulcer, with coccygectomy; with primary suture

15922 with flap closure

15931 Excision, sacral pressure ulcer, with primary suture;

15933 with ostectomy

15934 Excision, sacral pressure ulcer, with skin flap closure;

15935 with ostectomy

15936 Excision, sacral pressure ulcer, in preparation for muscle or myocutaneous flap or skin graft closure;

15937 with ostectomy

(For repair of defect using muscle or myocutaneous flap, use code(s) 15734 and/or 15738 in addition to 15936, 15937. For repair of defect using split skin graft, use codes 15100 and/or 15101 in addition to 15936, 15937)

Integumentary

Integumentary

15940 Excision, ischial pressure ulcer, with primary suture;

15941 with ostectomy (ischiectomy)

15944 Excision, ischial pressure ulcer, with skin flap closure;

15945 with ostectomy

15946 Excision, ischial pressure ulcer, with ostectomy, in preparation for muscle or myocutaneous flap or skin graft closure

(For repair of defect using muscle or myocutaneous flap, use code(s) 15734 and/or 15738 in addition to 15946. For repair of defect using split skin graft, use codes 15100 and/or 15101 in addition to 15946)

15950 Excision, trochanteric pressure ulcer, with primary suture;

15951 with ostectomy

15952 Excision, trochanteric pressure ulcer, with skin flap closure;

15953 with ostectomy

15956 Excision, trochanteric pressure ulcer, in preparation for muscle or myocutaneous flap or skin graft closure;

15958 with ostectomy

(For repair of defect using muscle or myocutaneous flap, use code(s) 15734 and/or 15738 in addition to 15956, 15958. For repair of defect using split skin graft, use codes 15100 and/or 15101 in addition to 15956, 15958)

15999 Unlisted procedure, excision pressure ulcer

(For free skin graft to close ulcer or donor site, see 15002 et seq)

Burns, Local Treatment

Procedures 16000-16036 refer to local treatment of burned surface only. Codes 16020-16030 include the application of materials (eg, dressings) not described in codes 15100-15278.

List percentage of body surface involved and depth of burn.

For necessary related medical services (eg, hospital visits, detention) in management of burned patients, see appropriate services in **Evaluation and Management** and **Medicine** sections.

For the application of skin grafts or skin substitutes, see codes 15100-15777.

16000 Initial treatment, first degree burn, when no more than local treatment is required

16020 Dressings and/or debridement of partial-thickness burns, initial or subsequent; small (less than 5% total body surface area)

16025 medium (eg, whole face or whole extremity, or 5% to 10% total body surface area)

16030 large (eg, more than 1 extremity, or greater than 10% total body surface area)

16035 Escharotomy; initial incision

+ 16036 each additional incision (List separately in addition to code for primary procedure)

(Use 16036 in conjunction with 16035)

(For debridement, curettement of burn wound, see 16020-16030)

Destruction

Destruction means the ablation of benign, premalignant or malignant tissues by any method, with or without curettement, including local anesthesia, and not usually requiring closure.

Any method includes electrosurgery, cryosurgery, laser and chemical treatment. Lesions include condylomata, papillomata, molluscum contagiosum, herpetic lesions, warts (ie, common, plantar, flat), milia, or other benign, premalignant (eg, actinic keratoses), or malignant lesions.

(For destruction of lesion(s) in specific anatomic sites, see 40820, 46900-46917, 46924, 54050-54057, 54065, 56501, 56515, 57061, 57065, 67850, 68135)

(For laser treatment for inflammatory skin disease, see 96920-96922)

(For paring or cutting of benign hyperkeratotic lesions (eg, corns or calluses), see 11055-11057)

(For sharp removal or electrosurgical destruction of skin tags and fibrocutaneous tags, see 11200, 11201)

(For cryotherapy of acne, use 17340)

(For initiation or follow-up care of topical chemotherapy (eg, 5-FU or similar agents), see appropriate office visits)

(For shaving of epidermal or dermal lesions, see 11300-11313)

Destruction, Benign or Premalignant Lesions

17000 Destruction (eg, laser surgery, electrosurgery, cryosurgery, chemosurgery, surgical curettement), premalignant lesions (eg, actinic keratoses); first lesion

+ 17003 second through 14 lesions, each (List separately in addition to code for first lesion)

(Use 17003 in conjunction with 17000)

(For destruction of common or plantar warts, see 17110, 17111)

⊘ **17004** Destruction (eg, laser surgery, electrosurgery, cryosurgery, chemosurgery, surgical curettement), premalignant lesions (eg, actinic keratoses), 15 or more lesions

(Do not report 17004 in conjunction with 17000-17003)

17106 Destruction of cutaneous vascular proliferative lesions (eg, laser technique); less than 10 sq cm

17107 10.0 to 50.0 sq cm

17108   over 50.0 sq cm

17110   Destruction (eg, laser surgery, electrosurgery, cryosurgery, chemosurgery, surgical curettement), of benign lesions other than skin tags or cutaneous vascular proliferative lesions; up to 14 lesions

17111   15 or more lesions

17250   Chemical cauterization of granulation tissue (proud flesh, sinus or fistula)

        (17250 is not to be used with removal or excision codes for the same lesion)

Destruction, Malignant Lesions, Any Method

17260   Destruction, malignant lesion (eg, laser surgery, electrosurgery, cryosurgery, chemosurgery, surgical curettement), trunk, arms or legs; lesion diameter 0.5 cm or less

17261   lesion diameter 0.6 to 1.0 cm

17262   lesion diameter 1.1 to 2.0 cm

17263   lesion diameter 2.1 to 3.0 cm

17264   lesion diameter 3.1 to 4.0 cm

17266   lesion diameter over 4.0 cm

17270   Destruction, malignant lesion (eg, laser surgery, electrosurgery, cryosurgery, chemosurgery, surgical curettement), scalp, neck, hands, feet, genitalia; lesion diameter 0.5 cm or less

17271   lesion diameter 0.6 to 1.0 cm

17272   lesion diameter 1.1 to 2.0 cm

17273   lesion diameter 2.1 to 3.0 cm

17274   lesion diameter 3.1 to 4.0 cm

17276   lesion diameter over 4.0 cm

17280   Destruction, malignant lesion (eg, laser surgery, electrosurgery, cryosurgery, chemosurgery, surgical curettement), face, ears, eyelids, nose, lips, mucous membrane; lesion diameter 0.5 cm or less

17281   lesion diameter 0.6 to 1.0 cm

17282   lesion diameter 1.1 to 2.0 cm

17283   lesion diameter 2.1 to 3.0 cm

17284   lesion diameter 3.1 to 4.0 cm

17286   lesion diameter over 4.0 cm

Mohs Micrographic Surgery

Mohs micrographic surgery is a technique for the removal of complex or ill-defined skin cancer with histologic examination of 100% of the surgical margins. It requires the integration of an individual functioning in two separate and distinct capacities: surgeon and pathologist. If either of these responsibilities is delegated to another

physician or other qualified health care professional who reports the services separately, these codes should not be reported. The Mohs surgeon removes the tumor tissue and maps and divides the tumor specimen into pieces, and each piece is embedded into an individual tissue block for histopathologic examination. Thus a tissue block in Mohs surgery is defined as an individual tissue piece embedded in a mounting medium for sectioning.

If repair is performed, use separate repair, flap, or graft codes. If a biopsy of a suspected skin cancer is performed on the same day as Mohs surgery because there was no prior pathology confirmation of a diagnosis, then report diagnostic skin biopsy (11100, 11101) and frozen section pathology (88331) with modifier 59 to distinguish from the subsequent definitive surgical procedure of Mohs surgery.

        (If additional special pathology procedures, stains or immunostains are required, see 88311-88314, 88342)

        (Do not report 88314 in conjunction with 17311-17315 for routine frozen section stain (eg, hematoxylin and eosin, toluidine blue) performed during Mohs surgery. When a nonroutine histochemical stain on frozen tissue is utilized, report 88314 with modifier 59)

        (Do not report 88302-88309 on the same specimen as part of the Mohs surgery)

17311   Mohs micrographic technique, including removal of all gross tumor, surgical excision of tissue specimens, mapping, color coding of specimens, microscopic examination of specimens by the surgeon, and histopathologic preparation including routine stain(s) (eg, hematoxylin and eosin, toluidine blue), head, neck, hands, feet, genitalia, or any location with surgery directly involving muscle, cartilage, bone, tendon, major nerves, or vessels; first stage, up to 5 tissue blocks

+ **17312**   each additional stage after the first stage, up to 5 tissue blocks (List separately in addition to code for primary procedure)

        (Use 17312 in conjunction with 17311)

17313   Mohs micrographic technique, including removal of all gross tumor, surgical excision of tissue specimens, mapping, color coding of specimens, microscopic examination of specimens by the surgeon, and histopathologic preparation including routine stain(s) (eg, hematoxylin and eosin, toluidine blue), of the trunk, arms, or legs; first stage, up to 5 tissue blocks

+ **17314**   each additional stage after the first stage, up to 5 tissue blocks (List separately in addition to code for primary procedure)

        (Use 17314 in conjunction with 17313)

Integumentary

▲=Revised code   ●=New code   ► ◄=Contains new or revised text   ⊘=Modifier 51 exempt

+ 17315 Mohs micrographic technique, including removal of all gross tumor, surgical excision of tissue specimens, mapping, color coding of specimens, microscopic examination of specimens by the surgeon, and histopathologic preparation including routine stain(s) (eg, hematoxylin and eosin, toluidine blue), each additional block after the first 5 tissue blocks, any stage (List separately in addition to code for primary procedure)

(Use 17315 in conjunction with 17311-17314)

Other Procedures

17340 Cryotherapy (CO2 slush, liquid N2) for acne

17360 Chemical exfoliation for acne (eg, acne paste, acid)

17380 Electrolysis epilation, each 30 minutes

(For actinotherapy, use 96900)

17999 Unlisted procedure, skin, mucous membrane and subcutaneous tissue

Breast

Incision

19000 Puncture aspiration of cyst of breast;

+ 19001 each additional cyst (List separately in addition to code for primary procedure)

(Use 19001 in conjunction with 19000)

(If imaging guidance is performed, see 76942, 77021)

19020 Mastotomy with exploration or drainage of abscess, deep

19030 Injection procedure only for mammary ductogram or galactogram

(For radiological supervision and interpretation, see 77053, 77054)

Excision

Excisional breast surgery includes certain biopsy procedures, the removal of cysts or other benign or malignant tumors or lesions, and the surgical treatment of breast and chest wall malignancies. Biopsy procedures may be percutaneous or open, and they involve the removal of differing amounts of tissue for diagnosis.

Breast biopsies, without image guidance are reported with 19100 and 19101. Image-guided breast biopsies, including the placement of localization devices when performed, are reported using codes 19081-19086. The image-guided placement of localization devices without image-guided biopsy are reported with 19281-19288. When more than one biopsy or localization device placement is performed using the same imaging modality, use an add-on code whether the additional service(s) is on the same or contra-lateral breast. If additional biopsies or

localization device placements are performed using different imaging modalities, report another primary code for each additional biopsy or localization device placement performed using a different image guidance modality. When an open incisional biopsy is performed after image-guided placement of a localization device, 19101 is reported and the appropriate image-guided localization device placement code is reported. The open excision of breast lesions (eg, lesions of the breast ducts, cysts, benign or malignant tumors), without specific attention to adequate surgical margins, with or without the preoperative placement of radiological markers, is reported using codes 19110-19126. Partial mastectomy procedures (eg, lumpectomy, tylectomy, quadrantectomy, or segmentectomy) describe open excisions of breast tissue with specific attention to adequate surgical margins.

Partial mastectomy procedures are reported using codes 19301 or 19302 as appropriate. Documentation for partial mastectomy procedures includes attention to the removal of adequate surgical margins surrounding the breast mass or lesion.

Total mastectomy procedures include simple mastectomy, complete mastectomy, subcutaneous mastectomy, modified radical mastectomy, radical mastectomy, and more extended procedures (eg, Urban type operation). Total mastectomy procedures are reported using codes 19303-19307 as appropriate.

Excisions or resections of chest wall tumors including ribs, with or without reconstruction, with or without mediastinal lymphadenectomy, are reported using codes 19260, 19271, or 19272. Codes 19260-19272 are not restricted to breast tumors and are used to report resections of chest wall tumors originating from any chest wall component. (For excision of lung or pleura, see 32310 et seq.)

When more than one breast biopsy is performed using the same imaging modality, use an add-on code whether the additional service(s) is on the same or contra-lateral breast. If additional biopsies are performed using different imaging modalities, report another primary code for each additional modality.

To report bilateral image-guided breast biopsies, report 19081, 19083, or 19085 for the initial biopsy. The contra-lateral and each additional breast image guided biopsy are then reported with code 19082, 19084 or 19086.

(To report bilateral procedures for codes 19100-19120, report modifier 50 with the procedure code)

19081 Biopsy, breast, with placement of breast localization device(s) (eg, clip, metallic pellet), when performed, and imaging of the biopsy specimen, when performed, percutaneous; first lesion, including stereotactic guidance

+ 19082   each additional lesion, including stereotactic guidance (List separately in addition to code for primary procedure)

(Use 19082 in conjunction with 19081)

19083   Biopsy, breast, with placement of breast localization device(s) (eg, clip, metallic pellet), when performed, and imaging of the biopsy specimen, when performed, percutaneous; first lesion, including ultrasound guidance

+ 19084   each additional lesion, including ultrasound guidance (List separately in addition to code for primary procedure)

(Use 19084 in conjunction with 19083)

19085   Biopsy, breast, with placement of breast localization device(s) (eg, clip, metallic pellet), when performed, and imaging of the biopsy specimen, when performed, percutaneous; first lesion, including magnetic resonance guidance

+ 19086   each additional lesion, including magnetic resonance guidance (List separately in addition to code for primary procedure)

(Use 19086 in conjunction with 19085)

(Do not report 19081-19086 in conjunction with 19281-19288, 76098, 76942, 77002, 77021 for same lesion)

19100   Biopsy of breast; percutaneous, needle core, not using imaging guidance (separate procedure)

(For fine needle aspiration, use 10021)

19101   open, incisional

(For placement of percutaneous localization clip with imaging guidance, see 19281-19288)

(19102, 19103 have been deleted. To report, see 19081-19086)

19105   Ablation, cryosurgical, of fibroadenoma, including ultrasound guidance, each fibroadenoma

(Do not report 19105 in conjunction with 76940, 76942)

(For adjacent lesions treated with 1 cryoprobe insertion, report once)

19110   Nipple exploration, with or without excision of a solitary lactiferous duct or a papilloma lactiferous duct

19112   Excision of lactiferous duct fistula

19120   Excision of cyst, fibroadenoma, or other benign or malignant tumor, aberrant breast tissue, duct lesion, nipple or areolar lesion (except 19300), open, male or female, 1 or more lesions

19125   Excision of breast lesion identified by preoperative placement of radiological marker, open; single lesion

+ 19126   each additional lesion separately identified by a preoperative radiological marker (List separately in addition to code for primary procedure)

(Use 19126 in conjunction with 19125)

19260   Excision of chest wall tumor including ribs

19271   Excision of chest wall tumor involving ribs, with plastic reconstruction; without mediastinal lymphadenectomy

19272   with mediastinal lymphadenectomy

(Do not report 19260, 19271, 19272 in conjunction with 32100, 32503, 32504, 32551, 32554, 32555)

Introduction

Breast biopsies without image guidance are reported with 19100 and 19101. Image-guided breast biopsies, including the placement of localization devices when performed, are reported using 19081-19086. The image-guided placement of localization devices without image-guided biopsy are reported with 19281-19288. When more than one biopsy or localization device placement is performed using the same imaging modality, use an add-on code whether the additional service(s) is on the same or contra-lateral breast. If additional biopsies or localization device placements are performed using different imaging modalities, report another primary code for each additional biopsy or localization device placement performed using a different image guidance modality. When an open incisional biopsy is performed after image-guided placement of a localization device, 19101 is reported and the appropriate image-guided localization device placement code is reported.

When more than one breast localization device placement is performed using the same imaging modality, use an add-on code whether the additional service(s) is on the same or contra-lateral breast. If additional localization devices are placed using different imaging modalities, report another primary code for each additional modality. When an open incisional biopsy is performed after image-guided placement of a localization device, 19101 is reported and the appropriate image-guided localization device placement code is reported.

To report bilateral image-guided placement of localization devices report 19281, 19283, 19285, or 19287 for the initial lesion localized. The contra-lateral and each additional breast image-guided localization device placement is reported with code 19282, 19284, 19286 or 19288.

19281   Placement of breast localization device(s) (eg, clip, metallic pellet, wire/needle, radioactive seeds), percutaneous; first lesion, including mammographic guidance

+ 19282   each additional lesion, including mammographic guidance (List separately in addition to code for primary procedure)

(Use 19282 in conjunction with 19281)

19283   Placement of breast localization device(s) (eg, clip, metallic pellet, wire/needle, radioactive seeds), percutaneous; first lesion, including stereotactic guidance

+ 19284 each additional lesion, including stereotactic guidance (List separately in addition to code for primary procedure)

(Use 19284 in conjunction with 19283)

19285 Placement of breast localization device(s) (eg, clip, metallic pellet, wire/needle, radioactive seeds), percutaneous; first lesion, including ultrasound guidance

+ 19286 each additional lesion, including ultrasound guidance (List separately in addition to code for primary procedure)

(Use 19286 in conjunction with 19285)

19287 Placement of breast localization device(s) (eg clip, metallic pellet, wire/needle, radioactive seeds), percutaneous; first lesion, including magnetic resonance guidance

+ 19288 each additional lesion, including magnetic resonance guidance (List separately in addition to code for primary procedure)

(Use 19288 in conjunction with 19287)

(Do not report 19281-19288 in conjunction with 19081-19086, 76942, 77002, 77021 for same lesion)

(For surgical specimen radiography, use 76098)

(19290, 19291 have been deleted)

(To report image-guided placement of breast localization devices during image-guided biopsy, see 19081-19086. To report image-guided placement of breast localization devices without image-guided biopsy, see 19281-19288)

(19295 has been deleted)

19296 Placement of radiotherapy afterloading expandable catheter (single or multichannel) into the breast for interstitial radioelement application following partial mastectomy, includes imaging guidance; on date separate from partial mastectomy

+ 19297 concurrent with partial mastectomy (List separately in addition to code for primary procedure)

(Use 19297 in conjunction with 19301 or 19302)

⊙ 19298 Placement of radiotherapy afterloading brachytherapy catheters (multiple tube and button type) into the breast for interstitial radioelement application following (at the time of or subsequent to) partial mastectomy, includes imaging guidance

Mastectomy Procedures

19300 Mastectomy for gynecomastia

19301 Mastectomy, partial (eg, lumpectomy, tylectomy, quadrantectomy, segmentectomy);

19302 with axillary lymphadenectomy

(For placement of radiotherapy afterloading balloon/brachytherapy catheters, see 19296-19298)

19303 Mastectomy, simple, complete

(For immediate or delayed insertion of implant, see 19340, 19342)

(For gynecomastia, use 19300)

19304 Mastectomy, subcutaneous

(For immediate or delayed insertion of implant, see 19340, 19342)

19305 Mastectomy, radical, including pectoral muscles, axillary lymph nodes

(For immediate or delayed insertion of implant, see 19340, 19342)

19306 Mastectomy, radical, including pectoral muscles, axillary and internal mammary lymph nodes (Urban type operation)

(For immediate or delayed insertion of implant, see 19340, 19342)

19307 Mastectomy, modified radical, including axillary lymph nodes, with or without pectoralis minor muscle, but excluding pectoralis major muscle

(For immediate or delayed insertion of implant, see 19340, 19342)

Repair and/or Reconstruction

(To report bilateral procedure, report modifier 50 with the procedure code)

(For biologic implant for soft tissue reinforcement, use 15777 in conjunction with primary procedure)

19316 Mastopexy

19318 Reduction mammaplasty

19324 Mammaplasty, augmentation; without prosthetic implant

19325 with prosthetic implant

(For flap or graft, use also appropriate number)

19328 Removal of intact mammary implant

19330 Removal of mammary implant material

19340 Immediate insertion of breast prosthesis following mastopexy, mastectomy or in reconstruction

19342 Delayed insertion of breast prosthesis following mastopexy, mastectomy or in reconstruction

(For supply of implant, use 99070)

(For preparation of custom breast implant, use 19396)

19350 Nipple/areola reconstruction

19355 Correction of inverted nipples

19357 Breast reconstruction, immediate or delayed, with tissue expander, including subsequent expansion

19361 Breast reconstruction with latissimus dorsi flap, without prosthetic implant

(For insertion of prosthesis, use also 19340)

Integumentary

19364   Breast reconstruction with free flap

(Do not report code 69990 in addition to code 19364)

(19364 includes harvesting of the flap, microvascular transfer, closure of the donor site, and inset shaping the flap into a breast)

19366   Breast reconstruction with other technique

(For operating microscope, use 69990)

(For insertion of prosthesis, use also 19340 or 19342)

19367   Breast reconstruction with transverse rectus abdominis myocutaneous flap (TRAM), single pedicle, including closure of donor site;

19368   with microvascular anastomosis (supercharging)

(Do not report code 69990 in addition to code 19368)

19369   Breast reconstruction with transverse rectus abdominis myocutaneous flap (TRAM), double pedicle, including closure of donor site

19370   Open periprosthetic capsulotomy, breast

19371   Periprosthetic capsulectomy, breast

19380   Revision of reconstructed breast

19396   Preparation of moulage for custom breast implant

Other Procedures

19499   Unlisted procedure, breast

Musculoskeletal System

Cast and strapping procedures appear at the end of this section.

The services listed below include the application and removal of the first cast or traction device only. Subsequent replacement of cast and/or traction device may require an additional listing.

Definitions

The terms "closed treatment," "open treatment," and "percutaneous skeletal fixation" have been carefully chosen to accurately reflect current orthopaedic procedural treatments.

Closed treatment specifically means that the fracture site is not surgically opened (exposed to the external environment and directly visualized). This terminology is used to describe procedures that treat fractures by three methods: (1) without manipulation; (2) with manipulation; or (3) with or without traction.

Open treatment is used when the fractured bone is either: (1) surgically opened (exposed to the external environment) and the fracture (bone ends) visualized and internal fixation may be used; or (2) the fractured bone is opened remote from the fracture site in order to insert an intramedullary nail across the fracture site (the fracture site is not opened and visualized).

Percutaneous skeletal fixation describes fracture treatment which is neither open nor closed. In this procedure, the fracture fragments are not visualized, but fixation (eg, pins) is placed across the fracture site, usually under X-ray imaging.

The type of fracture (eg, open, compound, closed) does not have any coding correlation with the type of treatment (eg, closed, open, or percutaneous) provided.

The codes for treatment of fractures and joint injuries (dislocations) are categorized by the type of manipulation (reduction) and stabilization (fixation or immobilization). These codes can apply to either open (compound) or closed fractures or joint injuries.

Skeletal traction is the application of a force (distracting or traction force) to a limb segment through a wire, pin, screw, or clamp that is attached (eg, penetrates) to bone.

Skin traction is the application of a force (longitudinal) to a limb using felt or strapping applied directly to skin only.

External fixation is the usage of skeletal pins plus an attaching mechanism/device used for temporary or definitive treatment of acute or chronic bony deformity.

Codes for obtaining autogenous bone grafts, cartilage, tendon, fascia lata grafts or other tissues through separate incisions are to be used only when the graft is not already listed as part of the basic procedure.

Re-reduction of a fracture and/or dislocation performed by the primary physician or other qualified health care professional may be identified by the addition of modifier 76 to the usual procedure number to indicate "Repeat Procedure or Service by Same Physician or Other Qualified Health Care Professional." (See Appendix A guidelines.)

Codes for external fixation are to be used only when external fixation is not already listed as part of the basic procedure.

All codes for suction irrigation have been deleted. To report, list only the primary surgical procedure performed (eg, sequestrectomy, deep incision).

Manipulation is used throughout the musculoskeletal fracture and dislocation subsections to specifically mean the attempted reduction or restoration of a fracture or joint dislocation to its normal anatomic alignment by the application of manually applied forces.

Excision of subcutaneous soft connective tissue tumors (including simple or intermediate repair) involves the simple or marginal resection of tumors confined to subcutaneous tissue below the skin but above the deep fascia. These tumors are usually benign and are resected without removing a significant amount of surrounding normal tissue. Code selection is based on the location and size of the tumor. Code selection is determined by measuring the greatest diameter of the tumor plus that margin required for complete excision of the tumor. The margins refer to the most narrow margin required to adequately excise the tumor, based on the physician's judgment. The measurement of the tumor plus margin is made at the time of the excision. Appreciable vessel exploration and/or neuroplasty should be reported separately. Extensive undermining or other techniques to close a defect created by skin excision may require a complex repair which should be reported separately. Dissection or elevation of tissue planes to permit resection of the tumor is included in the excision. For excision of benign lesions of cutaneous origin (eg, sebaceous cyst), see 11400-11446.

Excision of fascial or subfascial soft tissue tumors (including simple or intermediate repair) involves the resection of tumors confined to the tissue within or below the deep fascia, but not involving the bone. These tumors are usually benign, are often intramuscular, and are resected without removing a significant amount of surrounding normal tissue. Code selection is based on size and location of the tumor. Code selection is determined by measuring the greatest diameter of the tumor plus that margin required for complete excision of the tumor. The margins refer to the most narrow margin required to adequately excise the tumor, based on individual judgment. The measurement of the tumor plus margin is made at the time of the excision. Appreciable vessel exploration and/or neuroplasty should be reported separately. Extensive undermining or other techniques to close a defect created by skin excision may require a complex repair which should be reported separately.

Dissection or elevation of tissue planes to permit resection of the tumor is included in the excision.

Digital (ie, fingers and toes) subfascial tumors are defined as those tumors involving the tendons, tendon sheaths, or joints of the digit. Tumors which simply abut but do not breach the tendon, tendon sheath, or joint capsule are considered subcutaneous soft tissue tumors.

Radical resection of soft connective tissue tumors (including simple or intermediate repair) involves the resection of the tumor with wide margins of normal tissue. Appreciable vessel exploration and/or neuroplasty repair or reconstruction (eg, adjacent tissue transfer[s], flap[s]) should be reported separately. Extensive undermining or other techniques to close a defect created by skin excision may require a complex repair which should be reported separately. Dissection or elevation of tissue planes to permit resection of the tumor is included in the excision. Although these tumors may be confined to a specific layer (eg, subcutaneous, subfascial), radical resection may involve removal of tissue from one or more layers. Radical resection of soft tissue tumors is most commonly used for malignant connective tissue tumors or very aggressive benign connective tissue tumors. Code selection is based on size and location of the tumor. Code selection is determined by measuring the greatest diameter of the tumor plus that margin required for complete excision of the tumor. The margins refer to the most narrow margin required to adequately excise the tumor, based on individual judgment. The measurement of the tumor plus margin is made at the time of the excision. For radical resection of tumor(s) of cutaneous origin (eg, melanoma), see 11600-11646.

Radical resection of bone tumors (including simple or intermediate repair) involves the resection of the tumor with wide margins of normal tissue. Appreciable vessel exploration and/or neuroplasty and complex bone repair or reconstruction (eg, adjacent tissue transfer[s], flap[s]) should be reported separately. Extensive undermining or other techniques to close a defect created by skin excision may require a complex repair which should be reported separately. Dissection or elevation of tissue planes to permit resection of the tumor is included in the excision. It may require removal of the entire bone if tumor growth is extensive (eg, clavicle). Radical resection of bone tumors is usually performed for malignant tumors or very aggressive benign tumors. If surrounding soft tissue is removed during these procedures, the radical resection of soft tissue tumor codes should not be reported separately. Code selection is based solely on the location of the tumor, **not** on the size of the tumor or whether the tumor is benign or malignant, primary or metastatic.

General

Incision

(20000 has been deleted)

(For incision and drainage procedures, cutaneous/subcutaneous, see 10060, 10061)

20005   Incision and drainage of soft tissue abscess, subfascial (ie, involves the soft tissue below the deep fascia)

Wound Exploration—Trauma (eg, Penetrating Gunshot, Stab Wound)

20100-20103 relate to wound(s) resulting from penetrating trauma. These codes describe surgical exploration and enlargement of the wound, extension of dissection (to determine penetration), debridement, removal of foreign body(s), ligation or coagulation of minor subcutaneous and/or muscular blood vessel(s), of the subcutaneous tissue, muscle fascia, and/or muscle, not requiring thoracotomy or laparotomy. If a repair is done to major structure(s) or major blood vessel(s) requiring thoracotomy or laparotomy, then those specific code(s) would supersede the use of codes 20100-20103. To report simple, intermediate, or complex repair of wound(s) that do not require enlargement of the wound, extension of dissection, etc, as stated above, use specific Repair code(s) in the **Integumentary System** section.

20100   Exploration of penetrating wound (separate procedure); neck

20101   chest

20102   abdomen/flank/back

20103   extremity

Excision

20150   Excision of epiphyseal bar, with or without autogenous soft tissue graft obtained through same fascial incision

(For aspiration of bone marrow, use 38220)

20200   Biopsy, muscle; superficial

20205   deep

20206   Biopsy, muscle, percutaneous needle

(If imaging guidance is performed, see 76942, 77012, 77021)

(For fine needle aspiration, use 10021 or 10022)

(For evaluation of fine needle aspirate, see 88172-88173)

(For excision of muscle tumor, deep, see specific anatomic section)

20220   Biopsy, bone, trocar, or needle; superficial (eg, ilium, sternum, spinous process, ribs)

Musculoskeletal

Musculoskeletal

20225   deep (eg, vertebral body, femur)

(Do not report 20225 in conjunction with 22510, 22511, 22512, 22513, 22514, 22515, 0200T, 0201T, when performed at the same level)

(For bone marrow biopsy, use 38221)

(For radiologic supervision and interpretation, see 77002, 77012, 77021)

20240   Biopsy, bone, open; superficial (eg, ilium, sternum, spinous process, ribs, trochanter of femur)

20245   deep (eg, humerus, ischium, femur)

20250   Biopsy, vertebral body, open; thoracic

20251   lumbar or cervical

(For sequestrectomy, osteomyelitis or drainage of bone abscess, see anatomical area)

Introduction or Removal

(For injection procedure for arthrography, see anatomical area)

20500   Injection of sinus tract; therapeutic (separate procedure)

20501   diagnostic (sinogram)

(For radiological supervision and interpretation, use 76080)

(For contrast injection[s] and radiological assessment of gastrostomy, duodenostomy, jejunostomy, gastro-jejunostomy, or cecostomy [or other colonic] tube including fluoroscopic imaging guidance, use 49465)

20520   Removal of foreign body in muscle or tendon sheath; simple

20525   deep or complicated

20526   Injection, therapeutic (eg, local anesthetic, corticosteroid), carpal tunnel

20527   Injection, enzyme (eg, collagenase), palmar fascial cord (ie, Dupuytren's contracture)

(For manipulation of palmar fascial cord (ie, Dupuytren's cord) post enzyme injection (eg, collagenase), use 26341)

20550   Injection(s); single tendon sheath, or ligament, aponeurosis (eg, plantar "fascia")

(For injection of Morton's neuroma, see 64455, 64632)

20551   single tendon origin/insertion

(Do not report 20550, 20551 in conjunction with 0232T)

(For injection(s) of platelet rich plasma, use 0232T)

20552   Injection(s); single or multiple trigger point(s), 1 or 2 muscle(s)

20553   single or multiple trigger point(s), 3 or more muscles

(If imaging guidance is performed, see 76942, 77002, 77021)

20555   Placement of needles or catheters into muscle and/or soft tissue for subsequent interstitial radioelement application (at the time of or subsequent to the procedure)

(For placement of devices into the breast for interstitial radioelement application, see 19296-19298)

(For placement of needles, catheters, or devices into muscle or soft tissue of the head and neck, for interstitial radioelement application, use 41019)

(For placement of needles or catheters for interstitial radioelement application into prostate, use 55875)

(For placement of needles or catheters into the pelvic organs or genitalia [except prostate] for interstitial radioelement application, use 55920)

▶(For interstitial radioelement application, see 77770, 77771, 77772, 77778)◀

(For imaging guidance, see 76942, 77002, 77012, 77021)

20600   Arthrocentesis, aspiration and/or injection, small joint or bursa (eg, fingers, toes); without ultrasound guidance

20604   with ultrasound guidance, with permanent recording and reporting

(Do not report 20600, 20604 in conjunction with 76942)

(If fluoroscopic, CT, or MRI guidance is performed, see 77002, 77012, 77021)

20605   Arthrocentesis, aspiration and/or injection, intermediate joint or bursa (eg, temporomandibular, acromioclavicular, wrist, elbow or ankle, olecranon bursa); without ultrasound guidance

20606   with ultrasound guidance, with permanent recording and reporting

(Do not report 20605, 20606 in conjunction with 76942)

(If fluoroscopic, CT, or MRI guidance is performed, see 77002, 77012, 77021)

20610   Arthrocentesis, aspiration and/or injection, major joint or bursa (eg, shoulder, hip, knee, subacromial bursa); without ultrasound guidance

20611   with ultrasound guidance, with permanent recording and reporting

(Do not report 20610, 20611 in conjunction with 27370, 76942)

(If fluoroscopic, CT, or MRI guidance is performed, see 77002, 77012, 77021)

20612   Aspiration and/or injection of ganglion cyst(s) any location

(To report multiple ganglion cyst aspirations/injections, use 20612 and append modifier 59)

20615   Aspiration and injection for treatment of bone cyst

20650   Insertion of wire or pin with application of skeletal traction, including removal (separate procedure)

20660   Application of cranial tongs, caliper, or stereotactic frame, including removal (separate procedure)

20661   Application of halo, including removal; cranial

20662   pelvic

20663   femoral

20664   Application of halo, including removal, cranial, 6 or more pins placed, for thin skull osteology (eg, pediatric patients, hydrocephalus, osteogenesis imperfecta)

20665   Removal of tongs or halo applied by another individual

20670   Removal of implant; superficial (eg, buried wire, pin or rod) (separate procedure)

20680   deep (eg, buried wire, pin, screw, metal band, nail, rod or plate)

20690   Application of a uniplane (pins or wires in 1 plane), unilateral, external fixation system

20692   Application of a multiplane (pins or wires in more than 1 plane), unilateral, external fixation system (eg, Ilizarov, Monticelli type)

20693   Adjustment or revision of external fixation system requiring anesthesia (eg, new pin[s] or wire[s] and/or new ring[s] or bar[s])

20694   Removal, under anesthesia, of external fixation system

20696   Application of multiplane (pins or wires in more than 1 plane), unilateral, external fixation with stereotactic computer-assisted adjustment (eg, spatial frame), including imaging; initial and subsequent alignment(s), assessment(s), and computation(s) of adjustment schedule(s)

(Do not report 20696 in conjunction with 20692, 20697)

⊘ **20697**   exchange (ie, removal and replacement) of strut, each

(Do not report 20697 in conjunction with 20692, 20696)

Replantation

20802   Replantation, arm (includes surgical neck of humerus through elbow joint), complete amputation

(To report replantation of incomplete arm amputation, see specific code[s] for repair of bone[s], ligament[s], tendon[s], nerve[s], or blood vessel[s] with modifier 52)

20805   Replantation, forearm (includes radius and ulna to radial carpal joint), complete amputation

(To report replantation of incomplete forearm amputation, see specific code[s] for repair of bone[s], ligament[s], tendon[s], nerve[s], or blood vessel[s] with modifier 52)

20808   Replantation, hand (includes hand through metacarpophalangeal joints), complete amputation

(To report replantation of incomplete hand amputation, see specific code[s] for repair of bone[s], ligament[s], tendon[s], nerve[s], or blood vessel[s] with modifier 52)

20816   Replantation, digit, excluding thumb (includes metacarpophalangeal joint to insertion of flexor sublimis tendon), complete amputation

(To report replantation of incomplete digit amputation, excluding thumb, see specific code[s] for repair of bone[s], ligament[s], tendon[s], nerve[s], or blood vessel[s] with modifier 52)

20822   Replantation, digit, excluding thumb (includes distal tip to sublimis tendon insertion), complete amputation

(To report replantation of incomplete digit amputation, excluding thumb, see specific code[s] for repair of bone[s], ligament[s], tendon[s], nerve[s], or blood vessel[s] with modifier 52)

20824   Replantation, thumb (includes carpometacarpal joint to MP joint), complete amputation

(To report replantation of incomplete thumb amputation, see specific code[s] for repair of bone[s], ligament[s], tendon[s], nerve[s], or blood vessel[s] with modifier 52)

20827   Replantation, thumb (includes distal tip to MP joint), complete amputation

(To report replantation of incomplete thumb amputation, see specific code[s] for repair of bone[s], ligament[s], tendon[s], nerve[s], or blood vessel[s] with modifier 52)

(To report replantation of complete leg amputation, see specific code[s] for repair of bone[s], ligament[s], tendon[s], nerve[s], or blood vessel[s] with modifier 52)

(To report replantation of incomplete leg amputation, see specific code[s] for repair of bone[s], ligament[s], tendon[s], nerve[s], or blood vessel[s] with modifier 52)

20838   Replantation, foot, complete amputation

(To report replantation of incomplete foot amputation, see specific code[s] for repair of bone[s], ligament[s], tendon[s], nerve[s], or blood vessel[s] with modifier 52)

Grafts (or Implants)

Codes for obtaining autogenous bone, cartilage, tendon, fascia lata grafts, or other tissues through separate skin/fascial incisions should be reported separately unless the code descriptor references the harvesting of the graft or implant (eg, includes obtaining graft).

Do not append modifier 62 to bone graft codes 20900-20938.

(For spinal surgery bone graft[s] see codes 20930-20938)

20900   Bone graft, any donor area; minor or small (eg, dowel or button)

Musculoskeletal

20902	major or large
20910	Cartilage graft; costochondral
20912	nasal septum

(For ear cartilage, use 21235)

20920	Fascia lata graft; by stripper
20922	by incision and area exposure, complex or sheet
20924	Tendon graft, from a distance (eg, palmaris, toe extensor, plantaris)
20926	Tissue grafts, other (eg, paratenon, fat, dermis)

(For injection(s) of platelet rich plasma, use 0232T)

+ 20930 Allograft, morselized, or placement of osteopromotive material, for spine surgery only (List separately in addition to code for primary procedure)

(Use 20930 in conjunction with 22319, 22532, 22533, 22548-22558, 22590-22612, 22630, 22633, 22634, 22800-22812)

+ 20931 Allograft, structural, for spine surgery only (List separately in addition to code for primary procedure)

(Use 20931 in conjunction with 22319, 22532-22533, 22548-22558, 22590-22612, 22630, 22633, 22634, 22800-22812)

+ 20936 Autograft for spine surgery only (includes harvesting the graft); local (eg, ribs, spinous process, or laminar fragments) obtained from same incision (List separately in addition to code for primary procedure)

(Use 20936 in conjunction with 22319, 22532, 22533, 22548-22558, 22590-22612, 22630, 22633, 22634, 22800-22812)

+ 20937 morselized (through separate skin or fascial incision) (List separately in addition to code for primary procedure)

(Use 20937 in conjunction with 22319, 22532, 22533, 22548-22558, 22590-22612, 22630, 22633, 22634, 22800-22812)

+ 20938 structural, bicortical or tricortical (through separate skin or fascial incision) (List separately in addition to code for primary procedure)

(Use 20938 in conjunction with 22319, 22532, 22533, 22548-22558, 22590-22612, 22630, 22633, 22634, 22800-22812)

(For needle aspiration of bone marrow for the purpose of bone grafting, use 38220. Do not report 38220-38230 for bone marrow aspiration for platelet rich stem cell injection. For bone marrow aspiration for platelet rich stem cell injection, use 0232T)

Other Procedures

20950 Monitoring of interstitial fluid pressure (includes insertion of device, eg, wick catheter technique, needle manometer technique) in detection of muscle compartment syndrome

20955	Bone graft with microvascular anastomosis; fibula
20956	iliac crest
20957	metatarsal
20962	other than fibula, iliac crest, or metatarsal

(Do not report code 69990 in addition to codes 20955-20962)

20969 Free osteocutaneous flap with microvascular anastomosis; other than iliac crest, metatarsal, or great toe

20970	iliac crest
20972	metatarsal
20973	great toe with web space

(Do not report code 69990 in addition to codes 20969-20973)

(For great toe, wrap-around procedure, use 26551)

⊘ **20974** Electrical stimulation to aid bone healing; noninvasive (nonoperative)

⊘ **20975** invasive (operative)

20979 Low intensity ultrasound stimulation to aid bone healing, noninvasive (nonoperative)

⊙ **20982** Ablation therapy for reduction or eradication of 1 or more bone tumors (eg, metastasis) including adjacent soft tissue when involved by tumor extension, percutaneous, including imaging guidance when performed; radiofrequency

⊙ **20983** cryoablation

(Do not report 20982, 20983 in conjunction with 76940, 77002, 77013, 77022)

+ 20985 Computer-assisted surgical navigational procedure for musculoskeletal procedures, image-less (List separately in addition to code for primary procedure)

(Do not report 20985 in conjunction with 61781-61783)

(20986, 20987 have been deleted)

(For computer-assisted navigational procedures with image guidance based on pre-operative and intraoperatively obtained images, see 0054T, 0055T)

20999 Unlisted procedure, musculoskeletal system, general

Head

Skull, facial bones, and temporomandibular joint.

Incision

(For incision and drainage of superficial abscess and hematoma, see 10060, 10061)

(For incision and drainage of soft tissue abscess, use 20005)

(For removal of embedded foreign body from dentoalveolar structure, see 41805, 41806)

21010   Arthrotomy, temporomandibular joint

(To report bilateral procedure, report 21010 with modifier 50)

Excision

21011   Excision, tumor, soft tissue of face or scalp, subcutaneous; less than 2 cm

21012   2 cm or greater

(For excision of benign lesions of cutaneous origin [eg, sebaceous cyst], see 11420-11426)

21013   Excision, tumor, soft tissue of face and scalp, subfascial (eg, subgaleal, intramuscular); less than 2 cm

21014   2 cm or greater

21015   Radical resection of tumor (eg, sarcoma), soft tissue of face or scalp; less than 2 cm

(To report excision of skull tumor for osteomyelitis, use 61501)

21016   2 cm or greater

(For radical resection of tumor[s] of cutaneous origin [eg, melanoma], see 11620-11646)

21025   Excision of bone (eg, for osteomyelitis or bone abscess); mandible

21026   facial bone(s)

21029   Removal by contouring of benign tumor of facial bone (eg, fibrous dysplasia)

21030   Excision of benign tumor or cyst of maxilla or zygoma by enucleation and curettage

21031   Excision of torus mandibularis

21032   Excision of maxillary torus palatinus

21034   Excision of malignant tumor of maxilla or zygoma

21040   Excision of benign tumor or cyst of mandible, by enucleation and/or curettage

(For enucleation and/or curettage of benign cysts or tumors of mandible not requiring osteotomy, use 21040)

(For excision of benign tumor or cyst of mandible requiring osteotomy, see 21046-21047)

21044   Excision of malignant tumor of mandible;

21045   radical resection

(For bone graft, use 21215)

21046   Excision of benign tumor or cyst of mandible; requiring intra-oral osteotomy (eg, locally aggressive or destructive lesion[s])

21047   requiring extra-oral osteotomy and partial mandibulectomy (eg, locally aggressive or destructive lesion[s])

21048   Excision of benign tumor or cyst of maxilla; requiring intra-oral osteotomy (eg, locally aggressive or destructive lesion[s])

21049   requiring extra-oral osteotomy and partial maxillectomy (eg, locally aggressive or destructive lesion[s])

21050   Condylectomy, temporomandibular joint (separate procedure)

(For bilateral procedures, report 21050 with modifier 50)

21060   Meniscectomy, partial or complete, temporomandibular joint (separate procedure)

(For bilateral procedures, report 21060 with modifier 50)

21070   Coronoidectomy (separate procedure)

(For bilateral procedures, report 21070 with modifier 50)

Manipulation

21073   Manipulation of temporomandibular joint(s) (TMJ), therapeutic, requiring an anesthesia service (ie, general or monitored anesthesia care)

(For TMJ manipulation without an anesthesia service [ie, general or monitored anesthesia care], see 97140, 98925-98929, 98943)

(For closed treatment of temporomandibular dislocation, see 21480, 21485)

Head Prosthesis

Codes 21076-21089 describe professional services for the rehabilitation of patients with oral, facial, or other anatomical deficiencies by means of prostheses such as an artificial eye, ear, or nose or intraoral obturator to close a cleft. Codes 21076-21089 should only be used when the physician or other qualified health care professional actually designs and prepares the prosthesis (ie, not prepared by an outside laboratory).

(For application or removal of caliper or tongs, see 20660, 20665)

21076   Impression and custom preparation; surgical obturator prosthesis

21077   orbital prosthesis

21079   interim obturator prosthesis

21080   definitive obturator prosthesis

21081   mandibular resection prosthesis

21082   palatal augmentation prosthesis

21083   palatal lift prosthesis

21084   speech aid prosthesis

21085   oral surgical splint

21086   auricular prosthesis

21087   nasal prosthesis

21088   facial prosthesis

Musculoskeletal

Other Procedures

21089   Unlisted maxillofacial prosthetic procedure

Introduction or Removal

21100   Application of halo type appliance for maxillofacial fixation, includes removal (separate procedure)

21110   Application of interdental fixation device for conditions other than fracture or dislocation, includes removal

(For removal of interdental fixation by another individual, see 20670-20680)

21116   Injection procedure for temporomandibular joint arthrography

(For radiological supervision and interpretation, use 70332. Do not report 77002 in conjunction with 70332)

Repair, Revision, and/or Reconstruction

(For cranioplasty, see 21179, 21180 and 62120, 62140-62147)

21120   Genioplasty; augmentation (autograft, allograft, prosthetic material)

21121   sliding osteotomy, single piece

21122   sliding osteotomies, 2 or more osteotomies (eg, wedge excision or bone wedge reversal for asymmetrical chin)

21123   sliding, augmentation with interpositional bone grafts (includes obtaining autografts)

21125   Augmentation, mandibular body or angle; prosthetic material

21127   with bone graft, onlay or interpositional (includes obtaining autograft)

21137   Reduction forehead; contouring only

21138   contouring and application of prosthetic material or bone graft (includes obtaining autograft)

21139   contouring and setback of anterior frontal sinus wall

21141   Reconstruction midface, LeFort I; single piece, segment movement in any direction (eg, for Long Face Syndrome), without bone graft

21142   2 pieces, segment movement in any direction, without bone graft

21143   3 or more pieces, segment movement in any direction, without bone graft

21145   single piece, segment movement in any direction, requiring bone grafts (includes obtaining autografts)

21146   2 pieces, segment movement in any direction, requiring bone grafts (includes obtaining autografts) (eg, ungrafted unilateral alveolar cleft)

21147   3 or more pieces, segment movement in any direction, requiring bone grafts (includes obtaining autografts) (eg, ungrafted bilateral alveolar cleft or multiple osteotomies)

21150   Reconstruction midface, LeFort II; anterior intrusion (eg, Treacher-Collins Syndrome)

21151   any direction, requiring bone grafts (includes obtaining autografts)

21154   Reconstruction midface, LeFort III (extracranial), any type, requiring bone grafts (includes obtaining autografts); without LeFort I

21155   with LeFort I

21159   Reconstruction midface, LeFort III (extra and intracranial) with forehead advancement (eg, mono bloc), requiring bone grafts (includes obtaining autografts); without LeFort I

21160   with LeFort I

21172   Reconstruction superior-lateral orbital rim and lower forehead, advancement or alteration, with or without grafts (includes obtaining autografts)

(For frontal or parietal craniotomy performed for craniosynostosis, use 61556)

21175   Reconstruction, bifrontal, superior-lateral orbital rims and lower forehead, advancement or alteration (eg, plagiocephaly, trigonocephaly, brachycephaly), with or without grafts (includes obtaining autografts)

(For bifrontal craniotomy performed for craniosynostosis, use 61557)

21179   Reconstruction, entire or majority of forehead and/or supraorbital rims; with grafts (allograft or prosthetic material)

21180   with autograft (includes obtaining grafts)

(For extensive craniectomy for multiple suture craniosynostosis, use only 61558 or 61559)

21181   Reconstruction by contouring of benign tumor of cranial bones (eg, fibrous dysplasia), extracranial

21182   Reconstruction of orbital walls, rims, forehead, nasoethmoid complex following intra- and extracranial excision of benign tumor of cranial bone (eg, fibrous dysplasia), with multiple autografts (includes obtaining grafts); total area of bone grafting less than 40 sq cm

21183   total area of bone grafting greater than 40 sq cm but less than 80 sq cm

21184   total area of bone grafting greater than 80 sq cm

(For excision of benign tumor of cranial bones, see 61563, 61564)

21188   Reconstruction midface, osteotomies (other than LeFort type) and bone grafts (includes obtaining autografts)

21193   Reconstruction of mandibular rami, horizontal, vertical, C, or L osteotomy; without bone graft

21194　　　　with bone graft (includes obtaining graft)

21195　　Reconstruction of mandibular rami and/or body, sagittal split; without internal rigid fixation

21196　　　　with internal rigid fixation

21198　　Osteotomy, mandible, segmental;

21199　　　　with genioglossus advancement

　　　　(To report total osteotomy of the maxilla, see 21141-21160)

21206　　Osteotomy, maxilla, segmental (eg, Wassmund or Schuchard)

21208　　Osteoplasty, facial bones; augmentation (autograft, allograft, or prosthetic implant)

21209　　　　reduction

21210　　Graft, bone; nasal, maxillary or malar areas (includes obtaining graft)

　　　　(For cleft palate repair, see 42200-42225)

21215　　　　mandible (includes obtaining graft)

21230　　Graft; rib cartilage, autogenous, to face, chin, nose or ear (includes obtaining graft)

21235　　　　ear cartilage, autogenous, to nose or ear (includes obtaining graft)

　　　　(To report graft augmentation of facial bones, use 21208)

21240　　Arthroplasty, temporomandibular joint, with or without autograft (includes obtaining graft)

21242　　Arthroplasty, temporomandibular joint, with allograft

21243　　Arthroplasty, temporomandibular joint, with prosthetic joint replacement

21244　　Reconstruction of mandible, extraoral, with transosteal bone plate (eg, mandibular staple bone plate)

21245　　Reconstruction of mandible or maxilla, subperiosteal implant; partial

21246　　　　complete

21247　　Reconstruction of mandibular condyle with bone and cartilage autografts (includes obtaining grafts) (eg, for hemifacial microsomia)

21248　　Reconstruction of mandible or maxilla, endosteal implant (eg, blade, cylinder); partial

21249　　　　complete

　　　　(To report midface reconstruction, see 21141-21160)

21255　　Reconstruction of zygomatic arch and glenoid fossa with bone and cartilage (includes obtaining autografts)

21256　　Reconstruction of orbit with osteotomies (extracranial) and with bone grafts (includes obtaining autografts) (eg, micro-ophthalmia)

21260　　Periorbital osteotomies for orbital hypertelorism, with bone grafts; extracranial approach

21261　　　　combined intra- and extracranial approach

21263　　　　with forehead advancement

21267　　Orbital repositioning, periorbital osteotomies, unilateral, with bone grafts; extracranial approach

21268　　　　combined intra- and extracranial approach

21270　　Malar augmentation, prosthetic material

　　　　(For malar augmentation with bone graft, use 21210)

21275　　Secondary revision of orbitocraniofacial reconstruction

21280　　Medial canthopexy (separate procedure)

　　　　(For medial canthoplasty, use 67950)

21282　　Lateral canthopexy

21295　　Reduction of masseter muscle and bone (eg, for treatment of benign masseteric hypertrophy); extraoral approach

21296　　　　intraoral approach

Other Procedures

21299　　Unlisted craniofacial and maxillofacial procedure

Fracture and/or Dislocation

　　　　(For operative repair of skull fracture, see 62000-62010)

　　　　(To report closed treatment of skull fracture, use the appropriate Evaluation and Management code)

21310　　Closed treatment of nasal bone fracture without manipulation

21315　　Closed treatment of nasal bone fracture; without stabilization

21320　　　　with stabilization

21325　　Open treatment of nasal fracture; uncomplicated

21330　　　　complicated, with internal and/or external skeletal fixation

21335　　　　with concomitant open treatment of fractured septum

21336　　Open treatment of nasal septal fracture, with or without stabilization

21337　　Closed treatment of nasal septal fracture, with or without stabilization

21338　　Open treatment of nasoethmoid fracture; without external fixation

21339　　　　with external fixation

21340　　Percutaneous treatment of nasoethmoid complex fracture, with splint, wire or headcap fixation, including repair of canthal ligaments and/or the nasolacrimal apparatus

21343　　Open treatment of depressed frontal sinus fracture

21344　　Open treatment of complicated (eg, comminuted or involving posterior wall) frontal sinus fracture, via coronal or multiple approaches

Musculoskeletal

Musculoskeletal

21345 Closed treatment of nasomaxillary complex fracture (LeFort II type), with interdental wire fixation or fixation of denture or splint

21346 Open treatment of nasomaxillary complex fracture (LeFort II type); with wiring and/or local fixation

21347 requiring multiple open approaches

21348 with bone grafting (includes obtaining graft)

21355 Percutaneous treatment of fracture of malar area, including zygomatic arch and malar tripod, with manipulation

21356 Open treatment of depressed zygomatic arch fracture (eg, Gillies approach)

21360 Open treatment of depressed malar fracture, including zygomatic arch and malar tripod

21365 Open treatment of complicated (eg, comminuted or involving cranial nerve foramina) fracture(s) of malar area, including zygomatic arch and malar tripod; with internal fixation and multiple surgical approaches

21366 with bone grafting (includes obtaining graft)

21385 Open treatment of orbital floor blowout fracture; transantral approach (Caldwell-Luc type operation)

21386 periorbital approach

21387 combined approach

21390 periorbital approach, with alloplastic or other implant

21395 periorbital approach with bone graft (includes obtaining graft)

21400 Closed treatment of fracture of orbit, except blowout; without manipulation

21401 with manipulation

21406 Open treatment of fracture of orbit, except blowout; without implant

21407 with implant

21408 with bone grafting (includes obtaining graft)

21421 Closed treatment of palatal or maxillary fracture (LeFort I type), with interdental wire fixation or fixation of denture or splint

21422 Open treatment of palatal or maxillary fracture (LeFort I type);

21423 complicated (comminuted or involving cranial nerve foramina), multiple approaches

21431 Closed treatment of craniofacial separation (LeFort III type) using interdental wire fixation of denture or splint

21432 Open treatment of craniofacial separation (LeFort III type); with wiring and/or internal fixation

21433 complicated (eg, comminuted or involving cranial nerve foramina), multiple surgical approaches

21435 complicated, utilizing internal and/or external fixation techniques (eg, head cap, halo device, and/or intermaxillary fixation)

(For removal of internal or external fixation device, use 20670)

21436 complicated, multiple surgical approaches, internal fixation, with bone grafting (includes obtaining graft)

21440 Closed treatment of mandibular or maxillary alveolar ridge fracture (separate procedure)

21445 Open treatment of mandibular or maxillary alveolar ridge fracture (separate procedure)

21450 Closed treatment of mandibular fracture; without manipulation

21451 with manipulation

21452 Percutaneous treatment of mandibular fracture, with external fixation

21453 Closed treatment of mandibular fracture with interdental fixation

21454 Open treatment of mandibular fracture with external fixation

21461 Open treatment of mandibular fracture; without interdental fixation

21462 with interdental fixation

21465 Open treatment of mandibular condylar fracture

21470 Open treatment of complicated mandibular fracture by multiple surgical approaches including internal fixation, interdental fixation, and/or wiring of dentures or splints

21480 Closed treatment of temporomandibular dislocation; initial or subsequent

21485 complicated (eg, recurrent requiring intermaxillary fixation or splinting), initial or subsequent

21490 Open treatment of temporomandibular dislocation

(For interdental wire fixation, use 21497)

21495 Open treatment of hyoid fracture

(For laryngoplasty with open reduction of fracture, use 31584)

(To report treatment of closed fracture of larynx, use the applicable Evaluation and Management codes)

21497 Interdental wiring, for condition other than fracture

Other Procedures

21499 Unlisted musculoskeletal procedure, head

(For unlisted craniofacial or maxillofacial procedure, use 21299)

Neck (Soft Tissues) and Thorax

(For cervical spine and back, see 21920 et seq)

(For injection of fracture site or trigger point, use 20550)

Incision

(For incision and drainage of abscess or hematoma, superficial, see 10060, 10140)

21501   Incision and drainage, deep abscess or hematoma, soft tissues of neck or thorax;

(For posterior spine subfascial incision and drainage, see 22010-22015)

21502   with partial rib ostectomy

21510   Incision, deep, with opening of bone cortex (eg, for osteomyelitis or bone abscess), thorax

Excision

(For bone biopsy, see 20220-20251)

21550   Biopsy, soft tissue of neck or thorax

(For needle biopsy of soft tissue, use 20206)

21552   Code is out of numerical sequence. See 21550-21632

21554   Code is out of numerical sequence. See 21550-21632

21555   Excision, tumor, soft tissue of neck or anterior thorax, subcutaneous; less than 3 cm

 # 21552   3 cm or greater

(For excision of benign lesions of cutaneous origin [eg, sebaceous cyst], see 11420-11426)

21556   Excision, tumor, soft tissue of neck or anterior thorax, subfascial (eg, intramuscular); less than 5 cm

 # 21554   5 cm or greater

21557   Radical resection of tumor (eg, sarcoma), soft tissue of neck or anterior thorax; less than 5 cm

21558   5 cm or greater

(For radical resection of tumor[s] of cutaneous origin [eg, melanoma], see 11600-11620)

21600   Excision of rib, partial

(For radical resection of chest wall and rib cage for tumor, use 19260)

(For radical debridement of chest wall and rib cage for injury, see 11044, 11047)

21610   Costotransversectomy (separate procedure)

21615   Excision first and/or cervical rib;

21616   with sympathectomy

21620   Ostectomy of sternum, partial

21627   Sternal debridement

(For debridement and closure, use 21750)

21630   Radical resection of sternum;

21632   with mediastinal lymphadenectomy

Repair, Revision, and/or Reconstruction

(For superficial wound, see **Integumentary System** section under Repair—Simple)

21685   Hyoid myotomy and suspension

21700   Division of scalenus anticus; without resection of cervical rib

21705   with resection of cervical rib

21720   Division of sternocleidomastoid for torticollis, open operation; without cast application

(For transection of spinal accessory and cervical nerves, see 63191, 64722)

21725   with cast application

21740   Reconstructive repair of pectus excavatum or carinatum; open

21742   minimally invasive approach (Nuss procedure), without thoracoscopy

21743   minimally invasive approach (Nuss procedure), with thoracoscopy

21750   Closure of median sternotomy separation with or without debridement (separate procedure)

Fracture and/or Dislocation

(21800 has been deleted)

(To report closed treatment of an uncomplicated rib fracture, use the Evaluation and Management codes)

►(21805 has been deleted)◄

(21810 has been deleted. For external rib fixation, use 21899)

21811   Open treatment of rib fracture(s) with internal fixation, includes thoracoscopic visualization when performed, unilateral; 1-3 ribs

(For bilateral procedure, report 21811 with modifier 50)

21812   4-6 ribs

(For bilateral procedure, report 21812 with modifier 50)

21813   7 or more ribs

(For bilateral procedure, report 21813 with modifier 50)

21820   Closed treatment of sternum fracture

21825   Open treatment of sternum fracture with or without skeletal fixation

(For sternoclavicular dislocation, see 23520-23532)

Other Procedures

21899   Unlisted procedure, neck or thorax

Musculoskeletal

Back and Flank

Excision

21920   Biopsy, soft tissue of back or flank; superficial

21925   deep

      (For needle biopsy of soft tissue, use 20206)

21930   Excision, tumor, soft tissue of back or flank, subcutaneous; less than 3 cm

21931   3 cm or greater

      (For excision of benign lesions of cutaneous origin [eg, sebaceous cyst], see 11400-11406)

21932   Excision, tumor, soft tissue of back or flank, subfascial (eg, intramuscular); less than 5 cm

21933   5 cm or greater

21935   Radical resection of tumor (eg, sarcoma), soft tissue of back or flank; less than 5 cm

21936   5 cm or greater

      (For radical resection of tumor[s] of cutaneous origin [eg, melanoma], see 11600-11606)

Spine (Vertebral Column)

Cervical, thoracic, and lumbar spine.

Within the spine section, bone grafting procedures are reported separately and in addition to arthrodesis. For bone grafts in other Musculoskeletal sections, see specific code(s) descriptor(s) and/or accompanying guidelines.

To report bone grafts performed after arthrodesis, see 20930-20938. Do not append modifier 62 to bone graft codes 20900-20938.

Example:

Posterior arthrodesis of L5-S1 for degenerative disc disease utilizing morselized autogenous iliac bone graft harvested through a separate fascial incision.

Report as 22612 and 20937.

Within the spine section, instrumentation is reported separately and in addition to arthrodesis. To report instrumentation procedures performed with definitive vertebral procedure(s), see 22840-22855. Instrumentation procedure codes 22840-22848 and 22851 are reported in addition to the definitive procedure(s). Modifier 62 may not be appended to the definitive or add-on spinal instrumentation procedure code(s) 22840-22848 and 22850-22852.

Example:

Posterior arthrodesis of L4-S1, utilizing morselized autogenous iliac bone graft harvested through separate fascial incision, and pedicle screw fixation.

Report as 22612, 22614, 22842, and 20937.

Vertebral procedures are sometimes followed by arthrodesis and in addition may include bone grafts and instrumentation.

When arthrodesis is performed in addition to another procedure, the arthrodesis should be reported in addition to the original procedure with modifier 51 (multiple procedures). Examples are after osteotomy, fracture care, vertebral corpectomy, and laminectomy. Bone grafts and instrumentation are never performed without arthrodesis.

Example:

Treatment of a burst fracture of L2 by corpectomy followed by arthrodesis of L1-L3, utilizing anterior instrumentation L1-L3 and structural allograft.

Report as 63090, 22558-51, 22585, 22845, and 20931.

When two surgeons work together as primary surgeons performing distinct part(s) of a single reportable procedure, each surgeon should report his/her distinct operative work by appending modifier 62 to the single definitive procedure code. If additional procedure(s) (including add-on procedure[s]) are performed during the same surgical session, separate code(s) may be reported by each co-surgeon, with modifier 62 appended (see Appendix A).

Example:

A 42-year-old male with a history of posttraumatic degenerative disc disease at L3-4 and L4-5 (internal disc disruption) underwent surgical repair. Surgeon A performed an anterior exposure of the spine with mobilization of the great vessels. Surgeon B performed anterior (minimal) discectomy and fusion at L3-4 and L4-5 using anterior interbody technique.

Report surgeon A: 22558 append modifier 62, 22585 append modifier 62

Report surgeon B: 22558 append modifier 62, 22585 append modifier 62, 20931

      (Do not append modifier 62 to bone graft code 20931)

      (For injection procedure for myelography, use 62284)

      (For injection procedure for discography, see 62290, 62291)

      (For injection procedure, chemonucleolysis, single or multiple levels, use 62292)

      (For injection procedure for facet joints, see 64490-64495, 64633-64636)

      (For needle or trocar biopsy, see 20220-20225)

Incision

22010   Incision and drainage, open, of deep abscess (subfascial), posterior spine; cervical, thoracic, or cervicothoracic

22015   lumbar, sacral, or lumbosacral

      (Do not report 22015 in conjunction with 22010)

Musculoskeletal

(Do not report 22015 in conjunction with instrumentation removal, 10180, 22850, 22852)

(For incision and drainage of abscess or hematoma, superficial, see 10060, 10140)

Excision

For the following codes, when two surgeons work together as primary surgeons performing distinct part(s) of partial vertebral body excision, each surgeon should report his/her distinct operative work by appending modifier 62 to the procedure code. In this situation, modifier 62 may be appended to the procedure code(s) 22100-22102, 22110-22114 and, as appropriate, to the associated additional vertebral segment add-on code(s) 22103, 22116 as long as both surgeons continue to work together as primary surgeons.

(For bone biopsy, see 20220-20251)

(To report soft tissue biopsy of back or flank, see 21920-21925)

(For needle biopsy of soft tissue, use 20206)

(To report excision of soft tissue tumor of back or flank, use 21930)

22100   Partial excision of posterior vertebral component (eg, spinous process, lamina or facet) for intrinsic bony lesion, single vertebral segment; cervical

22101   thoracic

22102   lumbar

(For insertion of posterior spinous process distraction devices, see 0171T, 0172T)

+ 22103   each additional segment (List separately in addition to code for primary procedure)

(Use 22103 in conjunction with 22100, 22101, 22102)

22110   Partial excision of vertebral body, for intrinsic bony lesion, without decompression of spinal cord or nerve root(s), single vertebral segment; cervical

22112   thoracic

22114   lumbar

+ 22116   each additional vertebral segment (List separately in addition to code for primary procedure)

(Use 22116 in conjunction with 22110, 22112, 22114)

(For complete or near complete resection of vertebral body, see vertebral corpectomy, 63081-63091)

(For spinal reconstruction with bone graft [autograft, allograft] and/or methylmethacrylate of cervical vertebral body, use 63081 and 22554 and 20931 or 20938)

(For spinal reconstruction with bone graft [autograft, allograft] and/or methylmethacrylate of thoracic vertebral body, use 63085 or 63087 and 22556 and 20931 or 20938)

(For spinal reconstruction with bone graft [autograft, allograft] and/or methylmethacrylate of lumbar vertebral body, use 63087 or 63090 and 22558 and 20931 or 20938)

(For spinal reconstruction following vertebral body resection, use 63082 or 63086 or 63088 or 63091, and 22585)

(For harvest of bone autograft for vertebral reconstruction, see 20931 or 20938)

(For cervical spinal reconstruction with prosthetic replacement of resected vertebral bodies, see codes 63081 and 22554 and 20931 or 20938 and 22851)

(For thoracic spinal reconstruction with prosthetic replacement of resected vertebral bodies, see codes 63085 or 63087 and 22556 and 20931 or 20938 and 22851)

(For lumbar spinal reconstruction with prosthetic replacement of resected vertebral bodies, see codes 63087 or 63090 and 22558, and 20931 or 20938 and 22851)

(For osteotomy of spine, see 22210-22226)

Osteotomy

To report arthrodesis, see codes 22590-22632. (Report in addition to code[s] for the definitive procedure with modifier 51.)

To report instrumentation procedures, see 22840-22855. (Report in addition to code[s] for the definitive procedure[s].) Do not append modifier 62 to spinal instrumentation codes 22840-22848 and 22850-22852.

To report bone graft procedures, see 20930-20938. (Report in addition to code[s] for the definitive procedure[s].) Do not append modifier 62 to bone graft codes 20900-20938.

For the following codes, when two surgeons work together as primary surgeons performing distinct part(s) of an anterior spine osteotomy, each surgeon should report his/her distinct operative work by appending modifier 62 to the procedure code. In this situation, modifier 62 may be appended to the procedure code(s) 22210-22214, 22220-22224 and, as appropriate, to associated additional segment add-on code(s) 22216, 22226 as long as both surgeons continue to work together as primary surgeons.

Spinal osteotomy procedures are reported when a portion(s) of the vertebral segment(s) is cut and removed in preparation for re-aligning the spine as part of a spinal deformity correction. For excision of an intrinsic lesion of the vertebra without deformity correction, see 22100-22116. For decompression of the spinal cord and/or nerve roots, see 63001-63308.

The three columns are defined as anterior (anterior two-thirds of the vertebral body), middle (posterior third of the vertebral body and the pedicle), and posterior (articular facets, lamina, and spinous process).

Musculoskeletal

Musculoskeletal

22206 Osteotomy of spine, posterior or posterolateral approach, 3 columns, 1 vertebral segment (eg, pedicle/vertebral body subtraction); thoracic

(Do not report 22206 in conjunction with 22207)

22207 lumbar

(Do not report 22207 in conjunction with 22206)

+ 22208 each additional vertebral segment (List separately in addition to code for primary procedure)

(Use 22208 in conjunction with 22206, 22207)

(Do not report 22206, 22207, 22208 in conjunction with 22210-22226, 22830, 63001-63048, 63055-63066, 63075-63091, 63101-63103, when performed at the same level)

22210 Osteotomy of spine, posterior or posterolateral approach, 1 vertebral segment; cervical

22212 thoracic

22214 lumbar

+ 22216 each additional vertebral segment (List separately in addition to primary procedure)

(Use 22216 in conjunction with 22210, 22212, 22214)

22220 Osteotomy of spine, including discectomy, anterior approach, single vertebral segment; cervical

22222 thoracic

22224 lumbar

+ 22226 each additional vertebral segment (List separately in addition to code for primary procedure)

(Use 22226 in conjunction with 22220, 22222, 22224)

(For vertebral corpectomy, see 63081-63091)

Fracture and/or Dislocation

To report arthrodesis, see codes 22590-22632. (Report in addition to code[s] for the definitive procedure with modifier 51.)

To report instrumentation procedures, see 22840-22855. (Report in addition to code[s] for the definitive procedure[s].) Do not append modifier 62 to spinal instrumentation codes 22840-22848 and 22850-22852.

To report bone graft procedures, see 20930-20938. (Report in addition to code[s] for the definitive procedure[s].) Do not append modifier 62 to bone graft codes 20900-20938.

For the following codes, when two surgeons work together as primary surgeons performing distinct part(s) of open fracture and/or dislocation procedure(s), each surgeon should report his/her distinct operative work by appending modifier 62 to the procedure code. In this situation, modifier 62 may be appended to the procedure code(s) 22318-22327 and, as appropriate, the associated additional fracture vertebrae or dislocated segment add-on code 22328 as long as both surgeons continue to work together as primary surgeons.

22305 Closed treatment of vertebral process fracture(s)

22310 Closed treatment of vertebral body fracture(s), without manipulation, requiring and including casting or bracing

(Do not report 22310 in conjunction with 22510, 22511, 22512, 22513, 22514, 22515, when performed at the same level)

22315 Closed treatment of vertebral fracture(s) and/or dislocation(s) requiring casting or bracing, with and including casting and/or bracing by manipulation or traction

(Do not report 22315 in conjunction with 22510, 22511, 22512, 22513, 22514, 22515, when performed at the same level)

(For spinal subluxation, use 97140)

22318 Open treatment and/or reduction of odontoid fracture(s) and or dislocation(s) (including os odontoideum), anterior approach, including placement of internal fixation; without grafting

22319 with grafting

22325 Open treatment and/or reduction of vertebral fracture(s) and/or dislocation(s), posterior approach, 1 fractured vertebra or dislocated segment; lumbar

(Do not report 22325 in conjunction with 22511, 22512, 22514, 22515 when performed at the same level)

22326 cervical

(Do not report 22326 in conjunction with 22510, 22512, when performed at the same level)

22327 thoracic

(Do not report 22327 in conjunction with 22510, 22512, 22513, 22515 when performed at the same level)

+ 22328 each additional fractured vertebra or dislocated segment (List separately in addition to code for primary procedure)

(Use 22328 in conjunction with 22325-22327)

(For treatment of vertebral fracture by the anterior approach, see corpectomy 63081-63091, and appropriate arthrodesis, bone graft and instrument codes)

(For decompression of spine following fracture, see 63001-63091; for arthrodesis of spine following fracture, see 22548-22632)

Manipulation

(For spinal manipulation without anesthesia, use 97140)

22505 Manipulation of spine requiring anesthesia, any region

Percutaneous Vertebroplasty and Vertebral Augmentation

Codes 22510, 22511, 22512, 22513, 22514, 22515 describe procedures for percutaneous vertebral augmentation that include vertebroplasty of the cervical, thoracic, lumbar, and sacral spine and vertebral augmentation of the thoracic and lumbar spine.

For the purposes of reporting 22510, 22511, 22512, 22513, 22514, 22515, "vertebroplasty" is the process of injecting a material (cement) into the vertebral body to reinforce the structure of the body using image guidance. "Vertebral augmentation" is the process of cavity creation followed by the injection of the material (cement) under image guidance. For 0200T and 0201T, "sacral augmentation (sacroplasty)" refers to the creation of a cavity within a sacral vertebral body followed by injection of a material to fill that cavity.

The procedure codes are inclusive of bone biopsy when performed, moderate sedation, and imaging guidance necessary to perform the procedure. Use one primary procedure code and an add-on code for additional levels. When treating the sacrum, sacral procedures are reported only once per encounter.

⊙ **22510**   Percutaneous vertebroplasty (bone biopsy included when performed), 1 vertebral body, unilateral or bilateral injection, inclusive of all imaging guidance; cervicothoracic

⊙ **22511**   lumbosacral

⊙✚ **22512**   each additional cervicothoracic or lumbosacral vertebral body (List separately in addition to code for primary procedure)

(Use 22512 in conjunction with 22510, 22511)

(Do not report 22510, 22511, 22512 in conjunction with 20225, 22310, 22315, 22325, 22327, when performed at the same level as 22510, 22511, 22512)

⊙ **22513**   Percutaneous vertebral augmentation, including cavity creation (fracture reduction and bone biopsy included when performed) using mechanical device (eg, kyphoplasty), 1 vertebral body, unilateral or bilateral cannulation, inclusive of all imaging guidance; thoracic

⊙ **22514**   lumbar

⊙✚ **22515**   each additional thoracic or lumbar vertebral body (List separately in addition to code for primary procedure)

(Use 22515 in conjunction with 22513, 22514)

(Do not report 22513, 22514, 22515 in conjunction with 20225, 22310, 22315, 22325, 22327, when performed at the same level as 22513, 22514, 22515)

Percutaneous Augmentation and Annuloplasty

(22520, 22521, 22522, 22523, 22524, 22525 have been deleted. To report, see 22510, 22511, 22512, 22513, 22514, 22515)

⊙ **22526**   Percutaneous intradiscal electrothermal annuloplasty, unilateral or bilateral including fluoroscopic guidance; single level

⊙✚ **22527**   1 or more additional levels (List separately in addition to code for primary procedure)

(Use 22527 in conjunction with 22526)

(Do not report codes 22526, 22527 in conjunction with 77002, 77003)

(For percutaneous intradiscal annuloplasty using method other than electrothermal, use 22899)

Arthrodesis

Arthrodesis may be performed in the absence of other procedures and therefore when it is combined with another definitive procedure (eg, osteotomy, fracture care, vertebral corpectomy or laminectomy), modifier 51 is appropriate. However, arthrodesis codes 22585, 22614, and 22632 are considered add-on procedure codes and should not be used with modifier 51.

To report instrumentation procedures, see 22840-22855. (Codes 22840-22848, 22851 are reported in conjunction with code[s] for the definitive procedure[s]. When instrumentation reinsertion or removal is reported in conjunction with other definitive procedures including arthrodesis, decompression, and exploration of fusion, append modifier 51 to 22849, 22850, 22852, and 22855.) To report exploration of fusion, use 22830. (When exploration is reported in conjunction with other definitive procedures, including arthrodesis and decompression, append modifier 51 to 22830.) Do not append modifier 62 to spinal instrumentation codes 22840-22848 and 22850-22852.

To report bone graft procedures, see 20930-20938. (Report in addition to code[s] for the definitive procedure[s].) Do not append modifier 62 to bone graft codes 20900-20938.

Lateral Extracavitary Approach Technique

22532   Arthrodesis, lateral extracavitary technique, including minimal discectomy to prepare interspace (other than for decompression); thoracic

22533   lumbar

✚ **22534**   thoracic or lumbar, each additional vertebral segment (List separately in addition to code for primary procedure)

(Use 22534 in conjunction with 22532 and 22533)

Anterior or Anterolateral Approach Technique

Procedure codes 22554-22558 are for SINGLE interspace; for additional interspaces, use 22585. A vertebral interspace is the non-bony compartment between two adjacent vertebral bodies, which contains the intervertebral disc, and includes the nucleus pulposus, annulus fibrosus, and two cartilagenous endplates.

Musculoskeletal

For the following codes, when two surgeons work together as primary surgeons performing distinct part(s) of an anterior interbody arthrodesis, each surgeon should report his/her distinct operative work by appending modifier 62 to the procedure code. In this situation, modifier 62 may be appended to the procedure code(s) 22548-22558 and, as appropriate, to the associated additional interspace add-on code 22585 as long as both surgeons continue to work together as primary surgeons.

22548 Arthrodesis, anterior transoral or extraoral technique, clivus-C1-C2 (atlas-axis), with or without excision of odontoid process

(For intervertebral disc excision by laminotomy or laminectomy, see 63020-63042)

22551 Arthrodesis, anterior interbody, including disc space preparation, discectomy, osteophytectomy and decompression of spinal cord and/or nerve roots; cervical below C2

✛ **22552** cervical below C2, each additional interspace (List separately in addition to code for separate procedure)

(Use 22552 in conjunction with 22551)

22554 Arthrodesis, anterior interbody technique, including minimal discectomy to prepare interspace (other than for decompression); cervical below C2

(Do not report 22554 in conjunction with 63075, even if performed by a separate individual. To report anterior cervical discectomy and interbody fusion at the same level during the same session, use 22551)

22556 thoracic

22558 lumbar

(For arthrodesis using pre-sacral interbody technique, see 22586, 0195T)

✛ **22585** each additional interspace (List separately in addition to code for primary procedure)

(Use 22585 in conjunction with 22554, 22556, 22558)

(Do not report 22585 in conjunction with 63075, even if performed by a separate individual. To report anterior cervical discectomy and interbody fusion at the same level during the same session, use 22552)

22586 Arthrodesis, pre-sacral interbody technique, including disc space preparation, discectomy, with posterior instrumentation, with image guidance, includes bone graft when performed, L5-S1 interspace

(Do not report 22586 in conjunction with 20930-20938, 22840, 22848, 72275, 77002, 77003, 77011, 77012)

Posterior, Posterolateral or Lateral Transverse Process Technique

To report instrumentation procedures, see 22840-22855. (Report in addition to code[s] for the definitive procedure[s].) Do not append modifier 62 to spinal instrumentation codes 22840-22848 and 22850-22852.

To report bone graft procedures, see 20930-20938. (Report in addition to code[s] for the definitive procedure[s].) Do not append modifier 62 to bone graft codes 20900-20938.

A vertebral segment describes the basic constituent part into which the spine may be divided. It represents a single complete vertebral bone with its associated articular processes and laminae. A vertebral interspace is the non-bony compartment between two adjacent vertebral bodies which contains the intervertebral disc, and includes the nucleus pulposus, annulus fibrosus, and two cartilagenous endplates.

22590 Arthrodesis, posterior technique, craniocervical (occiput-C2)

22595 Arthrodesis, posterior technique, atlas-axis (C1-C2)

22600 Arthrodesis, posterior or posterolateral technique, single level; cervical below C2 segment

22610 thoracic (with lateral transverse technique, when performed)

22612 lumbar (with lateral transverse technique, when performed)

(Do not report 22612 in conjunction with 22630 for the same interspace and segment, use 22633)

✛ **22614** each additional vertebral segment (List separately in addition to code for primary procedure)

(Use 22614 in conjunction with 22600, 22610, 22612, 22630 or 22633 when performed at a different level. When performing a posterior or posterolateral technique for fusion/arthrodesis at an additional level, use 22614. When performing a posterior interbody fusion arthrodesis at an additional level, use 22632. When performing a combined posterior or posterolateral technique with posterior interbody arthrodesis at an additional level, use 22634)

(For facet joint fusion, see 0219T-0222T)

(For placement of a posterior intrafacet implant, see 0219T-0222T)

22630 Arthrodesis, posterior interbody technique, including laminectomy and/or discectomy to prepare interspace (other than for decompression), single interspace; lumbar

(Do not report 22630 in conjunction with 22612 for the same interspace and segment, use 22633)

✛ **22632** each additional interspace (List separately in addition to code for primary procedure)

(Use 22632 in conjunction with 22612, 22630, or 22633 when performed at a different level. When performing a posterior interbody fusion arthrodesis at an additional level, use 22632. When performing a posterior or posterolateral technique for fusion/arthrodesis at an additional level, use 22614. When performing a combined posterior or posterolateral technique with posterior interbody arthrodesis at an additional level, use 22634)

22633   Arthrodesis, combined posterior or posterolateral technique with posterior interbody technique including laminectomy and/or discectomy sufficient to prepare interspace (other than for decompression), single interspace and segment; lumbar

(Do not report with 22612 or 22630 at the same level)

+ 22634   each additional interspace and segment (List separately in addition to code for primary procedure)

(Use 22634 in conjunction with 22633)

Spine Deformity (eg, Scoliosis, Kyphosis)

To report instrumentation procedures, see 22840-22855. (Report in addition to code[s] for the definitive procedure[s].) Do not append modifier 62 to spinal instrumentation codes 22840-22848 and 22850-22852.

To report bone graft procedures, see 20930-20938. (Report in addition to code[s] for the definitive procedure[s].) Do not append modifier 62 to bone graft codes 20900-20938.

A vertebral segment describes the basic constituent part into which the spine may be divided. It represents a single complete vertebral bone with its associated articular processes and laminae.

For the following codes, when two surgeons work together as primary surgeons performing distinct part(s) of an arthrodesis for spinal deformity, each surgeon should report his/her distinct operative work by appending modifier 62 to the procedure code. In this situation, modifier 62 may be appended to procedure code(s) 22800-22819 as long as both surgeons continue to work together as primary surgeons.

22800   Arthrodesis, posterior, for spinal deformity, with or without cast; up to 6 vertebral segments

22802   7 to 12 vertebral segments

22804   13 or more vertebral segments

22808   Arthrodesis, anterior, for spinal deformity, with or without cast; 2 to 3 vertebral segments

22810   4 to 7 vertebral segments

22812   8 or more vertebral segments

22818   Kyphectomy, circumferential exposure of spine and resection of vertebral segment(s) (including body and posterior elements); single or 2 segments

22819   3 or more segments

(To report arthrodesis, see 22800-22804 and add modifier 51)

Exploration

To report instrumentation procedures, see 22840-22855. (Codes 22840-22848 and 22851 are reported in conjunction with code[s] for the definitive procedure[s].

When instrumentation reinsertion or removal is reported in conjunction with other definitive procedures including arthrodesis, decompression, and exploration of fusion, append modifier 51 to 22849, 22850, 22852 and 22855.) Code 22849 should not be reported with 22850, 22852, and 22855 at the same spinal levels. To report exploration of fusion, see 22830. (When exploration is reported in conjunction with other definitive procedures, including arthrodesis and decompression, append modifier 51 to 22830.)

(To report bone graft procedures, see 20930-20938)

22830   Exploration of spinal fusion

Spinal Instrumentation

Segmental instrumentation is defined as fixation at each end of the construct and at least one additional interposed bony attachment.

Non-segmental instrumentation is defined as fixation at each end of the construct and may span several vertebral segments without attachment to the intervening segments.

Insertion of spinal instrumentation is reported separately and in addition to arthrodesis. Instrumentation procedure codes 22840-22848 and 22851 are reported in addition to the definitive procedure(s). Do not append modifier 62 to spinal instrumentation codes 22840-22848 and 22850-22852.

To report bone graft procedures, see 20930-20938. (Report in addition to code[s] for definitive procedure[s].) Do not append modifier 62 to bone graft codes 20900-20938.

A vertebral segment describes the basic constituent part into which the spine may be divided. It represents a single complete vertebral bone with its associated articular processes and laminae. A vertebral interspace is the non-bony compartment between two adjacent vertebral bodies, which contains the intervertebral disc, and includes the nucleus pulposus, annulus fibrosus, and two cartilagenous endplates.

Codes 22849, 22850, 22852, and 22855 are subject to modifier 51 if reported with other definitive procedure(s), including arthrodesis, decompression, and exploration of fusion. Code 22849 should not be reported in conjunction with 22850, 22852, and 22855 at the same spinal levels. Only the appropriate insertion code (22840-22848) should be reported when previously placed spinal instrumentation is being removed or revised during the same session where new instrumentation is inserted at levels including all or part of the previously instrumented segments. Do not report the reinsertion (22849) or removal (22850, 22852, 22855) procedures in addition to the insertion of the new instrumentation (22840-22848).

Musculoskeletal

+ **22840** Posterior non-segmental instrumentation (eg, Harrington rod technique, pedicle fixation across 1 interspace, atlantoaxial transarticular screw fixation, sublaminar wiring at C1, facet screw fixation) (List separately in addition to code for primary procedure)

(Use 22840 in conjunction with 22100-22102, 22110-22114, 22206, 22207, 22210-22214, 22220-22224, 22305-22327, 22532, 22533, 22548-22558, 22590-22612, 22630, 22633, 22634, 22800-22812, 63001-63030, 63040-63042, 63045-63047, 63050-63056, 63064, 63075, 63077, 63081, 63085, 63087, 63090, 63101, 63102, 63170-63290, 63300-63307)

(For insertion of posterior spinous process distraction devices, see 0171T, 0172T)

+ **22841** Internal spinal fixation by wiring of spinous processes (List separately in addition to code for primary procedure)

(Use 22841 in conjunction with 22100-22102, 22110-22114, 22206, 22207, 22210-22214, 22220-22224, 22305-22327, 22532, 22533, 22548-22558, 22590-22612, 22630, 22633, 22634, 22800-22812, 63001-63030, 63040-63042, 63045-63047, 63050-63056, 63064, 63075, 63077, 63081, 63085, 63087, 63090, 63101, 63102, 63170-63290, 63300-63307)

+ **22842** Posterior segmental instrumentation (eg, pedicle fixation, dual rods with multiple hooks and sublaminar wires); 3 to 6 vertebral segments (List separately in addition to code for primary procedure)

(Use 22842 in conjunction with 22100-22102, 22110-22114, 22206, 22207, 22210-22214, 22220-22224, 22305-22327, 22532, 22533, 22548-22558, 22590-22612, 22630, 22633, 22634, 22800-22812, 63001-63030, 63040-63042, 63045-63047, 63050-63056, 63064, 63075, 63077, 63081, 63085, 63087, 63090, 63101, 63102, 63170-63290, 63300-63307)

+ **22843** 7 to 12 vertebral segments (List separately in addition to code for primary procedure)

(Use 22843 in conjunction with 22100-22102, 22110-22114, 22206, 22207, 22210-22214, 22220-22224, 22305-22327, 22532, 22533, 22548-22558, 22590-22612, 22630, 22633, 22634, 22800-22812, 63001-63030, 63040-63042, 63045-63047, 63050-63056, 63064, 63075, 63077, 63081, 63085, 63087, 63090, 63101, 63102, 63170-63290, 63300-63307)

+ **22844** 13 or more vertebral segments (List separately in addition to code for primary procedure)

(Use 22844 in conjunction with 22100-22102, 22110-22114, 22206, 22207, 22210-22214, 22220-22224, 22305-22327, 22532, 22533, 22548-22558, 22590-22612, 22630, 22633, 22634, 22800-22812, 63001-63030, 63040-63042, 63045-63047, 63050-63056, 63064, 63075, 63077, 63081, 63085, 63087, 63090, 63101, 63102, 63170-63290, 63300-63307)

+ **22845** Anterior instrumentation; 2 to 3 vertebral segments (List separately in addition to code for primary procedure)

(Use 22845 in conjunction with 22100-22102, 22110-22114, 22206, 22207, 22210-22214, 22220-22224, 22305-22327, 22532, 22533, 22548-22558, 22590-22612, 22630, 22633, 22634, 22800-22812, 63001-63030, 63040-63042, 63045-63047, 63050-63056, 63064, 63075, 63077, 63081, 63085, 63087, 63090, 63101, 63102, 63170-63290, 63300-63307)

+ **22846** 4 to 7 vertebral segments (List separately in addition to code for primary procedure)

(Use 22846 in conjunction with 22100-22102, 22110-22114, 22206, 22207, 22210-22214, 22220-22224, 22305-22327, 22532, 22533, 22548-22558, 22590-22612, 22630, 22633, 22634, 22800-22812, 63001-63030, 63040-63042, 63045-63047, 63050-63056, 63064, 63075, 63077, 63081, 63085, 63087, 63090, 63101, 63102, 63170-63290, 63300-63307)

+ **22847** 8 or more vertebral segments (List separately in addition to code for primary procedure)

(Use 22847 in conjunction with 22100-22102, 22110-22114, 22206, 22207, 22210-22214, 22220-22224, 22305-22327, 22532, 22533, 22548-22558, 22590-22612, 22630, 22633, 22634, 22800-22812, 63001-63030, 63040-63042, 63045-63047, 63050-63056, 63064, 63075, 63077, 63081, 63085, 63087, 63090, 63101, 63102, 63170-63290, 63300-63307)

+ **22848** Pelvic fixation (attachment of caudal end of instrumentation to pelvic bony structures) other than sacrum (List separately in addition to code for primary procedure)

(Use 22848 in conjunction with 22100-22102, 22110-22114, 22206, 22207, 22210-22214, 22220-22224, 22305-22327, 22532, 22533, 22548-22558, 22590-22612, 22630, 22633, 22634, 22800-22812, 63001-63030, 63040-63042, 63045-63047, 63050-63056, 63064, 63075, 63077, 63081, 63085, 63087, 63090, 63101, 63102, 63170-63290, 63300-63307)

22849 Reinsertion of spinal fixation device

22850 Removal of posterior nonsegmental instrumentation (eg, Harrington rod)

+ **22851** Application of intervertebral biomechanical device(s) (eg, synthetic cage(s), methylmethacrylate) to vertebral defect or interspace (List separately in addition to code for primary procedure)

(Use 22851 in conjunction with 22100-22102, 22110-22114, 22206, 22207, 22210-22214, 22220-22224, 22305-22327, 22532, 22533, 22548-22558, 22590-22612, 22630, 22633, 22634, 22800-22812, 63001-63030, 63040-63042, 63045-63047, 63050-63056, 63064, 63075, 63077, 63081, 63085, 63087, 63090, 63101, 63102, 63170-63290, 63300-63307)

(For application of an intervertebral bone device/graft, see 20930-20938)

(For insertion of posterior spinous process distraction devices, see 0171T, 0172T)

22852 Removal of posterior segmental instrumentation

22855   Removal of anterior instrumentation

22856   Total disc arthroplasty (artificial disc), anterior approach, including discectomy with end plate preparation (includes osteophytectomy for nerve root or spinal cord decompression and microdissection); single interspace, cervical

(Do not report 22856 in conjunction with 22554, 22845, 22851, 63075, 0375T, when performed at the same level)

(Do not report 22856 in conjunction with 69990)

(For additional interspace cervical total disc arthroplasty, see 22858, 0375T)

#+ 22858   second level, cervical (List separately in addition to code for primary procedure)

(Use 22858 in conjunction with 22856)

(Do not report 22858 in conjunction with 0375T, when performed at the same level)

22857   Total disc arthroplasty (artificial disc), anterior approach, including discectomy to prepare interspace (other than for decompression), single interspace, lumbar

(Do not report 22857 in conjunction with 22558, 22845, 22851, 49010 when performed at the same level)

(For additional interspace, use Category III code 0163T)

22858   Code is out of numerical sequence. See 22840-22865

22861   Revision including replacement of total disc arthroplasty (artificial disc), anterior approach, single interspace; cervical

(Do not report 22861 in conjunction with 22845, 22851, 22864, 63075 when performed at the same level)

(Do not report 22861 in conjunction with 69990)

(For additional interspace revision of cervical total disc arthroplasty, use 0098T)

22862   lumbar

(Do not report 22862 in conjunction with 22558, 22845, 22851, 22865, 49010 when performed at the same level)

(For additional interspace, use Category III code 0165T)

22864   Removal of total disc arthroplasty (artificial disc), anterior approach, single interspace; cervical

(Do not report 22864 in conjunction with 22861, 69990)

(For additional interspace removal of cervical total disc arthroplasty, use 0095T)

22865   lumbar

(Do not report 22865 in conjunction with 49010)

(For additional interspace, see Category III code 0164T)

(22856-22865 include fluoroscopy when performed)

(For decompression, see 63001-63048)

Other Procedures

22899   Unlisted procedure, spine

Abdomen

Excision

22900   Excision, tumor, soft tissue of abdominal wall, subfascial (eg, intramuscular); less than 5 cm

22901   5 cm or greater

22902   Excision, tumor, soft tissue of abdominal wall, subcutaneous; less than 3 cm

22903   3 cm or greater

(For excision of benign lesions of cutaneous origin [eg, sebaceous cyst], see 11400-11406)

22904   Radical resection of tumor (eg, sarcoma), soft tissue of abdominal wall; less than 5 cm

22905   5 cm or greater

(For radical resection of tumor[s] of cutaneous origin [eg, melanoma], see 11600-11606)

Other Procedures

22999   Unlisted procedure, abdomen, musculoskeletal system

Shoulder

The area known as the shoulder is made up of the clavicle, scapula, humerus head and neck, sterno-clavicular joint, acromioclavicular joint, and shoulder joint.

Incision

23000   Removal of subdeltoid calcareous deposits, open

(For arthroscopic removal of bursal deposits, use 29999)

23020   Capsular contracture release (eg, Sever type procedure)

(For incision and drainage procedures, superficial, see 10040-10160)

23030   Incision and drainage, shoulder area; deep abscess or hematoma

23031   infected bursa

23035   Incision, bone cortex (eg, osteomyelitis or bone abscess), shoulder area

23040   Arthrotomy, glenohumeral joint, including exploration, drainage, or removal of foreign body

23044   Arthrotomy, acromioclavicular, sternoclavicular joint, including exploration, drainage, or removal of foreign body

Musculoskeletal

Musculoskeletal

Excision

23065 Biopsy, soft tissue of shoulder area; superficial

23066 deep

(For needle biopsy of soft tissue, use 20206)

23071 Code is out of numerical sequence. See 23065-23220

23073 Code is out of numerical sequence. See 23065-23220

23075 Excision, tumor, soft tissue of shoulder area, subcutaneous; less than 3 cm

23071 3 cm or greater

(For excision of benign lesions of cutaneous origin [eg, sebaceous cyst], see 11400-11406)

23076 Excision, tumor, soft tissue of shoulder area, subfascial (eg, intramuscular); less than 5 cm

23073 5 cm or greater

23077 Radical resection of tumor (eg, sarcoma), soft tissue of shoulder area; less than 5 cm

23078 5 cm or greater

(For radical resection of tumor[s] of cutaneous origin [eg, melanoma], see 11600-11606)

23100 Arthrotomy, glenohumeral joint, including biopsy

23101 Arthrotomy, acromioclavicular joint or sternoclavicular joint, including biopsy and/or excision of torn cartilage

23105 Arthrotomy; glenohumeral joint, with synovectomy, with or without biopsy

23106 sternoclavicular joint, with synovectomy, with or without biopsy

23107 Arthrotomy, glenohumeral joint, with joint exploration, with or without removal of loose or foreign body

23120 Claviculectomy; partial

(For arthroscopic procedure, use 29824)

23125 total

23130 Acromioplasty or acromionectomy, partial, with or without coracoacromial ligament release

23140 Excision or curettage of bone cyst or benign tumor of clavicle or scapula;

23145 with autograft (includes obtaining graft)

23146 with allograft

23150 Excision or curettage of bone cyst or benign tumor of proximal humerus;

23155 with autograft (includes obtaining graft)

23156 with allograft

23170 Sequestrectomy (eg, for osteomyelitis or bone abscess), clavicle

23172 Sequestrectomy (eg, for osteomyelitis or bone abscess), scapula

23174 Sequestrectomy (eg, for osteomyelitis or bone abscess), humeral head to surgical neck

23180 Partial excision (craterization, saucerization, or diaphysectomy) bone (eg, osteomyelitis), clavicle

23182 Partial excision (craterization, saucerization, or diaphysectomy) bone (eg, osteomyelitis), scapula

23184 Partial excision (craterization, saucerization, or diaphysectomy) bone (eg, osteomyelitis), proximal humerus

23190 Ostectomy of scapula, partial (eg, superior medial angle)

23195 Resection, humeral head

(For replacement with implant, use 23470)

23200 Radical resection of tumor; clavicle

23210 scapula

23220 Radical resection of tumor, proximal humerus

(23221, 23222 have been deleted)

Introduction or Removal

(For arthrocentesis or needling of bursa, use 20610)

(For K-wire or pin insertion or removal, see 20650, 20670, 20680)

23330 Removal of foreign body, shoulder; subcutaneous

(23331, 23332 have been deleted)

(To report removal of foreign body, see 23330, 23333)

23333 deep (subfascial or intramuscular)

23334 Removal of prosthesis, includes debridement and synovectomy when performed; humeral **or** glenoid component

23335 humeral **and** glenoid components (eg, total shoulder)

(Do not report 23334, 23335 in conjunction with 23473, 23474 if a prosthesis [ie, humeral and/or glenoid component(s)] is being removed and replaced in the same shoulder during the same surgical session)

(To report removal of hardware, other than humeral and/or glenoid prosthesis, use 20680)

23350 Injection procedure for shoulder arthrography or enhanced CT/MRI shoulder arthrography

(For radiographic arthrography, radiological supervision and interpretation, use 73040. Fluoroscopy [77002] is inclusive of radiographic arthrography)

(When fluoroscopic guided injection is performed for enhanced CT arthrography, use 23350, 77002, and 73201 or 73202)

(When fluoroscopic guided injection is performed for enhanced MR arthrography, use 23350, 77002, and 73222 or 73223)

⊙=Moderate sedation   ✚=Add-on code   ✗=FDA approval pending   #=Resequenced code   ○=Recycled/reinstated code

(For enhanced CT or enhanced MRI arthrography, use 77002 and either 73201, 73202, 73222, or 73223)

(To report biopsy of the shoulder and joint, see 29805-29826)

Repair, Revision, and/or Reconstruction

23395 Muscle transfer, any type, shoulder or upper arm; single

23397   multiple

23400 Scapulopexy (eg, Sprengels deformity or for paralysis)

23405 Tenotomy, shoulder area; single tendon

23406   multiple tendons through same incision

23410 Repair of ruptured musculotendinous cuff (eg, rotator cuff) open; acute

23412   chronic

(For arthroscopic procedure, use 29827)

23415 Coracoacromial ligament release, with or without acromioplasty

(For arthroscopic procedure, use 29826)

23420 Reconstruction of complete shoulder (rotator) cuff avulsion, chronic (includes acromioplasty)

23430 Tenodesis of long tendon of biceps

(For arthroscopic biceps tenodesis, use 29828)

23440 Resection or transplantation of long tendon of biceps

23450 Capsulorrhaphy, anterior; Putti-Platt procedure or Magnuson type operation

(To report arthroscopic thermal capsulorrhaphy, use 29999)

23455   with labral repair (eg, Bankart procedure)

(For arthroscopic procedure, use 29806)

23460 Capsulorrhaphy, anterior, any type; with bone block

23462   with coracoid process transfer

(To report open thermal capsulorrhaphy, use 23929)

23465 Capsulorrhaphy, glenohumeral joint, posterior, with or without bone block

(For sternoclavicular and acromioclavicular reconstruction, see 23530, 23550)

23466 Capsulorrhaphy, glenohumeral joint, any type multi-directional instability

23470 Arthroplasty, glenohumeral joint; hemiarthroplasty

23472   total shoulder (glenoid and proximal humeral replacement (eg, total shoulder))

(For removal of total shoulder implants, see 23334, 23335)

(For osteotomy, proximal humerus, use 24400)

23473 Revision of total shoulder arthroplasty, including allograft when performed; humeral **or** glenoid component

23474   humeral **and** glenoid component

(Do not report 23473, 23474 in conjunction with 23334, 23335 if a prosthesis [ie, humeral and/or glenoid component(s)] is being removed and replaced in the same shoulder during the same surgical session)

23480 Osteotomy, clavicle, with or without internal fixation;

23485   with bone graft for nonunion or malunion (includes obtaining graft and/or necessary fixation)

23490 Prophylactic treatment (nailing, pinning, plating or wiring) with or without methylmethacrylate; clavicle

23491   proximal humerus

Fracture and/or Dislocation

23500 Closed treatment of clavicular fracture; without manipulation

23505   with manipulation

23515 Open treatment of clavicular fracture, includes internal fixation, when performed

23520 Closed treatment of sternoclavicular dislocation; without manipulation

23525   with manipulation

23530 Open treatment of sternoclavicular dislocation, acute or chronic;

23532   with fascial graft (includes obtaining graft)

23540 Closed treatment of acromioclavicular dislocation; without manipulation

23545   with manipulation

23550 Open treatment of acromioclavicular dislocation, acute or chronic;

23552   with fascial graft (includes obtaining graft)

23570 Closed treatment of scapular fracture; without manipulation

23575   with manipulation, with or without skeletal traction (with or without shoulder joint involvement)

23585 Open treatment of scapular fracture (body, glenoid or acromion) includes internal fixation, when performed

23600 Closed treatment of proximal humeral (surgical or anatomical neck) fracture; without manipulation

23605   with manipulation, with or without skeletal traction

23615 Open treatment of proximal humeral (surgical or anatomical neck) fracture, includes internal fixation, when performed, includes repair of tuberosity(s), when performed;

23616   with proximal humeral prosthetic replacement

23620 Closed treatment of greater humeral tuberosity fracture; without manipulation

23625   with manipulation

Musculoskeletal

23630 Open treatment of greater humeral tuberosity fracture, includes internal fixation, when performed

23650 Closed treatment of shoulder dislocation, with manipulation; without anesthesia

23655   requiring anesthesia

23660 Open treatment of acute shoulder dislocation

(Repairs for recurrent dislocations, see 23450-23466)

23665 Closed treatment of shoulder dislocation, with fracture of greater humeral tuberosity, with manipulation

23670 Open treatment of shoulder dislocation, with fracture of greater humeral tuberosity, includes internal fixation, when performed

23675 Closed treatment of shoulder dislocation, with surgical or anatomical neck fracture, with manipulation

23680 Open treatment of shoulder dislocation, with surgical or anatomical neck fracture, includes internal fixation, when performed

Manipulation

23700 Manipulation under anesthesia, shoulder joint, including application of fixation apparatus (dislocation excluded)

Arthrodesis

23800 Arthrodesis, glenohumeral joint;

23802   with autogenous graft (includes obtaining graft)

Amputation

23900 Interthoracoscapular amputation (forequarter)

23920 Disarticulation of shoulder;

23921   secondary closure or scar revision

Other Procedures

23929 Unlisted procedure, shoulder

Humerus (Upper Arm) and Elbow

The elbow area includes the head and neck of the radius and olecranon process.

Incision

(For incision and drainage procedures, superficial, see 10040-10160)

23930 Incision and drainage, upper arm or elbow area; deep abscess or hematoma

23931   bursa

23935 Incision, deep, with opening of bone cortex (eg, for osteomyelitis or bone abscess), humerus or elbow

24000 Arthrotomy, elbow, including exploration, drainage, or removal of foreign body

24006 Arthrotomy of the elbow, with capsular excision for capsular release (separate procedure)

Excision

24065 Biopsy, soft tissue of upper arm or elbow area; superficial

24066   deep (subfascial or intramuscular)

(For needle biopsy of soft tissue, use 20206)

24071 Code is out of numerical sequence. See 24065-24155

24073 Code is out of numerical sequence. See 24065-24155

24075 Excision, tumor, soft tissue of upper arm or elbow area, subcutaneous; less than 3 cm

 # 24071   3 cm or greater

(For excision of benign lesions of cutaneous origin [eg, sebaceous cyst], see 11400-11406)

24076 Excision, tumor, soft tissue of upper arm or elbow area, subfascial (eg, intramuscular); less than 5 cm

 # 24073   5 cm or greater

24077 Radical resection of tumor (eg, sarcoma), soft tissue of upper arm or elbow area; less than 5 cm

24079   5 cm or greater

(For radical resection of tumor[s] of cutaneous origin [eg, melanoma], see 11600-11606)

24100 Arthrotomy, elbow; with synovial biopsy only

24101   with joint exploration, with or without biopsy, with or without removal of loose or foreign body

24102   with synovectomy

24105 Excision, olecranon bursa

24110 Excision or curettage of bone cyst or benign tumor, humerus;

24115   with autograft (includes obtaining graft)

24116   with allograft

24120 Excision or curettage of bone cyst or benign tumor of head or neck of radius or olecranon process;

24125   with autograft (includes obtaining graft)

24126   with allograft

24130 Excision, radial head

(For replacement with implant, use 24366)

24134 Sequestrectomy (eg, for osteomyelitis or bone abscess), shaft or distal humerus

24136 Sequestrectomy (eg, for osteomyelitis or bone abscess), radial head or neck

24138 Sequestrectomy (eg, for osteomyelitis or bone abscess), olecranon process

24140   Partial excision (craterization, saucerization, or diaphysectomy) bone (eg, osteomyelitis), humerus

24145   Partial excision (craterization, saucerization, or diaphysectomy) bone (eg, osteomyelitis), radial head or neck

24147   Partial excision (craterization, saucerization, or diaphysectomy) bone (eg, osteomyelitis), olecranon process

24149   Radical resection of capsule, soft tissue, and heterotopic bone, elbow, with contracture release (separate procedure)

(For capsular and soft tissue release only, use 24006)

24150   Radical resection of tumor, shaft or distal humerus

24152   Radical resection of tumor, radial head or neck

24155   Resection of elbow joint (arthrectomy)

Introduction or Removal

(For K-wire or pin insertion or removal, see 20650, 20670, 20680)

(For arthrocentesis or needling of bursa or joint, use 20605)

24160   Removal of prosthesis, includes debridement and synovectomy when performed; humeral **and** ulnar components

(To report removal of foreign body, elbow, see 24200, 24201)

(To report removal of hardware from the distal humerus or proximal ulna, other than humeral and ulnar prosthesis, use 20680)

(Do not report 24160 in conjunction with 24370 or 24371 if a prosthesis [ie, humeral and/or ulnar component(s)] is being removed and replaced in the same elbow during the same surgical session)

24164   radial head

(To report removal of foreign body, elbow, see 24200, 24201)

(To report removal of hardware from proximal radius, other than radial head prosthesis, use 20680)

24200   Removal of foreign body, upper arm or elbow area; subcutaneous

24201   deep (subfascial or intramuscular)

24220   Injection procedure for elbow arthrography

(For radiological supervision and interpretation, use 73085. Do not report 77002 in conjunction with 73085)

(For injection for tennis elbow, use 20550)

Repair, Revision, and/or Reconstruction

24300   Manipulation, elbow, under anesthesia

(For application of external fixation, see 20690 or 20692)

24301   Muscle or tendon transfer, any type, upper arm or elbow, single (excluding 24320-24331)

24305   Tendon lengthening, upper arm or elbow, each tendon

24310   Tenotomy, open, elbow to shoulder, each tendon

24320   Tenoplasty, with muscle transfer, with or without free graft, elbow to shoulder, single (Seddon-Brookes type procedure)

24330   Flexor-plasty, elbow (eg, Steindler type advancement);

24331   with extensor advancement

24332   Tenolysis, triceps

24340   Tenodesis of biceps tendon at elbow (separate procedure)

24341   Repair, tendon or muscle, upper arm or elbow, each tendon or muscle, primary or secondary (excludes rotator cuff)

24342   Reinsertion of ruptured biceps or triceps tendon, distal, with or without tendon graft

24343   Repair lateral collateral ligament, elbow, with local tissue

24344   Reconstruction lateral collateral ligament, elbow, with tendon graft (includes harvesting of graft)

24345   Repair medial collateral ligament, elbow, with local tissue

24346   Reconstruction medial collateral ligament, elbow, with tendon graft (includes harvesting of graft)

24357   Tenotomy, elbow, lateral or medial (eg, epicondylitis, tennis elbow, golfer's elbow); percutaneous

24358   debridement, soft tissue and/or bone, open

24359   debridement, soft tissue and/or bone, open with tendon repair or reattachment

(Do not report 24357-24359 in conjunction with 29837, 29838)

24360   Arthroplasty, elbow; with membrane (eg, fascial)

24361   with distal humeral prosthetic replacement

24362   with implant and fascia lata ligament reconstruction

24363   with distal humerus and proximal ulnar prosthetic replacement (eg, total elbow)

(For revision of total elbow implant, see 24370, 24371)

24365   Arthroplasty, radial head;

24366   with implant

24370   Revision of total elbow arthroplasty, including allograft when performed; humeral **or** ulnar component

24371   humeral **and** ulnar component

(Do not report 24370, 24371 in conjunction with 24160 if a prosthesis [ie, humeral and/or ulnar component(s)] is being removed and replaced in the same elbow)

24400   Osteotomy, humerus, with or without internal fixation

Musculoskeletal

Musculoskeletal

24410 Multiple osteotomies with realignment on intramedullary rod, humeral shaft (Sofield type procedure)

24420 Osteoplasty, humerus (eg, shortening or lengthening) (excluding 64876)

24430 Repair of nonunion or malunion, humerus; without graft (eg, compression technique)

24435 with iliac or other autograft (includes obtaining graft)

(For proximal radius and/or ulna, see 25400-25420)

24470 Hemiepiphyseal arrest (eg, cubitus varus or valgus, distal humerus)

24495 Decompression fasciotomy, forearm, with brachial artery exploration

24498 Prophylactic treatment (nailing, pinning, plating or wiring), with or without methylmethacrylate, humeral shaft

Fracture and/or Dislocation

24500 Closed treatment of humeral shaft fracture; without manipulation

24505 with manipulation, with or without skeletal traction

24515 Open treatment of humeral shaft fracture with plate/screws, with or without cerclage

24516 Treatment of humeral shaft fracture, with insertion of intramedullary implant, with or without cerclage and/or locking screws

24530 Closed treatment of supracondylar or transcondylar humeral fracture, with or without intercondylar extension; without manipulation

24535 with manipulation, with or without skin or skeletal traction

24538 Percutaneous skeletal fixation of supracondylar or transcondylar humeral fracture, with or without intercondylar extension

24545 Open treatment of humeral supracondylar or transcondylar fracture, includes internal fixation, when performed; without intercondylar extension

24546 with intercondylar extension

24560 Closed treatment of humeral epicondylar fracture, medial or lateral; without manipulation

24565 with manipulation

24566 Percutaneous skeletal fixation of humeral epicondylar fracture, medial or lateral, with manipulation

24575 Open treatment of humeral epicondylar fracture, medial or lateral, includes internal fixation, when performed

24576 Closed treatment of humeral condylar fracture, medial or lateral; without manipulation

24577 with manipulation

24579 Open treatment of humeral condylar fracture, medial or lateral, includes internal fixation, when performed

(To report closed treatment of fractures without manipulation, see 24530, 24560, 24576, 24650, 24670)

(To report closed treatment of fractures with manipulation, see 24535, 24565, 24577, 24675)

24582 Percutaneous skeletal fixation of humeral condylar fracture, medial or lateral, with manipulation

24586 Open treatment of periarticular fracture and/or dislocation of the elbow (fracture distal humerus and proximal ulna and/or proximal radius);

24587 with implant arthroplasty

(See also 24361)

24600 Treatment of closed elbow dislocation; without anesthesia

24605 requiring anesthesia

24615 Open treatment of acute or chronic elbow dislocation

24620 Closed treatment of Monteggia type of fracture dislocation at elbow (fracture proximal end of ulna with dislocation of radial head), with manipulation

24635 Open treatment of Monteggia type of fracture dislocation at elbow (fracture proximal end of ulna with dislocation of radial head), includes internal fixation, when performed

24640 Closed treatment of radial head subluxation in child, nursemaid elbow, with manipulation

24650 Closed treatment of radial head or neck fracture; without manipulation

24655 with manipulation

24665 Open treatment of radial head or neck fracture, includes internal fixation or radial head excision, when performed;

24666 with radial head prosthetic replacement

24670 Closed treatment of ulnar fracture, proximal end (eg, olecranon or coronoid process[es]); without manipulation

24675 with manipulation

24685 Open treatment of ulnar fracture, proximal end (eg, olecranon or coronoid process[es]), includes internal fixation, when performed

(Do not report 24685 in conjunction with 24100-24102)

Arthrodesis

24800 Arthrodesis, elbow joint; local

24802 with autogenous graft (includes obtaining graft)

Amputation

24900 Amputation, arm through humerus; with primary closure

24920 open, circular (guillotine)

24925 secondary closure or scar revision

24930 re-amputation

24931	with implant
24935	Stump elongation, upper extremity
24940	Cineplasty, upper extremity, complete procedure

Other Procedures

24999	Unlisted procedure, humerus or elbow

Forearm and Wrist

Radius, ulna, carpal bones, and joints.

Incision

25000	Incision, extensor tendon sheath, wrist (eg, deQuervains disease)
	(For decompression median nerve or for carpal tunnel syndrome, use 64721)
25001	Incision, flexor tendon sheath, wrist (eg, flexor carpi radialis)
25020	Decompression fasciotomy, forearm and/or wrist, flexor OR extensor compartment; without debridement of nonviable muscle and/or nerve
25023	with debridement of nonviable muscle and/or nerve
	(For decompression fasciotomy with brachial artery exploration, use 24495)
	(For incision and drainage procedures, superficial, see 10060-10160)
	(For debridement, see also 11000-11044)
25024	Decompression fasciotomy, forearm and/or wrist, flexor AND extensor compartment; without debridement of nonviable muscle and/or nerve
25025	with debridement of nonviable muscle and/or nerve
25028	Incision and drainage, forearm and/or wrist; deep abscess or hematoma
25031	bursa
25035	Incision, deep, bone cortex, forearm and/or wrist (eg, osteomyelitis or bone abscess)
25040	Arthrotomy, radiocarpal or midcarpal joint, with exploration, drainage, or removal of foreign body

Excision

25065	Biopsy, soft tissue of forearm and/or wrist; superficial
25066	deep (subfascial or intramuscular)
	(For needle biopsy of soft tissue, use 20206)
25071	Code is out of numerical sequence. See 25065-25240
25073	Code is out of numerical sequence. See 25065-25240
25075	Excision, tumor, soft tissue of forearm and/or wrist area, subcutaneous; less than 3 cm

# 25071	3 cm or greater
	(For excision of benign lesions of cutaneous origin [eg, sebaceous cyst], see 11400-11406)
25076	Excision, tumor, soft tissue of forearm and/or wrist area, subfascial (eg, intramuscular); less than 3 cm
# 25073	3 cm or greater
25077	Radical resection of tumor (eg, sarcoma), soft tissue of forearm and/or wrist area; less than 3 cm
25078	3 cm or greater
	(For radical resection of tumor[s] of cutaneous origin [eg, melanoma], see 11600-11606)
25085	Capsulotomy, wrist (eg, contracture)
25100	Arthrotomy, wrist joint; with biopsy
25101	with joint exploration, with or without biopsy, with or without removal of loose or foreign body
25105	with synovectomy
25107	Arthrotomy, distal radioulnar joint including repair of triangular cartilage, complex
25109	Excision of tendon, forearm and/or wrist, flexor or extensor, each
25110	Excision, lesion of tendon sheath, forearm and/or wrist
25111	Excision of ganglion, wrist (dorsal or volar); primary
25112	recurrent
	(For hand or finger, use 26160)
25115	Radical excision of bursa, synovia of wrist, or forearm tendon sheaths (eg, tenosynovitis, fungus, Tbc, or other granulomas, rheumatoid arthritis); flexors
25116	extensors, with or without transposition of dorsal retinaculum
	(For finger synovectomies, use 26145)
25118	Synovectomy, extensor tendon sheath, wrist, single compartment;
25119	with resection of distal ulna
25120	Excision or curettage of bone cyst or benign tumor of radius or ulna (excluding head or neck of radius and olecranon process);
	(For head or neck of radius or olecranon process, see 24120-24126)
25125	with autograft (includes obtaining graft)
25126	with allograft
25130	Excision or curettage of bone cyst or benign tumor of carpal bones;
25135	with autograft (includes obtaining graft)
25136	with allograft
25145	Sequestrectomy (eg, for osteomyelitis or bone abscess), forearm and/or wrist

Musculoskeletal

Musculoskeletal

25150 Partial excision (craterization, saucerization, or diaphysectomy) of bone (eg, for osteomyelitis); ulna

25151   radius

(For head or neck of radius or olecranon process, see 24145, 24147)

25170 Radical resection of tumor, radius or ulna

25210 Carpectomy; 1 bone

(For carpectomy with implant, see 25441-25445)

25215   all bones of proximal row

25230 Radial styloidectomy (separate procedure)

25240 Excision distal ulna partial or complete (eg, Darrach type or matched resection)

(For implant replacement, distal ulna, use 25442)

(For obtaining fascia for interposition, see 20920, 20922)

Introduction or Removal

(For K-wire, pin or rod insertion or removal, see 20650, 20670, 20680)

25246 Injection procedure for wrist arthrography

(For radiological supervision and interpretation, use 73115. Do not report 77002 in conjunction with 73115)

(For foreign body removal, superficial use 20520)

25248 Exploration with removal of deep foreign body, forearm or wrist

25250 Removal of wrist prosthesis; (separate procedure)

25251   complicated, including total wrist

25259 Manipulation, wrist, under anesthesia

(For application of external fixation, see 20690 or 20692)

Repair, Revision, and/or Reconstruction

25260 Repair, tendon or muscle, flexor, forearm and/or wrist; primary, single, each tendon or muscle

25263   secondary, single, each tendon or muscle

25265   secondary, with free graft (includes obtaining graft), each tendon or muscle

25270 Repair, tendon or muscle, extensor, forearm and/or wrist; primary, single, each tendon or muscle

25272   secondary, single, each tendon or muscle

25274   secondary, with free graft (includes obtaining graft), each tendon or muscle

25275 Repair, tendon sheath, extensor, forearm and/or wrist, with free graft (includes obtaining graft) (eg, for extensor carpi ulnaris subluxation)

25280 Lengthening or shortening of flexor or extensor tendon, forearm and/or wrist, single, each tendon

25290 Tenotomy, open, flexor or extensor tendon, forearm and/or wrist, single, each tendon

25295 Tenolysis, flexor or extensor tendon, forearm and/or wrist, single, each tendon

25300 Tenodesis at wrist; flexors of fingers

25301   extensors of fingers

25310 Tendon transplantation or transfer, flexor or extensor, forearm and/or wrist, single; each tendon

25312   with tendon graft(s) (includes obtaining graft), each tendon

25315 Flexor origin slide (eg, for cerebral palsy, Volkmann contracture), forearm and/or wrist;

25316   with tendon(s) transfer

25320 Capsulorrhaphy or reconstruction, wrist, open (eg, capsulodesis, ligament repair, tendon transfer or graft) (includes synovectomy, capsulotomy and open reduction) for carpal instability

25332 Arthroplasty, wrist, with or without interposition, with or without external or internal fixation

(For obtaining fascia for interposition, see 20920, 20922)

(For prosthetic replacement arthroplasty, see 25441-25446)

25335 Centralization of wrist on ulna (eg, radial club hand)

25337 Reconstruction for stabilization of unstable distal ulna or distal radioulnar joint, secondary by soft tissue stabilization (eg, tendon transfer, tendon graft or weave, or tenodesis) with or without open reduction of distal radioulnar joint

(For harvesting of fascia lata graft, see 20920, 20922)

25350 Osteotomy, radius; distal third

25355   middle or proximal third

25360 Osteotomy; ulna

25365   radius AND ulna

25370 Multiple osteotomies, with realignment on intramedullary rod (Sofield type procedure); radius OR ulna

25375   radius AND ulna

25390 Osteoplasty, radius OR ulna; shortening

25391   lengthening with autograft

25392 Osteoplasty, radius AND ulna; shortening (excluding 64876)

25393   lengthening with autograft

25394 Osteoplasty, carpal bone, shortening

25400 Repair of nonunion or malunion, radius OR ulna; without graft (eg, compression technique)

25405   with autograft (includes obtaining graft)

25415 Repair of nonunion or malunion, radius AND ulna; without graft (eg, compression technique)

25420   with autograft (includes obtaining graft)

25425   Repair of defect with autograft; radius OR ulna

25426   radius AND ulna

25430   Insertion of vascular pedicle into carpal bone (eg, Hori procedure)

25431   Repair of nonunion of carpal bone (excluding carpal scaphoid (navicular)) (includes obtaining graft and necessary fixation), each bone

25440   Repair of nonunion, scaphoid carpal (navicular) bone, with or without radial styloidectomy (includes obtaining graft and necessary fixation)

25441   Arthroplasty with prosthetic replacement; distal radius

25442   distal ulna

25443   scaphoid carpal (navicular)

25444   lunate

25445   trapezium

25446   distal radius and partial or entire carpus (total wrist)

25447   Arthroplasty, interposition, intercarpal or carpometacarpal joints

   (For wrist arthroplasty, use 25332)

25449   Revision of arthroplasty, including removal of implant, wrist joint

25450   Epiphyseal arrest by epiphysiodesis or stapling; distal radius OR ulna

25455   distal radius AND ulna

25490   Prophylactic treatment (nailing, pinning, plating or wiring) with or without methylmethacrylate; radius

25491   ulna

25492   radius AND ulna

Fracture and/or Dislocation

   (For application of external fixation in addition to internal fixation, use 20690 and the appropriate internal fixation code)

25500   Closed treatment of radial shaft fracture; without manipulation

25505   with manipulation

25515   Open treatment of radial shaft fracture, includes internal fixation, when performed

25520   Closed treatment of radial shaft fracture and closed treatment of dislocation of distal radioulnar joint (Galeazzi fracture/dislocation)

25525   Open treatment of radial shaft fracture, includes internal fixation, when performed, and closed treatment of distal radioulnar joint dislocation (Galeazzi fracture/dislocation), includes percutaneous skeletal fixation, when performed

25526   Open treatment of radial shaft fracture, includes internal fixation, when performed, and open treatment of distal radioulnar joint dislocation (Galeazzi fracture/dislocation), includes internal fixation, when performed, includes repair of triangular fibrocartilage complex

25530   Closed treatment of ulnar shaft fracture; without manipulation

25535   with manipulation

25545   Open treatment of ulnar shaft fracture, includes internal fixation, when performed

25560   Closed treatment of radial and ulnar shaft fractures; without manipulation

25565   with manipulation

25574   Open treatment of radial AND ulnar shaft fractures, with internal fixation, when performed; of radius OR ulna

25575   of radius AND ulna

25600   Closed treatment of distal radial fracture (eg, Colles or Smith type) or epiphyseal separation, includes closed treatment of fracture of ulnar styloid, when performed; without manipulation

25605   with manipulation

   (Do not report 25600, 25605 in conjunction with 25650)

25606   Percutaneous skeletal fixation of distal radial fracture or epiphyseal separation

   (Do not report 25606 in conjunction with 25650)

   (For percutaneous treatment of ulnar styloid fracture, use 25651)

   (For open treatment of ulnar styloid fracture, use 25652)

25607   Open treatment of distal radial extra-articular fracture or epiphyseal separation, with internal fixation

   (Do not report 25607 in conjunction with 25650)

   (For percutaneous treatment of ulnar styloid fracture, use 25651)

   (For open treatment of ulnar styloid fracture, use 25652)

25608   Open treatment of distal radial intra-articular fracture or epiphyseal separation; with internal fixation of 2 fragments

   (Do not report 25608 in conjunction with 25609)

25609   with internal fixation of 3 or more fragments

   (Do not report 25608, 25609 in conjunction with 25650)

   (For percutaneous treatment of ulnar styloid fracture, use 25651)

   (For open treatment of ulnar styloid fracture, use 25652)

25622   Closed treatment of carpal scaphoid (navicular) fracture; without manipulation

25624   with manipulation

25628   Open treatment of carpal scaphoid (navicular) fracture, includes internal fixation, when performed

Musculoskeletal

25630	Closed treatment of carpal bone fracture (excluding carpal scaphoid [navicular]); without manipulation, each bone
25635	with manipulation, each bone
25645	Open treatment of carpal bone fracture (other than carpal scaphoid [navicular]), each bone
25650	Closed treatment of ulnar styloid fracture
	(Do not report 25650 in conjunction with 25600, 25605, 25607-25609)
25651	Percutaneous skeletal fixation of ulnar styloid fracture
25652	Open treatment of ulnar styloid fracture
25660	Closed treatment of radiocarpal or intercarpal dislocation, 1 or more bones, with manipulation
25670	Open treatment of radiocarpal or intercarpal dislocation, 1 or more bones
25671	Percutaneous skeletal fixation of distal radioulnar dislocation
25675	Closed treatment of distal radioulnar dislocation with manipulation
25676	Open treatment of distal radioulnar dislocation, acute or chronic
25680	Closed treatment of trans-scaphoperilunar type of fracture dislocation, with manipulation
25685	Open treatment of trans-scaphoperilunar type of fracture dislocation
25690	Closed treatment of lunate dislocation, with manipulation
25695	Open treatment of lunate dislocation

Arthrodesis

25800	Arthrodesis, wrist; complete, without bone graft (includes radiocarpal and/or intercarpal and/or carpometacarpal joints)
25805	with sliding graft
25810	with iliac or other autograft (includes obtaining graft)
25820	Arthrodesis, wrist; limited, without bone graft (eg, intercarpal or radiocarpal)
25825	with autograft (includes obtaining graft)
25830	Arthrodesis, distal radioulnar joint with segmental resection of ulna, with or without bone graft (eg, Sauve-Kapandji procedure)

Amputation

25900	Amputation, forearm, through radius and ulna;
25905	open, circular (guillotine)
25907	secondary closure or scar revision
25909	re-amputation
25915	Krukenberg procedure
25920	Disarticulation through wrist;
25922	secondary closure or scar revision
25924	re-amputation
25927	Transmetacarpal amputation;
25929	secondary closure or scar revision
25931	re-amputation

Other Procedures

25999	Unlisted procedure, forearm or wrist

Hand and Fingers

Incision

26010	Drainage of finger abscess; simple
26011	complicated (eg, felon)
26020	Drainage of tendon sheath, digit and/or palm, each
26025	Drainage of palmar bursa; single, bursa
26030	multiple bursa
26034	Incision, bone cortex, hand or finger (eg, osteomyelitis or bone abscess)
26035	Decompression fingers and/or hand, injection injury (eg, grease gun)
26037	Decompressive fasciotomy, hand (excludes 26035)
	(For injection injury, use 26035)
26040	Fasciotomy, palmar (eg, Dupuytren's contracture); percutaneous
26045	open, partial
	(For palmar fasciotomy by enzyme injection (eg, collagenase), see 20527, 26341)
	(For fasciectomy, see 26121-26125)
26055	Tendon sheath incision (eg, for trigger finger)
26060	Tenotomy, percutaneous, single, each digit
26070	Arthrotomy, with exploration, drainage, or removal of loose or foreign body; carpometacarpal joint
26075	metacarpophalangeal joint, each
26080	interphalangeal joint, each

Excision

26100	Arthrotomy with biopsy; carpometacarpal joint, each
26105	metacarpophalangeal joint, each
26110	interphalangeal joint, each
26111	Code is out of numerical sequence. See 26100-26262
26113	Code is out of numerical sequence. See 26100-26262

⊙=Moderate sedation ✛=Add-on code ✗=FDA approval pending #=Resequenced code ○=Recycled/reinstated code

26115   Excision, tumor or vascular malformation, soft tissue of hand or finger, subcutaneous; less than 1.5 cm

 # 26111   1.5 cm or greater

(For excision of benign lesions of cutaneous origin [eg, sebaceous cyst], see 11420-11426)

26116   Excision, tumor, soft tissue, or vascular malformation, of hand or finger, subfascial (eg, intramuscular); less than 1.5 cm

 # 26113   1.5 cm or greater

26117   Radical resection of tumor (eg, sarcoma), soft tissue of hand or finger; less than 3 cm

26118   3 cm or greater

(For radical resection of tumor[s] of cutaneous origin [eg, melanoma], see 11620-11626)

26121   Fasciectomy, palm only, with or without Z-plasty, other local tissue rearrangement, or skin grafting (includes obtaining graft)

26123   Fasciectomy, partial palmar with release of single digit including proximal interphalangeal joint, with or without Z-plasty, other local tissue rearrangement, or skin grafting (includes obtaining graft);

+ 26125   each additional digit (List separately in addition to code for primary procedure)

(Use 26125 in conjunction with 26123)

(For palmar fasciotomy by enzyme injection (eg, collagenase), see 20527, 26341)

(For fasciotomy, see 26040, 26045)

26130   Synovectomy, carpometacarpal joint

26135   Synovectomy, metacarpophalangeal joint including intrinsic release and extensor hood reconstruction, each digit

26140   Synovectomy, proximal interphalangeal joint, including extensor reconstruction, each interphalangeal joint

26145   Synovectomy, tendon sheath, radical (tenosynovectomy), flexor tendon, palm and/or finger, each tendon

(For tendon sheath synovectomies at wrist, see 25115, 25116)

26160   Excision of lesion of tendon sheath or joint capsule (eg, cyst, mucous cyst, or ganglion), hand or finger

(For wrist ganglion, see 25111, 25112)

(For trigger digit, use 26055)

26170   Excision of tendon, palm, flexor or extensor, single, each tendon

(Do not report 26170 in conjunction with 26390, 26415)

26180   Excision of tendon, finger, flexor or extensor, each tendon

(Do not report 26180 in conjunction with 26390, 26415)

26185   Sesamoidectomy, thumb or finger (separate procedure)

26200   Excision or curettage of bone cyst or benign tumor of metacarpal;

26205   with autograft (includes obtaining graft)

26210   Excision or curettage of bone cyst or benign tumor of proximal, middle, or distal phalanx of finger;

26215   with autograft (includes obtaining graft)

26230   Partial excision (craterization, saucerization, or diaphysectomy) bone (eg, osteomyelitis); metacarpal

26235   proximal or middle phalanx of finger

26236   distal phalanx of finger

26250   Radical resection of tumor, metacarpal

26260   Radical resection of tumor, proximal or middle phalanx of finger

26262   Radical resection of tumor, distal phalanx of finger

Introduction or Removal

26320   Removal of implant from finger or hand

(For removal of foreign body in hand or finger, see 20520, 20525)

Repair, Revision, and/or Reconstruction

26340   Manipulation, finger joint, under anesthesia, each joint

(For application of external fixation, see 20690 or 20692)

26341   Manipulation, palmar fascial cord (ie, Dupuytren's cord), post enzyme injection (eg, collagenase), single cord

(For enzyme injection (eg, collagenase), palmar fascial cord (eg, Dupuytren's contracture), use 20527)

(Report custom orthotic fabrication/application separately)

26350   Repair or advancement, flexor tendon, not in zone 2 digital flexor tendon sheath (eg, no man's land); primary or secondary without free graft, each tendon

26352   secondary with free graft (includes obtaining graft), each tendon

26356   Repair or advancement, flexor tendon, in zone 2 digital flexor tendon sheath (eg, no man's land); primary, without free graft, each tendon

26357   secondary, without free graft, each tendon

26358   secondary, with free graft (includes obtaining graft), each tendon

26370   Repair or advancement of profundus tendon, with intact superficialis tendon; primary, each tendon

26372   secondary with free graft (includes obtaining graft), each tendon

26373   secondary without free graft, each tendon

Musculoskeletal

Musculoskeletal

26390 Excision flexor tendon, with implantation of synthetic rod for delayed tendon graft, hand or finger, each rod

26392 Removal of synthetic rod and insertion of flexor tendon graft, hand or finger (includes obtaining graft), each rod

26410 Repair, extensor tendon, hand, primary or secondary; without free graft, each tendon

26412 with free graft (includes obtaining graft), each tendon

26415 Excision of extensor tendon, with implantation of synthetic rod for delayed tendon graft, hand or finger, each rod

26416 Removal of synthetic rod and insertion of extensor tendon graft (includes obtaining graft), hand or finger, each rod

26418 Repair, extensor tendon, finger, primary or secondary; without free graft, each tendon

26420 with free graft (includes obtaining graft) each tendon

26426 Repair of extensor tendon, central slip, secondary (eg, boutonniere deformity); using local tissue(s), including lateral band(s), each finger

26428 with free graft (includes obtaining graft), each finger

26432 Closed treatment of distal extensor tendon insertion, with or without percutaneous pinning (eg, mallet finger)

26433 Repair of extensor tendon, distal insertion, primary or secondary; without graft (eg, mallet finger)

26434 with free graft (includes obtaining graft)

(For tenovaginotomy for trigger finger, use 26055)

26437 Realignment of extensor tendon, hand, each tendon

26440 Tenolysis, flexor tendon; palm OR finger, each tendon

26442 palm AND finger, each tendon

26445 Tenolysis, extensor tendon, hand OR finger, each tendon

26449 Tenolysis, complex, extensor tendon, finger, including forearm, each tendon

26450 Tenotomy, flexor, palm, open, each tendon

26455 Tenotomy, flexor, finger, open, each tendon

26460 Tenotomy, extensor, hand or finger, open, each tendon

26471 Tenodesis; of proximal interphalangeal joint, each joint

26474 of distal joint, each joint

26476 Lengthening of tendon, extensor, hand or finger, each tendon

26477 Shortening of tendon, extensor, hand or finger, each tendon

26478 Lengthening of tendon, flexor, hand or finger, each tendon

26479 Shortening of tendon, flexor, hand or finger, each tendon

26480 Transfer or transplant of tendon, carpometacarpal area or dorsum of hand; without free graft, each tendon

26483 with free tendon graft (includes obtaining graft), each tendon

26485 Transfer or transplant of tendon, palmar; without free tendon graft, each tendon

26489 with free tendon graft (includes obtaining graft), each tendon

26490 Opponensplasty; superficialis tendon transfer type, each tendon

26492 tendon transfer with graft (includes obtaining graft), each tendon

26494 hypothenar muscle transfer

26496 other methods

(For thumb fusion in opposition, use 26820)

26497 Transfer of tendon to restore intrinsic function; ring and small finger

26498 all 4 fingers

26499 Correction claw finger, other methods

26500 Reconstruction of tendon pulley, each tendon; with local tissues (separate procedure)

26502 with tendon or fascial graft (includes obtaining graft) (separate procedure)

26508 Release of thenar muscle(s) (eg, thumb contracture)

26510 Cross intrinsic transfer, each tendon

26516 Capsulodesis, metacarpophalangeal joint; single digit

26517 2 digits

26518 3 or 4 digits

26520 Capsulectomy or capsulotomy; metacarpophalangeal joint, each joint

26525 interphalangeal joint, each joint

26530 Arthroplasty, metacarpophalangeal joint; each joint

(To report carpometacarpal joint arthroplasty, use 25447)

26531 with prosthetic implant, each joint

26535 Arthroplasty, interphalangeal joint; each joint

26536 with prosthetic implant, each joint

26540 Repair of collateral ligament, metacarpophalangeal or interphalangeal joint

26541 Reconstruction, collateral ligament, metacarpophalangeal joint, single; with tendon or fascial graft (includes obtaining graft)

26542 with local tissue (eg, adductor advancement)

26545 Reconstruction, collateral ligament, interphalangeal joint, single, including graft, each joint

26546 Repair non-union, metacarpal or phalanx (includes obtaining bone graft with or without external or internal fixation)

26548 Repair and reconstruction, finger, volar plate, interphalangeal joint

26550 Pollicization of a digit

26551   Transfer, toe-to-hand with microvascular anastomosis; great toe wrap-around with bone graft

      (For great toe with web space, use 20973)

26553   other than great toe, single

26554   other than great toe, double

      (Do not report code 69990 in addition to codes 26551-26554)

26555   Transfer, finger to another position without microvascular anastomosis

26556   Transfer, free toe joint, with microvascular anastomosis

      (Do not report code 69990 in addition to code 26556)

      (To report great toe-to-hand transfer, use 20973)

26560   Repair of syndactyly (web finger) each web space; with skin flaps

26561   with skin flaps and grafts

26562   complex (eg, involving bone, nails)

26565   Osteotomy; metacarpal, each

26567   phalanx of finger, each

26568   Osteoplasty, lengthening, metacarpal or phalanx

26580   Repair cleft hand

26587   Reconstruction of polydactylous digit, soft tissue and bone

      (For excision of polydactylous digit, soft tissue only, use 11200)

26590   Repair macrodactylia, each digit

26591   Repair, intrinsic muscles of hand, each muscle

26593   Release, intrinsic muscles of hand, each muscle

26596   Excision of constricting ring of finger, with multiple Z-plasties

      (To report release of scar contracture or graft repairs see 11042, 14040-14041, or 15120, 15240)

Fracture and/or Dislocation

26600   Closed treatment of metacarpal fracture, single; without manipulation, each bone

26605   with manipulation, each bone

26607   Closed treatment of metacarpal fracture, with manipulation, with external fixation, each bone

26608   Percutaneous skeletal fixation of metacarpal fracture, each bone

26615   Open treatment of metacarpal fracture, single, includes internal fixation, when performed, each bone

26641   Closed treatment of carpometacarpal dislocation, thumb, with manipulation

26645   Closed treatment of carpometacarpal fracture dislocation, thumb (Bennett fracture), with manipulation

26650   Percutaneous skeletal fixation of carpometacarpal fracture dislocation, thumb (Bennett fracture), with manipulation

26665   Open treatment of carpometacarpal fracture dislocation, thumb (Bennett fracture), includes internal fixation, when performed

26670   Closed treatment of carpometacarpal dislocation, other than thumb, with manipulation, each joint; without anesthesia

26675   requiring anesthesia

26676   Percutaneous skeletal fixation of carpometacarpal dislocation, other than thumb, with manipulation, each joint

26685   Open treatment of carpometacarpal dislocation, other than thumb; includes internal fixation, when performed, each joint

26686   complex, multiple, or delayed reduction

26700   Closed treatment of metacarpophalangeal dislocation, single, with manipulation; without anesthesia

26705   requiring anesthesia

26706   Percutaneous skeletal fixation of metacarpophalangeal dislocation, single, with manipulation

26715   Open treatment of metacarpophalangeal dislocation, single, includes internal fixation, when performed

26720   Closed treatment of phalangeal shaft fracture, proximal or middle phalanx, finger or thumb; without manipulation, each

26725   with manipulation, with or without skin or skeletal traction, each

26727   Percutaneous skeletal fixation of unstable phalangeal shaft fracture, proximal or middle phalanx, finger or thumb, with manipulation, each

26735   Open treatment of phalangeal shaft fracture, proximal or middle phalanx, finger or thumb, includes internal fixation, when performed, each

26740   Closed treatment of articular fracture, involving metacarpophalangeal or interphalangeal joint; without manipulation, each

26742   with manipulation, each

26746   Open treatment of articular fracture, involving metacarpophalangeal or interphalangeal joint, includes internal fixation, when performed, each

26750   Closed treatment of distal phalangeal fracture, finger or thumb; without manipulation, each

26755   with manipulation, each

26756   Percutaneous skeletal fixation of distal phalangeal fracture, finger or thumb, each

26765   Open treatment of distal phalangeal fracture, finger or thumb, includes internal fixation, when performed, each

Musculoskeletal

26770 Closed treatment of interphalangeal joint dislocation, single, with manipulation; without anesthesia

26775 requiring anesthesia

26776 Percutaneous skeletal fixation of interphalangeal joint dislocation, single, with manipulation

26785 Open treatment of interphalangeal joint dislocation, includes internal fixation, when performed, single

Arthrodesis

26820 Fusion in opposition, thumb, with autogenous graft (includes obtaining graft)

26841 Arthrodesis, carpometacarpal joint, thumb, with or without internal fixation;

26842 with autograft (includes obtaining graft)

26843 Arthrodesis, carpometacarpal joint, digit, other than thumb, each;

26844 with autograft (includes obtaining graft)

26850 Arthrodesis, metacarpophalangeal joint, with or without internal fixation;

26852 with autograft (includes obtaining graft)

26860 Arthrodesis, interphalangeal joint, with or without internal fixation;

+ 26861 each additional interphalangeal joint (List separately in addition to code for primary procedure)

(Use 26861 in conjunction with 26860)

26862 with autograft (includes obtaining graft)

+ 26863 with autograft (includes obtaining graft), each additional joint (List separately in addition to code for primary procedure)

(Use 26863 in conjunction with 26862)

Amputation

(For hand through metacarpal bones, use 25927)

26910 Amputation, metacarpal, with finger or thumb (ray amputation), single, with or without interosseous transfer

(For repositioning, see 26550, 26555)

26951 Amputation, finger or thumb, primary or secondary, any joint or phalanx, single, including neurectomies; with direct closure

26952 with local advancement flaps (V-Y, hood)

(For repair of soft tissue defect requiring split or full thickness graft or other pedicle flaps, see 15050-15758)

Other Procedures

26989 Unlisted procedure, hands or fingers

Pelvis and Hip Joint

Including head and neck of femur.

Incision

(For incision and drainage procedures, superficial, see 10040-10160)

26990 Incision and drainage, pelvis or hip joint area; deep abscess or hematoma

26991 infected bursa

26992 Incision, bone cortex, pelvis and/or hip joint (eg, osteomyelitis or bone abscess)

27000 Tenotomy, adductor of hip, percutaneous (separate procedure)

27001 Tenotomy, adductor of hip, open

(To report bilateral procedure, report 27001 with modifier 50)

27003 Tenotomy, adductor, subcutaneous, open, with obturator neurectomy

(To report bilateral procedure, report 27003 with modifier 50)

27005 Tenotomy, hip flexor(s), open (separate procedure)

27006 Tenotomy, abductors and/or extensor(s) of hip, open (separate procedure)

27025 Fasciotomy, hip or thigh, any type

(To report bilateral procedure, report 27025 with modifier 50)

27027 Decompression fasciotomy(ies), pelvic (buttock) compartment(s) (eg, gluteus medius-minimus, gluteus maximus, iliopsoas, and/or tensor fascia lata muscle), unilateral

(To report bilateral procedure, report 27027 with modifier 50)

27030 Arthrotomy, hip, with drainage (eg, infection)

27033 Arthrotomy, hip, including exploration or removal of loose or foreign body

27035 Denervation, hip joint, intrapelvic or extrapelvic intra-articular branches of sciatic, femoral, or obturator nerves

(For obturator neurectomy, see 64763, 64766)

27036 Capsulectomy or capsulotomy, hip, with or without excision of heterotopic bone, with release of hip flexor muscles (ie, gluteus medius, gluteus minimus, tensor fascia latae, rectus femoris, sartorius, iliopsoas)

Excision

27040 Biopsy, soft tissue of pelvis and hip area; superficial

27041 deep, subfascial or intramuscular

(For needle biopsy of soft tissue, use 20206)

Musculoskeletal

27043   Code is out of numerical sequence. See 27040-27080

27045   Code is out of numerical sequence. See 27040-27080

27047   Excision, tumor, soft tissue of pelvis and hip area, subcutaneous; less than 3 cm

 # 27043   3 cm or greater

(For excision of benign lesions of cutaneous origin [eg, sebaceous cyst], see 11400-11406)

27048   Excision, tumor, soft tissue of pelvis and hip area, subfascial (eg, intramuscular); less than 5 cm

 # 27045   5 cm or greater

27049   Radical resection of tumor (eg, sarcoma), soft tissue of pelvis and hip area; less than 5 cm

 # 27059   5 cm or greater

(For radical resection of tumor[s] of cutaneous origin [eg, melanoma], see 11600-11606)

27050   Arthrotomy, with biopsy; sacroiliac joint

27052   hip joint

27054   Arthrotomy with synovectomy, hip joint

27057   Decompression fasciotomy(ies), pelvic (buttock) compartment(s) (eg, gluteus medius-minimus, gluteus maximus, iliopsoas, and/or tensor fascia lata muscle) with debridement of nonviable muscle, unilateral

(To report bilateral procedure, report 27057 with modifier 50)

27059   Code is out of numerical sequence. See 27040-27080

27060   Excision; ischial bursa

27062   trochanteric bursa or calcification

(For arthrocentesis or needling of bursa, use 20610)

27065   Excision of bone cyst or benign tumor, wing of ilium, symphysis pubis, or greater trochanter of femur; superficial, includes autograft, when performed

27066   deep (subfascial), includes autograft, when performed

27067   with autograft requiring separate incision

27070   Partial excision, wing of ilium, symphysis pubis, or greater trochanter of femur, (craterization, saucerization) (eg, osteomyelitis or bone abscess); superficial

27071   deep (subfascial or intramuscular)

27075   Radical resection of tumor; wing of ilium, 1 pubic or ischial ramus or symphysis pubis

27076   ilium, including acetabulum, both pubic rami, or ischium and acetabulum

27077   innominate bone, total

27078   ischial tuberosity and greater trochanter of femur

27080   Coccygectomy, primary

(For pressure (decubitus) ulcer, see 15920, 15922 and 15931-15958)

Introduction or Removal

27086   Removal of foreign body, pelvis or hip; subcutaneous tissue

27087   deep (subfascial or intramuscular)

27090   Removal of hip prosthesis; (separate procedure)

27091   complicated, including total hip prosthesis, methylmethacrylate with or without insertion of spacer

27093   Injection procedure for hip arthrography; without anesthesia

(For radiological supervision and interpretation, use 73525. Do not report 77002 in conjunction with 73525)

27095   with anesthesia

(For radiological supervision and interpretation, use 73525. Do not report 77002 in conjunction with 73525)

27096   Injection procedure for sacroiliac joint, anesthetic/ steroid, with image guidance (fluoroscopy or CT) including arthrography when performed

(27096 is to be used only with CT or fluoroscopic imaging confirmation of intra-articular needle positioning)

(If CT or fluoroscopy imaging is not performed, use 20552)

(Code 27096 is a unilateral procedure. For bilateral procedure, use modifier 50)

Repair, Revision, and/or Reconstruction

27097   Release or recession, hamstring, proximal

27098   Transfer, adductor to ischium

27100   Transfer external oblique muscle to greater trochanter including fascial or tendon extension (graft)

27105   Transfer paraspinal muscle to hip (includes fascial or tendon extension graft)

27110   Transfer iliopsoas; to greater trochanter of femur

27111   to femoral neck

27120   Acetabuloplasty; (eg, Whitman, Colonna, Haygroves, or cup type)

27122   resection, femoral head (eg, Girdlestone procedure)

27125   Hemiarthroplasty, hip, partial (eg, femoral stem prosthesis, bipolar arthroplasty)

(For prosthetic replacement following fracture of the hip, use 27236)

27130   Arthroplasty, acetabular and proximal femoral prosthetic replacement (total hip arthroplasty), with or without autograft or allograft

27132   Conversion of previous hip surgery to total hip arthroplasty, with or without autograft or allograft

27134   Revision of total hip arthroplasty; both components, with or without autograft or allograft

Musculoskeletal

27137   acetabular component only, with or without autograft or allograft

27138   femoral component only, with or without allograft

27140   Osteotomy and transfer of greater trochanter of femur (separate procedure)

27146   Osteotomy, iliac, acetabular or innominate bone;

27147   with open reduction of hip

27151   with femoral osteotomy

27156   with femoral osteotomy and with open reduction of hip

27158   Osteotomy, pelvis, bilateral (eg, congenital malformation)

27161   Osteotomy, femoral neck (separate procedure)

27165   Osteotomy, intertrochanteric or subtrochanteric including internal or external fixation and/or cast

27170   Bone graft, femoral head, neck, intertrochanteric or subtrochanteric area (includes obtaining bone graft)

27175   Treatment of slipped femoral epiphysis; by traction, without reduction

27176   by single or multiple pinning, in situ

27177   Open treatment of slipped femoral epiphysis; single or multiple pinning or bone graft (includes obtaining graft)

27178   closed manipulation with single or multiple pinning

27179   osteoplasty of femoral neck (Heyman type procedure)

27181   osteotomy and internal fixation

27185   Epiphyseal arrest by epiphysiodesis or stapling, greater trochanter of femur

27187   Prophylactic treatment (nailing, pinning, plating or wiring) with or without methylmethacrylate, femoral neck and proximal femur

Fracture and/or Dislocation

27193   Closed treatment of pelvic ring fracture, dislocation, diastasis or subluxation; without manipulation

27194   with manipulation, requiring more than local anesthesia

27200   Closed treatment of coccygeal fracture

27202   Open treatment of coccygeal fracture

27215   Open treatment of iliac spine(s), tuberosity avulsion, or iliac wing fracture(s), unilateral, for pelvic bone fracture patterns that do not disrupt the pelvic ring, includes internal fixation, when performed

(To report bilateral procedure, report 27215 with modifier 50)

27216   Percutaneous skeletal fixation of posterior pelvic bone fracture and/or dislocation, for fracture patterns that disrupt the pelvic ring, unilateral (includes ipsilateral ilium, sacroiliac joint and/or sacrum)

(To report bilateral procedure, report 27216 with modifier 50)

(For percutaneous/minimally invasive arthrodesis of the sacroiliac joint without fracture and/or dislocation, use 27279)

27217   Open treatment of anterior pelvic bone fracture and/or dislocation for fracture patterns that disrupt the pelvic ring, unilateral, includes internal fixation, when performed (includes pubic symphysis and/or ipsilateral superior/inferior rami)

(To report bilateral procedure, report 27217 with modifier 50)

27218   Open treatment of posterior pelvic bone fracture and/or dislocation, for fracture patterns that disrupt the pelvic ring, unilateral, includes internal fixation, when performed (includes ipsilateral ilium, sacroiliac joint and/or sacrum)

(To report bilateral procedure, report 27218 with modifier 50)

(For percutaneous/minimally invasive arthrodesis of the sacroiliac joint without fracture and/or dislocation, use 27279)

27220   Closed treatment of acetabulum (hip socket) fracture(s); without manipulation

27222   with manipulation, with or without skeletal traction

27226   Open treatment of posterior or anterior acetabular wall fracture, with internal fixation

27227   Open treatment of acetabular fracture(s) involving anterior or posterior (one) column, or a fracture running transversely across the acetabulum, with internal fixation

27228   Open treatment of acetabular fracture(s) involving anterior and posterior (two) columns, includes T-fracture and both column fracture with complete articular detachment, or single column or transverse fracture with associated acetabular wall fracture, with internal fixation

27230   Closed treatment of femoral fracture, proximal end, neck; without manipulation

27232   with manipulation, with or without skeletal traction

27235   Percutaneous skeletal fixation of femoral fracture, proximal end, neck

27236   Open treatment of femoral fracture, proximal end, neck, internal fixation or prosthetic replacement

27238   Closed treatment of intertrochanteric, peritrochanteric, or subtrochanteric femoral fracture; without manipulation

27240   with manipulation, with or without skin or skeletal traction

27244   Treatment of intertrochanteric, peritrochanteric, or subtrochanteric femoral fracture; with plate/screw type implant, with or without cerclage

27245   with intramedullary implant, with or without interlocking screws and/or cerclage

27246 Closed treatment of greater trochanteric fracture, without manipulation

27248 Open treatment of greater trochanteric fracture, includes internal fixation, when performed

27250 Closed treatment of hip dislocation, traumatic; without anesthesia

27252   requiring anesthesia

27253 Open treatment of hip dislocation, traumatic, without internal fixation

27254 Open treatment of hip dislocation, traumatic, with acetabular wall and femoral head fracture, with or without internal or external fixation

(For treatment of acetabular fracture with fixation, see 27226, 27227)

27256 Treatment of spontaneous hip dislocation (developmental, including congenital or pathological), by abduction, splint or traction; without anesthesia, without manipulation

27257   with manipulation, requiring anesthesia

27258 Open treatment of spontaneous hip dislocation (developmental, including congenital or pathological), replacement of femoral head in acetabulum (including tenotomy, etc);

27259   with femoral shaft shortening

27265 Closed treatment of post hip arthroplasty dislocation; without anesthesia

27266   requiring regional or general anesthesia

27267 Closed treatment of femoral fracture, proximal end, head; without manipulation

27268   with manipulation

27269 Open treatment of femoral fracture, proximal end, head, includes internal fixation, when performed

(Do not report 27269 in conjunction with 27033, 27253)

Manipulation

27275 Manipulation, hip joint, requiring general anesthesia

Arthrodesis

27279 Arthrodesis, sacroiliac joint, percutaneous or minimally invasive (indirect visualization), with image guidance, includes obtaining bone graft when performed, and placement of transfixing device

(For bilateral procedure, report 27279 with modifier 50)

27280 Arthrodesis, open, sacroiliac joint, including obtaining bone graft, including instrumentation, when performed

(To report bilateral procedure, report 27280 with modifier 50)

(For percutaneous/minimally invasive arthrodesis of the sacroiliac joint without fracture and/or dislocation, use 27279)

27282 Arthrodesis, symphysis pubis (including obtaining graft)

27284 Arthrodesis, hip joint (including obtaining graft);

27286   with subtrochanteric osteotomy

Amputation

27290 Interpelviabdominal amputation (hindquarter amputation)

27295 Disarticulation of hip

Other Procedures

27299 Unlisted procedure, pelvis or hip joint

Femur (Thigh Region) and Knee Joint

Including tibial plateaus.

Incision

(For incision and drainage of abscess or hematoma, superficial, see 10040-10160)

27301 Incision and drainage, deep abscess, bursa, or hematoma, thigh or knee region

27303 Incision, deep, with opening of bone cortex, femur or knee (eg, osteomyelitis or bone abscess)

27305 Fasciotomy, iliotibial (tenotomy), open

(For combined Ober-Yount fasciotomy, use 27025)

27306 Tenotomy, percutaneous, adductor or hamstring; single tendon (separate procedure)

27307   multiple tendons

27310 Arthrotomy, knee, with exploration, drainage, or removal of foreign body (eg, infection)

Excision

27323 Biopsy, soft tissue of thigh or knee area; superficial

27324   deep (subfascial or intramuscular)

(For needle biopsy of soft tissue, use 20206)

27325 Neurectomy, hamstring muscle

27326 Neurectomy, popliteal (gastrocnemius)

27327 Excision, tumor, soft tissue of thigh or knee area, subcutaneous; less than 3 cm

\# **27337**   3 cm or greater

(For excision of benign lesions of cutaneous origin [eg, sebaceous cyst], see 11400-11406)

27328 Excision, tumor, soft tissue of thigh or knee area, subfascial (eg, intramuscular); less than 5 cm

Musculoskeletal

27329   Code is out of numerical sequence. See 27323-27365

\# 27339   5 cm or greater

27330   Arthrotomy, knee; with synovial biopsy only

27331   including joint exploration, biopsy, or removal of loose or foreign bodies

27332   Arthrotomy, with excision of semilunar cartilage (meniscectomy) knee; medial OR lateral

27333   medial AND lateral

27334   Arthrotomy, with synovectomy, knee; anterior OR posterior

27335   anterior AND posterior including popliteal area

27337   Code is out of numerical sequence. See 27323-27365

27339   Code is out of numerical sequence. See 27323-27365

27340   Excision, prepatellar bursa

27345   Excision of synovial cyst of popliteal space (eg, Baker's cyst)

27347   Excision of lesion of meniscus or capsule (eg, cyst, ganglion), knee

27350   Patellectomy or hemipatellectomy

27355   Excision or curettage of bone cyst or benign tumor of femur;

27356   with allograft

27357   with autograft (includes obtaining graft)

+ 27358   with internal fixation (List in addition to code for primary procedure)

(Use 27358 in conjunction with 27355, 27356, or 27357)

27360   Partial excision (craterization, saucerization, or diaphysectomy) bone, femur, proximal tibia and/or fibula (eg, osteomyelitis or bone abscess)

\# 27329   Radical resection of tumor (eg, sarcoma), soft tissue of thigh or knee area; less than 5 cm

27364   5 cm or greater

(For radical resection of tumor[s] of cutaneous origin [eg, melanoma], see 11600-11606)

27365   Radical resection of tumor, femur or knee

(For radical resection of tumor, soft tissue of thigh or knee area, see 27329, 27364)

Introduction or Removal

27370   Injection of contrast for knee arthrography

(For radiological supervision and interpretation, use 73580. Do not report 77002 in conjunction with 73580)

(Do not report 27370 in conjunction with 20610, 20611, 29871)

(For arthrocentesis of the knee or injection other than contrast, see 20610, 20611)

(For arthroscopic lavage and drainage of the knee, use 29871)

27372   Removal of foreign body, deep, thigh region or knee area

(For removal of knee prosthesis including "total knee," use 27488)

(For surgical arthroscopic knee procedures, see 29870-29887)

Repair, Revision, and/or Reconstruction

27380   Suture of infrapatellar tendon; primary

27381   secondary reconstruction, including fascial or tendon graft

27385   Suture of quadriceps or hamstring muscle rupture; primary

27386   secondary reconstruction, including fascial or tendon graft

27390   Tenotomy, open, hamstring, knee to hip; single tendon

27391   multiple tendons, 1 leg

27392   multiple tendons, bilateral

27393   Lengthening of hamstring tendon; single tendon

27394   multiple tendons, 1 leg

27395   multiple tendons, bilateral

27396   Transplant or transfer (with muscle redirection or rerouting), thigh (eg, extensor to flexor); single tendon

27397   multiple tendons

27400   Transfer, tendon or muscle, hamstrings to femur (eg, Egger's type procedure)

27403   Arthrotomy with meniscus repair, knee

(For arthroscopic repair, use 29882)

27405   Repair, primary, torn ligament and/or capsule, knee; collateral

27407   cruciate

(For cruciate ligament reconstruction, use 27427)

27409   collateral and cruciate ligaments

(For ligament reconstruction, see 27427-27429)

27412   Autologous chondrocyte implantation, knee

(Do not report 27412 in conjunction with 20926, 27331, 27570)

(For harvesting of chondrocytes, use 29870)

27415   Osteochondral allograft, knee, open

(For arthroscopic implant of osteochondral allograft, use 29867)

(Do not report 27415 in conjunction with 27416)

27416   Osteochondral autograft(s), knee, open (eg, mosaicplasty) (includes harvesting of autograft[s])

Musculoskeletal

(Do not report 27416 in conjunction with 27415, 29870, 29871, 29875, 29884 when performed at the same session and/or 29874, 29877, 29879, 29885-29887 when performed in the same compartment)

(For arthroscopic osteochondral autograft of knee, use 29866)

27418   Anterior tibial tubercleplasty (eg, Maquet type procedure)

27420   Reconstruction of dislocating patella; (eg, Hauser type procedure)

27422   with extensor realignment and/or muscle advancement or release (eg, Campbell, Goldwaite type procedure)

27424   with patellectomy

27425   Lateral retinacular release, open

(For arthroscopic lateral release, use 29873)

27427   Ligamentous reconstruction (augmentation), knee; extra-articular

27428   intra-articular (open)

27429   intra-articular (open) and extra-articular

(For primary repair of ligament(s) performed in conjunction with reconstruction, report 27405, 27407 or 27409 in conjunction with 27427, 27428 or 27429)

27430   Quadricepsplasty (eg, Bennett or Thompson type)

27435   Capsulotomy, posterior capsular release, knee

27437   Arthroplasty, patella; without prosthesis

27438   with prosthesis

27440   Arthroplasty, knee, tibial plateau;

27441   with debridement and partial synovectomy

27442   Arthroplasty, femoral condyles or tibial plateau(s), knee;

27443   with debridement and partial synovectomy

27445   Arthroplasty, knee, hinge prosthesis (eg, Walldius type)

27446   Arthroplasty, knee, condyle and plateau; medial OR lateral compartment

27447   medial AND lateral compartments with or without patella resurfacing (total knee arthroplasty)

(For revision of total knee arthroplasty, use 27487)

(For removal of total knee prosthesis, use 27488)

27448   Osteotomy, femur, shaft or supracondylar; without fixation

(To report bilateral procedure, report 27448 with modifier 50)

27450   with fixation

(To report bilateral procedure, report 27450 with modifier 50)

27454   Osteotomy, multiple, with realignment on intramedullary rod, femoral shaft (eg, Sofield type procedure)

27455   Osteotomy, proximal tibia, including fibular excision or osteotomy (includes correction of genu varus [bowleg] or genu valgus [knock-knee]); before epiphyseal closure

(To report bilateral procedure, report 27455 with modifier 50)

27457   after epiphyseal closure

(To report bilateral procedure, report 27457 with modifier 50)

27465   Osteoplasty, femur; shortening (excluding 64876)

27466   lengthening

27468   combined, lengthening and shortening with femoral segment transfer

27470   Repair, nonunion or malunion, femur, distal to head and neck; without graft (eg, compression technique)

27472   with iliac or other autogenous bone graft (includes obtaining graft)

27475   Arrest, epiphyseal, any method (eg, epiphysiodesis); distal femur

27477   tibia and fibula, proximal

27479   combined distal femur, proximal tibia and fibula

27485   Arrest, hemiepiphyseal, distal femur or proximal tibia or fibula (eg, genu varus or valgus)

27486   Revision of total knee arthroplasty, with or without allograft; 1 component

27487   femoral and entire tibial component

27488   Removal of prosthesis, including total knee prosthesis, methylmethacrylate with or without insertion of spacer, knee

27495   Prophylactic treatment (nailing, pinning, plating, or wiring) with or without methylmethacrylate, femur

27496   Decompression fasciotomy, thigh and/or knee, 1 compartment (flexor or extensor or adductor);

27497   with debridement of nonviable muscle and/or nerve

27498   Decompression fasciotomy, thigh and/or knee, multiple compartments;

27499   with debridement of nonviable muscle and/or nerve

Fracture and/or Dislocation

(For arthroscopic treatment of intercondylar spine[s] and tuberosity fracture[s] of the knee, see 29850, 29851)

(For arthroscopic treatment of tibial fracture, see 29855, 29856)

27500   Closed treatment of femoral shaft fracture, without manipulation

27501   Closed treatment of supracondylar or transcondylar femoral fracture with or without intercondylar extension, without manipulation

Musculoskeletal

Musculoskeletal

27502   Closed treatment of femoral shaft fracture, with manipulation, with or without skin or skeletal traction

27503   Closed treatment of supracondylar or transcondylar femoral fracture with or without intercondylar extension, with manipulation, with or without skin or skeletal traction

27506   Open treatment of femoral shaft fracture, with or without external fixation, with insertion of intramedullary implant, with or without cerclage and/or locking screws

27507   Open treatment of femoral shaft fracture with plate/screws, with or without cerclage

27508   Closed treatment of femoral fracture, distal end, medial or lateral condyle, without manipulation

27509   Percutaneous skeletal fixation of femoral fracture, distal end, medial or lateral condyle, or supracondylar or transcondylar, with or without intercondylar extension, or distal femoral epiphyseal separation

27510   Closed treatment of femoral fracture, distal end, medial or lateral condyle, with manipulation

27511   Open treatment of femoral supracondylar or transcondylar fracture without intercondylar extension, includes internal fixation, when performed

27513   Open treatment of femoral supracondylar or transcondylar fracture with intercondylar extension, includes internal fixation, when performed

27514   Open treatment of femoral fracture, distal end, medial or lateral condyle, includes internal fixation, when performed

27516   Closed treatment of distal femoral epiphyseal separation; without manipulation

27517   with manipulation, with or without skin or skeletal traction

27519   Open treatment of distal femoral epiphyseal separation, includes internal fixation, when performed

27520   Closed treatment of patellar fracture, without manipulation

27524   Open treatment of patellar fracture, with internal fixation and/or partial or complete patellectomy and soft tissue repair

27530   Closed treatment of tibial fracture, proximal (plateau); without manipulation

27532   with or without manipulation, with skeletal traction

(For arthroscopic treatment, see 29855, 29856)

27535   Open treatment of tibial fracture, proximal (plateau); unicondylar, includes internal fixation, when performed

27536   bicondylar, with or without internal fixation

(For arthroscopic treatment, see 29855, 29856)

27538   Closed treatment of intercondylar spine(s) and/or tuberosity fracture(s) of knee, with or without manipulation

(For arthroscopic treatment, see 29850, 29851)

27540   Open treatment of intercondylar spine(s) and/or tuberosity fracture(s) of the knee, includes internal fixation, when performed

27550   Closed treatment of knee dislocation; without anesthesia

27552   requiring anesthesia

27556   Open treatment of knee dislocation, includes internal fixation, when performed; without primary ligamentous repair or augmentation/reconstruction

27557   with primary ligamentous repair

27558   with primary ligamentous repair, with augmentation/reconstruction

27560   Closed treatment of patellar dislocation; without anesthesia

(For recurrent dislocation, see 27420-27424)

27562   requiring anesthesia

27566   Open treatment of patellar dislocation, with or without partial or total patellectomy

Manipulation

27570   Manipulation of knee joint under general anesthesia (includes application of traction or other fixation devices)

Arthrodesis

27580   Arthrodesis, knee, any technique

Amputation

27590   Amputation, thigh, through femur, any level;

27591   immediate fitting technique including first cast

27592   open, circular (guillotine)

27594   secondary closure or scar revision

27596   re-amputation

27598   Disarticulation at knee

Other Procedures

27599   Unlisted procedure, femur or knee

Leg (Tibia and Fibula) and Ankle Joint

Incision

27600   Decompression fasciotomy, leg; anterior and/or lateral compartments only

27601   posterior compartment(s) only

27602   anterior and/or lateral, and posterior compartment(s)

(For incision and drainage procedures, superficial, see 10040-10160)

⊙=Moderate sedation   ✚=Add-on code   ✒=FDA approval pending   #=Resequenced code   ○=Recycled/reinstated code

(For decompression fasciotomy with debridement, see 27892-27894)

27603 Incision and drainage, leg or ankle; deep abscess or hematoma

27604 infected bursa

27605 Tenotomy, percutaneous, Achilles tendon (separate procedure); local anesthesia

27606 general anesthesia

27607 Incision (eg, osteomyelitis or bone abscess), leg or ankle

27610 Arthrotomy, ankle, including exploration, drainage, or removal of foreign body

27612 Arthrotomy, posterior capsular release, ankle, with or without Achilles tendon lengthening

(See also 27685)

Excision

27613 Biopsy, soft tissue of leg or ankle area; superficial

27614 deep (subfascial or intramuscular)

(For needle biopsy of soft tissue, use 20206)

27615 Radical resection of tumor (eg, sarcoma), soft tissue of leg or ankle area; less than 5 cm

27616 5 cm or greater

(For radical resection of tumor[s] of cutaneous origin [eg, melanoma], see 11600-11606)

27618 Excision, tumor, soft tissue of leg or ankle area, subcutaneous; less than 3 cm

 # 27632 3 cm or greater

(For excision of benign lesions of cutaneous origin [eg, sebaceous cyst], see 11400-11406)

27619 Excision, tumor, soft tissue of leg or ankle area, subfascial (eg, intramuscular); less than 5 cm

 # 27634 5 cm or greater

27620 Arthrotomy, ankle, with joint exploration, with or without biopsy, with or without removal of loose or foreign body

27625 Arthrotomy, with synovectomy, ankle;

27626 including tenosynovectomy

27630 Excision of lesion of tendon sheath or capsule (eg, cyst or ganglion), leg and/or ankle

27632 Code is out of numerical sequence. See 27613-27647

27634 Code is out of numerical sequence. See 27613-27647

27635 Excision or curettage of bone cyst or benign tumor, tibia or fibula;

27637 with autograft (includes obtaining graft)

27638 with allograft

27640 Partial excision (craterization, saucerization, or diaphysectomy), bone (eg, osteomyelitis); tibia

(For exostosis excision, use 27635)

27641 fibula

(For exostosis excision, use 27635)

27645 Radical resection of tumor; tibia

27646 fibula

27647 talus or calcaneus

Introduction or Removal

27648 Injection procedure for ankle arthrography

(For radiological supervision and interpretation, use 73615. Do not report 77002 in conjunction with 73615)

(For ankle arthroscopy, see 29894-29898)

Repair, Revision, and/or Reconstruction

27650 Repair, primary, open or percutaneous, ruptured Achilles tendon;

27652 with graft (includes obtaining graft)

27654 Repair, secondary, Achilles tendon, with or without graft

27656 Repair, fascial defect of leg

27658 Repair, flexor tendon, leg; primary, without graft, each tendon

27659 secondary, with or without graft, each tendon

27664 Repair, extensor tendon, leg; primary, without graft, each tendon

27665 secondary, with or without graft, each tendon

27675 Repair, dislocating peroneal tendons; without fibular osteotomy

27676 with fibular osteotomy

27680 Tenolysis, flexor or extensor tendon, leg and/or ankle; single, each tendon

27681 multiple tendons (through separate incision[s])

27685 Lengthening or shortening of tendon, leg or ankle; single tendon (separate procedure)

27686 multiple tendons (through same incision), each

27687 Gastrocnemius recession (eg, Strayer procedure)

(Toe extensors are considered as a group to be a single tendon when transplanted into midfoot)

27690 Transfer or transplant of single tendon (with muscle redirection or rerouting); superficial (eg, anterior tibial extensors into midfoot)

27691 deep (eg, anterior tibial or posterior tibial through interosseous space, flexor digitorum longus, flexor hallucis longus, or peroneal tendon to midfoot or hindfoot)

Musculoskeletal

Musculoskeletal

+ **27692**   each additional tendon (List separately in addition to code for primary procedure)

(Use 27692 in conjunction with 27690, 27691)

27695   Repair, primary, disrupted ligament, ankle; collateral

27696   both collateral ligaments

27698   Repair, secondary, disrupted ligament, ankle, collateral (eg, Watson-Jones procedure)

27700   Arthroplasty, ankle;

27702   with implant (total ankle)

27703   revision, total ankle

27704   Removal of ankle implant

27705   Osteotomy; tibia

27707   fibula

27709   tibia and fibula

27712   multiple, with realignment on intramedullary rod (eg, Sofield type procedure)

(For osteotomy to correct genu varus [bowleg] or genu valgus [knock-knee], see 27455-27457)

27715   Osteoplasty, tibia and fibula, lengthening or shortening

27720   Repair of nonunion or malunion, tibia; without graft, (eg, compression technique)

27722   with sliding graft

27724   with iliac or other autograft (includes obtaining graft)

27725   by synostosis, with fibula, any method

27726   Repair of fibula nonunion and/or malunion with internal fixation

(Do not report 27726 in conjunction with 27707)

27727   Repair of congenital pseudarthrosis, tibia

27730   Arrest, epiphyseal (epiphysiodesis), open; distal tibia

27732   distal fibula

27734   distal tibia and fibula

27740   Arrest, epiphyseal (epiphysiodesis), any method, combined, proximal and distal tibia and fibula;

27742   and distal femur

(For epiphyseal arrest of proximal tibia and fibula, use 27477)

27745   Prophylactic treatment (nailing, pinning, plating or wiring) with or without methylmethacrylate, tibia

Fracture and/or Dislocation

27750   Closed treatment of tibial shaft fracture (with or without fibular fracture); without manipulation

27752   with manipulation, with or without skeletal traction

27756   Percutaneous skeletal fixation of tibial shaft fracture (with or without fibular fracture) (eg, pins or screws)

27758   Open treatment of tibial shaft fracture (with or without fibular fracture), with plate/screws, with or without cerclage

27759   Treatment of tibial shaft fracture (with or without fibular fracture) by intramedullary implant, with or without interlocking screws and/or cerclage

27760   Closed treatment of medial malleolus fracture; without manipulation

27762   with manipulation, with or without skin or skeletal traction

27766   Open treatment of medial malleolus fracture, includes internal fixation, when performed

27767   Closed treatment of posterior malleolus fracture; without manipulation

27768   with manipulation

27769   Open treatment of posterior malleolus fracture, includes internal fixation, when performed

(Do not report 27767-27769 in conjunction with 27808-27823)

27780   Closed treatment of proximal fibula or shaft fracture; without manipulation

27781   with manipulation

27784   Open treatment of proximal fibula or shaft fracture, includes internal fixation, when performed

27786   Closed treatment of distal fibular fracture (lateral malleolus); without manipulation

27788   with manipulation

27792   Open treatment of distal fibular fracture (lateral malleolus), includes internal fixation, when performed

(For treatment of tibia and fibula shaft fractures, see 27750-27759)

27808   Closed treatment of bimalleolar ankle fracture (eg, lateral and medial malleoli, or lateral and posterior malleoli or medial and posterior malleoli); without manipulation

27810   with manipulation

27814   Open treatment of bimalleolar ankle fracture (eg, lateral and medial malleoli, or lateral and posterior malleoli, or medial and posterior malleoli), includes internal fixation, when performed

27816   Closed treatment of trimalleolar ankle fracture; without manipulation

27818   with manipulation

27822   Open treatment of trimalleolar ankle fracture, includes internal fixation, when performed, medial and/or lateral malleolus; without fixation of posterior lip

27823   with fixation of posterior lip

27824   Closed treatment of fracture of weight bearing articular portion of distal tibia (eg, pilon or tibial plafond), with or without anesthesia; without manipulation

27825   with skeletal traction and/or requiring manipulation

27826   Open treatment of fracture of weight bearing articular surface/portion of distal tibia (eg, pilon or tibial plafond), with internal fixation, when performed; of fibula only

27827   of tibia only

27828   of both tibia and fibula

27829   Open treatment of distal tibiofibular joint (syndesmosis) disruption, includes internal fixation, when performed

27830   Closed treatment of proximal tibiofibular joint dislocation; without anesthesia

27831   requiring anesthesia

27832   Open treatment of proximal tibiofibular joint dislocation, includes internal fixation, when performed, or with excision of proximal fibula

27840   Closed treatment of ankle dislocation; without anesthesia

27842   requiring anesthesia, with or without percutaneous skeletal fixation

27846   Open treatment of ankle dislocation, with or without percutaneous skeletal fixation; without repair or internal fixation

27848   with repair or internal or external fixation

(For surgical or diagnostic arthroscopic procedures, see 29894-29898)

Manipulation

27860   Manipulation of ankle under general anesthesia (includes application of traction or other fixation apparatus)

Arthrodesis

27870   Arthrodesis, ankle, open

(For arthroscopic ankle arthrodesis, use 29899)

27871   Arthrodesis, tibiofibular joint, proximal or distal

Amputation

27880   Amputation, leg, through tibia and fibula;

27881   with immediate fitting technique including application of first cast

27882   open, circular (guillotine)

27884   secondary closure or scar revision

27886   re-amputation

27888   Amputation, ankle, through malleoli of tibia and fibula (eg, Syme, Pirogoff type procedures), with plastic closure and resection of nerves

27889   Ankle disarticulation

Other Procedures

27892   Decompression fasciotomy, leg; anterior and/or lateral compartments only, with debridement of nonviable muscle and/or nerve

(For decompression fasciotomy of the leg without debridement, use 27600)

27893   posterior compartment(s) only, with debridement of nonviable muscle and/or nerve

(For decompression fasciotomy of the leg without debridement, use 27601)

27894   anterior and/or lateral, and posterior compartment(s), with debridement of nonviable muscle and/or nerve

(For decompression fasciotomy of the leg without debridement, use 27602)

27899   Unlisted procedure, leg or ankle

Foot and Toes

Incision

(For incision and drainage procedures, superficial, see 10040-10160)

28001   Incision and drainage, bursa, foot

28002   Incision and drainage below fascia, with or without tendon sheath involvement, foot; single bursal space

28003   multiple areas

28005   Incision, bone cortex (eg, osteomyelitis or bone abscess), foot

28008   Fasciotomy, foot and/or toe

(See also 28060, 28062, 28250)

28010   Tenotomy, percutaneous, toe; single tendon

28011   multiple tendons

(For open tenotomy, see 28230-28234)

28020   Arthrotomy, including exploration, drainage, or removal of loose or foreign body; intertarsal or tarsometatarsal joint

28022   metatarsophalangeal joint

28024   interphalangeal joint

28035   Release, tarsal tunnel (posterior tibial nerve decompression)

(For other nerve entrapments, see 64704, 64722)

Excision

28039   Code is out of numerical sequence. See 28043-28175

28041   Code is out of numerical sequence. See 28043-28175

28043   Excision, tumor, soft tissue of foot or toe, subcutaneous; less than 1.5 cm

 # 28039   1.5 cm or greater

Musculoskeletal

(For excision of benign lesions of cutaneous origin [eg, sebaceous cyst], see 11420-11426)

28045 Excision, tumor, soft tissue of foot or toe, subfascial (eg, intramuscular); less than 1.5 cm

28041 1.5 cm or greater

28046 Radical resection of tumor (eg, sarcoma), soft tissue of foot or toe; less than 3 cm

28047 3 cm or greater

(For radical resection of tumor[s] of cutaneous origin [eg, melanoma], see 11620-11626)

28050 Arthrotomy with biopsy; intertarsal or tarsometatarsal joint

28052 metatarsophalangeal joint

28054 interphalangeal joint

28055 Neurectomy, intrinsic musculature of foot

28060 Fasciectomy, plantar fascia; partial (separate procedure)

28062 radical (separate procedure)

(For plantar fasciotomy, see 28008, 28250)

28070 Synovectomy; intertarsal or tarsometatarsal joint, each

28072 metatarsophalangeal joint, each

28080 Excision, interdigital (Morton) neuroma, single, each

28086 Synovectomy, tendon sheath, foot; flexor

28088 extensor

28090 Excision of lesion, tendon, tendon sheath, or capsule (including synovectomy) (eg, cyst or ganglion); foot

28092 toe(s), each

28100 Excision or curettage of bone cyst or benign tumor, talus or calcaneus;

28102 with iliac or other autograft (includes obtaining graft)

28103 with allograft

28104 Excision or curettage of bone cyst or benign tumor, tarsal or metatarsal, except talus or calcaneus;

28106 with iliac or other autograft (includes obtaining graft)

28107 with allograft

28108 Excision or curettage of bone cyst or benign tumor, phalanges of foot

(For ostectomy, partial (eg, hallux valgus, Silver type procedure), use 28290)

28110 Ostectomy, partial excision, fifth metatarsal head (bunionette) (separate procedure)

28111 Ostectomy, complete excision; first metatarsal head

28112 other metatarsal head (second, third or fourth)

28113 fifth metatarsal head

28114 all metatarsal heads, with partial proximal phalangectomy, excluding first metatarsal (eg, Clayton type procedure)

28116 Ostectomy, excision of tarsal coalition

28118 Ostectomy, calcaneus;

28119 for spur, with or without plantar fascial release

28120 Partial excision (craterization, saucerization, sequestrectomy, or diaphysectomy) bone (eg, osteomyelitis or bossing); talus or calcaneus

28122 tarsal or metatarsal bone, except talus or calcaneus

(For partial excision of talus or calcaneus, use 28120)

(For cheilectomy for hallux rigidus, use 28289)

28124 phalanx of toe

28126 Resection, partial or complete, phalangeal base, each toe

28130 Talectomy (astragalectomy)

(For calcanectomy, use 28118)

28140 Metatarsectomy

28150 Phalangectomy, toe, each toe

28153 Resection, condyle(s), distal end of phalanx, each toe

28160 Hemiphalangectomy or interphalangeal joint excision, toe, proximal end of phalanx, each

28171 Radical resection of tumor; tarsal (except talus or calcaneus)

28173 metatarsal

28175 phalanx of toe

(For talus or calcaneus, use 27647)

Introduction or Removal

28190 Removal of foreign body, foot; subcutaneous

28192 deep

28193 complicated

Repair, Revision, and/or Reconstruction

28200 Repair, tendon, flexor, foot; primary or secondary, without free graft, each tendon

28202 secondary with free graft, each tendon (includes obtaining graft)

28208 Repair, tendon, extensor, foot; primary or secondary, each tendon

28210 secondary with free graft, each tendon (includes obtaining graft)

28220 Tenolysis, flexor, foot; single tendon

28222 multiple tendons

28225 Tenolysis, extensor, foot; single tendon

28226 multiple tendons

28230 Tenotomy, open, tendon flexor; foot, single or multiple tendon(s) (separate procedure)

28232   toe, single tendon (separate procedure)

28234   Tenotomy, open, extensor, foot or toe, each tendon

(For tendon transfer to midfoot or hindfoot, see 27690, 27691)

28238   Reconstruction (advancement), posterior tibial tendon with excision of accessory tarsal navicular bone (eg, Kidner type procedure)

(For subcutaneous tenotomy, see 28010, 28011)

(For transfer or transplant of tendon with muscle redirection or rerouting, see 27690-27692)

(For extensor hallucis longus transfer with great toe IP fusion (Jones procedure), use 28760)

28240   Tenotomy, lengthening, or release, abductor hallucis muscle

28250   Division of plantar fascia and muscle (eg, Steindler stripping) (separate procedure)

28260   Capsulotomy, midfoot; medial release only (separate procedure)

28261   with tendon lengthening

28262   extensive, including posterior talotibial capsulotomy and tendon(s) lengthening (eg, resistant clubfoot deformity)

28264   Capsulotomy, midtarsal (eg, Heyman type procedure)

28270   Capsulotomy; metatarsophalangeal joint, with or without tenorrhaphy, each joint (separate procedure)

28272   interphalangeal joint, each joint (separate procedure)

28280   Syndactylization, toes (eg, webbing or Kelikian type procedure)

28285   Correction, hammertoe (eg, interphalangeal fusion, partial or total phalangectomy)

28286   Correction, cock-up fifth toe, with plastic skin closure (eg, Ruiz-Mora type procedure)

28288   Ostectomy, partial, exostectomy or condylectomy, metatarsal head, each metatarsal head

28289   Hallux rigidus correction with cheilectomy, debridement and capsular release of the first metatarsophalangeal joint

28290   Correction, hallux valgus (bunion), with or without sesamoidectomy; simple exostectomy (eg, Silver type procedure)

28292   Keller, McBride, or Mayo type procedure

28293   resection of joint with implant

28294   with tendon transplants (eg, Joplin type procedure)

28296   with metatarsal osteotomy (eg, Mitchell, Chevron, or concentric type procedures)

28297   Lapidus-type procedure

28298   by phalanx osteotomy

28299   by double osteotomy

28300   Osteotomy; calcaneus (eg, Dwyer or Chambers type procedure), with or without internal fixation

28302   talus

28304   Osteotomy, tarsal bones, other than calcaneus or talus;

28305   with autograft (includes obtaining graft) (eg, Fowler type)

28306   Osteotomy, with or without lengthening, shortening or angular correction, metatarsal; first metatarsal

28307   first metatarsal with autograft (other than first toe)

28308   other than first metatarsal, each

28309   multiple (eg, Swanson type cavus foot procedure)

28310   Osteotomy, shortening, angular or rotational correction; proximal phalanx, first toe (separate procedure)

28312   other phalanges, any toe

28313   Reconstruction, angular deformity of toe, soft tissue procedures only (eg, overlapping second toe, fifth toe, curly toes)

28315   Sesamoidectomy, first toe (separate procedure)

28320   Repair, nonunion or malunion; tarsal bones

28322   metatarsal, with or without bone graft (includes obtaining graft)

28340   Reconstruction, toe, macrodactyly; soft tissue resection

28341   requiring bone resection

28344   Reconstruction, toe(s); polydactyly

28345   syndactyly, with or without skin graft(s), each web

28360   Reconstruction, cleft foot

Fracture and/or Dislocation

28400   Closed treatment of calcaneal fracture; without manipulation

28405   with manipulation

28406   Percutaneous skeletal fixation of calcaneal fracture, with manipulation

28415   Open treatment of calcaneal fracture, includes internal fixation, when performed;

28420   with primary iliac or other autogenous bone graft (includes obtaining graft)

28430   Closed treatment of talus fracture; without manipulation

28435   with manipulation

28436   Percutaneous skeletal fixation of talus fracture, with manipulation

28445   Open treatment of talus fracture, includes internal fixation, when performed

28446   Open osteochondral autograft, talus (includes obtaining graft[s])

(Do not report 28446 in conjunction with 27705, 27707)

Musculoskeletal

(For arthroscopic osteochondral talus graft, use 29892)

(For open osteochondral allograft or repairs with industrial grafts, use 28899)

28450 Treatment of tarsal bone fracture (except talus and calcaneus); without manipulation, each

28455 with manipulation, each

28456 Percutaneous skeletal fixation of tarsal bone fracture (except talus and calcaneus), with manipulation, each

28465 Open treatment of tarsal bone fracture (except talus and calcaneus), includes internal fixation, when performed, each

28470 Closed treatment of metatarsal fracture; without manipulation, each

28475 with manipulation, each

28476 Percutaneous skeletal fixation of metatarsal fracture, with manipulation, each

28485 Open treatment of metatarsal fracture, includes internal fixation, when performed, each

28490 Closed treatment of fracture great toe, phalanx or phalanges; without manipulation

28495 with manipulation

28496 Percutaneous skeletal fixation of fracture great toe, phalanx or phalanges, with manipulation

28505 Open treatment of fracture, great toe, phalanx or phalanges, includes internal fixation, when performed

28510 Closed treatment of fracture, phalanx or phalanges, other than great toe; without manipulation, each

28515 with manipulation, each

28525 Open treatment of fracture, phalanx or phalanges, other than great toe, includes internal fixation, when performed, each

28530 Closed treatment of sesamoid fracture

28531 Open treatment of sesamoid fracture, with or without internal fixation

28540 Closed treatment of tarsal bone dislocation, other than talotarsal; without anesthesia

28545 requiring anesthesia

28546 Percutaneous skeletal fixation of tarsal bone dislocation, other than talotarsal, with manipulation

28555 Open treatment of tarsal bone dislocation, includes internal fixation, when performed

28570 Closed treatment of talotarsal joint dislocation; without anesthesia

28575 requiring anesthesia

28576 Percutaneous skeletal fixation of talotarsal joint dislocation, with manipulation

28585 Open treatment of talotarsal joint dislocation, includes internal fixation, when performed

28600 Closed treatment of tarsometatarsal joint dislocation; without anesthesia

28605 requiring anesthesia

28606 Percutaneous skeletal fixation of tarsometatarsal joint dislocation, with manipulation

28615 Open treatment of tarsometatarsal joint dislocation, includes internal fixation, when performed

28630 Closed treatment of metatarsophalangeal joint dislocation; without anesthesia

28635 requiring anesthesia

28636 Percutaneous skeletal fixation of metatarsophalangeal joint dislocation, with manipulation

28645 Open treatment of metatarsophalangeal joint dislocation, includes internal fixation, when performed

28660 Closed treatment of interphalangeal joint dislocation; without anesthesia

28665 requiring anesthesia

28666 Percutaneous skeletal fixation of interphalangeal joint dislocation, with manipulation

28675 Open treatment of interphalangeal joint dislocation, includes internal fixation, when performed

Arthrodesis

28705 Arthrodesis; pantalar

28715 triple

28725 subtalar

28730 Arthrodesis, midtarsal or tarsometatarsal, multiple or transverse;

28735 with osteotomy (eg, flatfoot correction)

28737 Arthrodesis, with tendon lengthening and advancement, midtarsal, tarsal navicular-cuneiform (eg, Miller type procedure)

28740 Arthrodesis, midtarsal or tarsometatarsal, single joint

28750 Arthrodesis, great toe; metatarsophalangeal joint

28755 interphalangeal joint

28760 Arthrodesis, with extensor hallucis longus transfer to first metatarsal neck, great toe, interphalangeal joint (eg, Jones type procedure)

(For hammertoe operation or interphalangeal fusion, use 28285)

Amputation

28800 Amputation, foot; midtarsal (eg, Chopart type procedure)

28805 transmetatarsal

28810 Amputation, metatarsal, with toe, single

28820 Amputation, toe; metatarsophalangeal joint

28825   interphalangeal joint

(For amputation of tuft of distal phalanx, use 11752)

Other Procedures

28890   Extracorporeal shock wave, high energy, performed by a physician or other qualified health care professional, requiring anesthesia other than local, including ultrasound guidance, involving the plantar fascia

(For extracorporeal shock wave therapy involving musculoskeletal system not otherwise specified, see 0019T, 0101T, 0102T)

(For extracorporeal shock wave therapy involving integumentary system not otherwise specified, see 0299T, 0300T)

(Do not report 28890 in conjunction with 0299T, 0300T when treating the same area)

28899   Unlisted procedure, foot or toes

Application of Casts and Strapping

The listed procedures apply when the cast application or strapping is a replacement procedure used during or after the period of follow-up care, or when the cast application or strapping is an initial service performed without a restorative treatment or procedure(s) to stabilize or protect a fracture, injury, or dislocation and/or to afford comfort to a patient. Restorative treatment or procedure(s) rendered by another individual following the application of the initial cast/splint/strap may be reported with a treatment of fracture and/or dislocation code.

An individual who applies the initial cast, strap, or splint and also assumes all of the subsequent fracture, dislocation, or injury care cannot use the application of casts and strapping codes as an initial service, since the first cast/splint or strap application is included in the treatment of fracture and/or dislocation codes. (See notes under Musculoskeletal System, page 72.) A temporary cast/splint/strap is not considered to be part of the preoperative care, and the use of the modifier 56 is not applicable. Additional evaluation and management services are reportable only if significant identifiable further services are provided at the time of the cast application or strapping.

If cast application or strapping is provided as an initial service (eg, casting of a sprained ankle or knee) in which no other procedure or treatment (eg, surgical repair, reduction of a fracture, or joint dislocation) is performed or is expected to be performed by an individual rendering the initial care only, use the casting, strapping, and/or supply code (99070) in addition to an evaluation and management code as appropriate.

Listed procedures include removal of cast or strapping.

(For orthotics management and training, see 97760-97762)

Body and Upper Extremity

Casts

29000   Application of halo type body cast (see 20661-20663 for insertion)

29010   Application of Risser jacket, localizer, body; only

29015   including head

(29020, 29025 have been deleted)

29035   Application of body cast, shoulder to hips;

29040   including head, Minerva type

29044   including 1 thigh

29046   including both thighs

29049   Application, cast; figure-of-eight

29055   shoulder spica

29058   plaster Velpeau

29065   shoulder to hand (long arm)

29075   elbow to finger (short arm)

29085   hand and lower forearm (gauntlet)

29086   finger (eg, contracture)

Splints

29105   Application of long arm splint (shoulder to hand)

29125   Application of short arm splint (forearm to hand); static

29126   dynamic

29130   Application of finger splint; static

29131   dynamic

Strapping—Any Age

29200   Strapping; thorax

(To report low back strapping, use 29799)

29240   shoulder (eg, Velpeau)

29260   elbow or wrist

29280   hand or finger

Lower Extremity

Casts

29305   Application of hip spica cast; 1 leg

29325   1 and one-half spica or both legs

(For hip spica (body) cast, including thighs only, use 29046)

Musculoskeletal

Musculoskeletal

29345	Application of long leg cast (thigh to toes);
29355	walker or ambulatory type
29358	Application of long leg cast brace
29365	Application of cylinder cast (thigh to ankle)
29405	Application of short leg cast (below knee to toes);
29425	walking or ambulatory type
29435	Application of patellar tendon bearing (PTB) cast
29440	Adding walker to previously applied cast
29445	Application of rigid total contact leg cast
29450	Application of clubfoot cast with molding or manipulation, long or short leg

(To report bilateral procedure, use 29450 with modifier 50)

Splints

29505	Application of long leg splint (thigh to ankle or toes)
29515	Application of short leg splint (calf to foot)

Strapping—Any Age

29520	Strapping; hip
29530	knee
29540	ankle and/or foot

(Do not report 29540 in conjunction with 29581, 29582)

29550	toes
29580	Unna boot

(Do not report 29580 in conjunction with 29581, 29582)

29581	Application of multi-layer compression system; leg (below knee), including ankle and foot

(Do not report 29581 in conjunction with 29540, 29580, 29582, 36475, 36476, 36478, 36479)

29582	thigh and leg, including ankle and foot, when performed

(Do not report 29582 in conjunction with 29540, 29580, 29581, 36475, 36476, 36478, 36479)

29583	upper arm and forearm

(Do not report 29583 in conjunction with 29584)

29584	upper arm, forearm, hand, and fingers

(Do not report 29584 in conjunction with 29583)

(29590 has been deleted)

Removal or Repair

Codes for cast removals should be employed only for casts applied by another individual.

29700	Removal or bivalving; gauntlet, boot or body cast
29705	full arm or full leg cast
29710	shoulder or hip spica, Minerva, or Risser jacket, etc.

(29715 has been deleted)

29720	Repair of spica, body cast or jacket
29730	Windowing of cast
29740	Wedging of cast (except clubfoot casts)
29750	Wedging of clubfoot cast

(To report bilateral procedure, use 29750 with modifier 50)

Other Procedures

29799	Unlisted procedure, casting or strapping

Endoscopy/Arthroscopy

Surgical endoscopy/arthroscopy always includes a diagnostic endoscopy/arthroscopy.

When arthroscopy is performed in conjunction with arthrotomy, add modifier 51.

29800	Arthroscopy, temporomandibular joint, diagnostic, with or without synovial biopsy (separate procedure)
29804	Arthroscopy, temporomandibular joint, surgical

(For open procedure, use 21010)

29805	Arthroscopy, shoulder, diagnostic, with or without synovial biopsy (separate procedure)

(For open procedure, see 23065-23066, 23100-23101)

29806	Arthroscopy, shoulder, surgical; capsulorrhaphy

(For open procedure, see 23450-23466)

(To report thermal capsulorrhaphy, use 29999)

29807	repair of SLAP lesion
29819	with removal of loose body or foreign body

(For open procedure, see 23040-23044, 23107)

29820	synovectomy, partial

(For open procedure, see 23105)

29821	synovectomy, complete

(For open procedure, see 23105)

29822	debridement, limited

(For open procedure, see specific open shoulder procedure performed)

29823	debridement, extensive

(For open procedure, see specific open shoulder procedure performed)

29824	distal claviculectomy including distal articular surface (Mumford procedure)

(For open procedure, use 23120)

29825   with lysis and resection of adhesions, with or without manipulation

(For open procedure, see specific open shoulder procedure performed)

+ 29826   decompression of subacromial space with partial acromioplasty, with coracoacromial ligament (ie, arch) release, when performed (List separately in addition to code for primary procedure)

(For open procedure, use 23130 or 23415)

(Use 29826 in conjunction with 29806-29825, 29827, 29828)

29827   with rotator cuff repair

(For open or mini-open rotator cuff repair, use 23412)

(When arthroscopic distal clavicle resection is performed at the same setting, use 29824 and append modifier 51)

29828   biceps tenodesis

(Do not report 29828 in conjunction with 29805, 29820, 29822)

(For open biceps tenodesis, use 23430)

29830   Arthroscopy, elbow, diagnostic, with or without synovial biopsy (separate procedure)

29834   Arthroscopy, elbow, surgical; with removal of loose body or foreign body

29835   synovectomy, partial

29836   synovectomy, complete

29837   debridement, limited

29838   debridement, extensive

29840   Arthroscopy, wrist, diagnostic, with or without synovial biopsy (separate procedure)

29843   Arthroscopy, wrist, surgical; for infection, lavage and drainage

29844   synovectomy, partial

29845   synovectomy, complete

29846   excision and/or repair of triangular fibrocartilage and/or joint debridement

29847   internal fixation for fracture or instability

29848   Endoscopy, wrist, surgical, with release of transverse carpal ligament

(For open procedure, use 64721)

29850   Arthroscopically aided treatment of intercondylar spine(s) and/or tuberosity fracture(s) of the knee, with or without manipulation; without internal or external fixation (includes arthroscopy)

29851   with internal or external fixation (includes arthroscopy)

(For bone graft, use 20900, 20902)

29855   Arthroscopically aided treatment of tibial fracture, proximal (plateau); unicondylar, includes internal fixation, when performed (includes arthroscopy)

29856   bicondylar, includes internal fixation, when performed (includes arthroscopy)

(For bone graft, use 20900, 20902)

29860   Arthroscopy, hip, diagnostic with or without synovial biopsy (separate procedure)

29861   Arthroscopy, hip, surgical; with removal of loose body or foreign body

29862   with debridement/shaving of articular cartilage (chondroplasty), abrasion arthroplasty, and/or resection of labrum

29863   with synovectomy

 # 29914   with femoroplasty (ie, treatment of cam lesion)

 # 29915   with acetabuloplasty (ie, treatment of pincer lesion)

(Do not report 29914, 29915 in conjunction with 29862, 29863)

 # 29916   with labral repair

(Do not report 29916 in conjunction with 29915, 29862, 29863)

29866   Arthroscopy, knee, surgical; osteochondral autograft(s) (eg, mosaicplasty) (includes harvesting of the autograft[s])

(Do not report 29866 in conjunction with 29870, 29871, 29875, 29884 when performed at the same session and/or 29874, 29877, 29879, 29885-29887 when performed in the same compartment)

(For open osteochondral autograft of knee, use 27416)

29867   osteochondral allograft (eg, mosaicplasty)

(Do not report 29867 in conjunction with 27570, 29870, 29871, 29875, 29884 when performed at the same session and/or 29874, 29877, 29879, 29885-29887 when performed in the same compartment)

(Do not report 29867 in conjunction with 27415)

29868   meniscal transplantation (includes arthrotomy for meniscal insertion), medial or lateral

(Do not report 29868 in conjunction with 29870, 29871, 29875, 29880, 29883, 29884 when performed at the same session or 29874, 29877, 29881, 29882 when performed in the same compartment)

29870   Arthroscopy, knee, diagnostic, with or without synovial biopsy (separate procedure)

(For open autologous chondrocyte implantation of the knee, use 27412)

29871   Arthroscopy, knee, surgical; for infection, lavage and drainage

(Do not report 29871 in conjunction with 27370)

(For implantation of osteochondral graft for treatment of articular surface defect, see 27412, 27415, 29866, 29867)

29873 with lateral release

(For open lateral release, use 27425)

29874 for removal of loose body or foreign body (eg, osteochondritis dissecans fragmentation, chondral fragmentation)

29875 synovectomy, limited (eg, plica or shelf resection) (separate procedure)

29876 synovectomy, major, 2 or more compartments (eg, medial or lateral)

29877 debridement/shaving of articular cartilage (chondroplasty)

(When performed with arthroscopic meniscectomy, see 29880 or 29881)

29879 abrasion arthroplasty (includes chondroplasty where necessary) or multiple drilling or microfracture

29880 with meniscectomy (medial AND lateral, including any meniscal shaving) including debridement/shaving of articular cartilage (chondroplasty), same or separate compartment(s), when performed

29881 with meniscectomy (medial OR lateral, including any meniscal shaving) including debridement/shaving of articular cartilage (chondroplasty), same or separate compartment(s), when performed

29882 with meniscus repair (medial OR lateral)

29883 with meniscus repair (medial AND lateral)

(For meniscal transplantation, medial or lateral, knee, use 29868)

29884 with lysis of adhesions, with or without manipulation (separate procedure)

29885 drilling for osteochondritis dissecans with bone grafting, with or without internal fixation (including debridement of base of lesion)

29886 drilling for intact osteochondritis dissecans lesion

29887 drilling for intact osteochondritis dissecans lesion with internal fixation

29888 Arthroscopically aided anterior cruciate ligament repair/ augmentation or reconstruction

29889 Arthroscopically aided posterior cruciate ligament repair/ augmentation or reconstruction

(Procedures 29888 and 29889 should not be used with reconstruction procedures 27427-27429)

29891 Arthroscopy, ankle, surgical, excision of osteochondral defect of talus and/or tibia, including drilling of the defect

29892 Arthroscopically aided repair of large osteochondritis dissecans lesion, talar dome fracture, or tibial plafond fracture, with or without internal fixation (includes arthroscopy)

29893 Endoscopic plantar fasciotomy

29894 Arthroscopy, ankle (tibiotalar and fibulotalar joints), surgical; with removal of loose body or foreign body

29895 synovectomy, partial

29897 debridement, limited

29898 debridement, extensive

29899 with ankle arthrodesis

(For open ankle arthrodesis, use 27870)

29900 Arthroscopy, metacarpophalangeal joint, diagnostic, includes synovial biopsy

(Do not report 29900 with 29901, 29902)

29901 Arthroscopy, metacarpophalangeal joint, surgical; with debridement

29902 with reduction of displaced ulnar collateral ligament (eg, Stenar lesion)

29904 Arthroscopy, subtalar joint, surgical; with removal of loose body or foreign body

29905 with synovectomy

29906 with debridement

29907 with subtalar arthrodesis

29914 Code is out of numerical sequence. See 29800-29999

29915 Code is out of numerical sequence. See 29800-29999

29916 Code is out of numerical sequence. See 29800-29999

29999 Unlisted procedure, arthroscopy

Respiratory System

Nose

Incision

30000   Drainage abscess or hematoma, nasal, internal approach

(For external approach, see 10060, 10140)

30020   Drainage abscess or hematoma, nasal septum

(For lateral rhinotomy, see specific application [eg, 30118, 30320])

Excision

30100   Biopsy, intranasal

(For biopsy skin of nose, see 11100, 11101)

30110   Excision, nasal polyp(s), simple

(30110 would normally be completed in an office setting)

(To report bilateral procedure, use 30110 with modifier 50)

30115   Excision, nasal polyp(s), extensive

(30115 would normally require the facilities available in a hospital setting)

(To report bilateral procedure, use 30115 with modifier 50)

30117   Excision or destruction (eg, laser), intranasal lesion; internal approach

30118   external approach (lateral rhinotomy)

30120   Excision or surgical planing of skin of nose for rhinophyma

30124   Excision dermoid cyst, nose; simple, skin, subcutaneous

30125   complex, under bone or cartilage

30130   Excision inferior turbinate, partial or complete, any method

(For excision of superior or middle turbinate, use 30999)

30140   Submucous resection inferior turbinate, partial or complete, any method

(Do not report 30130 or 30140 in conjunction with 30801, 30802, 30930)

(For submucous resection of superior or middle turbinate, use 30999)

(For endoscopic resection of concha bullosa of middle turbinate, use 31240)

(For submucous resection of nasal septum, use 30520)

30150   Rhinectomy; partial

30160   total

(For closure and/or reconstruction, primary or delayed, see **Integumentary System,** 13151-13160, 14060-14302, 15120, 15121, 15260, 15261, 15760, 20900-20912)

Introduction

30200   Injection into turbinate(s), therapeutic

30210   Displacement therapy (Proetz type)

30220   Insertion, nasal septal prosthesis (button)

Removal of Foreign Body

30300   Removal foreign body, intranasal; office type procedure

30310   requiring general anesthesia

30320   by lateral rhinotomy

Repair

(For obtaining tissues for graft, see 20900-20926, 21210)

30400   Rhinoplasty, primary; lateral and alar cartilages and/or elevation of nasal tip

(For columellar reconstruction, see 13151 et seq)

30410   complete, external parts including bony pyramid, lateral and alar cartilages, and/or elevation of nasal tip

30420   including major septal repair

30430   Rhinoplasty, secondary; minor revision (small amount of nasal tip work)

30435   intermediate revision (bony work with osteotomies)

30450   major revision (nasal tip work and osteotomies)

30460   Rhinoplasty for nasal deformity secondary to congenital cleft lip and/or palate, including columellar lengthening; tip only

30462   tip, septum, osteotomies

30465   Repair of nasal vestibular stenosis (eg, spreader grafting, lateral nasal wall reconstruction)

(30465 excludes obtaining graft. For graft procedure, see 20900-20926, 21210)

(30465 is used to report a bilateral procedure. For unilateral procedure, use modifier 52)

30520   Septoplasty or submucous resection, with or without cartilage scoring, contouring or replacement with graft

(For submucous resection of turbinates, use 30140)

30540   Repair choanal atresia; intranasal

30545   transpalatine

(Do not report modifier 63 in conjunction with 30540, 30545)

30560   Lysis intranasal synechia

Respiratory

Respiratory

30580 Repair fistula; oromaxillary (combine with 31030 if antrotomy is included)

30600 oronasal

30620 Septal or other intranasal dermatoplasty (does not include obtaining graft)

30630 Repair nasal septal perforations

Destruction

30801 Ablation, soft tissue of inferior turbinates, unilateral or bilateral, any method (eg, electrocautery, radiofrequency ablation, or tissue volume reduction); superficial

(For ablation of superior or middle turbinates, use 30999)

30802 intramural (ie, submucosal)

(Do not report 30801 in conjunction with 30802)

(Do not report 30801, 30802, 30930 in conjunction with 30130 or 30140)

(For cautery performed for control of nasal hemorrhage, see 30901-30906)

Other Procedures

30901 Control nasal hemorrhage, anterior, simple (limited cautery and/or packing) any method

(To report bilateral procedure, use 30901 with modifier 50)

30903 Control nasal hemorrhage, anterior, complex (extensive cautery and/or packing) any method

(To report bilateral procedure, use 30903 with modifier 50)

30905 Control nasal hemorrhage, posterior, with posterior nasal packs and/or cautery, any method; initial

30906 subsequent

30915 Ligation arteries; ethmoidal

30920 internal maxillary artery, transantral

(For ligation external carotid artery, use 37600)

30930 Fracture nasal inferior turbinate(s), therapeutic

(Do not report 30801, 30802, 30930 in conjunction with 30130 or 30140)

(For fracture of superior or middle turbinate[s], use 30999)

30999 Unlisted procedure, nose

Accessory Sinuses

Incision

31000 Lavage by cannulation; maxillary sinus (antrum puncture or natural ostium)

(To report bilateral procedure, use 31000 with modifier 50)

31002 sphenoid sinus

31020 Sinusotomy, maxillary (antrotomy); intranasal

(To report bilateral procedure, use 31020 with modifier 50)

31030 radical (Caldwell-Luc) without removal of antrochoanal polyps

(To report bilateral procedure, use 31030 with modifier 50)

31032 radical (Caldwell-Luc) with removal of antrochoanal polyps

(To report bilateral procedure, use 31032 with modifier 50)

31040 Pterygomaxillary fossa surgery, any approach

(For transantral ligation of internal maxillary artery, use 30920)

31050 Sinusotomy, sphenoid, with or without biopsy;

31051 with mucosal stripping or removal of polyp(s)

31070 Sinusotomy frontal; external, simple (trephine operation)

(For frontal intranasal sinusotomy, use 31276)

31075 transorbital, unilateral (for mucocele or osteoma, Lynch type)

31080 obliterative without osteoplastic flap, brow incision (includes ablation)

31081 obliterative, without osteoplastic flap, coronal incision (includes ablation)

31084 obliterative, with osteoplastic flap, brow incision

31085 obliterative, with osteoplastic flap, coronal incision

31086 nonobliterative, with osteoplastic flap, brow incision

31087 nonobliterative, with osteoplastic flap, coronal incision

31090 Sinusotomy, unilateral, 3 or more paranasal sinuses (frontal, maxillary, ethmoid, sphenoid)

Excision

31200 Ethmoidectomy; intranasal, anterior

31201 intranasal, total

31205 extranasal, total

31225 Maxillectomy; without orbital exenteration

31230 with orbital exenteration (en bloc)

(For orbital exenteration only, see 65110 et seq)

(For skin grafts, see 15120 et seq)

Endoscopy

A surgical sinus endoscopy includes a sinusotomy (when appropriate) and diagnostic endoscopy.

Codes 31295-31297 describe dilation of sinus ostia by displacement of tissue, any method, and include fluoroscopy if performed.

Codes 31233-31297 are used to report unilateral procedures unless otherwise specified.

Codes 31231-31235 for diagnostic evaluation refer to employing a nasal/sinus endoscope to inspect the interior of the nasal cavity and the middle and superior meatus, the turbinates, and the spheno-ethmoid recess. Any time a diagnostic evaluation is performed all these areas would be inspected and a separate code is not reported for each area.

31231   Nasal endoscopy, diagnostic, unilateral or bilateral (separate procedure)

31233   Nasal/sinus endoscopy, diagnostic with maxillary sinusoscopy (via inferior meatus or canine fossa puncture)

(Do not report 31233 in conjunction with 31295 when performed on the same sinus)

31235   Nasal/sinus endoscopy, diagnostic with sphenoid sinusoscopy (via puncture of sphenoidal face or cannulation of ostium)

(Do not report 31235 in conjunction with 31297 when performed on the same sinus)

31237   Nasal/sinus endoscopy, surgical; with biopsy, polypectomy or debridement (separate procedure)

31238   with control of nasal hemorrhage

31239   with dacryocystorhinostomy

31240   with concha bullosa resection

(For endoscopic osteomeatal complex [OMC] resection with antrostomy and/or anterior ethmoidectomy, with or without removal of polyp[s], use 31254 and 31256)

(For endoscopic osteomeatal complex [OMC] resection with antrostomy, removal of antral mucosal disease, and/or anterior ethmoidectomy, with or without removal of polyp[s], use 31254 and 31267)

(For endoscopic frontal sinus exploration, osteomeatal complex [OMC] resection and/or anterior ethmoidectomy, with or without removal of polyp[s], use 31254 and 31276)

(For endoscopic frontal sinus exploration, osteomeatal complex [OMC] resection, antrostomy, and/or anterior ethmoidectomy, with or without removal of polyp[s], use 31254, 31256, and 31276)

(For endoscopic nasal diagnostic endoscopy, see 31231-31235)

(For endoscopic osteomeatal complex [OMC] resection, frontal sinus exploration, antrostomy, removal of antral mucosal disease, and/or anterior ethmoidectomy, with or without removal of polyp[s], use 31254, 31267, and 31276)

31254   Nasal/sinus endoscopy, surgical; with ethmoidectomy, partial (anterior)

31255   with ethmoidectomy, total (anterior and posterior)

31256   Nasal/sinus endoscopy, surgical, with maxillary antrostomy;

(For endoscopic anterior and posterior ethmoidectomy [APE] and antrostomy, with or without removal of polyp[s], use 31255 and 31256)

(For endoscopic anterior and posterior ethmoidectomy [APE], antrostomy and removal of antral mucosal disease, with or without removal of polyp[s], use 31255 and 31267)

(For endoscopic anterior and posterior ethmoidectomy [APE], and frontal sinus exploration, with or without removal of polyp[s], use 31255 and 31276)

31267   with removal of tissue from maxillary sinus

(Do not report 31256, 31267 in conjunction with 31295 when performed on the same sinus)

(For endoscopic anterior and posterior ethmoidectomy [APE], and frontal sinus exploration and antrostomy, with or without removal of polyp[s], use 31255, 31256, and 31276)

(For endoscopic anterior and posterior ethmoidectomy [APE], frontal sinus exploration, antrostomy, and removal of antral mucosal disease, with or without removal of polyp[s], use 31255, 31267, and 31276)

31276   Nasal/sinus endoscopy, surgical with frontal sinus exploration, with or without removal of tissue from frontal sinus

(Do not report 31276 in conjunction with 31296 when performed on the same sinus)

(For endoscopic anterior and posterior ethmoidectomy and sphenoidotomy [APS], with or without removal of polyp[s], use 31255, 31287 or 31288)

(For endoscopic anterior and posterior ethmoidectomy and sphenoidotomy [APS], and antrostomy, with or without removal of polyp[s], use 31255, 31256, and 31287 or 31288)

(For endoscopic anterior and posterior ethmoidectomy and sphenoidotomy [APS], antrostomy and removal of antral mucosal disease, with or without removal of polyp[s], use 31255, 31267, and 31287 or 31288)

(For endoscopic anterior and posterior ethmoidectomy and sphenoidotomy [APS], and frontal sinus exploration with or without removal of polyp[s], use 31255, 31287 or 31288, and 31276)

Respiratory

Respiratory

(For endoscopic anterior and posterior ethmoidectomy and sphenoidotomy [APS], with or without removal of polyp[s], with frontal sinus exploration and antrostomy, use 31255, 31256, 31287 or 31288, and 31276)

(For unilateral endoscopy of 2 or more sinuses, see 31231-31235)

(For endoscopic anterior and posterior ethmoidectomy and sphenoidotomy [APS], frontal sinus exploration, antrostomy and removal of antral mucosal disease, with or without removal of polyp[s], see 31255, 31267, 31287 or 31288 and 31276)

31287 Nasal/sinus endoscopy, surgical, with sphenoidotomy;

31288 with removal of tissue from the sphenoid sinus

(Do not report 31287, 31288 in conjunction with 31297 when performed on the same sinus)

31290 Nasal/sinus endoscopy, surgical, with repair of cerebrospinal fluid leak; ethmoid region

31291 sphenoid region

31292 Nasal/sinus endoscopy, surgical; with medial or inferior orbital wall decompression

31293 with medial orbital wall and inferior orbital wall decompression

31294 with optic nerve decompression

31295 Nasal/sinus endoscopy, surgical; with dilation of maxillary sinus ostium (eg, balloon dilation), transnasal or via canine fossa

(Do not report 31295 in conjunction with 31233, 31256, 31267 when performed on the same sinus)

31296 with dilation of frontal sinus ostium (eg, balloon dilation)

(Do not report 31296 in conjunction with 31276 when performed on the same sinus)

31297 with dilation of sphenoid sinus ostium (eg, balloon dilation)

(Do not report 31297 in conjunction with 31235, 31287, 31288 when performed on the same sinus)

Other Procedures

(For hypophysectomy, transantral or transeptal approach, use 61548)

(For transcranial hypophysectomy, use 61546)

31299 Unlisted procedure, accessory sinuses

Larynx

Excision

31300 Laryngotomy (thyrotomy, laryngofissure); with removal of tumor or laryngocele, cordectomy

31320 diagnostic

31360 Laryngectomy; total, without radical neck dissection

31365 total, with radical neck dissection

31367 subtotal supraglottic, without radical neck dissection

31368 subtotal supraglottic, with radical neck dissection

31370 Partial laryngectomy (hemilaryngectomy); horizontal

31375 laterovertical

31380 anterovertical

31382 antero-latero-vertical

31390 Pharyngolaryngectomy, with radical neck dissection; without reconstruction

31395 with reconstruction

31400 Arytenoidectomy or arytenoidopexy, external approach

(For endoscopic arytenoidectomy, use 31560)

31420 Epiglottidectomy

Introduction

⊘ **31500** Intubation, endotracheal, emergency procedure

31502 Tracheotomy tube change prior to establishment of fistula tract

Endoscopy

For endoscopic procedures, report appropriate endoscopy of each anatomic site examined. Laryngoscopy includes examination of the tongue base, larynx, and hypopharynx. If using operating microscope, telescope, or both, use the applicable code only once per operative session.

31505 Laryngoscopy, indirect; diagnostic (separate procedure)

31510 with biopsy

31511 with removal of foreign body

31512 with removal of lesion

31513 with vocal cord injection

31515 Laryngoscopy direct, with or without tracheoscopy; for aspiration

31520 diagnostic, newborn

(Do not report modifier 63 in conjunction with 31520)

31525 diagnostic, except newborn

31526 diagnostic, with operating microscope or telescope

(Do not report 31526 in conjunction with 69990)

31527   with insertion of obturator

31528   with dilation, initial

31529   with dilation, subsequent

31530   Laryngoscopy, direct, operative, with foreign body removal;

31531   with operating microscope or telescope

(Do not report code 69990 in addition to code 31531)

31535   Laryngoscopy, direct, operative, with biopsy;

31536   with operating microscope or telescope

(Do not report code 69990 in addition to code 31536)

31540   Laryngoscopy, direct, operative, with excision of tumor and/or stripping of vocal cords or epiglottis;

31541   with operating microscope or telescope

(Do not report code 69990 in addition to code 31541)

31545   Laryngoscopy, direct, operative, with operating microscope or telescope, with submucosal removal of non-neoplastic lesion(s) of vocal cord; reconstruction with local tissue flap(s)

31546   reconstruction with graft(s) (includes obtaining autograft)

(Do not report 31546 in addition to 20926 for graft harvest)

(For reconstruction of vocal cord with allograft, use 31599)

(Do not report 31545 or 31546 in conjunction with 31540, 31541, 69990)

31560   Laryngoscopy, direct, operative, with arytenoidectomy;

31561   with operating microscope or telescope

(Do not report code 69990 in addition to code 31561)

31570   Laryngoscopy, direct, with injection into vocal cord(s), therapeutic;

31571   with operating microscope or telescope

(Do not report 31571 in conjunction with 69990)

31575   Laryngoscopy, flexible fiberoptic; diagnostic

(Do not report 31575 in conjunction with 43197, 43198)

31576   with biopsy

31577   with removal of foreign body

31578   with removal of lesion

(To report flexible fiberoptic endoscopic evaluation of swallowing, see 92612-92613)

(To report flexible fiberoptic endoscopic evaluation with sensory testing, see 92614-92615)

(To report flexible fiberoptic endoscopic evaluation of swallowing with sensory testing, see 92616-92617)

(For flexible fiberoptic laryngoscopy as part of flexible fiberoptic endoscopic evaluation of swallowing and/or laryngeal sensory testing by cine or video recording, see 92612-92617)

31579   Laryngoscopy, flexible or rigid fiberoptic, with stroboscopy

Repair

31580   Laryngoplasty; for laryngeal web, 2-stage, with keel insertion and removal

31582   for laryngeal stenosis, with graft or core mold, including tracheotomy

31584   with open reduction of fracture

31587   Laryngoplasty, cricoid split

31588   Laryngoplasty, not otherwise specified (eg, for burns, reconstruction after partial laryngectomy)

31590   Laryngeal reinnervation by neuromuscular pedicle

Destruction

31595   Section recurrent laryngeal nerve, therapeutic (separate procedure), unilateral

Other Procedures

31599   Unlisted procedure, larynx

Trachea and Bronchi

Incision

31600   Tracheostomy, planned (separate procedure);

31601   younger than 2 years

31603   Tracheostomy, emergency procedure; transtracheal

31605   cricothyroid membrane

31610   Tracheostomy, fenestration procedure with skin flaps

(For endotracheal intubation, use 31500)

(For tracheal aspiration under direct vision, use 31515)

31611   Construction of tracheoesophageal fistula and subsequent insertion of an alaryngeal speech prosthesis (eg, voice button, Blom-Singer prosthesis)

31612   Tracheal puncture, percutaneous with transtracheal aspiration and/or injection

31613   Tracheostoma revision; simple, without flap rotation

31614   complex, with flap rotation

Endoscopy

For endoscopy procedures, code appropriate endoscopy of each anatomic site examined. Surgical bronchoscopy always includes diagnostic bronchoscopy when performed

Respiratory

by the same physician. Codes 31622-31651, 31660, 31661 include fluoroscopic guidance, when performed.

►Codes 31652 and 31653 are complete services used for sampling (eg, aspiration/biopsy) lymph node(s) or adjacent structure(s) utilizing endobronchial ultrasound (EBUS) and are reported separately. Code 31654 is an add-on code and should be reported for identifying one or more peripheral lesion(s) with transendoscopic ultrasound.◄

⊙ **31615** Tracheobronchoscopy through established tracheostomy incision

►(For tracheoscopy, see laryngoscopy codes 31515-31578)◄

►(31620 has been deleted)◄

►(For bronchoscopy with endobronchial ultrasound [EBUS] guided transtracheal/transbronchial sampling of mediastinal and/or hilar lymph node stations or structures, see 31652, 31653. For transendoscopic ultrasound during bronchoscopic diagnostic or therapeutic intervention[s] for peripheral lesion[s], use 31654)◄

⊙ **31622** Bronchoscopy, rigid or flexible, including fluoroscopic guidance, when performed; diagnostic, with cell washing, when performed (separate procedure)

⊙ **31623**   with brushing or protected brushings

⊙ **31624**   with bronchial alveolar lavage

⊙ **31625**   with bronchial or endobronchial biopsy(s), single or multiple sites

⊙ **31626**   with placement of fiducial markers, single or multiple

(Report supply of device separately)

⊙➕ **31627**   with computer-assisted, image-guided navigation (List separately in addition to code for primary procedure[s])

(31627 includes 3D reconstruction. Do not report 31627 in conjunction with 76376, 76377)

(Use 31627 in conjunction with 31615, 31622-31626, 31628-31631, 31635, 31636, 31638-31643)

⊙ **31628**   with transbronchial lung biopsy(s), single lobe

(31628 should be reported only once regardless of how many transbronchial lung biopsies are performed in a lobe)

(To report transbronchial lung biopsies performed on additional lobe, use 31632)

⊙ **31629**   with transbronchial needle aspiration biopsy(s), trachea, main stem and/or lobar bronchus(i)

(31629 should be reported only once for upper airway biopsies regardless of how many transbronchial needle aspiration biopsies are performed in the upper airway or in a lobe)

(To report transbronchial needle aspiration biopsies performed on additional lobe[s], use 31633)

31630   with tracheal/bronchial dilation or closed reduction of fracture

31631   with placement of tracheal stent(s) (includes tracheal/bronchial dilation as required)

(For placement of bronchial stent, see 31636, 31637)

(For revision of tracheal/bronchial stent, use 31638)

⊙➕▲ **31632**   with transbronchial lung biopsy(s), each additional lobe (List separately in addition to code for primary procedure)

(Use 31632 in conjunction with 31628)

(31632 should be reported only once regardless of how many transbronchial lung biopsies are performed in a lobe)

⊙➕▲ **31633**   with transbronchial needle aspiration biopsy(s), each additional lobe (List separately in addition to code for primary procedure)

(Use 31633 in conjunction with 31629)

(31633 should be reported only once regardless of how many transbronchial needle aspiration biopsies are performed in the trachea or the additional lobe)

⊙ **31634**   with balloon occlusion, with assessment of air leak, with administration of occlusive substance (eg, fibrin glue), if performed

(Do not report 31634 in conjunction with 31647, 31651 at the same session)

⊙ **31635**   with removal of foreign body

(For removal of implanted bronchial valves, see 31648-31649)

31636   with placement of bronchial stent(s) (includes tracheal/bronchial dilation as required), initial bronchus

➕ **31637**   each additional major bronchus stented (List separately in addition to code for primary procedure)

(Use 31637 in conjunction with 31636)

31638   with revision of tracheal or bronchial stent inserted at previous session (includes tracheal/bronchial dilation as required)

31640   with excision of tumor

31641   with destruction of tumor or relief of stenosis by any method other than excision (eg, laser therapy, cryotherapy)

(For bronchoscopic photodynamic therapy, report 31641 in addition to 96570, 96571 as appropriate)

31643   with placement of catheter(s) for intracavitary radioelement application

►(For intracavitary radioelement application, see 77761-77763, 77770, 77771, 77772)◄

⊙ **31645**   with therapeutic aspiration of tracheobronchial tree, initial (eg, drainage of lung abscess)

⊙ **31646**   with therapeutic aspiration of tracheobronchial tree, subsequent

(For catheter aspiration of tracheobronchial tree at bedside, use 31725)

⊙ **31647**   with balloon occlusion, when performed, assessment of air leak, airway sizing, and insertion of bronchial valve(s), initial lobe

#⊙+ **31651**   with balloon occlusion, when performed, assessment of air leak, airway sizing, and insertion of bronchial valve(s), each additional lobe (List separately in addition to code for primary procedure[s])

(Use 31651 in conjunction with 31647)

⊙ **31648**   with removal of bronchial valve(s), initial lobe

(For removal and insertion of a bronchial valve at the same session, see 31647, 31648, and 31651)

⊙+ **31649**   with removal of bronchial valve(s), each additional lobe (List separately in addition to code for primary procedure)

(Use 31649 in conjunction with 31648)

31651   Code is out of numerical sequence. See 31615-31649

⊙● **31652**   with endobronchial ultrasound (EBUS) guided transtracheal and/or transbronchial sampling (eg, aspiration[s]/biopsy[ies]), one or two mediastinal and/or hilar lymph node stations or structures

⊙● **31653**   with endobronchial ultrasound (EBUS) guided transtracheal and/or transbronchial sampling (eg, aspiration[s]/biopsy[ies]), 3 or more mediastinal and/or hilar lymph node stations or structures

⊙+● **31654**   with transendoscopic endobronchial ultrasound (EBUS) during bronchoscopic diagnostic or therapeutic intervention(s) for peripheral lesion(s) (List separately in addition to code for primary procedure[s])

▶(Use 31654 in conjunction with 31622, 31623, 31624, 31625, 31626, 31628, 31629, 31640, 31643, 31645, 31646)◀

▶(For EBUS to access mediastinal or hilar lymph node station[s] or adjacent structure[s], see 31652, 31653)◀

▶(Report 31652, 31653, 31654 only once per session)◀

(31656 has been deleted. To report, use 31899)

Bronchial Thermoplasty

⊙ **31660**   Bronchoscopy, rigid or flexible, including fluoroscopic guidance, when performed; with bronchial thermoplasty, 1 lobe

⊙ **31661**   with bronchial thermoplasty, 2 or more lobes

Introduction

(For endotracheal intubation, use 31500)

(For tracheal aspiration under direct vision, see 31515)

(31715 has been deleted. To report, use 31899)

31717   Catheterization with bronchial brush biopsy

31720   Catheter aspiration (separate procedure); nasotracheal

⊙ **31725**   tracheobronchial with fiberscope, bedside

31730   Transtracheal (percutaneous) introduction of needle wire dilator/stent or indwelling tube for oxygen therapy

Excision, Repair

31750   Tracheoplasty; cervical

31755   tracheopharyngeal fistulization, each stage

31760   intrathoracic

31766   Carinal reconstruction

31770   Bronchoplasty; graft repair

31775   excision stenosis and anastomosis

(For lobectomy and bronchoplasty, use 32501)

31780   Excision tracheal stenosis and anastomosis; cervical

31781   cervicothoracic

31785   Excision of tracheal tumor or carcinoma; cervical

31786   thoracic

31800   Suture of tracheal wound or injury; cervical

31805   intrathoracic

31820   Surgical closure tracheostomy or fistula; without plastic repair

31825   with plastic repair

(For repair tracheoesophageal fistula, see 43305, 43312)

31830   Revision of tracheostomy scar

Other Procedures

31899   Unlisted procedure, trachea, bronchi

Lungs and Pleura

Pleural cavity or lung biopsy procedures may be accomplished using a percutaneous, thoracoscopic (Video-Assisted Thoracoscopic Surgery [VATS]), or thoracotomy approach. They involve the removal of differing amounts of tissue for diagnosis. A biopsy may be performed using different techniques such as incision or wedge. Lung resection procedures include diagnostic and therapeutic procedures, including the removal of blebs, bullae, cysts, and benign or malignant tumors or lesions. These procedures may involve the removal of small portions of the lung or even an entire lung. Additionally, lung resection procedures may require the removal of

Respiratory

Respiratory

adjacent structures. Both diagnostic lung biopsies and therapeutic lung resections can be performed utilizing a wedge technique. However, a diagnostic biopsy of a lung nodule using a wedge technique requires only that a tissue sample be obtained without particular attention to resection margins. A therapeutic wedge resection requires attention to margins and complete resection even when the wedge resection is ultimately followed by a more extensive resection. In the case of a wedge resection in which intraoperative pathology consultation determines that a more extensive resection is required in the same anatomic location, it becomes classified as a diagnostic wedge resection (32507, 32668). When no more extensive resection is required, the same procedure is a therapeutic wedge resection (32505, 32666).

Pleural or lung biopsies or diagnostic wedge resections should be reported using codes 32096, 32097, 32098, 32400, 32405, 32507, 32607, 32608, 32609, or 32668. The open or thoracoscopic (VATS) therapeutic resection of lung mass or nodules via a wedge resection is reported using codes 32505, 32506, 32666, and 32667. More extensive anatomic lung resection procedures, which can be performed with either thoracotomy or thoracoscopic (VATS) approaches, include: segmentectomy, lobectomy, bilobectomy, and pneumonectomy.

When diagnostic biopsy(ies) of the lung are performed, regardless of the approach (ie, open or thoracoscopic [VATS]) or technique (eg, incisional resection, cautery resection, or stapled wedge), and the specimen is sent for intraoperative pathology consultation, and during that same operative session the surgeon uses these results to determine the extent of the necessary surgical resection that includes the anatomical location biopsied, only the most extensive procedure performed (eg, segmentectomy, lobectomy, thoracoscopic [VATS] lobectomy) should be reported.

The therapeutic wedge resection codes (32505, 32506, 32666, or 32667) should not be reported in addition to the more extensive lung procedure (eg, lobectomy) unless the therapeutic wedge resection was performed on a different lobe or on the contralateral lung, whether or not an intraoperative pathology consultation is used to determine the extent of lung resection. When a diagnostic wedge resection is followed by a more extensive procedure in the same anatomical location, report add-on codes 32507 or 32668 with the more extensive procedure(s). When a therapeutic wedge resection (32505, 32506, 32666, or 32667) is performed in a different lobe than the more extensive lung resection (eg, lobectomy), report the therapeutic wedge resection with modifier 59.

Incision

32035	Thoracostomy; with rib resection for empyema
32036	with open flap drainage for empyema

(To report wound exploration due to penetrating trauma without thoracotomy, use 20101)

32096	Thoracotomy, with diagnostic biopsy(ies) of lung infiltrate(s) (eg, wedge, incisional), unilateral

(Do not report 32096 more than once per lung)

(Do not report 32096 in conjunction with 32440, 32442, 32445, 32488)

32097	Thoracotomy, with diagnostic biopsy(ies) of lung nodule(s) or mass(es) (eg, wedge, incisional), unilateral

(Do not report 32097 more than once per lung)

(Do not report 32097 in conjunction with 32440, 32442, 32445, 32488)

32098	Thoracotomy, with biopsy(ies) of pleura
32100	Thoracotomy; with exploration

(Do not report 32100 in conjunction with 19260, 19271, 19272, 32503, 32504, 33955, 33956, 33957, 33963, 33964)

32110	with control of traumatic hemorrhage and/or repair of lung tear
32120	for postoperative complications
32124	with open intrapleural pneumonolysis
32140	with cyst(s) removal, includes pleural procedure when performed
32141	with resection-plication of bullae, includes any pleural procedure when performed

(For lung volume reduction, use 32491)

32150	with removal of intrapleural foreign body or fibrin deposit
32151	with removal of intrapulmonary foreign body
32160	with cardiac massage

(For segmental or other resections of lung, see 32480-32504)

32200	Pneumonostomy, with open drainage of abscess or cyst

(32201 has been deleted)

(For percutaneous image-guided drainage of abscess or cyst of lungs or mediastinum by catheter placement, use 49405)

32215	Pleural scarification for repeat pneumothorax
32220	Decortication, pulmonary (separate procedure); total
32225	partial

Excision/Resection

32310	Pleurectomy, parietal (separate procedure)
32320	Decortication and parietal pleurectomy
32400	Biopsy, pleura, percutaneous needle

(If imaging guidance is performed, see 76942, 77002, 77012, 77021)

(For fine needle aspiration, use 10021 or 10022)

⊙ **32405** Biopsy, lung or mediastinum, percutaneous needle

(For open biopsy of lung, see 32096, 32097. For open biopsy of mediastinum, see 39000 or 39010. For thoracoscopic [VATS] biopsy of lung, pleura, pericardium, or mediastinal space structure, see 32604, 32606, 32607, 32608, 32609)

(For radiological supervision and interpretation, see 76942, 77002, 77012, 77021)

(For fine needle aspiration, use 10022)

Removal

(32420 has been deleted. To report, use 32405)

(32421 and 32422 have been deleted. To report, see 32554, 32555)

32440 Removal of lung, pneumonectomy;

32442 with resection of segment of trachea followed by broncho-tracheal anastomosis (sleeve pneumonectomy)

32445 extrapleural

(For extrapleural pneumonectomy, with empyemectomy, use 32445 and 32540)

(If lung resection is performed with chest wall tumor resection, report the appropriate chest wall tumor resection 19260-19272, in addition to lung resection 32440-32445)

32480 Removal of lung, other than pneumonectomy; single lobe (lobectomy)

32482 2 lobes (bilobectomy)

32484 single segment (segmentectomy)

(For removal of lung with bronchoplasty, use 32501)

32486 with circumferential resection of segment of bronchus followed by broncho-bronchial anastomosis (sleeve lobectomy)

32488 with all remaining lung following previous removal of a portion of lung (completion pneumonectomy)

(For lobectomy or segmentectomy, with concomitant decortication, use 32320 and the appropriate removal of lung code)

32491 with resection-plication of emphysematous lung(s) (bullous or non-bullous) for lung volume reduction, sternal split or transthoracic approach, includes any pleural procedure, when performed

(If lung resection is performed with chest wall tumor resection, report the appropriate chest wall tumor resection 19260-19272, in addition to lung resection 32480, 32482, 32484, 32486, 32488, 32505, 32506, 32507)

+ **32501** Resection and repair of portion of bronchus (bronchoplasty) when performed at time of lobectomy or segmentectomy (List separately in addition to code for primary procedure)

(Use 32501 in conjunction with 32480, 32482, 32484)

(32501 is to be used when a portion of the bronchus to preserved lung is removed and requires plastic closure to preserve function of that preserved lung. It is not to be used for closure for the proximal end of a resected bronchus)

32503 Resection of apical lung tumor (eg, Pancoast tumor), including chest wall resection, rib(s) resection(s), neurovascular dissection, when performed; without chest wall reconstruction(s)

32504 with chest wall reconstruction

(Do not report 32503, 32504 in conjunction with 19260, 19271, 19272, 32100, 32551, 32554, 32555)

32505 Thoracotomy; with therapeutic wedge resection (eg, mass, nodule), initial

(Do not report 32505 in conjunction with 32440, 32442, 32445, 32488)

+ **32506** with therapeutic wedge resection (eg, mass or nodule), each additional resection, ipsilateral (List separately in addition to code for primary procedure)

(Report 32506 only in conjunction with 32505)

(If lung resection is performed with chest wall tumor resection, report the appropriate chest wall tumor resection 19260-19272, in addition to lung resection 32480, 32482, 32484, 32486, 32488, 32505, 32506, 32507)

+ **32507** with diagnostic wedge resection followed by anatomic lung resection (List separately in addition to code for primary procedure)

(Report 32507 in conjunction with 32440, 32442, 32445, 32480, 32482, 32484, 32486, 32488, 32503, 32504)

32540 Extrapleural enucleation of empyema (empyemectomy)

(For extrapleural enucleation of empyema [empyemectomy] with lobectomy, use 32540 and the appropriate removal of lung code)

Introduction and Removal

⊙ **32550** Insertion of indwelling tunneled pleural catheter with cuff

(Do not report 32550 in conjunction with 32554, 32555, 32556, 32557 when performed on the same side of the chest)

(If imaging guidance is performed, use 75989)

⊙ **32551** Tube thoracostomy, includes connection to drainage system (eg, water seal), when performed, open (separate procedure)

32552 Removal of indwelling tunneled pleural catheter with cuff

⊙ **32553** Placement of interstitial device(s) for radiation therapy guidance (eg, fiducial markers, dosimeter), percutaneous, intra-thoracic, single or multiple

(Report supply of device separately)

Respiratory

(For imaging guidance, see 76942, 77002, 77012, 77021)

(For percutaneous placement of interstitial device[s] for intra-abdominal, intrapelvic, and/or retroperitoneal radiation therapy guidance, use 49411)

32554 Thoracentesis, needle or catheter, aspiration of the pleural space; without imaging guidance

32555 with imaging guidance

32556 Pleural drainage, percutaneous, with insertion of indwelling catheter; without imaging guidance

32557 with imaging guidance

(For insertion of indwelling tunneled pleural catheter with cuff, use 32550)

(For open procedure, use 32551)

(Do not report 32554-32557 in conjunction with 32550, 32551 when performed on the same side of the chest)

(Do not report 32554-32557 in conjunction with 75989, 76942, 77002, 77012, 77021)

Destruction

The instillation of a fibrinolytic agent may be performed multiple times per day over the course of several days. Code 32561 should be reported only once on the initial day treatment. Code 32562 should be reported only once on each subsequent day of treatment.

32560 Instillation, via chest tube/catheter, agent for pleurodesis (eg, talc for recurrent or persistent pneumothorax)

(For chest tube insertion, use 32551)

32561 Instillation(s), via chest tube/catheter, agent for fibrinolysis (eg, fibrinolytic agent for break up of multiloculated effusion); initial day

(For chest tube insertion, use 32551)

32562 subsequent day

(For chest tube insertion, use 32551)

Thoracoscopy (Video-assisted thoracic surgery [VATS])

Surgical thoracoscopy (video-assisted thoracic surgery [VATS]) always includes diagnostic thoracoscopy.

32601 Thoracoscopy, diagnostic (separate procedure); lungs, pericardial sac, mediastinal or pleural space, without biopsy

32604 pericardial sac, with biopsy

(For open pericardial biopsy, use 39010)

32606 mediastinal space, with biopsy

32607 Thoracoscopy; with diagnostic biopsy(ies) of lung infiltrate(s) (eg, wedge, incisional), unilateral

(Do not report 32607 more than once per lung)

(Do not report 32607 in conjunction with 32440, 32442, 32445, 32488, 32671)

32608 with diagnostic biopsy(ies) of lung nodule(s) or mass(es) (eg, wedge, incisional), unilateral

(Do not report 32608 more than once per lung)

(Do not report 32608 in conjunction with 32440, 32442, 32445, 32488, 32671)

32609 with biopsy(ies) of pleura

32650 Thoracoscopy, surgical; with pleurodesis (eg, mechanical or chemical)

32651 with partial pulmonary decortication

32652 with total pulmonary decortication, including intrapleural pneumonolysis

32653 with removal of intrapleural foreign body or fibrin deposit

32654 with control of traumatic hemorrhage

32655 with resection-plication of bullae, includes any pleural procedure when performed

(For thoracoscopic [VATS] lung volume reduction surgery, use 32672)

32656 with parietal pleurectomy

32658 with removal of clot or foreign body from pericardial sac

32659 with creation of pericardial window or partial resection of pericardial sac for drainage

(32660 has been deleted)

32661 with excision of pericardial cyst, tumor, or mass

32662 with excision of mediastinal cyst, tumor, or mass

32663 with lobectomy (single lobe)

(For thoracoscopic [VATS] segmentectomy, use 32669)

32664 with thoracic sympathectomy

32665 with esophagomyotomy (Heller type)

(For exploratory thoracoscopy, and exploratory thoracoscopy with biopsy, see 32601-32609)

32666 with therapeutic wedge resection (eg, mass, nodule), initial unilateral

(To report bilateral procedure, report 32666 with modifier 50)

(Do not report 32666 in conjunction with 32440, 32442, 32445, 32488, 32671)

+ **32667** with therapeutic wedge resection (eg, mass or nodule), each additional resection, ipsilateral (List separately in addition to code for primary procedure)

(Report 32667 only in conjunction with 32666)

(Do not report 32667 in conjunction with 32440, 32442, 32445, 32488, 32671)

+ **32668**   with diagnostic wedge resection followed by anatomic lung resection (List separately in addition to code for primary procedure)

(Report 32668 in conjunction with 32440, 32442, 32445, 32480, 32482, 32484, 32486, 32488, 32503, 32504, 32663, 32669, 32670, 32671)

32669   with removal of a single lung segment (segmentectomy)

32670   with removal of two lobes (bilobectomy)

32671   with removal of lung (pneumonectomy)

32672   with resection-plication for emphysematous lung (bullous or non-bullous) for lung volume reduction (LVRS), unilateral includes any pleural procedure, when performed

32673   with resection of thymus, unilateral or bilateral

(For open thymectomy see 60520, 60521, 60522)

(For open excision mediastinal cyst, see 39200; for open excision mediastinal tumor, use 39220)

(For exploratory thoracoscopy, and exploratory thoracoscopy with biopsy, see 32601-32609)

+ **32674**   with mediastinal and regional lymphadenectomy (List separately in addition to code for primary procedure)

(On the right, mediastinal lymph nodes include the paratracheal, subcarinal, paraesophageal, and inferior pulmonary ligament)

(On the left, mediastinal lymph nodes include the aortopulmonary window, subcarinal, paraesophageal, and inferior pulmonary ligament)

(Report 32674 in conjunction with 19260, 31760, 31766, 31786, 32096-32200, 32220-32320, 32440-32491, 32503-32505, 32601-32663, 32666, 32669-32673, 32815, 33025, 33030, 33050-33130, 39200-39220, 39560, 39561, 43101, 43112, 43117, 43118, 43122, 43123, 43351, 60270, 60505)

(To report mediastinal and regional lymphadenectomy via thoracotomy, use 38746)

Stereotactic Radiation Therapy

Thoracic stereotactic body radiation therapy (SRS/SBRT) is a distinct procedure which may involve collaboration between a surgeon and radiation oncologist. The surgeon identifies and delineates the target for therapy. The radiation oncologist reports the appropriate code(s) for clinical treatment planning, physics and dosimetry, treatment delivery and management from the Radiation Oncology section (see 77295, 77331, 77370, 77373, 77435). The same physician should not report target delineation services with radiation treatment management codes (77427-77499).

Target delineation involves specific determination of tumor borders to identify tumor volume and relationship

with adjacent structures (eg, chest wall, intraparenchymal vasculature and atelectatic lung) and previously placed fiducial markers, when present. Target delineation also includes availability to identify and validate the thoracic target prior to treatment delivery when a fiducial-less tracking system is utilized.

Do not report target delineation more than once per entire course of treatment when the treatment requires greater than one session.

32701   Thoracic target(s) delineation for stereotactic body radiation therapy (SRS/SBRT), (photon or particle beam), entire course of treatment

(Do not report 32701 in conjunction with 77261-77799)

(For placement of fiducial markers, see 31626, 32553)

Repair

32800   Repair lung hernia through chest wall

32810   Closure of chest wall following open flap drainage for empyema (Clagett type procedure)

32815   Open closure of major bronchial fistula

32820   Major reconstruction, chest wall (posttraumatic)

Lung Transplantation

Lung allotransplantation involves three distinct components of physician work:

1. *Cadaver donor pneumonectomy(s)*, which include(s) harvesting the allograft and cold preservation of the allograft (perfusing with cold preservation solution and cold maintenance) (use 32850).

2. *Backbench work*:

   Preparation of a cadaver donor single lung allograft prior to transplantation, including dissection of the allograft from surrounding soft tissues to prepare the pulmonary venous/atrial cuff, pulmonary artery, and bronchus unilaterally (use 32855).

   Preparation of a cadaver donor double lung allograft prior to transplantation, including dissection of the allograft from surrounding soft tissues to prepare the pulmonary venous/atrial cuff, pulmonary artery, and bronchus bilaterally (use 32856).

3. *Recipient lung allotransplantation*, which includes transplantation of a single or double lung allograft and care of the recipient (see 32851-32854).

32850   Donor pneumonectomy(s) (including cold preservation), from cadaver donor

32851   Lung transplant, single; without cardiopulmonary bypass

32852   with cardiopulmonary bypass

32853   Lung transplant, double (bilateral sequential or en bloc); without cardiopulmonary bypass

32854   with cardiopulmonary bypass

Respiratory

Respiratory

32855 Backbench standard preparation of cadaver donor lung allograft prior to transplantation, including dissection of allograft from surrounding soft tissues to prepare pulmonary venous/atrial cuff, pulmonary artery, and bronchus; unilateral

32856 bilateral

(For repair or resection procedures on the donor lung, see 32491, 32505, 32506, 32507, 35216, 35276)

Surgical Collapse Therapy; Thoracoplasty

(See also 32503, 32504)

32900 Resection of ribs, extrapleural, all stages

32905 Thoracoplasty, Schede type or extrapleural (all stages);

32906 with closure of bronchopleural fistula

(For open closure of major bronchial fistula, use 32815)

(For resection of first rib for thoracic outlet compression, see 21615, 21616)

32940 Pneumonolysis, extraperiosteal, including filling or packing procedures

32960 Pneumothorax, therapeutic, intrapleural injection of air

Other Procedures

32997 Total lung lavage (unilateral)

(For bronchoscopic bronchial alveolar lavage, use 31624)

32998 Ablation therapy for reduction or eradication of 1 or more pulmonary tumor(s) including pleura or chest wall when involved by tumor extension, percutaneous, radiofrequency, unilateral

(For imaging guidance and monitoring, see 76940, 77013, 77022)

32999 Unlisted procedure, lungs and pleura

Cardiovascular System

Selective vascular catheterizations should be coded to include introduction and all lesser order selective catheterizations used in the approach (eg, the description for a selective right middle cerebral artery catheterization includes the introduction and placement catheterization of the right common and internal carotid arteries).

Additional second and/or third order arterial catheterizations within the same family of arteries supplied by a single first order artery should be expressed by 36218 or 36248. Additional first order or higher catheterizations in vascular families supplied by a first order vessel different from a previously selected and coded family should be separately coded using the conventions described above.

(For monitoring, operation of pump and other nonsurgical services, see 99190-99192, 99291, 99292, 99354-99360)

(For other medical or laboratory related services, see appropriate section)

(For radiological supervision and interpretation, see 75600-75978)

Heart and Pericardium

Pericardium

(For thoracoscopic (VATS) pericardial procedures, see 32601, 32604, 32658, 32659, 32661)

⊙ **33010**   Pericardiocentesis; initial

(For radiological supervision and interpretation, use 76930)

⊙ **33011**   subsequent

(For radiological supervision and interpretation, use 76930)

33015   Tube pericardiostomy

33020   Pericardiotomy for removal of clot or foreign body (primary procedure)

33025   Creation of pericardial window or partial resection for drainage

(For thoracoscopic (VATS) pericardial window, use 32659)

33030   Pericardiectomy, subtotal or complete; without cardiopulmonary bypass

33031   with cardiopulmonary bypass

33050   Resection of pericardial cyst or tumor

(For open pericardial biopsy, use 39010)

(For thoracoscopic (VATS) resection of pericardial cyst, tumor or mass, use 32661)

Cardiac Tumor

33120   Excision of intracardiac tumor, resection with cardiopulmonary bypass

33130   Resection of external cardiac tumor

Transmyocardial Revascularization

33140   Transmyocardial laser revascularization, by thoracotomy; (separate procedure)

+ **33141**   performed at the time of other open cardiac procedure(s) (List separately in addition to code for primary procedure)

(Use 33141 in conjunction with 33400-33496, 33510-33536, 33542)

Pacemaker or Implantable Defibrillator

▶A pacemaker system with lead(s) includes a pulse generator containing electronics, a battery, and one or more leads. A lead consists of one or more electrodes, as well as conductor wires, insulation, and a fixation mechanism. Pulse generators are placed in a subcutaneous "pocket" created in either a subclavicular site or just above the abdominal muscles just below the ribcage. Leads may be inserted through a vein (transvenous) or they may be placed on the surface of the heart (epicardial). The epicardial location of leads requires a thoracotomy for insertion.

A single chamber pacemaker system with lead includes a pulse generator and one electrode inserted in either the atrium or ventricle. A dual chamber pacemaker system with two leads includes a pulse generator and one lead inserted in the right atrium and one lead inserted in the right ventricle. In certain circumstances, an additional lead may be required to achieve pacing of the left ventricle (bi-ventricular pacing). In this event, transvenous (cardiac vein) placement of the lead should be separately reported using code 33224 or 33225. Epicardial placement of the lead should be separately reported using 33202, 33203.

A leadless cardiac pacemaker system includes a pulse generator with built-in battery and electrode for implantation in a cardiac chamber via a transcatheter approach. For these services, see codes 0387T, 0388T, 0389T, 0390T, 0391T.◀

Like a pacemaker system, an implantable defibrillator system includes a pulse generator and electrodes. Two general categories of implantable defibrillators exist: transvenous implantable pacing cardioverter-defibrillator (ICD) and subcutaneous implantable defibrillator (S-ICD). Implantable pacing cardioverter-defibrillator devices use a combination of antitachycardia pacing, low-energy cardioversion or defibrillating shocks to treat ventricular tachycardia or ventricular fibrillation. The subcutaneous implantable defibrillator uses a single subcutaneous electrode to treat ventricular

Cardiovascular

tachyarrhythmias. Subcutaneous implantable defibrillators differ from transvenous implantable pacing cardioverter-defibrillators in that subcutaneous defibrillators do not provide antitachycardia pacing or chronic pacing.

Implantable defibrillator pulse generators may be implanted in a subcutaneous infraclavicular, axillary, or abdominal pocket. Removal of an implantable defibrillator pulse generator requires opening of the existing subcutaneous pocket and disconnection of the pulse generator from its electrode(s). A thoracotomy (or laparotomy in the case of abdominally placed pulse generators) is not required to remove the pulse generator.

The electrodes (leads) of an implantable defibrillator system may be positioned within the atrial and/or ventricular chambers of the heart via the venous system (transvenously), or placed on the surface of the heart (epicardial), or positioned under the skin overlying the heart (subcutaneous). Electrode positioning on the epicardial surface of the heart requires a thoracotomy or thoracoscopic placement of the leads. Epicardial placement of electrode(s) may be separately reported using 33202, 33203. The electrode (lead) of a subcutaneous implantable defibrillator system is tunneled under the skin to the left parasternal margin. Subcutaneous placement of electrode may be reported using 33270 or 33271. In certain circumstances, an additional electrode may be required to achieve pacing of the left ventricle (bi-ventricular pacing). In this event, transvenous (cardiac vein) placement of the electrode may be separately reported using 33224 or 33225.

▶Removal of a transvenous electrode(s) may first be attempted by transvenous extraction (33234, 33235, or 33244). However, if transvenous extraction is unsuccessful, a thoracotomy may be required to remove the electrodes (33238 or 33243). Use 33212, 33213, 33221, 33230, 33231, 33240 as appropriate, in addition to the thoracotomy or endoscopic epicardial lead placement codes (33202 or 33203) to report the insertion of the generator if done by the same physician during the same session. Removal of a subcutaneous implantable defibrillator electrode may be separately reported using 33272. For removal of a leadless pacemaker system, use 0388T.

When the "battery" of a pacemaker system with lead(s) or implantable defibrillator is changed, it is actually the pulse generator that is changed. Removal of only the pacemaker or implantable defibrillator pulse generator is reported with 33233 or 33241. If only a pulse generator is inserted or replaced without any right atrial and/or right ventricular lead(s) inserted or replaced, report the appropriate code for only pulse generator insertion or replacement based on the number of final existing lead(s) (33227, 33228, 33229 and 33262, 33263, 33264). Do not report removal of a pulse generator (33233 or 33241) separately for this service. Insertion of a new pulse generator, when existing lead(s) are already in place and

when no prior pulse generator is removed, is reported with 33212, 33213, 33221, 33230, 33231, 33240. When a pulse generator insertion involves the insertion or replacement of one or more right atrial and/or right ventricular lead(s) or subcutaneous lead(s), use system codes 33206, 33207, 33208 for pacemaker, 33249 for implantable pacing cardioverter-defibrillator, or 33270 for subcutaneous implantable defibrillator. When reporting the system insertion or replacement codes, removal of a pulse generator (33233 or 33241) may be reported separately, when performed. In addition, extraction of leads 33234, 33235 or 33244 for transvenous or 33272 for subcutaneous may be reported separately, when performed. An exception involves a pacemaker upgrade from single to dual system that includes removal of pulse generator, replacement of new pulse generator, and insertion of new lead, reported with 33214.◀

Revision of a skin pocket is included in 33206-33249, 33262, 33263, 33264, 33270, 33271, 33272, 33273. When revision of a skin pocket involves incision and drainage of a hematoma or complex wound infection, see 10140, 10180, 11042, 11043, 11044, 11045, 11046, 11047, as appropriate.

Relocation of a skin pocket for a pacemaker (33222) or implantable defibrillator (33223) is necessary for various clinical situations such as infection or erosion. Relocation of an existing pulse generator may be performed as a stand-alone procedure or at the time of a pulse generator or electrode insertion, replacement, or repositioning. When skin pocket relocation is performed as part of an explant of an existing generator followed by replacement with a new generator, the pocket relocation is reported separately. Skin pocket relocation includes all work associated with the initial pocket (eg, opening the pocket, incision and drainage of hematoma or abscess if performed, and any closure performed), in addition to the creation of a new pocket for the new generator to be placed.

Repositioning of a pacemaker electrode, implantable defibrillator electrode(s), or a left ventricular pacing electrode is reported using 33215, 33226, or 33273, as appropriate.

▶Device evaluation codes 93260, 93261, 93279-93299 for pacemaker system with lead(s) may not be reported in conjunction with pulse generator and lead insertion or revision codes 33206-33249, 33262, 33263, 33264, 33270, 33271, 33272, 33273. For leadless pacemaker systems, device evaluation codes 0389T, 0390T, 0391T may not be reported in conjunction with leadless pacemaker insertion and removal codes 0387T, 0388T. Defibrillator threshold testing (DFT) during transvenous implantable defibrillator insertion or replacement may be separately reported using 93640, 93641. DFT testing during subcutaneous implantable defibrillator system insertion is not separately reportable. DFT testing for transvenous or subcutaneous implantable defibrillator in

Cardiovascular

follow-up or at the time of replacement may be separately reported using 93642 or 93644.

Radiological supervision and interpretation related to the pacemaker or implantable defibrillator procedure is included in 33206-33249, 33262, 33263, 33264, 33270, 33271, 33272, 33273, 0387T, 0388T. To report fluoroscopic guidance for diagnostic lead evaluation without lead insertion, replacement, or revision procedures, use 76000.◄

The following definitions apply to 33206-33249, 33262, 33263, 33264, 33270, 33271, 33272, 33273.

Single lead: a pacemaker or implantable defibrillator with pacing and sensing function in only one chamber of the heart or a subcutaneous electrode.

Dual lead: a pacemaker or implantable defibrillator with pacing and sensing function in only two chambers of the heart.

Multiple lead: a pacemaker or implantable defibrillator with pacing and sensing function in three or more chambers of the heart. ◄

Procedure	System	
	Pacemaker	**Implantable Defibrillator**
Insert transvenous single lead only without pulse generator	33216	33216
Insert transvenous dual leads without pulse generator	33217	33217
Insert transvenous multiple leads without pulse generator	33217 + 33224	33217 + 33224
Insert subcutaneous defibrillator electrode only without pulse generator	N/A	33271
Initial pulse generator insertion only with existing single lead, includes transvenous or subcutaneous defibrillator lead	33212	33240
Initial pulse generator insertion only with existing dual leads	33213	33230
Initial pulse generator insertion only with existing multiple leads	33221	33231
Initial pulse generator insertion or replacement plus insertion of transvenous single lead	33206 (atrial) or 33207 (ventricular)	33249
Initial pulse generator insertion or replacement plus insertion of transvenous dual leads	33208	33249
Initial pulse generator insertion or replacement plus insertion of transvenous multiple leads	33208 + 33225	33249 + 33225
Initial pulse generator insertion or replacement plus insertion of subcutaneous defibrillator electrode	N/A	33270
Upgrade single chamber system to dual chamber system	33214 (includes removal of existing pulse generator)	33241 + 33249
Removal pulse generator only (without replacement)	33233	33241
Removal pulse generator with replacement pulse generator only single lead system, includes transvenous or subcutaneous defibrillator lead	33227	33262
Removal pulse generator with replacement pulse generator only dual lead system (transvenous)	33228	33263
Removal pulse generator with replacement pulse generator only multiple lead system (transvenous)	33229	33264
Removal transvenous electrode only single lead system	33234	33244
Removal transvenous electrode only dual lead system	33235	33244
Removal subcutaneous defibrillator lead only	N/A	33272
Removal and replacement of pulse generator and transvenous electrodes	33233 + (33234 or 33235) + (33206, 33207, or 33208) and 33225, when appropriate	33241 + 33244 + 33249 and 33225, when appropriate
Removal and replacement of implantable defibrillator pulse generator and subcutaneous electrode	N/A	33272 + 33241 + 33270
Conversion of existing system to bi-ventricular system (addition of LV lead and removal of current pulse generator with insertion of new pulse generator with bi-ventricular pacing capabilities)	33225 + 33228 or 33229	33225 + 33263 or 33264

Cardiovascular

33202 Insertion of epicardial electrode(s); open incision (eg, thoracotomy, median sternotomy, subxiphoid approach)

33203 endoscopic approach (eg, thoracoscopy, pericardioscopy)

(When epicardial lead placement is performed with insertion of the generator, report 33202, 33203 in conjunction with 33212, 33213, 33221, 33230, 33231, 33240)

⊙ **33206** Insertion of new or replacement of permanent pacemaker with transvenous electrode(s); atrial

⊙ **33207** ventricular

⊙ **33208** atrial and ventricular

(Do not report 33206-33208 in conjunction with 33227-33229)

(Do not report 33206, 33207, 33208 in conjunction with 33216, 33217)

(Codes 33206-33208 include subcutaneous insertion of the pulse generator and transvenous placement of electrode[s])

(For removal and replacement of pacemaker pulse generator and transvenous electrode(s), use 33233 in conjunction with either 33234 or 33235 and 33206-33208)

⊙ **33210** Insertion or replacement of temporary transvenous single chamber cardiac electrode or pacemaker catheter (separate procedure)

⊙ **33211** Insertion or replacement of temporary transvenous dual chamber pacing electrodes (separate procedure)

⊙ **33212** Insertion of pacemaker pulse generator only; with existing single lead

⊙ **33213** with existing dual leads

#⊙ **33221** with existing multiple leads

(Do not report 33212, 33213, 33221 in conjunction with 33216, 33217)

(Do not report 33212, 33213, 33221 in conjunction with 33233 for removal and replacement of the pacemaker pulse generator. Use 33227-33229, as appropriate, when pulse generator replacement is indicated)

(When epicardial lead placement is performed with insertion of generator, report 33202, 33203 in conjunction with 33212, 33213, 33221)

⊙ **33214** Upgrade of implanted pacemaker system, conversion of single chamber system to dual chamber system (includes removal of previously placed pulse generator, testing of existing lead, insertion of new lead, insertion of new pulse generator)

(Do not report 33214 in conjunction with 33216, 33217, 33227, 33228, 33229)

33215 Repositioning of previously implanted transvenous pacemaker or implantable defibrillator (right atrial or right ventricular) electrode

⊙ **33216** Insertion of a single transvenous electrode, permanent pacemaker or implantable defibrillator

(Do not report 33216 in conjunction with 33206, 33207, 33208, 33212, 33213, 33214, 33221, 33227, 33228, 33229, 33230, 33231, 33240, 33249, 33262, 33263, 33264)

⊙ **33217** Insertion of 2 transvenous electrodes, permanent pacemaker or implantable defibrillator

(Do not report 33217 in conjunction with 33206, 33207, 33208, 33212, 33213, 33214, 33221, 33227, 33228, 33229, 33230, 33231, 33240, 33249, 33262, 33263, 33264)

(For insertion or replacement of a cardiac venous system lead, see 33224, 33225)

⊙ **33218** Repair of single transvenous electrode, permanent pacemaker or implantable defibrillator

(For repair of single permanent pacemaker or implantable defibrillator electrode with replacement of pulse generator, see 33227, 33228, 33229 or 33262, 33263, 33264 and 33218)

⊙ **33220** Repair of 2 transvenous electrodes for permanent pacemaker or implantable defibrillator

(For repair of 2 transvenous electrodes for permanent pacemaker or implantable defibrillator with replacement of pulse generator, use 33220 in conjunction with 33228, 33229, 33263, 33264)

33221 Code is out of numerical sequence. See 33202-33249

⊙ **33222** Relocation of skin pocket for pacemaker

(Do not report 33222 in conjunction with 10140, 10180, 11042, 11043, 11044, 11045, 11046, 11047, 13100, 13101, 13102)

⊙ **33223** Relocation of skin pocket for implantable defibrillator

(Do not report 33223 in conjunction with 10140, 10180, 11042, 11043, 11044, 11045, 11046, 11047, 13100, 13101, 13102)

33224 Insertion of pacing electrode, cardiac venous system, for left ventricular pacing, with attachment to previously placed pacemaker or implantable defibrillator pulse generator (including revision of pocket, removal, insertion, and/or replacement of existing generator)

(When epicardial electrode placement is performed, report 33224 in conjunction with 33202, 33203)

+ **33225** Insertion of pacing electrode, cardiac venous system, for left ventricular pacing, at time of insertion of implantable defibrillator or pacemaker pulse generator (eg, for upgrade to dual chamber system) (List separately in addition to code for primary procedure)

(Use 33225 in conjunction with 33206, 33207, 33208, 33212, 33213, 33214, 33216, 33217, 33221, 33223, 33228, 33229, 33230, 33231, 33233, 33234, 33235, 33240, 33249, 33263, 33264)

(Use 33225 in conjunction with 33222 only with pacemaker pulse generator pocket relocation and with 33223 only with implantable defibrillator [ICD] pocket relocation)

33226 Repositioning of previously implanted cardiac venous system (left ventricular) electrode (including removal, insertion and/or replacement of existing generator)

33227 Code is out of numerical sequence. See 33202-33249

33228 Code is out of numerical sequence. See 33202-33249

33229 Code is out of numerical sequence. See 33202-33249

33230 Code is out of numerical sequence. See 33202-33249

33231 Code is out of numerical sequence. See 33202-33249

⊙ **33233** Removal of permanent pacemaker pulse generator only

#⊙ **33227** Removal of permanent pacemaker pulse generator with replacement of pacemaker pulse generator; single lead system

#⊙ **33228** dual lead system

#⊙ **33229** multiple lead system

(Do not report 33227, 33228, 33229 in conjunction with 33214, 33216, 33217, 33233)

(For removal and replacement of pacemaker pulse generator and transvenous electrode[s], use 33233 in conjunction with either 33234 or 33235 and 33206-33208)

⊙ **33234** Removal of transvenous pacemaker electrode(s); single lead system, atrial or ventricular

⊙ **33235** dual lead system

33236 Removal of permanent epicardial pacemaker and electrodes by thoracotomy; single lead system, atrial or ventricular

33237 dual lead system

33238 Removal of permanent transvenous electrode(s) by thoracotomy

⊙ **33240** Insertion of implantable defibrillator pulse generator only; with existing single lead

(Do not report 33240 in conjunction with 33271, 93260, 93261)

(Use 33240, as appropriate, in addition to the epicardial lead placement codes to report the insertion of the generator when done by the same physician during the same session)

#⊙ **33230** with existing dual leads

#⊙ **33231** with existing multiple leads

(Do not report 33230, 33231, 33240 in conjunction with 33216, 33217)

(Do not report 33230, 33231, 33240 in conjunction with 33241 for removal and replacement of the implantable defibrillator pulse generator. Use 33262, 33263, 33264, as appropriate, when pulse generator replacement is indicated)

(When epicardial lead placement is performed with insertion of generator, report 33202, 33203 in conjunction with 33230, 33231, 33240)

⊙ **33241** Removal of implantable defibrillator pulse generator only

(Do not report 33241 in conjunction with 93260, 93261)

(Do not report 33241 in conjunction with 33230, 33231, 33240 for removal and replacement of the implantable defibrillator pulse generator. Use 33262, 33263, 33264, as appropriate, when pulse generator replacement is indicated)

(For removal and replacement of an implantable defibrillator pulse generator and electrode[s], use 33241 in conjunction with either 33243 or 33244 and 33249 for transvenous electrode[s] or 33270 and 33272 for subcutaneous electrode)

#⊙ **33262** Removal of implantable defibrillator pulse generator with replacement of implantable defibrillator pulse generator; single lead system

(Do not report 33262 in conjunction with 33271, 93260, 93261)

#⊙ **33263** dual lead system

#⊙ **33264** multiple lead system

(Do not report 33262, 33263, 33264 in conjunction with 33216, 33217, 33241)

(For removal of electrode[s] by thoracotomy in conjunction with pulse generator removal or replacement, use 33243 in conjunction with 33241 or 33262, 33263, 33264)

(For removal of electrode[s] by transvenous extraction in conjunction with pulse generator removal or replacement, use 33244 in conjunction with 33241 or 33262, 33263, 33264)

(For repair of implantable defibrillator pulse generator and/or leads, see 33218, 33220)

(For removal of subcutaneous electrode in conjunction with implantable defibrillator pulse generator removal or replacement, use 33272 in conjunction with 33241 or 33262)

33243 Removal of single or dual chamber implantable defibrillator electrode(s); by thoracotomy

⊙ **33244** by transvenous extraction

⊙ **33249** Insertion or replacement of permanent implantable defibrillator system, with transvenous lead(s), single or dual chamber

(Do not report 33249 in conjunction with 33216, 33217)

Cardiovascular

(For removal and replacement of an implantable defibrillator pulse generator and transvenous electrode[s], use 33241 in conjunction with either 33243 or 33244 and 33249)

(For insertion of transvenous implantable defibrillator lead(s), without thoracotomy, use 33216 or 33217)

33270 Insertion or replacement of permanent subcutaneous implantable defibrillator system, with subcutaneous electrode, including defibrillation threshold evaluation, induction of arrhythmia, evaluation of sensing for arrhythmia termination, and programming or reprogramming of sensing or therapeutic parameters, when performed

(Do not report 33270 in conjunction with 33271, 93260, 93261, 93644)

(For removal and replacement of an implantable defibrillator pulse generator and subcutaneous electrode, use 33241 in conjunction with 33270 and 33272)

(For insertion of subcutaneous implantable defibrillator lead[s], use 33271)

33271 Insertion of subcutaneous implantable defibrillator electrode

(Do not report 33271 in conjunction with 33240, 33262, 33270, 93260, 93261)

(For insertion or replacement of a cardiac venous system lead, see 33224, 33225)

33272 Removal of subcutaneous implantable defibrillator electrode

33273 Repositioning of previously implanted subcutaneous implantable defibrillator electrode

(Do not report 33272, 33273 in conjunction with 93260, 93261)

Electrophysiologic Operative Procedures

This family of codes describes the surgical treatment of supraventricular dysrhythmias. Tissue ablation, disruption, and reconstruction can be accomplished by many methods including surgical incision or through the use of a variety of energy sources (eg, radiofrequency, cryotherapy, microwave, ultrasound, laser). If excision or isolation of the left atrial appendage by any method, including stapling, oversewing, ligation, or plication, is performed in conjunction with any of the atrial tissue ablation and reconstruction (maze) procedures (33254-33259, 33265-33266), it is considered part of the procedure. Codes 33254-33256 are only to be reported when there is no concurrently performed procedure that requires median sternotomy or cardiopulmonary bypass. The appropriate atrial tissue ablation add-on code, 33257, 33258, 33259 should be reported in addition to an open cardiac procedure requiring sternotomy or cardiopulmonary bypass if performed concurrently.

Definitions

Limited operative ablation and reconstruction includes:

Surgical isolation of triggers of supraventricular dysrhythmias by operative ablation that isolates the pulmonary veins or other anatomically defined triggers in the left or right atrium.

Extensive operative ablation and reconstruction includes:

1. The services included in *"limited"*

2. Additional ablation of atrial tissue to eliminate sustained supraventricular dysrhythmias. This must include operative ablation that involves either the right atrium, the atrial septum, or left atrium in continuity with the atrioventricular annulus.

Incision

33250 Operative ablation of supraventricular arrhythmogenic focus or pathway (eg, Wolff-Parkinson-White, atrioventricular node re-entry), tract(s) and/or focus (foci); without cardiopulmonary bypass

(For intraoperative pacing and mapping by a separate provider, use 93631)

33251 with cardiopulmonary bypass

33254 Operative tissue ablation and reconstruction of atria, limited (eg, modified maze procedure)

33255 Operative tissue ablation and reconstruction of atria, extensive (eg, maze procedure); without cardiopulmonary bypass

33256 with cardiopulmonary bypass

(Do not report 33254-33256 in conjunction with 32100, 32551, 33120, 33130, 33210, 33211, 33400-33507, 33510-33523, 33533-33548, 33600-33853, 33860-33864, 33910-33920)

+ 33257 Operative tissue ablation and reconstruction of atria, performed at the time of other cardiac procedure(s), limited (eg, modified maze procedure) (List separately in addition to code for primary procedure)

(Use 33257 in conjunction with 33120-33130, 33250-33251, 33261, 33300-33335, 33400-33496, 33500-33507, 33510-33516, 33533-33548, 33600-33619, 33641-33697, 33702-33732, 33735-33767, 33770-33814, 33840-33877, 33910-33922, 33925-33926, 33935, 33945, 33975-33980)

+ 33258 Operative tissue ablation and reconstruction of atria, performed at the time of other cardiac procedure(s), extensive (eg, maze procedure), without cardiopulmonary bypass (List separately in addition to code for primary procedure)

(Use 33258 in conjunction with 33130, 33250, 33300, 33310, 33320, 33321, 33330, 33401, 33414-33417, 33420, 33470, 33471, 33501-33503, 33510-33516, 33533-33536, 33690, 33735, 33737, 33800-33813, 33840-33852, 33915, 33925, when the procedure is performed without cardiopulmonary bypass)

+ 33259 Operative tissue ablation and reconstruction of atria, performed at the time of other cardiac procedure(s), extensive (eg, maze procedure), with cardiopulmonary bypass (List separately in addition to code for primary procedure)

(Use 33259 in conjunction with 33120, 33251, 33261, 33305, 33315, 33322, 33335, 33400, 33403-33413, 33422-33468, 33474-33478, 33496, 33500, 33504-33507, 33510-33516, 33533-33548, 33600-33688, 33692-33722, 33730, 33732, 33736, 33750-33767, 33770-33781, 33786-33788, 33814, 33853, 33860-33877, 33910, 33916-33922, 33926, 33935, 33945, 33975-33980 when the procedure is performed with cardiopulmonary bypass)

(Do not report 33257, 33258 and 33259 in conjunction with 32551, 33210, 33211, 33254-33256, 33265, 33266)

33261 Operative ablation of ventricular arrhythmogenic focus with cardiopulmonary bypass

33262 Code is out of numerical sequence. See 33202-33264

33263 Code is out of numerical sequence. See 33202-33264

33264 Code is out of numerical sequence. See 33202-33264

Endoscopy

33265 Endoscopy, surgical; operative tissue ablation and reconstruction of atria, limited (eg, modified maze procedure), without cardiopulmonary bypass

33266 operative tissue ablation and reconstruction of atria, extensive (eg, maze procedure), without cardiopulmonary bypass

(Do not report 33265-33266 in conjunction with 32551, 33210, 33211)

33270 Code is out of numerical sequence. See 33202-33270

33271 Code is out of numerical sequence. See 33202-33271

33272 Code is out of numerical sequence. See 33202-33272

33273 Code is out of numerical sequence. See 33202-33273

Patient-Activated Event Recorder

⊙ 33282 Implantation of patient-activated cardiac event recorder

(Initial implantation includes programming. For subsequent electronic analysis and/or reprogramming, use 93285, 93291, 93298, 93299)

⊙ 33284 Removal of an implantable, patient-activated cardiac event recorder

Heart (Including Valves) and Great Vessels

Patients receiving major cardiac procedures may require simultaneous cardiopulmonary bypass insertion of cannulae into the venous and arterial vasculatures with support of circulation and oxygenation by a heart-lung machine. Most services are described by codes in dyad

arrangements to allow distinct reporting of procedures with or without cardiopulmonary bypass. Cardiopulmonary bypass is distinct from support of cardiac output using devices (eg, ventricular assist or intra-aortic balloon). For cardiac assist services, see 33946, 33947, 33948, 33949, 33967-33983, 33990, 33991, 33992, 33993.

33300 Repair of cardiac wound; without bypass

33305 with cardiopulmonary bypass

33310 Cardiotomy, exploratory (includes removal of foreign body, atrial or ventricular thrombus); without bypass

33315 with cardiopulmonary bypass

(Do not report removal of thrombus [33310-33315] in conjunction with other cardiac procedures unless a separate incision in the heart is required to remove the atrial or ventricular thrombus)

(If removal of thrombus with cardiopulmonary bypass [33315] is reported in conjunction with 33120, 33130, 33420-33430, 33460-33468, 33496, 33542, 33545, 33641-33647, 33670, 33681, 33975-33980 which requires a separate heart incision, report 33315 with modifier 59)

33320 Suture repair of aorta or great vessels; without shunt or cardiopulmonary bypass

33321 with shunt bypass

33322 with cardiopulmonary bypass

33330 Insertion of graft, aorta or great vessels; without shunt, or cardiopulmonary bypass

(33332 has been deleted)

33335 with cardiopulmonary bypass

Cardiac Valves

(For multiple valve procedures, see 33400-33478 and add modifier 51 to the secondary valve procedure code)

Aortic Valve

Codes 33361, 33362, 33363, 33364, 33365, 33366 are used to report transcatheter aortic valve replacement (TAVR)/transcatheter aortic valve implantation (TAVI). TAVR/TAVI requires two physician operators and all components of the procedure are reported using modifier 62.

Codes 33361, 33362, 33363, 33364, 33365, 33366 include the work, when performed, of percutaneous access, placing the access sheath, balloon aortic valvuloplasty, advancing the valve delivery system into position, repositioning the valve as needed, deploying the valve, temporary pacemaker insertion for rapid pacing (33210), and closure of the arteriotomy when performed. Codes 33361, 33362, 33363, 33364, 33365, 33366 include open arterial or cardiac approach.

Cardiovascular

Cardiovascular

Angiography, radiological supervision, and interpretation performed to guide TAVR/TAVI (eg, guiding valve placement, documenting completion of the intervention, assessing the vascular access site for closure) are included in these codes.

Diagnostic left heart catheterization codes (93452, 93453, 93458-93461) and the supravalvular aortography code (93567) should **not** be used with TAVR/TAVI services (33361, 33362, 33363, 33364, 33365, 33366) to report:

1. Contrast injections, angiography, roadmapping, and/or fluoroscopic guidance for the TAVR/TAVI,

2. Aorta/left ventricular outflow tract measurement for the TAVR/TAVI, or

3. Post-TAVR/TAVI aortic or left ventricular angiography, as this work is captured in the TAVR/TAVI services codes (33361, 33362, 33363, 33364, 33365, 33366).

Diagnostic coronary angiography performed at the time of TAVR/TAVI may be separately reportable if:

1. No prior catheter-based coronary angiography study is available and a full diagnostic study is performed, or

2. A prior study is available, but as documented in the medical record:

   a. The patient's condition with respect to the clinical indication has changed since the prior study, or

   b. There is inadequate visualization of the anatomy and/or pathology, or

   c. There is a clinical change during the procedure that requires new evaluation.

   d. For same session/same day diagnostic coronary angiography services, report the appropriate diagnostic cardiac catheterization code(s) appended with modifier 59 indicating separate and distinct procedural service from TAVR/TAVI.

Diagnostic coronary angiography performed at a separate session from an interventional procedure may be separately reportable.

Other cardiac catheterization services may be reported separately when performed for diagnostic purposes not intrinsic to TAVR/TAVI.

Percutaneous coronary interventional procedures are reported separately, when performed.

When transcatheter ventricular support is required in conjunction with TAVR/TAVI, the appropriate code should be reported with the appropriate ventricular assist device (VAD) procedure code (33990-33993, 33975, 33976, 33999) or balloon pump insertion code (33967, 33970, 33973).

The TAVR/TAVI cardiovascular access and delivery procedures are reported with 33361, 33362, 33363, 33364, 33365, 33366. When cardiopulmonary bypass is performed in conjunction with TAVR/TAVI, codes

33361, 33362, 33363, 33364, 33365, 33366 should be reported with the appropriate add-on code for percutaneous peripheral bypass (33367), open peripheral bypass (33368), or central bypass (33369).

33361 Transcatheter aortic valve replacement (TAVR/TAVI) with prosthetic valve; percutaneous femoral artery approach

33362 open femoral artery approach

33363 open axillary artery approach

33364 open iliac artery approach

33365 transaortic approach (eg, median sternotomy, mediastinotomy)

33366 transapical exposure (eg, left thoracotomy)

+ 33367 cardiopulmonary bypass support with percutaneous peripheral arterial and venous cannulation (eg, femoral vessels) (List separately in addition to code for primary procedure)

►(Use 33367 in conjunction with 33361, 33362, 33363, 33364, 33365, 33366, 33418, 33477)◄

(Do not report 33367 in conjunction with 33368, 33369)

+ 33368 cardiopulmonary bypass support with open peripheral arterial and venous cannulation (eg, femoral, iliac, axillary vessels) (List separately in addition to code for primary procedure)

►(Use 33368 in conjunction with 33361, 33362, 33363, 33364, 33365, 33366, 33418, 33477)◄

(Do not report 33368 in conjunction with 33367, 33369)

+ 33369 cardiopulmonary bypass support with central arterial and venous cannulation (eg, aorta, right atrium, pulmonary artery) (List separately in addition to code for primary procedure)

►(Use 33369 in conjunction with 33361, 33362, 33363, 33364, 33365, 33366, 33418, 33477)◄

(Do not report 33369 in conjunction with 33367, 33368)

33400 Valvuloplasty, aortic valve; open, with cardiopulmonary bypass

33401 open, with inflow occlusion

33403 using transventricular dilation, with cardiopulmonary bypass

(Do not report modifier 63 in conjunction with 33401, 33403)

33404 Construction of apical-aortic conduit

33405 Replacement, aortic valve, with cardiopulmonary bypass; with prosthetic valve other than homograft or stentless valve

33406 with allograft valve (freehand)

(For aortic valve valvotomy, [commissurotomy] with inflow occlusion, use 33401)

(For aortic valve valvotomy, [commissurotomy] with cardiopulmonary bypass, use 33403)

33410   with stentless tissue valve

33411   Replacement, aortic valve; with aortic annulus enlargement, noncoronary sinus

33412   with transventricular aortic annulus enlargement (Konno procedure)

33413   by translocation of autologous pulmonary valve with allograft replacement of pulmonary valve (Ross procedure)

33414   Repair of left ventricular outflow tract obstruction by patch enlargement of the outflow tract

33415   Resection or incision of subvalvular tissue for discrete subvalvular aortic stenosis

33416   Ventriculomyotomy (-myectomy) for idiopathic hypertrophic subaortic stenosis (eg, asymmetric septal hypertrophy)

       (For percutaneous transcatheter septal reduction therapy, use 93583)

33417   Aortoplasty (gusset) for supravalvular stenosis

Mitral Valve

Codes 33418 and 33419 are used to report transcatheter mitral valve repair (TMVR). Code 33419 should only be reported once per session.

Codes 33418 and 33419 include the work, when performed, of percutaneous access, placing the access sheath, transseptal puncture, advancing the repair device delivery system into position, repositioning the device as needed, and deploying the device(s).

Angiography, radiological supervision, and interpretation performed to guide TMVR (eg, guiding device placement and documenting completion of the intervention) are included in these codes.

Diagnostic right and left heart catheterization codes (93451, 93452, 93453, 93456, 93457, 93458, 93459, 93460, 93461, 93530, 93531, 93532, 93533) should **not** be used with 33418, 33419 to report:

1. Contrast injections, angiography, road-mapping, and/or fluoroscopic guidance for the transcatheter mitral valve repair (TMVR),

2. Left ventricular angiography to assess mitral regurgitation for guidance of TMVR, or

3. Right and left heart catheterization for hemodynamic measurements before, during, and after TMVR for guidance of TMVR.

Diagnostic right and left heart catheterization codes (93451, 93452, 93453, 93456, 93457, 93458, 93459, 93460, 93461, 93530, 93531, 93532, 93533) and diagnostic coronary angiography codes (93454, 93455, 93456, 93457, 93458, 93459, 93460, 93461, 93563, 93564) may be reported with 33418, 33419, representing separate and distinct services from TMVR, if:

1. No prior study is available and a full diagnostic study is performed, or

2. A prior study is available, but as documented in the medical record:

    a. There is inadequate visualization of the anatomy and/or pathology, or

    b. The patient's condition with respect to the clinical indication has changed since the prior study, or

    c. There is a clinical change during the procedure that requires new evaluation.

Other cardiac catheterization services may be reported separately when performed for diagnostic purposes not intrinsic to TMVR.

For same session/same day diagnostic cardiac catheterization services, report the appropriate diagnostic cardiac catheterization code(s) appended with modifier 59 indicating separate and distinct procedural service from TMVR.

Diagnostic coronary angiography performed at a separate session from an interventional procedure may be separately reportable.

Percutaneous coronary interventional procedures may be reported separately, when performed.

When transcatheter ventricular support is required in conjunction with TMVR, the appropriate code may be reported with the appropriate ventricular assist device (VAD) procedure code (33990, 33991, 33992, 33993) or balloon pump insertion code (33967, 33970, 33973).

When cardiopulmonary bypass is performed in conjunction with TMVR, 33418, 33419 may be reported with the appropriate add-on code for percutaneous peripheral bypass (33367), open peripheral bypass (33368), or central bypass (33369).

33418   Transcatheter mitral valve repair, percutaneous approach, including transseptal puncture when performed; initial prosthesis

       (Do not report 33418 in conjunction with 93462 unless transapical puncture is performed)

+ 33419   additional prosthesis(es) during same session (List separately in addition to code for primary procedure)

       (Use 33419 in conjunction with 33418)

       (For transcatheter mitral valve percutaneous approach via the coronary sinus, use 0345T)

33420   Valvotomy, mitral valve; closed heart

33422   open heart, with cardiopulmonary bypass

33425   Valvuloplasty, mitral valve, with cardiopulmonary bypass;

33426   with prosthetic ring

33427   radical reconstruction, with or without ring

33430   Replacement, mitral valve, with cardiopulmonary bypass

Tricuspid Valve

33460   Valvectomy, tricuspid valve, with cardiopulmonary bypass

33463   Valvuloplasty, tricuspid valve; without ring insertion

33464   with ring insertion

33465   Replacement, tricuspid valve, with cardiopulmonary bypass

33468   Tricuspid valve repositioning and plication for Ebstein anomaly

Pulmonary Valve

►Code 33477 is used to report transcatheter pulmonary valve implantation (TPVI). Code 33477 should only be reported once per session.

Code 33477 includes the work, when performed, of percutaneous access, placing the access sheath, advancing the repair device delivery system into position, repositioning the device as needed, and deploying the device(s). Angiography, radiological supervision, and interpretation performed to guide TPVI (eg, guiding device placement and documenting completion of the intervention) are included in the code.

Code 33477 includes all cardiac catheterization(s), intraprocedural contrast injection(s), fluoroscopic radiological supervision and interpretation, and imaging guidance performed to complete the pulmonary valve procedure. Do not report 33477 in conjunction with 76000, 76001, 93451, 93453, 93454, 93455, 93456, 93457, 93458, 93459, 93460, 93461, 93530, 93531, 93532, 93533, 93563, 93566, 93567, 93568 for angiography intrinsic to the procedure.

Code 33477 includes percutaneous balloon angioplasty of the conduit/treatment zone, valvuloplasty of the pulmonary valve conduit, and stent deployment within the pulmonary conduit or an existing bioprosthetic pulmonary valve, when performed. Do not report 33477 in conjunction with 37236, 37237, 92997, 92998 for pulmonary artery angioplasty/valvuloplasty or stenting within the prosthetic valve delivery site.

Codes 92997, 92998 may be reported separately when pulmonary artery angioplasty is performed at a site separate from the prosthetic valve delivery site. Codes 37236, 37237 may be reported separately when pulmonary artery stenting is performed at a site separate from the prosthetic valve delivery site.

Diagnostic right heart catheterization and diagnostic coronary angiography codes (93451, 93453, 93454, 93455, 93456, 93457, 93458, 93459, 93460, 93461, 93530, 93531, 93532, 93533, 93563, 93566, 93567, 93568) should **not** be used with 33477 to report:

1. Contrast injections, angiography, roadmapping, and/or fluoroscopic guidance for the TPVI,

2. Pulmonary conduit angiography for guidance of TPVI, or

3. Right heart catheterization for hemodynamic measurements before, during, and after TPVI for guidance of TPVI.

Diagnostic right and left heart catheterization codes (93451, 93452, 93453, 93456, 93457, 93458, 93459, 93460, 93461, 93530, 93531, 93532, 93533), diagnostic coronary angiography codes (93454, 93455, 93456, 93457, 93458, 93459, 93460, 93461, 93563, 93564), and diagnostic pulmonary angiography code (93568) may be reported with 33477, representing separate and distinct services from TPVI, if:

1. No prior study is available and a full diagnostic study is performed, or

2. A prior study is available, but as documented in the medical record:

     a. There is inadequate visualization of the anatomy and/or pathology, or

     b. The patient's condition with respect to the clinical indication has changed since the prior study, or

     c. There is a clinical change during the procedure that requires new evaluation.

Other cardiac catheterization services may be reported separately when performed for diagnostic purposes not intrinsic to TPVI.

For same session/same day diagnostic cardiac catheterization services, report the appropriate diagnostic cardiac catheterization code(s) appended with modifier 59 to indicate separate and distinct procedural services from TPVI.

Diagnostic coronary angiography performed at a separate session from an interventional procedure may be separately reportable, when performed.

Percutaneous coronary interventional procedures may be reported separately, when performed.

Percutaneous pulmonary artery branch interventions may be reported separately, when performed.

When transcatheter ventricular support is required in conjunction with TPVI, the appropriate code may be reported with the appropriate percutaneous ventricular assist device (VAD) procedure codes (33990, 33991, 33992, 33993), extracorporeal membrane oxygenation (ECMO) or extracorporeal life support services (ECLS) procedure codes (33946-33989), or balloon pump insertion codes (33967, 33970, 33973).

When cardiopulmonary bypass is performed in conjunction with TPVI, code 33477 may be reported with the appropriate add-on code for percutaneous peripheral bypass (33367), open peripheral bypass (33368), or central bypass (33369).◄

33470   Valvotomy, pulmonary valve, closed heart; transventricular

(Do not report modifier 63 in conjunction with 33470)

33471   via pulmonary artery

(To report percutaneous valvuloplasty of pulmonary valve, use 92990)

(33472 has been deleted)

33474   Valvotomy, pulmonary valve, open heart, with cardiopulmonary bypass

33475   Replacement, pulmonary valve

33476   Right ventricular resection for infundibular stenosis, with or without commissurotomy

● 33477   Transcatheter pulmonary valve implantation, percutaneous approach, including pre-stenting of the valve delivery site, when performed

33478   Outflow tract augmentation (gusset), with or without commissurotomy or infundibular resection

(Use 33478 in conjunction with 33768 when a cavopulmonary anastomosis to a second superior vena cava is performed)

Other Valvular Procedures

33496   Repair of non-structural prosthetic valve dysfunction with cardiopulmonary bypass (separate procedure)

(For reoperation, use 33530 in addition to 33496)

Coronary Artery Anomalies

Basic procedures include endarterectomy or angioplasty.

33500   Repair of coronary arteriovenous or arteriocardiac chamber fistula; with cardiopulmonary bypass

33501   without cardiopulmonary bypass

33502   Repair of anomalous coronary artery from pulmonary artery origin; by ligation

33503   by graft, without cardiopulmonary bypass

(Do not report modifier 63 in conjunction with 33502, 33503)

33504   by graft, with cardiopulmonary bypass

33505   with construction of intrapulmonary artery tunnel (Takeuchi procedure)

33506   by translocation from pulmonary artery to aorta

(Do not report modifier 63 in conjunction with 33505, 33506)

33507   Repair of anomalous (eg, intramural) aortic origin of coronary artery by unroofing or translocation

Endoscopy

Surgical vascular endoscopy always includes diagnostic endoscopy.

+ 33508   Endoscopy, surgical, including video-assisted harvest of vein(s) for coronary artery bypass procedure (List separately in addition to code for primary procedure)

(Use 33508 in conjunction with 33510-33523)

(For open harvest of upper extremity vein procedure, use 35500)

Venous Grafting Only for Coronary Artery Bypass

The following codes are used to report coronary artery bypass procedures using venous grafts only. These codes should NOT be used to report the performance of coronary artery bypass procedures using arterial grafts and venous grafts during the same procedure. See 33517-33523 and 33533-33536 for reporting combined arterial-venous grafts.

Procurement of the saphenous vein graft is included in the description of the work for 33510-33516 and should not be reported as a separate service or co-surgery. To report harvesting of an upper extremity vein, use 35500 in addition to the bypass procedure. To report harvesting of a femoropopliteal vein segment, report 35572 in addition to the bypass procedure. When surgical assistant performs graft procurement, add modifier 80 to 33510-33516. For percutaneous ventricular assist device insertion, removal, repositioning, see 33990-33993.

33510   Coronary artery bypass, vein only; single coronary venous graft

33511   2 coronary venous grafts

33512   3 coronary venous grafts

33513   4 coronary venous grafts

33514   5 coronary venous grafts

33516   6 or more coronary venous grafts

Combined Arterial-Venous Grafting for Coronary Bypass

The following codes are used to report coronary artery bypass procedures using venous grafts and arterial grafts during the same procedure. These codes may NOT be used alone.

To report combined arterial-venous grafts it is necessary to report two codes: (1) the appropriate combined arterial-venous graft code (33517-33523); and (2) the appropriate arterial graft code (33533-33536).

Procurement of the saphenous vein graft is included in the description of the work for 33517-33523 and should not be reported as a separate service or co-surgery. Procurement of the artery for grafting is included in the description of the work for 33533-33536 and should not be reported as a separate service or co-surgery, except when an upper extremity artery (eg, radial artery) is procured. To report harvesting of an upper extremity artery, use 35600 in addition to the bypass procedure. To report harvesting of an upper extremity vein, use 35500 in addition to the bypass procedure. To report harvesting of a femoropopliteal vein segment, report 35572 in addition to the bypass procedure. When surgical assistant performs arterial and/or venous graft procurement, add modifier 80 to 33517-33523, 33533-33536, as appropriate. For percutaneous ventricular assist device insertion, removal, repositioning, see 33990-33993.

+ 33517   Coronary artery bypass, using venous graft(s) and arterial graft(s); single vein graft (List separately in addition to code for primary procedure)

(Use 33517 in conjunction with 33533-33536)

+ 33518   2 venous grafts (List separately in addition to code for primary procedure)

(Use 33518 in conjunction with 33533-33536)

+ 33519   3 venous grafts (List separately in addition to code for primary procedure)

(Use 33519 in conjunction with 33533-33536)

+ 33521   4 venous grafts (List separately in addition to code for primary procedure)

(Use 33521 in conjunction with 33533-33536)

+ 33522   5 venous grafts (List separately in addition to code for primary procedure)

(Use 33522 in conjunction with 33533-33536)

+ 33523   6 or more venous grafts (List separately in addition to code for primary procedure)

(Use 33523 in conjunction with 33533-33536)

+ 33530   Reoperation, coronary artery bypass procedure or valve procedure, more than 1 month after original operation (List separately in addition to code for primary procedure)

(Use 33530 in conjunction with 33400-33496; 33510-33536, 33863)

Arterial Grafting for Coronary Artery Bypass

The following codes are used to report coronary artery bypass procedures using either arterial grafts only or a combination of arterial-venous grafts. The codes include the use of the internal mammary artery, gastroepiploic artery, epigastric artery, radial artery, and arterial conduits procured from other sites.

To report combined arterial-venous grafts it is necessary to report two codes: (1) the appropriate arterial graft code (33533-33536); and (2) the appropriate combined arterial-venous graft code (33517-33523).

Procurement of the artery for grafting is included in the description of the work for 33533-33536 and should not be reported as a separate service or co-surgery, except when an upper extremity artery (eg, radial artery) is procured. To report harvesting of an upper extremity artery, use 35600 in addition to the bypass procedure. To report harvesting of an upper extremity vein, use 35500 in addition to the bypass procedure. To report harvesting of a femoropopliteal vein segment, report 35572 in addition to the bypass procedure. When surgical assistant performs arterial and/or venous graft procurement, add modifier 80 to 33517-33523, 33533-33536, as appropriate. For percutaneous ventricular assist device insertion, removal, repositioning, see 33990-33993.

33533   Coronary artery bypass, using arterial graft(s); single arterial graft

33534   2 coronary arterial grafts

33535   3 coronary arterial grafts

33536   4 or more coronary arterial grafts

33542   Myocardial resection (eg, ventricular aneurysmectomy)

33545   Repair of postinfarction ventricular septal defect, with or without myocardial resection

33548   Surgical ventricular restoration procedure, includes prosthetic patch, when performed (eg, ventricular remodeling, SVR, SAVER, Dor procedures)

(Do not report 33548 in conjunction with 32551, 33210, 33211, 33310, 33315)

(For Batista procedure or pachopexy, use 33999)

Coronary Endarterectomy

+ 33572   Coronary endarterectomy, open, any method, of left anterior descending, circumflex, or right coronary artery performed in conjunction with coronary artery bypass graft procedure, each vessel (List separately in addition to primary procedure)

(Use 33572 in conjunction with 33510-33516, 33533-33536)

Single Ventricle and Other Complex Cardiac Anomalies

33600   Closure of atrioventricular valve (mitral or tricuspid) by suture or patch

33602   Closure of semilunar valve (aortic or pulmonary) by suture or patch

33606   Anastomosis of pulmonary artery to aorta (Damus-Kaye-Stansel procedure)

33608   Repair of complex cardiac anomaly other than pulmonary atresia with ventricular septal defect by construction or replacement of conduit from right or left ventricle to pulmonary artery

(For repair of pulmonary artery arborization anomalies by unifocalization, see 33925-33926)

33610   Repair of complex cardiac anomalies (eg, single ventricle with subaortic obstruction) by surgical enlargement of ventricular septal defect

(Do not report modifier 63 in conjunction with 33610)

33611   Repair of double outlet right ventricle with intraventricular tunnel repair;

(Do not report modifier 63 in conjunction with 33611)

33612   with repair of right ventricular outflow tract obstruction

33615   Repair of complex cardiac anomalies (eg, tricuspid atresia) by closure of atrial septal defect and anastomosis of atria or vena cava to pulmonary artery (simple Fontan procedure)

33617   Repair of complex cardiac anomalies (eg, single ventricle) by modified Fontan procedure

(Use 33617 in conjunction with 33768 when a cavopulmonary anastomosis to a second superior vena cava is performed)

33619   Repair of single ventricle with aortic outflow obstruction and aortic arch hypoplasia (hypoplastic left heart syndrome) (eg, Norwood procedure)

(Do not report modifier 63 in conjunction with 33619)

33620   Application of right and left pulmonary artery bands (eg, hybrid approach stage 1)

(For banding of the main pulmonary artery related to septal defect, use 33690)

33621   Transthoracic insertion of catheter for stent placement with catheter removal and closure (eg, hybrid approach stage 1)

(For placement of stent, use 37236)

(Report both 33620, 33621 if performed in same session)

33622   Reconstruction of complex cardiac anomaly (eg, single ventricle or hypoplastic left heart) with palliation of single ventricle with aortic outflow obstruction and aortic arch hypoplasia, creation of cavopulmonary anastomosis, and removal of right and left pulmonary bands (eg, hybrid approach stage 2, Norwood, bidirectional Glenn, pulmonary artery debanding)

(Do not report 33622 in conjunction with 33619, 33767, 33822, 33840, 33845, 33851, 33853, 33917)

(For bilateral, bidirectional Glenn procedure, use 33622 in conjunction with 33768)

Septal Defect

33641   Repair atrial septal defect, secundum, with cardiopulmonary bypass, with or without patch

33645   Direct or patch closure, sinus venosus, with or without anomalous pulmonary venous drainage

(Do not report 33645 in conjunction with 33724, 33726)

33647   Repair of atrial septal defect and ventricular septal defect, with direct or patch closure

(Do not report modifier 63 in conjunction with 33647)

(For repair of tricuspid atresia (eg, Fontan, Gago procedures), use 33615)

33660   Repair of incomplete or partial atrioventricular canal (ostium primum atrial septal defect), with or without atrioventricular valve repair

33665   Repair of intermediate or transitional atrioventricular canal, with or without atrioventricular valve repair

33670   Repair of complete atrioventricular canal, with or without prosthetic valve

(Do not report modifier 63 in conjunction with 33670)

33675   Closure of multiple ventricular septal defects;

33676   with pulmonary valvotomy or infundibular resection (acyanotic)

33677   with removal of pulmonary artery band, with or without gusset

(Do not report 33675-33677 in conjunction with 32100, 32551, 32554, 32555, 33210, 33681, 33684, 33688)

(For percutaneous closure, use 93581)

33681   Closure of single ventricular septal defect, with or without patch;

33684   with pulmonary valvotomy or infundibular resection (acyanotic)

33688   with removal of pulmonary artery band, with or without gusset

(For pulmonary vein repair requiring creation of atrial septal defect, use 33724)

33690   Banding of pulmonary artery

(For right and left pulmonary artery banding in a single ventricle [eg, hybrid approach stage 1], use 33620)

(Do not report modifier 63 in conjunction with 33690)

33692   Complete repair tetralogy of Fallot without pulmonary atresia;

33694   with transannular patch

(Do not report modifier 63 in conjunction with 33694)

(For ligation and takedown of a systemic-to-pulmonary artery shunt, performed in conjunction with a congenital heart procedure; see 33924)

33697   Complete repair tetralogy of Fallot with pulmonary atresia including construction of conduit from right ventricle to pulmonary artery and closure of ventricular septal defect

(For ligation and takedown of a systemic-to-pulmonary artery shunt, performed in conjunction with a congenital heart procedure; see 33924)

Cardiovascular

Sinus of Valsalva

33702 Repair sinus of Valsalva fistula, with cardiopulmonary bypass;

33710   with repair of ventricular septal defect

33720 Repair sinus of Valsalva aneurysm, with cardiopulmonary bypass

33722 Closure of aortico-left ventricular tunnel

Venous Anomalies

33724 Repair of isolated partial anomalous pulmonary venous return (eg, Scimitar Syndrome)

(Do not report 33724 in conjunction with 32551, 33210, 33211)

33726 Repair of pulmonary venous stenosis

(Do not report 33726 in conjunction with 32551, 33210, 33211)

33730 Complete repair of anomalous pulmonary venous return (supracardiac, intracardiac, or infracardiac types)

(Do not report modifier 63 in conjunction with 33730)

(For partial anomalous pulmonary venous return, use 33724; for repair of pulmonary venous stenosis, use 33726)

33732 Repair of cor triatriatum or supravalvular mitral ring by resection of left atrial membrane

(Do not report modifier 63 in conjunction with 33732)

Shunting Procedures

33735 Atrial septectomy or septostomy; closed heart (Blalock-Hanlon type operation)

33736   open heart with cardiopulmonary bypass

(Do not report modifier 63 in conjunction with 33735, 33736)

33737   open heart, with inflow occlusion

(For transvenous method cardiac catheterization balloon atrial septectomy or septostomy (Rashkind type), use 92992)

(For blade method cardiac catheterization atrial septectomy or septostomy (Sang-Park septostomy), use 92993)

33750 Shunt; subclavian to pulmonary artery (Blalock-Taussig type operation)

33755   ascending aorta to pulmonary artery (Waterston type operation)

33762   descending aorta to pulmonary artery (Potts-Smith type operation)

(Do not report modifier 63 in conjunction with 33750, 33755, 33762)

33764   central, with prosthetic graft

33766   superior vena cava to pulmonary artery for flow to 1 lung (classical Glenn procedure)

33767   superior vena cava to pulmonary artery for flow to both lungs (bidirectional Glenn procedure)

+ 33768 Anastomosis, cavopulmonary, second superior vena cava (List separately in addition to primary procedure)

(Use 33768 in conjunction with 33478, 33617, 33622, 33767)

(Do not report 33768 in conjunction with 32551, 33210, 33211)

Transposition of the Great Vessels

33770 Repair of transposition of the great arteries with ventricular septal defect and subpulmonary stenosis; without surgical enlargement of ventricular septal defect

33771   with surgical enlargement of ventricular septal defect

33774 Repair of transposition of the great arteries, atrial baffle procedure (eg, Mustard or Senning type) with cardiopulmonary bypass;

33775   with removal of pulmonary band

33776   with closure of ventricular septal defect

33777   with repair of subpulmonic obstruction

33778 Repair of transposition of the great arteries, aortic pulmonary artery reconstruction (eg, Jatene type);

(Do not report modifier 63 in conjunction with 33778)

33779   with removal of pulmonary band

33780   with closure of ventricular septal defect

33781   with repair of subpulmonic obstruction

33782 Aortic root translocation with ventricular septal defect and pulmonary stenosis repair (ie, Nikaidoh procedure); without coronary ostium reimplantation

(Do not report 33782 in conjunction with 33412, 33413, 33608, 33681, 33770, 33771, 33778, 33780, 33920)

33783   with reimplantation of 1 or both coronary ostia

Truncus Arteriosus

33786 Total repair, truncus arteriosus (Rastelli type operation)

(Do not report modifier 63 in conjunction with 33786)

33788 Reimplantation of an anomalous pulmonary artery

(For pulmonary artery band, use 33690)

Aortic Anomalies

33800 Aortic suspension (aortopexy) for tracheal decompression (eg, for tracheomalacia) (separate procedure)

33802 Division of aberrant vessel (vascular ring);

33803　　　with reanastomosis

33813　　Obliteration of aortopulmonary septal defect; without cardiopulmonary bypass

33814　　　with cardiopulmonary bypass

33820　　Repair of patent ductus arteriosus; by ligation

33822　　　by division, younger than 18 years

33824　　　by division, 18 years and older

(For percutaneous transcatheter closure of patent ductus arteriosus, use 93582)

33840　　Excision of coarctation of aorta, with or without associated patent ductus arteriosus; with direct anastomosis

33845　　　with graft

33851　　　repair using either left subclavian artery or prosthetic material as gusset for enlargement

33852　　Repair of hypoplastic or interrupted aortic arch using autogenous or prosthetic material; without cardiopulmonary bypass

33853　　　with cardiopulmonary bypass

(For repair of hypoplastic left heart syndrome (eg, Norwood type), via excision of coarctation of aorta, use 33619)

Thoracic Aortic Aneurysm

33860　　Ascending aorta graft, with cardiopulmonary bypass, includes valve suspension, when performed

33863　　Ascending aorta graft, with cardiopulmonary bypass, with aortic root replacement using valved conduit and coronary reconstruction (eg, Bentall)

(Do not report 33863 in conjunction with 33405, 33406, 33410, 33411, 33412, 33413, 33860)

33864　　Ascending aorta graft, with cardiopulmonary bypass with valve suspension, with coronary reconstruction and valve-sparing aortic root remodeling (eg, David Procedure, Yacoub Procedure)

(Do not report 33864 in conjunction with 33400, 33860-33863)

33870　　Transverse arch graft, with cardiopulmonary bypass

33875　　Descending thoracic aorta graft, with or without bypass

33877　　Repair of thoracoabdominal aortic aneurysm with graft, with or without cardiopulmonary bypass

Endovascular Repair of Descending Thoracic Aorta

Codes 33880-33891 represent a family of procedures to report placement of an endovascular graft for repair of the descending thoracic aorta. These codes include all device introduction, manipulation, positioning, and deployment. All balloon angioplasty and/or stent deployment within the target treatment zone for the endoprosthesis, either before or after endograft deployment, are not separately reportable. Open arterial exposure and associated closure of the arteriotomy sites (eg, 34812, 34820, 34833, 34834), introduction of guidewires and catheters (eg, 36140, 36200-36218), and extensive repair or replacement of an artery (eg, 35226, 35286) should be additionally reported. Transposition of subclavian artery to carotid, and carotid-carotid bypass performed in conjunction with endovascular repair of the descending thoracic aorta (eg, 33889, 33891) should be separately reported. The primary codes, 33880 and 33881, include placement of all distal extensions, if required, in the distal thoracic aorta, while proximal extensions, if needed, are reported separately.

For fluoroscopic guidance in conjunction with endovascular repair of the thoracic aorta, see codes 75956-75959 as appropriate. Codes 75956 and 75957 include all angiography of the thoracic aorta and its branches for diagnostic imaging prior to deployment of the primary endovascular devices (including all routine components of modular devices), fluoroscopic guidance in the delivery of the endovascular components, and intraprocedural arterial angiography (eg, confirm position, detect endoleak, evaluate runoff). Code 75958 includes the analogous services for placement of each proximal thoracic endovascular extension. Code 75959 includes the analogous services for placement of a distal thoracic endovascular extension(s) placed during a procedure after the primary repair.

Other interventional procedures performed at the time of endovascular repair of the descending thoracic aorta should be additionally reported (eg, innominate, carotid, subclavian, visceral, or iliac artery transluminal angioplasty or stenting, arterial embolization, intravascular ultrasound) when performed before or after deployment of the aortic prostheses.

(For transcatheter placement of wireless physiologic sensor in aneurysmal sac, use 34806)

(For analysis, interpretation, and report of implanted wireless pressure sensor in aneurysmal sac, use 93982)

33880　　Endovascular repair of descending thoracic aorta (eg, aneurysm, pseudoaneurysm, dissection, penetrating ulcer, intramural hematoma, or traumatic disruption); involving coverage of left subclavian artery origin, initial endoprosthesis plus descending thoracic aortic extension(s), if required, to level of celiac artery origin

(For radiological supervision and interpretation, use 75956 in conjunction with 33880)

33881　　　not involving coverage of left subclavian artery origin, initial endoprosthesis plus descending thoracic aortic extension(s), if required, to level of celiac artery origin

(For radiological supervision and interpretation, use 75957 in conjunction with 33881)

Cardiovascular

Cardiovascular

33883   Placement of proximal extension prosthesis for endovascular repair of descending thoracic aorta (eg, aneurysm, pseudoaneurysm, dissection, penetrating ulcer, intramural hematoma, or traumatic disruption); initial extension

(For radiological supervision and interpretation, use 75958 in conjunction with 33883)

(Do not report 33881, 33883 when extension placement converts repair to cover left subclavian origin. Use only 33880)

+ 33884   each additional proximal extension (List separately in addition to code for primary procedure)

(Use 33884 in conjunction with 33883)

(For radiological supervision and interpretation, use 75958 in conjunction with 33884)

33886   Placement of distal extension prosthesis(s) delayed after endovascular repair of descending thoracic aorta

(Do not report 33886 in conjunction with 33880, 33881)

(Report 33886 once, regardless of number of modules deployed)

(For radiological supervision and interpretation, use 75959 in conjunction with 33886)

33889   Open subclavian to carotid artery transposition performed in conjunction with endovascular repair of descending thoracic aorta, by neck incision, unilateral

(Do not report 33889 in conjunction with 35694)

33891   Bypass graft, with other than vein, transcervical retropharyngeal carotid-carotid, performed in conjunction with endovascular repair of descending thoracic aorta, by neck incision

(Do not report 33891 in conjunction with 35509, 35601)

Pulmonary Artery

33910   Pulmonary artery embolectomy; with cardiopulmonary bypass

33915   without cardiopulmonary bypass

33916   Pulmonary endarterectomy, with or without embolectomy, with cardiopulmonary bypass

33917   Repair of pulmonary artery stenosis by reconstruction with patch or graft

33920   Repair of pulmonary atresia with ventricular septal defect, by construction or replacement of conduit from right or left ventricle to pulmonary artery

(For repair of other complex cardiac anomalies by construction or replacement of right or left ventricle to pulmonary artery conduit, use 33608)

33922   Transection of pulmonary artery with cardiopulmonary bypass

(Do not report modifier 63 in conjunction with 33922)

+ 33924   Ligation and takedown of a systemic-to-pulmonary artery shunt, performed in conjunction with a congenital heart procedure (List separately in addition to code for primary procedure)

(Use 33924 in conjunction with 33470-33478, 33600-33617, 33622, 33684-33688, 33692-33697, 33735-33767, 33770-33783, 33786, 33917, 33920, 33922, 33925, 33926, 33935, 33945)

33925   Repair of pulmonary artery arborization anomalies by unifocalization; without cardiopulmonary bypass

33926   with cardiopulmonary bypass

Heart/Lung Transplantation

Heart with or without lung allotransplantation involves three distinct components of physician work:

1. *Cadaver donor cardiectomy with or without pneumonectomy,* which includes harvesting the allograft and cold preservation of the allograft (perfusing with cold preservation solution and cold maintenance) (see 33930, 33940).

2. *Backbench work:*

Preparation of a cadaver donor heart and lung allograft prior to transplantation, including dissection of the allograft from surrounding soft tissues to prepare the aorta, superior vena cava, inferior vena cava, and trachea for implantation (use 33933).

Preparation of a cadaver donor heart allograft prior to transplantation, including dissection of the allograft from surrounding soft tissues to prepare aorta, superior vena cava, inferior vena cava, pulmonary artery, and left atrium for implantation (use 33944).

3. *Recipient heart with or without lung allotransplantation,* which includes transplantation of allograft and care of the recipient (see 33935, 33945).

(For implantation of a total replacement heart system (artificial heart) with recipient cardiectomy or heart replacement system components, see Category III codes 0051T-0053T)

33930   Donor cardiectomy-pneumonectomy (including cold preservation)

33933   Backbench standard preparation of cadaver donor heart/lung allograft prior to transplantation, including dissection of allograft from surrounding soft tissues to prepare aorta, superior vena cava, inferior vena cava, and trachea for implantation

33935   Heart-lung transplant with recipient cardiectomy-pneumonectomy

33940   Donor cardiectomy (including cold preservation)

33944   Backbench standard preparation of cadaver donor heart allograft prior to transplantation, including dissection of allograft from surrounding soft tissues to prepare aorta, superior vena cava, inferior vena cava, pulmonary artery, and left atrium for implantation

(For repair or resection procedures on the donor heart, see 33300, 33310, 33320, 33400, 33463, 33464, 33510, 33641, 35216, 35276 or 35685)

33945   Heart transplant, with or without recipient cardiectomy

Extracorporeal Membrane Oxygenation or Extracorporeal Life Support Services

Prolonged extracorporeal membrane oxygenation (ECMO) or extracorporeal life support (ECLS) is a procedure that provides cardiac and/or respiratory support to the heart and/or lungs, which allows them to rest and recover when sick or injured. ECMO/ECLS supports the function of the heart and/or lungs by continuously pumping some of the patient's blood out of the body to an oxygenator (membrane lung) where oxygen is added to the blood, carbon dioxide (CO_2) is removed, and the blood is warmed before it is returned to the patient. There are two methods that can be used to accomplish ECMO/ECLS. One method is veno-arterial extracorporeal life support, which will support both the heart and lungs. Veno-arterial ECMO/ECLS requires that two cannula(e) are placed—one in a large vein and one in a large artery. The other method is veno-venous extracorporeal life support. Veno-venous ECMO/ECLS is used for lung support only and requires one or two cannula(e), which are placed in a vein.

Services directly related to the cannulation, initiation, management, and discontinuation of the ECMO/ECLS circuit and parameters (33946, 33947, 33948, 33949) are distinct from the daily overall management of the patient. The daily overall management of the patient is a factor that will vary greatly depending on the patient's age, disease process, and condition. Daily overall management of the patient may be separately reported using the relevant hospital observation services, hospital inpatient services, or critical care evaluation and management codes (99218, 99219, 99220, 99221, 99222, 99223, 99231, 99232, 99233, 99234, 99235, 99236, 99291, 99292, 99468, 99469, 99471, 99472, 99475, 99476, 99477, 99478, 99479, 99480).

Services directly related to the ECMO/ECLS involve the initial cannulation and repositioning, removing, or adding cannula(e) while the patient is being supported by the ECMO/ECLS. Initiation of the ECMO/ECLS circuit and setting parameters (33946, 33947) is performed by the physician and involves determining the necessary ECMO/ECLS device components, blood flow, gas exchange, and other necessary parameters to manage the circuit. The daily management of the ECMO/ECLS circuit and monitoring parameters (33948, 33949) requires physician oversight to ensure that specific

features of the interaction of the circuit with the patient are met. Daily management of the circuit and parameters includes management of blood flow, oxygenation, CO_2 clearance by the membrane lung, systemic response, anticoagulation and treatment of bleeding, and cannula(e) positioning, alarms and safety. Once the patient's heart and/or lung function has sufficiently recovered, the physician will wean the patient from the ECMO/ECLS circuit and finally decannulate the patient. The basic management of the ECMO/ECLS circuit and parameters are similar, regardless of the patient's condition.

ECMO/ECLS commonly involves multiple physicians and supporting nonphysician personnel to manage each patient. Different physicians may insert the cannula(e) and initiate ECMO/ECLS, manage the ECMO/ECLS circuit, and decannulate the patient. In addition, it would be common for one physician to manage the ECMO/ECLS circuit and patient-related issues (eg, anticoagulation, complications related to the ECMO/ECLS devices), while another physician manages the overall patient medical condition and underlying disorders, all on a daily basis. The physicians involved in the patient's care are commonly of different specialties, and significant physician team interaction may be required. Depending on the type of circuit and the patient's condition, there is substantial nonphysician work by ECMO/ECLS specialists, cardiac perfusionists, respiratory therapists, and specially trained nurses who provide long periods of constant attention.

If the same physician provides any or all of the services for placing a patient on an ECMO/ECLS circuit, they may report the appropriate codes for the services they performed, which may include codes for the cannula(e) insertion (33951, 33952, 33953, 33954, 33955, 33956), ECMO/ECLS initiation (33946 or 33947), and overall patient management (99218, 99219, 99220, 99221, 99222, 99223, 99231, 99232, 99233, 99234, 99235, 99236, 99291, 99292, 99468, 99469, 99471, 99472, 99475, 99476, 99477, 99478, 99479, 99480).

ECMO/ECLS daily management (33948, 33949) and repositioning services (33957, 33958, 33959, 33962, 33963, 33964) may not be reported on the same day as initiation services (33946, 33947) by the same or different individuals.

If different physicians provide parts of the service, each physician may report the correct code(s) for the service(s) they provided, except as noted.

Repositioning of the ECMO/ECLS cannula(e) (33957, 33958, 33959, 33962, 33963, 33964) at the same session as insertion (33951, 33952, 33953, 33954, 33955, 33956) is not separately reportable. Replacement of ECMO/ECLS cannula(e) in the same vessel should only be reported using the insertion code (33951, 33952, 33953, 33954, 33955, 33956). If cannula(e) are removed from one vessel and new cannula(e) are placed in a different vessel, report the appropriate cannula(e) removal

(33965, 33966, 33969, 33984, 33985, 33986) and insertion (33951, 33952, 33953, 33954, 33955, 33956) codes. Extensive repair or replacement of an artery may be additionally reported (eg, 35266, 35286, 35371, and 35665). Fluoroscopic guidance used for cannula(e) repositioning (33957, 33958, 33959, 33962, 33963, 33964) is included in the procedure when performed and should not be separately reported.

Daily management codes (33948 and 33949) should not be reported on the same day as initiation of ECMO (33946 or 33947).

Initiation codes (33946 or 33947) should not be reported on the same day as repositioning codes (33957, 33958, 33959, 33962, 33963, 33964). See the CPT codes for ECMO/ECLS Procedure Chart.

33946 Extracorporeal membrane oxygenation (ECMO)/ extracorporeal life support (ECLS) provided by physician; initiation, veno-venous

(Do not report modifier 63 in conjunction with 33946, 33947, 33948, 33949)

(For insertion of cannula[e] for extracorporeal circulation, see 33951, 33952, 33953, 33954, 33955, 33956)

33947 initiation, veno-arterial

(Do not report modifier 63 in conjunction with 33946, 33947, 33948, 33949)

(Do not report 33946, 33947 in conjunction with 33948, 33949, 33957, 33958, 33959, 33962, 33963, 33964)

33948 daily management, each day, veno-venous

(Do not report modifier 63 in conjunction with 33946, 33947, 33948, 33949)

33949 daily management, each day, veno-arterial

(Do not report modifier 63 in conjunction with 33946, 33947, 33948, 33949)

(Do not report 33948, 33949 in conjunction with 33946, 33947)

CPT Codes For ECMO/ECLS Procedures

Abbreviation: Yrs indicates years; and ≥ indicates greater or equal to.

33951   insertion of peripheral (arterial and/or venous) cannula(e), percutaneous, birth through 5 years of age (includes fluoroscopic guidance, when performed)

(For initiation and daily management of extracorporeal circulation, see 33946, 33947, 33948, 33949)

33952   insertion of peripheral (arterial and/or venous) cannula(e), percutaneous, 6 years and older (includes fluoroscopic guidance, when performed)

(For maintenance of extracorporeal circulation, see 33946, 33947, 33948, 33949)

33953   insertion of peripheral (arterial and/or venous) cannula(e), open, birth through 5 years of age

(For maintenance of extracorporeal circulation, see 33946, 33947, 33948, 33949)

33954   insertion of peripheral (arterial and/or venous) cannula(e), open, 6 years and older

(Do not report 33953, 33954 in conjunction with 34812, 34820, 34834)

(For maintenance of extracorporeal circulation, see 33946, 33947, 33948, 33949)

33955   insertion of central cannula(e) by sternotomy or thoracotomy, birth through 5 years of age

(For maintenance of extracorporeal circulation, see 33946, 33947, 33948, 33949)

33956   insertion of central cannula(e) by sternotomy or thoracotomy, 6 years and older

(Do not report 33955, 33956 in conjunction with 32100, 39010)

(For maintenance of extracorporeal circulation, see 33946, 33947, 33948, 33949)

33957   reposition peripheral (arterial and/or venous) cannula(e), percutaneous, birth through 5 years of age (includes fluoroscopic guidance, when performed)

33958   reposition peripheral (arterial and/or venous) cannula(e), percutaneous, 6 years and older (includes fluoroscopic guidance, when performed)

(Do not report 33957, 33958 in conjunction with 34812, 34820, 34834)

33959   reposition peripheral (arterial and/or venous) cannula(e), open, birth through 5 years of age (includes fluoroscopic guidance, when performed)

33962   reposition peripheral (arterial and/or venous) cannula(e), open, 6 years and older (includes fluoroscopic guidance, when performed)

(Do not report 33959, 33962 in conjunction with 34812, 34820, 34834)

33963   reposition of central cannula(e) by sternotomy or thoracotomy, birth through 5 years of age (includes fluoroscopic guidance, when performed)

33964   reposition central cannula(e) by sternotomy or thoracotomy, 6 years and older (includes fluoroscopic guidance, when performed)

(Do not report 33963, 33964 in conjunction with 32100, 39010)

(Do not report 33957, 33958, 33959, 33962, 33963, 33964 in conjunction with 33946, 33947)

33965   removal of peripheral (arterial and/or venous) cannula(e), percutaneous, birth through 5 years of age

33966   removal of peripheral (arterial and/or venous) cannula(e), percutaneous, 6 years and older

33969   removal of peripheral (arterial and/or venous) cannula(e), open, birth through 5 years of age

(Do not report 33969 in conjunction with 34812, 34820, 34834, 35201, 35206, 35211, 35226)

33984   removal of peripheral (arterial and/or venous) cannula(e), open, 6 years and older

(Do not report 33984 in conjunction with 34812, 34820, 34834, 35201, 35206, 35211, 35226)

33985   removal of central cannula(e) by sternotomy or thoracotomy, birth through 5 years of age

(Do not report 33985 in conjunction with 35211)

33986   removal of central cannula(e) by sternotomy or thoracotomy, 6 years and older

(Do not report 33986 in conjunction with 35211)

#+ **33987**   Arterial exposure with creation of graft conduit (eg, chimney graft) to facilitate arterial perfusion for ECMO/ECLS (List separately in addition to code for primary procedure)

(Use 33987 in conjunction with 33953, 33954, 33955, 33956)

(Do not report 33987 in conjunction with 34833)

33988   Insertion of left heart vent by thoracic incision (eg, sternotomy, thoracotomy) for ECMO/ECLS

33989   Removal of left heart vent by thoracic incision (eg, sternotomy, thoracotomy) for ECMO/ECLS

Cardiac Assist

The insertion of a ventricular assist device (VAD) can be performed via percutaneous (33990, 33991) or transthoracic (33975, 33976, 33979) approach. The location of the ventricular assist device may be intracorporeal or extracorporeal.

Open arterial exposure when necessary to facilitate percutaneous ventricular assist device insertion (33990, 33991), may be reported separately (34812). Extensive repair or replacement of an artery may be additionally reported (eg, 35226 or 35286).

Removal of a ventricular assist device (33977, 33978, 33980, 33992) includes removal of the entire device, including the cannulas. Removal of a percutaneous ventricular assist device at the same session as insertion is not separately reportable. For removal of a percutaneous ventricular assist device at a separate and distinct session, but on the same day as insertion, report 33992 appended with modifier 59 indicating a distinct procedural service.

Repositioning of a percutaneous ventricular assist device at the same session as insertion is not separately reportable. Repositioning of percutaneous ventricular assist device not necessitating imaging guidance is not a reportable service. For repositioning of a percutaneous ventricular assist device necessitating imaging guidance at a separate and distinct session, but on the same day as insertion, report 33993 with modifier 59 indicating a distinct procedural service.

Replacement of a ventricular assist device pump (ie, 33981-33983) includes the removal of the pump and insertion of a new pump, connection, de-airing, and initiation of the new pump.

Replacement of the entire implantable ventricular assist device system, ie, pump(s) and cannulas, is reported using the insertion codes (ie, 33975, 33976, 33979). Removal (ie, 33977, 33978, 33980) of the ventricular assist device system being replaced is not separately reported. Replacement of a percutaneous ventricular assist device is reported using implantation codes (ie, 33990, 33991). Removal (ie, 33992) is not reported separately.

(33960 has been deleted. To report, see 33946, 33947, 33948, 33949)

(33961 has been deleted. To report, see 33948, 33949)

33962 Code is out of numerical sequence. See 33946-33993

33963 Code is out of numerical sequence. See 33946-33993

33964 Code is out of numerical sequence. See 33946-33993

33965 Code is out of numerical sequence. See 33946-33993

33966 Code is out of numerical sequence. See 33946-33993

33967 Insertion of intra-aortic balloon assist device, percutaneous

33968 Removal of intra-aortic balloon assist device, percutaneous

33969 Code is out of numerical sequence. See 33946-33993

33970 Insertion of intra-aortic balloon assist device through the femoral artery, open approach

33971 Removal of intra-aortic balloon assist device including repair of femoral artery, with or without graft

33973 Insertion of intra-aortic balloon assist device through the ascending aorta

33974 Removal of intra-aortic balloon assist device from the ascending aorta, including repair of the ascending aorta, with or without graft

33975 Insertion of ventricular assist device; extracorporeal, single ventricle

33976 extracorporeal, biventricular

33977 Removal of ventricular assist device; extracorporeal, single ventricle

33978 extracorporeal, biventricular

33979 Insertion of ventricular assist device, implantable intracorporeal, single ventricle

33980 Removal of ventricular assist device, implantable intracorporeal, single ventricle

33981 Replacement of extracorporeal ventricular assist device, single or biventricular, pump(s), single or each pump

33982 Replacement of ventricular assist device pump(s); implantable intracorporeal, single ventricle, without cardiopulmonary bypass

33983 implantable intracorporeal, single ventricle, with cardiopulmonary bypass

33984 Code is out of numerical sequence. See 33946-33993

33985 Code is out of numerical sequence. See 33946-33993

33986 Code is out of numerical sequence. See 33946-33993

33987 Code is out of numerical sequence. See 33946-33993

33988 Code is out of numerical sequence. See 33946-33993

33989 Code is out of numerical sequence. See 33946-33993

⊙ **33990** Insertion of ventricular assist device, percutaneous including radiological supervision and interpretation; arterial access only

⊙ **33991** both arterial and venous access, with transseptal puncture

⊙ **33992** Removal of percutaneous ventricular assist device at separate and distinct session from insertion

⊙ **33993** Repositioning of percutaneous ventricular assist device with imaging guidance at separate and distinct session from insertion

Other Procedures

33999 Unlisted procedure, cardiac surgery

Arteries and Veins

Primary vascular procedure listings include establishing both inflow and outflow by whatever procedures necessary. Also included is that portion of the operative arteriogram performed by the surgeon, as indicated. Sympathectomy, when done, is included in the listed aortic procedures. For unlisted vascular procedure, use 37799.

Embolectomy/Thrombectomy

Arterial, With or Without Catheter

34001 Embolectomy or thrombectomy, with or without catheter; carotid, subclavian or innominate artery, by neck incision

34051 innominate, subclavian artery, by thoracic incision

34101 axillary, brachial, innominate, subclavian artery, by arm incision

34111 radial or ulnar artery, by arm incision

34151 renal, celiac, mesentery, aortoiliac artery, by abdominal incision

34201 femoropopliteal, aortoiliac artery, by leg incision

34203 popliteal-tibio-peroneal artery, by leg incision

Venous, Direct or With Catheter

34401 Thrombectomy, direct or with catheter; vena cava, iliac vein, by abdominal incision

34421 vena cava, iliac, femoropopliteal vein, by leg incision

34451 vena cava, iliac, femoropopliteal vein, by abdominal and leg incision

34471 subclavian vein, by neck incision

34490 axillary and subclavian vein, by arm incision

Venous Reconstruction

34501 Valvuloplasty, femoral vein

34502 Reconstruction of vena cava, any method

34510 Venous valve transposition, any vein donor

34520 Cross-over vein graft to venous system

34530 Saphenopopliteal vein anastomosis

Endovascular Repair of Abdominal Aortic Aneurysm

Codes 34800-34826 represent a family of component procedures to report placement of an endovascular graft for abdominal aortic aneurysm repair. These codes describe open femoral or iliac artery exposure, device manipulation and deployment, and closure of the arteriotomy sites. Balloon angioplasty and/or stent deployment within the target treatment zone for the endoprosthesis, either before or after endograft deployment, are not separately reportable. Introduction of guide wires and catheters should be reported separately (eg, 36200, 36245-36248, 36140). Extensive repair or replacement of an artery should be additionally reported (eg, 35226 or 35286).

For fluoroscopic guidance in conjunction with endovascular aneurysm repair, see code 75952 or 75953, as appropriate. Code 75952 includes angiography of the aorta and its branches for diagnostic imaging prior to deployment of the endovascular device (including all routine components of modular devices), fluoroscopic guidance in the delivery of the endovascular components, and intraprocedural arterial angiography (eg, confirm position, detect endoleak, evaluate runoff). Code 75953 includes the analogous services for placement of additional extension prostheses (not for routine components of modular devices).

Other interventional procedures performed at the time of endovascular abdominal aortic aneurysm repair should be additionally reported (eg, renal transluminal angioplasty, arterial embolization, intravascular ultrasound, balloon angioplasty or stenting of native artery[s] outside the endoprosthesis target zone, when done before or after deployment of graft).

(For fenestrated endovascular repair of the visceral aorta, see 34841-34844. For fenestrated endovascular repair of the visceral aorta and concomitant infrarenal abdominal aorta, see 34845-34848)

(For transcatheter placement of wireless physiologic sensor in aneurysmal sac, use 34806)

(For analysis, interpretation and report of implanted wireless pressure sensor in aneurysmal sac, use 93982)

34800 Endovascular repair of infrarenal abdominal aortic aneurysm or dissection; using aorto-aortic tube prosthesis

34802 using modular bifurcated prosthesis (1 docking limb)

34803 using modular bifurcated prosthesis (2 docking limbs)

34804 using unibody bifurcated prosthesis

34805 using aorto-uniiliac or aorto-unifemoral prosthesis

(For radiological supervision and interpretation, use 75952 in conjunction with 34800-34805)

(Do not report 34800, 34802, 34803, 34804, 34805 in conjunction with 34841-34848)

+ 34806 Transcatheter placement of wireless physiologic sensor in aneurysmal sac during endovascular repair, including radiological supervision and interpretation, instrument calibration, and collection of pressure data (List separately in addition to code for primary procedure)

(Use 34806 in conjunction with 33880, 33881, 33886, 34800-34805, 34825, 34900)

(Do not report 34806 in conjunction with 93982)

+ 34808 Endovascular placement of iliac artery occlusion device (List separately in addition to code for primary procedure)

(Use 34808 in conjunction with 34800, 34805, 34813, 34825, 34826)

(For open arterial exposure, report 34812, 34820, 34833, 34834 as appropriate, in addition to 34800-34808)

Cardiovascular

34812 Open femoral artery exposure for delivery of endovascular prosthesis, by groin incision, unilateral

(Do not report 34812 in conjunction with 33953, 33954, 33959, 33962, 33969, 33984)

(For bilateral procedure, use modifier 50)

+ 34813 Placement of femoral-femoral prosthetic graft during endovascular aortic aneurysm repair (List separately in addition to code for primary procedure)

(Use 34813 in conjunction with 34812)

(For femoral artery grafting, see 35521, 35533, 35539, 35540, 35556, 35558, 35566, 35621, 35646, 35654-35661, 35666, 35700)

34820 Open iliac artery exposure for delivery of endovascular prosthesis or iliac occlusion during endovascular therapy, by abdominal or retroperitoneal incision, unilateral

(Do not report 34820 in conjunction with 33953, 33954, 33959, 33962, 33969, 33984)

(For bilateral procedure, use modifier 50)

34825 Placement of proximal or distal extension prosthesis for endovascular repair of infrarenal abdominal aortic or iliac aneurysm, false aneurysm, or dissection; initial vessel

+ 34826 each additional vessel (List separately in addition to code for primary procedure)

(Use 34826 in conjunction with 34825)

(Use 34825, 34826 in addition to 34800-34805, 34900 as appropriate)

(For radiological supervision and interpretation, use 75953)

34830 Open repair of infrarenal aortic aneurysm or dissection, plus repair of associated arterial trauma, following unsuccessful endovascular repair; tube prosthesis

34831 aorto-bi-iliac prosthesis

34832 aorto-bifemoral prosthesis

34833 Open iliac artery exposure with creation of conduit for delivery of aortic or iliac endovascular prosthesis, by abdominal or retroperitoneal incision, unilateral

(Do not report 34833 in conjunction with 33987, 34820)

(For bilateral procedure, use modifier 50)

34834 Open brachial artery exposure to assist in the deployment of aortic or iliac endovascular prosthesis by arm incision, unilateral

(Do not report 34834 in conjunction with 33953, 33954, 33959, 33962, 33969, 33984)

(For bilateral procedure, use modifier 50)

Fenestrated Endovascular Repair of the Visceral and Infrarenal Aorta

The upper abdominal aorta that contains the celiac, superior mesenteric, and renal arteries is termed the visceral aorta. For reporting purposes, the thoracic aorta extends from the aortic valve to the aortic segment just proximal to the celiac artery.

Code 34839 is used to report the physician planning and sizing for a patient-specific fenestrated visceral aortic endograft. The planning includes review of high-resolution cross-sectional images (eg, CT, CTA, MRI) and utilization of 3D software for iterative modeling of the aorta and device in multiplanar views and center line of flow analysis. Code 34839 may only be reported when the physician spends a minimum of 90 total minutes performing patient-specific fenestrated endograft planning. Physician planning time does not need to be continuous and should be clearly documented in the patient record. Code 34839 is reported on the date that planning work is complete and may not include time spent on the day before or the day of the fenestrated endovascular repair procedure (34841, 34842, 34843, 34844, 34845, 34846, 34847, 34848) nor be reported on the day before or the day of the fenestrated endovascular repair procedure.

Codes 34841, 34842, 34843, 34844, 34845, 34846, 34847, 34848 are used to report placement of a fenestrated endovascular graft in the visceral aorta, either alone or in combination with the infrarenal aorta for aneurysm, pseudoaneurysm, dissection, penetrating ulcer, intramural hematoma, or traumatic disruption. The fenestrated main body endoprosthesis is deployed within the visceral aorta. Fenestrations within the fabric allow for selective catheterization of the visceral and/or renal arteries and subsequent placement of an endoprosthesis (ie, bare metal or covered stent) to maintain flow to the visceral artery. Patient variation in the location and relative orientation of the renal and visceral artery origins requires use of a patient-specific fenestrated endograft for endovascular repair that preserves flow to essential visceral arteries and allows proximal seal and fixation to be achieved above the renal level as well as in the distal aorta or iliac vessel(s).

Fenestrated aortic repair is reported based on the extent of aorta treated. Codes 34841-34844 describe repair using proximal endoprostheses that span from the visceral aortic component to one, two, three, or four visceral artery origins and distal extent limited to the infrarenal aorta. These devices do not extend into the common iliac arteries. Codes 34845-34848 are used to report deployment of a fenestrated endoprosthesis that spans from the visceral aorta (including one, two, three, or four visceral artery origins) through the infrarenal aorta into the common iliac arteries. The infrarenal component may be a bifurcated unibody device, a modular bifurcated docking system with docking limb(s), or an aorto-uniiliac or aorta-unifemoral device. Codes 34845-34848 include placement of unilateral or bilateral docking limbs (depending on the device). Any additional stent graft extensions that terminate in the common iliac arteries are included in the work described by 34845-34848. Codes 34825 and 34826 may not be separately reported for

Cardiovascular

proximal abdominal aortic extension prosthesis(es) or for distal extension prosthesis(es) that terminate in the aorta or the common iliac arteries. However, codes 34825 and 34826 may be reported for distal extension prosthesis(es) that terminate in the internal iliac, external iliac, or common femoral artery(s).

Codes 34841-34844 and 34845-34848 define the total number of visceral and/or renal arteries (ie, celiac, superior mesenteric, and/or unilateral or bilateral renal artery[s]) requiring placement of an endoprosthesis (ie, bare metal or covered stent) through an aortic endograft fenestration.

Introduction of guide wires and catheters in the aorta and visceral and/or renal arteries is included in the work of 34841-34848 and is not separately reportable. However, catheterization of the hypogastric artery(s) and/or arterial families outside the treatment zone of the graft may be separately reported. Balloon angioplasty within the target treatment zone of the endograft, either before or after endograft deployment, is not separately reportable. Fluoroscopic guidance and radiological supervision and interpretation in conjunction with fenestrated endovascular aortic repair is not separately reportable and includes angiographic diagnostic imaging of the aorta and its branches prior to deployment of the fenestrated endovascular device, fluoroscopic guidance in the delivery of the fenestrated endovascular components, and intraprocedural arterial angiography (eg, confirm position, detect endoleak, evaluate runoff) done at the time of the endovascular aortic repair.

Exposure of the access vessels (eg, 34812) may be reported separately. Extensive repair of an artery (eg, 35226, 35286) may be reported separately. For concomitant endovascular treatment of the descending thoracic aorta, report 33880-33886 and 75956-75959 with 34841-34848. For isolated endovascular infrarenal abdominal aortic aneurysm repair that does not require placement of a fenestrated graft to preserve flow to the visceral branch(es), see 34800-34805.

Other interventional procedures performed at the time of fenestrated endovascular abdominal aortic aneurysm repair may be reported separately (eg, arterial embolization, intravascular ultrasound, balloon angioplasty or stenting of native artery[s] outside the endoprosthesis target zone, when done before or after deployment of endoprosthesis).

34839 Physician planning of a patient-specific fenestrated visceral aortic endograft requiring a minimum of 90 minutes of physician time

(Do not report 34839 in conjunction with 76376, 76377)

(Do not report 34839 in conjunction with 34841, 34842, 34843, 34844, 34845, 34846, 34847, 34848, when performed on the day before or the day of the fenestrated endovascular repair procedure)

34841 Endovascular repair of visceral aorta (eg, aneurysm, pseudoaneurysm, dissection, penetrating ulcer, intramural hematoma, or traumatic disruption) by deployment of a fenestrated visceral aortic endograft and all associated radiological supervision and interpretation, including target zone angioplasty, when performed; including one visceral artery endoprosthesis (superior mesenteric, celiac or renal artery)

34842 including two visceral artery endoprostheses (superior mesenteric, celiac and/or renal artery[s])

34843 including three visceral artery endoprostheses (superior mesenteric, celiac and/or renal artery[s])

34844 including four or more visceral artery endoprostheses (superior mesenteric, celiac and/or renal artery[s])

(Do not report 34841, 34842, 34843, 34844 in conjunction with 34800, 34802, 34803, 34804, 34805, 34845, 34846, 34847, 34848, 35452, 35472, 75952)

(Do not report 34841, 34842, 34843, 34844 in conjunction with 34839, when planning services are performed on the day before or the day of the fenestrated endovascular repair procedure)

34845 Endovascular repair of visceral aorta and infrarenal abdominal aorta (eg, aneurysm, pseudoaneurysm, dissection, penetrating ulcer, intramural hematoma, or traumatic disruption) with a fenestrated visceral aortic endograft and concomitant unibody or modular infrarenal aortic endograft and all associated radiological supervision and interpretation, including target zone angioplasty, when performed; including one visceral artery endoprosthesis (superior mesenteric, celiac or renal artery)

34846 including two visceral artery endoprostheses (superior mesenteric, celiac and/or renal artery[s])

34847 including three visceral artery endoprostheses (superior mesenteric, celiac and/or renal artery[s])

34848 including four or more visceral artery endoprostheses (superior mesenteric, celiac and/or renal artery[s])

(Do not report 34845, 34846, 34847, 34848 in conjunction with 34800, 34802, 34803, 34804, 34805, 34841, 34842, 34843, 34844, 35081, 35102, 35452, 35472, 75952)

(Do not report 34845, 34846, 34847, 34848 in conjunction with 34839, when planning services are performed on the day before or the day of the fenestrated endovascular repair procedure)

(Do not report 34841-34848 in conjunction with 37236, 37237 for bare metal or covered stents placed into the visceral branches within the endoprosthesis target zone)

(For placement of distal extension prosthesis[es] terminating in the internal iliac, external iliac, or common femoral artery[s], see 34825-34826, 75953, 0254T, 0255T)

(Use 34845, 34846, 34847, 34848 in conjunction with 37220, 37221, 37222, 37223, only when 37220, 37221, 37222, 37223 are performed outside the target treatment zone of the endoprosthesis)

Cardiovascular

Endovascular Repair of Iliac Aneurysm

Code 34900 represents a procedure to report introduction, positioning, and deployment of an endovascular graft for treatment of aneurysm, pseudoaneurysm, or arteriovenous malformation or trauma of the iliac artery (common, hypogastric, external). All balloon angioplasty and/or stent deployments within the target treatment zone for the endoprosthesis, either before or after endograft deployment, are included in the work of 34900 and are not separately reportable. Open femoral or iliac artery exposure (eg, 34812, 34820), introduction of guidewires and catheters (eg, 36200, 36245-36248), and extensive repair or replacement of an artery (eg, 35206-35286) should be additionally reported.

For fluoroscopic guidance in conjunction with endovascular iliac aneurysm repair, see code 75954. Code 75954 includes angiography of the aorta and iliac arteries for diagnostic imaging prior to deployment of the endovascular device (including all routine components), fluoroscopic guidance in the delivery of the endovascular components, and intraprocedural arterial angiography to confirm appropriate position of the graft, detect endoleaks, and evaluate the status of the runoff vessels (eg, evaluation for dissection, stenosis, thrombosis, distal embolization, or iatrogenic injury).

Other interventional procedures performed at the time of endovascular iliac aneurysm repair should be additionally reported (eg, transluminal angioplasty outside the aneurysm target zone, arterial embolization, intravascular ultrasound).

34900 Endovascular repair of iliac artery (eg, aneurysm, pseudoaneurysm, arteriovenous malformation, trauma) using ilio-iliac tube endoprosthesis

(For endovascular repair of iliac artery bifurcation [eg, aneurysm, pseudoaneurysm, arteriovenous malformation, trauma] using bifurcated endoprosthesis, use 0254T)

(For radiological supervision and interpretation, use 75954)

(For placement of extension prosthesis during endovascular iliac artery repair, use 34825)

(For bilateral procedure, use modifier 50)

Direct Repair of Aneurysm or Excision (Partial or Total) and Graft Insertion for Aneurysm, Pseudoaneurysm, Ruptured Aneurysm, and Associated Occlusive Disease

Procedures 35001-35152 include preparation of artery for anastomosis including endarterectomy.

(For direct repairs associated with occlusive disease only, see 35201-35286)

(For intracranial aneurysm, see 61700 et seq)

(For endovascular repair of abdominal aortic aneurysm, see 34800-34826)

(For endovascular repair of iliac artery aneurysm, see 34900)

(For thoracic aortic aneurysm, see 33860-33875)

(For endovascular repair of descending thoracic aorta, involving coverage of left subclavian artery origin, use 33880)

35001 Direct repair of aneurysm, pseudoaneurysm, or excision (partial or total) and graft insertion, with or without patch graft; for aneurysm and associated occlusive disease, carotid, subclavian artery, by neck incision

35002 for ruptured aneurysm, carotid, subclavian artery, by neck incision

35005 for aneurysm, pseudoaneurysm, and associated occlusive disease, vertebral artery

35011 for aneurysm and associated occlusive disease, axillary-brachial artery, by arm incision

35013 for ruptured aneurysm, axillary-brachial artery, by arm incision

35021 for aneurysm, pseudoaneurysm, and associated occlusive disease, innominate, subclavian artery, by thoracic incision

35022 for ruptured aneurysm, innominate, subclavian artery, by thoracic incision

35045 for aneurysm, pseudoaneurysm, and associated occlusive disease, radial or ulnar artery

35081 for aneurysm, pseudoaneurysm, and associated occlusive disease, abdominal aorta

35082 for ruptured aneurysm, abdominal aorta

35091 for aneurysm, pseudoaneurysm, and associated occlusive disease, abdominal aorta involving visceral vessels (mesenteric, celiac, renal)

35092 for ruptured aneurysm, abdominal aorta involving visceral vessels (mesenteric, celiac, renal)

35102 for aneurysm, pseudoaneurysm, and associated occlusive disease, abdominal aorta involving iliac vessels (common, hypogastric, external)

35103 for ruptured aneurysm, abdominal aorta involving iliac vessels (common, hypogastric, external)

35111 for aneurysm, pseudoaneurysm, and associated occlusive disease, splenic artery

35112 for ruptured aneurysm, splenic artery

35121 for aneurysm, pseudoaneurysm, and associated occlusive disease, hepatic, celiac, renal, or mesenteric artery

35122 for ruptured aneurysm, hepatic, celiac, renal, or mesenteric artery

⊙=Moderate sedation ✚=Add-on code ◢=FDA approval pending #=Resequenced code ○=Recycled/reinstated code

35131	for aneurysm, pseudoaneurysm, and associated occlusive disease, iliac artery (common, hypogastric, external)
35132	for ruptured aneurysm, iliac artery (common, hypogastric, external)
35141	for aneurysm, pseudoaneurysm, and associated occlusive disease, common femoral artery (profunda femoris, superficial femoral)
35142	for ruptured aneurysm, common femoral artery (profunda femoris, superficial femoral)
35151	for aneurysm, pseudoaneurysm, and associated occlusive disease, popliteal artery
35152	for ruptured aneurysm, popliteal artery

Repair Arteriovenous Fistula

35180	Repair, congenital arteriovenous fistula; head and neck
35182	thorax and abdomen
35184	extremities
35188	Repair, acquired or traumatic arteriovenous fistula; head and neck
35189	thorax and abdomen
35190	extremities

Repair Blood Vessel Other Than for Fistula, With or Without Patch Angioplasty

(For AV fistula repair, see 35180-35190)

35201	Repair blood vessel, direct; neck
	(Do not report 35201 in conjunction with 33969, 33984, 33985, 33986)
35206	upper extremity
	(Do not report 35206 in conjunction with 33969, 33984, 33985, 33986)
35207	hand, finger
35211	intrathoracic, with bypass
	(Do not report 35211 in conjunction with 33969, 33984, 33985, 33986)
35216	intrathoracic, without bypass
	(Do not report 35216 in conjunction with 33969, 33984, 33985, 33986)
35221	intra-abdominal
35226	lower extremity
	(Do not report 35226 in conjunction with 33969, 33984, 33985, 33986)
35231	Repair blood vessel with vein graft; neck
35236	upper extremity

35241	intrathoracic, with bypass
35246	intrathoracic, without bypass
35251	intra-abdominal
35256	lower extremity
35261	Repair blood vessel with graft other than vein; neck
35266	upper extremity
35271	intrathoracic, with bypass
35276	intrathoracic, without bypass
35281	intra-abdominal
35286	lower extremity

Thromboendarterectomy

(For coronary artery, see 33510-33536 and 33572)

(35301-35372 include harvest of saphenous or upper extremity vein when performed)

35301	Thromboendarterectomy, including patch graft, if performed; carotid, vertebral, subclavian, by neck incision
35302	superficial femoral artery
35303	popliteal artery
	(Do not report 35302, 35303 in conjunction with 35500, 37225, 37227)
35304	tibioperoneal trunk artery
35305	tibial or peroneal artery, initial vessel
+ 35306	each additional tibial or peroneal artery (List separately in addition to code for primary procedure)
	(Use 35306 in conjunction with 35305)
	(Do not report 35304, 35305, 35306 in conjunction with 35500, 37229, 37231, 37233, 37235)
35311	subclavian, innominate, by thoracic incision
35321	axillary-brachial
35331	abdominal aorta
35341	mesenteric, celiac, or renal
35351	iliac
35355	iliofemoral
35361	combined aortoiliac
35363	combined aortoiliofemoral
35371	common femoral
35372	deep (profunda) femoral
+ 35390	Reoperation, carotid, thromboendarterectomy, more than 1 month after original operation (List separately in addition to code for primary procedure)
	(Use 35390 in conjunction with 35301)

Cardiovascular

Angioscopy

+ 35400   Angioscopy (noncoronary vessels or grafts) during therapeutic intervention (List separately in addition to code for primary procedure)

Transluminal Angioplasty

If done as part of another operation, use modifier 51 or use modifier 52.

(For radiological supervision and interpretation, see 75962-75968 and 75978)

Open

35450   Transluminal balloon angioplasty, open; renal or other visceral artery

35452   aortic

(Do not report 35452 in conjunction with 34841-34848)

35458   brachiocephalic trunk or branches, each vessel

(Do not report 35458 in conjunction with 37217 for ipsilateral services)

35460   venous

Percutaneous

Codes for catheter placement and the radiologic supervision and interpretation should also be reported, in addition to the code(s) for the therapeutic aspect of the procedure.

⊙ **35471**   Transluminal balloon angioplasty, percutaneous; renal or visceral artery

⊙ **35472**   aortic

(Do not report 35472 in conjunction with 34841-34848)

⊙ **35475**   brachiocephalic trunk or branches, each vessel

⊙ **35476**   venous

(For radiological supervision and interpretation, use 75978)

Bypass Graft

Vein

Procurement of the saphenous vein graft is included in the description of the work for 35501-35587 and should not be reported as a separate service or co-surgery. To report harvesting of an upper extremity vein, use 35500 in addition to the bypass procedure. To report harvesting of a femoropopliteal vein segment, use 35572 in addition to the bypass procedure. To report harvesting and construction of an autogenous composite graft of two segments from two distant locations, report 35682 in

addition to the bypass procedure, for autogenous composite of three or more segments from distant sites, report 35683.

+ 35500   Harvest of upper extremity vein, 1 segment, for lower extremity or coronary artery bypass procedure (List separately in addition to code for primary procedure)

(Use 35500 in conjunction with 33510-33536, 35556, 35566, 35570, 35571, 35583-35587)

(For harvest of more than one vein segment, see 35682, 35683)

(For endoscopic procedure, use 33508)

35501   Bypass graft, with vein; common carotid-ipsilateral internal carotid

35506   carotid-subclavian or subclavian-carotid

35508   carotid-vertebral

35509   carotid-contralateral carotid

35510   carotid-brachial

35511   subclavian-subclavian

35512   subclavian-brachial

35515   subclavian-vertebral

35516   subclavian-axillary

35518   axillary-axillary

35521   axillary-femoral

(For bypass graft performed with synthetic graft, use 35621)

35522   axillary-brachial

35523   brachial-ulnar or -radial

(Do not report 35523 in conjunction with 35206, 35500, 35525, 36838)

(For bypass graft performed with synthetic conduit, use 37799)

35525   brachial-brachial

35526   aortosubclavian, aortoinnominate, or aortocarotid

(For bypass graft performed with synthetic graft, use 35626)

35531   aortoceliac or aortomesenteric

35533   axillary-femoral-femoral

(For bypass graft performed with synthetic graft, use 35654)

35535   hepatorenal

(Do not report 35535 in conjunction with 35221, 35251, 35281, 35500, 35536, 35560, 35631, 35636)

35536   splenorenal

35537   aortoiliac

(For bypass graft performed with synthetic graft, use 35637)

(Do not report 35537 in conjunction with 35538)

35538   aortobi-iliac

(For bypass graft performed with synthetic graft, use 35638)

(Do not report 35538 in conjunction with 35537)

35539   aortofemoral

(For bypass graft performed with synthetic graft, use 35647)

(Do not report 35539 in conjunction with 35540)

35540   aortobifemoral

(For bypass graft performed with synthetic graft, use 35646)

(Do not report 35540 in conjunction with 35539)

35556   femoral-popliteal

35558   femoral-femoral

35560   aortorenal

35563   ilioiliac

35565   iliofemoral

35566   femoral-anterior tibial, posterior tibial, peroneal artery or other distal vessels

35570   tibial-tibial, peroneal-tibial, or tibial/peroneal trunk-tibial

(Do not report 35570 in conjunction with 35256, 35286)

35571   popliteal-tibial, -peroneal artery or other distal vessels

+ 35572   Harvest of femoropopliteal vein, 1 segment, for vascular reconstruction procedure (eg, aortic, vena caval, coronary, peripheral artery) (List separately in addition to code for primary procedure)

(Use 35572 in conjunction with 33510-33516, 33517-33523, 33533-33536, 34502, 34520, 35001, 35002, 35011-35022, 35102, 35103, 35121-35152, 35231-35256, 35501-35587, 35879-35907)

(For bilateral procedure, use modifier 50)

In-Situ Vein

(To report aortobifemoral bypass using synthetic conduit, and femoral-popliteal bypass with vein conduit in-situ, use 35646 and 35583. To report aorto[uni]femoral bypass with synthetic conduit, and femoral-popliteal bypass with vein conduit in-situ, use 35647 and 35583. To report aortofemoral bypass using vein conduit, and femoral-popliteal bypass with vein conduit in-situ, use 35539 and 35583)

35583   In-situ vein bypass; femoral-popliteal

35585   femoral-anterior tibial, posterior tibial, or peroneal artery

35587   popliteal-tibial, peroneal

Other Than Vein

(For arterial transposition and/or reimplantation, see 35691-35695)

+ 35600   Harvest of upper extremity artery, 1 segment, for coronary artery bypass procedure (List separately in addition to code for primary procedure)

(Use 35600 in conjunction with 33533–33536)

35601   Bypass graft, with other than vein; common carotid-ipsilateral internal carotid

35606   carotid-subclavian

(For open transcervical common carotid-common carotid bypass performed in conjunction with endovascular repair of descending thoracic aorta, use 33891)

(For open subclavian to carotid artery transposition performed in conjunction with endovascular thoracic aneurysm repair by neck incision, use 33889)

35612   subclavian-subclavian

35616   subclavian-axillary

35621   axillary-femoral

35623   axillary-popliteal or -tibial

35626   aortosubclavian, aortoinnominate, or aortocarotid

35631   aortoceliac, aortomesenteric, aortorenal

35632   ilio-celiac

(Do not report 35632 in conjunction with 35221, 35251, 35281, 35531, 35631)

35633   ilio-mesenteric

(Do not report 35633 in conjunction with 35221, 35251, 35281, 35531, 35631)

35634   iliorenal

(Do not report 35634 in conjunction with 35221, 35251, 35281, 35560, 35536, 35631)

35636   splenorenal (splenic to renal arterial anastomosis)

35637   aortoiliac

(Do not report 35637 in conjunction with 35638, 35646)

35638   aortobi-iliac

(Do not report 35638 in conjunction with 35637, 35646)

(For open placement of aortobi-iliac prosthesis following unsuccessful endovascular repair, use 34831)

35642   carotid-vertebral

35645   subclavian-vertebral

Cardiovascular

35646	aortobifemoral

(For bypass graft performed with vein graft, use 35540)

(For open placement of aortobifemoral prosthesis following unsuccessful endovascular repair, use 34832)

35647	aortofemoral

(For bypass graft performed with vein graft, use 35539)

35650	axillary-axillary
35654	axillary-femoral-femoral
35656	femoral-popliteal
35661	femoral-femoral
35663	ilioiliac
35665	iliofemoral
35666	femoral-anterior tibial, posterior tibial, or peroneal artery
35671	popliteal-tibial or -peroneal artery

Composite Grafts

Codes 35682-35683 are used to report harvest and anastomosis of multiple vein segments from distant sites for use as arterial bypass graft conduits. These codes are intended for use when the two or more vein segments are harvested from a limb other than that undergoing bypass.

+ 35681 Bypass graft; composite, prosthetic and vein (List separately in addition to code for primary procedure)

(Do not report 35681 in addition to 35682, 35683)

+ 35682 autogenous composite, 2 segments of veins from 2 locations (List separately in addition to code for primary procedure)

(Use 35682 in conjunction with 35556, 35566, 35570, 35571, 35583-35587)

(Do not report 35682 in addition to 35681, 35683)

+ 35683 autogenous composite, 3 or more segments of vein from 2 or more locations (List separately in addition to code for primary procedure)

(Use 35683 in conjunction with 35556, 35566, 35570, 35571, 35583-35587)

(Do not report 35683 in addition to 35681, 35682)

Adjuvant Techniques

Adjuvant (additional) technique(s) may be required at the time a bypass graft is created to improve patency of the lower extremity autogenous or synthetic bypass graft (eg, femoral-popliteal, femoral-tibial, or popliteal-tibial arteries). Code 35685 should be reported in addition to the primary synthetic bypass graft procedure, when an interposition of venous tissue (vein patch or cuff) is placed at the anastomosis between the synthetic bypass conduit and the involved artery (includes harvest).

Code 35686 should be reported in addition to the primary bypass graft procedure, when autogenous vein is used to create a fistula between the tibial or peroneal artery and vein at or beyond the distal bypass anastomosis site of the involved artery.

(For composite graft(s), see 35681-35683)

+ 35685 Placement of vein patch or cuff at distal anastomosis of bypass graft, synthetic conduit (List separately in addition to code for primary procedure)

(Use 35685 in conjunction with 35656, 35666, or 35671)

+ 35686 Creation of distal arteriovenous fistula during lower extremity bypass surgery (non-hemodialysis) (List separately in addition to code for primary procedure)

(Use 35686 in conjunction with 35556, 35566, 35570, 35571, 35583-35587, 35623, 35656, 35666, 35671)

Arterial Transposition

35691	Transposition and/or reimplantation; vertebral to carotid artery
35693	vertebral to subclavian artery
35694	subclavian to carotid artery

(For open subclavian to carotid artery transposition performed in conjunction with endovascular repair of descending thoracic aorta, use 33889)

35695	carotid to subclavian artery

+ 35697 Reimplantation, visceral artery to infrarenal aortic prosthesis, each artery (List separately in addition to code for primary procedure)

(Do not report 35697 in conjunction with 33877)

Excision, Exploration, Repair, Revision

+ 35700 Reoperation, femoral-popliteal or femoral (popliteal)-anterior tibial, posterior tibial, peroneal artery, or other distal vessels, more than 1 month after original operation (List separately in addition to code for primary procedure)

(Use 35700 in conjunction with 35556, 35566, 35570, 35571, 35583, 35585, 35587, 35656, 35666, 35671)

35701	Exploration (not followed by surgical repair), with or without lysis of artery; carotid artery
35721	femoral artery
35741	popliteal artery
35761	other vessels
35800	Exploration for postoperative hemorrhage, thrombosis or infection; neck
35820	chest
35840	abdomen
35860	extremity
35870	Repair of graft-enteric fistula

Cardiovascular

35875   Thrombectomy of arterial or venous graft (other than hemodialysis graft or fistula);

35876   with revision of arterial or venous graft

        (For thrombectomy of hemodialysis graft or fistula, see 36831, 36833)

Codes 35879 and 35881 describe open revision of graft-threatening stenoses of lower extremity arterial bypass graft(s) (previously constructed with autogenous vein conduit) using vein patch angioplasty or segmental vein interposition techniques. For thrombectomy with revision of any noncoronary arterial or venous graft, including those of the lower extremity, (other than hemodialysis graft or fistula), use 35876. For direct repair (other than for fistula) of a lower extremity blood vessel (with or without patch angioplasty), use 35226. For repair (other than for fistula) of a lower extremity blood vessel using a vein graft, use 35256.

35879   Revision, lower extremity arterial bypass, without thrombectomy, open; with vein patch angioplasty

35881   with segmental vein interposition

        (For revision of femoral anastomosis of synthetic arterial bypass graft, see 35883, 35884)

        (For excision of infected graft, see 35901-35907 and appropriate revascularization code)

35883   Revision, femoral anastomosis of synthetic arterial bypass graft in groin, open; with nonautogenous patch graft (eg, Dacron, ePTFE, bovine pericardium)

        (For bilateral procedure, use modifier 50)

        (Do not report 35883 in conjunction with 35700, 35875, 35876, 35884)

35884   with autogenous vein patch graft

        (For bilateral procedure, use modifier 50)

        (Do not report 35884 in conjunction with 35700, 35875, 35876, 35883)

35901   Excision of infected graft; neck

35903   extremity

35905   thorax

35907   abdomen

Vascular Injection Procedures

Listed services for injection procedures include necessary local anesthesia, introduction of needles or catheter, injection of contrast media with or without automatic power injection, and/or necessary pre- and postinjection care specifically related to the injection procedure.

Selective vascular catheterization should be coded to include introduction and all lesser order selective catheterization used in the approach (eg, the description for a selective right middle cerebral artery catheterization

includes the introduction and placement catheterization of the right common and internal carotid arteries).

Additional second and/or third order arterial catheterization within the same family of arteries or veins supplied by a single first order vessel should be expressed by 36012, 36218, or 36248.

Additional first order or higher catheterization in vascular families supplied by a first order vessel different from a previously selected and coded family should be separately coded using the conventions described above.

        (For radiological supervision and interpretation, see **Radiology**)

        (For injection procedures in conjunction with cardiac catheterization, see 93452-93461, 93563-93568)

        (For chemotherapy of malignant disease, see 96401-96549)

Intravenous

An intracatheter is a sheathed combination of needle and short catheter.

36000   Introduction of needle or intracatheter, vein

36002   Injection procedures (eg, thrombin) for percutaneous treatment of extremity pseudoaneurysm

        (For imaging guidance, see 76942, 77002, 77012, 77021)

        (For ultrasound guided compression repair of pseudoaneurysms, use 76936)

        (Do not report 36002 for vascular sealant of an arteriotomy site)

36005   Injection procedure for extremity venography (including introduction of needle or intracatheter)

        (For radiological supervision and interpretation, see 75820, 75822)

⊙ 36010   Introduction of catheter, superior or inferior vena cava

36011   Selective catheter placement, venous system; first order branch (eg, renal vein, jugular vein)

36012   second order, or more selective, branch (eg, left adrenal vein, petrosal sinus)

36013   Introduction of catheter, right heart or main pulmonary artery

36014   Selective catheter placement, left or right pulmonary artery

36015   Selective catheter placement, segmental or subsegmental pulmonary artery

        (For insertion of flow directed catheter (eg, Swan-Ganz), use 93503)

        (For venous catheterization for selective organ blood sampling, use 36500)

Cardiovascular

Cardiovascular

Intra-Arterial—Intra-Aortic

(For radiological supervision and interpretation, see **Radiology**)

36100   Introduction of needle or intracatheter, carotid or vertebral artery

(For bilateral procedure, report 36100 with modifier 50)

36120   Introduction of needle or intracatheter; retrograde brachial artery

⊙ **36140**   extremity artery

(For insertion of arteriovenous cannula, see 36810-36821)

Diagnostic Studies of Arteriovenous (AV) Shunts for Dialysis: For diagnostic studies, the arteriovenous (AV) dialysis shunt (AV shunt) is defined as beginning with the arterial anastomosis and extending to the right atrium. This definition includes all upper and lower extremity AV shunts (arteriovenous fistulae [AVF] and arteriovenous grafts [AVG]). Code 36147 includes the work of directly accessing and imaging the entire AV shunt. Antegrade and/or retrograde punctures of the AV shunt are typically used for imaging, and contrast may be injected directly through a needle or through a catheter placed into the AV shunt. Occasionally the catheter needs to be advanced further into the shunt to adequately visualize the arterial anastomosis or the central veins, and all manipulation of the catheter for diagnostic imaging of the AV shunt is included in 36147. Advancement of the catheter to the vena cava to adequately image that segment of the AV shunt is included in 36147 and is not separately reported. Advancement of the catheter tip through the arterial anastomosis to adequately visualize the anastomosis is also considered integral to the work of 36147 and is not separately reported.

Ultrasound guidance for puncture of the AV shunt is not included in 36147. Particularly in the case of new or failing AVF, ultrasound may be necessary to safely and effectively puncture the AV access for evaluation, and this may be reported separately with 76937 if all the appropriate elements for reporting 76937 are performed.

Evaluation of the peri-anastomotic portion of the inflow is considered an integral part of the dialysis fistulagram and is included in the work of 36147. The peri-anastomotic portion of the vessel at the arterial anastomosis includes the short segment of the artery immediately adjacent to the anastomosis, the anastomosis itself, and the portion of the vessel or graft immediately distal to the anastomosis.

The arterial inflow to the AV access is considered a separate vessel. If a more proximal inflow problem separate from the peri-anastomotic segment is suspected and additional catheter work and imaging must be done for adequate evaluation, this work is not included in 36147. If a catheter is selectively advanced from the AV shunt puncture into the inflow artery, an additional catheterization code may be reported. In the typical case

of an upper extremity AV shunt, 36215 is used to report this work, and includes placement of the catheter retrograde into the inflow artery and into the aorta if necessary (ie, 36200 may not be also reported since that work is included in the work defined by 36215).

Interventions for Arteriovenous (AV) Shunts Created for Dialysis (AV Grafts and AV Fistulae): For the purposes of coding interventional procedures in arteriovenous (AV) shunts created for dialysis (both arteriovenous fistulae [AVF] and arteriovenous grafts [AVG]), the AV shunt is artificially divided into two vessel segments. The first segment is peripheral and extends from the peri-arterial anastomosis through the axillary vein (or entire cephalic vein in the case of cephalic venous outflow). The second segment includes the veins central to the axillary and cephalic veins, including the subclavian and innominate veins through the vena cava. Interventions performed in a single segment, regardless of the number of lesions treated, are coded as a single intervention.

The AV shunt is considered to be venous and most interventions are coded with the venous intervention codes (ie, angioplasty is reported with venous angioplasty codes 35476, 75978). Codes 35476 and 75978 would be reported once to describe all angioplasty work performed in one segment of the AV dialysis shunt, regardless of the number of distinct lesions treated within that segment, the number of times the balloon is inflated, or the number of balloon catheters required to open all lesions.

There is an exception to the use of venous interventional codes. When there is a stenosis at the arterial anastomosis, it typically extends across the anastomosis and involves the artery just proximal to and at the anastomosis as well as the outflow vessel or graft. This segment is called the peri-anastomotic (or juxta-anastomotic) region, and even though the stenosis can involve multiple vessels, it is typically a single lesion with a single etiology crossing the anastomosis, and treatment to open this lesion crosses from the artery into the vein or venous graft. An intervention treated in this peri-anastomotic segment is coded as an arterial intervention (35475, 75962). Since the entire segment of the AV shunt from the peri-arterial anastomosis through the axillary vein is considered a single vessel for coding of interventions, the arterial angioplasty codes include the work of opening the peri-anastomotic stenosis, as well as all other stenoses treated within this segment of the vessel. Codes 35475 and 75962 are reported once to describe all work done to angioplasty any lesion from the peri-arterial anastomosis through the axillary vein in procedures that involve angioplasty of the peri-arterial anastomosis of the AV shunt. In these special instances, venous angioplasty codes would not be reported additionally for this first or most peripheral shunt segment, even if balloon angioplasty is performed on segments of the AV dialysis shunt that are purely venous anatomy within this specific vessel segment.

It is never appropriate to report removal of the arterial plug during a declot/thrombectomy procedure as an arterial or venous angioplasty (35475, 35476). Removal of the arterial plug is included in the work of a fistula thrombectomy (36870), even if a balloon catheter is used to mechanically dislodge the resistant thrombus.

The central veins (eg, subclavian, innominate, and cava) are considered an additional, separate venous vessel segment for purposes of interventional coding for AV dialysis shunt interventions. If one or more central venous stenoses are treated with angioplasty, this is reported as a single venous angioplasty (35476, 75978), regardless of the number of discrete lesions treated within this segment, and also independent of the number of balloon inflations or number of balloon catheters or sizes required. This additional work should be clearly documented in the patient record and in the recorded images.

The same rules used for angioplasty apply to stent placements for AV dialysis shunts with respect to the number of interventions reported for each patient. Either 37236 or 37238 is reported once to describe all work of stenting lesions within the defined AV dialysis shunt segment from the peri-arterial anastomosis through the axillary and cephalic veins, regardless of the number of stents placed or the number of discrete lesions treated within that vessel segment. Code 37238 is reported for placement of AV access stent unless the treated lesion includes the peri-anastomotic region. This peri-anastomotic region is considered an artery and therefore 37236 is reported instead of 37238. If additional stenting is required for central venous stenosis, this may be reported as an additional stent placement (37239), describing all the work of stent placement within the central venous segment.

The work of catheterizing all the veins in the dialysis AV shunt is included in 36147 (and, if appropriate, 36148). Selective catheterization of the inferior/superior vena cava and central veins cannot be separately reported when performed from a direct puncture of the AVF/AVG.

However, if additional venous side branches off of the conduit, known as accessory veins, are separately catheterized for diagnosis or intervention such as embolization of a large competing accessory vein, this additional work may be separately reported using the appropriate selective venous catheterization codes (36011 and 36012). The embolization may be reported using 37241 once, irrespective of the number of branches embolized.

⊙ **36147**　Introduction of needle and/or catheter, arteriovenous shunt created for dialysis (graft/fistula); initial access with complete radiological evaluation of dialysis access, including fluoroscopy, image documentation and report (includes access of shunt, injection[s] of contrast, and all necessary imaging from the arterial anastomosis and adjacent artery through entire venous outflow including the inferior or superior vena cava)

(If 36147 indicates the need for a therapeutic intervention requiring a second catheterization of the shunt, use 36148)

(Do not report 36147 in conjunction with 75791)

⊙+ **36148**　additional access for therapeutic intervention (List separately in addition to code for primary procedure)

(Use 36148 in conjunction with 36147)

36160　Introduction of needle or intracatheter, aortic, translumbar

Diagnostic Studies of Cervicocerebral Arteries: Codes 36221-36228 describe non-selective and selective arterial catheter placement and diagnostic imaging of the aortic arch, carotid, and vertebral arteries. Codes 36221-36226 include the work of accessing the vessel, placement of catheter(s), contrast injection(s), fluoroscopy, radiological supervision and interpretation, and closure of the arteriotomy by pressure, or application of an arterial closure device. Codes 36221-36228 describe arterial contrast injections with arterial, capillary, and venous phase imaging, when performed.

Code 36227 is an add-on code to report unilateral selective arterial catheter placement and diagnostic imaging of the ipsilateral external carotid circulation and includes all the work of accessing the additional vessel, placement of catheter(s), contrast injection(s), fluoroscopy, radiological supervision and interpretation. Code 36227 is reported in conjunction with 36222, 36223, or 36224.

Code 36228 is an add-on code to report unilateral selective arterial catheter placement and diagnostic imaging of the initial and each additional intracranial branch of the internal carotid or vertebral arteries. Code 36228 is reported in conjunction with 36223, 36224, 36225 or 36226. This includes any additional second or third order catheter selective placement in the same primary branch of the internal carotid, vertebral, or basilar artery and includes all the work of accessing the additional vessel, placement of catheter(s), contrast injection(s), fluoroscopy, radiological supervision and interpretation. It is not reported more than twice per side, regardless of the number of additional branches selectively catheterized.

Codes 36221-36226 are built on progressive hierarchies with more intensive services inclusive of less intensive services. The code inclusive of all of the services provided for that vessel should be reported (ie, use the code inclusive of the most intensive services provided). Only one code in the range 36222-36224 may be reported for each ipsilateral carotid territory. Only one code in the range 36225-36226 may be reported for each ipsilateral vertebral territory.

Code 36221 is reported for non-selective arterial catheter placement in the thoracic aorta and diagnostic imaging of the aortic arch and great vessel origins. Codes 36222-36228 are reported for unilateral artery catheterization.

Do not report 36221 in conjunction with 36222-36226 as these selective codes include the work of 36221 when performed.

Do not report 36222, 36223, or 36224 together for ipsilateral angiography. Instead, select the code that represents the most comprehensive service using the following hierarchy of complexity (listed in descending order of complexity): 36224>36223>36222.

Do not report 36225 and 36226 together for ipsilateral angiography. Select the code that represents the more comprehensive service using the following hierarchy of complexity (listed in descending order of complexity): 36226>36225.

When bilateral carotid and/or vertebral arterial catheterization and imaging is performed, add modifier 50 to codes 36222-36228 if the same procedure is performed on both sides. For example, bilateral extracranial carotid angiography with selective catheterization of each common carotid artery would be reported with 36222 and modifier 50. However, when different territory(ies) is studied in the same session on both sides of the body, modifiers may be required to report the imaging performed. Use modifier 59 to denote that different carotid and/or vertebral arteries are being studied. For example, when selective right internal carotid artery catheterization accompanied by right extracranial and intracranial carotid angiography is followed by selective left common carotid artery catheterization with left extracranial carotid angiography, use 36224 to report the right side and 36222-59 to report the left side.

Diagnostic angiography of the cervicocerebral vessels may be followed by an interventional procedure at the same session. Interventional procedures may be separately reportable using standard coding conventions.

Do not report 36218 or 75774 as part of diagnostic angiography of the extracranial and intracranial cervicocerebral vessels. It may be appropriate to report 36218 and 75774 for diagnostic angiography of upper extremities and other vascular beds of the neck and/or shoulder girdle performed in the same session as vertebral angiography (eg, workup of a neck tumor that requires catheterization and angiography of the vertebral artery as well as other brachiocephalic arteries).

Report 76376 or 76377 for 3D rendering when performed in conjunction with 36221-36228.

Report 76937 for ultrasound guidance for vascular access, when performed in conjunction with 36221-36228.

⊙ **36200**   Introduction of catheter, aorta

(For non-selective angiography of the extracranial carotid and/or cerebral vessels and cervicocerebral arch, when performed, use 36221)

36215   Selective catheter placement, arterial system; each first order thoracic or brachiocephalic branch, within a vascular family

(For catheter placement for coronary angiography, see 93454-93461)

36216   initial second order thoracic or brachiocephalic branch, within a vascular family

36217   initial third order or more selective thoracic or brachiocephalic branch, within a vascular family

+ **36218**   additional second order, third order, and beyond, thoracic or brachiocephalic branch, within a vascular family (List in addition to code for initial second or third order vessel as appropriate)

(Use 36218 in conjunction with 36216, 36217, 36225, 36226)

(For angiography, see 36222-36228, 75600-75774, 75791)

(For angioplasty, see 35472, 35475)

▶(For transcatheter therapies, see 37200, 37211, 37213, 37214, 37236, 37237, 37238, 37239, 37241, 37242, 37243, 37244, 61624, 61626)◀

(When coronary artery, arterial conduit [eg, internal mammary, inferior epigastric or free radical artery] or venous bypass graft angiography is performed in conjunction with cardiac catheterization, see the appropriate cardiac catheterization, injection procedure, and imaging supervision code[s] [93455, 93457, 93459, 93461, 93530-93533, 93564] in the **Medicine** section. When internal mammary artery angiography only is performed without a concomitant cardiac catheterization, use 36216 or 36217 as appropriate)

⊙ **36221**   Non-selective catheter placement, thoracic aorta, with angiography of the extracranial carotid, vertebral, and/or intracranial vessels, unilateral or bilateral, and all associated radiological supervision and interpretation, includes angiography of the cervicocerebral arch, when performed

(Do not report 36221 with 36222-36226)

⊙ **36222**   Selective catheter placement, common carotid or innominate artery, unilateral, any approach, with angiography of the ipsilateral extracranial carotid circulation and all associated radiological supervision and interpretation, includes angiography of the cervicocerebral arch, when performed

(Do not report 36222 in conjunction with 37215, 37216, 37218 for the treated carotid artery)

⊙ **36223**   Selective catheter placement, common carotid or innominate artery, unilateral, any approach, with angiography of the ipsilateral intracranial carotid circulation and all associated radiological supervision and interpretation, includes angiography of the extracranial carotid and cervicocerebral arch, when performed

(Do not report 36223 in conjunction with 37215, 37216, 37218 for the treated carotid artery)

⊙ **36224**   Selective catheter placement, internal carotid artery, unilateral, with angiography of the ipsilateral intracranial carotid circulation and all associated radiological supervision and interpretation, includes angiography of the extracranial carotid and cervicocerebral arch, when performed

(Do not report 36224 in conjunction with 37215, 37216, 37218 for the treated carotid artery)

⊙ **36225**   Selective catheter placement, subclavian or innominate artery, unilateral, with angiography of the ipsilateral vertebral circulation and all associated radiological supervision and interpretation, includes angiography of the cervicocerebral arch, when performed

⊙ **36226**   Selective catheter placement, vertebral artery, unilateral, with angiography of the ipsilateral vertebral circulation and all associated radiological supervision and interpretation, includes angiography of the cervicocerebral arch, when performed

⊙+ **36227**   Selective catheter placement, external carotid artery, unilateral, with angiography of the ipsilateral external carotid circulation and all associated radiological supervision and interpretation (List separately in addition to code for primary procedure)

(Use 36227 in conjunction with 36222, 36223, or 36224)

(Do not report 36221-36227 in conjunction with 37217 for ipsilateral services)

⊙+ **36228**   Selective catheter placement, each intracranial branch of the internal carotid or vertebral arteries, unilateral, with angiography of the selected vessel circulation and all associated radiological supervision and interpretation (eg, middle cerebral artery, posterior inferior cerebellar artery) (List separately in addition to code for primary procedure)

(Use 36228 in conjunction with 36223, 36224, 36225 or 36226)

(Do not report 36228 more than twice per side)

⊙ **36245**   Selective catheter placement, arterial system; each first order abdominal, pelvic, or lower extremity artery branch, within a vascular family

⊙ **36246**   initial second order abdominal, pelvic, or lower extremity artery branch, within a vascular family

⊙ **36247**   initial third order or more selective abdominal, pelvic, or lower extremity artery branch, within a vascular family

⊙+ **36248**   additional second order, third order, and beyond, abdominal, pelvic, or lower extremity artery branch, within a vascular family (List in addition to code for initial second or third order vessel as appropriate)

(Use 36248 in conjunction with 36246, 36247)

⊙ **36251**   Selective catheter placement (first-order), main renal artery and any accessory renal artery(s) for renal angiography, including arterial puncture and catheter placement(s), fluoroscopy, contrast injection(s), image postprocessing, permanent recording of images, and radiological supervision and interpretation, including pressure gradient measurements when performed, and flush aortogram when performed; unilateral

⊙ **36252**   bilateral

⊙ **36253**   Superselective catheter placement (one or more second order or higher renal artery branches) renal artery and any accessory renal artery(s) for renal angiography, including arterial puncture, catheterization, fluoroscopy, contrast injection(s), image postprocessing, permanent recording of images, and radiological supervision and interpretation, including pressure gradient measurements when performed, and flush aortogram when performed; unilateral

(Do not report 36253 in conjunction with 36251 when performed for the same kidney)

⊙ **36254**   bilateral

(Do not report 36254 in conjunction with 36252)

(Placement of closure device at the vascular access site is not separately reported with 36251-36254)

(Do not report 36251, 36252, 36253, 36254 in conjunction with 0338T, 0339T)

36260   Insertion of implantable intra-arterial infusion pump (eg, for chemotherapy of liver)

36261   Revision of implanted intra-arterial infusion pump

36262   Removal of implanted intra-arterial infusion pump

36299   Unlisted procedure, vascular injection

Venous

Venipuncture, needle or catheter for diagnostic study or intravenous therapy, percutaneous. These codes are also used to report the therapy as specified. For collection of a specimen from an established catheter, use 36592. For collection of a specimen from a completely implantable venous access device, use 36591.

36400   Venipuncture, younger than age 3 years, necessitating the skill of a physician or other qualified health care professional, not to be used for routine venipuncture; femoral or jugular vein

36405   scalp vein

36406   other vein

36410   Venipuncture, age 3 years or older, necessitating the skill of a physician or other qualified health care professional (separate procedure), for diagnostic or therapeutic purposes (not to be used for routine venipuncture)

36415   Collection of venous blood by venipuncture

(Do not report modifier 63 in conjunction with 36415)

Cardiovascular

36416 Collection of capillary blood specimen (eg, finger, heel, ear stick)

36420 Venipuncture, cutdown; younger than age 1 year

(Do not report modifier 63 in conjunction with 36420)

36425 age 1 or over

(Do not report 36425 in conjunction with 36475, 36476, 36478)

36430 Transfusion, blood or blood components

36440 Push transfusion, blood, 2 years or younger

36450 Exchange transfusion, blood; newborn

(Do not report modifier 63 in conjunction with 36450)

36455 other than newborn

36460 Transfusion, intrauterine, fetal

(Do not report modifier 63 in conjunction with 36460)

(For radiological supervision and interpretation, use 76941)

36468 Single or multiple injections of sclerosing solutions, spider veins (telangiectasia), limb or trunk

(Do not report 36468 in conjunction with 37241 in the same surgical field)

(36469 has been deleted)

36470 Injection of sclerosing solution; single vein

36471 multiple veins, same leg

(For vascular embolization and occlusion procedures, see 37241, 37242, 37243, 37244)

(Do not report 36470, 36471 in conjunction with 37241 in the same surgical field)

36475 Endovenous ablation therapy of incompetent vein, extremity, inclusive of all imaging guidance and monitoring, percutaneous, radiofrequency; first vein treated

+ 36476 second and subsequent veins treated in a single extremity, each through separate access sites (List separately in addition to code for primary procedure)

(Use 36476 in conjunction with 36475)

(Do not report 36475, 36476 in conjunction with 29581, 29582, 36000, 36002, 36005, 36410, 36425, 36478, 36479, 37241-37244, 75894, 76000, 76001, 76937, 76942, 76998, 77022, 93970, 93971 in the same surgical field)

36478 Endovenous ablation therapy of incompetent vein, extremity, inclusive of all imaging guidance and monitoring, percutaneous, laser; first vein treated

+ 36479 second and subsequent veins treated in a single extremity, each through separate access sites (List separately in addition to code for primary procedure)

(Use 36479 in conjunction with 36478)

(Do not report 36478, 36479 in conjunction with 29581, 29582, 36000, 36002, 36005, 36410, 36425, 36475, 36476, 37241, 75894, 76000, 76001, 76937, 76942, 76998, 77022, 93970, 93971 in the same surgical field)

⊙ **36481** Percutaneous portal vein catheterization by any method

(For radiological supervision and interpretation, see 75885, 75887)

36500 Venous catheterization for selective organ blood sampling

(For catheterization in superior or inferior vena cava, use 36010)

(For radiological supervision and interpretation, use 75893)

36510 Catheterization of umbilical vein for diagnosis or therapy, newborn

(Do not report modifier 63 in conjunction with 36510)

36511 Therapeutic apheresis; for white blood cells

36512 for red blood cells

36513 for platelets

36514 for plasma pheresis

36515 with extracorporeal immunoadsorption and plasma reinfusion

36516 with extracorporeal selective adsorption or selective filtration and plasma reinfusion

(For professional evaluation, use modifier 26)

36522 Photopheresis, extracorporeal

Central Venous Access Procedures

To qualify as a central venous access catheter or device, the tip of the catheter/device must terminate in the subclavian, brachiocephalic (innominate) or iliac veins, the superior or inferior vena cava, or the right atrium. The venous access device may be either centrally inserted (jugular, subclavian, femoral vein or inferior vena cava catheter entry site) or peripherally inserted (eg, basilic or cephalic vein). The device may be accessed for use either via exposed catheter (external to the skin), via a subcutaneous port or via a subcutaneous pump.

The procedures involving these types of devices fall into five categories:

1. *Insertion* (placement of catheter through a newly established venous access)

2. *Repair* (fixing device without replacement of either catheter or port/pump, other than pharmacologic or mechanical correction of intracatheter or pericatheter occlusion [see 36595 or 36596])

3. *Partial replacement* of only the catheter component associated with a port/pump device, but not entire device

4. *Complete replacement* of entire device via same venous access site (complete exchange)

5. *Removal* of entire device.

There is no coding distinction between venous access achieved percutaneously versus by cutdown or based on catheter size.

For the repair, partial (catheter only) replacement, complete replacement, or removal of both catheters (placed from separate venous access sites) of a multi-catheter device, with or without subcutaneous ports/ pumps, use the appropriate code describing the service with a frequency of two.

If an existing central venous access device is removed and a new one placed via a separate venous access site, appropriate codes for both procedures (removal of old, if code exists, and insertion of new device) should be reported.

When imaging is used for these procedures, either for gaining access to the venous entry site or for manipulating the catheter into final central position, use 76937, 77001.

(For refilling and maintenance of an implantable pump or reservoir for intravenous or intra-arterial drug delivery, use 96522)

Insertion of Central Venous Access Device

⊙ **36555**   Insertion of non-tunneled centrally inserted central venous catheter; younger than 5 years of age

(For peripherally inserted non-tunneled central venous catheter, younger than 5 years of age, use 36568)

36556   age 5 years or older

(For peripherally inserted non-tunneled central venous catheter, age 5 years or older, use 36569)

⊙ **36557**   Insertion of tunneled centrally inserted central venous catheter, without subcutaneous port or pump; younger than 5 years of age

⊙ **36558**   age 5 years or older

(For peripherally inserted central venous catheter with port, 5 years or older, use 36571)

⊙ **36560**   Insertion of tunneled centrally inserted central venous access device, with subcutaneous port; younger than 5 years of age

(For peripherally inserted central venous access device with subcutaneous port, younger than 5 years of age, use 36570)

⊙ **36561**   age 5 years or older

(For peripherally inserted central venous catheter with subcutaneous port, 5 years or older, use 36571)

⊙ **36563**   Insertion of tunneled centrally inserted central venous access device with subcutaneous pump

⊙ **36565**   Insertion of tunneled centrally inserted central venous access device, requiring 2 catheters via 2 separate venous access sites; without subcutaneous port or pump (eg, Tesio type catheter)

⊙ **36566**   with subcutaneous port(s)

⊙ **36568**   Insertion of peripherally inserted central venous catheter (PICC), without subcutaneous port or pump; younger than 5 years of age

(For placement of centrally inserted non-tunneled central venous catheter, without subcutaneous port or pump, younger than 5 years of age, use 36555)

36569   age 5 years or older

(For placement of centrally inserted non-tunneled central venous catheter, without subcutaneous port or pump, age 5 years or older, use 36556)

⊙ **36570**   Insertion of peripherally inserted central venous access device, with subcutaneous port; younger than 5 years of age

(For insertion of tunneled centrally inserted central venous access device with subcutaneous port, younger than 5 years of age, use 36560)

⊙ **36571**   age 5 years or older

(For insertion of tunneled centrally inserted central venous access device with subcutaneous port, age 5 years or older, use 36561)

Repair of Central Venous Access Device

(For mechanical removal of pericatheter obstructive material, use 36595)

(For mechanical removal of intracatheter obstructive material, use 36596)

36575   Repair of tunneled or non-tunneled central venous access catheter, without subcutaneous port or pump, central or peripheral insertion site

⊙ **36576**   Repair of central venous access device, with subcutaneous port or pump, central or peripheral insertion site

Partial Replacement of Central Venous Access Device (Catheter Only)

⊙ **36578**   Replacement, catheter only, of central venous access device, with subcutaneous port or pump, central or peripheral insertion site

(For complete replacement of entire device through same venous access, use 36582 or 36583)

The Central Venous Access Procedures Table

	Non-tunneled	Tunneled Without Port or Pump	Central Tunneled	Tunneled With Port	Tunneled With Pump	Peripheral	<5 years	≥5 years	Any Age
Insertion									
Catheter	36555						36555		
	36556							36556	
		36557	36557				36557		
		36558	36558					36558	
	36568 (w/o port or pump)					36568 (w/o port or pump)	36568 (w/o port or pump)		
	36569 (w/o port or pump)					36569 (w/o port or pump)		36569 (w/o port or pump)	
Device			36560	36560			36560		
			36561	36561				36561	
			36563		36563				36563
		36565	36565						36565
			36566	36566					
	36570 (w port)			36570 (w port)		36570 (w port)	36570 (w port)		
	36571 (w port)			36571 (w port)		36571 (w port)		36571 (w port)	
Repair									
Catheter	36575 (w/o port or pump)	36575 (w/o port or pump)	36575 (w/o port or pump)			36575 (w/o port or pump)			36575
Device	36576 (w port or pump)					36576 (w port or pump)			36576
Partial Replacement - Central Venous Access Device (Catheter only)									
			36578	36578	36578	36578			36578
Complete Replacement - Central Venous Access Device (Through Same Venous Access Site)									
Catheter	36580 (w/o port or pump)								36580
		36581	36581						36581
	36584 (w/o port or pump)					36584 (w/o port or pump)			36584
Device			36582	36582					36582
			36583		36583				36583
				36585 (w port)		36585 (w port)			36585
Removal									
Catheter		36589							36589
Device			36590	36590	36590	36590			36590
Removal of Obstructive Material from Device									
	36595 (pericatheter)	36595 (pericatheter)	36595 (pericatheter)	36595 (pericatheter)	36595 (pericatheter)	36595 (pericatheter)			36595 (pericatheter)
	36596 (intraluminal)	36596 (intraluminal)	36596 (intraluminal)	36596 (intraluminal)	36596 (intraluminal)	36596 (intraluminal)			36596 (intraluminal)
Repositioning of Catheter									
	36597	36597	36597	36597	36597	36597	36597	36597	36597

⊙=Moderate sedation   ✚=Add-on code   ✗=FDA approval pending   #=Resequenced code   ○=Recycled/reinstated code

Complete Replacement of Central Venous Access Device Through Same Venous Access Site

36580   Replacement, complete, of a non-tunneled centrally inserted central venous catheter, without subcutaneous port or pump, through same venous access

⊙ **36581**   Replacement, complete, of a tunneled centrally inserted central venous catheter, without subcutaneous port or pump, through same venous access

⊙ **36582**   Replacement, complete, of a tunneled centrally inserted central venous access device, with subcutaneous port, through same venous access

⊙ **36583**   Replacement, complete, of a tunneled centrally inserted central venous access device, with subcutaneous pump, through same venous access

36584   Replacement, complete, of a peripherally inserted central venous catheter (PICC), without subcutaneous port or pump, through same venous access

⊙ **36585**   Replacement, complete, of a peripherally inserted central venous access device, with subcutaneous port, through same venous access

Removal of Central Venous Access Device

36589   Removal of tunneled central venous catheter, without subcutaneous port or pump

⊙ **36590**   Removal of tunneled central venous access device, with subcutaneous port or pump, central or peripheral insertion

(Do not report 36589 or 36590 for removal of non-tunneled central venous catheters)

Other Central Venous Access Procedures

36591   Collection of blood specimen from a completely implantable venous access device

(Do not report 36591 in conjunction with other services except a laboratory service)

(For collection of venous blood specimen by venipuncture, use 36415)

(For collection of capillary blood specimen, use 36416)

36592   Collection of blood specimen using established central or peripheral catheter, venous, not otherwise specified

(For blood collection from an established arterial catheter, use 37799)

(Do not report 36592 in conjunction with other services except a laboratory service)

36593   Declotting by thrombolytic agent of implanted vascular access device or catheter

36595   Mechanical removal of pericatheter obstructive material (eg, fibrin sheath) from central venous device via separate venous access

(Do not report 36595 in conjunction with 36593)

(For venous catheterization, see 36010-36012)

(For radiological supervision and interpretation, use 75901)

36596   Mechanical removal of intraluminal (intracatheter) obstructive material from central venous device through device lumen

(Do not report 36596 in conjunction with 36593)

(For venous catheterization, see 36010-36012)

(For radiological supervision and interpretation, use 75902)

36597   Repositioning of previously placed central venous catheter under fluoroscopic guidance

(For fluoroscopic guidance, use 76000)

36598   Contrast injection(s) for radiologic evaluation of existing central venous access device, including fluoroscopy, image documentation and report

(Do not report 36598 in conjunction with 76000)

(Do not report 36598 in conjunction with 36595, 36596)

(For complete diagnostic studies, see 75820, 75825, 75827)

Arterial

36600   Arterial puncture, withdrawal of blood for diagnosis

⊘ **36620**   Arterial catheterization or cannulation for sampling, monitoring or transfusion (separate procedure); percutaneous

36625   cutdown

36640   Arterial catheterization for prolonged infusion therapy (chemotherapy), cutdown

(See also 96420-96425)

(For arterial catheterization for occlusion therapy, see 75894)

36660   Catheterization, umbilical artery, newborn, for diagnosis or therapy

(Do not report modifier 63 in conjunction with 36660)

Intraosseous

36680   Placement of needle for intraosseous infusion

Cardiovascular

Hemodialysis Access, Intervascular Cannulation for Extracorporeal Circulation, or Shunt Insertion

36800 Insertion of cannula for hemodialysis, other purpose (separate procedure); vein to vein

36810 arteriovenous, external (Scribner type)

36815 arteriovenous, external revision, or closure

36818 Arteriovenous anastomosis, open; by upper arm cephalic vein transposition

(Do not report 36818 in conjunction with 36819, 36820, 36821, 36830 during a unilateral upper extremity procedure. For bilateral upper extremity open arteriovenous anastomoses performed at the same operative session, use modifier 50 or 59 as appropriate)

36819 by upper arm basilic vein transposition

(Do not report 36819 in conjunction with 36818, 36820, 36821, 36830 during a unilateral upper extremity procedure. For bilateral upper extremity open arteriovenous anastomoses performed at the same operative session, use modifier 50 or 59 as appropriate)

36820 by forearm vein transposition

36821 direct, any site (eg, Cimino type) (separate procedure)

(36822 has been deleted. To report, see 33951, 33952, 33953, 33954, 33955, 33956)

36823 Insertion of arterial and venous cannula(s) for isolated extracorporeal circulation including regional chemotherapy perfusion to an extremity, with or without hyperthermia, with removal of cannula(s) and repair of arteriotomy and venotomy sites

(36823 includes chemotherapy perfusion supported by a membrane oxygenator/perfusion pump. Do not report 96409-96425 in conjunction with 36823)

36825 Creation of arteriovenous fistula by other than direct arteriovenous anastomosis (separate procedure); autogenous graft

(For direct arteriovenous anastomosis, use 36821)

36830 nonautogenous graft (eg, biological collagen, thermoplastic graft)

(For direct arteriovenous anastomosis, use 36821)

36831 Thrombectomy, open, arteriovenous fistula without revision, autogenous or nonautogenous dialysis graft (separate procedure)

36832 Revision, open, arteriovenous fistula; without thrombectomy, autogenous or nonautogenous dialysis graft (separate procedure)

36833 with thrombectomy, autogenous or nonautogenous dialysis graft (separate procedure)

36835 Insertion of Thomas shunt (separate procedure)

36838 Distal revascularization and interval ligation (DRIL), upper extremity hemodialysis access (steal syndrome)

(Do not report 36838 in conjunction with 35512, 35522, 35523, 36832, 37607, 37618)

36860 External cannula declotting (separate procedure); without balloon catheter

36861 with balloon catheter

(If imaging guidance is performed, use 76000)

⊙ **36870** Thrombectomy, percutaneous, arteriovenous fistula, autogenous or nonautogenous graft (includes mechanical thrombus extraction and intra-graft thrombolysis)

(Do not report 36870 in conjunction with 36593)

(For catheterization, see 36147, 36148)

(For radiological supervision and interpretation, see 36147, 75791)

Portal Decompression Procedures

37140 Venous anastomosis, open; portocaval

(For peritoneal-venous shunt, use 49425)

37145 renoportal

37160 caval-mesenteric

37180 splenorenal, proximal

37181 splenorenal, distal (selective decompression of esophagogastric varices, any technique)

(For percutaneous procedure, use 37182)

37182 Insertion of transvenous intrahepatic portosystemic shunt(s) (TIPS) (includes venous access, hepatic and portal vein catheterization, portography with hemodynamic evaluation, intrahepatic tract formation/dilatation, stent placement and all associated imaging guidance and documentation)

(Do not report 75885 or 75887 in conjunction with 37182)

(For open procedure, use 37140)

⊙ **37183** Revision of transvenous intrahepatic portosystemic shunt(s) (TIPS) (includes venous access, hepatic and portal vein catheterization, portography with hemodynamic evaluation, intrahepatic tract recanulization/dilatation, stent placement and all associated imaging guidance and documentation)

(Do not report 75885 or 75887 in conjunction with 37183)

(For repair of arteriovenous aneurysm, use 36832)

Transcatheter Procedures

Codes for catheter placement and the radiologic supervision and interpretation should also be reported, in addition to the code(s) for the therapeutic aspect of the procedure.

Mechanical Thrombectomy

Code(s) for catheter placement(s), diagnostic studies, and other percutaneous interventions (eg, transluminal balloon angioplasty, stent placement) provided are separately reportable.

Codes 37184-37188 specifically include intraprocedural fluoroscopic radiological supervision and interpretation services for guidance of the procedure.

Intraprocedural injection(s) of a thrombolytic agent is an included service and not separately reportable in conjunction with mechanical thrombectomy. However, subsequent or prior continuous infusion of a thrombolytic is not an included service and is separately reportable (see 37211-37214).

For coronary mechanical thrombectomy, use 92973.

►For intracranial arterial mechanical thrombectomy, use 61645.◄

For mechanical thrombectomy for dialysis fistula, use 36870.

Transcatheter Thrombolytic Infusion

Codes 37211 or 37212 are used to report the initial day of transcatheter thrombolytic infusion(s) including follow-up arteriography/venography, and catheter position change or exchange, when performed. To report bilateral thrombolytic infusion through a separate access site(s), use modifier 50 in conjunction with 37211, 37212. Code 37213 is used to report continued transcatheter thrombolytic infusion(s) on subsequent day(s), other than initial day and final day of treatment. Code 37214 is used to report final day of transcatheter thrombolytic infusion(s). When initiation and completion of thrombolysis occur on the same day, report only 37211 or 37212.

Code(s) for catheter placement(s), diagnostic studies, and other percutaneous interventions (eg, transluminal balloon angioplasty, stent placement) provided may be separately reportable.

Codes 37211-37214 include fluoroscopic guidance and associated radiological supervision and interpretation.

Ongoing evaluation and management services on the day of the procedure related to thrombolysis are included in 37211-37214. If a significant, separately identifiable E/M service is performed by the same physician on the same day of the procedure, report the appropriate level of E/M service and append modifier 25.

Ultrasound guidance for vascular access is not included in 37211-37214. Code 76937 may be reported separately when performed if all the required elements are performed.

►For intracranial arterial mechanical thrombectomy and/or infusion for thrombolysis, use 61645.◄

Arterial Mechanical Thrombectomy

Arterial mechanical thrombectomy may be performed as a "primary" transcatheter procedure with pretreatment planning, performance of the procedure, and postprocedure evaluation focused on providing this service. Typically, the diagnosis of thrombus has been made prior to the procedure, and a mechanical thrombectomy is planned preoperatively. Primary mechanical thrombectomy is reported per vascular family using 37184 for the initial vessel treated and 37185 for second or all subsequent vessel(s) within the same vascular family. To report mechanical thrombectomy of an additional vascular family treated through a separate access site, use modifier 51 in conjunction with 37184-37185.

Primary mechanical thrombectomy may precede or follow another percutaneous intervention. Most commonly primary mechanical thrombectomy will precede another percutaneous intervention with the decision regarding the need for other services not made until after mechanical thrombectomy has been performed. Occasionally, the performance of primary mechanical thrombectomy may follow another percutaneous intervention.

Do **NOT** report 37184-37185 for mechanical thrombectomy performed for the retrieval of short segments of thrombus or embolus evident during other percutaneous interventional procedures. See 37186 for these procedures.

Arterial mechanical thrombectomy is considered a "secondary" transcatheter procedure for removal or retrieval of short segments of thrombus or embolus when performed either before or after another percutaneous intervention (eg, percutaneous transluminal balloon angioplasty, stent placement). Secondary mechanical thrombectomy is reported using 37186. Do **NOT** report 37186 in conjunction with 37184-37185.

Venous Mechanical Thrombectomy

Use 37187 to report the initial application of venous mechanical thrombectomy. To report bilateral venous mechanical thrombectomy performed through a separate access site(s), use modifier 50 in conjunction with 37187. For repeat treatment on a subsequent day during a course of thrombolytic therapy, use 37188.

Arterial Mechanical Thrombectomy

⊙▲ **37184**   Primary percutaneous transluminal mechanical thrombectomy, noncoronary, non-intracranial, arterial or arterial bypass graft, including fluoroscopic guidance and intraprocedural pharmacological thrombolytic injection(s); initial vessel

►(Do not report 37184 in conjunction with 61645, 76000, 76001, 96374, 99143-99150)◄

Cardiovascular

Cardiovascular

⊙+▲ **37185**   second and all subsequent vessel(s) within the same vascular family (List separately in addition to code for primary mechanical thrombectomy procedure)

(Do not report 37185 in conjunction with 76000, 76001, 96375)

▶(Do not report 37185 in conjunction with 61645 for treatment of the same vascular territory. See Nervous System Endovascular Therapy)◀

⊙+▲ **37186**   Secondary percutaneous transluminal thrombectomy (eg, nonprimary mechanical, snare basket, suction technique), noncoronary, non-intracranial, arterial or arterial bypass graft, including fluoroscopic guidance and intraprocedural pharmacological thrombolytic injections, provided in conjunction with another percutaneous intervention other than primary mechanical thrombectomy (List separately in addition to code for primary procedure)

(Do not report 37186 in conjunction with 76000, 76001, 96375)

▶(Do not report 37186 in conjunction with 61645 for treatment of the same vascular territory. See Nervous System Endovascular Therapy)◀

Venous Mechanical Thrombectomy

⊙ **37187**   Percutaneous transluminal mechanical thrombectomy, vein(s), including intraprocedural pharmacological thrombolytic injections and fluoroscopic guidance

(Do not report 37187 in conjunction with 76000, 76001, 96375)

⊙ **37188**   Percutaneous transluminal mechanical thrombectomy, vein(s), including intraprocedural pharmacological thrombolytic injections and fluoroscopic guidance, repeat treatment on subsequent day during course of thrombolytic therapy

(Do not report 37188 in conjunction with 76000, 76001, 96375)

Other Procedures

⊙ **37191**   Insertion of intravascular vena cava filter, endovascular approach including vascular access, vessel selection, and radiological supervision and interpretation, intraprocedural roadmapping, and imaging guidance (ultrasound and fluoroscopy), when performed

(For open surgical interruption of the inferior vena cava through a laparotomy or retroperitoneal exposure, use 37619)

⊙ **37192**   Repositioning of intravascular vena cava filter, endovascular approach including vascular access, vessel selection, and radiological supervision and interpretation, intraprocedural roadmapping, and imaging guidance (ultrasound and fluoroscopy), when performed

(Do not report 37192 in conjunction with 37191)

⊙ **37193**   Retrieval (removal) of intravascular vena cava filter, endovascular approach including vascular access, vessel selection, and radiological supervision and interpretation, intraprocedural roadmapping, and imaging guidance (ultrasound and fluoroscopy), when performed

(Do not report 37193 in conjunction with 37197)

37195   Thrombolysis, cerebral, by intravenous infusion

⊙ **37197**   Transcatheter retrieval, percutaneous, of intravascular foreign body (eg, fractured venous or arterial catheter), includes radiological supervision and interpretation, and imaging guidance (ultrasound or fluoroscopy), when performed

(For percutaneous retrieval of a vena cava filter, use 37193)

▶(For transcatheter removal of permanent leadless pacemaker, use 0388T)◀

37200   Transcatheter biopsy

(For radiological supervision and interpretation, use 75970)

(37201 has been deleted. To report see 37211-37214)

#⊙▲ **37211**   Transcatheter therapy, arterial infusion for thrombolysis other than coronary or intracranial, any method, including radiological supervision and interpretation, initial treatment day

▶(For intracranial arterial mechanical thrombectomy and/or infusion for thrombolysis, use 61645)◀

#⊙ **37212**   Transcatheter therapy, venous infusion for thrombolysis, any method, including radiological supervision and interpretation, initial treatment day

#⊙ **37213**   Transcatheter therapy, arterial or venous infusion for thrombolysis other than coronary, any method, including radiological supervision and interpretation, continued treatment on subsequent day during course of thrombolytic therapy, including follow-up catheter contrast injection, position change, or exchange, when performed;

#⊙ **37214**   cessation of thrombolysis including removal of catheter and vessel closure by any method

(Report 37211-37214 once per date of treatment)

(For declotting by thrombolytic agent of implanted vascular access device or catheter, use 36593)

(Do not report 37211-37214 in conjunction with 75898)

▶(37202 has been deleted. For intracranial arterial administration of pharmacological agent[s] other than for thrombolysis, see 61650, 61651)◀

37211   Code is out of numerical sequence. See 37191-37216

37212   Code is out of numerical sequence. See 37191-37216

37213   Code is out of numerical sequence. See 37191-37216

37214   Code is out of numerical sequence. See 37191-37216

⊙=Moderate sedation   ✚=Add-on code   ✗=FDA approval pending   #=Resequenced code   ○=Recycled/reinstated code

⊙ **37215**   Transcatheter placement of intravascular stent(s), cervical carotid artery, open or percutaneous, including angioplasty, when performed, and radiological supervision and interpretation; with distal embolic protection

⊙ **37216**   without distal embolic protection

(37215 and 37216 include all ipsilateral selective carotid catheterization, all diagnostic imaging for ipsilateral, cervical and cerebral carotid arteriography, and all related radiological supervision and interpretation. When ipsilateral carotid arteriogram (including imaging and selective catheterization) confirms the need for carotid stenting, 37215 and 37216 are inclusive of these services. If carotid stenting is not indicated, then the appropriate codes for carotid catheterization and imaging should be reported in lieu of 37215 and 37216)

(Do not report 37215, 37216 in conjunction with 36222-36224 for the treated carotid artery)

(For open or percutaneous transcatheter placement of extracranial vertebral artery stent[s], see Category III codes 0075T, 0076T)

37217   Transcatheter placement of intravascular stent(s), intrathoracic common carotid artery or innominate artery by retrograde treatment, open ipsilateral cervical carotid artery exposure, including angioplasty, when performed, and radiological supervision and interpretation

(37217 includes open vessel exposure and vascular access closure, all access and selective catheterization of the vessel, traversing the lesion, and any radiological supervision and interpretation directly related to the intervention when performed, standard closure of arteriotomy by suture, and imaging performed to document completion of the intervention in addition to the intervention[s] performed. Carotid artery revascularization services [eg, 33891, 35301, 35509, 35510, 35601, 35606] performed during the same session may be reported separately, when performed)

(Do not report 37217 in conjunction with 35201, 35458, 36221-36227, 75962 for ipsilateral services)

(For open or percutaneous transcatheter placement of intravascular cervical carotid artery stent[s], see 37215, 37216)

(For open or percutaneous antegrade transcatheter placement of innominate and/or intrathoracic carotid artery stent[s], use 37218)

(For open or percutaneous transcatheter placement of extracranial vertebral artery stent[s], see 0075T, 0076T)

(For transcatheter placement of intracranial stent[s], use 61635)

⊙ **37218**   Transcatheter placement of intravascular stent(s), intrathoracic common carotid artery or innominate artery, open or percutaneous antegrade approach, including angioplasty, when performed, and radiological supervision and interpretation

(37218 includes all ipsilateral extracranial intrathoracic selective innominate and carotid catheterization, all diagnostic imaging for ipsilateral extracranial intrathoracic innominate and/or carotid artery stenting, and all related radiologic supervision and interpretation. Report 37218 when the ipsilateral extracranial intrathoracic carotid arteriogram (including imaging and selective catheterization) confirms the need for stenting. If stenting is not indicated, report the appropriate codes for selective catheterization and imaging)

(Do not report 37218 in conjunction with 36222, 36223, 36224 for the treated carotid artery)

(For open or percutaneous transcatheter placement of intravascular cervical carotid artery stent[s], see 37215, 37216)

(For open or percutaneous transcatheter placement of extracranial vertebral artery stent[s], see 0075T, 0076T)

(For transcatheter placement of intracranial stent[s], use 61635)

Endovascular Revascularization (Open or Percutaneous, Transcatheter)

Codes 37220-37235 are to be used to describe lower extremity endovascular revascularization services performed for occlusive disease. These lower extremity codes are built on progressive hierarchies with more intensive services inclusive of lesser intensive services. The code inclusive of all of the services provided for that vessel should be reported (ie, use the code inclusive of the most intensive services provided). Only one code from this family (37220-37235) should be reported for each lower extremity vessel treated.

These lower extremity endovascular revascularization codes all include the work of accessing and selectively catheterizing the vessel, traversing the lesion, radiological supervision and interpretation directly related to the intervention(s) performed, embolic protection if used, closure of the arteriotomy by pressure and application of an arterial closure device or standard closure of the puncture by suture, and imaging performed to document completion of the intervention in addition to the intervention(s) performed. Extensive repair or replacement of an artery may be additionally reported (eg, 35226 or 35286). These codes describe endovascular procedures performed percutaneously and/or through an open surgical exposure. These codes include balloon angioplasty (eg, low-profile, cutting balloon, cryoplasty), atherectomy (eg, directional, rotational, laser), and stenting (eg, balloon-expandable, self-expanding, bare metal, covered, drug-eluting). Each code in this family (37220-37235) includes balloon angioplasty, when performed.

Cardiovascular

These codes describe revascularization therapies (ie, transluminal angioplasty, atherectomy, and stent placement) provided in three arterial vascular territories: iliac, femoral/popliteal, and tibial/peroneal.

When treating multiple vessels within a territory, report each additional vessel using an add-on code, as applicable. Select the base code that represents the most complex service using the following hierarchy of complexity (in descending order of complexity): atherectomy and stent> atherectomy>stent>angioplasty. When treating multiple lesions within the same vessel, report one service that reflects the combined procedures, whether done on one lesion or different lesions, using the same hierarchy.

1. *Iliac Vascular Territory*—The iliac territory is divided into 3 vessels: common iliac, internal iliac, and external iliac.

2. *Femoral/Popliteal Vascular Territory*—The entire femoral/popliteal territory in 1 lower extremity is considered a single vessel for CPT reporting specifically for the endovascular lower extremity revascularization codes 37224-37227.

3. *Tibial/Peroneal Territory*—The tibial/peroneal territory is divided into 3 vessels: anterior tibial, posterior tibial, and peroneal arteries.

There are specific coding guidelines for each of the 3 vascular territories.

1. *Iliac Vascular Territory*—A single primary code is used for the initial iliac artery treated in each leg (37220 or 37221). If other iliac vessels are also treated in that leg, these interventions are reported with the appropriate add-on code(s) (37222, 37223). Up to 2 add-on codes can be used in a unilateral iliac vascular territory since there are 3 vessels which could be treated. Add-on codes are used for different vessels, not distinct lesions within the same vessel.

2. *Femoral/Popliteal Territory*—A single interventional code is used no matter what combination of angioplasty/stent/atherectomy is applied to all segments, including the common, deep and superficial femoral arteries as well as the popliteal artery (37224, 37225, 37226, or 37227). There are no add-on codes for additional vessels treated within the femoral/popliteal territory. Because only 1 service is reported when 2 lesions are treated in this territory, report the most complex service (eg, use 37227 if a stent is placed for 1 lesion and an atherectomy is performed on a second lesion)

3. *Tibial/Peroneal Territory*—A single primary code is used for the initial tibial/peroneal artery treated in each leg (37228, 37229, 37230, or 37231). If other tibial/peroneal vessels are also treated in the same leg, these interventions are reported with the appropriate add-on code(s) (37232-37235). Up to 2 add-on codes could be used to describe services provided in a single leg since there are 3 tibial/peroneal vessels which could be treated. Add-on codes are used for different vessels, not distinct lesions within the same vessel. The common tibio-peroneal trunk is considered part of the tibial/peroneal territory, but is not considered a separate, fourth segment of vessel in the tibio-peroneal family for CPT reporting of endovascular lower extremity interventions. For instance, if lesions in the common tibio-peroneal trunk are treated in conjunction with lesions in the posterior tibial artery, a single code would be reported for treatment of this segment.

When treating multiple territories in the same leg, one primary lower extremity revascularization code is used for each territory treated. When second or third vessel(s) are treated in the iliac and/or tibial/peroneal territories, add-on code(s) are used to report the additional service(s). When more than one stent is placed in the same vessel, the code should be reported only once.

When multiple vessels in multiple territories in a single leg are treated at the same setting, the primary code for the treatment in the initial vessel in each vascular territory is reported. Add-on code(s) are reported when second and third iliac or tibial/peroneal arteries are treated in addition to the initial vessel in that vascular territory.

If a lesion extends across the margins of one vessel vascular territory into another, but can be opened with a single therapy, this intervention should be reported with a single code despite treating more than one vessel and/or vascular territory. For instance, if a stenosis extends from the common iliac artery into the proximal external iliac artery, and a single stent is placed to open the entire lesion, this therapy should be coded as a single stent placement in the iliac artery (37221). In this example, a code for an additional vessel treatment would not be used (do not report both 37221 and 37223).

For bifurcation lesions distal to the common iliac origins which require therapy of 2 distinct branches of the iliac or tibial/peroneal vascular territories, a primary code and an add-on code would be used to describe the intervention. In the femoral/popliteal territory, all branches are included in the primary code, so treatment of a bifurcation lesion would be reported as a single code.

When the same territor(ies) of both legs are treated in the same session, modifiers may be required to describe the interventions. Use modifier 59 to denote that different legs are being treated, even if the mode of therapy is different.

Mechanical thrombectomy and/or thrombolysis in the lower extremity vessels are sometimes necessary to aid in restoring flow to areas of occlusive disease, and are reported separately.

⊙ **37220** Revascularization, endovascular, open or percutaneous, iliac artery, unilateral, initial vessel; with transluminal angioplasty

⊙ **37221** with transluminal stent placement(s), includes angioplasty within the same vessel, when performed

(Use 37220, 37221 in conjunction with 34802-34805, 34825, 34826, 34845-34848, 34900, 0254T only when 37220 or 37221 are performed outside the target treatment zone of the endoprosthesis)

⊙+ **37222** Revascularization, endovascular, open or percutaneous, iliac artery, each additional ipsilateral iliac vessel; with transluminal angioplasty (List separately in addition to code for primary procedure)

(Use 37222 in conjunction with 37220, 37221)

⊙+ **37223** with transluminal stent placement(s), includes angioplasty within the same vessel, when performed (List separately in addition to code for primary procedure)

(Use 37223 in conjunction with 37221)

(Use 37222, 37223 in conjunction with 34802-34805, 34825, 34826, 34845-34848, 34900, 0254T only when 37222 or 37223 are performed outside the target treatment zone of the endoprosthesis)

⊙ **37224** Revascularization, endovascular, open or percutaneous, femoral, popliteal artery(s), unilateral; with transluminal angioplasty

⊙ **37225** with atherectomy, includes angioplasty within the same vessel, when performed

⊙ **37226** with transluminal stent placement(s), includes angioplasty within the same vessel, when performed

⊙ **37227** with transluminal stent placement(s) and atherectomy, includes angioplasty within the same vessel, when performed

⊙ **37228** Revascularization, endovascular, open or percutaneous, tibial, peroneal artery, unilateral, initial vessel; with transluminal angioplasty

⊙ **37229** with atherectomy, includes angioplasty within the same vessel, when performed

⊙ **37230** with transluminal stent placement(s), includes angioplasty within the same vessel, when performed

⊙ **37231** with transluminal stent placement(s) and atherectomy, includes angioplasty within the same vessel, when performed

⊙+ **37232** Revascularization, endovascular, open or percutaneous, tibial/peroneal artery, unilateral, each additional vessel; with transluminal angioplasty (List separately in addition to code for primary procedure)

(Use 37232 in conjunction with 37228-37231)

⊙+ **37233** with atherectomy, includes angioplasty within the same vessel, when performed (List separately in addition to code for primary procedure)

(Use 37233 in conjunction with 37229, 37231)

⊙+ **37234** with transluminal stent placement(s), includes angioplasty within the same vessel, when performed (List separately in addition to code for primary procedure)

(Use 37234 in conjunction with 37229, 37230, 37231)

⊙+ **37235** with transluminal stent placement(s) and atherectomy, includes angioplasty within the same vessel, when performed (List separately in addition to code for primary procedure)

(Use 37235 in conjunction with 37231)

Codes 37236-37239 are used to report endovascular revascularization for vessels other than lower extremity artery(s) for occlusive disease (ie, 37221, 37223, 37226, 37227, 37230, 37231, 37234, 37235), cervical carotid (ie, 37215, 37216), intracranial (ie, 61635), intracoronary (ie, 92928, 92929, 92933, 92934, 92937, 92938, 92941, 92943, 92944), innominate and/or intrathoracic carotid artery through an antegrade approach (37218), extracranial vertebral (ie, 0075T, 0076T) performed percutaneously and/or through an open surgical exposure, or open retrograde intrathoracic common carotid or innominate (37217).

Codes 37236, 37237 describe transluminal intravascular stent insertion in an artery while 37238, 37239 describe transluminal intravascular stent insertion in a vein. Multiple stents placed in a single vessel may only be reported with a single code. If a lesion extends across the margins of one vessel into another, but can be treated with a single therapy, the intervention should be reported only once. When additional, different vessels are treated in the same session, report 37237 and/or 37239 as appropriate. Each code in this family (37236-37239) includes any and all balloon angioplasty(s) performed in the treated vessel, including any pre-dilation (whether performed as a primary or secondary angioplasty), post-dilation following stent placement, treatment of a lesion outside the stented segment but in the same vessel, or use of larger/smaller balloon to achieve therapeutic result. Angioplasty in a separate and distinct vessel may be reported separately. Non-selective and/or selective catheterization(s) (eg, 36005, 36010-36015, 36200, 36215-36218, 36245-36248) is reported separately.

►Codes 37236-37239 include radiological supervision and interpretation directly related to the intervention(s) performed, closure of the arteriotomy by pressure, application of an arterial closure device or standard closure of the puncture by suture, and imaging performed to document completion of the intervention in addition to the intervention(s) performed. Extensive repair or replacement of an artery may be reported separately (eg, 35226 or 35286). Report 76937 for ultrasound guidance for vascular access, when performed in conjunction with 37236-37239. Intravascular ultrasound may be reported separately (ie, 37252, 37253). For mechanical thrombectomy and/or thrombolytic therapy, when performed, see 37184-37188, 37211-37214.◄

Cardiovascular

Intravascular stents, both covered and uncovered, are a class of devices that may be used as part of an embolization procedure. As such, there is the potential for overlap among codes used for placement of vascular stents and those used for embolization. When a stent is placed for the purpose of providing a latticework for deployment of embolization coils, such as for embolization of an aneurysm, the embolization code is reported and not the stent code. If a covered stent is deployed as the sole management of an aneurysm, pseudoaneurysm, or vascular extravasation, then the stent deployment code should be reported and not the embolization code.

⊙ **37236** Transcatheter placement of an intravascular stent(s) (except lower extremity artery(s) for occlusive disease, cervical carotid, extracranial vertebral or intrathoracic carotid, intracranial, or coronary), open or percutaneous, including radiological supervision and interpretation and including all angioplasty within the same vessel, when performed; initial artery

⊙+ **37237** each additional artery (List separately in addition to code for primary procedure)

(Use 37237 in conjunction with 37236)

(Do not report 37236, 37237 in conjunction with 34841-34848 for bare metal or covered stents placed into the visceral branches within the endoprosthesis target zone)

(For stent placement(s) in iliac, femoral, popliteal, or tibial/peroneal artery(s) for occlusive disease, see 37221, 37223, 37226, 37227, 37230, 37231, 37234, 37235)

(For transcatheter placement of intravascular cervical carotid artery stent(s), see 37215, 37216)

(For transcatheter placement of intracranial stent(s), use 61635)

(For transcatheter placement of intracoronary stent(s), see 92928, 92929, 92933, 92934, 92937, 92938, 92941, 92943, 92944)

(For stenting of visceral arteries in conjunction with fenestrated endovascular repair, see 34841-34848)

(For open or percutaneous antegrade transcatheter placement of intrathoracic carotid/innominate artery stent(s), use 37218)

(For open or percutaneous transcatheter placement of extracranial vertebral artery stent(s), see Category III codes 0075T, 0076T)

(For open retrograde transcatheter placement of intrathoracic common carotid/innominate artery stent(s), use 37217)

⊙ **37238** Transcatheter placement of an intravascular stent(s), open or percutaneous, including radiological supervision and interpretation and including angioplasty within the same vessel, when performed; initial vein

⊙+ **37239** each additional vein (List separately in addition to code for primary procedure)

(Use 37239 in conjunction with 37238)

Vascular Embolization and Occlusion

Codes 37241-37244 are used to describe the work of vascular embolization and occlusion procedures, excluding the central nervous system and the head and neck, which are reported using 61624, 61626, 61710, and 75894, and excluding the ablation/sclerotherapy procedures for venous insufficiency/telangiectasia of the extremities/skin, which are reported using 36468, 36470, and 36471. Embolization and occlusion procedures are performed for a wide variety of clinical indications and in a range of vascular territories. Arteries, veins, and lymphatics may all be the target of embolization.

The embolization codes include all associated radiological supervision and interpretation, intra-procedural guidance and road-mapping, and imaging necessary to document completion of the procedure. They do not include diagnostic angiography and all necessary catheter placement(s). Code(s) for catheter placement(s) may be separately reported using selective catheter placement code(s), if used consistent with guidelines. Code(s) for diagnostic angiography may also be separately reported, when performed according to guidelines for diagnostic angiography during endovascular procedures, using the appropriate diagnostic angiography codes. Report these services with an appropriate modifier (eg, modifier 59). Please see the guidelines on the reporting of diagnostic angiography preceding 75600 in the **Vascular Procedures, Aorta and Arteries** section.

Code 37241 is used to report vascular embolization or occlusion procedures performed for venous conditions other than hemorrhage. Examples include embolization of venous malformations, capillary hemangiomas, varicoceles, and visceral varices. Embolization of side branch(es) of an outflow vein from a hemodialysis access would be reported using 37241.

Code 37242 is used to report vascular embolization or occlusion performed for arterial conditions other than hemorrhage or tumor such as arteriovenous malformations and arteriovenous fistulas whether congenital or acquired. Embolizations of aneurysms and pseudoaneurysms are also reported with 37242. Tumor embolization is reported with 37243. Note that injection to treat an extremity pseudoaneurysm is correctly reported with 36002. Sometimes, embolization and occlusion of an artery are performed prior to another planned interventional procedure; an example is embolization of the left gastric artery prior to planned implantation of a hepatic artery chemotherapy port. The artery embolization is reported with 37242.

Code 37243 is used to report embolization for the purpose of tissue ablation and organ infarction or ischemia. This can be performed in many clinical circumstances, including embolization of benign or malignant tumors of the liver, kidney, uterus, or other organs. When chemotherapy is given as part of an embolization procedure, additional codes (eg, 96420)

Cardiovascular

may be separately reported. When a radioisotope (eg, Yttrium-90) is injected as part of an embolization, then additional codes (eg, 79445) may be separately reported. Uterine fibroid embolization is reported with 37243.

Code 37244 is used to report embolization for treatment of hemorrhage or vascular or lymphatic extravasation. Examples include embolization for management of gastrointestinal bleed, trauma-induced hemorrhage of the viscera or pelvis, embolization of the thoracic duct for chylous effusion and bronchial artery embolization for hemoptysis. Embolization of the uterine arteries for management of hemorrhage (eg, postpartum hemorrhage) is also reported with 37244.

Intravascular stents, both covered and uncovered, are a class of devices that may be used as part of an embolization procedure. As such, there is the potential for overlap among codes used for placement of vascular stents and those used for embolization. When a stent is placed for the purpose of providing a latticework for deployment of embolization coils, such as for embolization of an aneurysm, the embolization code is reported and not the stent code. If a stent is deployed as the sole management of an aneurysm, pseudoaneurysm, or vascular extravasation, then the stent deployment code should be reported and not the embolization code.

Only one embolization code should be reported for each surgical field (ie, the area immediately surrounding and directly involved in a treatment/procedure). For example, embolization of one or more venous side branches in a single arm for a patient with a dialysis arteriovenous fistula is reported with 37241 only once per session. Embolization procedures performed at a single setting and including multiple surgical fields (eg, a patient with multiple trauma and bleeding from the pelvis and the spleen) may be reported with multiple embolization codes with the appropriate modifier (eg, modifier 59).

There may be overlapping indications for an embolization procedure. The code for the immediate indication for the embolization should be used. For instance, if the immediate cause for embolization is bleeding in a patient with an aneurysm, report 37244.

⊙ **37241**   Vascular embolization or occlusion, inclusive of all radiological supervision and interpretation, intraprocedural roadmapping, and imaging guidance necessary to complete the intervention; venous, other than hemorrhage (eg, congenital or acquired venous malformations, venous and capillary hemangiomas, varices, varicoceles)

(For sclerosis of veins or endovenous ablation of incompetent extremity veins, see 36468-36479)

(Do not report 37241 in conjunction with 36468, 36470, 36471, 36475-36479, 75894, 75898 in the same surgical field)

⊙ **37242**   arterial, other than hemorrhage or tumor (eg, congenital or acquired arterial malformations, arteriovenous malformations, arteriovenous fistulas, aneurysms, pseudoaneurysms)

(For percutaneous treatment of extremity pseudoaneurysm, use 36002)

⊙ **37243**   for tumors, organ ischemia, or infarction

⊙ **37244**   for arterial or venous hemorrhage or lymphatic extravasation

(Do not report 37242-37244 in conjunction with 75894, 75898 in the same surgical field)

(For embolization procedures of the central nervous system or head and neck, see 61624, 61626, 61710)

Intravascular Ultrasound Services

▶Intravascular ultrasound (IVUS) services include all transducer manipulations and repositioning within the specific vessel being examined during a diagnostic procedure or before, during, and/or after therapeutic intervention (eg, stent or stent graft placement, angioplasty, atherectomy, embolization, thrombolysis, transcatheter biopsy).

IVUS is included in the work described by codes 37191, 37192, 37193, 37197 (intravascular vena cava [IVC] filter placement, repositioning and removal, and intravascular foreign body retrieval) and should not be separately reported with those procedures. If a lesion extends across the margins of one vessel into another, this should be reported with a single code despite imaging more than one vessel.

Non-selective and/or selective vascular catheterization may be separately reportable (eg, 36005-36248).◀

▶(37250, 37251 have been deleted. To report noncoronary intravascular ultrasound during diagnostic evaluation and/or therapeutic intervention, see 37252, 37253)◀

⊙+● **37252**   Intravascular ultrasound (noncoronary vessel) during diagnostic evaluation and/or therapeutic intervention, including radiological supervision and interpretation; initial noncoronary vessel (List separately in addition to code for primary procedure)

⊙+● **37253**   each additional noncoronary vessel (List separately in addition to code for primary procedure)

▶(Use 37253 in conjunction with 37252)◀

▶(Do not report 37252, 37253 in conjunction with 37191, 37192, 37193, 37197)◀

Endoscopy

Surgical vascular endoscopy always includes diagnostic endoscopy.

37500   Vascular endoscopy, surgical, with ligation of perforator veins, subfascial (SEPS)

(For open procedure, use 37760)

37501 Unlisted vascular endoscopy procedure

Ligation

(For phleborraphy and arteriorraphy, see 35201-35286)

37565 Ligation, internal jugular vein

37600 Ligation; external carotid artery

37605   internal or common carotid artery

37606   internal or common carotid artery, with gradual occlusion, as with Selverstone or Crutchfield clamp

(For transcatheter permanent arterial occlusion or embolization, see 61624-61626)

(For endovascular temporary arterial balloon occlusion, use 61623)

(For ligation treatment of intracranial aneurysm, use 61703)

37607 Ligation or banding of angioaccess arteriovenous fistula

37609 Ligation or biopsy, temporal artery

37615 Ligation, major artery (eg, post-traumatic, rupture); neck

37616   chest

37617   abdomen

37618   extremity

37619 Ligation of inferior vena cava

(For endovascular delivery of an inferior vena cava filter, use 37191)

37650 Ligation of femoral vein

(For bilateral procedure, report 37650 with modifier 50)

37660 Ligation of common iliac vein

37700 Ligation and division of long saphenous vein at saphenofemoral junction, or distal interruptions

(Do not report 37700 in conjunction with 37718, 37722)

(For bilateral procedure, report 37700 with modifier 50)

37718 Ligation, division, and stripping, short saphenous vein

(For bilateral procedure, use modifier 50)

(Do not report 37718 in conjunction with 37735, 37780)

37722 Ligation, division, and stripping, long (greater) saphenous veins from saphenofemoral junction to knee or below

(For ligation and stripping of the short saphenous vein, use 37718)

(For bilateral procedure, report 37722 with modifier 50)

(Do not report 37722 in conjunction with 37700, 37735)

(For ligation, division, and stripping of the greater saphenous vein, use 37722. For ligation, division, and stripping of the short saphenous vein, use 37718)

37735 Ligation and division and complete stripping of long or short saphenous veins with radical excision of ulcer and skin graft and/or interruption of communicating veins of lower leg, with excision of deep fascia

(Do not report 37735 in conjunction with 37700, 37718, 37722, 37780)

(For bilateral procedure, report 37735 with modifier 50)

37760 Ligation of perforator veins, subfascial, radical (Linton type), including skin graft, when performed, open,1 leg

(For endoscopic procedure, use 37500)

37761 Ligation of perforator vein(s), subfascial, open, including ultrasound guidance, when performed, 1 leg

(For bilateral procedure, report 37761 with modifier 50)

(Do not report 37760, 37761 in conjunction with 76937, 76942, 76998, 93971)

(For endoscopic ligation of subfascial perforator veins, use 37500)

37765 Stab phlebectomy of varicose veins, 1 extremity; 10-20 stab incisions

(For less than 10 incisions, use 37799)

(For more than 20 incisions, use 37766)

37766   more than 20 incisions

37780 Ligation and division of short saphenous vein at saphenopopliteal junction (separate procedure)

(For bilateral procedure, report 37780 with modifier 50)

37785 Ligation, division, and/or excision of varicose vein cluster(s), 1 leg

(For bilateral procedure, report 37785 with modifier 50)

Other Procedures

37788 Penile revascularization, artery, with or without vein graft

37790 Penile venous occlusive procedure

37799 Unlisted procedure, vascular surgery

Hemic and Lymphatic Systems

Spleen

Excision

38100 Splenectomy; total (separate procedure)

38101   partial (separate procedure)

+ 38102   total, en bloc for extensive disease, in conjunction with other procedure (List in addition to code for primary procedure)

⊙ =Moderate sedation   ✚ =Add-on code   ✗ =FDA approval pending   # =Resequenced code   ○ =Recycled/reinstated code

Repair

38115   Repair of ruptured spleen (splenorrhaphy) with or without partial splenectomy

Laparoscopy

Surgical laparoscopy always includes diagnostic laparoscopy. To report a diagnostic laparoscopy (peritoneoscopy) (separate procedure), use 49320.

38120   Laparoscopy, surgical, splenectomy

38129   Unlisted laparoscopy procedure, spleen

Introduction

38200   Injection procedure for splenoportography

(For radiological supervision and interpretation, use 75810)

General

Bone Marrow or Stem Cell Services/Procedures

Codes 38207-38215 describe various steps used to preserve, prepare and purify bone marrow/stem cells prior to transplantation or reinfusion. Each code may be reported only once per day regardless of the quantity of bone marrow/stem cells manipulated.

38204   Management of recipient hematopoietic progenitor cell donor search and cell acquisition

38205   Blood-derived hematopoietic progenitor cell harvesting for transplantation, per collection; allogeneic

38206   autologous

38207   Transplant preparation of hematopoietic progenitor cells; cryopreservation and storage

(For diagnostic cryopreservation and storage, use 88240)

38208   thawing of previously frozen harvest, without washing, per donor

(For diagnostic thawing and expansion of frozen cells, use 88241)

38209   thawing of previously frozen harvest, with washing, per donor

38210   specific cell depletion within harvest, T-cell depletion

38211   tumor cell depletion

38212   red blood cell removal

38213   platelet depletion

38214   plasma (volume) depletion

38215   cell concentration in plasma, mononuclear, or buffy coat layer

(Do not report 38207-38215 in conjunction with 88182, 88184-88189)

38220   Bone marrow; aspiration only

(For needle aspiration of bone marrow for the purpose of bone grafting, use 38220)

(Do not report 38220-38230 for bone marrow aspiration for platelet rich stem cell injection. For bone marrow aspiration for platelet rich stem cell injection, use 0232T)

38221   biopsy, needle or trocar

(For bone marrow biopsy interpretation, use 88305)

38230   Bone marrow harvesting for transplantation; allogeneic

38232   autologous

(For autologous and allogeneic blood-derived peripheral stem cell harvesting for transplantation, see 38205-38206)

(For bone marrow aspiration, use 38220)

Transplantation and Post-Transplantation Cellular Infusions

Hematopoietic cell transplantation (HCT) refers to the infusion of hematopoietic progenitor cells (HPC) obtained from bone marrow, peripheral blood apheresis, and/or umbilical cord blood. These procedure codes (38240-38243) include physician monitoring of multiple physiologic parameters, physician verification of cell processing, evaluation of the patient during as well as immediately before and after the HPC/lymphocyte infusion, physician presence during the HPC/lymphocyte infusion with associated direct physician supervision of clinical staff, and management of uncomplicated adverse events (eg, nausea, urticaria) during the infusion, which is not separately reportable.

HCT may be autologous (when the HPC donor and recipient are the same person) or allogeneic (when the HPC donor and recipient are not the same person). Code 38241 is used to report any autologous transplant while 38240 is used to report an allogeneic transplant. In some cases allogeneic transplants involve more than one donor and cells from each donor are infused sequentially whereby one unit of 38240 is reported for each donor infused. Code 38242 is used to report a donor lymphocyte infusion. Code 38243 is used to report a HPC boost from the original allogeneic HPC donor. A lymphocyte infusion or HPC boost can occur days, months or even years after the initial hematopoietic cell transplant. HPC boost represents an infusion of hematopoietic progenitor cells from the original donor that is being used to treat post-transplant cytopenia(s). Codes 38240, 38242, and 38243 should not be reported together on the same date of service.

Cardiovascular

If a separately identifiable evaluation and management service is performed on the same date of service, the appropriate E/M service code, including office or other outpatient services, established (99211-99215), hospital observation services (99217-99220, 99224-99226), hospital inpatient services (99221-99223, 99231-99239), and inpatient neonatal and pediatric critical care (99471, 99472, 99475, 99476) may be reported, using modifier 25, in addition to 38240, 38242 or 38243. Post-transplant infusion management of adverse reactions is reported separately using the appropriate E/M, prolonged service or critical care code(s). In accordance with place of service and facility reporting guidelines, the fluid used to administer the cells and other infusions for incidental hydration (eg, 96360, 96361) are not separately reportable. Similarly, infusion(s) of any medication(s) concurrently with the transplant infusion are not separately reportable. However, hydration or administration of medications (eg, antibiotics, narcotics) unrelated to the transplant are separately reportable using modifier 59.

38240	Hematopoietic progenitor cell (HPC); allogeneic transplantation per donor
38241	autologous transplantation
# 38243	HPC boost
38242	Allogeneic lymphocyte infusions

(For bone marrow aspiration, use 38220)

(For modification, treatment, and processing of hematopoietic progenitor cell specimens for transplantation, see 38210-38215)

(For cryopreservation, freezing, and storage of hematopoietic progenitor cells for transplantation, use 38207)

(For thawing and expansion of hematopoietic progenitor cells for transplantation, see 38208, 38209)

(For compatibility studies, see 81379-81383, 86812-86822)

38243	Code is out of numerical sequence. See 38240-38242

Lymph Nodes and Lymphatic Channels

Incision

38300	Drainage of lymph node abscess or lymphadenitis; simple
38305	extensive
38308	Lymphangiotomy or other operations on lymphatic channels
38380	Suture and/or ligation of thoracic duct; cervical approach
38381	thoracic approach
38382	abdominal approach

Excision

(For injection for sentinel node identification, use 38792)

38500	Biopsy or excision of lymph node(s); open, superficial

(Do not report 38500 with 38700-38780)

38505	by needle, superficial (eg, cervical, inguinal, axillary)

(If imaging guidance is performed, see 76942, 77012, 77021)

(For fine needle aspiration, use 10021 or 10022)

(For evaluation of fine needle aspirate, see 88172, 88173)

38510	open, deep cervical node(s)
38520	open, deep cervical node(s) with excision scalene fat pad
38525	open, deep axillary node(s)
38530	open, internal mammary node(s)

(Do not report 38530 with 38720-38746)

(For percutaneous needle biopsy, retroperitoneal lymph node or mass, use 49180. For fine needle aspiration, use 10022)

38542	Dissection, deep jugular node(s)

(For radical cervical neck dissection, use 38720)

38550	Excision of cystic hygroma, axillary or cervical; without deep neurovascular dissection
38555	with deep neurovascular dissection

Limited Lymphadenectomy for Staging

38562	Limited lymphadenectomy for staging (separate procedure); pelvic and para-aortic

(When combined with prostatectomy, use 55812 or 55842)

(When combined with insertion of radioactive substance into prostate, use 55862)

38564	retroperitoneal (aortic and/or splenic)

Laparoscopy

Surgical laparoscopy always includes diagnostic laparoscopy. To report a diagnostic laparoscopy (peritoneoscopy) (separate procedure), use 49320.

38570	Laparoscopy, surgical; with retroperitoneal lymph node sampling (biopsy), single or multiple
38571	with bilateral total pelvic lymphadenectomy
38572	with bilateral total pelvic lymphadenectomy and peri-aortic lymph node sampling (biopsy), single or multiple

(For drainage of lymphocele to peritoneal cavity, use 49323)

38589	Unlisted laparoscopy procedure, lymphatic system

Cardiovascular

Radical Lymphadenectomy (Radical Resection of Lymph Nodes)

(For limited pelvic and retroperitoneal lymphadenectomies, see 38562, 38564)

38700   Suprahyoid lymphadenectomy

(For bilateral procedure, report 38700 with modifier 50)

38720   Cervical lymphadenectomy (complete)

(For bilateral procedure, report 38720 with modifier 50)

38724   Cervical lymphadenectomy (modified radical neck dissection)

38740   Axillary lymphadenectomy; superficial

38745   complete

+ **38746**   Thoracic lymphadenectomy by thoracotomy, mediastinal and regional lymphadenectomy (List separately in addition to code for primary procedure)

(On the right, mediastinal lymph nodes include the paratracheal, subcarinal, paraesophageal, and inferior pulmonary ligament)

(On the left, mediastinal lymph nodes include the aortopulmonary window, subcarinal, paraesophageal, and inferior pulmonary ligament)

(Report 38746 in conjunction with 19260, 31760, 31766, 31786, 32096-32200, 32220-32320, 32440-32491, 32503-32505, 33025, 33030, 33050-33130, 39200-39220, 39560, 39561, 43101, 43112, 43117, 43118, 43122, 43123, 43351, 60270, 60505)

(To report mediastinal and regional lymphadenectomy via thoracoscopy [VATS], see 32674)

+ **38747**   Abdominal lymphadenectomy, regional, including celiac, gastric, portal, peripancreatic, with or without para-aortic and vena caval nodes (List separately in addition to code for primary procedure)

38760   Inguinofemoral lymphadenectomy, superficial, including Cloquets node (separate procedure)

(For bilateral procedure, report 38760 with modifier 50)

38765   Inguinofemoral lymphadenectomy, superficial, in continuity with pelvic lymphadenectomy, including external iliac, hypogastric, and obturator nodes (separate procedure)

(For bilateral procedure, report 38765 with modifier 50)

38770   Pelvic lymphadenectomy, including external iliac, hypogastric, and obturator nodes (separate procedure)

(For bilateral procedure, report 38770 with modifier 50)

38780   Retroperitoneal transabdominal lymphadenectomy, extensive, including pelvic, aortic, and renal nodes (separate procedure)

(For excision and repair of lymphedematous skin and subcutaneous tissue, see 15004-15005, 15570-15650)

Introduction

38790   Injection procedure; lymphangiography

(For bilateral procedure, report 38790 with modifier 50)

(For radiological supervision and interpretation, see 75801-75807)

38792   radioactive tracer for identification of sentinel node

(For excision of sentinel node, see 38500-38542)

(For nuclear medicine lymphatics and lymph gland imaging, use 78195)

(For intraoperative identification (eg, mapping) of sentinel lymph node(s) including injection of non-radioactive dye, see 38900)

38794   Cannulation, thoracic duct

Other Procedures

+ **38900**   Intraoperative identification (eg, mapping) of sentinel lymph node(s) includes injection of non-radioactive dye, when performed (List separately in addition to code for primary procedure)

(Use 38900 in conjunction with 19302, 19307, 38500, 38510, 38520, 38525, 38530, 38542, 38740, 38745)

(For injection of radioactive tracer for identification of sentinel node, use 38792)

38999   Unlisted procedure, hemic or lymphatic system

Mediastinum and Diaphragm

Mediastinum

Incision

39000   Mediastinotomy with exploration, drainage, removal of foreign body, or biopsy; cervical approach

39010   transthoracic approach, including either transthoracic or median sternotomy

(Do not report 39010 in conjunction with 33955, 33956, 33963, 33964)

(For VATS pericardial biopsy, use 32604)

Excision/Resection

39200   Resection of mediastinal cyst

39220   Resection of mediastinal tumor

(For substernal thyroidectomy, use 60270)

(For thymectomy, use 60520)

(For thoracoscopic [VATS] resection of mediastinal cyst, tumor, or mass, use 32662)

Cardiovascular

Endoscopy

▶(39400 has been deleted. To report mediastinoscopy with biopsy, see 39401, 39402)◀

● **39401** Mediastinoscopy; includes biopsy(ies) of mediastinal mass (eg, lymphoma), when performed

● **39402** with lymph node biopsy(ies) (eg, lung cancer staging)

Other Procedures

39499 Unlisted procedure, mediastinum

Diaphragm

Repair

(For transabdominal repair of diaphragmatic [esophageal hiatal] hernia, use 43325)

(For laparoscopic repair of diaphragmatic [esophageal hiatal] hernias and fundoplication, see 43280, 43281, 43282)

39501 Repair, laceration of diaphragm, any approach

(For laparoscopic paraesophageal hernia repair, see 43281, 43282)

39503 Repair, neonatal diaphragmatic hernia, with or without chest tube insertion and with or without creation of ventral hernia

(Do not report modifier 63 in conjunction with 39503)

(For laparoscopic paraesophageal hernia repair, see 43281, 43282)

(39530 has been deleted. To report thoracoabdominal diaphragmatic [esophageal hiatal] hernia repair, see 43336, 43337)

(39531 has been deleted. To report thoracoabdominal diaphragmatic [esophageal hiatal] hernia repair, see 43336, 43337)

39540 Repair, diaphragmatic hernia (other than neonatal), traumatic; acute

39541 chronic

39545 Imbrication of diaphragm for eventration, transthoracic or transabdominal, paralytic or nonparalytic

39560 Resection, diaphragm; with simple repair (eg, primary suture)

39561 with complex repair (eg, prosthetic material, local muscle flap)

Other Procedures

39599 Unlisted procedure, diaphragm

Cardiovascular

Digestive System

Lips

(For procedures on skin of lips, see 10040 et seq)

Excision

40490	Biopsy of lip
40500	Vermilionectomy (lip shave), with mucosal advancement
40510	Excision of lip; transverse wedge excision with primary closure
40520	V-excision with primary direct linear closure

(For excision of mucous lesions, see 40810-40816)

40525	full thickness, reconstruction with local flap (eg, Estlander or fan)
40527	full thickness, reconstruction with cross lip flap (Abbe-Estlander)
40530	Resection of lip, more than one-fourth, without reconstruction

(For reconstruction, see 13131 et seq)

Repair (Cheiloplasty)

40650	Repair lip, full thickness; vermilion only
40652	up to half vertical height
40654	over one-half vertical height, or complex
40700	Plastic repair of cleft lip/nasal deformity; primary, partial or complete, unilateral
40701	primary bilateral, 1-stage procedure
40702	primary bilateral, 1 of 2 stages
40720	secondary, by recreation of defect and reclosure

(For bilateral procedure, report 40720 with modifier 50)

(To report rhinoplasty only for nasal deformity secondary to congenital cleft lip, see 30460, 30462)

(For repair of cleft lip, with cross lip pedicle flap (Abbe-Estlander type), use 40527)

40761	with cross lip pedicle flap (Abbe-Estlander type), including sectioning and inserting of pedicle

(For repair cleft palate, see 42200 et seq)

(For other reconstructive procedures, see 14060, 14061, 15120-15261, 15574, 15576, 15630)

Other Procedures

40799	Unlisted procedure, lips

Vestibule of Mouth

The vestibule is the part of the oral cavity outside the dentoalveolar structures; it includes the mucosal and submucosal tissue of lips and cheeks.

Incision

40800	Drainage of abscess, cyst, hematoma, vestibule of mouth; simple
40801	complicated
40804	Removal of embedded foreign body, vestibule of mouth; simple
40805	complicated
40806	Incision of labial frenum (frenotomy)

Excision, Destruction

40808	Biopsy, vestibule of mouth
40810	Excision of lesion of mucosa and submucosa, vestibule of mouth; without repair
40812	with simple repair
40814	with complex repair
40816	complex, with excision of underlying muscle
40818	Excision of mucosa of vestibule of mouth as donor graft
40819	Excision of frenum, labial or buccal (frenumectomy, frenulectomy, frenectomy)
40820	Destruction of lesion or scar of vestibule of mouth by physical methods (eg, laser, thermal, cryo, chemical)

Repair

40830	Closure of laceration, vestibule of mouth; 2.5 cm or less
40831	over 2.5 cm or complex
40840	Vestibuloplasty; anterior
40842	posterior, unilateral
40843	posterior, bilateral
40844	entire arch
40845	complex (including ridge extension, muscle repositioning)

(For skin grafts, see 15002 et seq)

Other Procedures

40899	Unlisted procedure, vestibule of mouth

Digestive

Tongue and Floor of Mouth

Incision

41000 Intraoral incision and drainage of abscess, cyst, or hematoma of tongue or floor of mouth; lingual

41005 sublingual, superficial

41006 sublingual, deep, supramylohyoid

41007 submental space

41008 submandibular space

41009 masticator space

41010 Incision of lingual frenum (frenotomy)

41015 Extraoral incision and drainage of abscess, cyst, or hematoma of floor of mouth; sublingual

41016 submental

41017 submandibular

41018 masticator space

(For frenoplasty, use 41520)

41019 Placement of needles, catheters, or other device(s) into the head and/or neck region (percutaneous, transoral, or transnasal) for subsequent interstitial radioelement application

(For imaging guidance, see 76942, 77002, 77012, 77021)

(For stereotactic insertion of intracranial brachytherapy radiation sources, use 61770)

►(For interstitial radioelement application, see 77770, 77771, 77772, 77778)◄

Excision

41100 Biopsy of tongue; anterior two-thirds

41105 posterior one-third

41108 Biopsy of floor of mouth

41110 Excision of lesion of tongue without closure

41112 Excision of lesion of tongue with closure; anterior two-thirds

41113 posterior one-third

41114 with local tongue flap

(Do not report 41114 in conjunction with 41112 or 41113)

41115 Excision of lingual frenum (frenectomy)

41116 Excision, lesion of floor of mouth

41120 Glossectomy; less than one-half tongue

41130 hemiglossectomy

41135 partial, with unilateral radical neck dissection

41140 complete or total, with or without tracheostomy, without radical neck dissection

41145 complete or total, with or without tracheostomy, with unilateral radical neck dissection

41150 composite procedure with resection floor of mouth and mandibular resection, without radical neck dissection

41153 composite procedure with resection floor of mouth, with suprahyoid neck dissection

41155 composite procedure with resection floor of mouth, mandibular resection, and radical neck dissection (Commando type)

Repair

41250 Repair of laceration 2.5 cm or less; floor of mouth and/or anterior two-thirds of tongue

41251 posterior one-third of tongue

41252 Repair of laceration of tongue, floor of mouth, over 2.6 cm or complex

Other Procedures

41500 Fixation of tongue, mechanical, other than suture (eg, K-wire)

41510 Suture of tongue to lip for micrognathia (Douglas type procedure)

41512 Tongue base suspension, permanent suture technique

(For fixation of tongue, mechanical, other than suture, use 41500)

(For suture of tongue to lip for micrognathia, use 41510)

41520 Frenoplasty (surgical revision of frenum, eg, with Z-plasty)

(For frenotomy, see 40806, 41010)

41530 Submucosal ablation of the tongue base, radiofrequency, 1 or more sites, per session

41599 Unlisted procedure, tongue, floor of mouth

Dentoalveolar Structures

Incision

41800 Drainage of abscess, cyst, hematoma from dentoalveolar structures

41805 Removal of embedded foreign body from dentoalveolar structures; soft tissues

41806 bone

Excision, Destruction

41820 Gingivectomy, excision gingiva, each quadrant

41821 Operculectomy, excision pericoronal tissues

41822 Excision of fibrous tuberosities, dentoalveolar structures

41823   Excision of osseous tuberosities, dentoalveolar structures

41825   Excision of lesion or tumor (except listed above), dentoalveolar structures; without repair

41826   with simple repair

41827   with complex repair

(For nonexcisional destruction, use 41850)

41828   Excision of hyperplastic alveolar mucosa, each quadrant (specify)

41830   Alveolectomy, including curettage of osteitis or sequestrectomy

41850   Destruction of lesion (except excision), dentoalveolar structures

Other Procedures

41870   Periodontal mucosal grafting

41872   Gingivoplasty, each quadrant (specify)

41874   Alveoloplasty, each quadrant (specify)

(For closure of lacerations, see 40830, 40831)

(For segmental osteotomy, use 21206)

(For reduction of fractures, see 21421-21490)

41899   Unlisted procedure, dentoalveolar structures

Palate and Uvula

Incision

42000   Drainage of abscess of palate, uvula

Excision, Destruction

42100   Biopsy of palate, uvula

42104   Excision, lesion of palate, uvula; without closure

42106   with simple primary closure

42107   with local flap closure

(For skin graft, see 14040-14302)

(For mucosal graft, use 40818)

42120   Resection of palate or extensive resection of lesion

(For reconstruction of palate with extraoral tissue, see 14040-14302, 15050, 15120, 15240, 15576)

42140   Uvulectomy, excision of uvula

42145   Palatopharyngoplasty (eg, uvulopalatopharyngoplasty, uvulopharyngoplasty)

(For removal of exostosis of the bony palate, see 21031, 21032)

42160   Destruction of lesion, palate or uvula (thermal, cryo or chemical)

Repair

42180   Repair, laceration of palate; up to 2 cm

42182   over 2 cm or complex

42200   Palatoplasty for cleft palate, soft and/or hard palate only

42205   Palatoplasty for cleft palate, with closure of alveolar ridge; soft tissue only

42210   with bone graft to alveolar ridge (includes obtaining graft)

42215   Palatoplasty for cleft palate; major revision

42220   secondary lengthening procedure

42225   attachment pharyngeal flap

42226   Lengthening of palate, and pharyngeal flap

42227   Lengthening of palate, with island flap

42235   Repair of anterior palate, including vomer flap

(For repair of oronasal fistula, use 30600)

42260   Repair of nasolabial fistula

(For repair of cleft lip, see 40700 et seq)

42280   Maxillary impression for palatal prosthesis

42281   Insertion of pin-retained palatal prosthesis

Other Procedures

42299   Unlisted procedure, palate, uvula

Salivary Gland and Ducts

Incision

42300   Drainage of abscess; parotid, simple

42305   parotid, complicated

42310   Drainage of abscess; submaxillary or sublingual, intraoral

42320   submaxillary, external

42330   Sialolithotomy; submandibular (submaxillary), sublingual or parotid, uncomplicated, intraoral

42335   submandibular (submaxillary), complicated, intraoral

42340   parotid, extraoral or complicated intraoral

Excision

42400   Biopsy of salivary gland; needle

(For fine needle aspiration, see 10021, 10022)

(For evaluation of fine needle aspirate, see 88172, 88173)

(If imaging guidance is performed, see 76942, 77002, 77012, 77021)

42405   incisional

(If imaging guidance is performed, see 76942, 77002, 77012, 77021)

Digestive

42408 Excision of sublingual salivary cyst (ranula)

42409 Marsupialization of sublingual salivary cyst (ranula)

42410 Excision of parotid tumor or parotid gland; lateral lobe, without nerve dissection

42415 lateral lobe, with dissection and preservation of facial nerve

42420 total, with dissection and preservation of facial nerve

42425 total, en bloc removal with sacrifice of facial nerve

42426 total, with unilateral radical neck dissection

(For suture or grafting of facial nerve, see 64864, 64865, 69740, 69745)

42440 Excision of submandibular (submaxillary) gland

42450 Excision of sublingual gland

Repair

42500 Plastic repair of salivary duct, sialodochoplasty; primary or simple

42505 secondary or complicated

42507 Parotid duct diversion, bilateral (Wilke type procedure);

(42508 has been deleted)

42509 with excision of both submandibular glands

42510 with ligation of both submandibular (Wharton's) ducts

Other Procedures

42550 Injection procedure for sialography

(For radiological supervision and interpretation, use 70390)

42600 Closure salivary fistula

42650 Dilation salivary duct

42660 Dilation and catheterization of salivary duct, with or without injection

42665 Ligation salivary duct, intraoral

42699 Unlisted procedure, salivary glands or ducts

Pharynx, Adenoids, and Tonsils

Incision

42700 Incision and drainage abscess; peritonsillar

42720 retropharyngeal or parapharyngeal, intraoral approach

42725 retropharyngeal or parapharyngeal, external approach

Excision, Destruction

42800 Biopsy; oropharynx

(42802 has been deleted. To report biopsy of hypopharynx, see 31510, 31535, 31536, 31576)

42804 nasopharynx, visible lesion, simple

42806 nasopharynx, survey for unknown primary lesion

(For laryngoscopic biopsy, see 31510, 31535, 31536)

42808 Excision or destruction of lesion of pharynx, any method

42809 Removal of foreign body from pharynx

42810 Excision branchial cleft cyst or vestige, confined to skin and subcutaneous tissues

42815 Excision branchial cleft cyst, vestige, or fistula, extending beneath subcutaneous tissues and/or into pharynx

42820 Tonsillectomy and adenoidectomy; younger than age 12

42821 age 12 or over

42825 Tonsillectomy, primary or secondary; younger than age 12

42826 age 12 or over

42830 Adenoidectomy, primary; younger than age 12

42831 age 12 or over

42835 Adenoidectomy, secondary; younger than age 12

42836 age 12 or over

42842 Radical resection of tonsil, tonsillar pillars, and/or retromolar trigone; without closure

42844 closure with local flap (eg, tongue, buccal)

42845 closure with other flap

(For closure with other flap(s), use appropriate number for flap(s))

(When combined with radical neck dissection, use also 38720)

42860 Excision of tonsil tags

42870 Excision or destruction lingual tonsil, any method (separate procedure)

(For resection of the nasopharynx [eg, juvenile angiofibroma] by bicoronal and/or transzygomatic approach, see 61586 and 61600)

42890 Limited pharyngectomy

42892 Resection of lateral pharyngeal wall or pyriform sinus, direct closure by advancement of lateral and posterior pharyngeal walls

(When combined with radical neck dissection, use also 38720)

42894 Resection of pharyngeal wall requiring closure with myocutaneous or fasciocutaneous flap or free muscle, skin, or fascial flap with microvascular anastomosis

(When combined with radical neck dissection, use also 38720)

(For limited pharyngectomy with radical neck dissection, use 38720 with 42890)

(For flap used for reconstruction, see 15732, 15734, 15756, 15757, 15758)

Repair

42900　Suture pharynx for wound or injury

42950　Pharyngoplasty (plastic or reconstructive operation on pharynx)

　　　　(For pharyngeal flap, use 42225)

42953　Pharyngoesophageal repair

　　　　(For closure with myocutaneous or other flap, use appropriate number in addition)

Other Procedures

42955　Pharyngostomy (fistulization of pharynx, external for feeding)

42960　Control oropharyngeal hemorrhage, primary or secondary (eg, post-tonsillectomy); simple

42961　　complicated, requiring hospitalization

42962　　with secondary surgical intervention

42970　Control of nasopharyngeal hemorrhage, primary or secondary (eg, postadenoidectomy); simple, with posterior nasal packs, with or without anterior packs and/or cautery

42971　　complicated, requiring hospitalization

42972　　with secondary surgical intervention

42999　Unlisted procedure, pharynx, adenoids, or tonsils

Esophagus

Incision

　　　　(For esophageal intubation with laparotomy, use 43510)

43020　Esophagotomy, cervical approach, with removal of foreign body

43030　Cricopharyngeal myotomy

43045　Esophagotomy, thoracic approach, with removal of foreign body

Excision

　　　　(For gastrointestinal reconstruction for previous esophagectomy, see 43360, 43361)

43100　Excision of lesion, esophagus, with primary repair; cervical approach

43101　　thoracic or abdominal approach

　　　　(For wide excision of malignant lesion of cervical esophagus, with total laryngectomy without radical neck dissection, see 43107, 43116, 43124, and 31360)

　　　　(For wide excision of malignant lesion of cervical esophagus, with total laryngectomy with radical neck dissection, see 43107, 43116, 43124, and 31365)

43107　Total or near total esophagectomy, without thoracotomy; with pharyngogastrostomy or cervical esophagogastrostomy, with or without pyloroplasty (transhiatal)

43108　　with colon interposition or small intestine reconstruction, including intestine mobilization, preparation and anastomosis(es)

43112　Total or near total esophagectomy, with thoracotomy; with pharyngogastrostomy or cervical esophagogastrostomy, with or without pyloroplasty

43113　　with colon interposition or small intestine reconstruction, including intestine mobilization, preparation, and anastomosis(es)

43116　Partial esophagectomy, cervical, with free intestinal graft, including microvascular anastomosis, obtaining the graft and intestinal reconstruction

　　　　(Do not report 43116 in conjunction with 69990)

　　　　(Report 43116 with the modifier 52 appended if intestinal or free jejunal graft with microvascular anastomosis is performed by another physician)

　　　　(For free jejunal graft with microvascular anastomosis performed by another physician, use 43496)

43117　Partial esophagectomy, distal two-thirds, with thoracotomy and separate abdominal incision, with or without proximal gastrectomy; with thoracic esophagogastrostomy, with or without pyloroplasty (Ivor Lewis)

43118　　with colon interposition or small intestine reconstruction, including intestine mobilization, preparation, and anastomosis(es)

　　　　(For total esophagectomy with gastropharyngostomy, see 43107, 43124)

　　　　(For esophagogastrectomy (lower third) and vagotomy, use 43122)

43121　Partial esophagectomy, distal two-thirds, with thoracotomy only, with or without proximal gastrectomy, with thoracic esophagogastrostomy, with or without pyloroplasty

43122　Partial esophagectomy, thoracoabdominal or abdominal approach, with or without proximal gastrectomy; with esophagogastrostomy, with or without pyloroplasty

43123　　with colon interposition or small intestine reconstruction, including intestine mobilization, preparation, and anastomosis(es)

43124　Total or partial esophagectomy, without reconstruction (any approach), with cervical esophagostomy

43130　Diverticulectomy of hypopharynx or esophagus, with or without myotomy; cervical approach

43135　　thoracic approach

　　　　(For endoscopic diverticulectomy of hypopharynx or cervical esophagus, use 43180)

Digestive

Endoscopy

When bleeding occurs as a result of an endoscopic procedure, control of bleeding is not reported separately during the same operative session.

Esophagoscopy includes examination from the cricopharyngeus muscle (upper esophageal sphincter) to and including the gastroesophageal junction. It may also include examination of the proximal region of the stomach via retroflexion when performed.

Esophagoscopy

43180   Esophagoscopy, rigid, transoral with diverticulectomy of hypopharynx or cervical esophagus (eg, Zenker's diverticulum), with cricopharyngeal myotomy, includes use of telescope or operating microscope and repair, when performed

▶(Do not report 43180 in conjunction with 43210, 69990)◀

(For diverticulectomy of hypopharynx or esophagus [open], see 43130, 43135)

43191   Esophagoscopy, rigid, transoral; diagnostic, including collection of specimen(s) by brushing or washing when performed (separate procedure)

▶(Do not report 43191 in conjunction with 43192, 43193, 43194, 43195, 43196, 43197, 43198, 43210)◀

(For diagnostic transnasal esophagoscopy, see 43197, 43198)

(For diagnostic flexible transoral esophagoscopy, use 43200)

43192   with directed submucosal injection(s), any substance

(Do not report 43192 in conjunction with 43191, 43197, 43198)

(For flexible transoral esophagoscopy with directed submucosal injection(s), use 43201)

(For flexible transoral esophagoscopy with injection sclerosis of esophageal varices, use 43204)

(For rigid transoral esophagoscopy with injection sclerosis of esophageal varices, use 43499)

43193   with biopsy, single or multiple

(Do not report 43193 in conjunction with 43191, 43197, 43198)

(For flexible transoral esophagoscopy with biopsy, use 43202)

43194   with removal of foreign body(s)

(Do not report 43194 in conjunction with 43191, 43197, 43198)

(If fluoroscopic guidance is performed, use 76000)

(For flexible transoral esophagoscopy with removal of foreign body(s), use 43215)

43195   with balloon dilation (less than 30 mm diameter)

(Do not report 43195 in conjunction with 43191, 43197, 43198)

(If fluoroscopic guidance is performed, use 74360)

(For esophageal dilation with balloon 30 mm diameter or larger, see 43214, 43233)

(For dilation without endoscopic visualization, see 43450, 43453)

(For flexible transoral esophagoscopy with balloon dilation [less than 30 mm diameter], use 43220)

43196   with insertion of guide wire followed by dilation over guide wire

(Do not report 43196 in conjunction with 43191, 43197, 43198)

(If fluoroscopic guidance is performed, use 74360)

(For flexible transoral esophagoscopy with insertion of guide wire followed by dilation over guide wire, use 43226)

43197   Esophagoscopy, flexible, transnasal; diagnostic, including collection of specimen(s) by brushing or washing, when performed (separate procedure)

(Do not report 43197 in conjunction with 31575, 43191, 43192, 43193, 43194, 43195, 43196, 43198, 43200-43232, 43235-43259, 43266, 43270, 92511)

(Do not report 43197 in conjunction with 31231 unless separate type of endoscope [eg, rigid endoscope] is used)

(For transoral esophagoscopy, see 43191, 43200)

43198   with biopsy, single or multiple

(Do not report 43198 in conjunction with 31575, 43191, 43192, 43193, 43194, 43195, 43196, 43197, 43200-43232, 43235-43259, 43266, 43270, 92511)

(Do not report 43198 in conjunction with 31231 unless separate type of endoscope [eg, rigid endoscope] is used)

(For transoral esophagoscopy with biopsy, see 43193, 43202)

⊙ **43200**   Esophagoscopy, flexible, transoral; diagnostic, including collection of specimen(s) by brushing or washing, when performed (separate procedure)

(Do not report 43200 in conjunction with 43197, 43198, 43201-43232)

(For diagnostic rigid transoral esophagoscopy, use 43191)

(For diagnostic flexible transnasal esophagoscopy, use 43197)

(For diagnostic flexible esophagogastroduodenoscopy, use 43235)

⊙ **43201**   with directed submucosal injection(s), any substance

(Do not report 43201 in conjunction with 43204, 43211, 43227 for the same lesion)

(Do not report 43201 in conjunction with 43197, 43198, 43200)

(For rigid transoral esophagoscopy with directed submucosal injection[s], use 43192)

(For flexible transoral esophagoscopy with injection sclerosis of esophageal varices, use 43204)

(For rigid transoral esophagoscopy with injection sclerosis of esophageal varices, use 43499)

⊙ **43202**   with biopsy, single or multiple

(Do not report 43202 in conjunction with 43211 for the same lesion)

(Do not report 43202 in conjunction with 43197, 43198, 43200)

(For rigid transoral esophagoscopy with biopsy, use 43193)

(For flexible transnasal esophagoscopy with biopsy, use 43198)

⊙ **43204**   with injection sclerosis of esophageal varices

(Do not report 43204 in conjunction with 43201, 43227 for the same lesion)

(Do not report 43204 in conjunction with 43197, 43198, 43200)

(For rigid transoral esophagoscopy with injection sclerosis of esophageal varices, use 43499)

⊙ **43205**   with band ligation of esophageal varices

(Do not report 43205 in conjunction with 43227 for the same lesion)

(Do not report 43205 in conjunction with 43197, 43198, 43200)

(To report control of nonvariceal bleeding with band ligation, use 43227)

⊙ **43206**   with optical endomicroscopy

(Report supply of contrast agent separately)

(Do not report 43206 in conjunction with 43197, 43198, 43200, 88375)

43210   Code is out of numerical sequence. See 43235-43259

43211   Code is out of numerical sequence. See 43191-43232

43212   Code is out of numerical sequence. See 43191-43232

43213   Code is out of numerical sequence. See 43191-43232

43214   Code is out of numerical sequence. See 43191-43232

⊙ **43215**   with removal of foreign body(s)

(Do not report 43215 in conjunction with 43197, 43198, 43200)

(If fluoroscopic guidance is performed, use 76000)

(For rigid transoral esophagoscopy with removal of foreign body(s), use 43194)

⊙ **43216**   with removal of tumor(s), polyp(s), or other lesion(s) by hot biopsy forceps

(Do not report 43216 in conjunction with 43197, 43198, 43200)

⊙ **43217**   with removal of tumor(s), polyp(s), or other lesion(s) by snare technique

(Do not report 43217 in conjunction with 43211 for the same lesion)

(Do not report 43217 in conjunction with 43197, 43198, 43200)

(For esophagogastroduodenoscopy with removal of tumor[s], polyp[s], or other lesion[s] by snare technique, use 43251)

(For endoscopic mucosal resection, use 43211)

#⊙ **43211**   with endoscopic mucosal resection

(Do not report 43211 in conjunction with 43201, 43202, 43217 for the same lesion)

(Do not report 43211 in conjunction with 43197, 43198, 43200)

#⊙ **43212**   with placement of endoscopic stent (includes pre- and post-dilation and guide wire passage, when performed)

(Do not report 43212 in conjunction with 43197, 43198, 43200, 43220, 43226, 43241)

(If fluoroscopic guidance is performed, use 74360)

(43219 has been deleted. To report, use 43212)

⊙ **43220**   with transendoscopic balloon dilation (less than 30 mm diameter)

(Do not report 43220 in conjunction with 43197, 43198, 43200, 43212, 43226, 43229)

(If fluoroscopic guidance is performed, use 74360)

(For rigid transoral esophagoscopy with balloon dilation [less than 30 mm diameter], use 43195)

(For esophageal dilation with balloon 30 mm diameter or larger, use 43214)

(For dilation without endoscopic visualization, see 43450, 43453)

#⊙ **43213**   with dilation of esophagus, by balloon or dilator, retrograde (includes fluoroscopic guidance, when performed)

(Do not report 43213 in conjunction with 43197, 43198, 43200, 74360, 76000, 76001)

(For transendoscopic balloon dilation of multiple strictures during the same session, report 43213 with modifier 59 for each additional stricture dilated)

#⊙ **43214**   with dilation of esophagus with balloon (30 mm diameter or larger) (includes fluoroscopic guidance, when performed)

(Do not report 43214 in conjunction with 43197, 43198, 43200, 74360, 76000, 76001)

Digestive

⊙ **43226**   with insertion of guide wire followed by passage of dilator(s) over guide wire

(Do not report 43226 in conjunction with 43229 for the same lesion)

(Do not report 43226 in conjunction with 43197, 43198, 43200, 43212, 43220)

(If fluoroscopic guidance is performed, use 74360)

(For rigid transoral esophagoscopy with insertion of guide wire followed by dilation over guide wire, use 43196)

⊙ **43227**   with control of bleeding, any method

(Do not report 43227 in conjunction with 43201, 43204, 43205 for the same lesion)

(Do not report 43227 in conjunction with 43197, 43198, 43200)

(43228 has been deleted. To report, use 43229)

⊙ **43229**   with ablation of tumor(s), polyp(s), or other lesion(s) (includes pre- and post-dilation and guide wire passage, when performed)

(Do not report 43229 in conjunction with 43220, 43226 for the same lesion)

(Do not report 43229 in conjunction with 43197, 43198, 43200)

(For esophagoscopic photodynamic therapy, report 43229 in conjunction with 96570, 96571 as appropriate)

⊙ **43231**   with endoscopic ultrasound examination

(Do not report 43231 in conjunction with 43197, 43198, 43200, 43232, 76975)

(Do not report 43231 more than once per session)

⊙ **43232**   with transendoscopic ultrasound-guided intramural or transmural fine needle aspiration/biopsy(s)

(Do not report 43232 in conjunction with 43197, 43198, 43200, 43231, 76942, 76975)

(Do not report 43232 more than once per session)

43233   Code is out of numerical sequence. See 43249-43250

(43234 has been deleted. To report esophagogastroscopy, see 43197, 43200, 43235)

Esophagogastroduodenoscopy

(For examination of the esophagus from the cricopharyngeus muscle [upper esophageal sphincter] to and including the gastroesophageal junction, including examination of the proximal region of the stomach via retroflexion when performed, see 43197, 43198, 43200, 43201, 43202, 43204, 43205, 43206, 43211, 43212, 43213, 43214, 43215, 43216, 43217, 43220, 43226, 43227, 43229, 43231, 43232)

(Use 43233, 43235-43259, 43266, 43270 for examination of a surgically altered stomach where the jejunum is examined distal to the anastomosis [eg, gastric bypass, gastroenterostomy {Billroth II}])

To report esophagogastroscopy where the duodenum is deliberately not examined (eg, judged clinically not pertinent), or because the clinical situation precludes such exam (eg, significant gastric retention precludes safe exam of duodenum), append modifier 52 if repeat examination is not planned, or modifier 53 if repeat examination is planned.

⊙ **43235**   Esophagogastroduodenoscopy, flexible, transoral; diagnostic, including collection of specimen(s) by brushing or washing, when performed (separate procedure)

▶(Do not report 43235 in conjunction with 43197, 43198, 43210, 43236-43259, 43266, 43270, 44360, 44361, 44363, 44364, 44365, 44366, 44369, 44370, 44372, 44373, 44376, 44377, 44378, 44379)◀

⊙ **43236**   with directed submucosal injection(s), any substance

(Do not report 43236 in conjunction with 43243, 43254, 43255 for the same lesion)

(Do not report 43236 in conjunction with 43197, 43198, 43235, 44360, 44361, 44363, 44364, 44365, 44366, 44369, 44370, 44372, 44373, 44376, 44377, 44378, 44379)

(For flexible, transoral esophagogastroduodenoscopy with injection sclerosis of esophageal and/or gastric varices, use 43243)

⊙ **43237**   with endoscopic ultrasound examination limited to the esophagus, stomach or duodenum, and adjacent structures

(Do not report 43237 in conjunction with 43197, 43198, 43235, 43238, 43242, 43253, 43259, 44360, 44361, 44363, 44364, 44365, 44366, 44369, 44370, 44372, 44373, 44376, 44377, 44378, 44379, 76975)

(Do not report 43237 more than once per session)

⊙ **43238**   with transendoscopic ultrasound-guided intramural or transmural fine needle aspiration/biopsy(s), (includes endoscopic ultrasound examination limited to the esophagus, stomach or duodenum, and adjacent structures)

(Do not report 43238 in conjunction with 43197, 43198, 43235, 43237, 43242, 44360, 44361, 44363, 44364, 44365, 44366, 44369, 44370, 44372, 44373, 44376, 44377, 44378, 44379, 76942, 76975)

(Do not report 43238 more than once per session)

⊙ **43239**   with biopsy, single or multiple

(Do not report 43239 in conjunction with 43254 for the same lesion)

(Do not report 43239 in conjunction with 43197, 43198, 43235, 44360, 44361, 44363, 44364, 44365, 44366, 44369, 44370, 44372, 44373, 44376, 44377, 44378, 44379)

⊙ **43240**   with transmural drainage of pseudocyst (includes placement of transmural drainage catheter[s]/stent[s], when performed, and endoscopic ultrasound, when performed)

(Do not report 43240 in conjunction with 43253 for the same lesion)

(Do not report 43240 in conjunction with 43197, 43198, 43235, 43242, 43259, 43266, 44360, 44361, 44363, 44364, 44365, 44366, 44369, 44370, 44372, 44373, 44376, 44377, 44378, 44379)

(Do not report 43240 more than once per session)

(For endoscopic pancreatic necrosectomy, use 48999)

⊙ **43241**   with insertion of intraluminal tube or catheter

(Do not report 43241 in conjunction with 43197, 43198, 43212, 43235, 43266, 44360, 44361, 44363, 44364, 44365, 44366, 44369, 44370, 44372, 44373, 44376, 44377, 44378, 44379)

(For naso- or oro-gastric tube placement requiring physician's or other qualified health care professional's skill and fluoroscopic guidance, use 43752)

(For nonendoscopic enteric tube placement, see 44500, 74340)

⊙ **43242**   with transendoscopic ultrasound-guided intramural or transmural fine needle aspiration/biopsy(s) (includes endoscopic ultrasound examination of the esophagus, stomach, and either the duodenum or a surgically altered stomach where the jejunum is examined distal to the anastomosis)

(Do not report 43242 in conjunction with 43197, 43198, 43235, 43237, 43238, 43240, 43259, 44360, 44361, 44363, 44364, 44365, 44366, 44369, 44370, 44372, 44373, 44376, 44377, 44378, 44379, 76942, 76975)

(Do not report 43242 more than once per session)

(For transendoscopic ultrasound-guided transmural fine needle aspiration/biopsy limited to the esophagus, stomach, duodenum, or adjacent structure, use 43238)

⊙ **43243**   with injection sclerosis of esophageal/gastric varices

(Do not report 43243 in conjunction with 43236, 43255 for the same lesion)

(Do not report 43243 in conjunction with 43197, 43198, 43235, 44360, 44361, 44363, 44364, 44365, 44366, 44369, 44370, 44372, 44373, 44376, 44377, 44378, 44379)

⊙ **43244**   with band ligation of esophageal/gastric varices

(Do not report 43244 in conjunction with 43197, 43198, 43235, 43255, 44360, 44361, 44363, 44364, 44365, 44366, 44369, 44370, 44372, 44373, 44376, 44377, 44378, 44379)

(To report control of nonvariceal bleeding with band ligation, use 43255)

⊙ **43245**   with dilation of gastric/duodenal stricture(s) (eg, balloon, bougie)

(Do not report 43245 in conjunction with 43197, 43198, 43235, 43266, 44360, 44361, 44363, 44364, 44365, 44366, 44369, 44370, 44372, 44373, 44376, 44377, 44378, 44379)

(If fluoroscopic guidance is performed, use 74360)

⊙ **43246**   with directed placement of percutaneous gastrostomy tube

(Do not report 43246 in conjunction with 43197, 43198, 43235, 44360, 44361, 44363, 44364, 44365, 44366, 44369, 44370, 44372, 44376, 44377, 44378, 44379)

(For nonendoscopic percutaneous placement of gastrostomy tube, use 49440)

(For replacement of gastrostomy tube without imaging or endoscopy, use 43760)

⊙ **43247**   with removal of foreign body(s)

(Do not report 43247 in conjunction with 43197, 43198, 43235, 44360, 44361, 44363, 44364, 44365, 44366, 44369, 44370, 44372, 44373, 44376, 44377, 44378, 44379)

(If fluoroscopic guidance is performed, use 76000)

⊙ **43248**   with insertion of guide wire followed by passage of dilator(s) through esophagus over guide wire

(Do not report 43248 in conjunction with 43197, 43198, 43235, 43266, 43270, 44360, 44361, 44363, 44364, 44365, 44366, 44369, 44370, 44372, 44373, 44376, 44377, 44378, 44379)

(If fluoroscopic guidance is performed, use 74360)

⊙ **43249**   with transendoscopic balloon dilation of esophagus (less than 30 mm diameter)

(Do not report 43249 in conjunction with 43197, 43198, 43235, 43266, 43270, 44360, 44361, 44363, 44364, 44365, 44366, 44369, 44370, 44372, 44373, 44376, 44377, 44378, 44379)

(If fluoroscopic guidance is performed, use 74360)

#⊙ **43233**   with dilation of esophagus with balloon (30 mm diameter or larger) (includes fluoroscopic guidance, when performed)

(Do not report 43233 in conjunction with 43197, 43198, 43235, 44360, 44361, 44363, 44364, 44365, 44366, 44369, 44370, 44372, 44373, 44376, 44377, 44378, 44379, 74360, 76000, 76001)

⊙ **43250**   with removal of tumor(s), polyp(s), or other lesion(s) by hot biopsy forceps

(Do not report 43250 in conjunction with 43197, 43198, 43235, 44360, 44361, 44363, 44364, 44365, 44366, 44369, 44370, 44372, 44373, 44376, 44377, 44378, 44379)

⊙ **43251**   with removal of tumor(s), polyp(s), or other lesion(s) by snare technique

(Do not report 43251 in conjunction with 43254 for the same lesion)

Digestive

(Do not report 43251 in conjunction with 43197, 43198, 43235, 44360, 44361, 44363, 44364, 44365, 44366, 44369, 44370, 44372, 44373, 44376, 44377, 44378, 44379)

(For endoscopic mucosal resection, use 43254)

⊙ **43252**   with optical endomicroscopy

(Report supply of contrast agent separately)

(Do not report 43252 in conjunction with 43197, 43198, 43235, 44360, 44361, 44363, 44364, 44365, 44366, 44369, 44370, 44372, 44373, 44376, 44377, 44378, 44379, 88375)

⊙ **43253**   with transendoscopic ultrasound-guided transmural injection of diagnostic or therapeutic substance(s) (eg, anesthetic, neurolytic agent) or fiducial marker(s) (includes endoscopic ultrasound examination of the esophagus, stomach, and either the duodenum or a surgically altered stomach where the jejunum is examined distal to the anastomosis)

(Do not report 43253 in conjunction with 43240 for the same lesion)

(Do not report 43253 in conjunction with 43197, 43198, 43235, 43237, 43259, 44360, 44361, 44363, 44364, 44365, 44366, 44369, 44370, 44372, 44373, 44376, 44377, 44378, 44379, 76942, 76975)

(Do not report 43253 more than once per session)

(For transendoscopic ultrasound-guided transmural fine needle aspiration/biopsy, see 43238, 43242)

⊙ **43254**   with endoscopic mucosal resection

(Do not report 43254 in conjunction with 43236, 43239, 43251 for the same lesion)

(Do not report 43254 in conjunction with 43197, 43198, 43235, 44360, 44361, 44363, 44364, 44365, 44366, 44369, 44370, 44372, 44373, 44376, 44377, 44378, 44379)

⊙ **43255**   with control of bleeding, any method

(Do not report 43255 in conjunction with 43236, 43243, 43244 for the same lesion)

(Do not report 43255 in conjunction with 43197, 43198, 43235, 44360, 44361, 44363, 44364, 44365, 44366, 44369, 44370, 44372, 44373, 44376, 44377, 44378, 44379)

(43256 has been deleted. To report, use 43266)

#⊙ **43266**   with placement of endoscopic stent (includes pre- and post-dilation and guide wire passage, when performed)

(Do not report 43266 in conjunction with 43197, 43198, 43235, 43240, 43241, 43245, 43248, 43249, 44360, 44361, 44363, 44364, 44365, 44366, 44369, 44370, 44372, 44373, 44376, 44377, 44378, 44379)

(If fluoroscopic guidance is performed, use 74360)

⊙ **43257**   with delivery of thermal energy to the muscle of lower esophageal sphincter and/or gastric cardia, for treatment of gastroesophageal reflux disease

(Do not report 43257 in conjunction with 43197, 43198, 43235, 44360, 44361, 44363, 44364, 44365, 44366, 44369, 44370, 44372, 44373, 44376, 44377, 44378, 44379)

(For ablation of metaplastic/dysplastic esophageal lesion [eg, Barrett's esophagus], see 43229, 43270)

#⊙ **43270**   with ablation of tumor(s), polyp(s), or other lesion(s) (includes pre- and post-dilation and guide wire passage, when performed)

(43258 has been deleted. To report, use 43270)

(Do not report 43270 in conjunction with 43248, 43249 for the same lesion)

(Do not report 43270 in conjunction with 43197, 43198, 43235, 44360, 44361, 44363, 44364, 44365, 44366, 44369, 44370, 44372, 44373, 44376, 44377, 44378, 44379)

(For esophagoscopic photodynamic therapy, use 43270 in conjunction with 96570, 96571 as appropriate)

⊙ **43259**   with endoscopic ultrasound examination, including the esophagus, stomach, and either the duodenum or a surgically altered stomach where the jejunum is examined distal to the anastomosis

(Do not report 43259 in conjunction with 43197, 43198, 43235, 43237, 43240, 43242, 43253, 44360, 44361, 44363, 44364, 44365, 44366, 44369, 44370, 44372, 44373, 44376, 44377, 44378, 44379, 76975)

(Do not report 43259 more than once per session)

#● **43210**   with esophagogastric fundoplasty, partial or complete, includes duodenoscopy when performed

►(Do not report 43210 in conjunction with 43180, 43191, 43197, 43200, 43235)◄

Endoscopic Retrograde Cholangiopancreatography (ERCP)

Report the appropriate code(s) for each service performed. Therapeutic ERCP (43261, 43262, 43263, 43264, 43265, 43274, 43275, 43276, 43277, 43278) includes diagnostic ERCP (43260). ERCP includes guide wire passage when performed. An ERCP is considered complete if one or more of the ductal system(s), (pancreatic/biliary) is visualized. To report ERCP attempted but with unsuccessful cannulation of any ductal system, see 43235-43259, 43266, 43270.

►(For percutaneous biliary catheter procedures, see 47490-47544)◄

Codes 43274, 43275, 43276, and 43277 describe ERCP with stent placement, removal or replacement (exchange) of stent(s), and balloon dilation within the pancreaticobiliary system. For reporting purposes, ducts that may be reported as stented or subject to stent replacement (exchange) or to balloon dilation include:

Pancreas: major and minor ducts

Biliary tree: common bile duct, right hepatic duct, left hepatic duct, cystic duct/gallbladder

ERCP with stent placement includes any balloon dilation performed in that duct. ERCP with more than one stent placement (eg, different ducts or side by side in the same duct) performed during the same day/session may be reported with 43274 more than once with modifier 59 appended to the subsequent procedure(s). For ERCP with more than one stent exchanged during the same day/session, 43276 may be reported for the initial stent exchange, and 43276 with modifier 59 for each additional stent exchange. ERCP with balloon dilation of more than one duct during the same day/session may be reported with modifier 59 appended to the subsequent procedure(s). Sphincteroplasty, which is balloon dilation of the ampulla (sphincter of Oddi), is reported with 43277, and includes sphincterotomy (43262) when performed.

To report ERCP via altered postoperative anatomy, see 43260, 43262, 43263, 43264, 43265, 43273, 43274, 43275, 43276, 43277, 43278, for Billroth II gastroenterostomy. See 47999 (Unlisted procedure, biliary tract) or 48999 (Unlisted procedure, pancreas) for ERCP via gastrostomy (laparoscopic or open) or via Roux-en-Y anatomy (eg, post-bariatric gastric bypass, post-total gastrectomy).

►To report optical endomicroscopy of the biliary tract and pancreas, use 0397T. Do not report optical endomicroscopy more than once per session.◄

Stone destruction includes any stone removal in the same ductal system (biliary/pancreatic). Code 43277 may be separately reported if sphincteroplasty or dilation of a ductal stricture is required before proceeding to remove stones/debris from the duct during the same session. Dilation that is incidental to the passage of an instrument to clear stones or debris is not separately reported.

(Do not report 43277 for use of a balloon catheter to clear stones/debris from a duct. Any dilation of the duct that may occur during this maneuver is considered inherent to the work of 43264 and 43265)

(If imaging of the ductal systems is performed, including images saved to the permanent record and report of the imaging, see 74328, 74329, 74330)

⊙ **43260**   Endoscopic retrograde cholangiopancreatography (ERCP); diagnostic, including collection of specimen(s) by brushing or washing, when performed (separate procedure)

(Do not report 43260 in conjunction with 43261, 43262, 43263, 43264, 43265, 43274, 43275, 43276, 43277, 43278)

⊙ **43261**   with biopsy, single or multiple

(Do not report 43261 in conjunction with 43260)

►(For percutaneous endoluminal biopsy of biliary tree, use 47543)◄

⊙ **43262**   with sphincterotomy/papillotomy

(43262 may be reported when sphincterotomy is performed in addition to 43261, 43263, 43264, 43265, 43275, 43278)

(Do not report 43262 in conjunction with 43274 for stent placement or with 43276 for stent replacement [exchange] in the same location)

(Do not report 43262 in conjunction with 43260, 43277)

►(For percutaneous balloon dilation of biliary duct(s) or of ampulla, use 47542)◄

⊙ **43263**   with pressure measurement of sphincter of Oddi

(Do not report 43263 in conjunction with 43260)

(Do not report 43263 more than once per session)

⊙ **43264**   with removal of calculi/debris from biliary/pancreatic duct(s)

(Do not report 43264 if no calculi or debris are found, even if balloon catheter is deployed)

(Do not report 43264 in conjunction with 43260, 43265)

►(For percutaneous removal of calculi/debris, use 47544)◄

⊙ **43265**   with destruction of calculi, any method (eg, mechanical, electrohydraulic, lithotripsy)

(Do not report 43265 in conjunction with 43260, 43264)

►(For percutaneous removal of calculi/debris, use 47544)◄

43266   Code is out of numerical sequence. See 43235-43273

(43267 has been deleted. To report, use 43274)

(43268 has been deleted. To report, use 43274)

(43269 has been deleted. To report, see 43275, 43276)

43270   Code is out of numerical sequence. See 43235-43273

(43271 has been deleted. To report, use 43277)

(43272 has been deleted. To report, use 43278)

#⊙ **43274**   with placement of endoscopic stent into biliary or pancreatic duct, including pre- and post-dilation and guide wire passage, when performed, including sphincterotomy, when performed, each stent

(Do not report 43274 in conjunction with 43262, 43275, 43276, 43277 for stent placement or replacement [exchange] in the same duct)

Digestive

(For stent placement in both the pancreatic duct and the common bile duct during the same operative session, placement of separate stents in both the right and left hepatic ducts, or placement of two side-by-side stents in the same duct, 43274 may be reported for each additional stent placed, using modifier 59 with the subsequent procedure[s])

(To report naso-biliary or naso-pancreatic drainage tube placement, use 43274)

►(For percutaneous placement of biliary stent(s), see 47538, 47539, 47540)◄

#⊙ 43275　　with removal of foreign body(s) or stent(s) from biliary/pancreatic duct(s)

(Do not report 43275 in conjunction with 43260, 43274, 43276)

(For removal of stent from biliary or pancreatic duct without ERCP, use 43247)

(Report 43275 only once for removal of one or more stents or foreign bodies from biliary/pancreatic duct[s] during the same session)

►(For percutaneous removal of calculi/debris, use 47544)◄

#⊙ 43276　　with removal and exchange of stent(s), biliary or pancreatic duct, including pre- and post-dilation and guide wire passage, when performed, including sphincterotomy, when performed, each stent exchanged

(43276 includes removal and replacement [exchange] of one stent. For replacement [exchange] of additional stent[s] during the same session, report 43276 with modifier 59 for each additional replacement [exchange])

(Do not report 43276 in conjunction with 43260, 43275)

(Do not report 43276 in conjunction with 43262, 43274 for stent placement or exchange in the same duct)

#⊙ 43277　　with trans-endoscopic balloon dilation of biliary/pancreatic duct(s) or of ampulla (sphincteroplasty), including sphincterotomy, when performed, each duct

(Do not report 43277 in conjunction with 43278 for the same lesion)

(Do not report 43277 in conjunction with 43260, 43262)

(Do not report 43277 for incidental dilation using balloon for stone/debris removal performed with 43264, 43265)

(If sphincterotomy without sphincteroplasty is performed on a separate pancreatic duct orifice during the same session [ie, pancreas divisum], report 43262 with modifier 59)

(Do not report 43277 in conjunction with 43274, 43276 for dilation and stent placement/replacement [exchange] in the same duct)

(For transendoscopic balloon dilation of multiple strictures during the same session, use 43277 with modifier 59 for each additional stricture dilated)

(For bilateral balloon dilation [both right and left hepatic ducts], 43277 may be reported twice with modifier 59 appended to the second procedure)

►(For percutaneous balloon dilation of biliary duct(s) or of ampulla (sphincteroplasty), use 47542)◄

#⊙ 43278　　with ablation of tumor(s), polyp(s), or other lesion(s), including pre- and post-dilation and guide wire passage, when performed

(Do not report 43278 in conjunction with 43277 for the same lesion)

(Do not report 43278 in conjunction with 43260)

(For ampullectomy, use 43254)

⊙✚ 43273　　Endoscopic cannulation of papilla with direct visualization of pancreatic/common bile duct(s) (List separately in addition to code(s) for primary procedure)

(Report 43273 once per procedure)

(Use 43273 in conjunction with 43260, 43261, 43262, 43263, 43264, 43265, 43274, 43275, 43276, 43277, 43278)

43274　　Code is out of numerical sequence. See 43260-43273

43275　　Code is out of numerical sequence. See 43260-43273

43276　　Code is out of numerical sequence. See 43260-43273

43277　　Code is out of numerical sequence. See 43260-43273

43278　　Code is out of numerical sequence. See 43260-43273

Laparoscopy

Surgical laparoscopy always includes diagnostic laparoscopy. To report a diagnostic laparoscopy (peritoneoscopy) (separate procedure), use 49320.

43279　　Laparoscopy, surgical, esophagomyotomy (Heller type), with fundoplasty, when performed

(For open approach, see 43330, 43331)

(Do not report 43279 in conjunction with 43280)

43280　　Laparoscopy, surgical, esophagogastric fundoplasty (eg, Nissen, Toupet procedures)

(Do not report 43280 in conjunction with 43279)

(For open approach, see 43327, 43328)

►(For laparoscopy, surgical, esophageal sphincter augmentation procedure, placement of sphincter augmentation device, see 0392T, 0393T)◄

►(For esophagogastroduodenoscopy fundoplasty, partial or complete, transoral approach, use 43210)◄

43281　　Laparoscopy, surgical, repair of paraesophageal hernia, includes fundoplasty, when performed; without implantation of mesh

43282   with implantation of mesh

(To report transabdominal paraesophageal hiatal hernia repair, see 43332, 43333. To report transthoracic diaphragmatic hernia repair, see 43334, 43335)

(Do not report 43213, 43214, 43220, 43233, 43249, 43281, 43282 in conjunction with 43280, 43450, 43453, 49568)

+ 43283   Laparoscopy, surgical, esophageal lengthening procedure (eg, Collis gastroplasty or wedge gastroplasty) (List separately in addition to code for primary procedure)

(Use 43283 in conjunction with 43280, 43281, 43282)

43289   Unlisted laparoscopy procedure, esophagus

Repair

43300   Esophagoplasty (plastic repair or reconstruction), cervical approach; without repair of tracheoesophageal fistula

43305   with repair of tracheoesophageal fistula

43310   Esophagoplasty (plastic repair or reconstruction), thoracic approach; without repair of tracheoesophageal fistula

43312   with repair of tracheoesophageal fistula

43313   Esophagoplasty for congenital defect (plastic repair or reconstruction), thoracic approach; without repair of congenital tracheoesophageal fistula

43314   with repair of congenital tracheoesophageal fistula

(Do not report modifier 63 in conjunction with 43313, 43314)

43320   Esophagogastrostomy (cardioplasty), with or without vagotomy and pyloroplasty, transabdominal or transthoracic approach

(43324 has been deleted. To report esophagogastric fundoplasty, see 43327, 43328)

(For laparoscopic procedure, use 43280)

43325   Esophagogastric fundoplasty, with fundic patch (Thal-Nissen procedure)

(For cricopharyngeal myotomy, use 43030)

43327   Esophagogastric fundoplasty partial or complete; laparotomy

43328   thoracotomy

▶(For esophagogastroduodenoscopy fundoplasty, partial or complete, transoral approach, use 43210)◀

43330   Esophagomyotomy (Heller type); abdominal approach

(For laparoscopic esophagomyotomy procedure, use 43279)

43331   thoracic approach

(For thoracoscopic esophagomyotomy, use 32665)

43332   Repair, paraesophageal hiatal hernia (including fundoplication), via laparotomy, except neonatal; without implantation of mesh or other prosthesis

43333   with implantation of mesh or other prosthesis

(For neonatal diaphragmatic hernia repair, use 39503)

43334   Repair, paraesophageal hiatal hernia (including fundoplication), via thoracotomy, except neonatal; without implantation of mesh or other prosthesis

43335   with implantation of mesh or other prosthesis

(For neonatal diaphragmatic hernia repair, use 39503)

43336   Repair, paraesophageal hiatal hernia, (including fundoplication), via thoracoabdominal incision, except neonatal; without implantation of mesh or other prosthesis

43337   with implantation of mesh or other prosthesis

(For neonatal diaphragmatic hernia repair, use 39503)

+ 43338   Esophageal lengthening procedure (eg, Collis gastroplasty or wedge gastroplasty) (List separately in addition to code for primary procedure)

(Use 43338 in conjunction with 43280, 43327-43337)

43340   Esophagojejunostomy (without total gastrectomy); abdominal approach

43341   thoracic approach

(43350 has been deleted)

43351   Esophagostomy, fistulization of esophagus, external; thoracic approach

43352   cervical approach

43360   Gastrointestinal reconstruction for previous esophagectomy, for obstructing esophageal lesion or fistula, or for previous esophageal exclusion; with stomach, with or without pyloroplasty

43361   with colon interposition or small intestine reconstruction, including intestine mobilization, preparation, and anastomosis(es)

43400   Ligation, direct, esophageal varices

43401   Transection of esophagus with repair, for esophageal varices

43405   Ligation or stapling at gastroesophageal junction for pre-existing esophageal perforation

43410   Suture of esophageal wound or injury; cervical approach

43415   transthoracic or transabdominal approach

43420   Closure of esophagostomy or fistula; cervical approach

43425   transthoracic or transabdominal approach

(To report transabdominal paraesophageal hiatal hernia repair, see 43332, 43333. To report transthoracic diaphragmatic hernia repair, see 43334, 43335)

Digestive

Manipulation

(For associated esophagogram, use 74220)

43450   Dilation of esophagus, by unguided sound or bougie, single or multiple passes

(For radiological supervision and interpretation, use 74360)

⊙ **43453**   Dilation of esophagus, over guide wire

(For dilation with endoscopic visualization, see 43195, 43226)

(For dilation of esophagus, by balloon or dilator, see 43214, 43220, 43233, 43249)

(For radiological supervision and interpretation, use 74360)

(43456 has been deleted. To report, use 43213)

(43458 has been deleted. To report, see 43214, 43233)

(For endoscopic dilation of esophagus with balloon less than 30 mm diameter, see 43195, 43220, 43249)

(For endoscopic dilation of esophagus with balloon 30 mm diameter or larger, see 43214, 43233)

43460   Esophagogastric tamponade, with balloon (Sengstaken type)

(For removal of esophageal foreign body by balloon catheter, see 43499, 74235)

Other Procedures

43496   Free jejunum transfer with microvascular anastomosis

(Do not report code 69990 in addition to code 43496)

43499   Unlisted procedure, esophagus

Stomach

Incision

43500   Gastrotomy; with exploration or foreign body removal

43501   with suture repair of bleeding ulcer

43502   with suture repair of pre-existing esophagogastric laceration (eg, Mallory-Weiss)

43510   with esophageal dilation and insertion of permanent intraluminal tube (eg, Celestin or Mousseaux-Barbin)

43520   Pyloromyotomy, cutting of pyloric muscle (Fredet-Ramstedt type operation)

(Do not report modifier 63 in conjunction with 43520)

Excision

(43600 has been deleted)

43605   Biopsy of stomach, by laparotomy

43610   Excision, local; ulcer or benign tumor of stomach

43611   malignant tumor of stomach

43620   Gastrectomy, total; with esophagoenterostomy

43621   with Roux-en-Y reconstruction

43622   with formation of intestinal pouch, any type

43631   Gastrectomy, partial, distal; with gastroduodenostomy

43632   with gastrojejunostomy

43633   with Roux-en-Y reconstruction

43634   with formation of intestinal pouch

+ **43635**   Vagotomy when performed with partial distal gastrectomy (List separately in addition to code[s] for primary procedure)

(Use 43635 in conjunction with 43631, 43632, 43633, 43634)

43640   Vagotomy including pyloroplasty, with or without gastrostomy; truncal or selective

(For pyloroplasty, use 43800)

(For vagotomy, see 64755, 64760)

43641   parietal cell (highly selective)

(For upper gastrointestinal endoscopy, see 43235-43259)

Laparoscopy

Surgical laparoscopy always includes diagnostic laparoscopy. To report a diagnostic laparoscopy (peritoneoscopy) (separate procedure), use 49320.

(For upper gastrointestinal endoscopy including esophagus, stomach, and either the duodenum and/or jejunum, see 43235-43259)

43644   Laparoscopy, surgical, gastric restrictive procedure; with gastric bypass and Roux-en-Y gastroenterostomy (roux limb 150 cm or less)

(Do not report 43644 in conjunction with 43846, 49320)

(Esophagogastroduodenoscopy [EGD] performed for a separate condition should be reported with modifier 59)

(For greater than 150 cm, use 43645)

(For open procedure, use 43846)

43645   with gastric bypass and small intestine reconstruction to limit absorption

(Do not report 43645 in conjunction with 49320, 43847)

43647   Laparoscopy, surgical; implantation or replacement of gastric neurostimulator electrodes, antrum

43648   revision or removal of gastric neurostimulator electrodes, antrum

(For open approach, see 43881, 43882)

(For insertion of gastric neurostimulator pulse generator, use 64590)

(For revision or removal of gastric neurostimulator pulse generator, use 64595)

(For electronic analysis and programming of gastric neurostimulator pulse generator, see 95980-95982)

(For laparoscopic implantation, revision, or removal of gastric neurostimulator electrodes, lesser curvature [morbid obesity], use 43659)

(For laparoscopic implantation, revision, replacement, or removal of vagus nerve blocking neurostimulator electrode array and/or pulse generator at the esophagogastric junction, see 0312T-0317T)

43651 Laparoscopy, surgical; transection of vagus nerves, truncal

43652 transection of vagus nerves, selective or highly selective

43653 gastrostomy, without construction of gastric tube (eg, Stamm procedure) (separate procedure)

43659 Unlisted laparoscopy procedure, stomach

Introduction

43752 Naso- or oro-gastric tube placement, requiring physician's skill and fluoroscopic guidance (includes fluoroscopy, image documentation and report)

(Do not report 43752 in conjunction with critical care codes 99291-99292, neonatal critical care codes 99468, 99469, pediatric critical care codes 99471, 99472 or low birth weight intensive care service codes 99478, 99479)

(For percutaneous placement of gastrostomy tube, use 49440)

(For enteric tube placement, see 44500, 74340)

43753 Gastric intubation and aspiration(s) therapeutic, necessitating physician's skill (eg, for gastrointestinal hemorrhage), including lavage if performed

43754 Gastric intubation and aspiration, diagnostic; single specimen (eg, acid analysis)

43755 collection of multiple fractional specimens with gastric stimulation, single or double lumen tube (gastric secretory study) (eg, histamine, insulin, pentagastrin, calcium, secretin), includes drug administration

(For gastric acid analysis, use 82930)

(For naso- or oro-gastric tube placement by physician with fluoroscopic guidance, use 43752)

(Report the drug[s] or substance[s] administered. The fluid used to administer the drug[s] is not separately reported)

43756 Duodenal intubation and aspiration, diagnostic, includes image guidance; single specimen (eg, bile study for crystals or afferent loop culture)

43757 collection of multiple fractional specimens with pancreatic or gallbladder stimulation, single or double lumen tube, includes drug administration

(For appropriate chemical analysis procedures, see 89049-89240)

(Report the substances[s] or drug[s] administered. The fluid used to administer the drug[s] is not separately reported)

43760 Change of gastrostomy tube, percutaneous, without imaging or endoscopic guidance

(To report fluoroscopically guided replacement of gastrostomy tube, use 49450)

(For endoscopic placement of gastrostomy tube, use 43246)

43761 Repositioning of a naso- or oro-gastric feeding tube, through the duodenum for enteric nutrition

(Do not report 43761 in conjunction with 44500, 49446)

(If imaging guidance is performed, use 76000)

(For endoscopic conversion of a gastrostomy tube to jejunostomy tube, use 44373)

(For placement of a long gastrointestinal tube into the duodenum, use 44500)

Bariatric Surgery

Bariatric surgical procedures may involve the stomach, duodenum, jejunum, and/or the ileum.

Laparoscopy

Surgical laparoscopy always includes diagnostic laparoscopy. To report a diagnostic laparoscopy (separate procedure), use 49320.

Typical postoperative follow-up care (see Surgery Guidelines, CPT Surgical Package Definition) after gastric restriction using the adjustable gastric restrictive device includes subsequent restrictive device adjustment(s) through the postoperative period for the typical patient. Adjustment consists of changing the gastric restrictive device component diameter by injection or aspiration of fluid through the subcutaneous port component.

43770 Laparoscopy, surgical, gastric restrictive procedure; placement of adjustable gastric restrictive device (eg, gastric band and subcutaneous port components)

(For individual component placement, report 43770 with modifier 52)

43771 revision of adjustable gastric restrictive device component only

43772 removal of adjustable gastric restrictive device component only

43773 removal and replacement of adjustable gastric restrictive device component only

(Do not report 43773 in conjunction with 43772)

Digestive

43774   removal of adjustable gastric restrictive device and subcutaneous port components

(For removal and replacement of both gastric band and subcutaneous port components, use 43659)

43775   longitudinal gastrectomy (ie, sleeve gastrectomy)

(For open gastric restrictive procedure, without gastric bypass, for morbid obesity, other than vertical-banded gastroplasty, use 43843)

(For laparoscopic implantation, revision, replacement, removal or reprogramming of vagus nerve blocking neurostimulator electrode array and/or pulse generator at the esophagogastric junction, see 0312T-0317T)

Other Procedures

43800   Pyloroplasty

(For pyloroplasty and vagotomy, use 43640)

43810   Gastroduodenostomy

43820   Gastrojejunostomy; without vagotomy

43825   with vagotomy, any type

43830   Gastrostomy, open; without construction of gastric tube (eg, Stamm procedure) (separate procedure)

43831   neonatal, for feeding

(For change of gastrostomy tube, use 43760)

(Do not report modifier 63 in conjunction with 43831)

43832   with construction of gastric tube (eg, Janeway procedure)

(For percutaneous endoscopic gastrostomy, use 43246)

43840   Gastrorrhaphy, suture of perforated duodenal or gastric ulcer, wound, or injury

43842   Gastric restrictive procedure, without gastric bypass, for morbid obesity; vertical-banded gastroplasty

43843   other than vertical-banded gastroplasty

(For laparoscopic longitudinal gastrectomy [ie, sleeve gastrectomy], use 43775)

43845   Gastric restrictive procedure with partial gastrectomy, pylorus-preserving duodenoileostomy and ileoileostomy (50 to 100 cm common channel) to limit absorption (biliopancreatic diversion with duodenal switch)

(Do not report 43845 in conjunction with 43633, 43847, 44130, 49000)

43846   Gastric restrictive procedure, with gastric bypass for morbid obesity; with short limb (150 cm or less) Roux-en-Y gastroenterostomy

(For greater than 150 cm, use 43847)

(For laparoscopic procedure, use 43644)

43847   with small intestine reconstruction to limit absorption

43848   Revision, open, of gastric restrictive procedure for morbid obesity, other than adjustable gastric restrictive device (separate procedure)

(For laparoscopic adjustable gastric restrictive procedures, see 43770-43774)

(For gastric restrictive port procedures, see 43886-43888)

43850   Revision of gastroduodenal anastomosis (gastroduodenostomy) with reconstruction; without vagotomy

43855   with vagotomy

43860   Revision of gastrojejunal anastomosis (gastrojejunostomy) with reconstruction, with or without partial gastrectomy or intestine resection; without vagotomy

43865   with vagotomy

43870   Closure of gastrostomy, surgical

43880   Closure of gastrocolic fistula

43881   Implantation or replacement of gastric neurostimulator electrodes, antrum, open

43882   Revision or removal of gastric neurostimulator electrodes, antrum, open

(For laparoscopic approach, see 43647, 43648)

(For insertion of gastric neurostimulator pulse generator, use 64590)

(For revision or removal of gastric neurostimulator pulse generator, use 64595)

(For electronic analysis and programming of gastric neurostimulator pulse generator, see 95980-95982)

(For open implantation, revision, or removal of gastric neurostimulator electrodes, lesser curvature [morbid obesity], use 43999)

(For laparoscopic implantation, revision, replacement, removal or reprogramming of vagus nerve blocking neurostimulator electrode array and/or pulse generator at the esophagogastric junction, see 0312T-0317T)

(For open implantation, revision, or removal of gastric lesser curvature or vagal trunk (EGJ) neurostimulator electrodes, [morbid obesity], use 43999)

43886   Gastric restrictive procedure, open; revision of subcutaneous port component only

43887   removal of subcutaneous port component only

43888   removal and replacement of subcutaneous port component only

(Do not report 43888 in conjunction with 43774, 43887)

(For laparoscopic removal of both gastric restrictive device and subcutaneous port components, use 43774)

(For removal and replacement of both gastric restrictive device and subcutaneous port components, use 43659)

43999   Unlisted procedure, stomach

Intestines (Except Rectum)

Incision

44005   Enterolysis (freeing of intestinal adhesion) (separate procedure)

(Do not report 44005 in addition to 45136)

(For laparoscopic approach, use 44180)

44010   Duodenotomy, for exploration, biopsy(s), or foreign body removal

+ 44015   Tube or needle catheter jejunostomy for enteral alimentation, intraoperative, any method (List separately in addition to primary procedure)

44020   Enterotomy, small intestine, other than duodenum; for exploration, biopsy(s), or foreign body removal

44021   for decompression (eg, Baker tube)

44025   Colotomy, for exploration, biopsy(s), or foreign body removal

(For exteriorization of intestine (Mikulicz resection with crushing of spur), see 44602-44605)

44050   Reduction of volvulus, intussusception, internal hernia, by laparotomy

44055   Correction of malrotation by lysis of duodenal bands and/or reduction of midgut volvulus (eg, Ladd procedure)

(Do not report modifier 63 in conjunction with 44055)

Excision

Intestinal allotransplantation involves three distinct components of physician work:

1. **Cadaver donor enterectomy,** which includes harvesting the intestine graft and cold preservation of the graft (perfusing with cold preservation solution and cold maintenance) (use 44132). **Living donor enterectomy,** which includes harvesting the intestine graft, cold preservation of the graft (perfusing with cold preservation solution and cold maintenance), and care of the donor (use 44133).

2. **Backbench work:**

Standard preparation of an intestine allograft prior to transplantation includes mobilization and fashioning of the superior mesenteric artery and vein(see 44715).

Additional reconstruction of an intestine allograft prior to transplantation may include venous and/or arterial anastomosis(es) (see 44720-44721).

3. **Recipient intestinal allotransplantation with or without recipient enterectomy,** which includes transplantation of allograft and care of the recipient (see 44135, 44136).

44100   Biopsy of intestine by capsule, tube, peroral (1 or more specimens)

44110   Excision of 1 or more lesions of small or large intestine not requiring anastomosis, exteriorization, or fistulization; single enterotomy

44111   multiple enterotomies

44120   Enterectomy, resection of small intestine; single resection and anastomosis

(Do not report 44120 in addition to 45136)

+ 44121   each additional resection and anastomosis (List separately in addition to code for primary procedure)

(Use 44121 in conjunction with 44120)

44125   with enterostomy

44126   Enterectomy, resection of small intestine for congenital atresia, single resection and anastomosis of proximal segment of intestine; without tapering

44127   with tapering

+ 44128   each additional resection and anastomosis (List separately in addition to code for primary procedure)

(Use 44128 in conjunction with 44126, 44127)

(Do not report modifier 63 in conjunction with 44126, 44127, 44128)

44130   Enteroenterostomy, anastomosis of intestine, with or without cutaneous enterostomy (separate procedure)

44132   Donor enterectomy (including cold preservation), open; from cadaver donor

44133   partial, from living donor

(For backbench intestinal graft preparation or reconstruction, see 44715, 44720, 44721)

44135   Intestinal allotransplantation; from cadaver donor

44136   from living donor

44137   Removal of transplanted intestinal allograft, complete

(For partial removal of transplant allograft, see 44120, 44121, 44140)

+ 44139   Mobilization (take-down) of splenic flexure performed in conjunction with partial colectomy (List separately in addition to primary procedure)

(Use 44139 in conjunction with 44140-44147)

44140   Colectomy, partial; with anastomosis

(For laparoscopic procedure, use 44204)

44141   with skin level cecostomy or colostomy

44143   with end colostomy and closure of distal segment (Hartmann type procedure)

(For laparoscopic procedure, use 44206)

44144   with resection, with colostomy or ileostomy and creation of mucofistula

44145   with coloproctostomy (low pelvic anastomosis)

(For laparoscopic procedure, use 44207)

Digestive

44146   with coloproctostomy (low pelvic anastomosis), with colostomy

(For laparoscopic procedure, use 44208)

44147   abdominal and transanal approach

44150 Colectomy, total, abdominal, without proctectomy; with ileostomy or ileoproctostomy

(For laparoscopic procedure, use 44210)

44151   with continent ileostomy

44155 Colectomy, total, abdominal, with proctectomy; with ileostomy

(For laparoscopic procedure, use 44212)

44156   with continent ileostomy

44157   with ileoanal anastomosis, includes loop ileostomy, and rectal mucosectomy, when performed

44158   with ileoanal anastomosis, creation of ileal reservoir (S or J), includes loop ileostomy, and rectal mucosectomy, when performed

(For laparoscopic procedure, use 44211)

44160 Colectomy, partial, with removal of terminal ileum with ileocolostomy

(For laparoscopic procedure, use 44205)

Laparoscopy

Surgical laparoscopy always includes diagnostic laparoscopy. To report a diagnostic laparoscopy (peritoneoscopy) (separate procedure), use 49320.

Incision

44180 Laparoscopy, surgical, enterolysis (freeing of intestinal adhesion) (separate procedure)

(For laparoscopy with salpingolysis, ovariolysis, use 58660)

Enterostomy—External Fistulization of Intestines

44186 Laparoscopy, surgical; jejunostomy (eg, for decompression or feeding)

44187   ileostomy or jejunostomy, non-tube

(For open procedure, use 44310)

44188 Laparoscopy, surgical, colostomy or skin level cecostomy

(For open procedure, use 44320)

(Do not report 44188 in conjunction with 44970)

Excision

44202 Laparoscopy, surgical; enterectomy, resection of small intestine, single resection and anastomosis

+ 44203   each additional small intestine resection and anastomosis (List separately in addition to code for primary procedure)

(Use 44203 in conjunction with 44202)

(For open procedure, see 44120, 44121)

44204   colectomy, partial, with anastomosis

(For open procedure, use 44140)

44205   colectomy, partial, with removal of terminal ileum with ileocolostomy

(For open procedure, use 44160)

44206   colectomy, partial, with end colostomy and closure of distal segment (Hartmann type procedure)

(For open procedure, use 44143)

44207   colectomy, partial, with anastomosis, with coloproctostomy (low pelvic anastomosis)

(For open procedure, use 44145)

44208   colectomy, partial, with anastomosis, with coloproctostomy (low pelvic anastomosis) with colostomy

(For open procedure, use 44146)

44210   colectomy, total, abdominal, without proctectomy, with ileostomy or ileoproctostomy

(For open procedure, use 44150)

44211   colectomy, total, abdominal, with proctectomy, with ileoanal anastomosis, creation of ileal reservoir (S or J), with loop ileostomy, includes rectal mucosectomy, when performed

(For open procedure, see 44157, 44158)

44212   colectomy, total, abdominal, with proctectomy, with ileostomy

(For open procedure, use 44155)

+ 44213 Laparoscopy, surgical, mobilization (take-down) of splenic flexure performed in conjunction with partial colectomy (List separately in addition to primary procedure)

(Use 44213 in conjunction with 44204-44208)

(For open procedure, use 44139)

Repair

44227 Laparoscopy, surgical, closure of enterostomy, large or small intestine, with resection and anastomosis

(For open procedure, see 44625, 44626)

Other Procedures

44238 Unlisted laparoscopy procedure, intestine (except rectum)

Enterostomy—External Fistulization of Intestines

44300   Placement, enterostomy or cecostomy, tube open (eg, for feeding or decompression) (separate procedure)

(For percutaneous placement of duodenostomy, jejunostomy, gastro-jejunostomy or cecostomy [or other colonic] tube including fluoroscopic imaging guidance, see 49441-49442)

44310   Ileostomy or jejunostomy, non-tube

(For laparoscopic procedure, use 44187)

(Do not report 44310 in conjunction with 44144, 44150-44151, 44155, 44156, 45113, 45119, 45136)

44312   Revision of ileostomy; simple (release of superficial scar) (separate procedure)

44314   complicated (reconstruction in-depth) (separate procedure)

44316   Continent ileostomy (Kock procedure) (separate procedure)

(For fiberoptic evaluation, use 44385)

44320   Colostomy or skin level cecostomy;

(For laparoscopic procedure, use 44188)

(Do not report 44320 in conjunction with 44141, 44144, 44146, 44605, 45110, 45119, 45126, 45563, 45805, 45825, 50810, 51597, 57307, or 58240)

44322   with multiple biopsies (eg, for congenital megacolon) (separate procedure)

44340   Revision of colostomy; simple (release of superficial scar) (separate procedure)

44345   complicated (reconstruction in-depth) (separate procedure)

44346   with repair of paracolostomy hernia (separate procedure)

Endoscopy, Small Intestine

When bleeding occurs as the result of an endoscopic procedure, control of bleeding is not reported separately during the same operative session.

Antegrade transoral small intestinal endoscopy (enteroscopy) is defined by the most distal segment of small intestine that is examined. Codes 44360, 44361, 44363, 44364, 44365, 44366, 44369, 44370, 44372, 44373 are endoscopic procedures to visualize the esophagus through the jejunum using an antegrade approach. Codes 44376, 44377, 44378, 44379 are endoscopic procedures to visualize the esophagus through the ileum using an antegrade approach. If an endoscope cannot be advanced at least 50 cm beyond the pylorus, see 43233, 43235-43259, 43266, 43270; if an endoscope can be passed at least 50 cm beyond pylorus but only into jejunum, see 44360, 44361, 44363, 44364, 44365, 44366, 44369, 44370, 44372, 44373.

To report retrograde examination of small intestine via anus or colon stoma, use 44799, unlisted procedure, intestine.

(Do not report 44360, 44361, 44363, 44364, 44365, 44366, 44369, 44370, 44372, 44373 in conjunction with 43233, 43235-43259, 43266, 43270, 44376, 44377, 44378, 44379)

(Do not report 44376, 44377, 44378, 44379 in conjunction with 43233, 43235-43259, 43266, 43270, 44360, 44361, 44363, 44364, 44365, 44366, 44369, 44370, 44372, 44373)

(For esophagogastroduodenoscopy, see 43233, 43235-43259, 43266, 43270)

⊙ **44360**   Small intestinal endoscopy, enteroscopy beyond second portion of duodenum, not including ileum; diagnostic, including collection of specimen(s) by brushing or washing, when performed (separate procedure)

⊙ **44361**   with biopsy, single or multiple

⊙ **44363**   with removal of foreign body(s)

⊙ **44364**   with removal of tumor(s), polyp(s), or other lesion(s) by snare technique

⊙ **44365**   with removal of tumor(s), polyp(s), or other lesion(s) by hot biopsy forceps or bipolar cautery

⊙ **44366**   with control of bleeding (eg, injection, bipolar cautery, unipolar cautery, laser, heater probe, stapler, plasma coagulator)

⊙ **44369**   with ablation of tumor(s), polyp(s), or other lesion(s) not amenable to removal by hot biopsy forceps, bipolar cautery or snare technique

⊙ **44370**   with transendoscopic stent placement (includes predilation)

⊙ **44372**   with placement of percutaneous jejunostomy tube

⊙ **44373**   with conversion of percutaneous gastrostomy tube to percutaneous jejunostomy tube

(For fiberoptic jejunostomy through stoma, use 43235)

⊙ **44376**   Small intestinal endoscopy, enteroscopy beyond second portion of duodenum, including ileum; diagnostic, with or without collection of specimen(s) by brushing or washing (separate procedure)

(Do not report 44376 in conjunction with 44360, 44361, 44363, 44364, 44365, 44366, 44369, 44370, 44372, 44373)

⊙ **44377**   with biopsy, single or multiple

(Do not report 44377 in conjunction with 44360, 44361, 44363, 44364, 44365, 44366, 44369, 44370, 44372, 44373)

⊙ **44378**   with control of bleeding (eg, injection, bipolar cautery, unipolar cautery, laser, heater probe, stapler, plasma coagulator)

Digestive

(Do not report 44378 in conjunction with 44360, 44361, 44363, 44364, 44365, 44366, 44369, 44370, 44372, 44373)

⊙ **44379**   with transendoscopic stent placement (includes predilation)

(Do not report 44379 in conjunction with 44360, 44361, 44363, 44364, 44365, 44366, 44369, 44370, 44372, 44373)

Endoscopy, Stomal

Definitions

Proctosigmoidoscopy is the examination of the rectum and may include examination of a portion of the sigmoid colon.

Sigmoidoscopy is the examination of the entire rectum, sigmoid colon and may include examination of a portion of the descending colon.

Colonoscopy is the examination of the entire colon, from the rectum to the cecum, and may include examination of the terminal ileum or small intestine proximal to an anastomosis.

Colonoscopy through stoma is the examination of the colon, from the colostomy stoma to the cecum or colon-small intestine anastomosis, and may include examination of the terminal ileum or small intestine proximal to an anastomosis.

When performing a diagnostic or screening endoscopic procedure on a patient who is scheduled and prepared for a total colonoscopy, if the physician is unable to advance the colonoscope to the cecum or colon-small intestine anastomosis due to unforeseen circumstances, report 45378 (colonoscopy) or 44388 (colonoscopy through stoma) with modifier 53 and provide appropriate documentation.

If a therapeutic colonoscopy (44389-44407, 45379, 45380, 45381, 45382, 45384, 45388, 45398) is performed and does not reach the cecum or colon-small intestine anastomosis, report the appropriate therapeutic colonoscopy code with modifier 52 and provide appropriate documentation.

Report ileoscopy through stoma (44380, 44381, 44382, 44384) for endoscopic examination of a patient who has an ileostomy.

Report colonoscopy through stoma (44388-44408) for endoscopic examination of a patient who has undergone segmental resection of the colon (eg, hemicolectomy, sigmoid colectomy, low anterior resection) and has a colostomy.

For colonoscopy per rectum, see 45378, 45390, 45392, 45393, 45398.

Report proctosigmoidoscopy (45300-45327), flexible sigmoidoscopy (45330-45347), or anoscopy (46600,

46604, 46606, 46608, 46610, 46611, 46612, 46614, 46615), as appropriate for endoscopic examination of the defunctionalized rectum or distal colon in a patient who has undergone colectomy, in addition to colonoscopy through stoma (44388-44408) or ileoscopy through stoma (44380, 44381, 44382, 44384) if appropriate.

When bleeding occurs as the result of an endoscopic procedure, control of bleeding is not reported separately during the same operative session.

For computed tomographic colonography, see 74261, 74262, 74263.

⊙ **44380**   Ileoscopy, through stoma; diagnostic, including collection of specimen(s) by brushing or washing, when performed (separate procedure)

44381   Code is out of numerical sequence. See 44380-44394

(Do not report 44380 in conjunction with 44381, 44382, 44384)

⊙ **44382**   with biopsy, single or multiple

(Do not report 44382 in conjunction with 44380)

#⊙ **44381**   with transendoscopic balloon dilation

(Do not report 44381 in conjunction with 44380, 44384)

(If fluoroscopic guidance is performed, use 74360)

(For transendoscopic balloon dilation of multiple strictures during the same session, report 44381 with modifier 59 for each additional stricture dilated)

(44383 has been deleted. To report, use 44384)

⊙ **44384**   with placement of endoscopic stent (includes pre- and post-dilation and guide wire passage, when performed)

(Do not report 44384 in conjunction with 44380, 44381)

(If fluoroscopic guidance is performed, use 74360)

⊙ **44385**   Endoscopic evaluation of small intestinal pouch (eg, Kock pouch, ileal reservoir [S or J]); diagnostic, including collection of specimen(s) by brushing or washing, when performed (separate procedure)

(Do not report 44385 in conjunction with 44386)

⊙ **44386**   with biopsy, single or multiple

(Do not report 44386 in conjunction with 44385)

⊙ **44388**   Colonoscopy through stoma; diagnostic, including collection of specimen(s) by brushing or washing, when performed (separate procedure)

(Do not report 44388 in conjunction with 44389-44408)

⊙ **44389**   with biopsy, single or multiple

(Do not report 44389 in conjunction with 44403 for the same lesion)

(Do not report 44389 in conjunction with 44388)

⊙ **44390**   with removal of foreign body(s)

(Do not report 44390 in conjunction with 44388)

(If fluoroscopic guidance is performed, use 76000)

⊙ **44391**   with control of bleeding, any method

(Do not report 44391 in conjunction with 44404 for the same lesion)

(Do not report 44391 in conjunction with 44388)

⊙ **44392**   with removal of tumor(s), polyp(s), or other lesion(s) by hot biopsy forceps

(Do not report 44392 in conjunction with 44388)

(44393 has been deleted. To report, use 44401)

#⊙ **44401**   with ablation of tumor(s), polyp(s), or other lesion(s) (includes pre-and post-dilation and guide wire passage, when performed)

(Do not report 44401 in conjunction with 44405 for the same lesion)

(Do not report 44401 in conjunction with 44388)

⊙ **44394**   with removal of tumor(s), polyp(s), or other lesion(s) by snare technique

(Do not report 44394 in conjunction with 44403 for the same lesion)

(Do not report 44394 in conjunction with 44388)

(For endoscopic mucosal resection, use 44403)

(44397 has been deleted. To report, use 44402)

44401   Code is out of numerical sequence. See 44380-44408

⊙ **44402**   with endoscopic stent placement (including pre- and post-dilation and guide wire passage, when performed)

(Do not report 44402 in conjunction with 44388, 44405)

(If fluoroscopic guidance is performed, use 74360)

⊙ **44403**   with endoscopic mucosal resection

(Do not report 44403 in conjunction with 44389, 44394, 44404 for the same lesion)

(Do not report 44403 in conjunction with 44388)

⊙ **44404**   with directed submucosal injection(s), any substance

(Do not report 44404 in conjunction with 44391, 44403 for the same lesion)

(Do not report 44404 in conjunction with 44388)

⊙ **44405**   with transendoscopic balloon dilation

(Do not report 44405 in conjunction with 44388, 44401, 44402)

(If fluoroscopic guidance is performed, use 74360)

(For transendoscopic balloon dilation of multiple strictures during the same session, report 44405 with modifier 59 for each additional stricture dilated)

⊙ **44406**   with endoscopic ultrasound examination, limited to the sigmoid, descending, transverse, or ascending colon and cecum and adjacent structures

(Do not report 44406 in conjunction with 44388, 44407, 76975)

(Do not report 44406 more than once per session)

⊙ **44407**   with transendoscopic ultrasound guided intramural or transmural fine needle aspiration/biopsy(s), includes endoscopic ultrasound examination limited to the sigmoid, descending, transverse, or ascending colon and cecum and adjacent structures

(Do not report 44407 in conjunction with 44388, 44406, 76942, 76975)

(Do not report 44407 more than once per session)

⊙ **44408**   with decompression (for pathologic distention) (eg, volvulus, megacolon), including placement of decompression tube, when performed

(Do not report 44408 in conjunction with 44388)

(Do not report 44408 more than once per session)

Introduction

⊙⊘ **44500**   Introduction of long gastrointestinal tube (eg, Miller-Abbott) (separate procedure)

(For radiological supervision and interpretation, use 74340)

(For naso- or oro-gastric tube placement, use 43752)

Repair

44602   Suture of small intestine (enterorrhaphy) for perforated ulcer, diverticulum, wound, injury or rupture; single perforation

44603   multiple perforations

44604   Suture of large intestine (colorrhaphy) for perforated ulcer, diverticulum, wound, injury or rupture (single or multiple perforations); without colostomy

44605   with colostomy

44615   Intestinal stricturoplasty (enterotomy and enterorrhaphy) with or without dilation, for intestinal obstruction

44620   Closure of enterostomy, large or small intestine;

44625   with resection and anastomosis other than colorectal

44626   with resection and colorectal anastomosis (eg, closure of Hartmann type procedure)

(For laparoscopic procedure, use 44227)

44640   Closure of intestinal cutaneous fistula

44650   Closure of enteroenteric or enterocolic fistula

44660   Closure of enterovesical fistula; without intestinal or bladder resection

Digestive

44661 with intestine and/or bladder resection

(For closure of renocolic fistula, see 50525, 50526)

(For closure of gastrocolic fistula, use 43880)

(For closure of rectovesical fistula, see 45800, 45805)

44680 Intestinal plication (separate procedure)

Other Procedures

44700 Exclusion of small intestine from pelvis by mesh or other prosthesis, or native tissue (eg, bladder or omentum)

(For therapeutic radiation clinical treatment, see **Radiation Oncology** section)

+ 44701 Intraoperative colonic lavage (List separately in addition to code for primary procedure)

(Use 44701 in conjunction with 44140, 44145, 44150, or 44604 as appropriate)

(Do not report 44701 in conjunction with 44300, 44950-44960)

44705 Preparation of fecal microbiota for instillation, including assessment of donor specimen

(Do not report 44705 in conjunction with 74283)

(For fecal instillation by oro-nasogastric tube or enema, use 44799)

44715 Backbench standard preparation of cadaver or living donor intestine allograft prior to transplantation, including mobilization and fashioning of the superior mesenteric artery and vein

44720 Backbench reconstruction of cadaver or living donor intestine allograft prior to transplantation; venous anastomosis, each

44721 arterial anastomosis, each

44799 Unlisted procedure, small intestine

(For unlisted laparoscopic procedure, intestine except rectum, use 44238)

(For unlisted procedure, colon, use 45399)

Meckel's Diverticulum and the Mesentery

Excision

44800 Excision of Meckel's diverticulum (diverticulectomy) or omphalomesenteric duct

44820 Excision of lesion of mesentery (separate procedure)

(With intestine resection, see 44120 or 44140 et seq)

Suture

44850 Suture of mesentery (separate procedure)

(For reduction and repair of internal hernia, use 44050)

Other Procedures

44899 Unlisted procedure, Meckel's diverticulum and the mesentery

Appendix

Incision

44900 Incision and drainage of appendiceal abscess, open

(44901 has been deleted)

(For percutaneous image-guided drainage by catheter of appendiceal abscess, use 49406)

Excision

44950 Appendectomy;

(Incidental appendectomy during intra-abdominal surgery does not usually warrant a separate identification. If necessary to report, add modifier 52)

+ 44955 when done for indicated purpose at time of other major procedure (not as separate procedure) (List separately in addition to code for primary procedure)

44960 for ruptured appendix with abscess or generalized peritonitis

Laparoscopy

Surgical laparoscopy always includes diagnostic laparoscopy. To report a diagnostic laparoscopy (peritoneoscopy) (separate procedure), use 49320.

44970 Laparoscopy, surgical, appendectomy

44979 Unlisted laparoscopy procedure, appendix

Colon and Rectum

Incision

45000 Transrectal drainage of pelvic abscess

(For transrectal image-guided fluid collection drainage by catheter of pelvic abscess, use 49407)

45005 Incision and drainage of submucosal abscess, rectum

45020 Incision and drainage of deep supralevator, pelvirectal, or retrorectal abscess

(See also 46050, 46060)

Excision

45100 Biopsy of anorectal wall, anal approach (eg, congenital megacolon)

(For endoscopic biopsy, use 45305)

45108 Anorectal myomectomy

Digestive

45110   Proctectomy; complete, combined abdominoperineal, with colostomy

(For laparoscopic procedure, use 45395)

45111   partial resection of rectum, transabdominal approach

45112   Proctectomy, combined abdominoperineal, pull-through procedure (eg, colo-anal anastomosis)

(For colo-anal anastomosis with colonic reservoir or pouch, use 45119)

45113   Proctectomy, partial, with rectal mucosectomy, ileoanal anastomosis, creation of ileal reservoir (S or J), with or without loop ileostomy

45114   Proctectomy, partial, with anastomosis; abdominal and transsacral approach

45116   transsacral approach only (Kraske type)

45119   Proctectomy, combined abdominoperineal pull-through procedure (eg, colo-anal anastomosis), with creation of colonic reservoir (eg, J-pouch), with diverting enterostomy when performed

(For laparoscopic procedure, use 45397)

45120   Proctectomy, complete (for congenital megacolon), abdominal and perineal approach; with pull-through procedure and anastomosis (eg, Swenson, Duhamel, or Soave type operation)

45121   with subtotal or total colectomy, with multiple biopsies

45123   Proctectomy, partial, without anastomosis, perineal approach

45126   Pelvic exenteration for colorectal malignancy, with proctectomy (with or without colostomy), with removal of bladder and ureteral transplantations, and/or hysterectomy, or cervicectomy, with or without removal of tube(s), with or without removal of ovary(s), or any combination thereof

45130   Excision of rectal procidentia, with anastomosis; perineal approach

45135   abdominal and perineal approach

45136   Excision of ileoanal reservoir with ileostomy

(Do not report 45136 in addition to 44005, 44120, 44310)

45150   Division of stricture of rectum

45160   Excision of rectal tumor by proctotomy, transsacral or transcoccygeal approach

45171   Excision of rectal tumor, transanal approach; not including muscularis propria (ie, partial thickness)

45172   including muscularis propria (ie, full thickness)

(For destruction of rectal tumor, transanal approach, use 45190)

(For transanal endoscopic microsurgical [ie, TEMS] excision of rectal tumor, including muscularis propria [ie, full thickness], use 0184T)

Destruction

45190   Destruction of rectal tumor (eg, electrodesiccation, electrosurgery, laser ablation, laser resection, cryosurgery) transanal approach

(For excision of rectal tumor, transanal approach, see 45171, 45172)

(For transanal endoscopic microsurgical [ie, TEMS] excision of rectal tumor, including muscularis propria [ie, full thickness], use 0184T)

Endoscopy

Definitions

Proctosigmoidoscopy is the examination of the rectum and may include examination of a portion of the sigmoid colon.

Sigmoidoscopy is the examination of the entire rectum, sigmoid colon and may include examination of a portion of the descending colon.

Colonoscopy is the examination of the entire colon, from the rectum to the cecum, and may include examination of the terminal ileum or small intestine proximal to an anastomosis.

Colonoscopy through stoma is the examination of the colon, from the colostomy stoma to the cecum, and may include examination of the terminal ileum or small intestine proximal to an anastomosis.

When performing a diagnostic or screening endoscopic procedure on a patient who is scheduled and prepared for a total colonoscopy, if the physician is unable to advance the colonoscope to the cecum or colon-small intestine anastomosis due to unforeseen circumstances, report 45378 (colonoscopy) or 44388 (colonoscopy through stoma) with modifier 53 and provide appropriate documentation.

If a therapeutic colonoscopy (44389-44407, 45379, 45380, 45381, 45382, 45384, 45388, 45398) is performed and does not reach the cecum or colon-small intestine anastomosis, report the appropriate therapeutic colonoscopy code with modifier 52 and provide appropriate documentation.

Report flexible sigmoidoscopy (45330-45347) for endoscopic examination during which the endoscope is not advanced beyond the splenic flexure.

Report flexible sigmoidoscopy (45330-45347) for endoscopic examination of a patient who has undergone resection of the colon proximal to the sigmoid (eg, subtotal colectomy) and has an ileo-sigmoid or ileo-rectal anastomosis. Report pouch endoscopy codes (44385, 44386) for endoscopic examination of a patient who has undergone resection of colon with ileo-anal anastomosis (eg, J-pouch).

Digestive

Colonoscopy Decision Tree

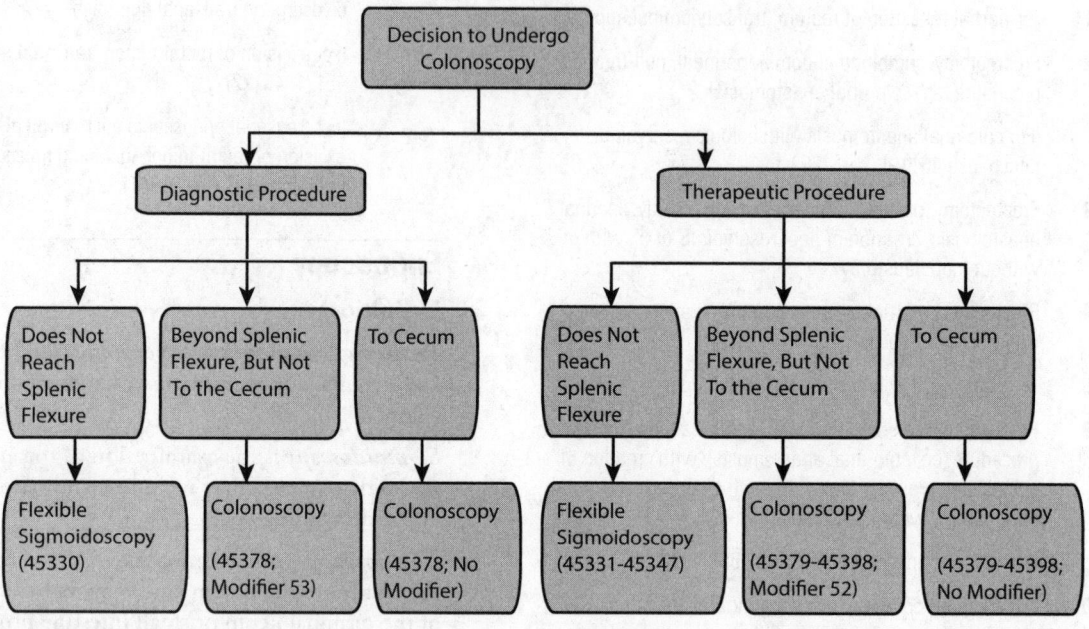

Colonoscopy Decision Tree

Report colonoscopy (45378-45398) for endoscopic examination of a patient who has undergone segmental resection of the colon (eg, hemicolectomy, sigmoid colectomy, low anterior resection).

For colonoscopy through stoma, see 44388-44408.

Report proctosigmoidoscopy (45300-45327), flexible sigmoidoscopy (45330-45347), or anoscopy (46600, 46604, 46606, 46608, 46610, 46611, 46612, 46614, 46615), as appropriate for endoscopic examination of the defunctionalized rectum or distal colon in a patient who has undergone colectomy, in addition to colonoscopy through stoma (44388-44408) or ileoscopy through stoma (44380, 44381, 44382, 44384) if appropriate.

When bleeding occurs as a result of an endoscopic procedure, control of bleeding is not reported separately during the same operative session.

For computed tomographic colonography, see 74261-74263.

45300   Proctosigmoidoscopy, rigid; diagnostic, with or without collection of specimen(s) by brushing or washing (separate procedure)

⊙ **45303**   with dilation (eg, balloon, guide wire, bougie)

     (For radiological supervision and interpretation, use 74360)

⊙ **45305**   with biopsy, single or multiple

⊙ **45307**   with removal of foreign body

⊙ **45308**   with removal of single tumor, polyp, or other lesion by hot biopsy forceps or bipolar cautery

⊙ **45309**   with removal of single tumor, polyp, or other lesion by snare technique

⊙ **45315**   with removal of multiple tumors, polyps, or other lesions by hot biopsy forceps, bipolar cautery or snare technique

⊙ **45317**   with control of bleeding (eg, injection, bipolar cautery, unipolar cautery, laser, heater probe, stapler, plasma coagulator)

⊙ **45320**   with ablation of tumor(s), polyp(s), or other lesion(s) not amenable to removal by hot biopsy forceps, bipolar cautery or snare technique (eg, laser)

⊙ **45321**   with decompression of volvulus

⊙ **45327**   with transendoscopic stent placement (includes predilation)

45330   Sigmoidoscopy, flexible; diagnostic, including collection of specimen(s) by brushing or washing, when performed (separate procedure)

     (Do not report 45330 in conjunction with 45331-45342, 45346, 45347, 45349, 45350)

45331   with biopsy, single or multiple

     (Do not report 45331 in conjunction with 45349 for the same lesion)

⊙ **45332**   with removal of foreign body(s)

     (Do not report 45332 in conjunction with 45330)

     (If fluoroscopic guidance is performed, use 76000)

⊙ **45333**   with removal of tumor(s), polyp(s), or other lesion(s) by hot biopsy forceps

     (Do not report 45333 in conjunction with 45330)

⊙ **45334**   with control of bleeding, any method

(Do not report 45334 in conjunction with 45335, 45350 for the same lesion)

(Do not report 45334 in conjunction with 45330)

⊙ **45335**   with directed submucosal injection(s), any substance

(Do not report 45335 in conjunction with 45334, 45349 for the same lesion)

(Do not report 45335 in conjunction with 45330)

⊙ **45337**   with decompression (for pathologic distention) (eg, volvulus, megacolon), including placement of decompression tube, when performed

(Do not report 45337 in conjunction with 45330)

(Do not report 45337 more than once per session)

⊙ **45338**   with removal of tumor(s), polyp(s), or other lesion(s) by snare technique

(Do not report 45338 in conjunction with 45349 for the same lesion)

(Do not report 45338 in conjunction with 45330)

(For endoscopic mucosal resection, use 45349)

(45339 has been deleted. To report, use 45346)

#⊙ **45346**   with ablation of tumor(s), polyp(s), or other lesion(s) (includes pre- and post-dilation and guide wire passage, when performed)

(Do not report 45346 in conjunction with 45330)

(Do not report 45346 in conjunction with 45340 for the same lesion)

⊙ **45340**   with transendoscopic balloon dilation

(Do not report 45340 in conjunction with 45330, 45346, 45347)

(If fluoroscopic guidance is performed, use 74360)

(For transendoscopic balloon dilation of multiple strictures during the same session, use 45340 with modifier 59 for each additional stricture dilated)

⊙ **45341**   with endoscopic ultrasound examination

(Do not report 45341 in conjunction with 45330, 45342, 76872, 76975)

(Do not report 45341 more than once per session)

⊙ **45342**   with transendoscopic ultrasound guided intramural or transmural fine needle aspiration/biopsy(s)

(Do not report 45342 in conjunction with 45330, 45341, 76872, 76942, 76975)

(Do not report 45342 more than once per session)

(45345 has been deleted. To report, use 45347)

45346   Code is out of numerical sequence. See 45330-45342

⊙ **45347**   with placement of endoscopic stent (includes pre- and post-dilation and guide wire passage, when performed)

(Do not report 45347 in conjunction with 45330, 45340)

(If fluoroscopic guidance is performed, use 74360)

⊙ **45349**   with endoscopic mucosal resection

(Do not report 45349 in conjunction with 45331, 45335, 45338, 45350 for the same lesion)

(Do not report 45349 in conjunction with 45330)

⊙ **45350**   with band ligation(s) (eg, hemorrhoids)

(Do not report 45350 in conjunction with 45334 for the same lesion)

(Do not report 45350 in conjunction with 45330, 45349, 46221)

(Do not report 45350 more than once per session)

(To report control of active bleeding with band ligation[s], use 45334)

(45355 has been deleted. To report, use 45399)

⊙ **45378**   Colonoscopy, flexible; diagnostic, including collection of specimen(s) by brushing or washing, when performed (separate procedure)

(Do not report 45378 in conjunction with 45379-45393, 45398)

(For colonoscopy with decompression [pathologic distention], use 45393)

⊙ **45379**   with removal of foreign body(s)

(Do not report 45379 in conjunction with 45378)

(If fluoroscopic guidance is performed, use 76000)

⊙ **45380**   with biopsy, single or multiple

(Do not report 45380 in conjunction with 45390 for the same lesion)

(Do not report 45380 in conjunction with 45378)

⊙ **45381**   with directed submucosal injection(s), any substance

(Do not report 45381 in conjunction with 45382, 45390 for the same lesion)

(Do not report 45381 in conjunction with 45378)

⊙ **45382**   with control of bleeding, any method

(Do not report 45382 in conjunction with 45381, 45398 for the same lesion)

(Do not report 45382 in conjunction with 45378)

(45383 has been deleted. To report, use 45388)

#⊙ **45388**   with ablation of tumor(s), polyp(s), or other lesion(s) (includes pre- and post-dilation and guide wire passage, when performed)

(Do not report 45388 in conjunction with 45386 for the same lesion)

(Do not report 45388 in conjunction with 45378)

Digestive

⊙ **45384**   with removal of tumor(s), polyp(s), or other lesion(s) by hot biopsy forceps

(Do not report 45384 in conjunction with 45378)

⊙ **45385**   with removal of tumor(s), polyp(s), or other lesion(s) by snare technique

(Do not report 45385 in conjunction with 45390 for the same lesion)

(Do not report 45385 in conjunction with 45378)

(For endoscopic mucosal resection, use 45390)

⊙ **45386**   with transendoscopic balloon dilation

(Do not report 45386 in conjunction with 45378, 45388, 45389)

(If fluoroscopic guidance is performed, use 74360)

(For transendoscopic balloon dilation of multiple strictures during the same session, report 45386 with modifier 59 for each additional stricture dilated)

(45387 has been deleted. To report, use 45389)

45388   Code is out of numerical sequence. See 45300-45393

⊙ **45389**   with endoscopic stent placement (includes pre- and post-dilation and guide wire passage, when performed)

(Do not report 45389 in conjunction with 45378, 45386)

(If fluoroscopic guidance is performed, use 74360)

45390   Code is out of numerical sequence. See 45300-45393

⊙ **45391**   with endoscopic ultrasound examination limited to the rectum, sigmoid, descending, transverse, or ascending colon and cecum, and adjacent structures

(Do not report 45391 in conjunction with 45378, 45392, 76872, 76975)

(Do not report 45391 more than once per session)

⊙ **45392**   with transendoscopic ultrasound guided intramural or transmural fine needle aspiration/biopsy(s), includes endoscopic ultrasound examination limited to the rectum, sigmoid, descending, transverse, or ascending colon and cecum, and adjacent structures

(Do not report 45392 in conjunction with 45378, 45391, 76872, 76942, 76975)

(Do not report 45392 more than once per session)

#⊙ **45390**   with endoscopic mucosal resection

(Do not report 45390 in conjunction with 45380, 45381, 45385, 45398 for the same lesion)

(Do not report 45390 in conjunction with 45378)

⊙ **45393**   with decompression (for pathologic distention) (eg, volvulus, megacolon), including placement of decompression tube, when performed

(Do not report 45393 in conjunction with 45378)

(Do not report 45393 more than once per session)

#⊙ **45398**   with band ligation(s) (eg, hemorrhoids)

(Do not report 45398 in conjunction with 45382 for the same lesion)

(Do not report 45398 in conjunction with 45378, 45390, 46221)

(Do not report 45398 more than once per session)

(To report control of active bleeding with band ligation[s], use 45382)

Laparoscopy

Surgical laparoscopy always includes diagnostic laparoscopy. To report a diagnostic laparoscopy (peritoneoscopy) (separate procedure), use 49320.

Excision

45395   Laparoscopy, surgical; proctectomy, complete, combined abdominoperineal, with colostomy

(For open procedure, use 45110)

45397   proctectomy, combined abdominoperineal pull-through procedure (eg, colo-anal anastomosis), with creation of colonic reservoir (eg, J-pouch), with diverting enterostomy, when performed

(For open procedure, use 45119)

45398   Code is out of numerical sequence. See 45395-45399

45399   Code is out of numerical sequence. See 45399-45999

Repair

45400   Laparoscopy, surgical; proctopexy (for prolapse)

(For open procedure, use 45540, 45541)

45402   proctopexy (for prolapse), with sigmoid resection

(For open procedure, use 45550)

45499   Unlisted laparoscopy procedure, rectum

Repair

45500   Proctoplasty; for stenosis

45505   for prolapse of mucous membrane

45520   Perirectal injection of sclerosing solution for prolapse

45540   Proctopexy (eg, for prolapse); abdominal approach

(For laparoscopic procedure, use 45400)

45541   perineal approach

45550   with sigmoid resection, abdominal approach

(For laparoscopic procedure, use 45402)

45560   Repair of rectocele (separate procedure)

(For repair of rectocele with posterior colporrhaphy, use 57250)

45562	Exploration, repair, and presacral drainage for rectal injury;
45563	with colostomy
45800	Closure of rectovesical fistula;
45805	with colostomy
45820	Closure of rectourethral fistula;
45825	with colostomy

(For rectovaginal fistula closure, see 57300-57308)

Manipulation

45900	Reduction of procidentia (separate procedure) under anesthesia
45905	Dilation of anal sphincter (separate procedure) under anesthesia other than local
45910	Dilation of rectal stricture (separate procedure) under anesthesia other than local
45915	Removal of fecal impaction or foreign body (separate procedure) under anesthesia

Other Procedures

Surgical diagnostic anorectal exam (45990) includes the following elements: external perineal exam, digital rectal exam, pelvic exam (when performed), diagnostic anoscopy, and diagnostic rigid proctoscopy.

# **45399**	Unlisted procedure, colon
45990	Anorectal exam, surgical, requiring anesthesia (general, spinal, or epidural), diagnostic

(Do not report 45990 in conjunction with 45300-45327, 46600, 57410, 99170)

45999	Unlisted procedure, rectum

(For unlisted laparoscopic procedure, rectum, use 45499)

Anus

▶For incision of thrombosed external hemorrhoid, use 46083. For ligation of internal hemorrhoid(s), see 46221, 46945, 46946. For excision of internal and/or external hemorrhoid(s), see 46250-46262, 46320. For injection of hemorrhoid(s), use 46500. For destruction of internal hemorrhoid(s) by thermal energy, use 46930. For destruction of hemorrhoid(s) by cryosurgery, use 46999. For hemorrhoidopexy, use 46947. Do not report 46600 in conjunction with 46020-46942, 0184T, 0249T, 0377T during the same operative session.◀

Incision

(For subcutaneous fistulotomy, use 46270)

46020	Placement of seton

(Do not report 46020 in addition to 46060, 46280, 46600, 0249T)

46030	Removal of anal seton, other marker
46040	Incision and drainage of ischiorectal and/or perirectal abscess (separate procedure)
46045	Incision and drainage of intramural, intramuscular, or submucosal abscess, transanal, under anesthesia
46050	Incision and drainage, perianal abscess, superficial

(See also 45020, 46060)

46060	Incision and drainage of ischiorectal or intramural abscess, with fistulectomy or fistulotomy, submuscular, with or without placement of seton

(Do not report 46060 in addition to 46020)

(See also 45020)

46070	Incision, anal septum (infant)

(For anoplasty, see 46700-46705)

(Do not report modifier 63 in conjunction with 46070)

46080	Sphincterotomy, anal, division of sphincter (separate procedure)
46083	Incision of thrombosed hemorrhoid, external

Excision

46200	Fissurectomy, including sphincterotomy, when performed

(46210, 46211 have been deleted. To report, use 46999)

46220	Code is out of numerical sequence. See 46200-46288
46221	Hemorrhoidectomy, internal, by rubber band ligation(s)

(Do not report 46221 in conjunction with 45350, 45398)

(For ligation, hemorrhoidal vascular bundle(s), including ultrasound guidance, use 0249T)

# **46945**	Hemorrhoidectomy, internal, by ligation other than rubber band; single hemorrhoid column/group
# **46946**	2 or more hemorrhoid columns/groups

(Do not report 46221, 46945, and 46946 in conjunction with 0249T)

# **46220**	Excision of single external papilla or tag, anus
46230	Excision of multiple external papillae or tags, anus
# **46320**	Excision of thrombosed hemorrhoid, external
46250	Hemorrhoidectomy, external, 2 or more columns/groups

(For hemorrhoidectomy, external, single column/group, use 46999)

46255	Hemorrhoidectomy, internal and external, single column/group;
46257	with fissurectomy
46258	with fistulectomy, including fissurectomy, when performed
46260	Hemorrhoidectomy, internal and external, 2 or more columns/groups;
46261	with fissurectomy

46262   with fistulectomy, including fissurectomy, when performed

         (Do not report 46250-46262 in conjunction with 0249T)

46270   Surgical treatment of anal fistula (fistulectomy/fistulotomy); subcutaneous

46275   intersphincteric

46280   transsphincteric, suprasphincteric, extrasphincteric or multiple, including placement of seton, when performed

         (Do not report 46280 in conjunction with 46020)

46285   second stage

46288   Closure of anal fistula with rectal advancement flap

46320   Code is out of numerical sequence. See 46200-46288

Introduction

46500   Injection of sclerosing solution, hemorrhoids

         (For anoscopy with directed submucosal injection of bulking agent for fecal incontinence, use 0377T)

46505   Chemodenervation of internal anal sphincter

         (For chemodenervation of other muscles, see 64612, 64616, 64617, 64642, 64643, 64644, 64645, 64646, 64647. For destruction of nerve by neurolytic agent, use 64630)

         (Report the specific service in conjunction with the specific substance(s) or drug(s) provided)

Endoscopy

Surgical endoscopy always includes diagnostic endoscopy.

         (For anoscopy with directed submucosal injection of bulking agent for fecal incontinence, use 0377T)

46600   Anoscopy; diagnostic, including collection of specimen(s) by brushing or washing, when performed (separate procedure)

         ▶(Do not report 46600 in conjunction with 46020-46942, 0184T, 0249T, 0377T during the same operative session)◀

         (For diagnostic high-resolution anoscopy [HRA], use 46601)

46601   diagnostic, with high-resolution magnification (HRA) (eg, colposcope, operating microscope) and chemical agent enhancement, including collection of specimen(s) by brushing or washing, when performed

         (Do not report 46601 in conjunction with 69990)

46604   with dilation (eg, balloon, guide wire, bougie)

46606   with biopsy, single or multiple

         (For high-resolution anoscopy [HRA] with biopsy, use 46607)

46607   with high-resolution magnification (HRA) (eg, colposcope, operating microscope) and chemical agent enhancement, with biopsy, single or multiple

         (Do not report 46607 in conjunction with 69990)

46608   with removal of foreign body

46610   with removal of single tumor, polyp, or other lesion by hot biopsy forceps or bipolar cautery

46611   with removal of single tumor, polyp, or other lesion by snare technique

46612   with removal of multiple tumors, polyps, or other lesions by hot biopsy forceps, bipolar cautery or snare technique

46614   with control of bleeding (eg, injection, bipolar cautery, unipolar cautery, laser, heater probe, stapler, plasma coagulator)

46615   with ablation of tumor(s), polyp(s), or other lesion(s) not amenable to removal by hot biopsy forceps, bipolar cautery or snare technique

         (For delivery of thermal energy to the muscle of the anal canal, use 0288T)

Repair

46700   Anoplasty, plastic operation for stricture; adult

46705   infant

         (Do not report modifier 63 in conjunction with 46705)

         (For simple incision of anal septum, use 46070)

46706   Repair of anal fistula with fibrin glue

46707   Repair of anorectal fistula with plug (eg, porcine small intestine submucosa [SIS])

46710   Repair of ileoanal pouch fistula/sinus (eg, perineal or vaginal), pouch advancement; transperineal approach

46712   combined transperineal and transabdominal approach

46715   Repair of low imperforate anus; with anoperineal fistula (cut-back procedure)

46716   with transposition of anoperineal or anovestibular fistula

         (Do not report modifier 63 in conjunction with 46715, 46716)

46730   Repair of high imperforate anus without fistula; perineal or sacroperineal approach

46735   combined transabdominal and sacroperineal approaches

         (Do not report modifier 63 in conjunction with 46730, 46735)

46740   Repair of high imperforate anus with rectourethral or rectovaginal fistula; perineal or sacroperineal approach

46742   combined transabdominal and sacroperineal approaches

(Do not report modifier 63 in conjunction with 46740, 46742)

46744 Repair of cloacal anomaly by anorectovaginoplasty and urethroplasty, sacroperineal approach

(Do not report modifier 63 in conjunction with 46744)

46746 Repair of cloacal anomaly by anorectovaginoplasty and urethroplasty, combined abdominal and sacroperineal approach;

46748 with vaginal lengthening by intestinal graft or pedicle flaps

46750 Sphincteroplasty, anal, for incontinence or prolapse; adult

46751 child

46753 Graft (Thiersch operation) for rectal incontinence and/or prolapse

46754 Removal of Thiersch wire or suture, anal canal

46760 Sphincteroplasty, anal, for incontinence, adult; muscle transplant

46761 levator muscle imbrication (Park posterior anal repair)

46762 implantation artificial sphincter

(For anoscopy with directed submucosal injection of bulking agent for fecal incontinence, use 0377T)

 # 46947 Hemorrhoidopexy (eg, for prolapsing internal hemorrhoids) by stapling

Destruction

46900 Destruction of lesion(s), anus (eg, condyloma, papilloma, molluscum contagiosum, herpetic vesicle), simple; chemical

46910 electrodesiccation

46916 cryosurgery

46917 laser surgery

46922 surgical excision

46924 Destruction of lesion(s), anus (eg, condyloma, papilloma, molluscum contagiosum, herpetic vesicle), extensive (eg, laser surgery, electrosurgery, cryosurgery, chemosurgery)

46930 Destruction of internal hemorrhoid(s) by thermal energy (eg, infrared coagulation, cautery, radiofrequency)

(46934-46936 have been deleted)

(46937, 46938 have been deleted. To report, use 45190)

46940 Curettage or cautery of anal fissure, including dilation of anal sphincter (separate procedure); initial

46942 subsequent

46945 Code is out of numerical sequence. See 46200-46288

46946 Code is out of numerical sequence. See 46200-46288

46947 Code is out of numerical sequence. See 46700-46947

Other Procedures

46999 Unlisted procedure, anus

Liver

Incision

⊙ **47000** Biopsy of liver, needle; percutaneous

(If imaging guidance is performed, see 76942, 77002, 77012, 77021)

+ **47001** when done for indicated purpose at time of other major procedure (List separately in addition to code for primary procedure)

(If imaging guidance is performed, see 76942, 77002)

(For fine needle aspiration in conjunction with 47000, 47001, see 10021, 10022)

(For evaluation of fine needle aspirate in conjunction with 47000, 47001, see 88172, 88173)

47010 Hepatotomy, for open drainage of abscess or cyst, 1 or 2 stages

(47011 has been deleted)

(For percutaneous image-guided fluid collection drainage by catheter of hepatic abscess or cyst, use 49405)

47015 Laparotomy, with aspiration and/or injection of hepatic parasitic (eg, amoebic or echinococcal) cyst(s) or abscess(es)

Excision

47100 Biopsy of liver, wedge

47120 Hepatectomy, resection of liver; partial lobectomy

47122 trisegmentectomy

47125 total left lobectomy

47130 total right lobectomy

Liver Transplantation

Liver allotransplantation involves three distinct components of physician work:

1. *Cadaver donor hepatectomy,* which includes harvesting the graft and cold preservation of the graft (perfusing with cold preservation solution and cold maintenance) (use 47133). *Living donor hepatectomy,* which includes harvesting the graft, cold preservation of the graft (perfusing with cold preservation solution and cold maintenance), and care of the donor (see 47140-47142).

2. *Backbench work:*

Standard preparation of the whole liver graft will include one of the following:

Digestive

Preparation of whole liver graft (including cholecystectomy, if necessary, and dissection and removal of surrounding soft tissues to prepare vena cava, portal vein, hepatic artery, and common bile duct for implantation) (use 47143).

Preparation as described for whole liver graft, plus trisegment split into two partial grafts (use 47144).

Preparation as described for whole liver graft, plus lobe split into two partial grafts (use 47145).

Additional reconstruction of the liver graft may include venous and/or arterial anastomosis(es) (see 47146, 47147).

►3. *Recipient liver allotransplantation,* which includes recipient hepatectomy (partial or whole), transplantation of the allograft (partial or whole), and care of the recipient (use 47135).◄

47133   Donor hepatectomy (including cold preservation), from cadaver donor

47135   Liver allotransplantation, orthotopic, partial or whole, from cadaver or living donor, any age

►(47136 has been deleted. To report, use 47399)◄

47140   Donor hepatectomy (including cold preservation), from living donor; left lateral segment only (segments II and III)

47141   total left lobectomy (segments II, III and IV)

47142   total right lobectomy (segments V, VI, VII and VIII)

47143   Backbench standard preparation of cadaver donor whole liver graft prior to allotransplantation, including cholecystectomy, if necessary, and dissection and removal of surrounding soft tissues to prepare the vena cava, portal vein, hepatic artery, and common bile duct for implantation; without trisegment or lobe split

47144   with trisegment split of whole liver graft into 2 partial liver grafts (ie, left lateral segment [segments II and III] and right trisegment [segments I and IV through VIII])

47145   with lobe split of whole liver graft into 2 partial liver grafts (ie, left lobe [segments II, III, and IV] and right lobe [segments I and V through VIII])

47146   Backbench reconstruction of cadaver or living donor liver graft prior to allotransplantation; venous anastomosis, each

47147   arterial anastomosis, each

(Do not report 47143-47147 in conjunction with 47120-47125, 47600, 47610)

Repair

47300   Marsupialization of cyst or abscess of liver

47350   Management of liver hemorrhage; simple suture of liver wound or injury

47360   complex suture of liver wound or injury, with or without hepatic artery ligation

47361   exploration of hepatic wound, extensive debridement, coagulation and/or suture, with or without packing of liver

47362   re-exploration of hepatic wound for removal of packing

Laparoscopy

Surgical laparoscopy always includes diagnostic laparoscopy. To report a diagnostic laparoscopy (peritoneoscopy) (separate procedure), use 49320.

47370   Laparoscopy, surgical, ablation of 1 or more liver tumor(s); radiofrequency

(For imaging guidance, use 76940)

47371   cryosurgical

(For imaging guidance, use 76940)

47379   Unlisted laparoscopic procedure, liver

Other Procedures

47380   Ablation, open, of 1 or more liver tumor(s); radiofrequency

(For imaging guidance, use 76940)

47381   cryosurgical

(For imaging guidance, use 76940)

⊙ **47382**   Ablation, 1 or more liver tumor(s), percutaneous, radiofrequency

(For imaging guidance and monitoring, see 76940, 77013, 77022)

⊙ **47383**   Ablation, 1 or more liver tumor(s), percutaneous, cryoablation

(For imaging guidance and monitoring, see 76940, 77013, 77022)

47399   Unlisted procedure, liver

Biliary Tract

Incision

47400   Hepaticotomy or hepaticostomy with exploration, drainage, or removal of calculus

47420   Choledochotomy or choledochostomy with exploration, drainage, or removal of calculus, with or without cholecystotomy; without transduodenal sphincterotomy or sphincteroplasty

47425   with transduodenal sphincterotomy or sphincteroplasty

47460   Transduodenal sphincterotomy or sphincteroplasty, with or without transduodenal extraction of calculus (separate procedure)

47480   Cholecystotomy or cholecystostomy, open, with exploration, drainage, or removal of calculus (separate procedure)

(For percutaneous cholecystostomy, use 47490)

Introduction

▶Percutaneous biliary procedures (eg, transhepatic, transcholecystic) are described by 47490 and 47531-47544, and are performed with imaging guidance. They are differentiated from endoscopic procedures that utilize an access to the biliary tree from a hollow viscus for diagnosis and therapy. Diagnostic cholangiography is typically performed with percutaneous biliary procedures, and is included in 47490, 47533, 47534, 47535, 47536, 47537, 47538, 47539, 47540, and 47541.

Codes 47531 and 47532 describe percutaneous diagnostic cholangiography that includes injection(s) of contrast material, all associated radiological supervision and interpretation, and procedural imaging guidance (eg, ultrasound and/or fluoroscopy). Code 47532 also includes accessing the biliary system with a needle or catheter. Codes 47531 and 47532 may not be reported with codes 47533, 47534, 47535, 47536, 47537, 47538, 47539, 47540, and 47541.

An external biliary drainage catheter is a catheter placed into a bile duct that does not terminate in bowel, and that drains bile externally only. An internal-external biliary drainage catheter is a single, externally accessible catheter that terminates in the small intestine, and may drain bile into the small intestine and/or externally. A "stent," as used in this code set, is a percutaneously placed device (eg, self-expanding metallic mesh stent, plastic tube) that is positioned within the biliary tree and is completely internal, with no portion extending outside the patient.

Codes 47533, 47534, 47535, 47536, 47537, 47538, 47539, and 47540 describe percutaneous therapeutic biliary procedures that include catheter or stent placement, catheter removal and replacement (exchange), and/or catheter removal. These codes include the elements of access, drainage catheter manipulations, diagnostic cholangiography, imaging guidance (eg, ultrasonography and/or fluoroscopy), and all associated radiological supervision and interpretation. Codes 47533, 47534, 47538, 47539, 47540 may be reported once for each catheter or stent placed (eg, bilobar placement, multi-segmental placement). Codes 47535, 47536, and 47537 may be reported once for each catheter conversion, exchange, or removal (eg, bilobar, bisegmental).

Codes 47538, 47539, 47540 may be reported only once per session to describe one or more overlapping or serial stent(s) placed within a single bile duct, or bridging more than one ductal segment (eg, left hepatic duct and common bile duct) through a single percutaneous access. Codes 47538, 47539, 47540 may be reported more than

once in the same session using modifier 59 for the additional procedures in the following circumstances: (i) placement of side-by-side (double-barrel) stents within a single bile duct; (ii) placement of two or more stents into separate bile ducts through a single percutaneous access; or (iii) placement of stents through two or more percutaneous access sites (eg, placement of one stent through the interstices of another stent). Code 47538 describes biliary stent placement through an existing access. Therefore, 47538 should not be reported together with 47536 if a biliary drainage catheter (eg, external or internal-external) is replaced after the biliary stent is placed. Code 47540 describes biliary stent placement with the additional service of placing a biliary drainage catheter (eg, external or internal-external). Therefore, 47540 should not be reported with 47533, 47534 for the same ductal system.

Code 47541 describes a procedure to assist with endoscopic procedures performed in conjunction with other physician specialists. Access placed may include wire and/or catheter. Code 47541 may not be reported if a wire is placed through existing percutaneous access.

Codes 47542, 47543, and 47544 describe procedures that may be performed in conjunction with other codes in this family, are add-on codes and do not include access, catheter placement, or diagnostic imaging. Do not report 47542 with 47538, 47539, 47540 because balloon dilation is included in 47538, 47539, and 47540. Code 47544 should not be reported with 47531-47543 for removal of incidental sludge and/or debris. Code 47542 should not be reported with 47544, if a balloon is used for removal of calculi, debris, and/or sludge rather than for dilation.◀

47490   Cholecystostomy, percutaneous, complete procedure, including imaging guidance, catheter placement, cholecystogram when performed, and radiological supervision and interpretation

▶(Do not report 47490 in conjunction with 47531, 47532, 75989, 76942, 77002, 77012, 77021)◀

▶(47500, 47505, 47510, 47511, 47525, 47530 have been deleted. To report, see 47531-47541)◀

● **47531**   Injection procedure for cholangiography, percutaneous, complete diagnostic procedure including imaging guidance (eg, ultrasound and/or fluoroscopy) and all associated radiological supervision and interpretation; existing access

⊙● **47532**   new access (eg, percutaneous transhepatic cholangiogram)

▶(Do not report 47531, 47532 in conjunction with 47490, 47533, 47534, 47535, 47536, 47537, 47538, 47539, 47540, 47541 for procedures performed through the same percutaneous access)◀

▶(For intraoperative cholangiography, see 74300, 74301)◀

Digestive

►**Exchanges/Conversions**

(Existing Access)

To

Do Not Report Exchange with Stent for Same Percutaneous Access

		Internal-External	External	Stent
From	External Drain	47535 Conversion	47536 Exchange	47538 Stent
	Internal-External Drain	47536 Exchange	47536 Exchange	47538 Stent ◄

⊙● **47533** Placement of biliary drainage catheter, percutaneous, including diagnostic cholangiography when performed, imaging guidance (eg, ultrasound and/or fluoroscopy), and all associated radiological supervision and interpretation; external

⊙● **47534**   internal-external

⊙● **47535** Conversion of external biliary drainage catheter to internal-external biliary drainage catheter, percutaneous, including diagnostic cholangiography when performed, imaging guidance (eg, fluoroscopy), and all associated radiological supervision and interpretation

⊙● **47536** Exchange of biliary drainage catheter (eg, external, internal-external, or conversion of internal-external to external only), percutaneous, including diagnostic cholangiography when performed, imaging guidance (eg, fluoroscopy), and all associated radiological supervision and interpretation

►(Do not report 47536 in conjunction with 47538 for the same access)◄

►(47536 includes exchange of one catheter. For exchange of additional catheter[s] during the same session, report 47536 with modifier 59 for each additional exchange)◄

● **47537** Removal of biliary drainage catheter, percutaneous, requiring fluoroscopic guidance (eg, with concurrent indwelling biliary stents), including diagnostic cholangiography when performed, imaging guidance (eg, fluoroscopy), and all associated radiological supervision and interpretation

►(Do not report 47537 in conjunction with 47538 for the same access)◄

►(For removal of biliary drainage catheter not requiring fluoroscopic guidance, see E/M services and report the appropriate level of service provided [eg 99201-99215, 99217, 99218, 99219, 99220, 99221, 99222, 99223, 99224, 99225, 99226, 99231, 99232, 99233])◄

⊙● **47538** Placement of stent(s) into a bile duct, percutaneous, including diagnostic cholangiography, imaging guidance (eg, fluoroscopy and/or ultrasound), balloon dilation, catheter exchange(s) and catheter removal(s) when performed, and all associated radiological supervision and interpretation, each stent; existing access

►(Do not report 47538 in conjunction with 47536, 47537 for the same percutaneous access)◄

⊙● **47539**   new access, without placement of separate biliary drainage catheter

⊙● **47540**   new access, with placement of separate biliary drainage catheter (eg, external or internal-external)

►(Do not report 47538, 47539, 47540 in conjunction with 43277, 47542, 47555, 47556 for the same lesion in the same session)◄

►(Do not report 47540 in conjunction with 47533, 47534 for the same percutaneous access)◄

⊙● **47541** Placement of access through the biliary tree and into small bowel to assist with an endoscopic biliary procedure (eg, rendezvous procedure), percutaneous, including diagnostic cholangiography when performed, imaging guidance (eg, ultrasound and/or fluoroscopy), and all associated radiological supervision and interpretation, new access

►(Do not report 47541 in conjunction with 47531, 47532, 47533, 47534, 47535, 47536, 47537, 47538, 47539, 47540)◄

►(Do not report 47541 when there is existing catheter access)◄

►(For use of existing access through the biliary tree into small bowel to assist with an endoscopic biliary procedure, see 47535, 47536, 47537)◄

⊙+● **47542** Balloon dilation of biliary duct(s) or of ampulla (sphincteroplasty), percutaneous, including imaging guidance (eg, fluoroscopy), and all associated radiological supervision and interpretation, each duct (List separately in addition to code for primary procedure)

►(Use 47542 in conjunction with 47531, 47532, 47533, 47534, 47535, 47536, 47537, 47541)◄

►(Do not report 47542 in conjunction with 43262, 43277, 47538, 47539, 47540, 47555, 47556)◄

►(Do not report 47542 in conjunction with 47544 if a balloon is used for removal of calculi, debris, and/or sludge rather than for dilation)◄

►(For percutaneous balloon dilation of multiple ducts during the same session, report an additional dilation once with 47542 and modifier 59, regardless of the number of additional ducts dilated)◄

►(For endoscopic balloon dilation, see 43277, 47555, 47556)◄

⊙+● **47543** Endoluminal biopsy(ies) of biliary tree, percutaneous, any method(s) (eg, brush, forceps, and/or needle), including imaging guidance (eg, fluoroscopy), and all associated radiological supervision and interpretation, single or multiple (List separately in addition to code for primary procedure)

►(Use 47543 in conjunction with 47531, 47532, 47533, 47534, 47535, 47536, 47537, 47538, 47539, 47540)◄

►(Report 47543 once per session)◄

►(For endoscopic brushings, see 43260, 47552)◄

►(For endoscopic biopsy, see 43261, 47553)◄

⊙+● **47544** Removal of calculi/debris from biliary duct(s) and/or gallbladder, percutaneous, including destruction of calculi by any method (eg, mechanical, electrohydraulic, lithotripsy) when performed, imaging guidance (eg, fluoroscopy), and all associated radiological supervision and interpretation (List separately in addition to code for primary procedure)

►(Use 47544 in conjunction with 47531, 47532, 47533, 47534, 47535, 47536, 47537, 47538, 47539, 47540)◄

►(Do not report 47544 if no calculi or debris are found, even if removal device is deployed)◄

►(Do not report 47544 in conjunction with 43264, 47554)◄

►(Do not report 47544 in conjunction with 47531-47543 for removal of incidental sludge and/or debris)◄

►(For endoscopic removal of calculi, see 43264, 47554)◄

►(For endoscopic destruction of calculi, use 43265)◄

Endoscopy

Surgical endoscopy always includes diagnostic endoscopy.

+ **47550** Biliary endoscopy, intraoperative (choledochoscopy) (List separately in addition to code for primary procedure)

47552 Biliary endoscopy, percutaneous via T-tube or other tract; diagnostic, with collection of specimen(s) by brushing and/or washing, when performed (separate procedure)

47553   with biopsy, single or multiple

47554   with removal of calculus/calculi

47555   with dilation of biliary duct stricture(s) without stent

47556   with dilation of biliary duct stricture(s) with stent

►(For ERCP, see 43260-43278, 74328, 74329, 74330, 74363)◄

►(If imaging guidance is performed, use 74363)◄

Laparoscopy

Surgical laparoscopy always includes diagnostic laparoscopy. To report a diagnostic laparoscopy (peritoneoscopy) (separate procedure), use 49320.

►(47560, 47561 have been deleted. To report laparoscopically guided transhepatic cholangiography with biopsy, use 47579)◄

►(For percutaneous cholangiography, see 47531 or 47532)◄

47562 Laparoscopy, surgical; cholecystectomy

47563   cholecystectomy with cholangiography

►(For intraoperative cholangiography radiological supervision and interpretation, see 74300, 74301)◄

►(For percutaneous cholangiography, see 47531, 47532)◄

47564   cholecystectomy with exploration of common duct

47570   cholecystoenterostomy

47579 Unlisted laparoscopy procedure, biliary tract

Excision

47600 Cholecystectomy;

47605   with cholangiography

(For laparoscopic approach, see 47562-47564)

47610 Cholecystectomy with exploration of common duct;

(For cholecystectomy with exploration of common duct with biliary endoscopy, use 47610 with 47550)

47612   with choledochoenterostomy

47620   with transduodenal sphincterotomy or sphincteroplasty, with or without cholangiography

►(47630 has been deleted. For percutaneous biliary duct stone extraction, use 47544)◄

47700 Exploration for congenital atresia of bile ducts, without repair, with or without liver biopsy, with or without cholangiography

(Do not report modifier 63 in conjunction with 47700)

47701 Portoenterostomy (eg, Kasai procedure)

(Do not report modifier 63 in conjunction with 47701)

47711 Excision of bile duct tumor, with or without primary repair of bile duct; extrahepatic

47712   intrahepatic

(For anastomosis, see 47760-47800)

47715 Excision of choledochal cyst

Digestive

Repair

47720 Cholecystoenterostomy; direct

(For laparoscopic approach, use 47570)

47721 with gastroenterostomy

47740 Roux-en-Y

47741 Roux-en-Y with gastroenterostomy

47760 Anastomosis, of extrahepatic biliary ducts and gastrointestinal tract

47765 Anastomosis, of intrahepatic ducts and gastrointestinal tract

47780 Anastomosis, Roux-en-Y, of extrahepatic biliary ducts and gastrointestinal tract

47785 Anastomosis, Roux-en-Y, of intrahepatic biliary ducts and gastrointestinal tract

47800 Reconstruction, plastic, of extrahepatic biliary ducts with end-to-end anastomosis

47801 Placement of choledochal stent

47802 U-tube hepaticoenterostomy

47900 Suture of extrahepatic biliary duct for pre-existing injury (separate procedure)

Other Procedures

47999 Unlisted procedure, biliary tract

Pancreas

(For peroral pancreatic endoscopic procedures, see 43260-43265, 43274-43278)

Incision

48000 Placement of drains, peripancreatic, for acute pancreatitis;

48001 with cholecystostomy, gastrostomy, and jejunostomy

48020 Removal of pancreatic calculus

Excision

48100 Biopsy of pancreas, open (eg, fine needle aspiration, needle core biopsy, wedge biopsy)

48102 Biopsy of pancreas, percutaneous needle

(For radiological supervision and interpretation, see 76942, 77002, 77012, 77021)

(For fine needle aspiration, use 10022)

(For evaluation of fine needle aspirate, see 88172, 88173)

48105 Resection or debridement of pancreas and peripancreatic tissue for acute necrotizing pancreatitis

48120 Excision of lesion of pancreas (eg, cyst, adenoma)

48140 Pancreatectomy, distal subtotal, with or without splenectomy; without pancreaticojejunostomy

48145 with pancreaticojejunostomy

48146 Pancreatectomy, distal, near-total with preservation of duodenum (Child-type procedure)

48148 Excision of ampulla of Vater

48150 Pancreatectomy, proximal subtotal with total duodenectomy, partial gastrectomy, choledochoenterostomy and gastrojejunostomy (Whipple-type procedure); with pancreatojejunostomy

48152 without pancreatojejunostomy

48153 Pancreatectomy, proximal subtotal with near-total duodenectomy, choledochoenterostomy and duodenojejunostomy (pylorus-sparing, Whipple-type procedure); with pancreatojejunostomy

48154 without pancreatojejunostomy

48155 Pancreatectomy, total

48160 Pancreatectomy, total or subtotal, with autologous transplantation of pancreas or pancreatic islet cells

Introduction

+ 48400 Injection procedure for intraoperative pancreatography (List separately in addition to code for primary procedure)

►(For radiological supervision and interpretation, see 74300, 74301)◄

►(For intraoperative pancreatography radiological supervision and interpretation, see 74300, 74301)◄

Repair

48500 Marsupialization of pancreatic cyst

48510 External drainage, pseudocyst of pancreas, open

(48511 has been deleted)

(For percutaneous image-guided fluid collection drainage by catheter of pancreatic pseudocyst, use 49405)

48520 Internal anastomosis of pancreatic cyst to gastrointestinal tract; direct

48540 Roux-en-Y

48545 Pancreatorrhaphy for injury

48547 Duodenal exclusion with gastrojejunostomy for pancreatic injury

48548 Pancreaticojejunostomy, side-to-side anastomosis (Puestow-type operation)

Pancreas Transplantation

Pancreas allotransplantation involves three distinct components of physician work:

1. *Cadaver donor pancreatectomy,* which includes harvesting the pancreas graft, with or without duodenal segment, and cold preservation of the graft (perfusing with cold preservation solution and cold maintenance) (use 48550).

2. *Backbench work:*

Standard preparation of a cadaver donor pancreas allograft prior to transplantation includes dissection of the allograft from surrounding soft tissues, splenectomy, duodenotomy, ligation of bile duct, ligation of mesenteric vessels, and Y-graft arterial anastomoses from the iliac artery to the superior mesenteric artery and to the splenic artery (use 48551).

Additional reconstruction of a cadaver donor pancreas allograft prior to transplantation may include venous anastomosis(es) (use 48552).

3. *Recipient pancreas allotransplantation,* which includes transplantation of allograft, and care of the recipient (use 48554).

48550   Donor pancreatectomy (including cold preservation), with or without duodenal segment for transplantation

48551   Backbench standard preparation of cadaver donor pancreas allograft prior to transplantation, including dissection of allograft from surrounding soft tissues, splenectomy, duodenotomy, ligation of bile duct, ligation of mesenteric vessels, and Y-graft arterial anastomoses from iliac artery to superior mesenteric artery and to splenic artery

48552   Backbench reconstruction of cadaver donor pancreas allograft prior to transplantation, venous anastomosis, each

►(Do not report 48551 and 48552 in conjunction with 35531, 35563, 35685, 38100-38102, 44010, 44820, 44850, 47460, 47550-47556, 48100-48120, 48545)◄

48554   Transplantation of pancreatic allograft

48556   Removal of transplanted pancreatic allograft

Other Procedures

48999   Unlisted procedure, pancreas

Abdomen, Peritoneum, and Omentum

Incision

49000   Exploratory laparotomy, exploratory celiotomy with or without biopsy(s) (separate procedure)

(To report wound exploration due to penetrating trauma without laparotomy, use 20102)

49002   Reopening of recent laparotomy

(To report re-exploration of hepatic wound for removal of packing, use 47362)

49010   Exploration, retroperitoneal area with or without biopsy(s) (separate procedure)

(To report wound exploration due to penetrating trauma without laparotomy, use 20102)

49020   Drainage of peritoneal abscess or localized peritonitis, exclusive of appendiceal abscess, open

(For appendiceal abscess, use 44900)

(49021 has been deleted)

►(For percutaneous image-guided drainage of peritoneal abscess or localized peritonitis by catheter, use 49406)◄

►(For transrectal or transvaginal image-guided drainage of peritoneal abscess by catheter, use 49407)◄

49040   Drainage of subdiaphragmatic or subphrenic abscess, open

(49041 has been deleted)

►(For percutaneous image-guided drainage of subdiaphragmatic or subphrenic abscess by catheter, use 49406)◄

49060   Drainage of retroperitoneal abscess, open

(49061 has been deleted)

►(For percutaneous image-guided drainage of retroperitoneal abscess by catheter, use 49406)◄

►(For transrectal or transvaginal image-guided drainage of retroperitoneal abscess by catheter, use 49407)◄

49062   Drainage of extraperitoneal lymphocele to peritoneal cavity, open

►(For laparoscopic drainage of lymphocele to peritoneal cavity, use 49323)◄

►(For percutaneous image-guided drainage of peritoneal or retroperitoneal lymphocele by catheter, use 49406)◄

49082   Abdominal paracentesis (diagnostic or therapeutic); without imaging guidance

49083   with imaging guidance

(Do not report 49083 in conjunction with 76942, 77002, 77012, 77021)

►(For percutaneous image-guided drainage of retroperitoneal abscess by catheter, use 49406)◄

49084   Peritoneal lavage, including imaging guidance, when performed

(Do not report 49084 in conjunction with 76942, 77002, 77012, 77021)

►(For percutaneous image-guided drainage of retroperitoneal abscess by catheter, use 49406)◄

Excision, Destruction

▶Code 49185 describes sclerotherapy of a fluid collection (eg, lymphocele, cyst, or seroma) through a percutaneous access. It includes contrast injection(s), sclerosant injection(s), sclerosant dwell time, diagnostic study, imaging guidance (eg, ultrasound, fluoroscopy), and radiological supervision and interpretation, when performed. Code 49185 may be reported once per day for each lesion treated through a separate catheter. Do not report 49185 more than once if treating multiple lesions through the same catheter. Codes for access to and drainage of the collection may be separately reportable according to location (eg, 10030, 10160, 49405, 49406, 49407, 50390).◀

(For lysis of intestinal adhesions, use 44005)

49180 Biopsy, abdominal or retroperitoneal mass, percutaneous needle

(If imaging guidance is performed, see 76942, 77002, 77012, 77021)

(For fine needle aspiration, use 10021 or 10022)

(For evaluation of fine needle aspirate, see 88172, 88173)

● **49185** Sclerotherapy of a fluid collection (eg, lymphocele, cyst, or seroma), percutaneous, including contrast injection(s), sclerosant injection(s), diagnostic study, imaging guidance (eg, ultrasound, fluoroscopy) and radiological supervision and interpretation when performed

▶(For treatment of multiple lesions in a single day requiring separate access, use modifier 59 for each additional treated lesion)◀

▶(For treatment of multiple interconnected lesions treated through a single access, report 49185 once)◀

▶(For access/drainage with needle, see 10160, 50390)◀

▶(For access/drainage with catheter, see 10030, 49405, 49406, 49407, 50390)◀

▶(For exchange of existing catheter, before or after injection of sclerosant, see 49423, 75984)◀

▶(For sclerotherapy of a lymphatic/vascular malformation, use 37241)◀

▶(For sclerosis of veins or endovenous ablation of incompetent extremity veins, see 36468, 36470, 36471, 36475, 36476, 36478, 36479)◀

▶(For pleurodesis, use 32560)◀

▶(Do not report 49185 in conjunction with 49424, 76080)◀

49203 Excision or destruction, open, intra-abdominal tumors, cysts or endometriomas, 1 or more peritoneal, mesenteric, or retroperitoneal primary or secondary tumors; largest tumor 5 cm diameter or less

49204   largest tumor 5.1-10.0 cm diameter

49205   largest tumor greater than 10.0 cm diameter

(Do not report 49203-49205 in conjunction with 38770, 38780, 49000, 49010, 49215, 50010, 50205, 50225, 50236, 50250, 50290, 58900-58960)

(For partial or total nephrectomy, use 50220 or 50240 in conjunction with 49203-49205)

(For colectomy, use 44140 in conjunction with 49203-49205)

(For small bowel resection, use 44120 in conjunction with 49203-49205)

(For vena caval resection with reconstruction, use 49203-49205 in conjunction with 37799)

(For resection of recurrent ovarian, tubal, primary peritoneal, or uterine malignancy, see 58957, 58958)

(For cryoablation of renal tumors, see 50250, 50593)

49215 Excision of presacral or sacrococcygeal tumor

(Do not report modifier 63 in conjunction with 49215)

49220 Staging laparotomy for Hodgkins disease or lymphoma (includes splenectomy, needle or open biopsies of both liver lobes, possibly also removal of abdominal nodes, abdominal node and/or bone marrow biopsies, ovarian repositioning)

49250 Umbilectomy, omphalectomy, excision of umbilicus (separate procedure)

49255 Omentectomy, epiploectomy, resection of omentum (separate procedure)

Laparoscopy

Surgical laparoscopy always includes diagnostic laparoscopy. To report a diagnostic laparoscopy (peritoneoscopy), (separate procedure), use 49320.

For laparoscopic fulguration or excision of lesions of the ovary, pelvic viscera, or peritoneal surface use 58662.

49320 Laparoscopy, abdomen, peritoneum, and omentum, diagnostic, with or without collection of specimen(s) by brushing or washing (separate procedure)

49321 Laparoscopy, surgical; with biopsy (single or multiple)

49322   with aspiration of cavity or cyst (eg, ovarian cyst) (single or multiple)

49323   with drainage of lymphocele to peritoneal cavity

▶(For open drainage of lymphocele to peritoneal cavity, use 49062)◀

49324   with insertion of tunneled intraperitoneal catheter

(For subcutaneous extension of intraperitoneal catheter with remote chest exit site, use 49435 in conjunction with 49324)

(For open insertion of tunneled intraperitoneal catheter, use 49421)

49325   with revision of previously placed intraperitoneal cannula or catheter, with removal of intraluminal obstructive material if performed

⊙=Moderate sedation   ✚=Add-on code   ✇=FDA approval pending   #=Resequenced code   ○=Recycled/reinstated code

+ 49326   with omentopexy (omental tacking procedure) (List separately in addition to code for primary procedure)

(Use 49326 in conjunction with 49324, 49325)

+ 49327   with placement of interstitial device(s) for radiation therapy guidance (eg, fiducial markers, dosimeter), intra-abdominal, intrapelvic, and/or retroperitoneum, including imaging guidance, if performed, single or multiple (List separately in addition to code for primary procedure)

(Use 49327 in conjunction with laparoscopic abdominal, pelvic, or retroperitoneal procedure[s] performed concurrently)

(For placement of interstitial device[s] for intra-abdominal, intrapelvic, and/or retroperitoneal radiation therapy guidance concurrent with open procedure, use 49412)

(For percutaneous placement of interstitial device[s] for intra-abdominal, intrapelvic, and/or retroperitoneal radiation therapy guidance, use 49411)

49329   Unlisted laparoscopy procedure, abdomen, peritoneum and omentum

Introduction, Revision, Removal

49400   Injection of air or contrast into peritoneal cavity (separate procedure)

(For radiological supervision and interpretation, use 74190)

49402   Removal of peritoneal foreign body from peritoneal cavity

(For lysis of intestinal adhesions, use 44005)

(For open or percutaneous peritoneal drainage or lavage, see 49406, 49020, 49040, 49082-49084, as appropriate)

(For percutaneous insertion of a tunneled intraperitoneal catheter without subcutaneous port, use 49418)

⊙ 49405   Image-guided fluid collection drainage by catheter (eg, abscess, hematoma, seroma, lymphocele, cyst); visceral (eg, kidney, liver, spleen, lung/mediastinum), percutaneous

(Do not report 49405 in conjunction with 75989, 76942, 77002, 77003, 77012, 77021)

(For percutaneous cholecystostomy, use 47490)

(For pneumonostomy, use 32200)

(For thoracentesis, see 32554, 32555)

►(For percutaneous pleural drainage, see 32556, 32557)◄

►(For open visceral drainage, see 32200 [lung abscess or cyst], 47010 [liver abscess or cyst], 48510 [pseudocyst of pancreas], 50020 [perirenal or renal abscess])◄

⊙ 49406   peritoneal or retroperitoneal, percutaneous

(Do not report 49406 in conjunction with 75989, 76942, 77002, 77003, 77012, 77021)

(For abdominal paracentesis [diagnostic or therapeutic], see 49082, 49083)

►(For transrectal or transvaginal image-guided peritoneal or retroperitoneal fluid collection drainage by catheter, use 49407)◄

►(For open transrectal drainage of pelvic abscess, use 45000)◄

►(For open peritoneal or retroperitoneal drainage, see 44900 [appendiceal abscess], 49020 [peritoneal abscess or localized peritonitis], 49040 [subdiaphragmatic or subphrenic abscess], 49060 [retroperitoneal abscess], 49062 [extraperitoneal lymphocele], 49084 [peritoneal lavage], 50020 [perirenal or renal abscess], 58805 [ovarian cyst], 58822 [ovarian abscess])◄

►(For percutaneous paracentesis, see 49082, 49083)◄

(For percutaneous insertion of a tunneled intraperitoneal catheter without subcutaneous port, use 49418)

⊙ 49407   peritoneal or retroperitoneal, transvaginal or transrectal

(Do not report 49407 in conjunction with 75989, 76942, 77002, 77003, 77012, 77021)

(Report 49405, 49406, 49407 separately for each individual collection drained with a separate catheter)

►(For open transrectal or transvaginal drainage, see 45000 [pelvic abscess], 58800 [ovarian cyst], 58820 [ovarian abscess])◄

(For percutaneous image-guided fluid collection drainage by catheter [eg, abscess, hematoma, seroma, lymphocele, cyst] for soft tissue [eg, extremity, abdominal wall, neck], use 10030)

⊙ 49411   Placement of interstitial device(s) for radiation therapy guidance (eg, fiducial markers, dosimeter), percutaneous, intra-abdominal, intra-pelvic (except prostate), and/or retroperitoneum, single or multiple

(Report supply of device separately)

(For imaging guidance, see 76942, 77002, 77012, 77021)

(For percutaneous placement of interstitial device[s] for intra-thoracic radiation therapy guidance, use 32553)

+ 49412   Placement of interstitial device(s) for radiation therapy guidance (eg, fiducial markers, dosimeter), open, intra-abdominal, intrapelvic, and/or retroperitoneum, including image guidance, if performed, single or multiple (List separately in addition to code for primary procedure)

(Use 49412 in conjunction with open abdominal, pelvic, or retroperitoneal procedure[s] performed concurrently)

(For placement of interstitial device[s] for intra-abdominal, intrapelvic, and/or retroperitoneal radiation therapy guidance concurrent with laparoscopic procedure, use 49327)

(For percutaneous placement of interstitial device[s] for intra-abdominal, intrapelvic, and/or retroperitoneal radiation therapy guidance, use 49411)

⊙ **49418**   Insertion of tunneled intraperitoneal catheter (eg, dialysis, intraperitoneal chemotherapy instillation, management of ascites), complete procedure, including imaging guidance, catheter placement, contrast injection when performed, and radiological supervision and interpretation, percutaneous

49419   Insertion of tunneled intraperitoneal catheter, with subcutaneous port (ie, totally implantable)

(For removal, use 49422)

(49420 has been deleted. To report open placement of a tunneled intraperitoneal catheter for dialysis, use 49421. To report open or percutaneous peritoneal drainage or lavage, see 49406, 49020, 49040, 49082-49084, as appropriate. To report percutaneous insertion of a tunneled intraperitoneal catheter without subcutaneous port, use 49418)

49421   Insertion of tunneled intraperitoneal catheter for dialysis, open

(For laparoscopic insertion of tunneled intraperitoneal catheter, use 49324)

(For subcutaneous extension of intraperitoneal catheter with remote chest exit site, use 49435 in conjunction with 49421)

49422   Removal of tunneled intraperitoneal catheter

(For removal of a non-tunneled catheter, use appropriate E/M code)

49423   Exchange of previously placed abscess or cyst drainage catheter under radiological guidance (separate procedure)

(For radiological supervision and interpretation, use 75984)

49424   Contrast injection for assessment of abscess or cyst via previously placed drainage catheter or tube (separate procedure)

(For radiological supervision and interpretation, use 76080)

49425   Insertion of peritoneal-venous shunt

49426   Revision of peritoneal-venous shunt

(For shunt patency test, use 78291)

49427   Injection procedure (eg, contrast media) for evaluation of previously placed peritoneal-venous shunt

(For radiological supervision and interpretation, see 75809, 78291)

49428   Ligation of peritoneal-venous shunt

49429   Removal of peritoneal-venous shunt

+ **49435**   Insertion of subcutaneous extension to intraperitoneal cannula or catheter with remote chest exit site (List separately in addition to code for primary procedure)

(Use 49435 in conjunction with 49324, 49421)

49436   Delayed creation of exit site from embedded subcutaneous segment of intraperitoneal cannula or catheter

Initial Placement

Do not additionally report 43752 for placement of a nasogastric (NG) or orogastric (OG) tube to insufflate the stomach prior to percutaneous gastrointestinal tube placement. NG or OG tube placement is considered part of the procedure in this family of codes.

⊙ **49440**   Insertion of gastrostomy tube, percutaneous, under fluoroscopic guidance including contrast injection(s), image documentation and report

(For conversion to a gastro-jejunostomy tube at the time of initial gastrostomy tube placement, use 49440 in conjunction with 49446)

⊙ **49441**   Insertion of duodenostomy or jejunostomy tube, percutaneous, under fluoroscopic guidance including contrast injection(s), image documentation and report

(For conversion of gastrostomy tube to gastro-jejunostomy tube, use 49446)

⊙ **49442**   Insertion of cecostomy or other colonic tube, percutaneous, under fluoroscopic guidance including contrast injection(s), image documentation and report

Conversion

⊙ **49446**   Conversion of gastrostomy tube to gastro-jejunostomy tube, percutaneous, under fluoroscopic guidance including contrast injection(s), image documentation and report

(For conversion to a gastro-jejunostomy tube at the time of initial gastrostomy tube placement, use 49446 in conjunction with 49440)

Replacement

If an existing gastrostomy, duodenostomy, jejunostomy, gastro-jejunostomy, or cecostomy (or other colonic) tube is removed and a new tube is placed via a separate percutaneous access site, the placement of the new tube is not considered a replacement and would be reported using the appropriate initial placement codes 49440-49442.

49450   Replacement of gastrostomy or cecostomy (or other colonic) tube, percutaneous, under fluoroscopic guidance including contrast injection(s), image documentation and report

(To report a percutaneous change of a gastrostomy tube without imaging or endoscopic guidance, use 43760)

49451   Replacement of duodenostomy or jejunostomy tube, percutaneous, under fluoroscopic guidance including contrast injection(s), image documentation and report

49452   Replacement of gastro-jejunostomy tube, percutaneous, under fluoroscopic guidance including contrast injection(s), image documentation and report

Mechanical Removal of Obstructive Material

49460   Mechanical removal of obstructive material from gastrostomy, duodenostomy, jejunostomy, gastro-jejunostomy, or cecostomy (or other colonic) tube, any method, under fluoroscopic guidance including contrast injection(s), if performed, image documentation and report

(Do not report 49460 in conjunction with 49450-49452, 49465)

Other

49465   Contrast injection(s) for radiological evaluation of existing gastrostomy, duodenostomy, jejunostomy, gastro-jejunostomy, or cecostomy (or other colonic) tube, from a percutaneous approach including image documentation and report

(Do not report 49465 in conjunction with 49450-49460)

Repair

Hernioplasty, Herniorrhaphy, Herniotomy

The hernia repair codes in this section are categorized primarily by the type of hernia (inguinal, femoral, incisional, etc).

Some types of hernias are further categorized as "initial" or "recurrent" based on whether or not the hernia has required previous repair(s).

Additional variables accounted for by some of the codes include patient age and clinical presentation (reducible vs. incarcerated or strangulated).

With the exception of the incisional hernia repairs (see 49560-49566) the use of mesh or other prostheses is not separately reported.

The excision/repair of strangulated organs or structures such as testicle(s), intestine, ovaries are reported by using the appropriate code for the excision/repair (eg, 44120, 54520, and 58940) in addition to the appropriate code for the repair of the strangulated hernia.

(For reduction and repair of intra-abdominal hernia, use 44050)

(For debridement of abdominal wall, see 11042, 11043)

(Codes 49491-49651 are unilateral procedures. To report bilateral procedure, report modifier 50 with the appropriate procedure code)

49491   Repair, initial inguinal hernia, preterm infant (younger than 37 weeks gestation at birth), performed from birth up to 50 weeks postconception age, with or without hydrocelectomy; reducible

49492   incarcerated or strangulated

(Do not report modifier 63 in conjunction with 49491, 49492)

(Postconception age equals gestational age at birth plus age of infant in weeks at the time of the hernia repair. Initial inguinal hernia repairs that are performed on preterm infants who are older than 50 weeks postconception age and younger than age 6 months at the time of surgery, should be reported using codes 49495, 49496)

49495   Repair, initial inguinal hernia, full term infant younger than age 6 months, or preterm infant older than 50 weeks postconception age and younger than age 6 months at the time of surgery, with or without hydrocelectomy; reducible

49496   incarcerated or strangulated

(Do not report modifier 63 in conjunction with 49495, 49496)

(Postconception age equals gestational age at birth plus age in weeks at the time of the hernia repair. Initial inguinal hernia repairs that are performed on preterm infants who are younger than or up to 50 weeks postconception age but younger than 6 months of age since birth, should be reported using codes 49491, 49492. Inguinal hernia repairs on infants age 6 months to younger than 5 years should be reported using codes 49500-49501)

49500   Repair initial inguinal hernia, age 6 months to younger than 5 years, with or without hydrocelectomy; reducible

49501   incarcerated or strangulated

49505   Repair initial inguinal hernia, age 5 years or older; reducible

49507   incarcerated or strangulated

(For inguinal hernia repair, with simple orchiectomy, see 49505 or 49507 and 54520)

(For inguinal hernia repair, with excision of hydrocele or spermatocele, see 49505 or 49507 and 54840 or 55040)

49520   Repair recurrent inguinal hernia, any age; reducible

49521   incarcerated or strangulated

49525   Repair inguinal hernia, sliding, any age

(For incarcerated or strangulated inguinal hernia repair, see 49496, 49501, 49507, 49521)

49540   Repair lumbar hernia

49550   Repair initial femoral hernia, any age; reducible

49553   incarcerated or strangulated

49555   Repair recurrent femoral hernia; reducible

Digestive

49557   incarcerated or strangulated

49560   Repair initial incisional or ventral hernia; reducible

49561   incarcerated or strangulated

49565   Repair recurrent incisional or ventral hernia; reducible

49566   incarcerated or strangulated

+ 49568   Implantation of mesh or other prosthesis for open incisional or ventral hernia repair or mesh for closure of debridement for necrotizing soft tissue infection (List separately in addition to code for the incisional or ventral hernia repair)

(Use 49568 in conjunction with 11004-11006, 49560-49566)

49570   Repair epigastric hernia (eg, preperitoneal fat); reducible (separate procedure)

49572   incarcerated or strangulated

49580   Repair umbilical hernia, younger than age 5 years; reducible

49582   incarcerated or strangulated

49585   Repair umbilical hernia, age 5 years or older; reducible

49587   incarcerated or strangulated

49590   Repair spigelian hernia

49600   Repair of small omphalocele, with primary closure

(Do not report modifier 63 in conjunction with 49600)

49605   Repair of large omphalocele or gastroschisis; with or without prosthesis

49606   with removal of prosthesis, final reduction and closure, in operating room

(Do not report modifier 63 in conjunction with 49605, 49606)

49610   Repair of omphalocele (Gross type operation); first stage

49611   second stage

(Do not report modifier 63 in conjunction with 49610, 49611)

(For diaphragmatic or hiatal hernia repair, see 39503, 43332)

(For surgical repair of omentum, use 49999)

Laparoscopy

Surgical laparoscopy always includes diagnostic laparoscopy. To report a diagnostic laparoscopy (peritoneoscopy) (separate procedure), use 49320.

49650   Laparoscopy, surgical; repair initial inguinal hernia

49651   repair recurrent inguinal hernia

49652   Laparoscopy, surgical, repair, ventral, umbilical, spigelian or epigastric hernia (includes mesh insertion, when performed); reducible

(Do not report 49652 in conjunction with 44180, 49568)

49653   incarcerated or strangulated

(Do not report 49653 in conjunction with 44180, 49568)

49654   Laparoscopy, surgical, repair, incisional hernia (includes mesh insertion, when performed); reducible

(Do not report 49654 in conjunction with 44180, 49568)

49655   incarcerated or strangulated

(Do not report 49655 in conjunction with 44180, 49568)

49656   Laparoscopy, surgical, repair, recurrent incisional hernia (includes mesh insertion, when performed); reducible

(Do not report 49656 in conjunction with 44180, 49568)

49657   incarcerated or strangulated

(Do not report 49657 in conjunction with 44180, 49568)

49659   Unlisted laparoscopy procedure, hernioplasty, herniorrhaphy, herniotomy

Suture

49900   Suture, secondary, of abdominal wall for evisceration or dehiscence

(For suture of ruptured diaphragm, see 39540, 39541)

(For debridement of abdominal wall, see 11042, 11043)

Other Procedures

49904   Omental flap, extra-abdominal (eg, for reconstruction of sternal and chest wall defects)

(Code 49904 includes harvest and transfer. If a second surgeon harvests the omental flap, then the 2 surgeons should code 49904 as co-surgeons, using modifier 62)

+ 49905   Omental flap, intra-abdominal (List separately in addition to code for primary procedure)

(Do not report 49905 in conjunction with 44700)

49906   Free omental flap with microvascular anastomosis

(Do not report code 69990 in addition to 49906)

49999   Unlisted procedure, abdomen, peritoneum and omentum

Urinary System

(For provision of chemotherapeutic agents, report both the specific service in addition to code(s) for the specific substance(s) or drug(s) provided)

Kidney

Incision

(For retroperitoneal exploration, abscess, tumor, or cyst, see 49010, 49060, 49203-49205)

50010   Renal exploration, not necessitating other specific procedures

(For laparoscopic ablation of renal mass lesion(s), use 50542)

50020   Drainage of perirenal or renal abscess, open

(50021 has been deleted)

(For percutaneous image-guided fluid collection drainage by catheter of perirenal/renal abscess, use 49405)

50040   Nephrostomy, nephrotomy with drainage

50045   Nephrotomy, with exploration

(For renal endoscopy performed in conjunction with this procedure, see 50570-50580)

50060   Nephrolithotomy; removal of calculus

50065   secondary surgical operation for calculus

50070   complicated by congenital kidney abnormality

50075   removal of large staghorn calculus filling renal pelvis and calyces (including anatrophic pyelolithotomy)

50080   Percutaneous nephrostolithotomy or pyelostolithotomy, with or without dilation, endoscopy, lithotripsy, stenting, or basket extraction; up to 2 cm

50081   over 2 cm

(For establishment of nephrostomy without nephrostolithotomy, see 50040, 50395, 52334)

(For fluoroscopic guidance, see 76000, 76001)

50100   Transection or repositioning of aberrant renal vessels (separate procedure)

50120   Pyelotomy; with exploration

(For renal endoscopy performed in conjunction with this procedure, see 50570-50580)

50125   with drainage, pyelostomy

50130   with removal of calculus (pyelolithotomy, pelviolithotomy, including coagulum pyelolithotomy)

50135   complicated (eg, secondary operation, congenital kidney abnormality)

(For supply of anticarcinogenic agents, use 99070 in addition to code for primary procedure)

Excision

(For excision of retroperitoneal tumor or cyst, see 49203-49205)

(For laparoscopic ablation of renal mass lesion(s), use 50542)

⊙ **50200**   Renal biopsy; percutaneous, by trocar or needle

(For radiological supervision and interpretation, see 76942, 77002, 77012, 77021)

(For fine needle aspiration, use 10022)

(For evaluation of fine needle aspirate, see 88172, 88173)

50205   by surgical exposure of kidney

50220   Nephrectomy, including partial ureterectomy, any open approach including rib resection;

50225   complicated because of previous surgery on same kidney

50230   radical, with regional lymphadenectomy and/or vena caval thrombectomy

(When vena caval resection with reconstruction is necessary, use 37799)

50234   Nephrectomy with total ureterectomy and bladder cuff; through same incision

50236   through separate incision

50240   Nephrectomy, partial

(For laparoscopic partial nephrectomy, use 50543)

50250   Ablation, open, 1 or more renal mass lesion(s), cryosurgical, including intraoperative ultrasound guidance and monitoring, if performed

(For laparoscopic ablation of renal mass lesions, use 50542)

(For percutaneous ablation of renal tumors, see 50592, 50593)

50280   Excision or unroofing of cyst(s) of kidney

(For laparoscopic ablation of renal cysts, use 50541)

50290   Excision of perinephric cyst

Renal Transplantation

Renal *auto*transplantation includes reimplantation of the autograft as the primary procedure, along with secondary extra-corporeal procedure(s) (eg, partial nephrectomy, nephrolithotomy) reported with modifier 51 (see 50380 and applicable secondary procedure(s)).

Renal *allo*transplantation involves three distinct components of physician work:

1. ***Cadaver donor nephrectomy, unilateral or bilateral,*** which includes harvesting the graft(s) and cold preservation of the graft(s) (perfusing with cold preservation solution and cold maintenance) (use 50300). ***Living donor nephrectomy,*** which includes

harvesting the graft, cold preservation of the graft (perfusing with cold preservation solution and cold maintenance), and care of the donor (see 50320, 50547).

2. ***Backbench work:***

Standard preparation of a cadaver donor renal allograft prior to transplantation including dissection and removal of perinephric fat, diaphragmatic and retroperitoneal attachments; excision of adrenal gland; and preparation of ureter(s), renal vein(s), and renal artery(s), ligating branches, as necessary (use 50323).

Standard preparation of a living donor renal allograft (open or laparoscopic) prior to transplantation including dissection and removal of perinephric fat and preparation of ureter(s), renal vein(s), and renal artery(s), ligating branches, as necessary (use 50325).

Additional reconstruction of a cadaver or living donor renal allograft prior to transplantation may include venous, arterial, and/or ureteral anastomosis(es) necessary for implantation (see 50327-50329).

3. ***Recipient renal allotransplantation,*** which includes transplantation of the allograft (with or without recipient nephrectomy) and care of the recipient (see 50360, 50365).

(For dialysis, see 90935-90999)

(For laparoscopic donor nephrectomy, use 50547)

(For laparoscopic drainage of lymphocele to peritoneal cavity, use 49323)

50300 Donor nephrectomy (including cold preservation); from cadaver donor, unilateral or bilateral

50320 open, from living donor

50323 Backbench standard preparation of cadaver donor renal allograft prior to transplantation, including dissection and removal of perinephric fat, diaphragmatic and retroperitoneal attachments, excision of adrenal gland, and preparation of ureter(s), renal vein(s), and renal artery(s), ligating branches, as necessary

(Do not report 50323 in conjunction with 60540, 60545)

50325 Backbench standard preparation of living donor renal allograft (open or laparoscopic) prior to transplantation, including dissection and removal of perinephric fat and preparation of ureter(s), renal vein(s), and renal artery(s), ligating branches, as necessary

50327 Backbench reconstruction of cadaver or living donor renal allograft prior to transplantation; venous anastomosis, each

50328 arterial anastomosis, each

50329 ureteral anastomosis, each

50340 Recipient nephrectomy (separate procedure)

(For bilateral procedure, report 50340 with modifier 50)

50360 Renal allotransplantation, implantation of graft; without recipient nephrectomy

50365 with recipient nephrectomy

(For bilateral procedure, report 50365 with modifier 50)

50370 Removal of transplanted renal allograft

50380 Renal autotransplantation, reimplantation of kidney

(For renal autotransplantation extra-corporeal [bench] surgery, use autotransplantation as the primary procedure and report secondary procedure[s] [eg, partial nephrectomy, nephrolithotomy] with modifier 51)

Introduction

Renal Pelvis Catheter Procedures

Internally Dwelling

⊙ **50382** Removal (via snare/capture) and replacement of internally dwelling ureteral stent via percutaneous approach, including radiological supervision and interpretation

(For bilateral procedure, use modifier 50)

(For removal and replacement of an internally dwelling ureteral stent via a transurethral approach, use 50385)

⊙ **50384** Removal (via snare/capture) of internally dwelling ureteral stent via percutaneous approach, including radiological supervision and interpretation

(For bilateral procedure, use modifier 50)

(Do not report 50382, 50384 in conjunction with 50395)

(For removal of an internally dwelling ureteral stent via a transurethral approach, use 50386)

⊙ **50385** Removal (via snare/capture) and replacement of internally dwelling ureteral stent via transurethral approach, without use of cystoscopy, including radiological supervision and interpretation

⊙ **50386** Removal (via snare/capture) of internally dwelling ureteral stent via transurethral approach, without use of cystoscopy, including radiological supervision and interpretation

Externally Accessible

⊙▲ **50387** Removal and replacement of externally accessible nephroureteral catheter (eg, external/internal stent) requiring fluoroscopic guidance, including radiological supervision and interpretation

(For bilateral procedure, use modifier 50)

(For removal and replacement of externally accessible ureteral stent via ureterostomy or ileal conduit, use 50688)

(For removal without replacement of an externally accessible ureteral stent not requiring fluoroscopic guidance, see Evaluation and Management services codes)

50389   Removal of nephrostomy tube, requiring fluoroscopic guidance (eg, with concurrent indwelling ureteral stent)

(Removal of nephrostomy tube not requiring fluoroscopic guidance is considered inherent to E/M services. Report the appropriate level of E/M service provided)

▶Other Introduction (Injection/Change/ Removal) Procedures◀

▶Percutaneous genitourinary procedures are performed with imaging guidance (eg, fluoroscopy and/or ultrasound). Diagnostic nephrostogram and/or ureterogram are typically performed with percutaneous genitourinary procedures and are included in 50432, 50433, 50434, 50435, 50693, 50694, 50695.

Codes 50430 and 50431 are diagnostic procedure codes that include injection(s) of contrast material, all associated radiological supervision and interpretation, and procedural imaging guidance (eg, ultrasound and/or fluoroscopy). Code 50430 also includes accessing the collecting system and/or associated ureter with a needle and/or catheter. Code 50430 or 50431 may not be reported together with 50432, 50433, 50434, 50435, 50693, 50694, 50695.

Codes 50432, 50433, 50434, 50435 represent therapeutic procedures describing catheter placement or exchange, and include the elements of access, drainage catheter manipulations, and imaging guidance (eg, ultra-sonography and/or fluoroscopy), as well as diagnostic imaging supervision and interpretation, when performed.

Code 50433 describes percutaneous nephrostomy with the additional accessing of the ureter/bladder to ultimately place a nephroureteral catheter (a single transnephric catheter with nephrostomy and ureteral components that allows drainage internally, externally, or both).

For codes 50430, 50431, 50432, 50433, 50434, 50435, 50606, 50693, 50694, 50695, 50705, and 50706, the renal pelvis and its associated ureter are considered a single entity for reporting purposes. Codes 50430, 50431, 50432, 50433, 50434, 50435, 50606, 50693, 50694, 50695, 50705, and 50706 may be reported once for each renal collecting system/ureter accessed (eg, two separate codes would be reported for bilateral nephrostomy tube placement or for unilateral duplicated collecting system/ureter requiring two separate procedures.◀

50390   Aspiration and/or injection of renal cyst or pelvis by needle, percutaneous

(For radiological supervision and interpretation, see 74425, 74470, 76942, 77002, 77012, 77021)

▶(For antegrade nephrostogram and/or antegrade pyelogram, see 50430, 50431)◀

50391   Instillation(s) of therapeutic agent into renal pelvis and/or ureter through established nephrostomy, pyelostomy or ureterostomy tube (eg, anticarcinogenic or antifungal agent)

▶(50392 has been deleted. To report nephrostomy tube placement, use 50432)◀

▶(50393 has been deleted. To report ureteral catheter placement, see 50693, 50694, 50695)◀

▶(50394 has been deleted. To report injection procedures for antegrade nephrostogram and/or antegrade pyelogram, see 50430, 50431)◀

50395   Introduction of guide into renal pelvis and/or ureter with dilation to establish nephrostomy tract, percutaneous

▶(For radiological supervision and interpretation, use 74485)◀

(For nephrostolithotomy, see 50080, 50081)

(For retrograde percutaneous nephrostomy, use 52334)

(For endoscopic surgery, see 50551-50561)

50396   Manometric studies through nephrostomy or pyelostomy tube, or indwelling ureteral catheter

▶(For radiological supervision and interpretation, use 74425)◀

▶(50398 has been deleted. To report exchange of a percutaneous nephrostomy catheter, use 50435)◀

#⊙● **50430**   Injection procedure for antegrade nephrostogram and/or ureterogram, complete diagnostic procedure including imaging guidance (eg, ultrasound and fluoroscopy) and all associated radiological supervision and interpretation; new access

#● **50431**   existing access

▶(Do not report 50430, 50431 in conjunction with 50432, 50433, 50434, 50435, 50693, 50694, 50695, 74425 for the same renal collecting system and/or associated ureter)◀

#⊙● **50432**   Placement of nephrostomy catheter, percutaneous, including diagnostic nephrostogram and/or ureterogram when performed, imaging guidance (eg, ultrasound and/or fluoroscopy) and all associated radiological supervision and interpretation

▶(Do not report 50432 in conjunction with 50430, 50431, 50433, 50694, 50695, 74425 for the same renal collecting system and/or associated ureter)◀

▶(Do not report 50432 in conjunction with 50395 for dilation of the nephrostomy tube tract)◀

#⊙● **50433**   Placement of nephroureteral catheter, percutaneous, including diagnostic nephrostogram and/or ureterogram when performed, imaging guidance (eg, ultrasound and/or fluoroscopy) and all associated radiological supervision and interpretation, new access

Urinary

▶(Do not report 50433 in conjunction with 50430, 50431, 50432, 50693, 50694, 50695, 74425 for the same renal collecting system and/or associated ureter)◀

▶(Do not report 50433 in conjunction with 50395 for dilation of the nephroureteral catheter tract)◀

▶(For nephroureteral catheter removal and replacement, use 50387)◀

#⊙● 50434 Convert nephrostomy catheter to nephroureteral catheter, percutaneous, including diagnostic nephrostogram and/or ureterogram when performed, imaging guidance (eg, ultrasound and/or fluoroscopy) and all associated radiological supervision and interpretation, via pre-existing nephrostomy tract

▶(Do not report 50434 in conjunction with 50430, 50431, 50435, 50684, 50693, 74425 for the same renal collecting system and/or associated ureter)◀

#● 50435 Exchange nephrostomy catheter, percutaneous, including diagnostic nephrostogram and/or ureterogram when performed, imaging guidance (eg, ultrasound and/or fluoroscopy) and all associated radiological supervision and interpretation

▶(Do not report 50435 in conjunction with 50430, 50431, 50434, 50693, 74425 for the same renal collecting system and/or associated ureter)◀

▶(For removal of nephrostomy catheter requiring fluoroscopic guidance, use 50389)◀

Repair

50400 Pyeloplasty (Foley Y-pyeloplasty), plastic operation on renal pelvis, with or without plastic operation on ureter, nephropexy, nephrostomy, pyelostomy, or ureteral splinting; simple

50405 complicated (congenital kidney abnormality, secondary pyeloplasty, solitary kidney, calycoplasty)

(For laparoscopic approach, use 50544)

50430 Code is out of numerical sequence. See 50390-50435

50431 Code is out of numerical sequence. See 50390-50435

50432 Code is out of numerical sequence. See 50390-50435

50433 Code is out of numerical sequence. See 50390-50435

50434 Code is out of numerical sequence. See 50390-50435

50435 Code is out of numerical sequence. See 50390-50435

50500 Nephrorrhaphy, suture of kidney wound or injury

50520 Closure of nephrocutaneous or pyelocutaneous fistula

50525 Closure of nephrovisceral fistula (eg, renocolic), including visceral repair; abdominal approach

50526 thoracic approach

50540 Symphysiotomy for horseshoe kidney with or without pyeloplasty and/or other plastic procedure, unilateral or bilateral (1 operation)

Laparoscopy

Surgical laparoscopy always includes diagnostic laparoscopy. To report a diagnostic laparoscopy (peritoneoscopy) (separate procedure), use 49320.

50541 Laparoscopy, surgical; ablation of renal cysts

50542 ablation of renal mass lesion(s), including intraoperative ultrasound guidance and monitoring, when performed

(For open procedure, use 50250)

(For percutaneous ablation of renal tumors, see 50592, 50593)

50543 partial nephrectomy

(For open procedure, use 50240)

50544 pyeloplasty

50545 radical nephrectomy (includes removal of Gerota's fascia and surrounding fatty tissue, removal of regional lymph nodes, and adrenalectomy)

(For open procedure, use 50230)

50546 nephrectomy, including partial ureterectomy

50547 donor nephrectomy (including cold preservation), from living donor

(For open procedure, use 50320)

(For backbench renal allograft standard preparation prior to transplantation, use 50325)

(For backbench renal allograft reconstruction prior to transplantation, see 50327-50329)

50548 nephrectomy with total ureterectomy

(For open procedure, see 50234, 50236)

50549 Unlisted laparoscopy procedure, renal

(For laparoscopic drainage of lymphocele to peritoneal cavity, use 49323)

Endoscopy

(For supplies and materials, use 99070)

50551 Renal endoscopy through established nephrostomy or pyelostomy, with or without irrigation, instillation, or ureteropyelography, exclusive of radiologic service;

50553 with ureteral catheterization, with or without dilation of ureter

▶(For image-guided dilation of ureter without endoscopic guidance, use 50706)◀

50555 with biopsy

▶(For image-guided biopsy of ureter and/or renal pelvis without endoscopic guidance, use 50606)◀

50557 with fulguration and/or incision, with or without biopsy

50561 with removal of foreign body or calculus

50562   with resection of tumor

(When procedures 50570-50580 provide a significant identifiable service, they may be added to 50045 and 50120)

50570   Renal endoscopy through nephrotomy or pyelotomy, with or without irrigation, instillation, or ureteropyelography, exclusive of radiologic service;

(For nephrotomy, use 50045)

(For pyelotomy, use 50120)

50572   with ureteral catheterization, with or without dilation of ureter

►(For image-guided dilation of ureter without endoscopic guidance, use 50706)◄

50574   with biopsy

►(For image-guided biopsy of ureter and/or renal pelvis without endoscopic guidance, use 50606)◄

50575   with endopyelotomy (includes cystoscopy, ureteroscopy, dilation of ureter and ureteral pelvic junction, incision of ureteral pelvic junction and insertion of endopyelotomy stent)

50576   with fulguration and/or incision, with or without biopsy

50580   with removal of foreign body or calculus

Other Procedures

50590   Lithotripsy, extracorporeal shock wave

⊙ **50592**   Ablation, 1 or more renal tumor(s), percutaneous, unilateral, radiofrequency

(50592 is a unilateral procedure. For bilateral procedure, report 50592 with modifier 50)

(For imaging guidance and monitoring, see 76940, 77013, 77022)

⊙ **50593**   Ablation, renal tumor(s), unilateral, percutaneous, cryotherapy

(50593 is a unilateral procedure. For bilateral procedure, report 50593 with modifier 50)

(For imaging guidance and monitoring, see codes 76940, 77013, 77022)

Ureter

►Incision/Biopsy◄

►Code 50606 is an add-on code describing endoluminal biopsy (eg, brush) using non-endoscopic imaging guidance, which may be reported once per ureter per day. This code includes the work of the biopsy and the imaging guidance and radiological supervision and interpretation required to accomplish the biopsy. The biopsy may be performed through *de novo* transrenal access, an existing renal/ureteral access, transurethral

access, an ileal conduit, or ureterostomy. The service of gaining access may be reported separately. Diagnostic pyelography/ureterography is not included in the work of 50606 and may be reported separately. Other interventions or catheter placements performed at the same setting as the biopsy may be reported separately.

For codes 50430, 50431, 50432, 50433, 50434, 50435, 50606, 50693, 50694, 50695, 50705, and 50706, the renal pelvis and its associated ureter are considered a single entity for reporting purposes. Codes 50430, 50431, 50432, 50433, 50434, 50435, 50606, 50693, 50694, 50695, 50705, and 50706 may be reported once for each renal collecting system/ureter accessed (eg, two separate codes would be reported for bilateral nephrostomy tube placement or for unilateral duplicated collecting system/ureter requiring two separate procedures.◄

50600   Ureterotomy with exploration or drainage (separate procedure)

(For ureteral endoscopy performed in conjunction with this procedure, see 50970-50980)

50605   Ureterotomy for insertion of indwelling stent, all types

⊙+● **50606**   Endoluminal biopsy of ureter and/or renal pelvis, non-endoscopic, including imaging guidance (eg, ultrasound and/or fluoroscopy) and all associated radiological supervision and interpretation (List separately in addition to code for primary procedure)

►(Use 50606 in conjunction with 50382, 50384, 50385, 50386, 50387, 50389, 50430, 50431, 50432, 50433, 50434, 50435, 50684, 50688, 50690, 50693, 50694, 50695, 51610)◄

►(Do not report 50606 in conjunction with 50555, 50574, 50955, 50974, 52007, 74425 for the same renal collecting system and/or associated ureter)◄

50610   Ureterolithotomy; upper one-third of ureter

50620   middle one-third of ureter

50630   lower one-third of ureter

(For laparoscopic approach, use 50945)

(For transvesical ureterolithotomy, use 51060)

(For cystotomy with stone basket extraction of ureteral calculus, use 51065)

(For endoscopic extraction or manipulation of ureteral calculus, see 50080, 50081, 50561, 50961, 50980, 52320-52330, 52352, 52353, 52356)

Excision

(For ureterocele, see 51535, 52300)

50650   Ureterectomy, with bladder cuff (separate procedure)

50660   Ureterectomy, total, ectopic ureter, combination abdominal, vaginal and/or perineal approach

Introduction

▶Other Introduction (Injection/Change/ Removal) Procedures◀

▶Codes 50693, 50694, 50695 are therapeutic procedure codes describing percutaneous placement of ureteral stents. These codes include access, drainage, catheter manipulations, diagnostic nephrostogram and/or ureterogram, when performed, imaging guidance (eg, ultrasonography and/or fluoroscopy), and all associated radiological supervision and interpretation. When a separate ureteral stent and a nephrostomy catheter are placed into a ureter and its associated renal pelvis during the same session through a new percutaneous renal access, use 50695 to report the procedure.◀

50684 Injection procedure for ureterography or ureteropyelography through ureterostomy or indwelling ureteral catheter

▶(Do not report 50684 in conjunction with 50433, 50434, 50693, 50694, 50695)◀

(For radiological supervision and interpretation, use 74425)

50686 Manometric studies through ureterostomy or indwelling ureteral catheter

50688 Change of ureterostomy tube or externally accessible ureteral stent via ileal conduit

(If imaging guidance is performed, use 75984)

50690 Injection procedure for visualization of ileal conduit and/ or ureteropyelography, exclusive of radiologic service

(For radiological supervision and interpretation, use 74425)

⊙● **50693** Placement of ureteral stent, percutaneous, including diagnostic nephrostogram and/or ureterogram when performed, imaging guidance (eg, ultrasound and/or fluoroscopy), and all associated radiological supervision and interpretation; pre-existing nephrostomy tract

⊙● **50694** new access, without separate nephrostomy catheter

⊙● **50695** new access, with separate nephrostomy catheter

▶(Do not report 50693, 50694, 50695 in conjunction with 50430, 50431, 50432, 50433, 50434, 50435, 50684, 74425 for the same renal collecting system and/or associated ureter)◀

Repair

▶Codes 50705, 50706 are add-on codes describing embolization and balloon dilation of the ureter using non-endoscopic imaging guidance, and each may be reported once per ureter per day. These codes include embolization or dilation plus imaging guidance and radiological supervision and interpretation required to accomplish the embolization or dilation. These procedures may be performed through *de novo* transrenal access, an existing renal/ureteral access, transurethral access, an ileal conduit, or ureterostomy. The service of gaining access may be reported separately. Diagnostic pyelography/ureterography is not included in 50705 and 50706 and may be reported separately. Other interventions or catheter placements performed at the same setting as the embolization/dilation may be reported separately.◀

50700 Ureteroplasty, plastic operation on ureter (eg, stricture)

⊙+● **50705** Ureteral embolization or occlusion, including imaging guidance (eg, ultrasound and/or fluoroscopy) and all associated radiological supervision and interpretation (List separately in addition to code for primary procedure)

▶(Use 50705 in conjunction with 50382, 50384, 50385, 50386, 50387, 50389, 50430, 50431, 50432, 50433, 50434, 50435, 50684, 50688, 50690, 50693, 50694, 50695, 51610)◀

⊙+● **50706** Balloon dilation, ureteral stricture, including imaging guidance (eg, ultrasound and/or fluoroscopy) and all associated radiological supervision and interpretation (List separately in addition to code for primary procedure)

▶(Use 50706 in conjunction with 50382, 50384, 50385, 50386, 50387, 50389, 50430, 50431, 50432, 50433, 50434, 50435, 50684, 50688, 50690, 50693, 50694, 50695, 51610)◀

▶(Do not report 50706 in conjunction with 50553, 50572, 50953, 50972, 52341, 52344, 52345, 74485)◀

▶(For percutaneous nephrostomy, nephroureteral catheter, and/or ureteral catheter placement use 50385, 50387, 50432, 50433, 50434, 50435, 50693, 50694, 50695)◀

50715 Ureterolysis, with or without repositioning of ureter for retroperitoneal fibrosis

(For bilateral procedure, report 50715 with modifier 50)

50722 Ureterolysis for ovarian vein syndrome

50725 Ureterolysis for retrocaval ureter, with reanastomosis of upper urinary tract or vena cava

50727 Revision of urinary-cutaneous anastomosis (any type urostomy);

50728 with repair of fascial defect and hernia

50740 Ureteropyelostomy, anastomosis of ureter and renal pelvis

50750 Ureterocalycostomy, anastomosis of ureter to renal calyx

50760 Ureteroureterostomy

50770 Transureteroureterostomy, anastomosis of ureter to contralateral ureter

(Codes 50780-50785 include minor procedures to prevent vesicoureteral reflux)

50780 Ureteroneocystostomy; anastomosis of single ureter to bladder

(For bilateral procedure, report 50780 with modifier 50)

(When combined with cystourethroplasty or vesical neck revision, use 51820)

50782 anastomosis of duplicated ureter to bladder

50783 with extensive ureteral tailoring

50785 with vesico-psoas hitch or bladder flap

(For bilateral procedure, report 50785 with modifier 50)

50800 Ureteroenterostomy, direct anastomosis of ureter to intestine

(For bilateral procedure, report 50800 with modifier 50)

50810 Ureterosigmoidostomy, with creation of sigmoid bladder and establishment of abdominal or perineal colostomy, including intestine anastomosis

50815 Ureterocolon conduit, including intestine anastomosis

(For bilateral procedure, report 50815 with modifier 50)

50820 Ureteroileal conduit (ileal bladder), including intestine anastomosis (Bricker operation)

(For bilateral procedure, report 50820 with modifier 50)

(For combination of 50800-50820 with cystectomy, see 51580-51595)

50825 Continent diversion, including intestine anastomosis using any segment of small and/or large intestine (Kock pouch or Camey enterocystoplasty)

50830 Urinary undiversion (eg, taking down of ureteroileal conduit, ureterosigmoidostomy or ureteroenterostomy with ureteroureterostomy or ureteroneocystostomy)

50840 Replacement of all or part of ureter by intestine segment, including intestine anastomosis

(For bilateral procedure, report 50840 with modifier 50)

50845 Cutaneous appendico-vesicostomy

50860 Ureterostomy, transplantation of ureter to skin

(For bilateral procedure, report 50860 with modifier 50)

50900 Ureterorrhaphy, suture of ureter (separate procedure)

50920 Closure of ureterocutaneous fistula

50930 Closure of ureterovisceral fistula (including visceral repair)

50940 Deligation of ureter

(For ureteroplasty, ureterolysis, see 50700-50860)

Laparoscopy

Surgical laparoscopy always includes diagnostic laparoscopy. To report a diagnostic laparoscopy (peritoneoscopy) (separate procedure), use 49320.

50945 Laparoscopy, surgical; ureterolithotomy

50947 ureteroneocystostomy with cystoscopy and ureteral stent placement

50948 ureteroneocystostomy without cystoscopy and ureteral stent placement

(For open ureteroneocystostomy, see 50780-50785)

50949 Unlisted laparoscopy procedure, ureter

Endoscopy

50951 Ureteral endoscopy through established ureterostomy, with or without irrigation, instillation, or ureteropyelography, exclusive of radiologic service;

50953 with ureteral catheterization, with or without dilation of ureter

►(For image-guided dilation of ureter without endoscopic guidance, use 50706)◄

50955 with biopsy

►(For image-guided biopsy of ureter and/or renal pelvis without endoscopic guidance, use 50606)◄

50957 with fulguration and/or incision, with or without biopsy

50961 with removal of foreign body or calculus

50970 Ureteral endoscopy through ureterotomy, with or without irrigation, instillation, or ureteropyelography, exclusive of radiologic service;

(For ureterotomy, use 50600)

50972 with ureteral catheterization, with or without dilation of ureter

►(For image-guided dilation of ureter without endoscopic guidance, use 50706)◄

50974 with biopsy

►(For image-guided biopsy of ureter and/or renal pelvis without endoscopic guidance, use 50606)◄

50976 with fulguration and/or incision, with or without biopsy

50980 with removal of foreign body or calculus

Bladder

Incision

51020 Cystotomy or cystostomy; with fulguration and/or insertion of radioactive material

51030 with cryosurgical destruction of intravesical lesion

51040 Cystostomy, cystotomy with drainage

51045 Cystotomy, with insertion of ureteral catheter or stent (separate procedure)

51050 Cystolithotomy, cystotomy with removal of calculus, without vesical neck resection

51060 Transvesical ureterolithotomy

Urinary

51065   Cystotomy, with calculus basket extraction and/or ultrasonic or electrohydraulic fragmentation of ureteral calculus

51080   Drainage of perivesical or prevesical space abscess

(For percutaneous image-guided fluid collection drainage by catheter of perivesicular or prevesicular space abscess, use 49406)

Removal

51100   Aspiration of bladder; by needle

51101   by trocar or intracatheter

51102   with insertion of suprapubic catheter

(For imaging guidance, see 76942, 77002, 77012)

Excision

51500   Excision of urachal cyst or sinus, with or without umbilical hernia repair

51520   Cystotomy; for simple excision of vesical neck (separate procedure)

51525   for excision of bladder diverticulum, single or multiple (separate procedure)

51530   for excision of bladder tumor

(For transurethral resection, see 52234-52240, 52305)

51535   Cystotomy for excision, incision, or repair of ureterocele

(For bilateral procedure, report 51535 with modifier 50)

(For transurethral excision, use 52300)

51550   Cystectomy, partial; simple

51555   complicated (eg, postradiation, previous surgery, difficult location)

51565   Cystectomy, partial, with reimplantation of ureter(s) into bladder (ureteroneocystostomy)

51570   Cystectomy, complete; (separate procedure)

51575   with bilateral pelvic lymphadenectomy, including external iliac, hypogastric, and obturator nodes

51580   Cystectomy, complete, with ureterosigmoidostomy or ureterocutaneous transplantations;

51585   with bilateral pelvic lymphadenectomy, including external iliac, hypogastric, and obturator nodes

51590   Cystectomy, complete, with ureteroileal conduit or sigmoid bladder, including intestine anastomosis;

51595   with bilateral pelvic lymphadenectomy, including external iliac, hypogastric, and obturator nodes

51596   Cystectomy, complete, with continent diversion, any open technique, using any segment of small and/or large intestine to construct neobladder

51597   Pelvic exenteration, complete, for vesical, prostatic or urethral malignancy, with removal of bladder and ureteral transplantations, with or without hysterectomy and/or abdominoperineal resection of rectum and colon and colostomy, or any combination thereof

(For pelvic exenteration for gynecologic malignancy, use 58240)

Introduction

51600   Injection procedure for cystography or voiding urethrocystography

(For radiological supervision and interpretation, see 74430, 74455)

51605   Injection procedure and placement of chain for contrast and/or chain urethrocystography

(For radiological supervision and interpretation, use 74430)

51610   Injection procedure for retrograde urethrocystography

(For radiological supervision and interpretation, use 74450)

51700   Bladder irrigation, simple, lavage and/or instillation

(Codes 51701-51702 are reported only when performed independently. Do not report 51701-51702 when catheter insertion is an inclusive component of another procedure.)

51701   Insertion of non-indwelling bladder catheter (eg, straight catheterization for residual urine)

51702   Insertion of temporary indwelling bladder catheter; simple (eg, Foley)

(Do not report 51702 in conjunction with 0071T, 0072T)

51703   complicated (eg, altered anatomy, fractured catheter/balloon)

51705   Change of cystostomy tube; simple

51710   complicated

(If imaging guidance is performed, use 75984)

51715   Endoscopic injection of implant material into the submucosal tissues of the urethra and/or bladder neck

(For anoscopy with directed submucosal injection of bulking agent for fecal incontinence, use 0377T)

51720   Bladder instillation of anticarcinogenic agent (including retention time)

Urodynamics

The following section (51725-51798) lists procedures that may be used separately or in many and varied combinations.

When multiple procedures are performed in the same investigative session, modifier 51 should be employed.

All procedures in this section imply that these services are performed by, or are under the direct supervision of, a physician or other qualified health care professional and that all instruments, equipment, fluids, gases, probes, catheters, technician's fees, medications, gloves, trays, tubing, and other sterile supplies be provided by that individual. When the individual only interprets the results and/or operates the equipment, a professional component, modifier 26, should be used to identify these services.

51725   Simple cystometrogram (CMG) (eg, spinal manometer)

51726   Complex cystometrogram (ie, calibrated electronic equipment);

51727   with urethral pressure profile studies (ie, urethral closure pressure profile), any technique

51728   with voiding pressure studies (ie, bladder voiding pressure), any technique

51729   with voiding pressure studies (ie, bladder voiding pressure) and urethral pressure profile studies (ie, urethral closure pressure profile), any technique

#+ **51797**   Voiding pressure studies, intra-abdominal (ie, rectal, gastric, intraperitoneal) (List separately in addition to code for primary procedure)

            (Use 51797 in conjunction with 51728, 51729)

51736   Simple uroflowmetry (UFR) (eg, stop-watch flow rate, mechanical uroflowmeter)

51741   Complex uroflowmetry (eg, calibrated electronic equipment)

51784   Electromyography studies (EMG) of anal or urethral sphincter, other than needle, any technique

            (Do not report 51784 in conjunction with 51792)

51785   Needle electromyography studies (EMG) of anal or urethral sphincter, any technique

51792   Stimulus evoked response (eg, measurement of bulbocavernosus reflex latency time)

            (Do not report 51792 in conjunction with 51784)

51797   Code is out of numerical sequence. See 51725-51798

51798   Measurement of post-voiding residual urine and/or bladder capacity by ultrasound, non-imaging

Repair

51800   Cystoplasty or cystourethroplasty, plastic operation on bladder and/or vesical neck (anterior Y-plasty, vesical fundus resection), any procedure, with or without wedge resection of posterior vesical neck

51820   Cystourethroplasty with unilateral or bilateral ureteroneocystostomy

51840   Anterior vesicourethropexy, or urethropexy (eg, Marshall-Marchetti-Krantz, Burch); simple

51841   complicated (eg, secondary repair)

            (For urethropexy (Pereyra type), use 57289)

51845   Abdomino-vaginal vesical neck suspension, with or without endoscopic control (eg, Stamey, Raz, modified Pereyra)

51860   Cystorrhaphy, suture of bladder wound, injury or rupture; simple

51865   complicated

51880   Closure of cystostomy (separate procedure)

51900   Closure of vesicovaginal fistula, abdominal approach

            (For vaginal approach, see 57320-57330)

51920   Closure of vesicouterine fistula;

51925   with hysterectomy

            (For closure of vesicoenteric fistula, see 44660, 44661)

            (For closure of rectovesical fistula, see 45800-45805)

51940   Closure, exstrophy of bladder

            (See also 54390)

51960   Enterocystoplasty, including intestinal anastomosis

51980   Cutaneous vesicostomy

Laparoscopy

Surgical laparoscopy always includes diagnostic laparoscopy. To report a diagnostic laparoscopy (peritoneoscopy) (separate procedure), use 49320.

51990   Laparoscopy, surgical; urethral suspension for stress incontinence

51992   sling operation for stress incontinence (eg, fascia or synthetic)

            (For open sling operation for stress incontinence, use 57288)

            (For reversal or removal of sling operation for stress incontinence, use 57287)

51999   Unlisted laparoscopy procedure, bladder

Endoscopy—Cystoscopy, Urethroscopy, Cystourethroscopy

Endoscopic descriptions are listed so that the main procedure can be identified without having to list all the minor related functions performed at the same time. For example: meatotomy, urethral calibration and/or dilation, urethroscopy, and cystoscopy prior to a transurethral resection of prostate; ureteral catheterization following extraction of ureteral calculus; internal urethrotomy and bladder neck fulguration when performing a cystourethroscopy for the female urethral syndrome. When the secondary procedure requires significant additional time and effort, it may be identified by the addition of modifier 22.

For example: urethrotomy performed for a documented pre-existing stricture or bladder neck contracture.

Urinary

▶Because cutaneous urinary diversions utilizing ileum or colon serve as functional replacements of a native bladder, endoscopy of such bowel segments, as well as performance of secondary procedures can be captured by using the cystourethroscopy codes. For example, endoscopy of an ileal loop with removal of ureteral calculus would be coded as cystourethroscopy (including ureteral catheterization); with removal of ureteral calculus (52320).◀

52000   Cystourethroscopy (separate procedure)

(Do not report 52000 in conjunction with 52001, 52320, 52325, 52327, 52330, 52332, 52334, 52341, 52342, 52343, 52356)

52001   Cystourethroscopy with irrigation and evacuation of multiple obstructing clots

(Do not report 52001 in conjunction with 52000)

52005   Cystourethroscopy, with ureteral catheterization, with or without irrigation, instillation, or ureteropyelography, exclusive of radiologic service;

52007   with brush biopsy of ureter and/or renal pelvis

▶(For image-guided biopsy of ureter and/or renal pelvis without endoscopic guidance, use 50606)◀

52010   Cystourethroscopy, with ejaculatory duct catheterization, with or without irrigation, instillation, or duct radiography, exclusive of radiologic service

(For radiological supervision and interpretation, use 74440)

Transurethral Surgery

Urethra and Bladder

52204   Cystourethroscopy, with biopsy(s)

52214   Cystourethroscopy, with fulguration (including cryosurgery or laser surgery) of trigone, bladder neck, prostatic fossa, urethra, or periurethral glands

(For transurethral fulguration of prostate tissue performed within the postoperative period of 52601 or 52630 performed by the same physician, append modifier 78)

(For transurethral fulguration of prostate tissue performed within the postoperative period of a related procedure performed by the same physician, append modifier 78)

(For transurethral fulguration of prostate for postoperative bleeding performed by the same physician, append modifier 78)

52224   Cystourethroscopy, with fulguration (including cryosurgery or laser surgery) or treatment of MINOR (less than 0.5 cm) lesion(s) with or without biopsy

52234   Cystourethroscopy, with fulguration (including cryosurgery or laser surgery) and/or resection of; SMALL bladder tumor(s) (0.5 up to 2.0 cm)

52235   MEDIUM bladder tumor(s) (2.0 to 5.0 cm)

52240   LARGE bladder tumor(s)

52250   Cystourethroscopy with insertion of radioactive substance, with or without biopsy or fulguration

52260   Cystourethroscopy, with dilation of bladder for interstitial cystitis; general or conduction (spinal) anesthesia

52265   local anesthesia

52270   Cystourethroscopy, with internal urethrotomy; female

52275   male

52276   Cystourethroscopy with direct vision internal urethrotomy

52277   Cystourethroscopy, with resection of external sphincter (sphincterotomy)

52281   Cystourethroscopy, with calibration and/or dilation of urethral stricture or stenosis, with or without meatotomy, with or without injection procedure for cystography, male or female

52282   Cystourethroscopy, with insertion of permanent urethral stent

(For placement of temporary prostatic urethral stent, use 53855)

52283   Cystourethroscopy, with steroid injection into stricture

52285   Cystourethroscopy for treatment of the female urethral syndrome with any or all of the following: urethral meatotomy, urethral dilation, internal urethrotomy, lysis of urethrovaginal septal fibrosis, lateral incisions of the bladder neck, and fulguration of polyp(s) of urethra, bladder neck, and/or trigone

52287   Cystourethroscopy, with injection(s) for chemodenervation of the bladder

(The supply of the chemodenervation agent is reported separately)

52290   Cystourethroscopy; with ureteral meatotomy, unilateral or bilateral

52300   with resection or fulguration of orthotopic ureterocele(s), unilateral or bilateral

52301   with resection or fulguration of ectopic ureterocele(s), unilateral or bilateral

52305   with incision or resection of orifice of bladder diverticulum, single or multiple

52310   Cystourethroscopy, with removal of foreign body, calculus, or ureteral stent from urethra or bladder (separate procedure); simple

52315   complicated

52317   Litholapaxy: crushing or fragmentation of calculus by any means in bladder and removal of fragments; simple or small (less than 2.5 cm)

52318   complicated or large (over 2.5 cm)

Urinary

Ureter and Pelvis

Therapeutic cystourethroscopy always includes diagnostic cystourethroscopy. To report a diagnostic cystourethroscopy, use 52000. Therapeutic cystourethroscopy with ureteroscopy and/or pyeloscopy always includes diagnostic cystourethroscopy with ureteroscopy and/or pyeloscopy. To report a diagnostic cystourethroscopy with ureteroscopy and/or pyeloscopy, use 52351.

Do not report 52000 in conjunction with 52320-52343, 52356.

Do not report 52351 in conjunction with 52344-52346, 52352-52356.

The insertion and removal of a temporary ureteral catheter (52005) during diagnostic or therapeutic cystourethroscopy with ureteroscopy and/or pyeloscopy is included in 52320-52356 and should not be reported separately.

To report insertion of a self-retaining, indwelling stent performed during diagnostic or therapeutic cystourethroscopy with ureteroscopy and/or pyeloscopy, report 52332, in addition to primary procedure(s) performed (52320-52330, 52334-52352, 52354, 52355), and append modifier 51. Code 52332 is used to report a unilateral procedure unless otherwise specified.

For bilateral insertion of self-retaining, indwelling ureteral stents, use code 52332, and append modifier 50.

To report cystourethroscopic removal of a self-retaining, indwelling ureteral stent, see 52310, 52315, and append modifier 58, if appropriate.

52320 Cystourethroscopy (including ureteral catheterization); with removal of ureteral calculus

52325 with fragmentation of ureteral calculus (eg, ultrasonic or electro-hydraulic technique)

52327 with subureteric injection of implant material

52330 with manipulation, without removal of ureteral calculus

(Do not report 52320, 52325, 52327, 52330 in conjunction with 52000)

52332 Cystourethroscopy, with insertion of indwelling ureteral stent (eg, Gibbons or double-J type)

(Do not report 52332 in conjunction with 52000, 52353, 52356 when performed together on the same side)

52334 Cystourethroscopy with insertion of ureteral guide wire through kidney to establish a percutaneous nephrostomy, retrograde

(For percutaneous nephrostolithotomy, see 50080, 50081; for establishment of nephrostomy tract only, use 50395)

(For cystourethroscopy, with ureteroscopy and/or pyeloscopy, see 52351-52356)

(For cystourethroscopy with incision, fulguration, or resection of congenital posterior urethral valves or obstructive hypertrophic mucosal folds, use 52400)

(Do not report 52334 in conjunction with 52000, 52351)

52341 Cystourethroscopy; with treatment of ureteral stricture (eg, balloon dilation, laser, electrocautery, and incision)

52342 with treatment of ureteropelvic junction stricture (eg, balloon dilation, laser, electrocautery, and incision)

52343 with treatment of intra-renal stricture (eg, balloon dilation, laser, electrocautery, and incision)

(Do not report 52341, 52342, 52343 in conjunction with 52000, 52351)

►(For image-guided dilation of ureter, ureteropelvic junction stricture without endoscopic guidance, use 50706)◄

52344 Cystourethroscopy with ureteroscopy; with treatment of ureteral stricture (eg, balloon dilation, laser, electrocautery, and incision)

52345 with treatment of ureteropelvic junction stricture (eg, balloon dilation, laser, electrocautery, and incision)

52346 with treatment of intra-renal stricture (eg, balloon dilation, laser, electrocautery, and incision)

(For transurethral resection or incision of ejaculatory ducts, use 52402)

(Do not report 52344, 52345, 52346 in conjunction with 52351)

►(For image-guided dilation of ureter, ureteropelvic junction stricture without endoscopic guidance, use 50706)◄

52351 Cystourethroscopy, with ureteroscopy and/or pyeloscopy; diagnostic

(For radiological supervision and interpretation, use 74485)

(Do not report 52351 in conjunction with 52341, 52342, 52343, 52344, 52345, 52346, 52352-52356)

52352 with removal or manipulation of calculus (ureteral catheterization is included)

52353 with lithotripsy (ureteral catheterization is included)

(Do not report 52353 in conjunction with 52332, 52356 when performed together on the same side)

 # 52356 with lithotripsy including insertion of indwelling ureteral stent (eg, Gibbons or double-J type)

(Do not report 52356 in conjunction with 52332, 52353 when performed together on the same side)

52354 with biopsy and/or fulguration of ureteral or renal pelvic lesion

►(For image-guided biopsy of ureter and/or renal pelvis without endoscopic guidance, use 50606)◄

Urinary

52355   with resection of ureteral or renal pelvic tumor

52356   Code is out of numerical sequence. See 52320-52355

Vesical Neck and Prostate

52400   Cystourethroscopy with incision, fulguration, or resection of congenital posterior urethral valves, or congenital obstructive hypertrophic mucosal folds

52402   Cystourethroscopy with transurethral resection or incision of ejaculatory ducts

52441   Cystourethroscopy, with insertion of permanent adjustable transprostatic implant; single implant

+ 52442   each additional permanent adjustable transprostatic implant (List separately in addition to code for primary procedure)

(Use 52442 in conjunction with 52441)

(To report removal of implant[s], use 52310)

(For insertion of a permanent urethral stent, use 52282. For insertion of a temporary prostatic urethral stent, use 53855)

52450   Transurethral incision of prostate

52500   Transurethral resection of bladder neck (separate procedure)

52601   Transurethral electrosurgical resection of prostate, including control of postoperative bleeding, complete (vasectomy, meatotomy, cystourethroscopy, urethral calibration and/or dilation, and internal urethrotomy are included)

(For other approaches, see 55801-55845)

(52612, 52614, 52620 have been deleted. For first stage transurethral partial resection of prostate, use 52601. For second stage partial resection of prostate, use 52601 with modifier 58. For transurethral resection of residual or regrowth of obstructive prostate tissue, use 52630)

52630   Transurethral resection; residual or regrowth of obstructive prostate tissue including control of postoperative bleeding, complete (vasectomy, meatotomy, cystourethroscopy, urethral calibration and/ or dilation, and internal urethrotomy are included)

(For resection of residual prostate tissue performed within the postoperative period of a related procedure performed by the same physician, append modifier 78)

52640   of postoperative bladder neck contracture

52647   Laser coagulation of prostate, including control of postoperative bleeding, complete (vasectomy, meatotomy, cystourethroscopy, urethral calibration and/ or dilation, and internal urethrotomy are included if performed)

52648   Laser vaporization of prostate, including control of postoperative bleeding, complete (vasectomy, meatotomy, cystourethroscopy, urethral calibration and/ or dilation, internal urethrotomy and transurethral resection of prostate are included if performed)

52649   Laser enucleation of the prostate with morcellation, including control of postoperative bleeding, complete (vasectomy, meatotomy, cystourethroscopy, urethral calibration and/or dilation, internal urethrotomy and transurethral resection of prostate are included if performed)

(Do not report 52649 in conjunction with 52000, 52276, 52281, 52601, 52647, 52648, 53020, 55250)

52700   Transurethral drainage of prostatic abscess

(For litholapaxy, use 52317, 52318)

Urethra

(For endoscopy, see cystoscopy, urethroscopy, cystourethroscopy, 52000-52700)

(For injection procedure for urethrocystography, see 51600-51610)

Incision

53000   Urethrotomy or urethrostomy, external (separate procedure); pendulous urethra

53010   perineal urethra, external

53020   Meatotomy, cutting of meatus (separate procedure); except infant

53025   infant

(Do not report modifier 63 in conjunction with 53025)

53040   Drainage of deep periurethral abscess

(For subcutaneous abscess, see 10060, 10061)

53060   Drainage of Skene's gland abscess or cyst

53080   Drainage of perineal urinary extravasation; uncomplicated (separate procedure)

53085   complicated

Excision

53200   Biopsy of urethra

53210   Urethrectomy, total, including cystostomy; female

53215   male

53220   Excision or fulguration of carcinoma of urethra

53230   Excision of urethral diverticulum (separate procedure); female

53235   male

53240   Marsupialization of urethral diverticulum, male or female

53250   Excision of bulbourethral gland (Cowper's gland)

53260   Excision or fulguration; urethral polyp(s), distal urethra

(For endoscopic approach, see 52214, 52224)

53265   urethral caruncle

53270   Skene's glands

53275   urethral prolapse

Urinary

Repair

(For hypospadias, see 54300-54352)

53400   Urethroplasty; first stage, for fistula, diverticulum, or stricture (eg, Johannsen type)

53405   second stage (formation of urethra), including urinary diversion

53410   Urethroplasty, 1-stage reconstruction of male anterior urethra

53415   Urethroplasty, transpubic or perineal, 1-stage, for reconstruction or repair of prostatic or membranous urethra

53420   Urethroplasty, 2-stage reconstruction or repair of prostatic or membranous urethra; first stage

53425   second stage

53430   Urethroplasty, reconstruction of female urethra

53431   Urethroplasty with tubularization of posterior urethra and/or lower bladder for incontinence (eg, Tenago, Leadbetter procedure)

53440   Sling operation for correction of male urinary incontinence (eg, fascia or synthetic)

53442   Removal or revision of sling for male urinary incontinence (eg, fascia or synthetic)

53444   Insertion of tandem cuff (dual cuff)

53445   Insertion of inflatable urethral/bladder neck sphincter, including placement of pump, reservoir, and cuff

53446   Removal of inflatable urethral/bladder neck sphincter, including pump, reservoir, and cuff

53447   Removal and replacement of inflatable urethral/bladder neck sphincter including pump, reservoir, and cuff at the same operative session

53448   Removal and replacement of inflatable urethral/bladder neck sphincter including pump, reservoir, and cuff through an infected field at the same operative session including irrigation and debridement of infected tissue

(Do not report 11042, 11043 in addition to 53448)

53449   Repair of inflatable urethral/bladder neck sphincter, including pump, reservoir, and cuff

53450   Urethromeatoplasty, with mucosal advancement

(For meatotomy, see 53020, 53025)

53460   Urethromeatoplasty, with partial excision of distal urethral segment (Richardson type procedure)

53500   Urethrolysis, transvaginal, secondary, open, including cystourethroscopy (eg, postsurgical obstruction, scarring)

(For urethrolysis by retropubic approach, use 53899)

(Do not report 53500 in conjunction with 52000)

53502   Urethrorrhaphy, suture of urethral wound or injury, female

53505   Urethrorrhaphy, suture of urethral wound or injury; penile

53510   perineal

53515   prostatomembranous

53520   Closure of urethrostomy or urethrocutaneous fistula, male (separate procedure)

(For closure of urethrovaginal fistula, use 57310)

(For closure of urethrorectal fistula, see 45820, 45825)

Manipulation

(For radiological supervision and interpretation, use 74485)

53600   Dilation of urethral stricture by passage of sound or urethral dilator, male; initial

53601   subsequent

53605   Dilation of urethral stricture or vesical neck by passage of sound or urethral dilator, male, general or conduction (spinal) anesthesia

(For dilation of urethral stricture, male, performed under local anesthesia, see 53600, 53601, 53620, 53621)

53620   Dilation of urethral stricture by passage of filiform and follower, male; initial

53621   subsequent

53660   Dilation of female urethra including suppository and/or instillation; initial

53661   subsequent

53665   Dilation of female urethra, general or conduction (spinal) anesthesia

(For urethral catheterization, see 51701-51703)

(For dilation of urethra performed under local anesthesia, female, see 53660, 53661)

Other Procedures

(For 2 or 3 glass urinalysis, use 81020)

53850   Transurethral destruction of prostate tissue; by microwave thermotherapy

53852   by radiofrequency thermotherapy

53855   Insertion of a temporary prostatic urethral stent, including urethral measurement

(For insertion of permanent urethral stent, use 52282)

53860   Transurethral radiofrequency micro-remodeling of the female bladder neck and proximal urethra for stress urinary incontinence

53899   Unlisted procedure, urinary system

Urinary

Male Genital System

Penis

Incision

(For abdominal perineal gangrene debridement, see 11004-11006)

54000 Slitting of prepuce, dorsal or lateral (separate procedure); newborn

(Do not report modifier 63 in conjunction with 54000)

54001 except newborn

54015 Incision and drainage of penis, deep

(For skin and subcutaneous abscess, see 10060-10160)

Destruction

54050 Destruction of lesion(s), penis (eg, condyloma, papilloma, molluscum contagiosum, herpetic vesicle), simple; chemical

54055 electrodesiccation

54056 cryosurgery

54057 laser surgery

54060 surgical excision

54065 Destruction of lesion(s), penis (eg, condyloma, papilloma, molluscum contagiosum, herpetic vesicle), extensive (eg, laser surgery, electrosurgery, cryosurgery, chemosurgery)

(For destruction or excision of other lesions, see **Integumentary System**)

Excision

54100 Biopsy of penis; (separate procedure)

54105 deep structures

54110 Excision of penile plaque (Peyronie disease);

54111 with graft to 5 cm in length

54112 with graft greater than 5 cm in length

54115 Removal foreign body from deep penile tissue (eg, plastic implant)

54120 Amputation of penis; partial

54125 complete

54130 Amputation of penis, radical; with bilateral inguinofemoral lymphadenectomy

54135 in continuity with bilateral pelvic lymphadenectomy, including external iliac, hypogastric and obturator nodes

(For lymphadenectomy [separate procedure], see 38760-38770)

54150 Circumcision, using clamp or other device with regional dorsal penile or ring block

(Do not report modifier 63 in conjunction with 54150)

(Report 54150 with modifier 52 when performed without dorsal penile or ring block)

54160 Circumcision, surgical excision other than clamp, device, or dorsal slit; neonate (28 days of age or less)

(Do not report modifier 63 in conjunction with 54160)

54161 older than 28 days of age

54162 Lysis or excision of penile post-circumcision adhesions

54163 Repair incomplete circumcision

54164 Frenulotomy of penis

(Do not report 54164 with circumcision codes 54150-54161, 54162, 54163)

Introduction

54200 Injection procedure for Peyronie disease;

54205 with surgical exposure of plaque

54220 Irrigation of corpora cavernosa for priapism

54230 Injection procedure for corpora cavernosography

(For radiological supervision and interpretation, use 74445)

54231 Dynamic cavernosometry, including intracavernosal injection of vasoactive drugs (eg, papaverine, phentolamine)

54235 Injection of corpora cavernosa with pharmacologic agent(s) (eg, papaverine, phentolamine)

54240 Penile plethysmography

54250 Nocturnal penile tumescence and/or rigidity test

Repair

(For other urethroplasties, see 53400-53430)

(For penile revascularization, use 37788)

54300 Plastic operation of penis for straightening of chordee (eg, hypospadias), with or without mobilization of urethra

54304 Plastic operation on penis for correction of chordee or for first stage hypospadias repair with or without transplantation of prepuce and/or skin flaps

54308 Urethroplasty for second stage hypospadias repair (including urinary diversion); less than 3 cm

54312 greater than 3 cm

54316 Urethroplasty for second stage hypospadias repair (including urinary diversion) with free skin graft obtained from site other than genitalia

54318 Urethroplasty for third stage hypospadias repair to release penis from scrotum (eg, third stage Cecil repair)

Male Genital

54322 1-stage distal hypospadias repair (with or without chordee or circumcision); with simple meatal advancement (eg, Magpi, V-flap)

54324 with urethroplasty by local skin flaps (eg, flip-flap, prepucial flap)

54326 with urethroplasty by local skin flaps and mobilization of urethra

54328 with extensive dissection to correct chordee and urethroplasty with local skin flaps, skin graft patch, and/or island flap

(For urethroplasty and straightening of chordee, use 54308)

54332 1-stage proximal penile or penoscrotal hypospadias repair requiring extensive dissection to correct chordee and urethroplasty by use of skin graft tube and/or island flap

54336 1-stage perineal hypospadias repair requiring extensive dissection to correct chordee and urethroplasty by use of skin graft tube and/or island flap

54340 Repair of hypospadias complications (ie, fistula, stricture, diverticula); by closure, incision, or excision, simple

54344 requiring mobilization of skin flaps and urethroplasty with flap or patch graft

54348 requiring extensive dissection and urethroplasty with flap, patch or tubed graft (includes urinary diversion)

54352 Repair of hypospadias cripple requiring extensive dissection and excision of previously constructed structures including re-release of chordee and reconstruction of urethra and penis by use of local skin as grafts and island flaps and skin brought in as flaps or grafts

54360 Plastic operation on penis to correct angulation

54380 Plastic operation on penis for epispadias distal to external sphincter;

54385 with incontinence

54390 with exstrophy of bladder

54400 Insertion of penile prosthesis; non-inflatable (semi-rigid)

54401 inflatable (self-contained)

(For removal or replacement of penile prosthesis, see 54415, 54416)

54405 Insertion of multi-component, inflatable penile prosthesis, including placement of pump, cylinders, and reservoir

(For reduced services, report 54405 with modifier 52)

54406 Removal of all components of a multi-component, inflatable penile prosthesis without replacement of prosthesis

(For reduced services, report 54406 with modifier 52)

54408 Repair of component(s) of a multi-component, inflatable penile prosthesis

54410 Removal and replacement of all component(s) of a multi-component, inflatable penile prosthesis at the same operative session

54411 Removal and replacement of all components of a multi-component inflatable penile prosthesis through an infected field at the same operative session, including irrigation and debridement of infected tissue

(For reduced services, report 54411 with modifier 52)

(Do not report 11042, 11043 in addition to 54411)

54415 Removal of non-inflatable (semi-rigid) or inflatable (self-contained) penile prosthesis, without replacement of prosthesis

54416 Removal and replacement of non-inflatable (semi-rigid) or inflatable (self-contained) penile prosthesis at the same operative session

54417 Removal and replacement of non-inflatable (semi-rigid) or inflatable (self-contained) penile prosthesis through an infected field at the same operative session, including irrigation and debridement of infected tissue

(Do not report 11042, 11043 in addition to 54417)

54420 Corpora cavernosa-saphenous vein shunt (priapism operation), unilateral or bilateral

54430 Corpora cavernosa-corpus spongiosum shunt (priapism operation), unilateral or bilateral

54435 Corpora cavernosa-glans penis fistulization (eg, biopsy needle, Winter procedure, rongeur, or punch) for priapism

● **54437** Repair of traumatic corporeal tear(s)

►(For repair of urethra, see 53410, 53415)◄

● **54438** Replantation, penis, complete amputation including urethral repair

►(To report replantation of incomplete penile amputation, see 54437 for repair of corporeal tear[s], and 53410, 53415 for repair of the urethra)◄

54440 Plastic operation of penis for injury

Manipulation

54450 Foreskin manipulation including lysis of preputial adhesions and stretching

Testis

Excision

(For abdominal perineal gangrene debridement, see 11004-11006)

54500 Biopsy of testis, needle (separate procedure)

(For fine needle aspiration, see 10021, 10022)

(For evaluation of fine needle aspirate, see 88172, 88173)

Male Genital

54505 Biopsy of testis, incisional (separate procedure)

(For bilateral procedure, report 54505 with modifier 50)

(When combined with vasogram, seminal vesiculogram, or epididymogram, use 55300)

54512 Excision of extraparenchymal lesion of testis

54520 Orchiectomy, simple (including subcapsular), with or without testicular prosthesis, scrotal or inguinal approach

(For bilateral procedure, report 54520 with modifier 50)

54522 Orchiectomy, partial

54530 Orchiectomy, radical, for tumor; inguinal approach

54535   with abdominal exploration

(For orchiectomy with repair of hernia, see 49505 or 49507 and 54520)

(For radical retroperitoneal lymphadenectomy, use 38780)

Exploration

54550 Exploration for undescended testis (inguinal or scrotal area)

(For bilateral procedure, report 54550 with modifier 50)

54560 Exploration for undescended testis with abdominal exploration

(For bilateral procedure, report 54560 with modifier 50)

Repair

54600 Reduction of torsion of testis, surgical, with or without fixation of contralateral testis

54620 Fixation of contralateral testis (separate procedure)

54640 Orchiopexy, inguinal approach, with or without hernia repair

(For bilateral procedure, report 54640 with modifier 50)

(For inguinal hernia repair performed in conjunction with inguinal orchiopexy, see 49495-49525)

54650 Orchiopexy, abdominal approach, for intra-abdominal testis (eg, Fowler-Stephens)

(For laparoscopic approach, use 54692)

54660 Insertion of testicular prosthesis (separate procedure)

(For bilateral procedure, report 54660 with modifier 50)

54670 Suture or repair of testicular injury

54680 Transplantation of testis(es) to thigh (because of scrotal destruction)

Laparoscopy

Surgical laparoscopy always includes diagnostic laparoscopy. To report a diagnostic laparoscopy (peritoneoscopy) (separate procedure), use 49320.

54690 Laparoscopy, surgical; orchiectomy

54692   orchiopexy for intra-abdominal testis

54699 Unlisted laparoscopy procedure, testis

Epididymis

Incision

54700 Incision and drainage of epididymis, testis and/or scrotal space (eg, abscess or hematoma)

(For debridement of necrotizing soft tissue infection of external genitalia, see 11004-11006)

Excision

54800 Biopsy of epididymis, needle

(For fine needle aspiration, see 10021, 10022)

(For evaluation of fine needle aspirate, see 88172, 88173)

54830 Excision of local lesion of epididymis

54840 Excision of spermatocele, with or without epididymectomy

54860 Epididymectomy; unilateral

54861   bilateral

Exploration

54865 Exploration of epididymis, with or without biopsy

Repair

54900 Epididymovasostomy, anastomosis of epididymis to vas deferens; unilateral

54901   bilateral

(For operating microscope, use 69990)

Tunica Vaginalis

Incision

55000 Puncture aspiration of hydrocele, tunica vaginalis, with or without injection of medication

Excision

55040 Excision of hydrocele; unilateral

55041   bilateral

(With hernia repair, see 49495-49501)

Repair

55060 Repair of tunica vaginalis hydrocele (Bottle type)

⊙=Moderate sedation   ✚=Add-on code   ✗=FDA approval pending   #=Resequenced code   ○=Recycled/reinstated code

Male Genital

Scrotum

Incision

55100   Drainage of scrotal wall abscess

(See also 54700)

(For debridement of necrotizing soft tissue infection of external genitalia, see 11004-11006)

55110   Scrotal exploration

55120   Removal of foreign body in scrotum

Excision

(For excision of local lesion of skin of scrotum, see **Integumentary System**)

55150   Resection of scrotum

Repair

55175   Scrotoplasty; simple

55180   complicated

Vas Deferens

Incision

55200   Vasotomy, cannulization with or without incision of vas, unilateral or bilateral (separate procedure)

Excision

55250   Vasectomy, unilateral or bilateral (separate procedure), including postoperative semen examination(s)

Introduction

55300   Vasotomy for vasograms, seminal vesiculograms, or epididymograms, unilateral or bilateral

(For radiological supervision and interpretation, use 74440)

(When combined with biopsy of testis, see 54505 and use modifier 51)

Repair

55400   Vasovasostomy, vasovasorrhaphy

(For bilateral procedure, report 55400 with modifier 50)

(For operating microscope, use 69990)

Suture

55450   Ligation (percutaneous) of vas deferens, unilateral or bilateral (separate procedure)

Spermatic Cord

Excision

55500   Excision of hydrocele of spermatic cord, unilateral (separate procedure)

55520   Excision of lesion of spermatic cord (separate procedure)

55530   Excision of varicocele or ligation of spermatic veins for varicocele; (separate procedure)

55535   abdominal approach

55540   with hernia repair

Laparoscopy

Surgical laparoscopy always includes diagnostic laparoscopy. To report a diagnostic laparoscopy (peritoneoscopy) (separate procedure), use 49320.

55550   Laparoscopy, surgical, with ligation of spermatic veins for varicocele

55559   Unlisted laparoscopy procedure, spermatic cord

Seminal Vesicles

Incision

55600   Vesiculotomy;

(For bilateral procedure, report 55600 with modifier 50)

55605   complicated

Excision

55650   Vesiculectomy, any approach

(For bilateral procedure, report 55650 with modifier 50)

55680   Excision of Mullerian duct cyst

(For injection procedure, see 52010, 55300)

Prostate

Incision

55700   Biopsy, prostate; needle or punch, single or multiple, any approach

(If imaging guidance is performed, use 76942)

(For fine needle aspiration, see 10021, 10022)

(For evaluation of fine needle aspirate, see 88172, 88173)

(For transperineal stereotactic template guided saturation prostate biopsies, use 55706)

55705   incisional, any approach

55706 Biopsies, prostate, needle, transperineal, stereotactic template guided saturation sampling, including imaging guidance

(Do not report 55706 in conjunction with 55700)

55720 Prostatotomy, external drainage of prostatic abscess, any approach; simple

55725   complicated

(For transurethral drainage, use 52700)

Excision

(For transurethral removal of prostate, see 52601-52640)

(For transurethral destruction of prostate, see 53850-53852)

(For limited pelvic lymphadenectomy for staging [separate procedure], use 38562)

(For independent node dissection, see 38770-38780)

55801 Prostatectomy, perineal, subtotal (including control of postoperative bleeding, vasectomy, meatotomy, urethral calibration and/or dilation, and internal urethrotomy)

55810 Prostatectomy, perineal radical;

55812   with lymph node biopsy(s) (limited pelvic lymphadenectomy)

55815   with bilateral pelvic lymphadenectomy, including external iliac, hypogastric and obturator nodes

(If 55815 is carried out on separate days, use 38770 with modifier 50 and 55810)

55821 Prostatectomy (including control of postoperative bleeding, vasectomy, meatotomy, urethral calibration and/or dilation, and internal urethrotomy); suprapubic, subtotal, 1 or 2 stages

55831   retropubic, subtotal

55840 Prostatectomy, retropubic radical, with or without nerve sparing;

55842   with lymph node biopsy(s) (limited pelvic lymphadenectomy)

55845   with bilateral pelvic lymphadenectomy, including external iliac, hypogastric, and obturator nodes

(If 55845 is carried out on separate days, use 38770 with modifier 50 and 55840)

(For laparoscopic retropubic radical prostatectomy, use 55866)

55860 Exposure of prostate, any approach, for insertion of radioactive substance;

►(For application of interstitial radioelement, see 77770, 77771, 77772, 77778)◄

55862   with lymph node biopsy(s) (limited pelvic lymphadenectomy)

55865   with bilateral pelvic lymphadenectomy, including external iliac, hypogastric and obturator nodes

Laparoscopy

Surgical laparoscopy always includes diagnostic laparoscopy. To report a diagnostic laparoscopy (peritoneoscopy) (separate procedure), use 49320.

55866 Laparoscopy, surgical prostatectomy, retropubic radical, including nerve sparing, includes robotic assistance, when performed

(For open procedure, use 55840)

Other Procedures

(For artificial insemination, see 58321, 58322)

55870 Electroejaculation

55873 Cryosurgical ablation of the prostate (includes ultrasonic guidance and monitoring)

55875 Transperineal placement of needles or catheters into prostate for interstitial radioelement application, with or without cystoscopy

(For placement of needles or catheters into pelvic organs and/or genitalia [except prostate] for interstitial radioelement application, use 55920)

►(For interstitial radioelement application, see 77770, 77771, 77772, 77778)◄

(For ultrasonic guidance for interstitial radioelement application, use 76965)

55876 Placement of interstitial device(s) for radiation therapy guidance (eg, fiducial markers, dosimeter), prostate (via needle, any approach), single or multiple

(Report supply of device separately)

(For imaging guidance, see 76942, 77002, 77012, 77021)

55899 Unlisted procedure, male genital system

Reproductive System Procedures

55920 Placement of needles or catheters into pelvic organs and/or genitalia (except prostate) for subsequent interstitial radioelement application

(For placement of needles or catheters into prostate, use 55875)

(For insertion of uterine tandems and/or vaginal ovoids for clinical brachytherapy, use 57155)

(For insertion of Heyman capsules for clinical brachytherapy, use 58346)

Intersex Surgery

55970 Intersex surgery; male to female

55980   female to male

Male Genital

Female Genital System

(For pelvic laparotomy, use 49000)

(For excision or destruction of endometriomas, open method, see 49203-49205, 58957, 58958)

(For paracentesis, see 49082, 49083, 49084)

(For secondary closure of abdominal wall evisceration or disruption, use 49900)

(For fulguration or excision of lesions, laparoscopic approach, use 58662)

(For chemotherapy, see 96401-96549)

Vulva, Perineum, and Introitus

Definitions

The following definitions apply to the vulvectomy codes (56620-56640):

A *simple* procedure is the removal of skin and superficial subcutaneous tissues.

A *radical* procedure is the removal of skin and deep subcutaneous tissue.

A *partial* procedure is the removal of less than 80% of the vulvar area.

A *complete* procedure is the removal of greater than 80% of the vulvar area.

Incision

(For incision and drainage of sebaceous cyst, furuncle, or abscess, see 10040, 10060, 10061)

56405   Incision and drainage of vulva or perineal abscess

56420   Incision and drainage of Bartholin's gland abscess

(For incision and drainage of Skene's gland abscess or cyst, use 53060)

56440   Marsupialization of Bartholin's gland cyst

56441   Lysis of labial adhesions

56442   Hymenotomy, simple incision

Destruction

56501   Destruction of lesion(s), vulva; simple (eg, laser surgery, electrosurgery, cryosurgery, chemosurgery)

56515   extensive (eg, laser surgery, electrosurgery, cryosurgery, chemosurgery)

(For destruction of Skene's gland cyst or abscess, use 53270)

(For cautery destruction of urethral caruncle, use 53265)

Excision

56605   Biopsy of vulva or perineum (separate procedure); 1 lesion

+ 56606   each separate additional lesion (List separately in addition to code for primary procedure)

(Use 56606 in conjunction with 56605)

(For excision of local lesion, see 11420-11426, 11620-11626)

56620   Vulvectomy simple; partial

56625   complete

(For skin graft, see 15002 et seq)

56630   Vulvectomy, radical, partial;

(For skin graft, if used, see 15004-15005, 15120, 15121, 15240, 15241)

56631   with unilateral inguinofemoral lymphadenectomy

56632   with bilateral inguinofemoral lymphadenectomy

56633   Vulvectomy, radical, complete;

56634   with unilateral inguinofemoral lymphadenectomy

56637   with bilateral inguinofemoral lymphadenectomy

56640   Vulvectomy, radical, complete, with inguinofemoral, iliac, and pelvic lymphadenectomy

(For bilateral procedure, report 56640 with modifier 50)

(For lymphadenectomy, see 38760-38780)

56700   Partial hymenectomy or revision of hymenal ring

56740   Excision of Bartholin's gland or cyst

(For excision of Skene's gland, use 53270)

(For excision of urethral caruncle, use 53265)

(For excision or fulguration of urethral carcinoma, use 53220)

(For excision or marsupialization of urethral diverticulum, see 53230, 53240)

Repair

(For repair of urethra for mucosal prolapse, use 53275)

56800   Plastic repair of introitus

56805   Clitoroplasty for intersex state

56810   Perineoplasty, repair of perineum, nonobstetrical (separate procedure)

(See also 56800)

(For repair of wounds to genitalia, see 12001-12007, 12041-12047, 13131-13133)

(For repair of recent injury of vagina and perineum, nonobstetrical, use 57210)

Female Genital

(For anal sphincteroplasty, see 46750, 46751)

(For episiorrhaphy, episioperineorrhaphy for recent injury of vulva and/or perineum, nonobstetrical, use 57210)

Endoscopy

56820 Colposcopy of the vulva;

56821 with biopsy(s)

(For colposcopic examinations/procedures involving the vagina, see 57420, 57421; cervix, see 57452-57461)

Vagina

Incision

57000 Colpotomy; with exploration

57010 with drainage of pelvic abscess

57020 Colpocentesis (separate procedure)

57022 Incision and drainage of vaginal hematoma; obstetrical/ postpartum

57023 non-obstetrical (eg, post-trauma, spontaneous bleeding)

Destruction

57061 Destruction of vaginal lesion(s); simple (eg, laser surgery, electrosurgery, cryosurgery, chemosurgery)

57065 extensive (eg, laser surgery, electrosurgery, cryosurgery, chemosurgery)

Excision

57100 Biopsy of vaginal mucosa; simple (separate procedure)

57105 extensive, requiring suture (including cysts)

57106 Vaginectomy, partial removal of vaginal wall;

57107 with removal of paravaginal tissue (radical vaginectomy)

57109 with removal of paravaginal tissue (radical vaginectomy) with bilateral total pelvic lymphadenectomy and para-aortic lymph node sampling (biopsy)

57110 Vaginectomy, complete removal of vaginal wall;

57111 with removal of paravaginal tissue (radical vaginectomy)

57112 with removal of paravaginal tissue (radical vaginectomy) with bilateral total pelvic lymphadenectomy and para-aortic lymph node sampling (biopsy)

57120 Colpocleisis (Le Fort type)

57130 Excision of vaginal septum

57135 Excision of vaginal cyst or tumor

Introduction

57150 Irrigation of vagina and/or application of medicament for treatment of bacterial, parasitic, or fungoid disease

⊙ **57155** Insertion of uterine tandem and/or vaginal ovoids for clinical brachytherapy

(For placement of needles or catheters into pelvic organs and/or genitalia [except prostate] for interstitial radioelement application, use 55920)

►(For insertion of radioelement sources or ribbons, see 77761-77763, 77770, 77771, 77772)◄

57156 Insertion of a vaginal radiation afterloading apparatus for clinical brachytherapy

57160 Fitting and insertion of pessary or other intravaginal support device

57170 Diaphragm or cervical cap fitting with instructions

57180 Introduction of any hemostatic agent or pack for spontaneous or traumatic nonobstetrical vaginal hemorrhage (separate procedure)

Repair

(For urethral suspension, Marshall-Marchetti-Krantz type, abdominal approach, see 51840, 51841)

(For laparoscopic suspension, use 51990)

57200 Colporrhaphy, suture of injury of vagina (nonobstetrical)

57210 Colpoperineorrhaphy, suture of injury of vagina and/or perineum (nonobstetrical)

57220 Plastic operation on urethral sphincter, vaginal approach (eg, Kelly urethral plication)

57230 Plastic repair of urethrocele

57240 Anterior colporrhaphy, repair of cystocele with or without repair of urethrocele

57250 Posterior colporrhaphy, repair of rectocele with or without perineorrhaphy

(For repair of rectocele [separate procedure] without posterior colporrhaphy, use 45560)

57260 Combined anteroposterior colporrhaphy;

57265 with enterocele repair

✚ **57267** Insertion of mesh or other prosthesis for repair of pelvic floor defect, each site (anterior, posterior compartment), vaginal approach (List separately in addition to code for primary procedure)

(Use 57267 in conjunction with 45560, 57240-57265, 57285)

57268 Repair of enterocele, vaginal approach (separate procedure)

57270 Repair of enterocele, abdominal approach (separate procedure)

57280 Colpopexy, abdominal approach

Female Genital

57282   Colpopexy, vaginal; extra-peritoneal approach (sacrospinous, iliococcygeus)

57283   intra-peritoneal approach (uterosacral, levator myorrhaphy)

(Do not report 57283 in conjunction with 57556, 58263, 58270, 58280, 58292, 58294)

57284   Paravaginal defect repair (including repair of cystocele, if performed); open abdominal approach

(Do not report 57284 in conjunction with 51840, 51841, 51990, 57240, 57260, 57265, 58152, 58267)

57285   vaginal approach

(Do not report 57285 in conjunction with 51990, 57240, 57260, 57265, 58267)

57287   Removal or revision of sling for stress incontinence (eg, fascia or synthetic)

57288   Sling operation for stress incontinence (eg, fascia or synthetic)

(For laparoscopic approach, use 51992)

57289   Pereyra procedure, including anterior colporrhaphy

57291   Construction of artificial vagina; without graft

57292   with graft

57295   Revision (including removal) of prosthetic vaginal graft; vaginal approach

57296   open abdominal approach

(For laparoscopic approach, use 57426)

57300   Closure of rectovaginal fistula; vaginal or transanal approach

57305   abdominal approach

57307   abdominal approach, with concomitant colostomy

57308   transperineal approach, with perineal body reconstruction, with or without levator plication

57310   Closure of urethrovaginal fistula;

57311   with bulbocavernosus transplant

57320   Closure of vesicovaginal fistula; vaginal approach

(For concomitant cystostomy, see 51020-51040, 51101, 51102)

57330   transvesical and vaginal approach

(For abdominal approach, use 51900)

57335   Vaginoplasty for intersex state

Manipulation

57400   Dilation of vagina under anesthesia (other than local)

57410   Pelvic examination under anesthesia (other than local)

57415   Removal of impacted vaginal foreign body (separate procedure) under anesthesia (other than local)

(For removal without anesthesia of an impacted vaginal foreign body, use the appropriate E/M code)

Endoscopy/Laparoscopy

57420   Colposcopy of the entire vagina, with cervix if present;

57421   with biopsy(s) of vagina/cervix

(For colposcopic visualization of cervix and adjacent upper vagina, use 57452)

(When reporting colposcopies of multiple sites, use modifier 51 as appropriate. For colposcopic examinations/procedures involving the vulva, see 56820, 56821; cervix, see 57452-57461)

(For endometrial sampling [biopsy] performed in conjunction with colposcopy, use 58110)

57423   Paravaginal defect repair (including repair of cystocele, if performed), laparoscopic approach

(Do not report 57423 in conjunction with 49320, 51840, 51841, 51990, 57240, 57260, 58152, 58267)

57425   Laparoscopy, surgical, colpopexy (suspension of vaginal apex)

57426   Revision (including removal) of prosthetic vaginal graft, laparoscopic approach

(For vaginal approach, see 57295. For open abdominal approach, see 57296)

Cervix Uteri

Endoscopy

(For colposcopic examinations/procedures involving the vulva, see 56820, 56821; vagina, see 57420, 57421)

57452   Colposcopy of the cervix including upper/adjacent vagina;

(Do not report 57452 in addition to 57454-57461)

57454   with biopsy(s) of the cervix and endocervical curettage

57455   with biopsy(s) of the cervix

57456   with endocervical curettage

57460   with loop electrode biopsy(s) of the cervix

57461   with loop electrode conization of the cervix

(Do not report 57461 in addition to 57456)

(For endometrial sampling [biopsy] performed in conjunction with colposcopy, use 58110)

Female Genital

Excision

(For radical surgical procedures, see 58200-58240)

57500   Biopsy of cervix, single or multiple, or local excision of lesion, with or without fulguration (separate procedure)

57505   Endocervical curettage (not done as part of a dilation and curettage)

57510   Cautery of cervix; electro or thermal

57511   cryocautery, initial or repeat

57513   laser ablation

57520   Conization of cervix, with or without fulguration, with or without dilation and curettage, with or without repair; cold knife or laser

(See also 58120)

57522   loop electrode excision

57530   Trachelectomy (cervicectomy), amputation of cervix (separate procedure)

57531   Radical trachelectomy, with bilateral total pelvic lymphadenectomy and para-aortic lymph node sampling biopsy, with or without removal of tube(s), with or without removal of ovary(s)

(For radical abdominal hysterectomy, use 58210)

57540   Excision of cervical stump, abdominal approach;

57545   with pelvic floor repair

57550   Excision of cervical stump, vaginal approach;

57555   with anterior and/or posterior repair

57556   with repair of enterocele

(For insertion of intrauterine device, use 58300)

(For insertion of any hemostatic agent or pack for control of spontaneous non-obstetrical hemorrhage, see 57180)

57558   Dilation and curettage of cervical stump

Repair

57700   Cerclage of uterine cervix, nonobstetrical

57720   Trachelorrhaphy, plastic repair of uterine cervix, vaginal approach

Manipulation

57800   Dilation of cervical canal, instrumental (separate procedure)

Corpus Uteri

Excision

58100   Endometrial sampling (biopsy) with or without endocervical sampling (biopsy), without cervical dilation, any method (separate procedure)

(For endocervical curettage only, use 57505)

(For endometrial sampling [biopsy] performed in conjunction with colposcopy [57420, 57421, 57452-57461], use 58110)

+ 58110   Endometrial sampling (biopsy) performed in conjunction with colposcopy (List separately in addition to code for primary procedure)

(Use 58110 in conjunction with 57420, 57421, 57452-57461)

58120   Dilation and curettage, diagnostic and/or therapeutic (nonobstetrical)

(For postpartum hemorrhage, use 59160)

58140   Myomectomy, excision of fibroid tumor(s) of uterus, 1 to 4 intramural myoma(s) with total weight of 250 g or less and/or removal of surface myomas; abdominal approach

58145   vaginal approach

58146   Myomectomy, excision of fibroid tumor(s) of uterus, 5 or more intramural myomas and/or intramural myomas with total weight greater than 250 g, abdominal approach

(Do not report 58146 in addition to 58140-58145, 58150-58240)

Hysterectomy Procedures

58150   Total abdominal hysterectomy (corpus and cervix), with or without removal of tube(s), with or without removal of ovary(s);

58152   with colpo-urethrocystopexy (eg, Marshall-Marchetti-Krantz, Burch)

(For urethrocystopexy without hysterectomy, see 51840, 51841)

58180   Supracervical abdominal hysterectomy (subtotal hysterectomy), with or without removal of tube(s), with or without removal of ovary(s)

58200   Total abdominal hysterectomy, including partial vaginectomy, with para-aortic and pelvic lymph node sampling, with or without removal of tube(s), with or without removal of ovary(s)

58210   Radical abdominal hysterectomy, with bilateral total pelvic lymphadenectomy and para-aortic lymph node sampling (biopsy), with or without removal of tube(s), with or without removal of ovary(s)

(For radical hysterectomy with ovarian transposition, use also 58825)

58240   Pelvic exenteration for gynecologic malignancy, with total abdominal hysterectomy or cervicectomy, with or without removal of tube(s), with or without removal of ovary(s), with removal of bladder and ureteral transplantations, and/or abdominoperineal resection of rectum and colon and colostomy, or any combination thereof

(For pelvic exenteration for lower urinary tract or male genital malignancy, use 51597)

Female Genital

58260 Vaginal hysterectomy, for uterus 250 g or less;

58262 with removal of tube(s), and/or ovary(s)

58263 with removal of tube(s), and/or ovary(s), with repair of enterocele

58267 with colpo-urethrocystopexy (Marshall-Marchetti-Krantz type, Pereyra type) with or without endoscopic control

58270 with repair of enterocele

(For repair of enterocele with removal of tubes and/or ovaries, use 58263)

58275 Vaginal hysterectomy, with total or partial vaginectomy;

58280 with repair of enterocele

58285 Vaginal hysterectomy, radical (Schauta type operation)

58290 Vaginal hysterectomy, for uterus greater than 250 g;

58291 with removal of tube(s) and/or ovary(s)

58292 with removal of tube(s) and/or ovary(s), with repair of enterocele

58293 with colpo-urethrocystopexy (Marshall-Marchetti-Krantz type, Pereyra type) with or without endoscopic control

58294 with repair of enterocele

Introduction

(To report insertion of non-biodegradable drug delivery implant for contraception, use 11981. To report removal of implantable contraceptive capsules with subsequent insertion of non-biodegradable drug delivery implant, use 11976 and 11981)

58300 Insertion of intrauterine device (IUD)

58301 Removal of intrauterine device (IUD)

58321 Artificial insemination; intra-cervical

58322 intra-uterine

58323 Sperm washing for artificial insemination

58340 Catheterization and introduction of saline or contrast material for saline infusion sonohysterography (SIS) or hysterosalpingography

(For radiological supervision and interpretation of saline infusion sonohysterography, use 76831)

(For radiological supervision and interpretation of hysterosalpingography, use 74740)

58345 Transcervical introduction of fallopian tube catheter for diagnosis and/or re-establishing patency (any method), with or without hysterosalpingography

(For radiological supervision and interpretation, use 74742)

58346 Insertion of Heyman capsules for clinical brachytherapy

(For placement of needles or catheters into pelvic organs and/or genitalia [except prostate] for interstitial radioelement application, use 55920)

►(For insertion of radioelement sources or ribbons, see 77761-77763, 77770, 77771, 77772)◄

58350 Chromotubation of oviduct, including materials

(To report the supply of any materials, use 99070)

58353 Endometrial ablation, thermal, without hysteroscopic guidance

(For hysteroscopic procedure, use 58563)

58356 Endometrial cryoablation with ultrasonic guidance, including endometrial curettage, when performed

(Do not report 58356 in conjunction with 58100, 58120, 58340, 76700, 76856)

Repair

58400 Uterine suspension, with or without shortening of round ligaments, with or without shortening of sacrouterine ligaments; (separate procedure)

58410 with presacral sympathectomy

(For anastomosis of tubes to uterus, use 58752)

58520 Hysterorrhaphy, repair of ruptured uterus (nonobstetrical)

58540 Hysteroplasty, repair of uterine anomaly (Strassman type)

(For closure of vesicouterine fistula, use 51920)

Laparoscopy/Hysteroscopy

Surgical laparoscopy always includes diagnostic laparoscopy. To report a diagnostic laparoscopy (peritoneoscopy) (separate procedure), use 49320. To report a diagnostic hysteroscopy (separate procedure), use 58555.

58541 Laparoscopy, surgical, supracervical hysterectomy, for uterus 250 g or less;

58542 with removal of tube(s) and/or ovary(s)

(Do not report 58541, 58542 in conjunction with 49320, 57000, 57180, 57410, 58140-58146, 58545, 58546, 58561, 58661, 58670, 58671)

58543 Laparoscopy, surgical, supracervical hysterectomy, for uterus greater than 250 g;

58544 with removal of tube(s) and/or ovary(s)

(Do not report 58543-58544 in conjunction with 49320, 57000, 57180, 57410, 58140-58146, 58545, 58546, 58561, 58661, 58670, 58671)

58545 Laparoscopy, surgical, myomectomy, excision; 1 to 4 intramural myomas with total weight of 250 g or less and/or removal of surface myomas

Female Genital

58546   5 or more intramural myomas and/or intramural myomas with total weight greater than 250 g

58548   Laparoscopy, surgical, with radical hysterectomy, with bilateral total pelvic lymphadenectomy and para-aortic lymph node sampling (biopsy), with removal of tube(s) and ovary(s), if performed

(Do not report 58548 in conjunction with 38570-38572, 58210, 58285, 58550-58554)

58550   Laparoscopy, surgical, with vaginal hysterectomy, for uterus 250 g or less;

58552   with removal of tube(s) and/or ovary(s)

(Do not report 58550-58552 in conjunction with 49320, 57000, 57180, 57410, 58140-58146, 58545, 58546, 58561, 58661, 58670, 58671)

58553   Laparoscopy, surgical, with vaginal hysterectomy, for uterus greater than 250 g;

58554   with removal of tube(s) and/or ovary(s)

(Do not report 58553-58554 in conjunction with 49320, 57000, 57180, 57410, 58140-58146, 58545, 58546, 58561, 58661, 58670, 58671)

58555   Hysteroscopy, diagnostic (separate procedure)

58558   Hysteroscopy, surgical; with sampling (biopsy) of endometrium and/or polypectomy, with or without D & C

58559   with lysis of intrauterine adhesions (any method)

58560   with division or resection of intrauterine septum (any method)

58561   with removal of leiomyomata

58562   with removal of impacted foreign body

58563   with endometrial ablation (eg, endometrial resection, electrosurgical ablation, thermoablation)

58565   with bilateral fallopian tube cannulation to induce occlusion by placement of permanent implants

(Do not report 58565 in conjunction with 58555 or 57800)

(For unilateral procedure, use modifier 52)

58570   Laparoscopy, surgical, with total hysterectomy, for uterus 250 g or less;

58571   with removal of tube(s) and/or ovary(s)

58572   Laparoscopy, surgical, with total hysterectomy, for uterus greater than 250 g;

58573   with removal of tube(s) and/or ovary(s)

(Do not report 58570-58573 in conjunction with 49320, 57000, 57180, 57410, 58140-58146, 58150, 58545, 58546, 58561, 58661, 58670, 58671)

58578   Unlisted laparoscopy procedure, uterus

58579   Unlisted hysteroscopy procedure, uterus

Oviduct/Ovary

Incision

58600   Ligation or transection of fallopian tube(s), abdominal or vaginal approach, unilateral or bilateral

58605   Ligation or transection of fallopian tube(s), abdominal or vaginal approach, postpartum, unilateral or bilateral, during same hospitalization (separate procedure)

(For laparoscopic procedures, use 58670, 58671)

+ 58611   Ligation or transection of fallopian tube(s) when done at the time of cesarean delivery or intra-abdominal surgery (not a separate procedure) (List separately in addition to code for primary procedure)

58615   Occlusion of fallopian tube(s) by device (eg, band, clip, Falope ring) vaginal or suprapubic approach

(For laparoscopic approach, use 58671)

(For lysis of adnexal adhesions, use 58740)

Laparoscopy

Surgical laparoscopy always includes diagnostic laparoscopy. To report a diagnostic laparoscopy (peritoneoscopy) (separate procedure), use 49320.

58660   Laparoscopy, surgical; with lysis of adhesions (salpingolysis, ovariolysis) (separate procedure)

58661   with removal of adnexal structures (partial or total oophorectomy and/or salpingectomy)

58662   with fulguration or excision of lesions of the ovary, pelvic viscera, or peritoneal surface by any method

58670   with fulguration of oviducts (with or without transection)

58671   with occlusion of oviducts by device (eg, band, clip, or Falope ring)

58672   with fimbrioplasty

58673   with salpingostomy (salpingoneostomy)

(Codes 58672 and 58673 are used to report unilateral procedures. For bilateral procedure, use modifier 50)

58679   Unlisted laparoscopy procedure, oviduct, ovary

(For laparoscopic aspiration of ovarian cyst, use 49322)

(For laparoscopic biopsy of the ovary or fallopian tube, use 49321)

Excision

58700   Salpingectomy, complete or partial, unilateral or bilateral (separate procedure)

58720   Salpingo-oophorectomy, complete or partial, unilateral or bilateral (separate procedure)

Repair

58740   Lysis of adhesions (salpingolysis, ovariolysis)

(For laparoscopic approach, use 58660)

(For excision or destruction of endometriomas, open method, see 49203-49205, 58957, 58958)

(For fulguration or excision of lesions, laparoscopic approach, use 58662)

58750   Tubotubal anastomosis

58752   Tubouterine implantation

58760   Fimbrioplasty

(For laparoscopic approach, use 58672)

58770   Salpingostomy (salpingoneostomy)

(For laparoscopic approach, use 58673)

Ovary

Incision

58800   Drainage of ovarian cyst(s), unilateral or bilateral (separate procedure); vaginal approach

58805   abdominal approach

58820   Drainage of ovarian abscess; vaginal approach, open

58822   abdominal approach

(58823 has been deleted)

(For transrectal image-guided fluid collection drainage by catheter of pelvic abscess, use 49407)

58825   Transposition, ovary(s)

Excision

58900   Biopsy of ovary, unilateral or bilateral (separate procedure)

(For laparoscopic biopsy of the ovary or fallopian tube, use 49321)

58920   Wedge resection or bisection of ovary, unilateral or bilateral

58925   Ovarian cystectomy, unilateral or bilateral

58940   Oophorectomy, partial or total, unilateral or bilateral;

(For oophorectomy with concomitant debulking for ovarian malignancy, use 58952)

58943   for ovarian, tubal or primary peritoneal malignancy, with para-aortic and pelvic lymph node biopsies, peritoneal washings, peritoneal biopsies, diaphragmatic assessments, with or without salpingectomy(s), with or without omentectomy

58950   Resection (initial) of ovarian, tubal or primary peritoneal malignancy with bilateral salpingo-oophorectomy and omentectomy;

58951   with total abdominal hysterectomy, pelvic and limited para-aortic lymphadenectomy

58952   with radical dissection for debulking (ie, radical excision or destruction, intra-abdominal or retroperitoneal tumors)

(For resection of recurrent ovarian, tubal, primary peritoneal, or uterine malignancy, see 58957, 58958)

58953   Bilateral salpingo-oophorectomy with omentectomy, total abdominal hysterectomy and radical dissection for debulking;

58954   with pelvic lymphadenectomy and limited para-aortic lymphadenectomy

58956   Bilateral salpingo-oophorectomy with total omentectomy, total abdominal hysterectomy for malignancy

(Do not report 58956 in conjunction with 49255, 58150, 58180, 58262, 58263, 58550, 58661, 58700, 58720, 58900, 58925, 58940, 58957, 58958)

58957   Resection (tumor debulking) of recurrent ovarian, tubal, primary peritoneal, uterine malignancy (intra-abdominal, retroperitoneal tumors), with omentectomy, if performed;

58958   with pelvic lymphadenectomy and limited para-aortic lymphadenectomy

(Do not report 58957, 58958 in conjunction with 38770, 38780, 44005, 49000, 49203-49215, 49255, 58900-58960)

58960   Laparotomy, for staging or restaging of ovarian, tubal, or primary peritoneal malignancy (second look), with or without omentectomy, peritoneal washing, biopsy of abdominal and pelvic peritoneum, diaphragmatic assessment with pelvic and limited para-aortic lymphadenectomy

(Do not report 58960 in conjunction with 58957, 58958)

In Vitro Fertilization

58970   Follicle puncture for oocyte retrieval, any method

(For radiological supervision and interpretation, use 76948)

58974   Embryo transfer, intrauterine

58976   Gamete, zygote, or embryo intrafallopian transfer, any method

(For laparoscopic adnexal procedures, see 58660-58673)

Other Procedures

58999   Unlisted procedure, female genital system (nonobstetrical)

Female Genital

Maternity Care and Delivery

The services normally provided in uncomplicated maternity cases include antepartum care, delivery, and postpartum care. Pregnancy confirmation during a problem oriented or preventive visit is not considered a part of antepartum care and should be reported using the appropriate E/M service codes 99201, 99202, 99203, 99204, 99205, 99211, 99212, 99213, 99214, 99215, 99241, 99242, 99243, 99244, 99245, 99281, 99282, 99283, 99284, 99285, 99384, 99385, 99386, 99394, 99395, 99396 for that visit.

Antepartum care includes the initial prenatal history and physical examination; subsequent prenatal history and physical examinations; recording of weight, blood pressures, fetal heart tones, routine chemical urinalysis, and monthly visits up to 28 weeks gestation; biweekly visits to 36 weeks gestation; and weekly visits until delivery. Any other visits or services within this time period should be coded separately.

Delivery services include admission to the hospital, the admission history and physical examination, management of uncomplicated labor, vaginal delivery (with or without episiotomy, with or without forceps), or cesarean delivery. When reporting delivery only services (59409, 59514, 59612, 59620), report inpatient postdelivery management and discharge services using Evaluation and Management Services codes (99217-99239). Delivery and postpartum services (59410, 59515, 59614, 59622) include delivery services and all inpatient and outpatient postpartum services. Medical complications of pregnancy (eg, cardiac problems, neurological problems, diabetes, hypertension, toxemia, hyperemesis, preterm labor, premature rupture of membranes, trauma) and medical problems complicating labor and delivery management may require additional resources and may be reported separately.

Postpartum care only services (59430) include office or other outpatient visits following vaginal or cesarean section delivery.

For surgical complications of pregnancy (eg, appendectomy, hernia, ovarian cyst, Bartholin cyst), see services in the **Surgery** section.

If all or part of the antepartum and/or postpartum patient care is provided except delivery due to termination of pregnancy by abortion or referral to another physician or other qualified health care professional for delivery, see the antepartum and postpartum care codes 59425, 59426, and 59430.

(For circumcision of newborn, see 54150, 54160)

Antepartum and Fetal Invasive Services

(For fetal intrauterine transfusion, use 36460)

(For unlisted fetal invasive procedure, use 59897)

59000	Amniocentesis; diagnostic
	(For radiological supervision and interpretation, use 76946)
59001	therapeutic amniotic fluid reduction (includes ultrasound guidance)
59012	Cordocentesis (intrauterine), any method
	(For radiological supervision and interpretation, use 76941)
59015	Chorionic villus sampling, any method
	(For radiological supervision and interpretation, use 76945)
59020	Fetal contraction stress test
59025	Fetal non-stress test
59030	Fetal scalp blood sampling
	(For repeat fetal scalp blood sampling, use 59030 and see modifiers 76 and 77)
59050	Fetal monitoring during labor by consulting physician (ie, non-attending physician) with written report; supervision and interpretation
59051	interpretation only
59070	Transabdominal amnioinfusion, including ultrasound guidance
59072	Fetal umbilical cord occlusion, including ultrasound guidance
59074	Fetal fluid drainage (eg, vesicocentesis, thoracocentesis, paracentesis), including ultrasound guidance
59076	Fetal shunt placement, including ultrasound guidance

Excision

59100	Hysterotomy, abdominal (eg, for hydatidiform mole, abortion)
	(When tubal ligation is performed at the same time as hysterotomy, use 58611 in addition to 59100)
59120	Surgical treatment of ectopic pregnancy; tubal or ovarian, requiring salpingectomy and/or oophorectomy, abdominal or vaginal approach
59121	tubal or ovarian, without salpingectomy and/or oophorectomy
59130	abdominal pregnancy
59135	interstitial, uterine pregnancy requiring total hysterectomy
59136	interstitial, uterine pregnancy with partial resection of uterus
59140	cervical, with evacuation
59150	Laparoscopic treatment of ectopic pregnancy; without salpingectomy and/or oophorectomy
59151	with salpingectomy and/or oophorectomy
59160	Curettage, postpartum

Female Genital

Introduction

(For intrauterine fetal transfusion, use 36460)

(For introduction of hypertonic solution and/or prostaglandins to initiate labor, see 59850-59857)

59200   Insertion of cervical dilator (eg, laminaria, prostaglandin) (separate procedure)

Repair

(For tracheloplasty, use 57700)

59300   Episiotomy or vaginal repair, by other than attending

59320   Cerclage of cervix, during pregnancy; vaginal

59325   abdominal

59350   Hysterorrhaphy of ruptured uterus

Vaginal Delivery, Antepartum and Postpartum Care

59400   Routine obstetric care including antepartum care, vaginal delivery (with or without episiotomy, and/or forceps) and postpartum care

59409   Vaginal delivery only (with or without episiotomy and/or forceps);

59410   including postpartum care

59412   External cephalic version, with or without tocolysis

(Use 59412 in addition to code[s] for delivery)

59414   Delivery of placenta (separate procedure)

(For antepartum care only, see 59425, 59426 or appropriate E/M code[s])

(For 1-3 antepartum care visits, see appropriate E/M code[s])

59425   Antepartum care only; 4-6 visits

59426   7 or more visits

59430   Postpartum care only (separate procedure)

Cesarean Delivery

(For standby attendance for infant, use 99360)

(For low cervical cesarean section, see 59510, 59515, 59525)

59510   Routine obstetric care including antepartum care, cesarean delivery, and postpartum care

59514   Cesarean delivery only;

59515   including postpartum care

(For classic cesarean section, see 59510, 59515, 59525)

+ 59525   Subtotal or total hysterectomy after cesarean delivery (List separately in addition to code for primary procedure)

(Use 59525 in conjunction with 59510, 59514, 59515, 59618, 59620, 59622)

(For extraperitoneal cesarean section, or cesarean section with subtotal or total hysterectomy, see 59510, 59515, 59525)

Delivery After Previous Cesarean Delivery

Patients who have had a previous cesarean delivery and now present with the expectation of a vaginal delivery are coded using codes 59610-59622. If the patient has a successful vaginal delivery after a previous cesarean delivery (VBAC), use codes 59610-59614. If the attempt is unsuccessful and another cesarean delivery is carried out, use codes 59618-59622. To report elective cesarean deliveries use code 59510, 59514 or 59515.

59610   Routine obstetric care including antepartum care, vaginal delivery (with or without episiotomy, and/or forceps) and postpartum care, after previous cesarean delivery

59612   Vaginal delivery only, after previous cesarean delivery (with or without episiotomy and/or forceps);

59614   including postpartum care

59618   Routine obstetric care including antepartum care, cesarean delivery, and postpartum care, following attempted vaginal delivery after previous cesarean delivery

59620   Cesarean delivery only, following attempted vaginal delivery after previous cesarean delivery;

59622   including postpartum care

Abortion

(For medical treatment of spontaneous complete abortion, any trimester, use E/M codes 99201-99233)

(For surgical treatment of spontaneous abortion, use 59812)

59812   Treatment of incomplete abortion, any trimester, completed surgically

59820   Treatment of missed abortion, completed surgically; first trimester

59821   second trimester

59830   Treatment of septic abortion, completed surgically

59840   Induced abortion, by dilation and curettage

59841   Induced abortion, by dilation and evacuation

59850   Induced abortion, by 1 or more intra-amniotic injections (amniocentesis-injections), including hospital admission and visits, delivery of fetus and secundines;

Female Genital

59851	with dilation and curettage and/or evacuation
59852	with hysterotomy (failed intra-amniotic injection)
	(For insertion of cervical dilator, use 59200)
59855	Induced abortion, by 1 or more vaginal suppositories (eg, prostaglandin) with or without cervical dilation (eg, laminaria), including hospital admission and visits, delivery of fetus and secundines;
59856	with dilation and curettage and/or evacuation
59857	with hysterotomy (failed medical evacuation)

Other Procedures

59866	Multifetal pregnancy reduction(s) (MPR)
59870	Uterine evacuation and curettage for hydatidiform mole
59871	Removal of cerclage suture under anesthesia (other than local)
59897	Unlisted fetal invasive procedure, including ultrasound guidance, when performed
59898	Unlisted laparoscopy procedure, maternity care and delivery
59899	Unlisted procedure, maternity care and delivery

Endocrine System

(For pituitary and pineal surgery, see **Nervous System**)

Thyroid Gland

Incision

60000	Incision and drainage of thyroglossal duct cyst, infected

Excision

60100	Biopsy thyroid, percutaneous core needle
	(If imaging guidance is performed, see 76942, 77002, 77012, 77021)
	(For fine needle aspiration, use 10021 or 10022)
	(For evaluation of fine needle aspirate, see 88172, 88173)
60200	Excision of cyst or adenoma of thyroid, or transection of isthmus
60210	Partial thyroid lobectomy, unilateral; with or without isthmusectomy
60212	with contralateral subtotal lobectomy, including isthmusectomy
60220	Total thyroid lobectomy, unilateral; with or without isthmusectomy

60225	with contralateral subtotal lobectomy, including isthmusectomy
60240	Thyroidectomy, total or complete
	(For thyroidectomy, subtotal or partial, use 60271)
60252	Thyroidectomy, total or subtotal for malignancy; with limited neck dissection
60254	with radical neck dissection
60260	Thyroidectomy, removal of all remaining thyroid tissue following previous removal of a portion of thyroid
	(For bilateral procedure, report 60260 with modifier 50)
60270	Thyroidectomy, including substernal thyroid; sternal split or transthoracic approach
60271	cervical approach
60280	Excision of thyroglossal duct cyst or sinus;
60281	recurrent
	(For thyroid ultrasonography, use 76536)

Removal

60300	Aspiration and/or injection, thyroid cyst
	(For fine needle aspiration, see 10021, 10022)
	(If imaging guidance is performed, see 76942, 77012)

Parathyroid, Thymus, Adrenal Glands, Pancreas, and Carotid Body

Excision

(For pituitary and pineal surgery, see **Nervous System**)

60500	Parathyroidectomy or exploration of parathyroid(s);
60502	re-exploration
60505	with mediastinal exploration, sternal split or transthoracic approach
+ 60512	Parathyroid autotransplantation (List separately in addition to code for primary procedure)
	(Use 60512 in conjunction with 60500, 60502, 60505, 60212, 60225, 60240, 60252, 60254, 60260, 60270, 60271)
60520	Thymectomy, partial or total; transcervical approach (separate procedure)
60521	sternal split or transthoracic approach, without radical mediastinal dissection (separate procedure)
60522	sternal split or transthoracic approach, with radical mediastinal dissection (separate procedure)
	(For thoracoscopic [VATS] thymectomy, see 32673)

60540   Adrenalectomy, partial or complete, or exploration of adrenal gland with or without biopsy, transabdominal, lumbar or dorsal (separate procedure);

60545   with excision of adjacent retroperitoneal tumor

(Do not report 60540, 60545 in conjunction with 50323)

(For bilateral procedure, report 60540 with modifier 50)

(For excision of remote or disseminated pheochromocytoma, see 49203-49205)

(For laparoscopic approach, use 60650)

60600   Excision of carotid body tumor; without excision of carotid artery

60605   with excision of carotid artery

Laparoscopy

Surgical laparoscopy always includes diagnostic laparoscopy. To report a diagnostic laparoscopy (peritoneoscopy) (separate procedure), use 49320.

60650   Laparoscopy, surgical, with adrenalectomy, partial or complete, or exploration of adrenal gland with or without biopsy, transabdominal, lumbar or dorsal

60659   Unlisted laparoscopy procedure, endocrine system

Other Procedures

60699   Unlisted procedure, endocrine system

Female Genital

Nervous System

Skull, Meninges, and Brain

(For injection procedure for cerebral angiography, see 36100-36218)

(For injection procedure for ventriculography, see 61026, 61120)

(For injection procedure for pneumoencephalography, use 61055)

Injection, Drainage, or Aspiration

61000   Subdural tap through fontanelle, or suture, infant, unilateral or bilateral; initial

61001   subsequent taps

61020   Ventricular puncture through previous burr hole, fontanelle, suture, or implanted ventricular catheter/reservoir; without injection

61026   with injection of medication or other substance for diagnosis or treatment

61050   Cisternal or lateral cervical (C1-C2) puncture; without injection (separate procedure)

61055   with injection of medication or other substance for diagnosis or treatment

(Do not report 61055 in conjunction with 62302, 62303, 62304, 62305)

(For radiological supervision and interpretation by a different physician or qualified health care professional, see **Radiology**)

61070   Puncture of shunt tubing or reservoir for aspiration or injection procedure

(For radiological supervision and interpretation, use 75809)

Twist Drill, Burr Hole(s), or Trephine

61105   Twist drill hole for subdural or ventricular puncture

⊘ **61107**   Twist drill hole(s) for subdural, intracerebral, or ventricular puncture; for implanting ventricular catheter, pressure recording device, or other intracerebral monitoring device

(For intracranial neuroendoscopic ventricular catheter placement, use 62160)

61108   for evacuation and/or drainage of subdural hematoma

61120   Burr hole(s) for ventricular puncture (including injection of gas, contrast media, dye, or radioactive material)

61140   Burr hole(s) or trephine; with biopsy of brain or intracranial lesion

61150   with drainage of brain abscess or cyst

61151   with subsequent tapping (aspiration) of intracranial abscess or cyst

61154   Burr hole(s) with evacuation and/or drainage of hematoma, extradural or subdural

(For bilateral procedure, report 61154 with modifier 50)

61156   Burr hole(s); with aspiration of hematoma or cyst, intracerebral

61210   for implanting ventricular catheter, reservoir, EEG electrode(s), pressure recording device, or other cerebral monitoring device (separate procedure)

(For intracranial neuroendoscopic ventricular catheter placement, use 62160)

61215   Insertion of subcutaneous reservoir, pump or continuous infusion system for connection to ventricular catheter

(For refilling and maintenance of an implantable infusion pump for spinal or brain drug therapy, use 95990)

(For chemotherapy, use 96450)

61250   Burr hole(s) or trephine, supratentorial, exploratory, not followed by other surgery

(For bilateral procedure, report 61250 with modifier 50)

61253   Burr hole(s) or trephine, infratentorial, unilateral or bilateral

(If burr hole[s] or trephine are followed by craniotomy at same operative session, use 61304-61321; do not use 61250 or 61253)

Craniectomy or Craniotomy

61304   Craniectomy or craniotomy, exploratory; supratentorial

61305   infratentorial (posterior fossa)

61312   Craniectomy or craniotomy for evacuation of hematoma, supratentorial; extradural or subdural

61313   intracerebral

61314   Craniectomy or craniotomy for evacuation of hematoma, infratentorial; extradural or subdural

61315   intracerebellar

+ **61316**   Incision and subcutaneous placement of cranial bone graft (List separately in addition to code for primary procedure)

(Use 61316 in conjunction with 61304, 61312, 61313, 61322, 61323, 61340, 61570, 61571, 61680-61705)

61320   Craniectomy or craniotomy, drainage of intracranial abscess; supratentorial

61321   infratentorial

61322   Craniectomy or craniotomy, decompressive, with or without duraplasty, for treatment of intracranial hypertension, without evacuation of associated intraparenchymal hematoma; without lobectomy

(Do not report 61313 in addition to 61322)

(For subtemporal decompression, use 61340)

61323   with lobectomy

(Do not report 61313 in addition to 61323)

(For subtemporal decompression, use 61340)

61330   Decompression of orbit only, transcranial approach

(For bilateral procedure, report 61330 with modifier 50)

61332   Exploration of orbit (transcranial approach); with biopsy

61333   with removal of lesion

(61334 has been deleted)

61340   Subtemporal cranial decompression (pseudotumor cerebri, slit ventricle syndrome)

(For bilateral procedure, report 61340 with modifier 50)

(For decompressive craniotomy or craniectomy for intracranial hypertension, without hematoma evacuation, see 61322, 61323)

61343   Craniectomy, suboccipital with cervical laminectomy for decompression of medulla and spinal cord, with or without dural graft (eg, Arnold-Chiari malformation)

61345   Other cranial decompression, posterior fossa

(For orbital decompression by lateral wall approach, Kroenlein type, use 67445)

(61440 has been deleted)

61450   Craniectomy, subtemporal, for section, compression, or decompression of sensory root of gasserian ganglion

61458   Craniectomy, suboccipital; for exploration or decompression of cranial nerves

61460   for section of 1 or more cranial nerves

(61470 has been deleted)

61480   for mesencephalic tractotomy or pedunculotomy

(61490 has been deleted)

61500   Craniectomy; with excision of tumor or other bone lesion of skull

61501   for osteomyelitis

61510   Craniectomy, trephination, bone flap craniotomy; for excision of brain tumor, supratentorial, except meningioma

61512   for excision of meningioma, supratentorial

61514   for excision of brain abscess, supratentorial

61516   for excision or fenestration of cyst, supratentorial

(For excision of pituitary tumor or craniopharyngioma, see 61545, 61546, 61548)

+ 61517   Implantation of brain intracavitary chemotherapy agent (List separately in addition to code for primary procedure)

(Use 61517 only in conjunction with 61510 or 61518)

▶(Do not report 61517 for brachytherapy insertion. For intracavitary insertion of radioelement sources or ribbons, see 77770, 77771, 77772)◀

61518   Craniectomy for excision of brain tumor, infratentorial or posterior fossa; except meningioma, cerebellopontine angle tumor, or midline tumor at base of skull

61519   meningioma

61520   cerebellopontine angle tumor

61521   midline tumor at base of skull

61522   Craniectomy, infratentorial or posterior fossa; for excision of brain abscess

61524   for excision or fenestration of cyst

61526   Craniectomy, bone flap craniotomy, transtemporal (mastoid) for excision of cerebellopontine angle tumor;

61530   combined with middle/posterior fossa craniotomy/ craniectomy

61531   Subdural implantation of strip electrodes through 1 or more burr or trephine hole(s) for long-term seizure monitoring

(For stereotactic implantation of electrodes, use 61760)

(For craniotomy for excision of intracranial arteriovenous malformation, see 61680-61692)

61533   Craniotomy with elevation of bone flap; for subdural implantation of an electrode array, for long-term seizure monitoring

(For continuous EEG monitoring, see 95950-95954)

61534   for excision of epileptogenic focus without electrocorticography during surgery

61535   for removal of epidural or subdural electrode array, without excision of cerebral tissue (separate procedure)

61536   for excision of cerebral epileptogenic focus, with electrocorticography during surgery (includes removal of electrode array)

61537   for lobectomy, temporal lobe, without electrocorticography during surgery

61538   for lobectomy, temporal lobe, with electrocorticography during surgery

61539   for lobectomy, other than temporal lobe, partial or total, with electrocorticography during surgery

61540   for lobectomy, other than temporal lobe, partial or total, without electrocorticography during surgery

61541   for transection of corpus callosum

(61542 has been deleted)

61543   for partial or subtotal (functional) hemispherectomy

61544   for excision or coagulation of choroid plexus

61545   for excision of craniopharyngioma

(For craniotomy for selective amygdalohippocampectomy, use 61566)

(For craniotomy for multiple subpial transections during surgery, use 61567)

Nervous

61546 Craniotomy for hypophysectomy or excision of pituitary tumor, intracranial approach

61548 Hypophysectomy or excision of pituitary tumor, transnasal or transseptal approach, nonstereotactic

(Do not report code 69990 in addition to code 61548)

61550 Craniectomy for craniosynostosis; single cranial suture

61552   multiple cranial sutures

(For cranial reconstruction for orbital hypertelorism, see 21260-21263)

(For reconstruction, see 21172-21180)

61556 Craniotomy for craniosynostosis; frontal or parietal bone flap

61557   bifrontal bone flap

61558 Extensive craniectomy for multiple cranial suture craniosynostosis (eg, cloverleaf skull); not requiring bone grafts

61559   recontouring with multiple osteotomies and bone autografts (eg, barrel-stave procedure) (includes obtaining grafts)

(For reconstruction, see 21172-21180)

61563 Excision, intra and extracranial, benign tumor of cranial bone (eg, fibrous dysplasia); without optic nerve decompression

61564   with optic nerve decompression

(For reconstruction, see 21181-21183)

61566 Craniotomy with elevation of bone flap; for selective amygdalohippocampectomy

61567   for multiple subpial transections, with electrocorticography during surgery

61570 Craniectomy or craniotomy; with excision of foreign body from brain

61571   with treatment of penetrating wound of brain

(For sequestrectomy for osteomyelitis, use 61501)

61575 Transoral approach to skull base, brain stem or upper spinal cord for biopsy, decompression or excision of lesion;

61576   requiring splitting of tongue and/or mandible (including tracheostomy)

(For arthrodesis, use 22548)

Surgery of Skull Base

The surgical management of lesions involving the skull base (base of anterior, middle, and posterior cranial fossae) often requires the skills of several surgeons of different surgical specialties working together or in tandem during the operative session. These operations are usually not staged because of the need for definitive

closure of dura, subcutaneous tissues, and skin to avoid serious infections such as osteomyelitis and/or meningitis.

The procedures are categorized according to:

(1) *approach procedure* necessary to obtain adequate exposure to the lesion (pathologic entity), (2) *definitive procedure(s)* necessary to biopsy, excise or otherwise treat the lesion, and (3) *repair/reconstruction* of the defect present following the definitive procedure(s).

The *approach procedure* is described according to anatomical area involved, ie, anterior cranial fossa, middle cranial fossa, posterior cranial fossa, and brain stem or upper spinal cord.

The *definitive procedure(s)* describes the repair, biopsy, resection, or excision of various lesions of the skull base and, when appropriate, primary closure of the dura, mucous membranes, and skin.

The *repair/reconstruction procedure(s)* is reported separately if extensive dural grafting, cranioplasty, local or regional myocutaneous pedicle flaps, or extensive skin grafts are required.

For primary closure, see the appropriate codes (ie, 15732, 15756-15758).

When one surgeon performs the approach procedure, another surgeon performs the definitive procedure, and another surgeon performs the repair/reconstruction procedure, each surgeon reports only the code for the specific procedure performed.

If one surgeon performs more than one procedure (ie, approach procedure and definitive procedure), then both codes are reported, adding modifier 51 to the secondary, additional procedure(s).

Approach Procedures

Anterior Cranial Fossa

61580 Craniofacial approach to anterior cranial fossa; extradural, including lateral rhinotomy, ethmoidectomy, sphenoidectomy, without maxillectomy or orbital exenteration

61581   extradural, including lateral rhinotomy, orbital exenteration, ethmoidectomy, sphenoidectomy and/or maxillectomy

61582   extradural, including unilateral or bifrontal craniotomy, elevation of frontal lobe(s), osteotomy of base of anterior cranial fossa

61583   intradural, including unilateral or bifrontal craniotomy, elevation or resection of frontal lobe, osteotomy of base of anterior cranial fossa

61584 Orbitocranial approach to anterior cranial fossa, extradural, including supraorbital ridge osteotomy and elevation of frontal and/or temporal lobe(s); without orbital exenteration

Nervous

61585   with orbital exenteration

61586   Bicoronal, transzygomatic and/or LeFort I osteotomy approach to anterior cranial fossa with or without internal fixation, without bone graft

Middle Cranial Fossa

61590   Infratemporal pre-auricular approach to middle cranial fossa (parapharyngeal space, infratemporal and midline skull base, nasopharynx), with or without disarticulation of the mandible, including parotidectomy, craniotomy, decompression and/or mobilization of the facial nerve and/or petrous carotid artery

61591   Infratemporal post-auricular approach to middle cranial fossa (internal auditory meatus, petrous apex, tentorium, cavernous sinus, parasellar area, infratemporal fossa) including mastoidectomy, resection of sigmoid sinus, with or without decompression and/or mobilization of contents of auditory canal or petrous carotid artery

61592   Orbitocranial zygomatic approach to middle cranial fossa (cavernous sinus and carotid artery, clivus, basilar artery or petrous apex) including osteotomy of zygoma, craniotomy, extra- or intradural elevation of temporal lobe

Posterior Cranial Fossa

61595   Transtemporal approach to posterior cranial fossa, jugular foramen or midline skull base, including mastoidectomy, decompression of sigmoid sinus and/or facial nerve, with or without mobilization

61596   Transcochlear approach to posterior cranial fossa, jugular foramen or midline skull base, including labyrinthectomy, decompression, with or without mobilization of facial nerve and/or petrous carotid artery

61597   Transcondylar (far lateral) approach to posterior cranial fossa, jugular foramen or midline skull base, including occipital condylectomy, mastoidectomy, resection of C1-C3 vertebral body(s), decompression of vertebral artery, with or without mobilization

61598   Transpetrosal approach to posterior cranial fossa, clivus or foramen magnum, including ligation of superior petrosal sinus and/or sigmoid sinus

Definitive Procedures
Base of Anterior Cranial Fossa

61600   Resection or excision of neoplastic, vascular or infectious lesion of base of anterior cranial fossa; extradural

61601   intradural, including dural repair, with or without graft

Base of Middle Cranial Fossa

61605   Resection or excision of neoplastic, vascular or infectious lesion of infratemporal fossa, parapharyngeal space, petrous apex; extradural

61606   intradural, including dural repair, with or without graft

61607   Resection or excision of neoplastic, vascular or infectious lesion of parasellar area, cavernous sinus, clivus or midline skull base; extradural

61608   intradural, including dural repair, with or without graft

Codes 61610, 61611, 61612 are reported in addition to code(s) for primary procedure(s) 61605-61608. Report only one transection or ligation of carotid artery code per operative session.

(61609 has been deleted)

+ 61610   Transection or ligation, carotid artery in cavernous sinus, with repair by anastomosis or graft (List separately in addition to code for primary procedure)

+ 61611   Transection or ligation, carotid artery in petrous canal; without repair (List separately in addition to code for primary procedure)

+ 61612   with repair by anastomosis or graft (List separately in addition to code for primary procedure)

61613   Obliteration of carotid aneurysm, arteriovenous malformation, or carotid-cavernous fistula by dissection within cavernous sinus

Base of Posterior Cranial Fossa

61615   Resection or excision of neoplastic, vascular or infectious lesion of base of posterior cranial fossa, jugular foramen, foramen magnum, or C1-C3 vertebral bodies; extradural

61616   intradural, including dural repair, with or without graft

Repair and/or Reconstruction of Surgical Defects of Skull Base

61618   Secondary repair of dura for cerebrospinal fluid leak, anterior, middle or posterior cranial fossa following surgery of the skull base; by free tissue graft (eg, pericranium, fascia, tensor fascia lata, adipose tissue, homologous or synthetic grafts)

61619   by local or regionalized vascularized pedicle flap or myocutaneous flap (including galea, temporalis, frontalis or occipitalis muscle)

Nervous

Endovascular Therapy

61623   Endovascular temporary balloon arterial occlusion, head or neck (extracranial/intracranial) including selective catheterization of vessel to be occluded, positioning and inflation of occlusion balloon, concomitant neurological monitoring, and radiologic supervision and interpretation of all angiography required for balloon occlusion and to exclude vascular injury post occlusion

(If selective catheterization and angiography of arteries other than artery to be occluded is performed, use appropriate catheterization and radiologic supervision and interpretation codes)

(If complete diagnostic angiography of the artery to be occluded is performed immediately prior to temporary occlusion, use appropriate radiologic supervision and interpretation codes only)

61624   Transcatheter permanent occlusion or embolization (eg, for tumor destruction, to achieve hemostasis, to occlude a vascular malformation), percutaneous, any method; central nervous system (intracranial, spinal cord)

(For non-central nervous system and non-head or neck embolization, see 37241-37244)

(For radiological supervision and interpretation, use 75894)

61626   non-central nervous system, head or neck (extracranial, brachiocephalic branch)

(For non-central nervous system and non-head or neck embolization, see 37241-37244)

(For radiological supervision and interpretation, use 75894)

61630   Balloon angioplasty, intracranial (eg, atherosclerotic stenosis), percutaneous

61635   Transcatheter placement of intravascular stent(s), intracranial (eg, atherosclerotic stenosis), including balloon angioplasty, if performed

(61630 and 61635 include all selective vascular catheterization of the target vascular family, all diagnostic imaging for arteriography of the target vascular family, and all related radiological supervision and interpretation. When diagnostic arteriogram (including imaging and selective catheterization) confirms the need for angioplasty or stent placement, 61630 and 61635 are inclusive of these services. If angioplasty or stenting are not indicated, then the appropriate codes for selective catheterization and imaging should be reported in lieu of 61630 and 61635)

▶(Do not report 61630 or 61635 in conjunction with 61645 for the same vascular territory)◀

▶(For definition of vascular territory, see the Nervous System Endovascular Therapy guidelines)◀

61640   Balloon dilatation of intracranial vasospasm, percutaneous; initial vessel

+ 61641   each additional vessel in same vascular family (List separately in addition to code for primary procedure)

+ 61642   each additional vessel in different vascular family (List separately in addition to code for primary procedure)

(Use 61641 and 61642 in conjunction with 61640)

(61640, 61641, 61642 include all selective vascular catheterization of the target vessel, contrast injection[s], vessel measurement, roadmapping, postdilatation angiography, and fluoroscopic guidance for the balloon dilatation)

▶(Do not report 61640, 61642 in conjunction with 61650 or 61651 for the same vascular territory)◀

▶(For definition of vascular territory, see the Nervous System Endovascular Therapy guidelines)◀

▶Codes 61645, 61650, 61651 describe cerebral endovascular therapeutic interventions in any intracranial artery. They include selective catheterization, diagnostic angiography, and all subsequent angiography including associated radiological supervision and interpretation within the treated vascular territory, fluoroscopic guidance, neurologic and hemodynamic monitoring of the patient, and closure of the arteriotomy by manual pressure, an arterial closure device, or suture.

For purposes of reporting services described by 61645, 61650, 61651, the intracranial arteries are divided into three vascular territories: 1) right carotid circulation; 2) left carotid circulation; 3) vertebro-basilar circulation. Code 61645 may be reported once for each intracranial vascular territory treated. Code 61650 is reported once for the first intracranial vascular territory treated with intra-arterial prolonged administration of pharmacologic agent(s). If additional intracranial vascular territory(ies) is also treated with intra-arterial prolonged administration of pharmacologic agent(s) during the same session, the treatment of each additional vascular territory(ies) is reported using 61651 (may be reported maximally two times per day).

Code 61645 describes endovascular revascularization of thrombotic/embolic occlusion of intracranial arterial vessel(s) via any method, including mechanical thrombectomy (eg, mechanical retrieval device, aspiration catheter) and/or the administration of any agent(s) for the purpose of revascularization, such as thrombolytics or IIB/IIIA inhibitors.

Codes 61650, 61651 describe the cerebral endovascular continuous or intermittent therapeutic prolonged administration of any non-thrombolytic agent(s) (eg, spasmolytics or chemotherapy) into an artery to treat non-iatrogenic central nervous system diseases or sequelae thereof. These codes should not be used to report administration of agents (eg, heparin, nitroglycerin, saline) usually administered during endovascular interventions. These codes are used for prolonged

Nervous

administrations, ie, of at least 10 minutes continuous or intermittent duration.

Do not report 61645, 61650, or 61651 in conjunction with 36221, 36226, 36228, 37184, or 37186 for the treated vascular territory. Do not report 61645 in conjunction with 61650 or 61651 for the same vascular distribution. Diagnostic angiography of a non-treated vascular territory may be reported separately. For example, angiography of the left carotid and/or the vertebral circulations may be reported if the intervention is performed in the right carotid circulation.◄

● **61645** Percutaneous arterial transluminal mechanical thrombectomy and/or infusion for thrombolysis, intracranial, any method, including diagnostic angiography, fluoroscopic guidance, catheter placement, and intraprocedural pharmacological thrombolytic injection(s)

►(Do not report 61645 in conjunction with 36221, 36222, 36223, 36224, 36225, 36226, 37184, 61630, 61635, 61650, 61651 for the same vascular territory)◄

►(To report venous mechanical thrombectomy and/or thrombolysis, see 37187, 37188, 37212, 37214)◄

● **61650** Endovascular intracranial prolonged administration of pharmacologic agent(s) other than for thrombolysis, arterial, including catheter placement, diagnostic angiography, and imaging guidance; initial vascular territory

+● **61651** each additional vascular territory (List separately in addition to code for primary procedure)

►(Use 61651 in conjunction with 61650)◄

►(Do not report 61650 or 61651 in conjunction with 36221, 36222, 36223, 36224, 36225, 36226, 61640, 61641, 61642, 61645 for the same vascular territory)◄

►(Do not report 61650 or 61651 in conjunction with 96420, 96422, 96423, 96425 for the same vascular territory)◄

Surgery for Aneurysm, Arteriovenous Malformation, or Vascular Disease

Includes craniotomy when appropriate for procedure.

61680 Surgery of intracranial arteriovenous malformation; supratentorial, simple

61682 supratentorial, complex

61684 infratentorial, simple

61686 infratentorial, complex

61690 dural, simple

61692 dural, complex

61697 Surgery of complex intracranial aneurysm, intracranial approach; carotid circulation

61698 vertebrobasilar circulation

(61697, 61698 involve aneurysms that are larger than 15 mm or with calcification of the aneurysm neck, or with incorporation of normal vessels into the aneurysm neck, or a procedure requiring temporary vessel occlusion, trapping, or cardiopulmonary bypass to successfully treat the aneurysm)

61700 Surgery of simple intracranial aneurysm, intracranial approach; carotid circulation

61702 vertebrobasilar circulation

61703 Surgery of intracranial aneurysm, cervical approach by application of occluding clamp to cervical carotid artery (Selverstone-Crutchfield type)

(For cervical approach for direct ligation of carotid artery, see 37600-37606)

61705 Surgery of aneurysm, vascular malformation or carotid-cavernous fistula; by intracranial and cervical occlusion of carotid artery

61708 by intracranial electrothrombosis

(For ligation or gradual occlusion of internal/common carotid artery, see 37605, 37606)

61710 by intra-arterial embolization, injection procedure, or balloon catheter

61711 Anastomosis, arterial, extracranial-intracranial (eg, middle cerebral/cortical) arteries

(For carotid or vertebral thromboendarterectomy, use 35301)

(Use 69990 when the surgical microscope is employed for the microsurgical procedure. Do not use 69990 for visualization with magnifying loupes or corrected vision)

Stereotaxis

61720 Creation of lesion by stereotactic method, including burr hole(s) and localizing and recording techniques, single or multiple stages; globus pallidus or thalamus

61735 subcortical structure(s) other than globus pallidus or thalamus

61750 Stereotactic biopsy, aspiration, or excision, including burr hole(s), for intracranial lesion;

61751 with computed tomography and/or magnetic resonance guidance

(For radiological supervision and interpretation of computerized tomography, see 70450, 70460, or 70470 as appropriate)

(For radiological supervision and interpretation of magnetic resonance imaging, see 70551, 70552, or 70553 as appropriate)

61760 Stereotactic implantation of depth electrodes into the cerebrum for long-term seizure monitoring

Nervous

61770 Stereotactic localization, including burr hole(s), with insertion of catheter(s) or probe(s) for placement of radiation source

+ 61781 Stereotactic computer-assisted (navigational) procedure; cranial, intradural (List separately in addition to code for primary procedure)

(Do not report 61781 in conjunction with 61720-61791, 61796-61799, 61863-61868, 62201, 77371-77373, 77432)

+ 61782 cranial, extradural (List separately in addition to code for primary procedure)

(Do not report 61781, 61782 by the same individual during the same surgical session)

+ 61783 spinal (List separately in addition to code for primary procedure)

(Do not report 61783 in conjunction with 63620, 63621)

61790 Creation of lesion by stereotactic method, percutaneous, by neurolytic agent (eg, alcohol, thermal, electrical, radiofrequency); gasserian ganglion

61791 trigeminal medullary tract

Stereotactic Radiosurgery (Cranial)

Cranial stereotactic radiosurgery is a distinct procedure that utilizes externally generated ionizing radiation to inactivate or eradicate defined target(s) in the head without the need to make an incision. The target is defined by and the treatment is delivered using high-resolution stereotactic imaging. Stereotactic radiosurgery codes and headframe application procedures are reported by the neurosurgeon. The radiation oncologist reports the appropriate code(s) for clinical treatment planning, physics and dosimetry, treatment delivery, and management from the **Radiation Oncology** section (77261-77790). Any necessary planning, dosimetry, targeting, positioning, or blocking by the neurosurgeon is included in the stereotactic radiation surgery services. The same individual should not report stereotactic radiosurgery services with radiation treatment management codes (77427-77435).

Cranial stereotactic radiosurgery is typically performed in a single planning and treatment session, using a rigidly attached stereotactic guiding device, other immobilization technology and/or a stereotactic image-guidance system, but can be performed with more than one planning session and in a limited number of treatment sessions, up to a maximum of five sessions. Do not report stereotactic radiosurgery more than once per lesion per course of treatment when the treatment requires more than one session.

Codes 61796 and 61797 involve stereotactic radiosurgery for simple cranial lesions. Simple cranial lesions are lesions less than 3.5 cm in maximum dimension that do not meet the definition of a complex lesion provided below. Report code 61796 when all lesions are simple.

Codes 61798 and 61799 involve stereotactic radiosurgery for complex cranial lesions and procedures that create therapeutic lesions (eg, thalamotomy or pallidotomy). All lesions 3.5 cm in maximum dimension or greater are complex. When performing therapeutic lesion creation procedures, report code 61798 only once regardless of the number of lesions created. Schwannomas, arterio-venous malformations, pituitary tumors, glomus tumors, pineal region tumors and cavernous sinus/parasellar/petroclival tumors are complex. Any lesion that is adjacent (5mm or less) to the optic nerve/optic chasm/optic tract or within the brainstem is complex. If treating multiple lesions, and any single lesion treated is complex, use 61798.

Do not report codes 61796-61800 in conjunction with code 20660.

Codes 61796-61799 include computer-assisted planning. Do not report codes 61796-61799 in conjunction with 61781-61783.

(For intensity modulated beam delivery plan and treatment, see 77301, 77385, 77386. For stereotactic body radiation therapy, see 77373, 77435)

61796 Stereotactic radiosurgery (particle beam, gamma ray, or linear accelerator); 1 simple cranial lesion

(Do not report 61796 more than once per course of treatment)

(Do not report 61796 in conjunction with 61798)

+ 61797 each additional cranial lesion, simple (List separately in addition to code for primary procedure)

(Use 61797 in conjunction with 61796, 61798)

(For each course of treatment, 61797 and 61799 may be reported no more than once per lesion. Do not report any combination of 61797 and 61799 more than 4 times for entire course of treatment regardless of number of lesions treated)

61798 1 complex cranial lesion

(Do not report 61798 more than once per course of treatment)

(Do not report 61798 in conjunction with 61796)

+ 61799 each additional cranial lesion, complex (List separately in addition to code for primary procedure)

(Use 61799 in conjunction with 61798)

(For each course of treatment, 61797 and 61799 may be reported no more than once per lesion. Do not report any combination of 61797 and 61799 more than 4 times for entire course of treatment regardless of number of lesions treated)

+ 61800 Application of stereotactic headframe for stereotactic radiosurgery (List separately in addition to code for primary procedure)

(Use 61800 in conjunction with 61796, 61798)

Neurostimulators (Intracranial)

Codes 61850-61888 apply to both simple and complex neurostimulators. For initial or subsequent electronic analysis and programming of neurostimulator pulse generators, see codes 95970-95975.

Microelectrode recording, when performed by the operating surgeon in association with implantation of neurostimulator electrode arrays, is an inclusive service and should not be reported separately. If another individual participates in neurophysiological mapping during a deep brain stimulator implantation procedure, this service may be reported by the second individual with codes 95961-95962.

61850 Twist drill or burr hole(s) for implantation of neurostimulator electrodes, cortical

61860 Craniectomy or craniotomy for implantation of neurostimulator electrodes, cerebral, cortical

61863 Twist drill, burr hole, craniotomy, or craniectomy with stereotactic implantation of neurostimulator electrode array in subcortical site (eg, thalamus, globus pallidus, subthalamic nucleus, periventricular, periaqueductal gray), without use of intraoperative microelectrode recording; first array

+ 61864 each additional array (List separately in addition to primary procedure)

(Use 61864 in conjunction with 61863)

61867 Twist drill, burr hole, craniotomy, or craniectomy with stereotactic implantation of neurostimulator electrode array in subcortical site (eg, thalamus, globus pallidus, subthalamic nucleus, periventricular, periaqueductal gray), with use of intraoperative microelectrode recording; first array

+ 61868 each additional array (List separately in addition to primary procedure)

(Use 61868 in conjunction with 61867)

61870 Craniectomy for implantation of neurostimulator electrodes, cerebellar, cortical

(61875 has been deleted)

61880 Revision or removal of intracranial neurostimulator electrodes

61885 Insertion or replacement of cranial neurostimulator pulse generator or receiver, direct or inductive coupling; with connection to a single electrode array

61886 with connection to 2 or more electrode arrays

(For percutaneous placement of cranial nerve (eg, vagus, trigeminal) neurostimulator electrode(s), use 64553)

(For revision or removal of cranial nerve (eg, vagus, trigeminal) neurostimulator electrode array, use 64569)

61888 Revision or removal of cranial neurostimulator pulse generator or receiver

(Do not report 61888 in conjunction with 61885 or 61886 for the same pulse generator)

Repair

62000 Elevation of depressed skull fracture; simple, extradural

62005 compound or comminuted, extradural

62010 with repair of dura and/or debridement of brain

62100 Craniotomy for repair of dural/cerebrospinal fluid leak, including surgery for rhinorrhea/otorrhea

(For repair of spinal dural/CSF leak, see 63707, 63709)

62115 Reduction of craniomegalic skull (eg, treated hydrocephalus); not requiring bone grafts or cranioplasty

(62116 has been deleted)

62117 requiring craniotomy and reconstruction with or without bone graft (includes obtaining grafts)

62120 Repair of encephalocele, skull vault, including cranioplasty

62121 Craniotomy for repair of encephalocele, skull base

62140 Cranioplasty for skull defect; up to 5 cm diameter

62141 larger than 5 cm diameter

62142 Removal of bone flap or prosthetic plate of skull

62143 Replacement of bone flap or prosthetic plate of skull

62145 Cranioplasty for skull defect with reparative brain surgery

62146 Cranioplasty with autograft (includes obtaining bone grafts); up to 5 cm diameter

62147 larger than 5 cm diameter

+ 62148 Incision and retrieval of subcutaneous cranial bone graft for cranioplasty (List separately in addition to code for primary procedure)

(Use 62148 in conjunction with 62140-62147)

Neuroendoscopy

Surgical endoscopy always includes diagnostic endoscopy.

+ 62160 Neuroendoscopy, intracranial, for placement or replacement of ventricular catheter and attachment to shunt system or external drainage (List separately in addition to code for primary procedure)

(Use 62160 only in conjunction with 61107, 61210, 62220-62230, 62258)

62161 Neuroendoscopy, intracranial; with dissection of adhesions, fenestration of septum pellucidum or intraventricular cysts (including placement, replacement, or removal of ventricular catheter)

Nervous

62162   with fenestration or excision of colloid cyst, including placement of external ventricular catheter for drainage

62163   with retrieval of foreign body

62164   with excision of brain tumor, including placement of external ventricular catheter for drainage

62165   with excision of pituitary tumor, transnasal or transsphenoidal approach

Cerebrospinal Fluid (CSF) Shunt

62180   Ventriculocisternostomy (Torkildsen type operation)

62190   Creation of shunt; subarachnoid/subdural-atrial, -jugular, -auricular

62192   subarachnoid/subdural-peritoneal, -pleural, other terminus

62194   Replacement or irrigation, subarachnoid/subdural catheter

62200   Ventriculocisternostomy, third ventricle;

62201   stereotactic, neuroendoscopic method

(For intracranial neuroendoscopic procedures, see 62161-62165)

62220   Creation of shunt; ventriculo-atrial, -jugular, -auricular

(For intracranial neuroendoscopic ventricular catheter placement, use 62160)

62223   ventriculo-peritoneal, -pleural, other terminus

(For intracranial neuroendoscopic ventricular catheter placement, use 62160)

62225   Replacement or irrigation, ventricular catheter

(For intracranial neuroendoscopic ventricular catheter placement, use 62160)

62230   Replacement or revision of cerebrospinal fluid shunt, obstructed valve, or distal catheter in shunt system

(For intracranial neuroendoscopic ventricular catheter placement, use 62160)

62252   Reprogramming of programmable cerebrospinal shunt

62256   Removal of complete cerebrospinal fluid shunt system; without replacement

62258   with replacement by similar or other shunt at same operation

(For percutaneous irrigation or aspiration of shunt reservoir, use 61070)

(For reprogramming of programmable CSF shunt, use 62252)

(For intracranial neuroendoscopic ventricular catheter placement, use 62160)

Spine and Spinal Cord

(For application of caliper or tongs, use 20660)

(For treatment of fracture or dislocation of spine, see 22305-22327)

Injection, Drainage, or Aspiration

Injection of contrast during fluoroscopic guidance and localization is an inclusive component of 62263, 62264, 62267, 62270, 62272, 62273, 62280, 62281, 62282, 62302, 62303, 62304, 62305, 62310-62319. Fluoroscopic guidance and localization is reported with 77003, unless a formal contrast study (myelography, epidurography, or arthrography) is performed, in which case the use of fluoroscopy is included in the supervision and interpretation codes or the myelography via lumbar injection code. Image guidance and the injection of contrast are inclusive components and are required for the performance of myelography, as described by codes 62302, 62303, 62304, 62305.

For radiologic supervision and interpretation of epidurography, use 72275. Code 72275 is only to be used when an epidurogram is performed, images documented, and a formal radiologic report is issued.

Code 62263 describes a catheter-based treatment involving targeted injection of various substances (eg, hypertonic saline, steroid, anesthetic) via an indwelling epidural catheter. Code 62263 includes percutaneous insertion and removal of an epidural catheter (remaining in place over a several-day period), for the administration of multiple injections of a neurolytic agent(s) performed during serial treatment sessions (ie, spanning two or more treatment days). If required, adhesions or scarring may also be lysed by mechanical means. Code 62263 is **not** reported for each adhesiolysis treatment, but should be reported **once** to describe the entire series of injections/infusions spanning two or more treatment days.

Code 62264 describes multiple adhesiolysis treatment sessions performed on the same day. Adhesions or scarring may be lysed by injections of neurolytic agent(s). If required, adhesions or scarring may also be lysed mechanically using a percutaneously-deployed catheter.

Codes 62263 and 62264 include the procedure of injections of contrast for epidurography (72275) and fluoroscopic guidance and localization (77003) during initial or subsequent sessions.

Fluoroscopy (for localization) may be used in the placement of injections reported with 62310-62319, but is not required. If used, fluoroscopy should be reported with 77003. For epidurography, use 72275.

The placement and use of a catheter to administer one or more epidural or subarachnoid injections on a single calendar day should be reported in the same manner as if

Nervous

a needle had been used, ie, as a single injection using either 62310 or 62311. Such injections should not be reported with 62318 or 62319.

Threading a catheter into the epidural space, injecting substances at one or more levels and then removing the catheter should be treated as a single injection (62310, 62311). If the catheter is left in place to deliver substance(s) over a prolonged period (ie, more than a single calendar day) either continuously or via intermittent bolus, use 62318, 62319 as appropriate.

When reporting 62310-62319, code choice is based on the region at which the needle or catheter entered the body (eg, lumbar). Codes 62310-62319 should be reported only once, when the substance injected spreads or catheter tip insertion moves into another spinal region (eg, 62311 is reported only once for injection or catheter insertion at L3-4 with spread of the substance or placement of the catheter tip to the thoracic region).

Percutaneous spinal procedures are done with indirect visualization (eg, image guidance or endoscopic approaches) and without direct visualization (including through a microscope). Endoscopic assistance during an open procedure with direct visualization is reported using excision codes (eg, 63020-63035).

(Report 01996 for daily hospital management of continuous epidural or subarachnoid drug administration performed in conjunction with 62318-62319)

62263   Percutaneous lysis of epidural adhesions using solution injection (eg, hypertonic saline, enzyme) or mechanical means (eg, catheter) including radiologic localization (includes contrast when administered), multiple adhesiolysis sessions; 2 or more days

(62263 includes codes 72275 and 77003)

62264   1 day

(Do not report 62264 with 62263)

(62264 includes codes 72275 and 77003)

62267   Percutaneous aspiration within the nucleus pulposus, intervertebral disc, or paravertebral tissue for diagnostic purposes

(For imaging, use 77003)

(Do not report 62267 in conjunction with 10022, 20225, 62287, 62290, 62291)

62268   Percutaneous aspiration, spinal cord cyst or syrinx

(For radiological supervision and interpretation, see 76942, 77002, 77012)

62269   Biopsy of spinal cord, percutaneous needle

(For radiological supervision and interpretation, see 76942, 77002, 77012)

(For fine needle aspiration, see 10021, 10022)

(For evaluation of fine needle aspirate, see 88172, 88173)

62270   Spinal puncture, lumbar, diagnostic

62272   Spinal puncture, therapeutic, for drainage of cerebrospinal fluid (by needle or catheter)

62273   Injection, epidural, of blood or clot patch

(For injection of diagnostic or therapeutic substance(s), see 62310, 62311, 62318, 62319)

62280   Injection/infusion of neurolytic substance (eg, alcohol, phenol, iced saline solutions), with or without other therapeutic substance; subarachnoid

62281   epidural, cervical or thoracic

62282   epidural, lumbar, sacral (caudal)

62284   Injection procedure for myelography and/or computed tomography, lumbar

(Do not report 62284 in conjunction with 62302, 62303, 62304, 62305, 72240, 72255, 72265, 72270)

(When both 62284 and 72240, 72255, 72265, 72270 are performed by the same physician or other qualified health care professional for myelography, see 62302, 62303, 62304, 62305)

(For injection procedure at C1-C2, use 61055)

(For radiological supervision and interpretation, see **Radiology**)

62287   Decompression procedure, percutaneous, of nucleus pulposus of intervertebral disc, any method utilizing needle based technique to remove disc material under fluoroscopic imaging or other form of indirect visualization, with the use of an endoscope, with discography and/or epidural injection(s) at the treated level(s), when performed, single or multiple levels, lumbar

(This includes endoscopic approach)

(Do not report 62287 in conjunction with 62267, 62290, 62311, 77003, 77012, 72295, when performed at same level)

(For non-needle based technique for percutaneous decompression of nucleus pulposus of intervertebral disc, see 0274T, 0275T)

62290   Injection procedure for discography, each level; lumbar

62291   cervical or thoracic

(For radiological supervision and interpretation, see 72285, 72295)

62292   Injection procedure for chemonucleolysis, including discography, intervertebral disc, single or multiple levels, lumbar

62294   Injection procedure, arterial, for occlusion of arteriovenous malformation, spinal

62302   Myelography via lumbar injection, including radiological supervision and interpretation; cervical

(Do not report 62302 in conjunction with 62284, 62303, 62304, 62305, 72240, 72255, 72265, 72270)

Nervous

62303   thoracic

(Do not report 62303 in conjunction with 62284, 62302, 62304, 62305, 72240, 72255, 72265, 72270)

62304   lumbosacral

(Do not report 62304 in conjunction with 62284, 62302, 62303, 62305, 72240, 72255, 72265, 72270)

62305   2 or more regions (eg, lumbar/thoracic, cervical/thoracic, lumbar/cervical, lumbar/thoracic/cervical)

(Do not report 62305 in conjunction with 62284, 62302, 62303, 62304, 72240, 72255, 72265, 72270)

(For myelography lumbar injection and imaging performed by different physicians or other qualified health care professionals, see 62284 or 72240, 72255, 72265, 72270)

(For injection procedure at C1-C2, use 61055)

62310   Injection(s), of diagnostic or therapeutic substance(s) (including anesthetic, antispasmodic, opioid, steroid, other solution), not including neurolytic substances, including needle or catheter placement, includes contrast for localization when performed, epidural or subarachnoid; cervical or thoracic

62311   lumbar or sacral (caudal)

62318   Injection(s), including indwelling catheter placement, continuous infusion or intermittent bolus, of diagnostic or therapeutic substance(s) (including anesthetic, antispasmodic, opioid, steroid, other solution), not including neurolytic substances, includes contrast for localization when performed, epidural or subarachnoid; cervical or thoracic

62319   lumbar or sacral (caudal)

(For transforaminal epidural injection, see 64479-64484)

(Report 01996 for daily hospital management of continuous epidural or subarachnoid drug administration performed in conjunction with 62318-62319)

Catheter Implantation

(For percutaneous placement of intrathecal or epidural catheter, see codes 62270-62273, 62280-62284, 62310-62319)

62350   Implantation, revision or repositioning of tunneled intrathecal or epidural catheter, for long-term medication administration via an external pump or implantable reservoir/infusion pump; without laminectomy

62351   with laminectomy

(For refilling and maintenance of an implantable infusion pump for spinal or brain drug therapy, see 95990, 95991)

62355   Removal of previously implanted intrathecal or epidural catheter

Reservoir/Pump Implantation

62360   Implantation or replacement of device for intrathecal or epidural drug infusion; subcutaneous reservoir

62361   nonprogrammable pump

62362   programmable pump, including preparation of pump, with or without programming

62365   Removal of subcutaneous reservoir or pump, previously implanted for intrathecal or epidural infusion

62367   Electronic analysis of programmable, implanted pump for intrathecal or epidural drug infusion (includes evaluation of reservoir status, alarm status, drug prescription status); without reprogramming or refill

62368   with reprogramming

(For refilling and maintenance of an implantable infusion pump for spinal or brain drug therapy, see 95990-95991)

62369   with reprogramming and refill

62370   with reprogramming and refill (requiring skill of a physician or other qualified health care professional)

(Do not report 62367-62370 in conjunction with 95990, 95991. For refilling and maintenance of a reservoir or an implantable infusion pump for spinal or brain drug delivery without reprogramming, see 95990, 95991)

Posterior Extradural Laminotomy or Laminectomy for Exploration/Decompression of Neural Elements or Excision of Herniated Intervertebral Discs

Endoscopically assisted laminotomy (hemilaminectomy) requires open and direct visualization. When visualization is only endoscopic and/or image guidance, the procedure is percutaneous and reported using 0274T, 0275T.

(When 63001-63048 are followed by arthrodesis, see 22590-22614)

63001   Laminectomy with exploration and/or decompression of spinal cord and/or cauda equina, without facetectomy, foraminotomy or discectomy (eg, spinal stenosis), 1 or 2 vertebral segments; cervical

63003   thoracic

63005   lumbar, except for spondylolisthesis

63011   sacral

63012   Laminectomy with removal of abnormal facets and/or pars inter-articularis with decompression of cauda equina and nerve roots for spondylolisthesis, lumbar (Gill type procedure)

63015   Laminectomy with exploration and/or decompression of spinal cord and/or cauda equina, without facetectomy, foraminotomy or discectomy (eg, spinal stenosis), more than 2 vertebral segments; cervical

63016   thoracic

63017   lumbar

63020   Laminotomy (hemilaminectomy), with decompression of nerve root(s), including partial facetectomy, foraminotomy and/or excision of herniated intervertebral disc; 1 interspace, cervical

(For bilateral procedure, report 63020 with modifier 50)

63030   1 interspace, lumbar

(For bilateral procedure, report 63030 with modifier 50)

+ 63035   each additional interspace, cervical or lumbar (List separately in addition to code for primary procedure)

(Use 63035 in conjunction with 63020-63030)

(For bilateral procedure, report 63035 with modifier 50)

(For percutaneous endoscopic approach, see 0274T, 0275T)

63040   Laminotomy (hemilaminectomy), with decompression of nerve root(s), including partial facetectomy, foraminotomy and/or excision of herniated intervertebral disc, reexploration, single interspace; cervical

(For bilateral procedure, report 63040 with modifier 50)

63042   lumbar

(For bilateral procedure, report 63042 with modifier 50)

+ 63043   each additional cervical interspace (List separately in addition to code for primary procedure)

(Use 63043 in conjunction with 63040)

(For bilateral procedure, report 63043 with modifier 50)

+ 63044   each additional lumbar interspace (List separately in addition to code for primary procedure)

(Use 63044 in conjunction with 63042)

(For bilateral procedure, report 63044 with modifier 50)

63045   Laminectomy, facetectomy and foraminotomy (unilateral or bilateral with decompression of spinal cord, cauda equina and/or nerve root[s], [eg, spinal or lateral recess stenosis]), single vertebral segment; cervical

63046   thoracic

63047   lumbar

+ 63048   each additional segment, cervical, thoracic, or lumbar (List separately in addition to code for primary procedure)

(Use 63048 in conjunction with 63045-63047)

63050   Laminoplasty, cervical, with decompression of the spinal cord, 2 or more vertebral segments;

63051   with reconstruction of the posterior bony elements (including the application of bridging bone graft and non-segmental fixation devices [eg, wire, suture, mini-plates], when performed)

(Do not report 63050 or 63051 in conjunction with 22600, 22614, 22840-22842, 63001, 63015, 63045, 63048, 63295 for the same vertebral segment(s))

Transpedicular or Costovertebral Approach for Posterolateral Extradural Exploration/Decompression

63055   Transpedicular approach with decompression of spinal cord, equina and/or nerve root(s) (eg, herniated intervertebral disc), single segment; thoracic

63056   lumbar (including transfacet, or lateral extraforaminal approach) (eg, far lateral herniated intervertebral disc)

+ 63057   each additional segment, thoracic or lumbar (List separately in addition to code for primary procedure)

(Use 63057 in conjunction with 63055, 63056)

63064   Costovertebral approach with decompression of spinal cord or nerve root(s) (eg, herniated intervertebral disc), thoracic; single segment

+ 63066   each additional segment (List separately in addition to code for primary procedure)

(Use 63066 in conjunction with 63064)

(For excision of thoracic intraspinal lesions by laminectomy, see 63266, 63271, 63276, 63281, 63286)

Anterior or Anterolateral Approach for Extradural Exploration/Decompression

For the following codes, when two surgeons work together as primary surgeons performing distinct part(s) of spinal cord exploration/decompression operation, each surgeon should report his/her distinct operative work by appending modifier 62 to the procedure code (and any associated add-on codes for that procedure code as long as both surgeons continue to work together as primary surgeons). In this situation, modifier 62 may be appended to the definitive procedure code(s) 63075, 63077, 63081, 63085, 63087, 63090 and, as appropriate, to associated additional interspace add-on code(s) 63076, 63078 or additional segment add-on code(s) 63082, 63086, 63088, 63091 as long as both surgeons continue to work together as primary surgeons.

63075   Discectomy, anterior, with decompression of spinal cord and/or nerve root(s), including osteophytectomy; cervical, single interspace

(Do not report 63075 in conjunction with 22554, even if performed by separate individuals. To report anterior cervical discectomy and interbody fusion at the same level during the same session, use 22551)

+ 63076   cervical, each additional interspace (List separately in addition to code for primary procedure)

(Do not report 63076 in conjunction with 22554, even if performed by separate individuals. To report anterior cervical discectomy and interbody fusion at the same level during the same session, use 22552)

(Use 63076 in conjunction with 63075)

63077   thoracic, single interspace

Nervous

+ **63078**   thoracic, each additional interspace (List separately in addition to code for primary procedure)

(Use 63078 in conjunction with 63077)

(Do not report code 69990 in addition to codes 63075-63078)

63081   Vertebral corpectomy (vertebral body resection), partial or complete, anterior approach with decompression of spinal cord and/or nerve root(s); cervical, single segment

+ **63082**   cervical, each additional segment (List separately in addition to code for primary procedure)

(Use 63082 in conjunction with 63081)

(For transoral approach, see 61575, 61576)

63085   Vertebral corpectomy (vertebral body resection), partial or complete, transthoracic approach with decompression of spinal cord and/or nerve root(s); thoracic, single segment

+ **63086**   thoracic, each additional segment (List separately in addition to code for primary procedure)

(Use 63086 in conjunction with 63085)

63087   Vertebral corpectomy (vertebral body resection), partial or complete, combined thoracolumbar approach with decompression of spinal cord, cauda equina or nerve root(s), lower thoracic or lumbar; single segment

+ **63088**   each additional segment (List separately in addition to code for primary procedure)

(Use 63088 in conjunction with 63087)

63090   Vertebral corpectomy (vertebral body resection), partial or complete, transperitoneal or retroperitoneal approach with decompression of spinal cord, cauda equina or nerve root(s), lower thoracic, lumbar, or sacral; single segment

+ **63091**   each additional segment (List separately in addition to code for primary procedure)

(Use 63091 in conjunction with 63090)

(Procedures 63081-63091 include discectomy above and/or below vertebral segment)

(If followed by arthrodesis, see 22548-22812)

(For reconstruction of spine, use appropriate vertebral corpectomy codes 63081-63091, bone graft codes 20930-20938, arthrodesis codes 22548-22812, and spinal instrumentation codes 22840-22855)

Lateral Extracavitary Approach for Extradural Exploration/Decompression

63101   Vertebral corpectomy (vertebral body resection), partial or complete, lateral extracavitary approach with decompression of spinal cord and/or nerve root(s) (eg, for tumor or retropulsed bone fragments); thoracic, single segment

63102   lumbar, single segment

+ **63103**   thoracic or lumbar, each additional segment (List separately in addition to code for primary procedure)

(Use 63103 in conjunction with 63101 and 63102)

Incision

63170   Laminectomy with myelotomy (eg, Bischof or DREZ type), cervical, thoracic, or thoracolumbar

63172   Laminectomy with drainage of intramedullary cyst/syrinx; to subarachnoid space

63173   to peritoneal or pleural space

63180   Laminectomy and section of dentate ligaments, with or without dural graft, cervical; 1 or 2 segments

63182   more than 2 segments

63185   Laminectomy with rhizotomy; 1 or 2 segments

63190   more than 2 segments

63191   Laminectomy with section of spinal accessory nerve

(For bilateral procedure, report 63191 with modifier 50)

(For resection of sternocleidomastoid muscle, use 21720)

63194   Laminectomy with cordotomy, with section of 1 spinothalamic tract, 1 stage; cervical

63195   thoracic

63196   Laminectomy with cordotomy, with section of both spinothalamic tracts, 1 stage; cervical

63197   thoracic

63198   Laminectomy with cordotomy with section of both spinothalamic tracts, 2 stages within 14 days; cervical

63199   thoracic

63200   Laminectomy, with release of tethered spinal cord, lumbar

Excision by Laminectomy of Lesion Other Than Herniated Disc

63250   Laminectomy for excision or occlusion of arteriovenous malformation of spinal cord; cervical

63251   thoracic

63252   thoracolumbar

63265   Laminectomy for excision or evacuation of intraspinal lesion other than neoplasm, extradural; cervical

63266   thoracic

63267   lumbar

63268   sacral

63270   Laminectomy for excision of intraspinal lesion other than neoplasm, intradural; cervical

63271   thoracic

63272   lumbar

Nervous

63273   sacral

63275   Laminectomy for biopsy/excision of intraspinal neoplasm; extradural, cervical

63276   extradural, thoracic

63277   extradural, lumbar

63278   extradural, sacral

63280   intradural, extramedullary, cervical

63281   intradural, extramedullary, thoracic

63282   intradural, extramedullary, lumbar

63283   intradural, sacral

63285   intradural, intramedullary, cervical

63286   intradural, intramedullary, thoracic

63287   intradural, intramedullary, thoracolumbar

63290   combined extradural-intradural lesion, any level

(For drainage of intramedullary cyst/syrinx, use 63172, 63173)

+ **63295**   Osteoplastic reconstruction of dorsal spinal elements, following primary intraspinal procedure (List separately in addition to code for primary procedure)

(Use 63295 in conjunction with 63172, 63173, 63185, 63190, 63200-63290)

(Do not report 63295 in conjunction with 22590-22614, 22840-22844, 63050, 63051 for the same vertebral segment(s))

Excision, Anterior or Anterolateral Approach, Intraspinal Lesion

For the following codes, when two surgeons work together as primary surgeons performing distinct part(s) of an anterior approach for an intraspinal excision, each surgeon should report his/her distinct operative work by appending modifier 62 to the single definitive procedure code. In this situation, modifier 62 may be appended to the definitive procedure code(s) 63300-63307 and, as appropriate, to the associated additional segment add-on code 63308 as long as both surgeons continue to work together as primary surgeons.

(For arthrodesis, see 22548-22585)

(For reconstruction of spine, see 20930-20938)

63300   Vertebral corpectomy (vertebral body resection), partial or complete, for excision of intraspinal lesion, single segment; extradural, cervical

63301   extradural, thoracic by transthoracic approach

63302   extradural, thoracic by thoracolumbar approach

63303   extradural, lumbar or sacral by transperitoneal or retroperitoneal approach

63304   intradural, cervical

63305   intradural, thoracic by transthoracic approach

63306   intradural, thoracic by thoracolumbar approach

63307   intradural, lumbar or sacral by transperitoneal or retroperitoneal approach

+ **63308**   each additional segment (List separately in addition to codes for single segment)

(Use 63308 in conjunction with 63300-63307)

Stereotaxis

63600   Creation of lesion of spinal cord by stereotactic method, percutaneous, any modality (including stimulation and/or recording)

63610   Stereotactic stimulation of spinal cord, percutaneous, separate procedure not followed by other surgery

63615   Stereotactic biopsy, aspiration, or excision of lesion, spinal cord

Stereotactic Radiosurgery (Spinal)

Spinal stereotactic radiosurgery is a distinct procedure that utilizes externally generated ionizing radiation to inactivate or eradicate defined target(s) in the spine without the need to make an incision. The target is defined by and the treatment is delivered using high-resolution stereotactic imaging. These codes are reported by the surgeon. The radiation oncologist reports the appropriate code(s) for clinical treatment planning, physics and dosimetry, treatment delivery and management from the **Radiation Oncology** section (77261-77790). Any necessary planning, dosimetry, targeting, positioning, or blocking by the neurosurgeon is included in the stereotactic radiation surgery services. The same individual should not report stereotactic radiosurgery services with radiation treatment management codes (77427-77432).

Spinal stereotactic radiosurgery is typically performed in a single planning and treatment session using a stereotactic image-guidance system, but can be performed with a planning session and in a limited number of treatment sessions, up to a maximum of five sessions. Do not report stereotactic radiosurgery more than once per lesion per course of treatment when the treatment requires greater than one session.

Stereotactic spinal surgery is only used when the tumor being treated affects spinal neural tissue or abuts the dura mater. Arteriovenous malformations must be subdural. For other radiation services of the spine, see **Radiation Oncology** services.

Codes 63620, 63621 include computer-assisted planning. Do not report 63620, 63621 in conjunction with 61781-61783.

(For intensity modulated beam delivery plan and treatment, see 77301, 77385, 77386. For stereotactic body radiation therapy, see 77373, 77435)

Nervous

63620 Stereotactic radiosurgery (particle beam, gamma ray, or linear accelerator); 1 spinal lesion

(Do not report 63620 more than once per course of treatment)

+ **63621** each additional spinal lesion (List separately in addition to code for primary procedure)

(Report 63621 in conjunction with 63620)

(For each course of treatment, 63621 may be reported no more than once per lesion. Do not report 63621 more than 2 times for entire course of treatment regardless of number of lesions treated)

Neurostimulators (Spinal)

Codes 63650-63688 apply to both simple and complex neurostimulators. For initial or subsequent electronic analysis and programming of neurostimulator pulse generators, see codes 95970-95975.

Codes 63650, 63655, and 63661-63664 describe the operative placement, revision, replacement, or removal of the spinal neurostimulator system components to provide spinal electrical stimulation. A neurostimulator system includes an implanted neurostimulator, external controller, extension, and collection of contacts. Multiple contacts or electrodes (4 or more) provide the actual electrical stimulation in the epidural space.

For percutaneously placed neurostimulator systems (63650, 63661, 63663), the contacts are on a catheter-like lead. An array defines the collection of contacts that are on one catheter.

For systems placed via an open surgical exposure (63655, 63662, 63664), the contacts are on a plate or paddle-shaped surface.

Do not report 63661 or 63663 when removing or replacing a temporary percutaneously placed array for an external generator.

63650 Percutaneous implantation of neurostimulator electrode array, epidural

63655 Laminectomy for implantation of neurostimulator electrodes, plate/paddle, epidural

63661 Removal of spinal neurostimulator electrode percutaneous array(s), including fluoroscopy, when performed

63662 Removal of spinal neurostimulator electrode plate/paddle(s) placed via laminotomy or laminectomy, including fluoroscopy, when performed

63663 Revision including replacement, when performed, of spinal neurostimulator electrode percutaneous array(s), including fluoroscopy, when performed

(Do not report 63663 in conjunction with 63661, 63662 for the same spinal level)

63664 Revision including replacement, when performed, of spinal neurostimulator electrode plate/paddle(s) placed via laminotomy or laminectomy, including fluoroscopy, when performed

(Do not report 63664 in conjunction with 63661, 63662 for the same spinal level)

63685 Insertion or replacement of spinal neurostimulator pulse generator or receiver, direct or inductive coupling

(Do not report 63685 in conjunction with 63688 for the same pulse generator or receiver)

63688 Revision or removal of implanted spinal neurostimulator pulse generator or receiver

(For electronic analysis of implanted neurostimulator pulse generator system, see 95970-95975)

Repair

63700 Repair of meningocele; less than 5 cm diameter

63702 larger than 5 cm diameter

(Do not use modifier 63 in conjunction with 63700, 63702)

63704 Repair of myelomeningocele; less than 5 cm diameter

63706 larger than 5 cm diameter

(Do not use modifier 63 in conjunction with 63704, 63706)

(For complex skin closure, see **Integumentary System**)

63707 Repair of dural/cerebrospinal fluid leak, not requiring laminectomy

63709 Repair of dural/cerebrospinal fluid leak or pseudomeningocele, with laminectomy

63710 Dural graft, spinal

(For laminectomy and section of dentate ligaments, with or without dural graft, cervical, see 63180, 63182)

Shunt, Spinal CSF

63740 Creation of shunt, lumbar, subarachnoid-peritoneal, -pleural, or other; including laminectomy

63741 percutaneous, not requiring laminectomy

63744 Replacement, irrigation or revision of lumbosubarachnoid shunt

63746 Removal of entire lumbosubarachnoid shunt system without replacement

(For insertion of subarachnoid catheter with reservoir and/or pump for intermittent or continuous infusion of drug including laminectomy, see 62351 and 62360, 62361 or 62362)

(For insertion or replacement of subarachnoid or epidural catheter, with reservoir and/or pump for drug infusion without laminectomy, see 62350 and 62360, 62361 or 62362)

Nervous

Extracranial Nerves, Peripheral Nerves, and Autonomic Nervous System

(For intracranial surgery on cranial nerves, see 61450, 61460, 61790)

Introduction/Injection of Anesthetic Agent (Nerve Block), Diagnostic or Therapeutic

(For destruction by neurolytic agent or chemodenervation, see 62280-62282, 64600-64681)

(For epidural or subarachnoid injection, see 62310-62319)

(64479-64487, 64490-64495 are unilateral procedures. For bilateral procedures, use modifier 50)

Somatic Nerves

64400	Injection, anesthetic agent; trigeminal nerve, any division or branch
64402	facial nerve
64405	greater occipital nerve
64408	vagus nerve
64410	phrenic nerve

►(64412 has been deleted. To report, use 64999)◄

64413	cervical plexus
64415	brachial plexus, single
64416	brachial plexus, continuous infusion by catheter (including catheter placement)

(Do not report 64416 in conjunction with 01996)

64417	axillary nerve
64418	suprascapular nerve
64420	intercostal nerve, single
64421	intercostal nerves, multiple, regional block
64425	ilioinguinal, iliohypogastric nerves
64430	pudendal nerve
64435	paracervical (uterine) nerve
64445	sciatic nerve, single
64446	sciatic nerve, continuous infusion by catheter (including catheter placement)

(Do not report 64446 in conjunction with 01996)

64447	femoral nerve, single

(Do not report 64447 in conjunction with 01996)

64448	femoral nerve, continuous infusion by catheter (including catheter placement)

(Do not report 64448 in conjunction with 01996)

64449	lumbar plexus, posterior approach, continuous infusion by catheter (including catheter placement)

(Do not report 64449 in conjunction with 01996)

64450	other peripheral nerve or branch
64455	Injection(s), anesthetic agent and/or steroid, plantar common digital nerve(s) (eg, Morton's neuroma)

(Do not report 64455 in conjunction with 64632)

(Imaging guidance [fluoroscopy or CT] and any injection of contrast are inclusive components of 64479-64484. Imaging guidance and localization are required for the performance of 64479-64484.)

(64470-64476 have been deleted. To report, see 64490-64495)

64461	Code is out of numerical sequence. See 64400-64489
64462	Code is out of numerical sequence. See 64400-64489
64463	Code is out of numerical sequence. See 64400-64489
64479	Injection(s), anesthetic agent and/or steroid, transforaminal epidural, with imaging guidance (fluoroscopy or CT); cervical or thoracic, single level

(For transforaminal epidural injection under ultrasound guidance, use 0228T)

+ 64480	cervical or thoracic, each additional level (List separately in addition to code for primary procedure)

(Use 64480 in conjunction with 64479)

(For transforaminal epidural injection under ultrasound guidance, use 0229T)

(For transforaminal epidural injection at the T12-L1 level, use 64479)

64483	lumbar or sacral, single level

(For transforaminal epidural injection under ultrasound guidance, use 0230T)

+ 64484	lumbar or sacral, each additional level (List separately in addition to code for primary procedure)

(Use 64484 in conjunction with 64483)

(For transforaminal epidural injection under ultrasound guidance, use 0231T)

(64479-64484 are unilateral procedures. For bilateral procedures, use modifier 50)

#● 64461	Paravertebral block (PVB) (paraspinous block), thoracic; single injection site (includes imaging guidance, when performed)
#+● 64462	second and any additional injection site(s) (includes imaging guidance, when performed) (List separately in addition to code for primary procedure)

►(Use 64462 in conjunction with 64461)◄

►(Do not report 64462 more than once per day)◄

Nervous

#● **64463**   continuous infusion by catheter (includes imaging guidance, when performed)

►(Do not report 64461, 64462, 64463 in conjunction with 62310, 62318, 64420, 64421, 64479, 64480, 64490, 64491, 64492, 76942, 77002, 77003)◄

64486   Transversus abdominis plane (TAP) block (abdominal plane block, rectus sheath block) unilateral; by injection(s) (includes imaging guidance, when performed)

64487   by continuous infusion(s) (includes imaging guidance, when performed)

64488   Transversus abdominis plane (TAP) block (abdominal plane block, rectus sheath block) bilateral; by injections (includes imaging guidance, when performed)

64489   by continuous infusions (includes imaging guidance, when performed)

Paravertebral Spinal Nerves and Branches

(Image guidance [fluoroscopy or CT] and any injection of contrast are inclusive components of 64490-64495. Imaging guidance and localization are required for the performance of paravertebral facet joint injections described by codes 64490-64495. If imaging is not used, report 20552-20553. If ultrasound guidance is used, report 0213T-0218T)

(For bilateral paravertebral facet injection procedures, use modifier 50)

(For paravertebral facet injection of the T12-L1 joint, or nerves innervating that joint, use 64490)

64490   Injection(s), diagnostic or therapeutic agent, paravertebral facet (zygapophyseal) joint (or nerves innervating that joint) with image guidance (fluoroscopy or CT), cervical or thoracic; single level

+ 64491   second level (List separately in addition to code for primary procedure)

(Use 64491 in conjunction with 64490)

+ 64492   third and any additional level(s) (List separately in addition to code for primary procedure)

(Do not report 64492 more than once per day)

(Use 64492 in conjunction with 64490, 64491)

64493   Injection(s), diagnostic or therapeutic agent, paravertebral facet (zygapophyseal) joint (or nerves innervating that joint) with image guidance (fluoroscopy or CT), lumbar or sacral; single level

+ 64494   second level (List separately in addition to code for primary procedure)

(Use 64494 in conjunction with 64493)

+ 64495   third and any additional level(s) (List separately in addition to code for primary procedure)

(Do not report 64495 more than once per day)

(Use 64495 in conjunction with 64493, 64494)

Autonomic Nerves

64505   Injection, anesthetic agent; sphenopalatine ganglion

64508   carotid sinus (separate procedure)

64510   stellate ganglion (cervical sympathetic)

64517   superior hypogastric plexus

64520   lumbar or thoracic (paravertebral sympathetic)

64530   celiac plexus, with or without radiologic monitoring

(For transendoscopic ultrasound-guided transmural injection, anesthetic, celiac plexus, use 43253)

Neurostimulators (Peripheral Nerve)

Codes 64553-64595 apply to both simple and complex neurostimulators. For initial or subsequent electronic analysis and programming of neurostimulator pulse generators, see codes 95970-95975. An electrode array is a catheter or other device with more than one contact. The function of each contact may be capable of being adjusted during programming services.

(For implantation of trial or permanent electrode arrays or pulse generators for peripheral subcutaneous field stimulation, see 0282T-0284T)

64550   Application of surface (transcutaneous) neurostimulator

64553   Percutaneous implantation of neurostimulator electrode array; cranial nerve

(For open placement of cranial nerve (eg, vagus, trigeminal) neurostimulator pulse generator or receiver, see 61885, 61886, as appropriate)

64555   peripheral nerve (excludes sacral nerve)

(Do not report 64555 in conjunction with 64566)

(64560 has been deleted)

64561   sacral nerve (transforaminal placement) including image guidance, if performed

64565   neuromuscular

64566   Posterior tibial neurostimulation, percutaneous needle electrode, single treatment, includes programming

(Do not report 64566 in conjunction with 64555, 95970-95972)

64568   Incision for implantation of cranial nerve (eg, vagus nerve) neurostimulator electrode array and pulse generator

(Do not report 64568 in conjunction with 61885, 61886, 64570)

64569   Revision or replacement of cranial nerve (eg, vagus nerve) neurostimulator electrode array, including connection to existing pulse generator

(Do not report 64569 in conjunction with 64570 or 61888)

(For replacement of pulse generator, use 61885)

64570   Removal of cranial nerve (eg, vagus nerve) neurostimulator electrode array and pulse generator

(Do not report 64570 in conjunction with 61888)

(For laparoscopic implantation, revision, replacement, or removal of vagus nerve blocking neurostimulator electrode array and/or pulse generator at the esophagogastric junction, see 0312T-0317T)

(64573 has been deleted)

64575   Incision for implantation of neurostimulator electrode array; peripheral nerve (excludes sacral nerve)

(64577 has been deleted)

64580   neuromuscular

64581   sacral nerve (transforaminal placement)

64585   Revision or removal of peripheral neurostimulator electrode array

64590   Insertion or replacement of peripheral or gastric neurostimulator pulse generator or receiver, direct or inductive coupling

(Do not report 64590 in conjunction with 64595)

64595   Revision or removal of peripheral or gastric neurostimulator pulse generator or receiver

Destruction by Neurolytic Agent (eg, Chemical, Thermal, Electrical or Radiofrequency), Chemodenervation

Codes 64600-64681 include the injection of other therapeutic agents (eg, corticosteroids). Do not report diagnostic/therapeutic injections separately. Do not report a code labeled as destruction when using therapies that are not destructive of the target nerve (eg, pulsed radiofrequency), use 64999. For codes labeled as chemodenervation, the supply of the chemodenervation agent is reported separately.

(For chemodenervation of internal anal sphincter, use 46505)

(For chemodenervation of the bladder, use 52287)

(For chemodenervation for strabismus involving the extraocular muscles, use 67345)

(For chemodenervation guided by needle electromyography or muscle electrical stimulation, see 95873, 95874)

Somatic Nerves

64600   Destruction by neurolytic agent, trigeminal nerve; supraorbital, infraorbital, mental, or inferior alveolar branch

64605   second and third division branches at foramen ovale

64610   second and third division branches at foramen ovale under radiologic monitoring

64611   Chemodenervation of parotid and submandibular salivary glands, bilateral

(Report 64611 with modifier 52 if fewer than four salivary glands are injected)

64612   Chemodenervation of muscle(s); muscle(s) innervated by facial nerve, unilateral (eg, for blepharospasm, hemifacial spasm)

(For bilateral procedure, report 64612 with modifier 50)

(64613 has been deleted. To report, use 64616)

(64614 has been deleted. To report, see 64642, 64643, 64644, 64645, 64646, 64647)

64615   muscle(s) innervated by facial, trigeminal, cervical spinal and accessory nerves, bilateral (eg, for chronic migraine)

(Report 64615 only once per session)

(Do not report 64615 in conjunction with 64612, 64616, 64617, 64642, 64643, 64644, 64645, 64646, 64647)

(For guidance see 95873, 95874. Do not report more than one guidance code for 64615)

64616   neck muscle(s), excluding muscles of the larynx, unilateral (eg, for cervical dystonia, spasmodic torticollis)

(For bilateral procedure, report 64616 with modifier 50)

(For chemodenervation guided by needle electromyography or muscle electrical stimulation, see 95873, 95874. Do not report more than one guidance code for any unit of 64616)

64617   larynx, unilateral, percutaneous (eg, for spasmodic dysphonia), includes guidance by needle electromyography, when performed

(For bilateral procedure, report 64617 with modifier 50)

(Do not report 64617 in conjunction with 95873, 95874)

(For diagnostic needle electromyography of the larynx, use 95865)

(For chemodenervation of the larynx performed with direct laryngoscopy, see 31570, 31571)

64620   Destruction by neurolytic agent, intercostal nerve

(64622-64627 have been deleted. For image-guided neurolysis of facet joint nerve(s), see 64633-64636)

(Imaging guidance [fluoroscopy or CT] are inclusive components of 64633-64636)

(Image guidance [fluoroscopy or CT] and any injection of contrast are inclusive components of 64633-64636. Image guidance and localization are required for the performance of paravertebral facet joint nerve destruction by neurolytic agent described by 64633-64636. If CT or fluoroscopic imaging is not used, report 64999)

Nervous

▶Report 64633, 64634, 64635, 64636 per joint, not per nerve. Although two nerves innervate each facet joint, only one code may be reported for each joint denervated, regardless of the number of nerves treated. Use 64634 or 64636 to report each additional facet joint at a different vertebral level in the same spinal region.

For neurolytic destruction of the nerves innervating the T12-L1 paravertebral facet joint, use 64633.

Do not report 64633, 64634, 64635, 64636 for non-thermal facet joint denervation including chemical, low-grade thermal energy (<80 degrees Celsius), or any form of pulsed radiofrequency. To appropriately report any of these modalities, use 64999.◀

64633 Destruction by neurolytic agent, paravertebral facet joint nerve(s), with imaging guidance (fluoroscopy or CT); cervical or thoracic, single facet joint

(For bilateral procedure, report 64633 with modifier 50)

#+ **64634** cervical or thoracic, each additional facet joint (List separately in addition to code for primary procedure)

(Use 64634 in conjunction with 64633)

(For bilateral procedure, report 64634 with modifier 50)

64635 lumbar or sacral, single facet joint

(For bilateral procedure, report 64635 with modifier 50)

#+ **64636** lumbar or sacral, each additional facet joint (List separately in addition to code for primary procedure)

(Use 64636 in conjunction with 64635)

(For bilateral procedure, report 64636 with modifier 50)

(Do not report 64633-64636 in conjunction with 77003, 77012)

▶(For destruction by neurolytic agent, individual nerves, sacroiliac joint, use 64640)◀

64630 Destruction by neurolytic agent; pudendal nerve

64632 plantar common digital nerve

(Do not report 64632 in conjunction with 64455)

64633 Code is out of numerical sequence. See 64600-64640

64634 Code is out of numerical sequence. See 64600-64640

64635 Code is out of numerical sequence. See 64600-64640

64636 Code is out of numerical sequence. See 64600-64640

64640 other peripheral nerve or branch

Report 64642, 64643, 64644, 64645 once per extremity. Codes 64642, 64643, 64644, 64645 can be reported together up to a combined total of four units of service per patient when all four extremities are injected. Report only one base code (64642 or 64644) per session. Report one unit of additional extremity code(s) (64643 or 64645) for each additional extremity injected.

Report 64646 or 64647 for chemodenervation of muscles of the trunk.

Trunk muscles include the erector spinae and paraspinal muscles, rectus abdominus and obliques. All other somatic muscles are extremity muscles, head muscles, or neck muscles.

(For chemodenervation guided by needle electromyography or muscle electrical stimulation, see 95873, 95874. Do not report more than one guidance code for each corresponding chemodenervation of extremity or trunk code)

(Do not report modifier 50 in conjunction with 64642, 64643, 64644, 64645, 64646, 64647)

64642 Chemodenervation of one extremity; 1-4 muscle(s)

+ **64643** each additional extremity, 1-4 muscle(s) (List separately in addition to code for primary procedure)

(Use 64643 in conjunction with 64642, 64644)

64644 Chemodenervation of one extremity; 5 or more muscles

+ **64645** each additional extremity, 5 or more muscles (List separately in addition to code for primary procedure)

(Use 64645 in conjunction with 64644)

64646 Chemodenervation of trunk muscle(s); 1-5 muscle(s)

64647 6 or more muscles

(Report either 64646 or 64647 only once per session)

Sympathetic Nerves

64650 Chemodenervation of eccrine glands; both axillae

64653 other area(s) (eg, scalp, face, neck), per day

(Report the specific service in conjunction with code(s) for the specific substance(s) or drug(s) provided)

(For chemodenervation of extremities (eg, hands or feet), use 64999)

(For chemodenervation of bladder, use 52287)

64680 Destruction by neurolytic agent, with or without radiologic monitoring; celiac plexus

(For transendoscopic ultrasound-guided transmural injection, neurolytic agent, celiac plexus, use 43253)

64681 superior hypogastric plexus

Neuroplasty (Exploration, Neurolysis or Nerve Decompression)

Neuroplasty is the surgical decompression or freeing of intact nerve from scar tissue, including external neurolysis and/or transposition to repair or restore the nerve.

(For percutaneous neurolysis, see 62263, 62264, 62280-62282)

(For internal neurolysis requiring use of operating microscope, use 64727)

(For facial nerve decompression, use 69720)

(For neuroplasty with nerve wrapping, see 64702-64727, 64999)

64702 Neuroplasty; digital, 1 or both, same digit

64704   nerve of hand or foot

64708 Neuroplasty, major peripheral nerve, arm or leg, open; other than specified

64712   sciatic nerve

64713   brachial plexus

64714   lumbar plexus

64716 Neuroplasty and/or transposition; cranial nerve (specify)

64718   ulnar nerve at elbow

64719   ulnar nerve at wrist

64721   median nerve at carpal tunnel

(For arthroscopic procedure, use 29848)

64722 Decompression; unspecified nerve(s) (specify)

64726   plantar digital nerve

+ 64727 Internal neurolysis, requiring use of operating microscope (List separately in addition to code for neuroplasty)

(Neuroplasty includes external neurolysis)

(Do not report code 69990 in addition to code 64727)

Transection or Avulsion

(For stereotactic lesion of gasserian ganglion, use 61790)

64732 Transection or avulsion of; supraorbital nerve

64734   infraorbital nerve

64736   mental nerve

64738   inferior alveolar nerve by osteotomy

64740   lingual nerve

64742   facial nerve, differential or complete

64744   greater occipital nerve

64746   phrenic nerve

(For section of recurrent laryngeal nerve, use 31595)

(64752 has been deleted)

64755   vagus nerves limited to proximal stomach (selective proximal vagotomy, proximal gastric vagotomy, parietal cell vagotomy, supra- or highly selective vagotomy)

(For laparoscopic approach, use 43652)

64760   vagus nerve (vagotomy), abdominal

(For laparoscopic approach, use 43651)

(64761 has been deleted)

64763 Transection or avulsion of obturator nerve, extrapelvic, with or without adductor tenotomy

(For bilateral procedure, report 64763 with modifier 50)

64766 Transection or avulsion of obturator nerve, intrapelvic, with or without adductor tenotomy

(For bilateral procedure, report 64766 with modifier 50)

64771 Transection or avulsion of other cranial nerve, extradural

64772 Transection or avulsion of other spinal nerve, extradural

(For excision of tender scar, skin and subcutaneous tissue, with or without tiny neuroma, see 11400-11446, 13100-13153)

Excision

Somatic Nerves

(For Morton neurectomy, use 28080)

64774 Excision of neuroma; cutaneous nerve, surgically identifiable

64776   digital nerve, 1 or both, same digit

+ 64778   digital nerve, each additional digit (List separately in addition to code for primary procedure)

(Use 64778 in conjunction with 64776)

64782   hand or foot, except digital nerve

+ 64783   hand or foot, each additional nerve, except same digit (List separately in addition to code for primary procedure)

(Use 64783 in conjunction with 64782)

64784   major peripheral nerve, except sciatic

64786   sciatic nerve

+ 64787 Implantation of nerve end into bone or muscle (List separately in addition to neuroma excision)

(Use 64787 in conjunction with 64774-64786)

64788 Excision of neurofibroma or neurolemmoma; cutaneous nerve

64790   major peripheral nerve

64792   extensive (including malignant type)

64795 Biopsy of nerve

Sympathetic Nerves

64802 Sympathectomy, cervical

(For bilateral procedure, report 64802 with modifier 50)

64804 Sympathectomy, cervicothoracic

(For bilateral procedure, report 64804 with modifier 50)

64809 Sympathectomy, thoracolumbar

(For bilateral procedure, report 64809 with modifier 50)

Nervous

64818 Sympathectomy, lumbar

(For bilateral procedure, report 64818 with modifier 50)

64820 Sympathectomy; digital arteries, each digit

(Do not report 69990 in addition to code 64820)

64821 radial artery

(Do not report 69990 in addition to code 64821)

64822 ulnar artery

(Do not report 69990 in addition to code 64822)

64823 superficial palmar arch

(Do not report 69990 in addition to code 64823)

Neurorrhaphy

64831 Suture of digital nerve, hand or foot; 1 nerve

+ 64832 each additional digital nerve (List separately in addition to code for primary procedure)

(Use 64832 in conjunction with 64831)

64834 Suture of 1 nerve; hand or foot, common sensory nerve

64835 median motor thenar

64836 ulnar motor

+ 64837 Suture of each additional nerve, hand or foot (List separately in addition to code for primary procedure)

(Use 64837 in conjunction with 64834-64836)

64840 Suture of posterior tibial nerve

64856 Suture of major peripheral nerve, arm or leg, except sciatic; including transposition

64857 without transposition

64858 Suture of sciatic nerve

+ 64859 Suture of each additional major peripheral nerve (List separately in addition to code for primary procedure)

(Use 64859 in conjunction with 64856, 64857)

64861 Suture of; brachial plexus

64862 lumbar plexus

64864 Suture of facial nerve; extracranial

64865 infratemporal, with or without grafting

64866 Anastomosis; facial-spinal accessory

64868 facial-hypoglossal

(64870 has been deleted)

+ 64872 Suture of nerve; requiring secondary or delayed suture (List separately in addition to code for primary neurorrhaphy)

(Use 64872 in conjunction with 64831-64865)

+ 64874 requiring extensive mobilization, or transposition of nerve (List separately in addition to code for nerve suture)

(Use 64874 in conjunction with 64831-64865)

+ 64876 requiring shortening of bone of extremity (List separately in addition to code for nerve suture)

(Use 64876 in conjunction with 64831-64865)

Neurorrhaphy With Nerve Graft, Vein Graft, or Conduit

64885 Nerve graft (includes obtaining graft), head or neck; up to 4 cm in length

64886 more than 4 cm length

64890 Nerve graft (includes obtaining graft), single strand, hand or foot; up to 4 cm length

64891 more than 4 cm length

64892 Nerve graft (includes obtaining graft), single strand, arm or leg; up to 4 cm length

64893 more than 4 cm length

64895 Nerve graft (includes obtaining graft), multiple strands (cable), hand or foot; up to 4 cm length

64896 more than 4 cm length

64897 Nerve graft (includes obtaining graft), multiple strands (cable), arm or leg; up to 4 cm length

64898 more than 4 cm length

+ 64901 Nerve graft, each additional nerve; single strand (List separately in addition to code for primary procedure)

(Use 64901 in conjunction with 64885-64893)

+ 64902 multiple strands (cable) (List separately in addition to code for primary procedure)

(Use 64902 in conjunction with 64885, 64886, 64895-64898)

64905 Nerve pedicle transfer; first stage

64907 second stage

64910 Nerve repair; with synthetic conduit or vein allograft (eg, nerve tube), each nerve

64911 with autogenous vein graft (includes harvest of vein graft), each nerve

(Do not report 69990 in addition to 64910, 64911)

Other Procedures

64999 Unlisted procedure, nervous system

Eye and Ocular Adnexa

(For diagnostic and treatment ophthalmological services, see **Medicine, Ophthalmology,** and 92002 et seq)

(Do not report code 69990 in addition to codes 65091-68850)

Eyeball

Removal of Eye

65091 Evisceration of ocular contents; without implant

65093 with implant

65101 Enucleation of eye; without implant

65103 with implant, muscles not attached to implant

65105 with implant, muscles attached to implant

(For conjunctivoplasty after enucleation, see 68320 et seq)

65110 Exenteration of orbit (does not include skin graft), removal of orbital contents; only

65112 with therapeutic removal of bone

65114 with muscle or myocutaneous flap

(For skin graft to orbit (split skin), see 15120, 15121; free, full thickness, see 15260, 15261)

(For eyelid repair involving more than skin, see 67930 et seq)

Secondary Implant(s) Procedures

An ocular implant is an implant inside muscular cone; an orbital implant is an implant outside muscular cone.

65125 Modification of ocular implant with placement or replacement of pegs (eg, drilling receptacle for prosthesis appendage) (separate procedure)

65130 Insertion of ocular implant secondary; after evisceration, in scleral shell

65135 after enucleation, muscles not attached to implant

65140 after enucleation, muscles attached to implant

65150 Reinsertion of ocular implant; with or without conjunctival graft

65155 with use of foreign material for reinforcement and/or attachment of muscles to implant

65175 Removal of ocular implant

(For orbital implant (implant outside muscle cone) insertion, use 67550; removal, use 67560)

Removal of Foreign Body

(For removal of implanted material: ocular implant, use 65175; anterior segment implant, use 65920; posterior segment implant, use 67120; orbital implant, use 67560)

(For diagnostic x-ray for foreign body, use 70030)

(For diagnostic echography for foreign body, use 76529)

(For removal of foreign body from orbit: frontal approach, use 67413; lateral approach, use 67430)

(For removal of foreign body from eyelid, embedded, use 67938)

(For removal of foreign body from lacrimal system, use 68530)

65205 Removal of foreign body, external eye; conjunctival superficial

65210 conjunctival embedded (includes concretions), subconjunctival, or scleral nonperforating

65220 corneal, without slit lamp

65222 corneal, with slit lamp

(For repair of corneal laceration with foreign body, use 65275)

65235 Removal of foreign body, intraocular; from anterior chamber of eye or lens

(For removal of implanted material from anterior segment, use 65920)

65260 from posterior segment, magnetic extraction, anterior or posterior route

65265 from posterior segment, nonmagnetic extraction

(For removal of implanted material from posterior segment, use 67120)

Repair of Laceration

(For fracture of orbit, see 21385 et seq)

(For repair of wound of eyelid, skin, linear, simple, see 12011-12018; intermediate, layered closure, see 12051-12057; linear, complex, see 13151-13160; other, see 67930, 67935)

(For repair of wound of lacrimal system, use 68700)

(For repair of operative wound, use 66250)

65270 Repair of laceration; conjunctiva, with or without nonperforating laceration sclera, direct closure

65272 conjunctiva, by mobilization and rearrangement, without hospitalization

65273 conjunctiva, by mobilization and rearrangement, with hospitalization

Eye/Ocular Adnexa

65275 cornea, nonperforating, with or without removal foreign body

65280 cornea and/or sclera, perforating, not involving uveal tissue

65285 cornea and/or sclera, perforating, with reposition or resection of uveal tissue

(65280 and 65285 are not used for repair of a surgical wound)

65286 application of tissue glue, wounds of cornea and/or sclera

(Repair of laceration includes use of conjunctival flap and restoration of anterior chamber, by air or saline injection when indicated)

(For repair of iris or ciliary body, use 66680)

65290 Repair of wound, extraocular muscle, tendon and/or Tenon's capsule

Anterior Segment

Cornea

Excision

65400 Excision of lesion, cornea (keratectomy, lamellar, partial), except pterygium

65410 Biopsy of cornea

65420 Excision or transposition of pterygium; without graft

65426 with graft

Removal or Destruction

65430 Scraping of cornea, diagnostic, for smear and/or culture

65435 Removal of corneal epithelium; with or without chemocauterization (abrasion, curettage)

►(Do not report 65435 in conjunction with 0402T)◄

65436 with application of chelating agent (eg, EDTA)

65450 Destruction of lesion of cornea by cryotherapy, photocoagulation or thermocauterization

65600 Multiple punctures of anterior cornea (eg, for corneal erosion, tattoo)

Keratoplasty

Corneal transplant includes use of fresh or preserved grafts. The preparation of donor material is included for penetrating or anterior lamellar keratoplasty, but reported separately for endothelial keratoplasty. Do not report 65710-65757 in conjunction with 92025.

(Keratoplasty excludes refractive keratoplasty procedures, 65760, 65765, and 65767)

65710 Keratoplasty (corneal transplant); anterior lamellar

65730 penetrating (except in aphakia or pseudophakia)

65750 penetrating (in aphakia)

65755 penetrating (in pseudophakia)

65756 endothelial

+ 65757 Backbench preparation of corneal endothelial allograft prior to transplantation (List separately in addition to code for primary procedure)

(Use 65757 in conjunction with 65756)

Other Procedures

Do not report 65760-65771 in conjunction with 92025.

65760 Keratomileusis

65765 Keratophakia

65767 Epikeratoplasty

65770 Keratoprosthesis

65771 Radial keratotomy

65772 Corneal relaxing incision for correction of surgically induced astigmatism

65775 Corneal wedge resection for correction of surgically induced astigmatism

(For fitting of contact lens for treatment of disease, see 92071, 92072)

(For unlisted procedures on cornea, use 66999)

65778 Placement of amniotic membrane on the ocular surface; without sutures

65779 single layer, sutured

(Do not report 65778, 65779 in conjunction with 65430, 65435, 65780)

(For placement of amniotic membrane using tissue glue, use 66999)

65780 Ocular surface reconstruction; amniotic membrane transplantation, multiple layers

(For placement of amniotic membrane without reconstruction using no sutures or single layer suture technique, see 65778, 65779)

65781 limbal stem cell allograft (eg, cadaveric or living donor)

65782 limbal conjunctival autograft (includes obtaining graft)

(For harvesting conjunctival allograft, living donor, use 68371)

● 65785 Implantation of intrastromal corneal ring segments

Anterior Chamber

Incision

65800 Paracentesis of anterior chamber of eye (separate procedure); with removal of aqueous

(65805 has been deleted. To report, use 65800)

65810   with removal of vitreous and/or discission of anterior hyaloid membrane, with or without air injection

65815   with removal of blood, with or without irrigation and/or air injection

(For injection, see 66020-66030)

(For removal of blood clot, use 65930)

65820 Goniotomy

(Do not report modifier 63 in conjunction with 65820)

(For use of ophthalmic endoscope with 65820, use 66990)

65850 Trabeculotomy ab externo

▲ **65855** Trabeculoplasty by laser surgery

►(Do not report 65855 in conjunction with 65860, 65865, 65870, 65875, 65880)◄

(For trabeculectomy, use 66170)

65860 Severing adhesions of anterior segment, laser technique (separate procedure)

65865 Severing adhesions of anterior segment of eye, incisional technique (with or without injection of air or liquid) (separate procedure); goniosynechiae

(For trabeculoplasty by laser surgery, use 65855)

65870   anterior synechiae, except goniosynechiae

65875   posterior synechiae

(For use of ophthalmic endoscope with 65875, use 66990)

65880   corneovitreal adhesions

(For laser surgery, use 66821)

Removal

65900 Removal of epithelial downgrowth, anterior chamber of eye

65920 Removal of implanted material, anterior segment of eye

(For use of ophthalmic endoscope with 65920, use 66990)

65930 Removal of blood clot, anterior segment of eye

Introduction

66020 Injection, anterior chamber of eye (separate procedure); air or liquid

66030   medication

(For unlisted procedures on anterior segment, use 66999)

Anterior Sclera

Excision

(For removal of intraocular foreign body, use 65235)

(For operations on posterior sclera, use 67250, 67255)

66130 Excision of lesion, sclera

66150 Fistulization of sclera for glaucoma; trephination with iridectomy

66155   thermocauterization with iridectomy

66160   sclerectomy with punch or scissors, with iridectomy

(66165 has been deleted)

66170   trabeculectomy ab externo in absence of previous surgery

(For trabeculotomy ab externo, use 65850)

(For repair of operative wound, use 66250)

66172   trabeculectomy ab externo with scarring from previous ocular surgery or trauma (includes injection of antifibrotic agents)

66174 Transluminal dilation of aqueous outflow canal; without retention of device or stent

66175   with retention of device or stent

Aqueous Shunt

66179 Aqueous shunt to extraocular equatorial plate reservoir, external approach; without graft

66180   with graft

(Do not report 66180 in conjunction with 67255)

66183 Insertion of anterior segment aqueous drainage device, without extraocular reservoir, external approach

66184 Revision of aqueous shunt to extraocular equatorial plate reservoir; without graft

66185   with graft

(Do not report 66185 in conjunction with 67255)

(For removal of implanted shunt, use 67120)

Repair or Revision

(For scleral procedures in retinal surgery, see 67101 et seq)

66220 Repair of scleral staphyloma; without graft

66225   with graft

(For scleral reinforcement, see 67250, 67255)

66250 Revision or repair of operative wound of anterior segment, any type, early or late, major or minor procedure

(For unlisted procedures on anterior sclera, use 66999)

Eye/Ocular Adnexa

Iris, Ciliary Body

Incision

66500 Iridotomy by stab incision (separate procedure); except transfixion

66505 with transfixion as for iris bombe

(For iridotomy by photocoagulation, use 66761)

Excision

66600 Iridectomy, with corneoscleral or corneal section; for removal of lesion

66605 with cyclectomy

66625 peripheral for glaucoma (separate procedure)

66630 sector for glaucoma (separate procedure)

66635 optical (separate procedure)

(For coreoplasty by photocoagulation, use 66762)

Repair

66680 Repair of iris, ciliary body (as for iridodialysis)

(For reposition or resection of uveal tissue with perforating wound of cornea or sclera, use 65285)

66682 Suture of iris, ciliary body (separate procedure) with retrieval of suture through small incision (eg, McCannel suture)

Destruction

66700 Ciliary body destruction; diathermy

66710 cyclophotocoagulation, transscleral

66711 cyclophotocoagulation, endoscopic

(Do not report 66711 in conjunction with 66990)

⊙ **66720** cryotherapy

66740 cyclodialysis

66761 Iridotomy/iridectomy by laser surgery (eg, for glaucoma) (per session)

66762 Iridoplasty by photocoagulation (1 or more sessions) (eg, for improvement of vision, for widening of anterior chamber angle)

66770 Destruction of cyst or lesion iris or ciliary body (nonexcisional procedure)

(For excision lesion iris, ciliary body, see 66600, 66605; for removal of epithelial downgrowth, use 65900)

(For unlisted procedures on iris, ciliary body, use 66999)

Lens

Incision

66820 Discission of secondary membranous cataract (opacified posterior lens capsule and/or anterior hyaloid); stab incision technique (Ziegler or Wheeler knife)

66821 laser surgery (eg, YAG laser) (1 or more stages)

66825 Repositioning of intraocular lens prosthesis, requiring an incision (separate procedure)

Removal

Lateral canthotomy, iridectomy, iridotomy, anterior capsulotomy, posterior capsulotomy, the use of viscoelastic agents, enzymatic zonulysis, use of other pharmacologic agents, and subconjunctival or sub-tenon injections are included as part of the code for the extraction of lens.

66830 Removal of secondary membranous cataract (opacified posterior lens capsule and/or anterior hyaloid) with corneo-scleral section, with or without iridectomy (iridocapsulotomy, iridocapsulectomy)

66840 Removal of lens material; aspiration technique, 1 or more stages

66850 phacofragmentation technique (mechanical or ultrasonic) (eg, phacoemulsification), with aspiration

66852 pars plana approach, with or without vitrectomy

66920 intracapsular

66930 intracapsular, for dislocated lens

66940 extracapsular (other than 66840, 66850, 66852)

(For removal of intralenticular foreign body without lens extraction, use 65235)

(For repair of operative wound, use 66250)

Intraocular Lens Procedures

66982 Extracapsular cataract removal with insertion of intraocular lens prosthesis (1-stage procedure), manual or mechanical technique (eg, irrigation and aspiration or phacoemulsification), complex, requiring devices or techniques not generally used in routine cataract surgery (eg, iris expansion device, suture support for intraocular lens, or primary posterior capsulorrhexis) or performed on patients in the amblyogenic developmental stage

(For insertion of ocular telescope prosthesis including removal of crystalline lens, use 0308T)

66983 Intracapsular cataract extraction with insertion of intraocular lens prosthesis (1 stage procedure)

(Do not report 66983 in conjunction with 0308T)

⊙=Moderate sedation ✚=Add-on code ⊬=FDA approval pending #=Resequenced code ○=Recycled/reinstated code

66984 Extracapsular cataract removal with insertion of intraocular lens prosthesis (1 stage procedure), manual or mechanical technique (eg, irrigation and aspiration or phacoemulsification)

(For complex extracapsular cataract removal, use 66982)

(For insertion of ocular telescope prosthesis including removal of crystalline lens, use 0308T)

66985 Insertion of intraocular lens prosthesis (secondary implant), not associated with concurrent cataract removal

(To code implant at time of concurrent cataract surgery, see 66982, 66983, 66984)

(To report supply of intraocular lens prosthesis, use 99070)

(For ultrasonic determination of intraocular lens power, use 76519)

(For removal of implanted material from anterior segment, use 65920)

(For secondary fixation (separate procedure), use 66682)

(For use of ophthalmic endoscope with 66985, use 66990)

66986 Exchange of intraocular lens

(For use of ophthalmic endoscope with 66986, use 66990)

Other Procedures

+ 66990 Use of ophthalmic endoscope (List separately in addition to code for primary procedure)

▶(66990 may be used only with codes 65820, 65875, 65920, 66985, 66986, 67036, 67039, 67040, 67041, 67042, 67043, 67113)◀

66999 Unlisted procedure, anterior segment of eye

Posterior Segment

Vitreous

67005 Removal of vitreous, anterior approach (open sky technique or limbal incision); partial removal

67010   subtotal removal with mechanical vitrectomy

(For removal of vitreous by paracentesis of anterior chamber, use 65810)

(For removal of corneovitreal adhesions, use 65880)

67015 Aspiration or release of vitreous, subretinal or choroidal fluid, pars plana approach (posterior sclerotomy)

67025 Injection of vitreous substitute, pars plana or limbal approach (fluid-gas exchange), with or without aspiration (separate procedure)

67027 Implantation of intravitreal drug delivery system (eg, ganciclovir implant), includes concomitant removal of vitreous

(For removal, use 67121)

67028 Intravitreal injection of a pharmacologic agent (separate procedure)

67030 Discission of vitreous strands (without removal), pars plana approach

67031 Severing of vitreous strands, vitreous face adhesions, sheets, membranes or opacities, laser surgery (1 or more stages)

67036 Vitrectomy, mechanical, pars plana approach;

(For application of intraocular epiretinal radiation with 67036, use 0190T)

67039   with focal endolaser photocoagulation

67040   with endolaser panretinal photocoagulation

67041   with removal of preretinal cellular membrane (eg, macular pucker)

67042   with removal of internal limiting membrane of retina (eg, for repair of macular hole, diabetic macular edema), includes, if performed, intraocular tamponade (ie, air, gas or silicone oil)

67043   with removal of subretinal membrane (eg, choroidal neovascularization), includes, if performed, intraocular tamponade (ie, air, gas or silicone oil) and laser photocoagulation

(For use of ophthalmic endoscope with 67036, 67039, 67040-67043, use 66990)

(For associated lensectomy, use 66850)

(For use of vitrectomy in retinal detachment surgery, see 67108, 67113)

(For associated removal of foreign body, see 65260, 65265)

(For unlisted procedures on vitreous, use 67299)

Retina or Choroid

Repair

(If diathermy, cryotherapy and/or photocoagulation are combined, report under principal modality used)

▲ **67101** Repair of retinal detachment, 1 or more sessions; cryotherapy or diathermy, including drainage of subretinal fluid, when performed

▲ **67105**   photocoagulation, including drainage of subretinal fluid, when performed

▲ **67107** Repair of retinal detachment; scleral buckling (such as lamellar scleral dissection, imbrication or encircling procedure), including, when performed, implant, cryotherapy, photocoagulation, and drainage of subretinal fluid

▲ **67108**   with vitrectomy, any method, including, when performed, air or gas tamponade, focal endolaser photocoagulation, cryotherapy, drainage of subretinal fluid, scleral buckling, and/or removal of lens by same technique

Eye/Ocular Adnexa

67110   by injection of air or other gas (eg, pneumatic retinopexy)

▶(67112 has been deleted. To report, see 67107, 67108, 67110, 67113)◀

(For aspiration or drainage of subretinal or subchoroidal fluid, use 67015)

▲ **67113**   Repair of complex retinal detachment (eg, proliferative vitreoretinopathy, stage C-1 or greater, diabetic traction retinal detachment, retinopathy of prematurity, retinal tear of greater than 90 degrees), with vitrectomy and membrane peeling, including, when performed, air, gas, or silicone oil tamponade, cryotherapy, endolaser photocoagulation, drainage of subretinal fluid, scleral buckling, and/or removal of lens

(To report vitrectomy, pars plana approach, other than in retinal detachment surgery, see 67036-67043)

(For use of ophthalmic endoscope with 67113, use 66990)

67115   Release of encircling material (posterior segment)

67120   Removal of implanted material, posterior segment; extraocular

67121   intraocular

(For removal from anterior segment, use 65920)

(For removal of foreign body, see 65260, 65265)

Prophylaxis

Codes 67141, 67145 include treatment at one or more sessions that may occur at different encounters. These codes should be reported once during a defined treatment period.

Repetitive services. The services listed below are often performed in multiple sessions or groups of sessions. The methods of reporting vary.

The following descriptors are intended to include all sessions in a defined treatment period.

67141   Prophylaxis of retinal detachment (eg, retinal break, lattice degeneration) without drainage, 1 or more sessions; cryotherapy, diathermy

67145   photocoagulation (laser or xenon arc)

Destruction

▶Codes 67208, 67210, 67218, 67220, 67229 include treatment at one or more sessions that may occur at different encounters. These codes should be reported once during a defined treatment period.◀

67208   Destruction of localized lesion of retina (eg, macular edema, tumors), 1 or more sessions; cryotherapy, diathermy

67210   photocoagulation

67218   radiation by implantation of source (includes removal of source)

67220   Destruction of localized lesion of choroid (eg, choroidal neovascularization); photocoagulation (eg, laser), 1 or more sessions

67221   photodynamic therapy (includes intravenous infusion)

+ **67225**   photodynamic therapy, second eye, at single session (List separately in addition to code for primary eye treatment)

(Use 67225 in conjunction with 67221)

▲ **67227**   Destruction of extensive or progressive retinopathy (eg, diabetic retinopathy), cryotherapy, diathermy

▲ **67228**   Treatment of extensive or progressive retinopathy (eg, diabetic retinopathy), photocoagulation

67229   Treatment of extensive or progressive retinopathy, 1 or more sessions, preterm infant (less than 37 weeks gestation at birth), performed from birth up to 1 year of age (eg, retinopathy of prematurity), photocoagulation or cryotherapy

▶(For bilateral procedure, use modifier 50 with 67208, 67210, 67218, 67220, 67227, 67228, 67229)◀

(For unlisted procedures on retina, use 67299)

Posterior Sclera

Repair

(For excision lesion sclera, use 66130)

67250   Scleral reinforcement (separate procedure); without graft

67255   with graft

(Do not report 67255 in conjunction with 66180, 66185)

(For repair scleral staphyloma, see 66220, 66225)

Other Procedures

67299   Unlisted procedure, posterior segment

Ocular Adnexa

Extraocular Muscles

67311   Strabismus surgery, recession or resection procedure; 1 horizontal muscle

67312   2 horizontal muscles

67314   1 vertical muscle (excluding superior oblique)

67316   2 or more vertical muscles (excluding superior oblique)

(For adjustable sutures, use 67335 in addition to codes 67311-67334 for primary procedure reflecting number of muscles operated on)

67318   Strabismus surgery, any procedure, superior oblique muscle

Eye/Ocular Adnexa

+ 67320 Transposition procedure (eg, for paretic extraocular muscle), any extraocular muscle (specify) (List separately in addition to code for primary procedure)

(Use 67320 in conjunction with 67311-67318)

+ 67331 Strabismus surgery on patient with previous eye surgery or injury that did not involve the extraocular muscles (List separately in addition to code for primary procedure)

(Use 67331 in conjunction with 67311-67318)

+ 67332 Strabismus surgery on patient with scarring of extraocular muscles (eg, prior ocular injury, strabismus or retinal detachment surgery) or restrictive myopathy (eg, dysthyroid ophthalmopathy) (List separately in addition to code for primary procedure)

(Use 67332 in conjunction with 67311-67318)

+ 67334 Strabismus surgery by posterior fixation suture technique, with or without muscle recession (List separately in addition to code for primary procedure)

(Use 67334 in conjunction with 67311-67318)

+ 67335 Placement of adjustable suture(s) during strabismus surgery, including postoperative adjustment(s) of suture(s) (List separately in addition to code for specific strabismus surgery)

(Use 67335 in conjunction with 67311-67334)

+ 67340 Strabismus surgery involving exploration and/or repair of detached extraocular muscle(s) (List separately in addition to code for primary procedure)

(Use 67340 in conjunction with 67311-67334)

67343 Release of extensive scar tissue without detaching extraocular muscle (separate procedure)

(Use 67343 in conjunction with 67311-67340, when such procedures are performed other than on the affected muscle)

67345 Chemodenervation of extraocular muscle

(For chemodenervation for blepharospasm and other neurological disorders, see 64612 and 64616)

67346 Biopsy of extraocular muscle

(For repair of wound, extraocular muscle, tendon or Tenon's capsule, use 65290)

Other Procedures

67399 Unlisted procedure, extraocular muscle

Orbit

Exploration, Excision, Decompression

67400 Orbitotomy without bone flap (frontal or transconjunctival approach); for exploration, with or without biopsy

67405 with drainage only

67412 with removal of lesion

67413 with removal of foreign body

67414 with removal of bone for decompression

67415 Fine needle aspiration of orbital contents

(For exenteration, enucleation, and repair, see 65101 et seq; for optic nerve decompression, use 67570)

67420 Orbitotomy with bone flap or window, lateral approach (eg, Kroenlein); with removal of lesion

67430 with removal of foreign body

67440 with drainage

67445 with removal of bone for decompression

(For optic nerve sheath decompression, use 67570)

67450 for exploration, with or without biopsy

(For orbitotomy, transcranial approach, see 61330, 61332, 61333)

(For orbital implant, see 67550, 67560)

(For removal of eyeball or for repair after removal, see 65091-65175)

Other Procedures

67500 Retrobulbar injection; medication (separate procedure, does not include supply of medication)

67505 alcohol

67515 Injection of medication or other substance into Tenon's capsule

(For subconjunctival injection, use 68200)

67550 Orbital implant (implant outside muscle cone); insertion

67560 removal or revision

(For ocular implant (implant inside muscle cone), see 65093-65105, 65130-65175)

(For treatment of fractures of malar area, orbit, see 21355 et seq)

67570 Optic nerve decompression (eg, incision or fenestration of optic nerve sheath)

67599 Unlisted procedure, orbit

Eyelids

Incision

67700 Blepharotomy, drainage of abscess, eyelid

67710 Severing of tarsorrhaphy

67715 Canthotomy (separate procedure)

(For canthoplasty, use 67950)

(For division of symblepharon, use 68340)

67810 Incisional biopsy of eyelid skin including lid margin

(For biopsy of skin of the eyelid, see 11100, 11101, 11310-11313)

Excision, Destruction

Codes for removal of lesion include more than skin (ie, involving lid margin, tarsus, and/or palpebral conjunctiva).

(For removal of lesion, involving mainly skin of eyelid, see 11310-11313; 11440-11446; 11640-11646; 17000-17004)

(For repair of wounds, blepharoplasty, grafts, reconstructive surgery, see 67930-67975)

67800 Excision of chalazion; single

67801 multiple, same lid

67805 multiple, different lids

67808 under general anesthesia and/or requiring hospitalization, single or multiple

67810 Code is out of numerical sequence. See 67700-67810

67820 Correction of trichiasis; epilation, by forceps only

67825 epilation by other than forceps (eg, by electrosurgery, cryotherapy, laser surgery)

67830 incision of lid margin

67835 incision of lid margin, with free mucous membrane graft

67840 Excision of lesion of eyelid (except chalazion) without closure or with simple direct closure

(For excision and repair of eyelid by reconstructive surgery, see 67961, 67966)

67850 Destruction of lesion of lid margin (up to 1 cm)

(For Mohs micrographic surgery, see 17311-17315)

(For initiation or follow-up care of topical chemotherapy (eg, 5-FU or similar agents), see appropriate office visits)

Tarsorrhaphy

67875 Temporary closure of eyelids by suture (eg, Frost suture)

67880 Construction of intermarginal adhesions, median tarsorrhaphy, or canthorrhaphy;

67882 with transposition of tarsal plate

(For severing of tarsorrhaphy, use 67710)

(For canthoplasty, reconstruction canthus, use 67950)

(For canthotomy, use 67715)

Repair (Brow Ptosis, Blepharoptosis, Lid Retraction, Ectropion, Entropion)

67900 Repair of brow ptosis (supraciliary, mid-forehead or coronal approach)

(For forehead rhytidectomy, use 15824)

67901 Repair of blepharoptosis; frontalis muscle technique with suture or other material (eg, banked fascia)

67902 frontalis muscle technique with autologous fascial sling (includes obtaining fascia)

67903 (tarso) levator resection or advancement, internal approach

67904 (tarso) levator resection or advancement, external approach

67906 superior rectus technique with fascial sling (includes obtaining fascia)

67908 conjunctivo-tarso-Muller's muscle-levator resection (eg, Fasanella-Servat type)

67909 Reduction of overcorrection of ptosis

67911 Correction of lid retraction

(For obtaining autogenous graft materials, see 20920, 20922 or 20926)

(For correction of trichiasis by mucous membrane graft, use 67835)

67912 Correction of lagophthalmos, with implantation of upper eyelid lid load (eg, gold weight)

67914 Repair of ectropion; suture

67915 thermocauterization

67916 excision tarsal wedge

67917 extensive (eg, tarsal strip operations)

(For correction of everted punctum, use 68705)

67921 Repair of entropion; suture

67922 thermocauterization

67923 excision tarsal wedge

67924 extensive (eg, tarsal strip or capsulopalpebral fascia repairs operation)

(For repair of cicatricial ectropion or entropion requiring scar excision or skin graft, see also 67961 et seq)

Reconstruction

Codes for blepharoplasty involve more than skin (ie, involving lid margin, tarsus, and/or palpebral conjunctiva).

67930 Suture of recent wound, eyelid, involving lid margin, tarsus, and/or palpebral conjunctiva direct closure; partial thickness

67935   full thickness

67938   Removal of embedded foreign body, eyelid

(For repair of skin of eyelid, see 12011-12018, 12051-12057, 13151-13153)

(For tarsorrhaphy, canthorrhaphy, see 67880, 67882)

(For repair of blepharoptosis and lid retraction, see 67901-67911)

(For blepharoplasty for entropion, ectropion, see 67916, 67917, 67923, 67924)

(For correction of blepharochalasis (blepharorhytidectomy), see 15820-15823)

(For repair of skin of eyelid, adjacent tissue transfer, see 14060, 14061; preparation for graft, use 15004; free graft, see 15120, 15121, 15260, 15261)

(For excision of lesion of eyelid, use 67800 et seq)

(For repair of lacrimal canaliculi, use 68700)

67950   Canthoplasty (reconstruction of canthus)

67961   Excision and repair of eyelid, involving lid margin, tarsus, conjunctiva, canthus, or full thickness, may include preparation for skin graft or pedicle flap with adjacent tissue transfer or rearrangement; up to one-fourth of lid margin

67966   over one-fourth of lid margin

(For canthoplasty, use 67950)

(For free skin grafts, see 15120, 15121, 15260, 15261)

(For tubed pedicle flap preparation, use 15576; for delay, use 15630; for attachment, use 15650)

67971   Reconstruction of eyelid, full thickness by transfer of tarsoconjunctival flap from opposing eyelid; up to two-thirds of eyelid, 1 stage or first stage

67973   total eyelid, lower, 1 stage or first stage

67974   total eyelid, upper, 1 stage or first stage

67975   second stage

Other Procedures

67999   Unlisted procedure, eyelids

Conjunctiva

(For removal of foreign body, see 65205 et seq)

Incision and Drainage

68020   Incision of conjunctiva, drainage of cyst

68040   Expression of conjunctival follicles (eg, for trachoma)

(To report automated evacuation of Meibomian glands, use 0207T)

Excision and/or Destruction

68100   Biopsy of conjunctiva

68110   Excision of lesion, conjunctiva; up to 1 cm

68115   over 1 cm

68130   with adjacent sclera

68135   Destruction of lesion, conjunctiva

Injection

(For injection into Tenon's capsule or retrobulbar injection, see 67500-67515)

68200   Subconjunctival injection

Conjunctivoplasty

(For wound repair, see 65270-65273)

68320   Conjunctivoplasty; with conjunctival graft or extensive rearrangement

68325   with buccal mucous membrane graft (includes obtaining graft)

68326   Conjunctivoplasty, reconstruction cul-de-sac; with conjunctival graft or extensive rearrangement

68328   with buccal mucous membrane graft (includes obtaining graft)

68330   Repair of symblepharon; conjunctivoplasty, without graft

68335   with free graft conjunctiva or buccal mucous membrane (includes obtaining graft)

68340   division of symblepharon, with or without insertion of conformer or contact lens

Other Procedures

68360   Conjunctival flap; bridge or partial (separate procedure)

68362   total (such as Gunderson thin flap or purse string flap)

(For conjunctival flap for perforating injury, see 65280, 65285)

(For repair of operative wound, use 66250)

(For removal of conjunctival foreign body, see 65205, 65210)

68371   Harvesting conjunctival allograft, living donor

68399   Unlisted procedure, conjunctiva

Lacrimal System

Incision

68400   Incision, drainage of lacrimal gland

68420   Incision, drainage of lacrimal sac (dacryocystotomy or dacryocystostomy)

Eye/Ocular Adnexa

68440 Snip incision of lacrimal punctum

Excision

68500 Excision of lacrimal gland (dacryoadenectomy), except for tumor; total

68505   partial

68510 Biopsy of lacrimal gland

68520 Excision of lacrimal sac (dacryocystectomy)

68525 Biopsy of lacrimal sac

68530 Removal of foreign body or dacryolith, lacrimal passages

68540 Excision of lacrimal gland tumor; frontal approach

68550   involving osteotomy

Repair

68700 Plastic repair of canaliculi

68705 Correction of everted punctum, cautery

68720 Dacryocystorhinostomy (fistulization of lacrimal sac to nasal cavity)

68745 Conjunctivorhinostomy (fistulization of conjunctiva to nasal cavity); without tube

68750   with insertion of tube or stent

68760 Closure of the lacrimal punctum; by thermocauterization, ligation, or laser surgery

68761   by plug, each

(For insertion and removal of drug-eluting implant into lacrimal canaliculus for intra-ocular pressure, use 0356T)

68770 Closure of lacrimal fistula (separate procedure)

Probing and/or Related Procedures

68801 Dilation of lacrimal punctum, with or without irrigation

(To report a bilateral procedure, use 68801 with modifier 50)

68810 Probing of nasolacrimal duct, with or without irrigation;

(For bilateral procedure, report 68810 with modifier 50)

68811   requiring general anesthesia

(For bilateral procedure, report 68811 with modifier 50)

68815   with insertion of tube or stent

(See also 92018)

(For bilateral procedure, report 68815 with modifier 50)

(For insertion and removal of drug-eluting implant into lacrimal canaliculus for intra-ocular pressure, use 0356T)

68816   with transluminal balloon catheter dilation

(Do not report 68816 in conjunction with 68810, 68811, 68815)

(For bilateral procedure, report 68816 with modifier 50)

68840 Probing of lacrimal canaliculi, with or without irrigation

68850 Injection of contrast medium for dacryocystography

(For radiological supervision and interpretation, see 70170, 78660)

Other Procedures

68899 Unlisted procedure, lacrimal system

Auditory System

(For diagnostic services (eg, audiometry, vestibular tests), see 92502 et seq)

External Ear

Incision

69000   Drainage external ear, abscess or hematoma; simple

69005   complicated

69020   Drainage external auditory canal, abscess

69090   Ear piercing

Excision

69100   Biopsy external ear

69105   Biopsy external auditory canal

69110   Excision external ear; partial, simple repair

69120   complete amputation

(For reconstruction of ear, see 15120 et seq)

69140   Excision exostosis(es), external auditory canal

69145   Excision soft tissue lesion, external auditory canal

69150   Radical excision external auditory canal lesion; without neck dissection

69155   with neck dissection

(For resection of temporal bone, use 69535)

(For skin grafting, see 15004-15261)

Removal

69200   Removal foreign body from external auditory canal; without general anesthesia

69205   with general anesthesia

● **69209**   Removal impacted cerumen using irrigation/lavage, unilateral

►(Do not report 69209 in conjunction with 69210 when performed on the same ear)◄

►(For bilateral procedure, report 69209 with modifier 50)◄

►(For removal of impacted cerumen requiring instrumentation, use 69210)◄

►(For cerumen removal that is not impacted, see E/M service code, which may include new or established patient office or other outpatient services [99201-99215], hospital observation services [99217-99220, 99224-99226], hospital care [99221-99223, 99231-99233], consultations [99241-99255], emergency department services [99281-99285], nursing facility services [99304-99318], domiciliary, rest home, or custodial care services [99324-99337], home services [99341-99350])◄

69210   Removal impacted cerumen requiring instrumentation, unilateral

►(Do not report 69210 in conjunction with 69209 when performed on the same ear)◄

(For bilateral procedure, report 69210 with modifier 50)

►(For removal of impacted cerumen achieved with irrigation and/or lavage but without instrumentation, use 69209)◄

►(For cerumen removal that is not impacted, see E/M service code, which may include new or established patient office or other outpatient services [99201-99215], hospital observation services [99217-99220, 99224-99226], hospital care [99221-99223, 99231-99233], consultations [99241-99255], emergency department services [99281-99285], nursing facility services [99304-99318], domiciliary, rest home, or custodial care services [99324-99337], home services [99341-99350])◄

69220   Debridement, mastoidectomy cavity, simple (eg, routine cleaning)

(For bilateral procedure, report 69220 with modifier 50)

69222   Debridement, mastoidectomy cavity, complex (eg, with anesthesia or more than routine cleaning)

(For bilateral procedure, report 69222 with modifier 50)

Repair

(For suture of wound or injury of external ear, see 12011-14302)

⊙ **69300**   Otoplasty, protruding ear, with or without size reduction

(For bilateral procedure, report 69300 with modifier 50)

69310   Reconstruction of external auditory canal (meatoplasty) (eg, for stenosis due to injury, infection) (separate procedure)

69320   Reconstruction external auditory canal for congenital atresia, single stage

(For combination with middle ear reconstruction, see 69631, 69641)

(For other reconstructive procedures with grafts (eg, skin, cartilage, bone), see 13151-15760, 21230-21235)

Other Procedures

(For otoscopy under general anesthesia, use 92502)

69399   Unlisted procedure, external ear

Auditory

Middle Ear

Introduction

(69400 has been deleted. To report, use 69799)

(69401 has been deleted. To report, see the appropriate Evaluation and Management code 99201, 99202, 99203, 99204, 99205, 99211, 99212, 99213, 99214, 99215)

(69405 has been deleted. To report, use 69799)

Incision

69420 Myringotomy including aspiration and/or eustachian tube inflation

69421 Myringotomy including aspiration and/or eustachian tube inflation requiring general anesthesia

69424 Ventilating tube removal requiring general anesthesia

(For bilateral procedure, report 69424 with modifier 50)

(Do not report code 69424 in conjunction with 69205, 69210, 69420, 69421, 69433-69676, 69710-69745, 69801-69930)

69433 Tympanostomy (requiring insertion of ventilating tube), local or topical anesthesia

(For bilateral procedure, report 69433 with modifier 50)

69436 Tympanostomy (requiring insertion of ventilating tube), general anesthesia

(For bilateral procedure, report 69436 with modifier 50)

69440 Middle ear exploration through postauricular or ear canal incision

(For atticotomy, see 69601 et seq)

69450 Tympanolysis, transcanal

Excision

69501 Transmastoid antrotomy (simple mastoidectomy)

69502 Mastoidectomy; complete

69505 modified radical

69511 radical

(For skin graft, see 15004 et seq)

(For mastoidectomy cavity debridement, see 69220, 69222)

69530 Petrous apicectomy including radical mastoidectomy

69535 Resection temporal bone, external approach

(For middle fossa approach, see 69950-69970)

69540 Excision aural polyp

69550 Excision aural glomus tumor; transcanal

69552 transmastoid

69554 extended (extratemporal)

Repair

69601 Revision mastoidectomy; resulting in complete mastoidectomy

69602 resulting in modified radical mastoidectomy

69603 resulting in radical mastoidectomy

69604 resulting in tympanoplasty

(For planned secondary tympanoplasty after mastoidectomy, see 69631, 69632)

69605 with apicectomy

(For skin graft, see 15120, 15121, 15260, 15261)

69610 Tympanic membrane repair, with or without site preparation of perforation for closure, with or without patch

69620 Myringoplasty (surgery confined to drumhead and donor area)

69631 Tympanoplasty without mastoidectomy (including canalplasty, atticotomy and/or middle ear surgery), initial or revision; without ossicular chain reconstruction

69632 with ossicular chain reconstruction (eg, postfenestration)

69633 with ossicular chain reconstruction and synthetic prosthesis (eg, partial ossicular replacement prosthesis [PORP], total ossicular replacement prosthesis [TORP])

69635 Tympanoplasty with antrotomy or mastoidotomy (including canalplasty, atticotomy, middle ear surgery, and/or tympanic membrane repair); without ossicular chain reconstruction

69636 with ossicular chain reconstruction

69637 with ossicular chain reconstruction and synthetic prosthesis (eg, partial ossicular replacement prosthesis [PORP], total ossicular replacement prosthesis [TORP])

69641 Tympanoplasty with mastoidectomy (including canalplasty, middle ear surgery, tympanic membrane repair); without ossicular chain reconstruction

69642 with ossicular chain reconstruction

69643 with intact or reconstructed wall, without ossicular chain reconstruction

69644 with intact or reconstructed canal wall, with ossicular chain reconstruction

69645 radical or complete, without ossicular chain reconstruction

69646 radical or complete, with ossicular chain reconstruction

69650 Stapes mobilization

69660 Stapedectomy or stapedotomy with reestablishment of ossicular continuity, with or without use of foreign material;

Auditory

69661   with footplate drill out

69662   Revision of stapedectomy or stapedotomy

69666   Repair oval window fistula

69667   Repair round window fistula

69670   Mastoid obliteration (separate procedure)

69676   Tympanic neurectomy

(For bilateral procedure, report 69676 with modifier 50)

Other Procedures

69700   Closure postauricular fistula, mastoid (separate procedure)

69710   Implantation or replacement of electromagnetic bone conduction hearing device in temporal bone

(Replacement procedure includes removal of old device)

69711   Removal or repair of electromagnetic bone conduction hearing device in temporal bone

69714   Implantation, osseointegrated implant, temporal bone, with percutaneous attachment to external speech processor/cochlear stimulator; without mastoidectomy

69715   with mastoidectomy

69717   Replacement (including removal of existing device), osseointegrated implant, temporal bone, with percutaneous attachment to external speech processor/ cochlear stimulator; without mastoidectomy

69718   with mastoidectomy

69720   Decompression facial nerve, intratemporal; lateral to geniculate ganglion

69725   including medial to geniculate ganglion

69740   Suture facial nerve, intratemporal, with or without graft or decompression; lateral to geniculate ganglion

69745   including medial to geniculate ganglion

(For extracranial suture of facial nerve, use 64864)

69799   Unlisted procedure, middle ear

Inner Ear

Incision and/or Destruction

69801   Labyrinthotomy, with perfusion of vestibuloactive drug(s), transcanal

(Do not report 69801 more than once per day)

(Do not report 69801 in conjunction with 69420, 69421, 69433, 69436 when performed on the same ear)

(69802 has been deleted)

69805   Endolymphatic sac operation; without shunt

69806   with shunt

69820   Fenestration semicircular canal

69840   Revision fenestration operation

Excision

69905   Labyrinthectomy; transcanal

69910   with mastoidectomy

69915   Vestibular nerve section, translabyrinthine approach

(For transcranial approach, use 69950)

Introduction

69930   Cochlear device implantation, with or without mastoidectomy

Other Procedures

69949   Unlisted procedure, inner ear

Temporal Bone, Middle Fossa Approach

(For external approach, use 69535)

69950   Vestibular nerve section, transcranial approach

69955   Total facial nerve decompression and/or repair (may include graft)

69960   Decompression internal auditory canal

69970   Removal of tumor, temporal bone

Other Procedures

69979   Unlisted procedure, temporal bone, middle fossa approach

Operating Microscope

►The surgical microscope is employed when the surgical services are performed using the techniques of microsurgery. Code 69990 should be reported (without modifier 51 appended) in addition to the code for the primary procedure performed. Do not use 69990 for visualization with magnifying loupes or corrected vision. Do not report 69990 in addition to procedures where use of the operating microscope is an inclusive component (15756-15758, 15842, 19364, 19368, 20955-20962, 20969-20973, 22551, 22552, 22856-22861, 26551- 26554, 26556, 31526, 31531, 31536, 31541, 31545, 31546, 31561, 31571, 43116, 43180, 43496, 46601, 46607, 49906, 61548, 63075-63078, 64727, 64820- 64823, 65091-68850, 0184T, 0308T, 0402T).◄

+ 69990   Microsurgical techniques, requiring use of operating microscope (List separately in addition to code for primary procedure)

Auditory

Notes

⊙=Moderate sedation ✚=Add-on code ⊿=FDA approval pending #=Resequenced code ○=Recycled/reinstated code

Radiology Guidelines (Including Nuclear Medicine and Diagnostic Ultrasound)

Guidelines to direct general reporting of services are presented in the **Introduction.** Some of the commonalities are repeated here for the convenience of those referring to this section on **Radiology (Including Nuclear Medicine and Diagnostic Ultrasound).** Other definitions and items unique to Radiology are also listed.

Subject Listings

Subject listings apply when radiological services are performed by or under the responsible supervision of a physician or other qualified health care professional.

Separate Procedures

Some of the procedures or services listed in the CPT codebook that are commonly carried out as an integral component of a total service or procedure have been identified by the inclusion of the term "separate procedure." The codes designated as "separate procedure" should not be reported in addition to the code for the total procedure or service of which it is considered an integral component.

However, when a procedure or service that is designated as a "separate procedure" is carried out independently or considered to be unrelated or distinct from other procedures/services provided at that time, it may be reported by itself, or in addition to other procedures/services by appending modifier 59 to the specific "separate procedure" code to indicate that the procedure is not considered to be a component of another procedure, but is a distinct, independent procedure. This may represent a different session or patient encounter, different procedure or surgery, different site or organ system, separate incision/excision, separate lesion, separate injury, or area of injury in extensive injuries.

Unlisted Service or Procedure

A service or procedure may be provided that is not listed in this edition of the CPT codebook. When reporting such a service, the appropriate "Unlisted Procedure" code may be used to indicate the service, identifying it by "Special Report" as discussed below. The "Unlisted Procedures" and accompanying codes for **Radiology (Including Nuclear Medicine and Diagnostic Ultrasound)** are as follows:

76496	Unlisted fluoroscopic procedure (eg, diagnostic, interventional)
76497	Unlisted computed tomography procedure (eg, diagnostic, interventional)
76498	Unlisted magnetic resonance procedure (eg, diagnostic, interventional)
76499	Unlisted diagnostic radiographic procedure
76999	Unlisted ultrasound procedure (eg, diagnostic, interventional)
77299	Unlisted procedure, therapeutic radiology clinical treatment planning
77399	Unlisted procedure, medical radiation physics, dosimetry and treatment devices, and special services
77499	Unlisted procedure, therapeutic radiology treatment management
77799	Unlisted procedure, clinical brachytherapy
78099	Unlisted endocrine procedure, diagnostic nuclear medicine
78199	Unlisted hematopoietic, reticuloendothelial and lymphatic procedure, diagnostic nuclear medicine
78299	Unlisted gastrointestinal procedure, diagnostic nuclear medicine
78399	Unlisted musculoskeletal procedure, diagnostic nuclear medicine
78499	Unlisted cardiovascular procedure, diagnostic nuclear medicine
78599	Unlisted respiratory procedure, diagnostic nuclear medicine

Radiology

78699	Unlisted nervous system procedure, diagnostic nuclear medicine
78799	Unlisted genitourinary procedure, diagnostic nuclear medicine
78999	Unlisted miscellaneous procedure, diagnostic nuclear medicine
79999	Radiopharmaceutical therapy, unlisted procedure

Special Report

A service that is rarely provided, unusual, variable, or new may require a special report. Pertinent information should include an adequate definition or description of the nature, extent, and need for the procedure; and the time, effort, and equipment necessary to provide the service.

Supervision and Interpretation

Imaging may be required during the performance of certain procedures or certain imaging procedures may require surgical procedures to access the imaged area. Many services include image guidance, which is not separately reportable and is so stated in the descriptor or guidelines. When imaging is not included in a surgical procedure or procedure from the **Medicine** section, image guidance codes or codes labeled "radiological supervision and interpretation" may be reported for the portion of the service that requires imaging. Both services require image documentation and radiological supervision, interpretation, and report services require a separate interpretation.

(The Radiological Supervision and Interpretation codes are not applicable to the Radiation Oncology subsection.)

Administration of Contrast Material(s)

The phrase "with contrast" used in the codes for procedures performed using contrast for imaging enhancement represents contrast material administered intravascularly, intra-articularly, or intrathecally.

For intra-articular injection, use the appropriate joint injection code. If radiographic arthrography is performed, also use the arthrography supervision and interpretation code for the appropriate joint (which includes fluoroscopy). If computed tomography (CT) or magnetic resonance (MR) arthrography are performed without radiographic arthrography, use the appropriate joint injection code, the appropriate CT or MR code ("with contrast" or "without followed by contrast"), and the appropriate imaging guidance code for needle placement for contrast injection.

For spine examinations using computed tomography, magnetic resonance imaging, magnetic resonance angiography, "with contrast" includes intrathecal or intravascular injection. For intrathecal injection, use also 61055 or 62284.

Injection of intravascular contrast material is part of the "with contrast" CT, computed tomographic angiography (CTA), magnetic resonance imaging (MRI), and magnetic resonance angiography (MRA) procedures.

Oral and/or rectal contrast administration alone does not qualify as a study "with contrast."

Written Report(s)

►A written report (eg, handwritten or electronic) signed by the interpreting individual should be considered an integral part of a radiologic procedure or interpretation.

With regard to CPT descriptors for radiography services, "images" refer to those acquired in either an analog (ie, film) or digital (ie, electronic) manner.◄

Radiology

Radiology

Diagnostic Radiology (Diagnostic Imaging)

Head and Neck

70010   Myelography, posterior fossa, radiological supervision and interpretation

70015   Cisternography, positive contrast, radiological supervision and interpretation

70030   Radiologic examination, eye, for detection of foreign body

70100   Radiologic examination, mandible; partial, less than 4 views

70110   complete, minimum of 4 views

70120   Radiologic examination, mastoids; less than 3 views per side

70130   complete, minimum of 3 views per side

70134   Radiologic examination, internal auditory meati, complete

70140   Radiologic examination, facial bones; less than 3 views

70150   complete, minimum of 3 views

70160   Radiologic examination, nasal bones, complete, minimum of 3 views

70170   Dacryocystography, nasolacrimal duct, radiological supervision and interpretation

70190   Radiologic examination; optic foramina

70200   orbits, complete, minimum of 4 views

70210   Radiologic examination, sinuses, paranasal, less than 3 views

70220   Radiologic examination, sinuses, paranasal, complete, minimum of 3 views

70240   Radiologic examination, sella turcica

70250   Radiologic examination, skull; less than 4 views

70260   complete, minimum of 4 views

70300   Radiologic examination, teeth; single view

70310   partial examination, less than full mouth

70320   complete, full mouth

70328   Radiologic examination, temporomandibular joint, open and closed mouth; unilateral

70330   bilateral

70332   Temporomandibular joint arthrography, radiological supervision and interpretation

     (Do not report 70332 in conjunction with 77002)

70336   Magnetic resonance (eg, proton) imaging, temporomandibular joint(s)

70350   Cephalogram, orthodontic

70355   Orthopantogram (eg, panoramic x-ray)

70360   Radiologic examination; neck, soft tissue

70370   pharynx or larynx, including fluoroscopy and/or magnification technique

70371   Complex dynamic pharyngeal and speech evaluation by cine or video recording

     ▶(70373 has been deleted. For contrast laryngography, use 76499)◀

     ▶(For laryngeal computed tomography, see 70490, 70491, 70492)◀

70380   Radiologic examination, salivary gland for calculus

70390   Sialography, radiological supervision and interpretation

70450   Computed tomography, head or brain; without contrast material

70460   with contrast material(s)

70470   without contrast material, followed by contrast material(s) and further sections

     (To report 3D rendering, see 76376, 76377)

70480   Computed tomography, orbit, sella, or posterior fossa or outer, middle, or inner ear; without contrast material

70481   with contrast material(s)

70482   without contrast material, followed by contrast material(s) and further sections

     (To report 3D rendering, see 76376, 76377)

70486   Computed tomography, maxillofacial area; without contrast material

70487   with contrast material(s)

70488   without contrast material, followed by contrast material(s) and further sections

     (To report 3D rendering, see 76376, 76377)

70490   Computed tomography, soft tissue neck; without contrast material

70491   with contrast material(s)

70492   without contrast material followed by contrast material(s) and further sections

     (To report 3D rendering, see 76376, 76377)

     (For cervical spine, see 72125, 72126)

70496   Computed tomographic angiography, head, with contrast material(s), including noncontrast images, if performed, and image postprocessing

Radiology

70498 Computed tomographic angiography, neck, with contrast material(s), including noncontrast images, if performed, and image postprocessing

70540 Magnetic resonance (eg, proton) imaging, orbit, face, and/or neck; without contrast material(s)

(For head or neck magnetic resonance angiography studies, see 70544-70546, 70547-70549)

70542   with contrast material(s)

70543   without contrast material(s), followed by contrast material(s) and further sequences

(Report 70540-70543 once per imaging session)

70544 Magnetic resonance angiography, head; without contrast material(s)

70545   with contrast material(s)

70546   without contrast material(s), followed by contrast material(s) and further sequences

70547 Magnetic resonance angiography, neck; without contrast material(s)

70548   with contrast material(s)

70549   without contrast material(s), followed by contrast material(s) and further sequences

70551 Magnetic resonance (eg, proton) imaging, brain (including brain stem); without contrast material

70552   with contrast material(s)

70553   without contrast material, followed by contrast material(s) and further sequences

(For magnetic spectroscopy, use 76390)

Functional MRI involves identification and mapping of stimulation of brain function. When neurofunctional tests are administered by a technologist or other non-physician or non-psychologist, use 70554. When neurofunctional tests are entirely administered by a physician or psychologist, use 70555.

70554 Magnetic resonance imaging, brain, functional MRI; including test selection and administration of repetitive body part movement and/or visual stimulation, not requiring physician or psychologist administration

(Do not report 70554 in conjunction with 96020)

70555   requiring physician or psychologist administration of entire neurofunctional testing

(Do not report 70555 unless 96020 is performed)

(Do not report 70554, 70555 in conjunction with 70551-70553 unless a separate diagnostic MRI is performed)

70557 Magnetic resonance (eg, proton) imaging, brain (including brain stem and skull base), during open intracranial procedure (eg, to assess for residual tumor or residual vascular malformation); without contrast material

70558   with contrast material(s)

70559   without contrast material(s), followed by contrast material(s) and further sequences

(For stereotactic biopsy of intracranial lesion with magnetic resonance guidance, use 61751.70557, 70558, or 70559 may be reported only if a separate report is generated. Report only 1 of the above codes once per operative session. Do not use these codes in conjunction with 61751, 77021, 77022)

Chest

(For fluoroscopic or ultrasonic guidance for needle placement procedures (eg, biopsy, aspiration, injection, localization device) of the thorax, see 76942, 77002)

71010 Radiologic examination, chest; single view, frontal

71015   stereo, frontal

71020 Radiologic examination, chest, 2 views, frontal and lateral;

71021   with apical lordotic procedure

71022   with oblique projections

71023   with fluoroscopy

71030 Radiologic examination, chest, complete, minimum of 4 views;

(For concurrent computer-aided detection [CAD] performed in addition to codes 71010, 71020, 71021, 71022, and 71030, use 0174T. Do not report 71010, 71020, 71021, 71022, and 71030 in conjunction with 0175T for CAD performed remotely from the primary interpretation)

71034   with fluoroscopy

(For separate chest fluoroscopy, use 76000)

71035 Radiologic examination, chest, special views (eg, lateral decubitus, Bucky studies)

(71040, 71060 have been deleted. To report, use 76499)

71100 Radiologic examination, ribs, unilateral; 2 views

71101   including posteroanterior chest, minimum of 3 views

71110 Radiologic examination, ribs, bilateral; 3 views

71111   including posteroanterior chest, minimum of 4 views

71120 Radiologic examination; sternum, minimum of 2 views

71130   sternoclavicular joint or joints, minimum of 3 views

71250 Computed tomography, thorax; without contrast material

71260   with contrast material(s)

71270   without contrast material, followed by contrast material(s) and further sections

(For cardiac computed tomography of the heart, see 75571-75574)

(To report 3D rendering, see 76376, 76377)

Radiology

71275 Computed tomographic angiography, chest (noncoronary), with contrast material(s), including noncontrast images, if performed, and image postprocessing

(For coronary artery computed tomographic angiography including calcification score and/or cardiac morphology, use 75574)

71550 Magnetic resonance (eg, proton) imaging, chest (eg, for evaluation of hilar and mediastinal lymphadenopathy); without contrast material(s)

71551   with contrast material(s)

71552   without contrast material(s), followed by contrast material(s) and further sequences

(For breast MRI, see 77058, 77059)

71555 Magnetic resonance angiography, chest (excluding myocardium), with or without contrast material(s)

Spine and Pelvis

►(72010 has been deleted. To report, use 72082)◄

72020 Radiologic examination, spine, single view, specify level

►(For a single view that includes the entire thoracic and lumbar spine, use 72081)◄

72040 Radiologic examination, spine, cervical; 2 or 3 views

72050   4 or 5 views

72052   6 or more views

►(72069 has been deleted. To report, see 72081, 72082, 72083, 72084)◄

72070 Radiologic examination, spine; thoracic, 2 views

72072   thoracic, 3 views

72074   thoracic, minimum of 4 views

▲ **72080**   thoracolumbar junction, minimum of 2 views

►(For a single view examination of the thoracolumbar junction, use 72020)◄

● **72081** Radiologic examination, spine, entire thoracic and lumbar, including skull, cervical and sacral spine if performed (eg, scoliosis evaluation); one view

● **72082**   2 or 3 views

● **72083**   4 or 5 views

● **72084**   minimum of 6 views

►(72090 has been deleted. To report, see 72081, 72082, 72083, 72084)◄

72100 Radiologic examination, spine, lumbosacral; 2 or 3 views

72110   minimum of 4 views

72114   complete, including bending views, minimum of 6 views

72120   bending views only, 2 or 3 views

(Contrast material in CT of spine is either by intrathecal or intravenous injection. For intrathecal injection, use also 61055 or 62284. IV injection of contrast material is part of the CT procedure)

72125 Computed tomography, cervical spine; without contrast material

72126   with contrast material

72127   without contrast material, followed by contrast material(s) and further sections

(For intrathecal injection procedure, see 61055, 62284)

72128 Computed tomography, thoracic spine; without contrast material

72129   with contrast material

(For intrathecal injection procedure, see 61055, 62284)

72130   without contrast material, followed by contrast material(s) and further sections

(For intrathecal injection procedure, see 61055, 62284)

72131 Computed tomography, lumbar spine; without contrast material

72132   with contrast material

72133   without contrast material, followed by contrast material(s) and further sections

(For intrathecal injection procedure, see 61055, 62284)

(To report 3D rendering, see 76376, 76377)

72141 Magnetic resonance (eg, proton) imaging, spinal canal and contents, cervical; without contrast material

72142   with contrast material(s)

(For cervical spinal canal imaging without contrast material followed by contrast material, use 72156)

72146 Magnetic resonance (eg, proton) imaging, spinal canal and contents, thoracic; without contrast material

72147   with contrast material(s)

(For thoracic spinal canal imaging without contrast material followed by contrast material, use 72157)

72148 Magnetic resonance (eg, proton) imaging, spinal canal and contents, lumbar; without contrast material

72149   with contrast material(s)

(For lumbar spinal canal imaging without contrast material followed by contrast material, use 72158)

72156 Magnetic resonance (eg, proton) imaging, spinal canal and contents, without contrast material, followed by contrast material(s) and further sequences; cervical

72157   thoracic

72158   lumbar

72159 Magnetic resonance angiography, spinal canal and contents, with or without contrast material(s)

72170 Radiologic examination, pelvis; 1 or 2 views

72190 complete, minimum of 3 views

(For pelvimetry, use 74710)

(For a combined computed tomography [CT] or computed tomographic angiography abdomen and pelvis study, see 74174, 74176-74178)

72191 Computed tomographic angiography, pelvis, with contrast material(s), including noncontrast images, if performed, and image postprocessing

(Do not report 72191 in conjunction with 73706 or 75635. For CTA aorto-iliofemoral runoff, use 75635)

(Do not report 72191 in conjunction with 74175. For a combined computed tomographic angiography abdomen and pelvis study, use 74174)

72192 Computed tomography, pelvis; without contrast material

72193 with contrast material(s)

72194 without contrast material, followed by contrast material(s) and further sections

(For a combined CT abdomen and pelvis study, see 74176-74178)

(To report 3D rendering, see 76376, 76377)

(For computed tomographic colonography, diagnostic, see 74261-74262. For computed tomographic colonography, screening, use 74263)

(Do not report 72192-72194 in conjunction with 74261-74263)

72195 Magnetic resonance (eg, proton) imaging, pelvis; without contrast material(s)

72196 with contrast material(s)

72197 without contrast material(s), followed by contrast material(s) and further sequences

►(Do not report 72195, 72196, 72197 in conjunction with 74712, 74713)◄

►(For magnetic resonance imaging of a fetus[es], see 74712, 74713)◄

72198 Magnetic resonance angiography, pelvis, with or without contrast material(s)

72200 Radiologic examination, sacroiliac joints; less than 3 views

72202 3 or more views

72220 Radiologic examination, sacrum and coccyx, minimum of 2 views

72240 Myelography, cervical, radiological supervision and interpretation

(Do not report 72240 in conjunction with 62284, 62302, 62303, 62304, 62305)

(When both 62284 and 72240 are performed by the same physician or other qualified health care professional for cervical myelography, use 62302)

(For complete cervical myelography via injection procedure at C1-C2, see 61055, 72240)

72255 Myelography, thoracic, radiological supervision and interpretation

(Do not report 72255 in conjunction with 62284, 62302, 62303, 62304, 62305)

(When both 62284 and 72255 are performed by the same physician or other qualified health care professional for thoracic myelography, use 62303)

(For complete thoracic myelography via injection procedure at C1-C2, see 61055, 72255)

72265 Myelography, lumbosacral, radiological supervision and interpretation

(Do not report 72265 in conjunction with 62284, 62302, 62303, 62304, 62305)

(When both 62284 and 72265 are performed by the same physician or other qualified health care professional for lumbosacral myelography, use 62304)

(For complete lumbosacral myelography via injection procedure at C1-C2, see 61055, 72265)

72270 Myelography, 2 or more regions (eg, lumbar/thoracic, cervical/thoracic, lumbar/cervical, lumbar/thoracic/cervical), radiological supervision and interpretation

(Do not report 72270 in conjunction with 62284, 62302, 62303, 62304, 62305)

(When both 62284 and 72270 are performed by the same physician or other qualified health care professional for myelography of 2 or more regions, use 62305)

(For complete myelography of 2 or more regions via injection procedure at C1-C2, see 61055, 72270)

72275 Epidurography, radiological supervision and interpretation

(72275 includes 77003)

(For injection procedure, see 62280-62282, 62310-62319, 64479-64484)

(Use 72275 only when an epidurogram is performed, images documented, and a formal radiologic report is issued)

(Do not report 72275 in conjunction with 22586, 0195T, 0196T, 0309T)

72285 Discography, cervical or thoracic, radiological supervision and interpretation

(72291 and 72292 have been deleted. To report, see 22510, 22511, 22512, 22513, 22514, 22515, 0200T, 0201T)

72295 Discography, lumbar, radiological supervision and interpretation

Radiology

Upper Extremities

(For stress views, any joint, use 77071)

73000   Radiologic examination; clavicle, complete

73010   scapula, complete

73020   Radiologic examination, shoulder; 1 view

73030   complete, minimum of 2 views

73040   Radiologic examination, shoulder, arthrography, radiological supervision and interpretation

(Do not report 77002 in conjunction with 73040)

73050   Radiologic examination; acromioclavicular joints, bilateral, with or without weighted distraction

73060   humerus, minimum of 2 views

73070   Radiologic examination, elbow; 2 views

73080   complete, minimum of 3 views

73085   Radiologic examination, elbow, arthrography, radiological supervision and interpretation

(Do not report 77002 in conjunction with 73085)

73090   Radiologic examination; forearm, 2 views

73092   upper extremity, infant, minimum of 2 views

73100   Radiologic examination, wrist; 2 views

73110   complete, minimum of 3 views

73115   Radiologic examination, wrist, arthrography, radiological supervision and interpretation

(Do not report 77002 in conjunction with 73115)

73120   Radiologic examination, hand; 2 views

73130   minimum of 3 views

73140   Radiologic examination, finger(s), minimum of 2 views

73200   Computed tomography, upper extremity; without contrast material

73201   with contrast material(s)

73202   without contrast material, followed by contrast material(s) and further sections

(To report 3D rendering, see 76376, 76377)

73206   Computed tomographic angiography, upper extremity, with contrast material(s), including noncontrast images, if performed, and image postprocessing

73218   Magnetic resonance (eg, proton) imaging, upper extremity, other than joint; without contrast material(s)

73219   with contrast material(s)

73220   without contrast material(s), followed by contrast material(s) and further sequences

73221   Magnetic resonance (eg, proton) imaging, any joint of upper extremity; without contrast material(s)

73222   with contrast material(s)

73223   without contrast material(s), followed by contrast material(s) and further sequences

73225   Magnetic resonance angiography, upper extremity, with or without contrast material(s)

Lower Extremities

(For stress views, any joint, use 77071)

►(73500 has been deleted. To report, use 73501)◄

● **73501**   Radiologic examination, hip, unilateral, with pelvis when performed; 1 view

● **73502**   2-3 views

● **73503**   minimum of 4 views

►(73510 has been deleted. To report, see 73502, 73503)◄

►(73520 has been deleted. To report, see 73521, 73522, 73523)◄

● **73521**   Radiologic examination, hips, bilateral, with pelvis when performed; 2 views

● **73522**   3-4 views

● **73523**   minimum of 5 views

73525   Radiologic examination, hip, arthrography, radiological supervision and interpretation

(Do not report 73525 in conjunction with 77002)

►(73530, 73540 have been deleted. To report, see 73501, 73502, 73503)◄

►(73550 has been deleted. To report, see 73551, 73552)◄

● **73551**   Radiologic examination, femur; 1 view

● **73552**   minimum 2 views

73560   Radiologic examination, knee; 1 or 2 views

73562   3 views

73564   complete, 4 or more views

73565   both knees, standing, anteroposterior

73580   Radiologic examination, knee, arthrography, radiological supervision and interpretation

(Do not report 73580 in conjunction with 77002)

73590   Radiologic examination; tibia and fibula, 2 views

73592   lower extremity, infant, minimum of 2 views

73600   Radiologic examination, ankle; 2 views

73610   complete, minimum of 3 views

73615   Radiologic examination, ankle, arthrography, radiological supervision and interpretation

(Do not report 73615 in conjunction with 77002)

73620   Radiologic examination, foot; 2 views

73630   complete, minimum of 3 views

Radiology

73650 Radiologic examination; calcaneus, minimum of 2 views

73660   toe(s), minimum of 2 views

73700 Computed tomography, lower extremity; without contrast material

73701   with contrast material(s)

73702   without contrast material, followed by contrast material(s) and further sections

(To report 3D rendering, see 76376, 76377)

73706 Computed tomographic angiography, lower extremity, with contrast material(s), including noncontrast images, if performed, and image postprocessing

(For CTA aorto-iliofemoral runoff, use 75635)

73718 Magnetic resonance (eg, proton) imaging, lower extremity other than joint; without contrast material(s)

73719   with contrast material(s)

73720   without contrast material(s), followed by contrast material(s) and further sequences

73721 Magnetic resonance (eg, proton) imaging, any joint of lower extremity; without contrast material

73722   with contrast material(s)

73723   without contrast material(s), followed by contrast material(s) and further sequences

73725 Magnetic resonance angiography, lower extremity, with or without contrast material(s)

Abdomen

74000 Radiologic examination, abdomen; single anteroposterior view

74010   anteroposterior and additional oblique and cone views

74020   complete, including decubitus and/or erect views

74022   complete acute abdomen series, including supine, erect, and/or decubitus views, single view chest

74150 Computed tomography, abdomen; without contrast material

74160   with contrast material(s)

74170   without contrast material, followed by contrast material(s) and further sections

(For a combined CT abdomen and pelvis study, see 74176-74178)

(To report 3D rendering, see 76376, 76377)

(For computed tomographic colonography, diagnostic, see 74261-74262. For computed tomographic colonography, screening, use 74263)

(Do not report 74150-74170 in conjunction with 74261-74263)

74174 Computed tomographic angiography, abdomen and pelvis, with contrast material(s), including noncontrast images, if performed, and image postprocessing

(Do not report 74174 in conjunction with 72191, 73706, 74175, 75635, 76376, 76377)

(For CTA aorto-iliofemoral runoff, use 75635)

74175 Computed tomographic angiography, abdomen, with contrast material(s), including noncontrast images, if performed, and image postprocessing

(Do not report 74175 in conjunction with 73706 or 75635. For CTA aorto-iliofemoral runoff, use 75635)

(Do not report 74175 in conjunction with 72191. For a combined computed tomographic angiography abdomen and pelvis study, use 74174)

For combinations of CT of the abdomen with CT of the pelvis performed at the same session, use the following table. Do not report more than one CT of the abdomen or CT of the pelvis for any session.

Stand Alone Code	74150 CT Abdomen WO Contrast	74160 CT Abdomen W Contrast	74170 CT Abdomen WO/W Contrast
72192 CT Pelvis WO Contrast	74176	74178	74178
72193 CT Pelvis W Contrast	74178	74177	74178
72194 CT Pelvis WO/W Contrast	74178	74178	74178

74176 Computed tomography, abdomen and pelvis; without contrast material

74177   with contrast material(s)

74178   without contrast material in one or both body regions, followed by contrast material(s) and further sections in one or both body regions

(Do not report 74176-74178 in conjunction with 72192-72194, 74150-74170)

(Report 74176, 74177, or 74178 only once per CT abdomen and pelvis examination)

74181 Magnetic resonance (eg, proton) imaging, abdomen; without contrast material(s)

74182   with contrast material(s)

74183   without contrast material(s), followed by with contrast material(s) and further sequences

74185 Magnetic resonance angiography, abdomen, with or without contrast material(s)

74190 Peritoneogram (eg, after injection of air or contrast), radiological supervision and interpretation

(For procedure, use 49400)

(For computed tomography, see 72192 or 74150)

Gastrointestinal Tract

(For percutaneous placement of gastrostomy tube, use 43246)

74210   Radiologic examination; pharynx and/or cervical esophagus

74220   esophagus

74230   Swallowing function, with cineradiography/videoradiography

74235   Removal of foreign body(s), esophageal, with use of balloon catheter, radiological supervision and interpretation

(For procedure, use 43499)

▲ **74240**   Radiologic examination, gastrointestinal tract, upper; with or without delayed images, without KUB

▲ **74241**   with or without delayed images, with KUB

▲ **74245**   with small intestine, includes multiple serial images

▲ **74246**   Radiological examination, gastrointestinal tract, upper, air contrast, with specific high density barium, effervescent agent, with or without glucagon; with or without delayed images, without KUB

▲ **74247**   with or without delayed images, with KUB

74249   with small intestine follow-through

▲ **74250**   Radiologic examination, small intestine, includes multiple serial images;

▲ **74251**   via enteroclysis tube

74260   Duodenography, hypotonic

74261   Computed tomographic (CT) colonography, diagnostic, including image postprocessing; without contrast material

74262   with contrast material(s) including non-contrast images, if performed

(Do not report 74261, 74262 in conjunction with 72192-72194, 74150-74170, 74263, 76376, 76377)

74263   Computed tomographic (CT) colonography, screening, including image postprocessing

(Do not report 74263 in conjunction with 72192-72194, 74150-74170, 74261, 74262, 76376, 76377)

74270   Radiologic examination, colon; contrast (eg, barium) enema, with or without KUB

74280   air contrast with specific high density barium, with or without glucagon

74283   Therapeutic enema, contrast or air, for reduction of intussusception or other intraluminal obstruction (eg, meconium ileus)

74290   Cholecystography, oral contrast

(74291 has been deleted)

74300   Cholangiography and/or pancreatography; intraoperative, radiological supervision and interpretation

+ **74301**   additional set intraoperative, radiological supervision and interpretation (List separately in addition to code for primary procedure)

(Use 74301 in conjunction with 74300)

▶(74305 has been deleted. To report, use 47531)◀

▶(74320 has been deleted. To report, use 47532)◀

▶(74327 has been deleted. For percutaneous biliary stone extraction, use 47544)◀

74328   Endoscopic catheterization of the biliary ductal system, radiological supervision and interpretation

(For procedure, see 43260-43278 as appropriate)

74329   Endoscopic catheterization of the pancreatic ductal system, radiological supervision and interpretation

(For procedure, see 43260-43278 as appropriate)

74330   Combined endoscopic catheterization of the biliary and pancreatic ductal systems, radiological supervision and interpretation

(For procedure, see 43260-43278 as appropriate)

▲ **74340**   Introduction of long gastrointestinal tube (eg, Miller-Abbott), including multiple fluoroscopies and images, radiological supervision and interpretation

(For tube placement, use 44500)

74355   Percutaneous placement of enteroclysis tube, radiological supervision and interpretation

74360   Intraluminal dilation of strictures and/or obstructions (eg, esophagus), radiological supervision and interpretation

(Do not report 74360 in conjunction with 43213, 43214, 43233)

74363   Percutaneous transhepatic dilation of biliary duct stricture with or without placement of stent, radiological supervision and interpretation

▶(For procedure, see 47555, 47556)◀

Urinary Tract

74400   Urography (pyelography), intravenous, with or without KUB, with or without tomography

74410   Urography, infusion, drip technique and/or bolus technique;

74415   with nephrotomography

74420   Urography, retrograde, with or without KUB

74425   Urography, antegrade (pyelostogram, nephrostogram, loopogram), radiological supervision and interpretation

▶(Do not report 74425 in conjunction with 50430, 50431, 50432, 50433, 50434, 50435, 50693, 50694, 50695)◀

74430   Cystography, minimum of 3 views, radiological supervision and interpretation

74440   Vasography, vesiculography, or epididymography, radiological supervision and interpretation

Radiology

74445   Corpora cavernosography, radiological supervision and interpretation

74450   Urethrocystography, retrograde, radiological supervision and interpretation

74455   Urethrocystography, voiding, radiological supervision and interpretation

74470   Radiologic examination, renal cyst study, translumbar, contrast visualization, radiological supervision and interpretation

        ▶(74475, 74480 have been deleted. To report, see 50432, 50433, 50434, 50435, 50606, 50693, 50694, 50695)◀

74485   Dilation of nephrostomy, ureters, or urethra, radiological supervision and interpretation

        (For dilation of ureter without radiologic guidance, use 52341, 52344)

        ▶(For change of nephrostomy or pyelostomy tube, use 50435)◀

Gynecological and Obstetrical

        (For abdomen and pelvis, see 72170-72190, 74000-74170)

74710   Pelvimetry, with or without placental localization

● **74712**   Magnetic resonance (eg, proton) imaging, fetal, including placental and maternal pelvic imaging when performed; single or first gestation

+● **74713**   each additional gestation (List separately in addition to code for primary procedure)

        ▶(Use 74713 in conjunction with 74712)◀

        ▶(Do not report 74712, 74713 in conjunction with 72195, 72196, 72197)◀

        ▶(If only placenta or maternal pelvis is imaged without fetal imaging, see 72195, 72196, 72197)◀

74740   Hysterosalpingography, radiological supervision and interpretation

        (For introduction of saline or contrast for hysterosalpingography, see 58340)

74742   Transcervical catheterization of fallopian tube, radiological supervision and interpretation

        (For procedure, use 58345)

74775   Perineogram (eg, vaginogram, for sex determination or extent of anomalies)

Heart

Cardiac magnetic imaging differs from traditional magnetic resonance imaging (MRI) in its ability to provide a physiologic evaluation of cardiac function. Traditional MRI relies on static images to obtain clinical diagnoses based upon anatomic information. Improvement in spatial and temporal resolution has expanded the application from an anatomic test and includes physiologic evaluation of cardiac function. Flow and velocity assessment for valves and intracardiac shunts

is performed in addition to a function and morphologic evaluation. Use 75559 with 75565 to report flow with pharmacologic wall motion stress evaluation without contrast. Use 75563 with 75565 to report flow with pharmacologic perfusion stress with contrast.

Cardiac MRI for velocity flow mapping can be reported in conjunction with 75557, 75559, 75561, or 75563.

Listed procedures may be performed independently or in the course of overall medical care. If the individual providing these services is also responsible for diagnostic workup and/or follow-up care of the patient, also see appropriate sections. Only one procedure in the series 75557-75563 is appropriately reported per session. Only one add-on code for flow velocity can be reported per session.

Cardiac MRI studies may be performed at rest and/or during pharmacologic stress. Therefore, the appropriate stress testing code from the 93015-93018 series should be reported in addition to 75559 or 75563.

Cardiac computed tomography (CT) and coronary computed tomographic angiography (CTA) include the axial source images of the pre-contrast, arterial phase sequence, and venous phase sequence (if performed), as well as the two-dimensional and three-dimensional reformatted images resulting from the study, including cine review. Contrast enhanced cardiac CT and coronary CTA codes 75571-75574 include any quantitative assessment when performed as part of the same encounter. Report only one computed tomography heart service per encounter.

        (For separate injection procedures for vascular radiology, see **Surgery** section, 36000-36299)

        (For cardiac catheterization procedures, see 93451-93572)

        (75552-75556 have been deleted. To report, see 75557, 75559, 75561, 75563, 75565)

75557   Cardiac magnetic resonance imaging for morphology and function without contrast material;

75559   with stress imaging

75561   Cardiac magnetic resonance imaging for morphology and function without contrast material(s), followed by contrast material(s) and further sequences;

75563   with stress imaging

        (75558, 75560, 75562, 75564 have been deleted. To report flow velocity, use 75565)

+ **75565**   Cardiac magnetic resonance imaging for velocity flow mapping (List separately in addition to code for primary procedure)

        (Use 75565 in conjunction with 75557, 75559, 75561, 75563)

        (Do not report 75557, 75559, 75561, 75563, 75565 in conjunction with 76376, 76377)

Radiology

75571   Computed tomography, heart, without contrast material, with quantitative evaluation of coronary calcium

75572   Computed tomography, heart, with contrast material, for evaluation of cardiac structure and morphology (including 3D image postprocessing, assessment of cardiac function, and evaluation of venous structures, if performed)

75573   Computed tomography, heart, with contrast material, for evaluation of cardiac structure and morphology in the setting of congenital heart disease (including 3D image postprocessing, assessment of LV cardiac function, RV structure and function and evaluation of venous structures, if performed)

75574   Computed tomographic angiography, heart, coronary arteries and bypass grafts (when present), with contrast material, including 3D image postprocessing (including evaluation of cardiac structure and morphology, assessment of cardiac function, and evaluation of venous structures, if performed)

Vascular Procedures

Aorta and Arteries

Selective vascular catheterizations should be coded to include introduction and all lesser order selective catheterizations used in the approach (eg, the description for a selective right middle cerebral artery catheterization includes the introduction and placement catheterization of the right common and internal carotid arteries).

Additional second and/or third order arterial catheterizations within the same family of arteries supplied by a single first order artery should be expressed by 36218 or 36248. Additional first order or higher catheterizations in vascular families supplied by a first order vessel different from a previously selected and coded family should be separately coded using the conventions described above.

The lower extremity endovascular revascularization codes describing services performed for occlusive disease (37220-37235) include catheterization (36200, 36140, 36245-36248) in the work described by the codes. Catheterization codes are not additionally reported for diagnostic lower extremity angiography when performed through the same access site as the therapy (37220-37235) performed in the same session. However, catheterization for the diagnostic lower extremity angiogram may be reported separately if a different arterial puncture site is necessary.

For angiography performed in conjunction with therapeutic transcatheter radiological supervision and interpretation services, see the **Radiology Transcatheter Procedures** guidelines.

Diagnostic angiography (radiological supervision and interpretation) codes should NOT be used with interventional procedures for:

1. Contrast injections, angiography, roadmapping, and/or fluoroscopic guidance for the intervention,

2. Vessel measurement, and

3. Post-angioplasty/stent/atherectomy angiography, as this work is captured in the radiological supervision and interpretation code(s). In those therapeutic codes that include radiological supervision and interpretation, this work is captured in the therapeutic code.

Diagnostic angiography performed at the time of an interventional procedure is separately reportable if:

1. No prior catheter-based angiographic study is available and a full diagnostic study is performed, and the decision to intervene is based on the diagnostic study, OR

2. A prior study is available, but as documented in the medical record:

   a. The patient's condition with respect to the clinical indication has changed since the prior study, OR

   b. There is inadequate visualization of the anatomy and/or pathology, OR

   c. There is a clinical change during the procedure that requires new evaluation outside the target area of intervention.

Diagnostic angiography performed at a separate sessions from an interventional procedure is separately reported.

If diagnostic angiography is necessary, is performed at the same session as the interventional procedure and meets the above criteria, modifier 59 must be appended to the diagnostic radiological supervision and interpretation code(s) to denote that diagnostic work has been done following these guidelines.

Diagnostic angiography performed at the time of an interventional procedure is NOT separately reportable if it is specifically included in the interventional code descriptor.

> (For intravenous procedure, see 36000, 36005-36015, and for intra-arterial procedure, see 36100-36248)
>
> (For radiological supervision and interpretation, see 75600-75893)

75600   Aortography, thoracic, without serialography, radiological supervision and interpretation

> (For supravalvular aortography performed at the time of cardiac catheterization, use 93567, which includes imaging supervision, interpretation, and report)

75605   Aortography, thoracic, by serialography, radiological supervision and interpretation

> (For supravalvular aortography performed at the time of cardiac catheterization, use 93567, which includes imaging supervision, interpretation, and report)

75625   Aortography, abdominal, by serialography, radiological supervision and interpretation

Radiology

75630 Aortography, abdominal plus bilateral iliofemoral lower extremity, catheter, by serialography, radiological supervision and interpretation

75635 Computed tomographic angiography, abdominal aorta and bilateral iliofemoral lower extremity runoff, with contrast material(s), including noncontrast images, if performed, and image postprocessing

(Do not report 75635 in conjunction with 72191, 73706, 74174 or 74175)

(75650 has been deleted. To report, see 36221-36226)

75658 Angiography, brachial, retrograde, radiological supervision and interpretation

(75660 has been deleted. To report, use 36227)

(75662 has been deleted. To report, use 36227 and append modifier 50)

(75665 has been deleted. To report, see 36223, 36224)

(75671 has been deleted. To report, see 36223 and 36224 and append modifier 50 as appropriate)

(75676 has been deleted. To report, see 36222-36224)

(75680 has been deleted. To report, see 36222-36224 and append modifier 50 as appropriate)

75705 Angiography, spinal, selective, radiological supervision and interpretation

75710 Angiography, extremity, unilateral, radiological supervision and interpretation

75716 Angiography, extremity, bilateral, radiological supervision and interpretation

75726 Angiography, visceral, selective or supraselective (with or without flush aortogram), radiological supervision and interpretation

(For selective angiography, each additional visceral vessel studied after basic examination, use 75774)

75731 Angiography, adrenal, unilateral, selective, radiological supervision and interpretation

75733 Angiography, adrenal, bilateral, selective, radiological supervision and interpretation

75736 Angiography, pelvic, selective or supraselective, radiological supervision and interpretation

75741 Angiography, pulmonary, unilateral, selective, radiological supervision and interpretation

75743 Angiography, pulmonary, bilateral, selective, radiological supervision and interpretation

75746 Angiography, pulmonary, by nonselective catheter or venous injection, radiological supervision and interpretation

(For pulmonary angiography by nonselective catheter or venous injection performed at the time of cardiac catheterization, use 93568, which includes imaging supervision, interpretation, and report)

75756 Angiography, internal mammary, radiological supervision and interpretation

(For internal mammary angiography performed at the time of cardiac catheterization, see 93455, 93457, 93459, 93461, 93564, which include imaging supervision, interpretation, and report)

+ 75774 Angiography, selective, each additional vessel studied after basic examination, radiological supervision and interpretation (List separately in addition to code for primary procedure)

(Use 75774 in addition to code for specific initial vessel studied)

(Do not report 75774 as part of diagnostic angiography of the extracranial and intracranial cervicocerebral vessels. It may be appropriate to report 75774 for diagnostic angiography of upper extremities and other vascular beds performed in the same session)

(For angiography, see 36147, 75600-75756, 75791)

(For catheterizations, see codes 36215-36248)

(For cardiac catheterization procedures, see 93452-93462, 93531-93533, 93563-93568)

75791 Angiography, arteriovenous shunt (eg, dialysis patient fistula/graft), complete evaluation of dialysis access, including fluoroscopy, image documentation and report (includes injections of contrast and all necessary imaging from the arterial anastomosis and adjacent artery through entire venous outflow including the inferior or superior vena cava), radiological supervision and interpretation

(Do not report 75791 in conjunction with 36147, 36148)

(For introduction of catheter, if necessary, see 36140, 36215-36217, 36245-36247)

(Use 75791 only if radiological evaluation is performed through an already existing access into the shunt or from an access that is not a direct puncture of the shunt)

(For radiological evaluation with needle/catheter introduction, AV dialysis shunt, complete procedure, use 36147)

Veins and Lymphatics

For venography performed in conjunction with therapeutic transcatheter radiological supervision and interpretation services, see the **Radiology Transcatheter Procedures** guidelines.

Diagnostic venography (radiological supervision and interpretation) codes should NOT be used with interventional procedures for:

1. Contrast injections, venography, roadmapping, and/or fluoroscopic guidance for the intervention,

2. Vessel measurement, and

3. Post-angioplasty/stent venography, as this work is captured in the radiological supervision and intrepetation code(s).

Diagnostic venography performed at the time of an interventional procedure is separately reportable if:

1. No prior catheter-based venographic study is available and a full diagnostic study is performed, and decision to intervene is based on the diagnostic study, OR

2. A prior study is available, but as documented in the medical record:

   a. The patient's condition with respect to the clinical indication has changed since the prior study, OR

   b. There is inadequate visualization of the anatomy and/or pathology, OR

   c. There is a clinical change during the procedure that requires new evaluation outside the target area of intervention.

Diagnostic venography performed at a separate setting from an interventional procedure is separately reported.

Diagnostic venography performed at the time of an interventional procedure is NOT separately reportable if it is specifically included in the interventional code descriptor.

> (For injection procedure for venous system, see 36000-36015, 36400-36510)

> (For injection procedure for lymphatic system, use 38790)

75801　Lymphangiography, extremity only, unilateral, radiological supervision and interpretation

75803　Lymphangiography, extremity only, bilateral, radiological supervision and interpretation

75805　Lymphangiography, pelvic/abdominal, unilateral, radiological supervision and interpretation

75807　Lymphangiography, pelvic/abdominal, bilateral, radiological supervision and interpretation

75809　Shuntogram for investigation of previously placed indwelling nonvascular shunt (eg, LeVeen shunt, ventriculoperitoneal shunt, indwelling infusion pump), radiological supervision and interpretation

> (For procedure, see 49427 or 61070)

75810　Splenoportography, radiological supervision and interpretation

75820　Venography, extremity, unilateral, radiological supervision and interpretation

75822　Venography, extremity, bilateral, radiological supervision and interpretation

75825　Venography, caval, inferior, with serialography, radiological supervision and interpretation

75827　Venography, caval, superior, with serialography, radiological supervision and interpretation

75831　Venography, renal, unilateral, selective, radiological supervision and interpretation

75833　Venography, renal, bilateral, selective, radiological supervision and interpretation

75840　Venography, adrenal, unilateral, selective, radiological supervision and interpretation

75842　Venography, adrenal, bilateral, selective, radiological supervision and interpretation

75860　Venography, venous sinus (eg, petrosal and inferior sagittal) or jugular, catheter, radiological supervision and interpretation

75870　Venography, superior sagittal sinus, radiological supervision and interpretation

75872　Venography, epidural, radiological supervision and interpretation

75880　Venography, orbital, radiological supervision and interpretation

75885　Percutaneous transhepatic portography with hemodynamic evaluation, radiological supervision and interpretation

75887　Percutaneous transhepatic portography without hemodynamic evaluation, radiological supervision and interpretation

75889　Hepatic venography, wedged or free, with hemodynamic evaluation, radiological supervision and interpretation

75891　Hepatic venography, wedged or free, without hemodynamic evaluation, radiological supervision and interpretation

75893　Venous sampling through catheter, with or without angiography (eg, for parathyroid hormone, renin), radiological supervision and interpretation

> (For procedure, use 36500)

Transcatheter Procedures

Therapeutic transcatheter radiological supervision and interpretation code(s) include the following services associated with that intervention:

1. Contrast injections, angiography/venography, roadmapping, and fluoroscopic guidance for the intervention,

2. Vessel measurement, and

3. Completion angiography/venography (except for those uses permitted by 75898).

Unless specifically included in the code descriptor, diagnostic angiography/venography performed at the time of transcatheter therapeutic radiological and interpretation service(s) is separately reportable (eg, no prior catheter-based diagnostic angiography/venography study of the target vessel is available, prior diagnostic study is inadequate, patient's condition with respect to the clinical indication has changed since the prior study or during the intervention). See 75600-75893.

Radiology

Codes 75956 and 75957 include all angiography of the thoracic aorta and its branches for diagnostic imaging prior to deployment of the primary endovascular devices (including all routine components of modular devices), fluoroscopic guidance in the delivery of the endovascular components, and intraprocedural arterial angiography (eg, confirm position, detect endoleak, evaluate runoff).

Code 75958 includes the analogous services for placement of each proximal thoracic endovascular extension. Code 75959 includes the analogous services for placement of a distal thoracic endovascular extension(s) placed during a procedure after the primary repair.

75894   Transcatheter therapy, embolization, any method, radiological supervision and interpretation

(Do not report 75894 in conjunction with 36475, 36476, 36478, 36479, 37241-37244)

►(75896 has been deleted. For radiological supervision and interpretation for thrombolysis other than coronary, see 37211, 37212, 37213, 37214. For radiological supervision and interpretation for intracranial arterial administration of pharmacological agent(s) other than for thrombolysis, see 61650, 61651)◄

75898   Angiography through existing catheter for follow-up study for transcatheter therapy, embolization or infusion, other than for thrombolysis

►(For thrombolysis infusion management other than coronary, see 37211-37214, 61645)◄

►(For non-thrombolysis infusion management other than coronary, see 61650, 61651)◄

►(Do not report 75898 in conjunction with 37211-37214, 37241-37244, 61645, 61650, 61651)◄

75901   Mechanical removal of pericatheter obstructive material (eg, fibrin sheath) from central venous device via separate venous access, radiologic supervision and interpretation

(For procedure, use 36595)

(For venous catheterization, see 36010-36012)

75902   Mechanical removal of intraluminal (intracatheter) obstructive material from central venous device through device lumen, radiologic supervision and interpretation

(For procedure, use 36596)

(For venous catheterization, see 36010-36012)

►(75945, 75946 have been deleted. To report noncoronary intravascular ultrasound during diagnostic evaluation and/or therapeutic intervention, see 37252, 37253)◄

75952   Endovascular repair of infrarenal abdominal aortic aneurysm or dissection, radiological supervision and interpretation

(For implantation of endovascular grafts, see 34800-34805)

(For radiologic supervision and interpretation of fenestrated endovascular repair of the visceral aorta with or without concomitant infrarenal abdominal aorta and common iliac artery[s], see 34841-34848)

(Do not report 75952 in conjunction with 34841-34848)

75953   Placement of proximal or distal extension prosthesis for endovascular repair of infrarenal aortic or iliac artery aneurysm, pseudoaneurysm, or dissection, radiological supervision and interpretation

(For implantation of endovascular extension prostheses, see 34825, 34826)

75954   Endovascular repair of iliac artery aneurysm, pseudoaneurysm, arteriovenous malformation, or trauma, using ilio-iliac tube endoprosthesis, radiological supervision and interpretation

(For implantation of endovascular graft, see 34900)

(For endovascular repair of iliac artery bifurcation [eg, aneurysm, pseudoaneurysm, arteriovenous malformation, trauma] using bifurcated endoprosthesis, radiological supervision and interpretation, use 0255T)

75956   Endovascular repair of descending thoracic aorta (eg, aneurysm, pseudoaneurysm, dissection, penetrating ulcer, intramural hematoma, or traumatic disruption); involving coverage of left subclavian artery origin, initial endoprosthesis plus descending thoracic aortic extension(s), if required, to level of celiac artery origin, radiological supervision and interpretation

(For implantation of endovascular graft, use 33880)

75957   not involving coverage of left subclavian artery origin, initial endoprosthesis plus descending thoracic aortic extension(s), if required, to level of celiac artery origin, radiological supervision and interpretation

(For implantation of endovascular graft, use 33881)

75958   Placement of proximal extension prosthesis for endovascular repair of descending thoracic aorta (eg, aneurysm, pseudoaneurysm, dissection, penetrating ulcer, intramural hematoma, or traumatic disruption), radiological supervision and interpretation

(Report 75958 for each proximal extension)

(For implantation of proximal endovascular extension, see 33883, 33884)

75959   Placement of distal extension prosthesis(s) (delayed) after endovascular repair of descending thoracic aorta, as needed, to level of celiac origin, radiological supervision and interpretation

(Do not report 75959 in conjunction with 75956, 75957)

(Report 75959 once, regardless of number of modules deployed)

(For implantation of distal endovascular extension, use 33886)

(75960 has been deleted)

(Radiologic supervision for transcatheter placement of stent[s] is included in the therapeutic service codes)

(75961 has been deleted. To report, use 37197)

(For removal of a vena cava filter, use 37193)

75962 Transluminal balloon angioplasty, peripheral artery other than renal, or other visceral artery, iliac or lower extremity, radiological supervision and interpretation

(For radiological supervision and interpretation for transluminal balloon angioplasty in iliac, femoral, popliteal, and tibial/peroneal arteries, see 37220-37235)

(For procedure, see 35458, 35475)

(Do not report 75962 in conjunction with 37217 for ipsilateral services)

+ 75964 Transluminal balloon angioplasty, each additional peripheral artery other than renal or other visceral artery, iliac or lower extremity, radiological supervision and interpretation (List separately in addition to code for primary procedure)

(Use 75964 in conjunction with 75962)

75966 Transluminal balloon angioplasty, renal or other visceral artery, radiological supervision and interpretation

+ 75968 Transluminal balloon angioplasty, each additional visceral artery, radiological supervision and interpretation (List separately in addition to code for primary procedure)

(Use 75968 in conjunction with 75966)

(For percutaneous transluminal coronary angioplasty, see 92920-92944)

75970 Transcatheter biopsy, radiological supervision and interpretation

(For injection procedure only for transcatheter therapy or biopsy, see 36100-36299)

(For transcatheter renal and ureteral biopsy, use 52007)

(For percutaneous needle biopsy of pancreas, use 48102; of retroperitoneal lymph node or mass, use 49180)

75978 Transluminal balloon angioplasty, venous (eg, subclavian stenosis), radiological supervision and interpretation

▶(75980 has been deleted. To report, see 47533, 47534, 47535, 47536, 47537)◀

▶(75982 has been deleted. To report, see 47533, 47534, 47535, 47536, 47537, 47538, 47539, 47540)◀

75984 Change of percutaneous tube or drainage catheter with contrast monitoring (eg, genitourinary system, abscess), radiological supervision and interpretation

(For percutaneous replacement of gastrostomy, duodenostomy, jejunostomy, gastro-jejunostomy, or cecostomy [or other colonic] tube including fluoroscopic imaging guidance, see 49450-49452)

▶(To report exchange of a percutaneous nephrostomy catheter, use 50435)◀

(For percutaneous cholecystostomy, use 47490)

▶(For percutaneous biliary procedures, including radiological supervision and interpretation, see 47531-47544)◀

(For percutaneous nephrostolithotomy or pyelostolithotomy, see 50080, 50081)

(For removal and/or replacement of an internally dwelling ureteral stent via a transurethral approach, see 50385-50386)

75989 Radiological guidance (ie, fluoroscopy, ultrasound, or computed tomography), for percutaneous drainage (eg, abscess, specimen collection), with placement of catheter, radiological supervision and interpretation

(Do not report 75989 in conjunction with 10030, 32554, 32555, 32556, 32557, 47490, 49405, 49406, 49407)

Other Procedures

(For computed tomography cerebral perfusion analysis, see Category III code 0042T)

(For arthrography of shoulder, use 73040; elbow, use 73085; wrist, use 73115; hip, use 73525; knee, use 73580; ankle, use 73615)

76000 Fluoroscopy (separate procedure), up to 1 hour physician or other qualified health care professional time, other than 71023 or 71034 (eg, cardiac fluoroscopy)

(Do not report 76000 in conjunction with 33957, 33958, 33959, 33962, 33963, 33964)

76001 Fluoroscopy, physician or other qualified health care professional time more than 1 hour, assisting a nonradiologic physician or other qualified health care professional (eg, nephrostolithotomy, ERCP, bronchoscopy, transbronchial biopsy)

(Do not report 76001 in conjunction with 33957, 33958, 33959, 33962, 33963, 33964)

76010 Radiologic examination from nose to rectum for foreign body, single view, child

76080 Radiologic examination, abscess, fistula or sinus tract study, radiological supervision and interpretation

(For contrast injection[s] and radiological assessment of gastrostomy, duodenostomy, jejunostomy, gastro-jejunostomy, or cecostomy [or other colonic] tube including fluoroscopic imaging guidance, use 49465)

76098 Radiological examination, surgical specimen

(Do not report 76098 in conjunction with 19081-19086)

76100 Radiologic examination, single plane body section (eg, tomography), other than with urography

76101 Radiologic examination, complex motion (ie, hypercycloidal) body section (eg, mastoid polytomography), other than with urography; unilateral

Radiology

76102   bilateral

(Do not report 76101, 76102 more than once per day)

(For panoramic X-ray, use 70355)

(For nephrotomography, use 74415)

76120   Cineradiography/videoradiography, except where specifically included

+ 76125   Cineradiography/videoradiography to complement routine examination (List separately in addition to code for primary procedure)

76140   Consultation on X-ray examination made elsewhere, written report

(76150 has been deleted)

(76350 has been deleted)

(2D reformatting is no longer separately reported. To report 3D rendering, see 76376, 76377)

76376   3D rendering with interpretation and reporting of computed tomography, magnetic resonance imaging, ultrasound, or other tomographic modality with image postprocessing under concurrent supervision; not requiring image postprocessing on an independent workstation

(Use 76376 in conjunction with code[s] for base imaging procedure[s])

(Do not report 76376 in conjunction with 31627, 34839, 70496, 70498, 70544, 70545, 70546, 70547, 70548, 70549, 71275, 71555, 72159, 72191, 72198, 73206, 73225, 73706, 73725, 74174, 74175, 74185, 74261, 74262, 74263, 75557, 75559, 75561, 75563, 75565, 75571, 75572, 75573, 75574, 75635, 76377, 77061, 77062, 77063, 78012-78999, 93355, 0159T)

76377   requiring image postprocessing on an independent workstation

(Use 76377 in conjunction with code[s] for base imaging procedure[s])

(Do not report 76377 in conjunction with 34839, 70496, 70498, 70544, 70545, 70546, 70547, 70548, 70549, 71275, 71555, 72159, 72191, 72198, 73206, 73225, 73706, 73725, 74174, 74175, 74185, 74261, 74262, 74263, 75557, 75559, 75561, 75563, 75565, 75571, 75572, 75573, 75574, 75635, 76376, 77061, 77062, 77063, 78012-78999, 93355, 0159T)

(To report computer-aided detection, including computer algorithm analysis of MRI data for lesion detection/characterization, pharmacokinetic analysis, breast MRI, use Category III code 0159T)

(76376, 76377 require concurrent supervision of image postprocessing 3D manipulation of volumetric data set and image rendering)

76380   Computed tomography, limited or localized follow-up study

76390   Magnetic resonance spectroscopy

(For magnetic resonance imaging, use appropriate MRI body site code)

76496   Unlisted fluoroscopic procedure (eg, diagnostic, interventional)

76497   Unlisted computed tomography procedure (eg, diagnostic, interventional)

76498   Unlisted magnetic resonance procedure (eg, diagnostic, interventional)

76499   Unlisted diagnostic radiographic procedure

Diagnostic Ultrasound

All diagnostic ultrasound examinations require permanently recorded images with measurements, when such measurements are clinically indicated. For those codes whose sole diagnostic goal is a biometric measure (ie, 76514, 76516, and 76519), permanently recorded images are not required. A final, written report should be issued for inclusion in the patient's medical record. The prescription form for the intraocular lens satisfies the written report requirement for 76519. For those anatomic regions that have "complete" and "limited" ultrasound codes, note the elements that comprise a "complete" exam. The report should contain a description of these elements or the reason that an element could not be visualized (eg, obscured by bowel gas, surgically absent).

If less than the required elements for a "complete" exam are reported (eg, limited number of organs or limited portion of region evaluated), the "limited" code for that anatomic region should be used once per patient exam session. A "limited" exam of an anatomic region should not be reported for the same exam session as a "complete" exam of that same region.

Evaluation of vascular structures using both color and spectral Doppler is separately reportable. To report, see **Noninvasive Vascular Diagnostic Studies** (93880-93990). However, color Doppler alone, when performed for anatomic structure identification in conjunction with a real-time ultrasound examination, is not reported separately.

Ultrasound guidance procedures also require permanently recorded images of the site to be localized, as well as a documented description of the localization process, either separately or within the report of the procedure for which the guidance is utilized.

Use of ultrasound, without thorough evaluation of organ(s) or anatomic region, image documentation, and final, written report, is not separately reportable.

Definitions

A-mode implies a one-dimensional ultrasonic measurement procedure.

M-mode implies a one-dimensional ultrasonic measurement procedure with movement of the trace to record amplitude and velocity of moving echo-producing structures.

B-scan implies a two-dimensional ultrasonic scanning procedure with a two-dimensional display.

Real-time scan implies a two-dimensional ultrasonic scanning procedure with display of both two-dimensional structure and motion with time.

> (To report diagnostic vascular ultrasound studies, see 93880-93990)

> (For focused ultrasound ablation treatment of uterine leiomyomata, see Category III codes 0071T, 0072T)

Head and Neck

76506 Echoencephalography, real time with image documentation (gray scale) (for determination of ventricular size, delineation of cerebral contents, and detection of fluid masses or other intracranial abnormalities), including A-mode encephalography as secondary component where indicated

76510 Ophthalmic ultrasound, diagnostic; B-scan and quantitative A-scan performed during the same patient encounter

76511 quantitative A-scan only

76512 B-scan (with or without superimposed non-quantitative A-scan)

76513 anterior segment ultrasound, immersion (water bath) B-scan or high resolution biomicroscopy

> (For scanning computerized ophthalmic diagnostic imaging of the anterior and posterior segments using technology other than ultrasound, see 92132, 92133, 92134)

76514 corneal pachymetry, unilateral or bilateral (determination of corneal thickness)

> ►(Do not report 76514 in conjunction with 0402T)◄

76516 Ophthalmic biometry by ultrasound echography, A-scan;

76519 with intraocular lens power calculation

> (For partial coherence interferometry, use 92136)

76529 Ophthalmic ultrasonic foreign body localization

76536 Ultrasound, soft tissues of head and neck (eg, thyroid, parathyroid, parotid), real time with image documentation

Chest

Code 76641 represents a complete ultrasound examination of the breast. Code 76641 consists of an ultrasound examination of all four quadrants of the breast and the retroareolar region. It also includes ultrasound examination of the axilla, if performed.

Code 76642 consists of a focused ultrasound examination of the breast limited to the assessment of one or more, but not all of the elements listed in code 76641. It also includes ultrasound examination of the axilla, if performed.

Use of ultrasound, without thorough evaluation of organ(s) or anatomic region, image documentation, and final written report, is not separately reportable.

76604 Ultrasound, chest (includes mediastinum), real time with image documentation

76641 Ultrasound, breast, unilateral, real time with image documentation, including axilla when performed; complete

76642 limited

> (Report 76641, 76642 only once per breast, per session)

> (For axillary ultrasound only, use 76882)

> (76645 has been deleted. To report, see 76641, 76642)

Abdomen and Retroperitoneum

A complete ultrasound examination of the abdomen (76700) consists of real time scans of the liver, gall bladder, common bile duct, pancreas, spleen, kidneys, and the upper abdominal aorta and inferior vena cava including any demonstrated abdominal abnormality.

A complete ultrasound examination of the retroperitoneum (76770) consists of real time scans of the kidneys, abdominal aorta, common iliac artery origins, and inferior vena cava, including any demonstrated retroperitoneal abnormality. Alternatively, if clinical history suggests urinary tract pathology, complete evaluation of the kidneys and urinary bladder also comprises a complete retroperitoneal ultrasound.

Use of ultrasound, without thorough evaluation of organ(s) or anatomic region, image documentation and final, written report, is not separately reportable.

76700 Ultrasound, abdominal, real time with image documentation; complete

76705 limited (eg, single organ, quadrant, follow-up)

76770 Ultrasound, retroperitoneal (eg, renal, aorta, nodes), real time with image documentation; complete

76775 limited

76776   Ultrasound, transplanted kidney, real time and duplex Doppler with image documentation

(For ultrasound of transplanted kidney without duplex Doppler, use 76775)

(For ultrasound and duplex Doppler of a transplanted kidney, do not report 76776 in conjunction with 93975, 93976)

Spinal Canal

76800   Ultrasound, spinal canal and contents

Pelvis

Obstetrical

Codes 76801 and 76802 include determination of the number of gestational sacs and fetuses, gestational sac/ fetal measurements appropriate for gestation (younger than 14 weeks 0 days), survey of visible fetal and placental anatomic structure, qualitative assessment of amniotic fluid volume/gestational sac shape and examination of the maternal uterus and adnexa.

Codes 76805 and 76810 include determination of number of fetuses and amniotic/chorionic sacs, measurements appropriate for gestational age (older than or equal to 14 weeks 0 days), survey of intracranial/ spinal/abdominal anatomy, 4 chambered heart, umbilical cord insertion site, placenta location and amniotic fluid assessment and, when visible, examination of maternal adnexa.

Codes 76811 and 76812 include all elements of codes 76805 and 76810 plus detailed anatomic evaluation of the fetal brain/ventricles, face, heart/outflow tracts and chest anatomy, abdominal organ specific anatomy, number/length/architecture of limbs and detailed evaluation of the umbilical cord and placenta and other fetal anatomy as clinically indicated.

Report should document the results of the evaluation of each element described above or the reason for non-visualization.

Code 76815 represents a focused "quick look" exam limited to the assessment of one or more of the elements listed in code 76815.

Code 76816 describes an examination designed to reassess fetal size and interval growth or reevaluate one or more anatomic abnormalities of a fetus previously demonstrated on ultrasound, and should be coded once for each fetus requiring reevaluation using modifier 59 for each fetus after the first.

Code 76817 describes a transvaginal obstetric ultrasound performed separately or in addition to one of the transabdominal examinations described above. For transvaginal examinations performed for non-obstetrical purposes, use code 76830.

76801   Ultrasound, pregnant uterus, real time with image documentation, fetal and maternal evaluation, first trimester (< 14 weeks 0 days), transabdominal approach; single or first gestation

(To report first trimester fetal nuchal translucency measurement, use 76813)

+ 76802   each additional gestation (List separately in addition to code for primary procedure)

(Use 76802 in conjunction with 76801)

(To report first trimester fetal nuchal translucency measurement, use 76814)

76805   Ultrasound, pregnant uterus, real time with image documentation, fetal and maternal evaluation, after first trimester (> or = 14 weeks 0 days), transabdominal approach; single or first gestation

+ 76810   each additional gestation (List separately in addition to code for primary procedure)

(Use 76810 in conjunction with 76805)

76811   Ultrasound, pregnant uterus, real time with image documentation, fetal and maternal evaluation plus detailed fetal anatomic examination, transabdominal approach; single or first gestation

+ 76812   each additional gestation (List separately in addition to code for primary procedure)

(Use 76812 in conjunction with 76811)

76813   Ultrasound, pregnant uterus, real time with image documentation, first trimester fetal nuchal translucency measurement, transabdominal or transvaginal approach; single or first gestation

+ 76814   each additional gestation (List separately in addition to code for primary procedure)

(Use 76814 in conjunction with 76813)

76815   Ultrasound, pregnant uterus, real time with image documentation, limited (eg, fetal heart beat, placental location, fetal position and/or qualitative amniotic fluid volume), 1 or more fetuses

(Use 76815 only once per exam and not per element)

(To report first trimester fetal nuchal translucency measurement, see 76813, 76814)

76816   Ultrasound, pregnant uterus, real time with image documentation, follow-up (eg, re-evaluation of fetal size by measuring standard growth parameters and amniotic fluid volume, re-evaluation of organ system(s) suspected or confirmed to be abnormal on a previous scan), transabdominal approach, per fetus

(Report 76816 with modifier 59 for each additional fetus examined in a multiple pregnancy)

76817   Ultrasound, pregnant uterus, real time with image documentation, transvaginal

(For non-obstetrical transvaginal ultrasound, use 76830)

(If transvaginal examination is done in addition to transabdominal obstetrical ultrasound exam, use 76817 in addition to appropriate transabdominal exam code)

76818   Fetal biophysical profile; with non-stress testing

76819   without non-stress testing

(Fetal biophysical profile assessments for the second and any additional fetuses, should be reported separately by code 76818 or 76819 with the modifier 59 appended)

(For amniotic fluid index without non-stress test, use 76815)

76820   Doppler velocimetry, fetal; umbilical artery

76821   middle cerebral artery

76825   Echocardiography, fetal, cardiovascular system, real time with image documentation (2D), with or without M-mode recording;

76826   follow-up or repeat study

76827   Doppler echocardiography, fetal, pulsed wave and/or continuous wave with spectral display; complete

76828   follow-up or repeat study

(To report the use of color mapping, use 93325)

Nonobstetrical

Code 76856 includes the complete evaluation of the female pelvic anatomy. Elements of this examination include a description and measurements of the uterus and adnexal structures, measurement of the endometrium, measurement of the bladder (when applicable), and a description of any pelvic pathology (eg, ovarian cysts, uterine leiomyomata, free pelvic fluid).

Code 76856 is also applicable to a complete evaluation of the male pelvis. Elements of the examination include evaluation and measurement (when applicable) of the urinary bladder, evaluation of the prostate and seminal vesicles to the extent that they are visualized transabdominally, and any pelvic pathology (eg, bladder tumor, enlarged prostate, free pelvic fluid, pelvic abscess).

Code 76857 represents a focused examination limited to the assessment of one or more elements listed in code 76856 and/or the reevaluation of one or more pelvic abnormalities previously demonstrated on ultrasound. Code 76857, rather than 76770, should be utilized if the urinary bladder alone (ie, not including the kidneys) is imaged, whereas code 51798 should be utilized if a bladder volume or post-void residual measurement is obtained without imaging the bladder.

Use of ultrasound, without thorough evaluation of organ(s) or anatomic region, image documentation, and final, written report, is not separately reportable.

76830   Ultrasound, transvaginal

(For obstetrical transvaginal ultrasound, use 76817)

(If transvaginal examination is done in addition to transabdominal non-obstetrical ultrasound exam, use 76830 in addition to appropriate transabdominal exam code)

76831   Saline infusion sonohysterography (SIS), including color flow Doppler, when performed

(For introduction of saline for saline infusion sonohysterography, use 58340)

76856   Ultrasound, pelvic (nonobstetric), real time with image documentation; complete

76857   limited or follow-up (eg, for follicles)

Genitalia

76870   Ultrasound, scrotum and contents

76872   Ultrasound, transrectal;

(Do not report 76872 in conjunction with 45341, 45342, 45391, 45392, 0249T)

76873   prostate volume study for brachytherapy treatment planning (separate procedure)

Extremities

A complete ultrasound examination of an extremity (76881) consists of real time scans of a specific joint that includes examination of the muscles, tendons, joint, other soft tissue structures, and any identifiable abnormality.

Code 76882 refers to an examination of an extremity that would be performed primarily for evaluation of muscles, tendons, joints, and/or soft tissues. This is a limited examination of the extremity where a specific anatomic structure such as a tendon or muscle is assessed. In addition, the code would be used to evaluate a soft-tissue mass that may be present in an extremity where knowledge of its cystic or solid characteristics is needed.

For spectral and color Doppler evaluation of the extremities, use 93925, 93926, 93930, 93931, 93970, or 93971 as appropriate.

76881   Ultrasound, extremity, nonvascular, real-time with image documentation; complete

76882   limited, anatomic specific

76885   Ultrasound, infant hips, real time with imaging documentation; dynamic (requiring physician or other qualified health care professional manipulation)

76886   limited, static (not requiring physician or other qualified health care professional manipulation)

Radiology

Ultrasonic Guidance Procedures

76930 Ultrasonic guidance for pericardiocentesis, imaging supervision and interpretation

76932 Ultrasonic guidance for endomyocardial biopsy, imaging supervision and interpretation

76936 Ultrasound guided compression repair of arterial pseudoaneurysm or arteriovenous fistulae (includes diagnostic ultrasound evaluation, compression of lesion and imaging)

+ 76937 Ultrasound guidance for vascular access requiring ultrasound evaluation of potential access sites, documentation of selected vessel patency, concurrent realtime ultrasound visualization of vascular needle entry, with permanent recording and reporting (List separately in addition to code for primary procedure)

(Do not report 76937 in conjunction with 37191, 37192, 37193, 37760, 37761, 76942)

(If extremity venous non-invasive vascular diagnostic study is performed separate from venous access guidance, use 93965, 93970 or 93971)

76940 Ultrasound guidance for, and monitoring of, parenchymal tissue ablation

(Do not report 76940 in conjunction with 20982, 20983, 50250, 50542, 76942, 76998, 0340T)

(For ablation, see 32998, 47370-47382, 47383, 50592, 50593)

76941 Ultrasonic guidance for intrauterine fetal transfusion or cordocentesis, imaging supervision and interpretation

(For procedure, see 36460, 59012)

76942 Ultrasonic guidance for needle placement (eg, biopsy, aspiration, injection, localization device), imaging supervision and interpretation

(Do not report 76942 in conjunction with 10030, 19083, 19285, 20604, 20606, 20611, 27096, 32554, 32555, 32556, 32557, 37760, 37761, 43232, 43237, 43242, 45341, 45342, 64479-64484, 64490-64495, 76975, 0213T-0218T, 0228T-0231T, 0232T, 0249T, 0301T)

(For injection(s) of platelet rich plasma, use 0232T)

76945 Ultrasonic guidance for chorionic villus sampling, imaging supervision and interpretation

(For procedure, use 59015)

76946 Ultrasonic guidance for amniocentesis, imaging supervision and interpretation

76948 Ultrasonic guidance for aspiration of ova, imaging supervision and interpretation

(76950 has been deleted. To report, use 77387)

(For placement of interstitial device[s] for radiation therapy guidance, see 31627, 32553, 49411, 55876)

76965 Ultrasonic guidance for interstitial radioelement application

Other Procedures

76970 Ultrasound study follow-up (specify)

76975 Gastrointestinal endoscopic ultrasound, supervision and interpretation

(Do not report 76975 in conjunction with 43231, 43232, 43237, 43238, 43240, 43242, 43259, 44406, 44407, 45341, 45342, 45391, 45392, 76942)

76977 Ultrasound bone density measurement and interpretation, peripheral site(s), any method

76998 Ultrasonic guidance, intraoperative

(Do not report 76998 in conjunction with 36475, 36479, 37760, 37761, 47370-47382, 0249T, 0301T)

(For ultrasound guidance for open and laparoscopic radiofrequency tissue ablation, use 76940)

76999 Unlisted ultrasound procedure (eg, diagnostic, interventional)

Radiologic Guidance

Fluoroscopic Guidance

(Do not report guidance codes 77001, 77002, 77003 for services in which fluoroscopic guidance is included in the descriptor)

+ 77001 Fluoroscopic guidance for central venous access device placement, replacement (catheter only or complete), or removal (includes fluoroscopic guidance for vascular access and catheter manipulation, any necessary contrast injections through access site or catheter with related venography radiologic supervision and interpretation, and radiographic documentation of final catheter position) (List separately in addition to code for primary procedure)

(Do not report 77001 in conjunction with 33957, 33958, 33959, 33962, 33963, 33964, 77002)

(If formal extremity venography is performed from separate venous access and separately interpreted, use 36005 and 75820, 75822, 75825, or 75827)

77002 Fluoroscopic guidance for needle placement (eg, biopsy, aspiration, injection, localization device)

(See appropriate surgical code for procedure and anatomic location)

(77002 is included in all arthrography radiological supervision and interpretation codes. See **Administration of Contrast Material[s]** introductory guidelines for reporting of arthrography procedures)

(Do not report 77002 in conjunction with 10030, 19081-19086, 19281-19288, 20982, 20983, 32554, 32555, 32556, 32557, 70332, 73040, 73085, 73115, 73525, 73580, 73615, 0232T)

(For injection(s) of platelet rich plasma, use 0232T)

⊙=Moderate sedation ✚=Add-on code ✗=FDA approval pending #=Resequenced code ○=Recycled/reinstated code

Radiology

▶(77002 is included in the organ/anatomic specific radiological supervision and interpretation procedures 49440, 74355, 74445, 74470, 75809, 75810, 75885, 75887, 75989)◀

77003 Fluoroscopic guidance and localization of needle or catheter tip for spine or paraspinous diagnostic or therapeutic injection procedures (epidural or subarachnoid)

(Injection of contrast during fluoroscopic guidance and localization [77003] is included in 22526, 22527, 27096, 62263, 62264, 62267, 62270-62282, 62310-62319)

(Fluoroscopic guidance for subarachnoid puncture for diagnostic radiographic myelography is included in supervision and interpretation codes 72240-72270)

(For epidural or subarachnoid needle or catheter placement and injection, see 62270-62282, 62310-62319)

(For sacroiliac joint arthrography, see 27096)

(For paravertebral facet joint injection, see 64490-64495. For paravertebral facet joint nerve destruction by neurolysis, see 64633-64636. For transforaminal epidural needle placement and injection, see 64479-64484)

(Do not report 77002, 77003 in conjunction with 10030, 22586, 27096, 64479–64484, 64490-64495, 64633-64636, 0195T, 0196T, 0309T)

(For percutaneous or endoscopic lysis of epidural adhesions, 62263, 62264 include fluoroscopic guidance and localization)

Computed Tomography Guidance

77011 Computed tomography guidance for stereotactic localization

77012 Computed tomography guidance for needle placement (eg, biopsy, aspiration, injection, localization device), radiological supervision and interpretation

(Do not report 77011, 77012 in conjunction with 22586, 0195T, 0196T, 0309T)

(Do not report 77012 in conjunction with 10030, 27096, 32554, 32555, 32556, 32557, 64479-64484, 64490-64495, 64633-64636, 0232T)

(For injection(s) of platelet rich plasma, use 0232T)

77013 Computed tomography guidance for, and monitoring of, parenchymal tissue ablation

(Do not report 77013 in conjunction with 20982, 20983, 0340T)

(For percutaneous ablation, see 32998, 47382, 47383, 50592, 50593)

77014 Computed tomography guidance for placement of radiation therapy fields

(For placement of interstitial device[s] for radiation therapy guidance, see 31627, 32553, 49411, 55876)

Magnetic Resonance Guidance

77021 Magnetic resonance guidance for needle placement (eg, for biopsy, needle aspiration, injection, or placement of localization device) radiological supervision and interpretation

(For procedure, see appropriate organ or site)

(Do not report 77021 in conjunction with 10030, 19085, 19287, 32554, 32555, 32556, 32557, 0232T)

(For injection(s) of platelet rich plasma, use 0232T)

77022 Magnetic resonance guidance for, and monitoring of, parenchymal tissue ablation

(Do not report 77022 in conjunction with 0071T, 0072T, 20982, 20983, 0340T)

(For percutaneous ablation, see 32998, 47382, 47383, 50592, 50593)

(For focused ultrasound ablation treatment of uterine leiomyomata, see Category III codes 0071T, 0072T)

(77031 has been deleted)

(To report stereotactic localization guidance for breast biopsy or for placement of breast localization device[s], see 19081, 19283)

(77032 has been deleted)

(To report mammographic guidance for placement of breast localization device[s], use 19281)

Breast, Mammography

+ 77051 Computer-aided detection (computer algorithm analysis of digital image data for lesion detection) with further review for interpretation, with or without digitization of film radiographic images; diagnostic mammography (List separately in addition to code for primary procedure)

(Use 77051 in conjunction with 77055, 77056)

+ 77052 screening mammography (List separately in addition to code for primary procedure)

(Use 77052 in conjunction with 77057)

77053 Mammary ductogram or galactogram, single duct, radiological supervision and interpretation

(For mammary ductogram or galactogram injection, use 19030)

77054 Mammary ductogram or galactogram, multiple ducts, radiological supervision and interpretation

77055 Mammography; unilateral

77056 bilateral

(Do not report 77055, 77056 in conjunction with 77063)

(Use 77055, 77056 in conjunction with 77051 for computer-aided detection applied to a diagnostic mammogram)

▲ **77057**   Screening mammography, bilateral (2-view study of each breast)

(Do not report 77057 in conjunction with 77061, 77062)

(Use 77057 in conjunction with 77052 for computer-aided detection applied to a screening mammogram)

(For electrical impedance breast scan, use 76499)

77058   Magnetic resonance imaging, breast, without and/or with contrast material(s); unilateral

77059   bilateral

77061   Digital breast tomosynthesis; unilateral

77062   bilateral

(Do not report 77061, 77062 in conjunction with 76376, 76377, 77057)

✚ **77063**   Screening digital breast tomosynthesis, bilateral (List separately in addition to code for primary procedure)

(Do not report 77063 in conjunction with 76376, 76377, 77055, 77056)

(Use 77063 in conjunction with 77057)

Bone/Joint Studies

77071   Manual application of stress performed by physician or other qualified health care professional for joint radiography, including contralateral joint if indicated

(For radiographic interpretation of stressed images, see appropriate anatomic site and number of views)

77072   Bone age studies

77073   Bone length studies (orthoroentgenogram, scanogram)

77074   Radiologic examination, osseous survey; limited (eg, for metastases)

77075   complete (axial and appendicular skeleton)

77076   Radiologic examination, osseous survey, infant

77077   Joint survey, single view, 2 or more joints (specify)

77078   Computed tomography, bone mineral density study, 1 or more sites, axial skeleton (eg, hips, pelvis, spine)

(77079 has been deleted)

77080   Dual-energy X-ray absorptiometry (DXA), bone density study, 1 or more sites; axial skeleton (eg, hips, pelvis, spine)

(Do not report 77080 in conjunction with 77085, 77086)

77081   appendicular skeleton (peripheral) (eg, radius, wrist, heel)

(77082 has been deleted. To report, use 77086)

(For dual energy x-ray absorptiometry [DXA] body composition study, use 76499)

(77083 has been deleted)

\# **77085**   axial skeleton (eg, hips, pelvis, spine), including vertebral fracture assessment

(Do not report 77085 in conjunction with 77080, 77086)

\# **77086**   Vertebral fracture assessment via dual-energy X-ray absorptiometry (DXA)

(Do not report 77086 in conjunction with 77080, 77085)

77084   Magnetic resonance (eg, proton) imaging, bone marrow blood supply

77085   Code is out of numerical sequence. See 77071-77086

77086   Code is out of numerical sequence. See 77071-77086

Radiation Oncology

Listings for Radiation Oncology provide for teletherapy and brachytherapy to include initial consultation, clinical treatment planning, simulation, medical radiation physics, dosimetry, treatment devices, special services, and clinical treatment management procedures. They include normal follow-up care during course of treatment and for three months following its completion.

When a service or procedure is provided that is not listed in this edition of the CPT codebook it should be identified by a Special Report (see page 407) and one of the following unlisted procedure codes:

77299 Unlisted procedure, therapeutic radiology clinical treatment planning

77399 Unlisted procedure, medical radiation physics, dosimetry and treatment devices, and special services

77499 Unlisted procedure, therapeutic radiology treatment management

77799 Unlisted procedure, clinical brachytherapy

For treatment by injectable or ingestible isotopes, see subsection Nuclear Medicine.

Consultation: Clinical Management

Preliminary consultation, evaluation of patient prior to decision to treat, or full medical care (in addition to treatment management) when provided by the therapeutic radiologist may be identified by the appropriate procedure codes from **Evaluation and Management, Medicine,** or **Surgery** sections.

Clinical Treatment Planning (External and Internal Sources)

The clinical treatment planning process is a complex service including interpretation of special testing, tumor localization, treatment volume determination, treatment time/dosage determination, choice of treatment modality, determination of number and size of treatment ports, selection of appropriate treatment devices, and other procedures.

⊙=Moderate sedation   ✚=Add-on code   ✗=FDA approval pending   #=Resequenced code   ○=Recycled/reinstated code

Definitions

Simple planning requires a single treatment area of interest encompassed in a single port or simple parallel opposed ports with simple or no blocking.

Intermediate planning requires 3 or more converging ports, 2 separate treatment areas, multiple blocks, or special time dose constraints.

Complex planning requires highly complex blocking, custom shielding blocks, tangential ports, special wedges or compensators, three or more separate treatment areas, rotational or special beam considerations, combination of therapeutic modalities.

77261   Therapeutic radiology treatment planning; simple

77262   intermediate

77263   complex

Simulation is the process of defining relevant normal and abnormal target anatomy, and acquiring the images and data necessary to develop the optimal radiation treatment process for the patient. A simulation is defined as complex if any of these criteria are met: particle, rotation or arc therapy, complex or custom blocking, brachytherapy simulation, hyperthermia probe verification, or any use of contrast material. If a simulation does not meet any of these criteria, the complexity is defined by the number of treatment areas: one treatment area is simple, two treatment areas are intermediate, and three or more treatment areas are complex.

A treatment area is a contiguous anatomic location that will be treated with radiation therapy. Generally, this includes the primary tumor organ or the resection bed and the draining lymph node chains, if indicated. An example is a breast cancer patient for whom a single treatment area could be the breast alone or the breast, adjacent supraclavicular fossa, and internal mammary nodes. In some cases, a patient might receive radiation therapy to more than one discontinuous anatomic location. An example would be a patient with multiple bone metastases in separate sites (eg, femur and cervical spine); in this case, each distinct and separate anatomic site to be irradiated is a separate treatment area.

Definitions

Simple: simulation of a single treatment area.

Intermediate: two separate treatment areas.

Complex: three or more treatment areas, or any number of treatment areas if any of the following are involved: particle, rotation or arc therapy, complex blocking, custom shielding blocks, brachytherapy simulation, hyperthermia probe verification, any use of contrast materials.

77280   Therapeutic radiology simulation-aided field setting; simple

77285   intermediate

77290   complex

+ 77293   Respiratory motion management simulation (List separately in addition to code for primary procedure)

(Use 77293 in conjunction with 77295, 77301)

77295   Code is out of numerical sequence. See 77295-77370

77299   Unlisted procedure, therapeutic radiology clinical treatment planning

Medical Radiation Physics, Dosimetry, Treatment Devices, and Special Services

 # 77295   3-dimensional radiotherapy plan, including dose-volume histograms

77300   Basic radiation dosimetry calculation, central axis depth dose calculation, TDF, NSD, gap calculation, off axis factor, tissue inhomogeneity factors, calculation of non-ionizing radiation surface and depth dose, as required during course of treatment, only when prescribed by the treating physician

►(Do not report 77300 in conjunction with 77306, 77307, 77316, 77317, 77318, 77321, 77767, 77768, 77770, 77771, 77772, 0394T, 0395T)◄

77301   Intensity modulated radiotherapy plan, including dose-volume histograms for target and critical structure partial tolerance specifications

(Dose plan is optimized using inverse or forward planning technique for modulated beam delivery [eg, binary, dynamic MLC] to create highly conformal dose distribution. Computer plan distribution must be verified for positional accuracy based on dosimetric verification of the intensity map with verification of treatment set-up and interpretation of verification methodology)

(77305 has been deleted. To report, use 77306)

77306   Teletherapy isodose plan; simple (1 or 2 unmodified ports directed to a single area of interest), includes basic dosimetry calculation(s)

77307   complex (multiple treatment areas, tangential ports, the use of wedges, blocking, rotational beam, or special beam considerations), includes basic dosimetry calculation(s)

(Only 1 teletherapy isodose plan may be reported for a given course of therapy to a specific treatment area)

(Do not report 77306, 77307 in conjunction with 77300)

(77310 has been deleted. To report, see 77306, 77307)

(77315 has been deleted. To report, use 77307)

77316   Brachytherapy isodose plan; simple (calculation[s] made from 1 to 4 sources, or remote afterloading brachytherapy, 1 channel), includes basic dosimetry calculation(s)

(For definition of source, see clinical brachytherapy introductory guidelines)

Radiology

77317   intermediate (calculation[s] made from 5 to 10 sources, or remote afterloading brachytherapy, 2-12 channels), includes basic dosimetry calculation(s)

77318   complex (calculation[s] made from over 10 sources, or remote afterloading brachytherapy, over 12 channels), includes basic dosimetry calculation(s)

(Do not report 77316, 77317, 77318 in conjunction with 77300)

77321   Special teletherapy port plan, particles, hemibody, total body

(77326 has been deleted. To report, use 77316)

(77327 has been deleted. To report, use 77317)

(77328 has been deleted. To report, use 77318)

77331   Special dosimetry (eg, TLD, microdosimetry) (specify), only when prescribed by the treating physician

77332   Treatment devices, design and construction; simple (simple block, simple bolus)

77333   intermediate (multiple blocks, stents, bite blocks, special bolus)

77334   complex (irregular blocks, special shields, compensators, wedges, molds or casts)

77336   Continuing medical physics consultation, including assessment of treatment parameters, quality assurance of dose delivery, and review of patient treatment documentation in support of the radiation oncologist, reported per week of therapy

77338   Multi-leaf collimator (MLC) device(s) for intensity modulated radiation therapy (IMRT), design and construction per IMRT plan

(Do not report 77338 in conjunction with 77385 for compensator based IMRT)

(Do not report 77338 more than once per IMRT plan)

(For immobilization in IMRT treatment, see 77332-77334)

77370   Special medical radiation physics consultation

Stereotactic Radiation Treatment Delivery

⊙ 77371   Radiation treatment delivery, stereotactic radiosurgery (SRS), complete course of treatment of cranial lesion(s) consisting of 1 session; multi-source Cobalt 60 based

77372   linear accelerator based

(For radiation treatment management, use 77432)

77373   Stereotactic body radiation therapy, treatment delivery, per fraction to 1 or more lesions, including image guidance, entire course not to exceed 5 fractions

(Do not report 77373 in conjunction with 77385, 77386, 77401, 77402, 77407, 77412)

(For single fraction cranial lesion[s], see 77371, 77372)

77385   Code is out of numerical sequence. See 77401-77425

77386   Code is out of numerical sequence. See 77401-77425

77387   Code is out of numerical sequence. See 77401-77425

Other Procedures

77399   Unlisted procedure, medical radiation physics, dosimetry and treatment devices, and special services

Radiation Treatment Delivery

Following dosimetry calculations, there are a number of alternative methods to deliver external radiation treatments, which are described with specific CPT codes:

- X-ray (photon), including conventional and intensity modulated radiation therapy (IMRT) beams;

- Electron beams;

- Neutron beams;

- Proton beams.

All treatment delivery codes are reported once per treatment session. The treatment delivery codes recognize technical-only services and contain no physician work (the professional component). In contrast, the treatment management codes contain only the professional component.

Radiation treatment delivery with conventional X-ray or electron beams is assigned levels of complexity based on the number of treatment sites and complexity of the treatment fields, blocking, wedges, and physical or virtual tissue compensators. A simple block is straight-edged or an approximation of a straight edge created by a multileaf collimator (MLC). Energy of the megavoltage (≥ 1 MeV) beam does not contribute to complexity. Techniques such as treating a field-in-field to ensure dose homogeneity reflect added complexity.

▶Energies below the megavoltage range may be used in the treatment of skin lesions. Superficial radiation energies (up to 200 kV) may be generated by a variety of technologies and should not be reported with megavoltage (77402, 77407, 77412) for surface application. Do not report clinical treatment planning (77261, 77262, 77263), treatment devices (77332, 77333, 77334), isodose planning (77306, 77307, 77316, 77317, 77318), physics consultation (77336), or radiation treatment management (77427, 77431, 77432, 77435, 77469, 77470, 77499) with 77401, 0394T, or 0395T. When reporting 77401 alone, evaluation and management, when performed, may be reported with the appropriate E/M codes.◀

Intensity modulated radiation therapy (IMRT) uses computer-based optimization techniques with non-uniform radiation beam intensities to create highly conformal dose distributions that can be delivered by a radiotherapy treatment machine. A number of technologies, including spatially and temporally modulated beams, cylindrical beamlets, dynamic MLC, single or multiple fields or arcs, or compensators, may be

Radiology

used to generate IMRT. The complexity of IMRT may vary depending on the area being treated or the technique being used.

Image guided radiation therapy (IGRT) may be used to direct the radiation beam and to reflect motion during treatment. A variety of techniques may be used to perform this guidance including imaging (eg, ultrasound, CT, MRI, stereoscopic imaging) and non-imaging (eg, electromagnetic or infrared) techniques. Guidance may be used with any radiation treatment delivery technique and is typically used with IMRT delivery. IMRT delivery codes include the technical component of guidance or tracking, if performed. Because only the technical portion of IGRT is bundled into IMRT, the physician involvement in guidance or tracking may be reported separately. When guidance is required with conventional radiation treatment delivery, both the professional and technical components are reported because neither component of guidance is bundled into conventional radiation treatment delivery services.

The technical and professional components of guidance are handled differently with each radiation delivery code depending on the type of radiation being administered. The **Radiation Management and Treatment Table** is provided for clarity.

Definitions

Radiation Treatment Delivery, megavoltage (≥ 1 MeV), any energy

Simple: All of the following criteria are met (and none of the complex or intermediate criteria are met): single treatment area, one or two ports, and two or fewer simple blocks.

Intermediate: Any of the following criteria are met (and none of the complex criteria are met): 2 separate treatment areas, 3 or more ports on a single treatment area, or 3 or more simple blocks.

Complex: Any of the following criteria are met: 3 or more separate treatment areas, custom blocking, tangential ports, wedges, rotational beam, field-in-field or other tissue compensation that does not meet IMRT guidelines, or electron beam.

Intensity Modulated Radiation Therapy (IMRT), any energy, includes the technical services for guidance

Simple: Any of the following: prostate, breast, and all sites using physical compensator based IMRT.

Complex: Includes all other sites if not using physical compensator based IMRT.

77401   Radiation treatment delivery, superficial and/or ortho voltage, per day

(Do not report 77401 in conjunction with 77373)

77402   Radiation treatment delivery, ≥1 MeV; simple

(Do not report 77402 in conjunction with 77373)

(77403, 77404, 77406 have been deleted. To report, use 77402)

77407   intermediate

(Do not report 77407 in conjunction with 77373)

(77408, 77409, 77411 have been deleted. To report, use 77407)

77412   complex

(Do not report 77412 in conjunction with 77373)

(77413, 77414, 77416 have been deleted. To report, use 77412)

▲ **77417**   Therapeutic radiology port image(s)

(77418 has been deleted)

(For intensity modulated treatment planning, use 77301)

77385   Intensity modulated radiation treatment delivery (IMRT), includes guidance and tracking, when performed; simple

(To report professional component [PC] of guidance and tracking, use 77387 with modifier 26)

77386   complex

(To report professional component [PC] of guidance and tracking, use 77387 with modifier 26)

(Do not report 77385, 77386 in conjunction with 77371, 77372, 77373)

77387   Guidance for localization of target volume for delivery of radiation treatment delivery, includes intrafraction tracking, when performed

(Do not report technical component [TC] with 77385, 77386, 77371, 77372, 77373)

(77421 has been deleted. To report, use 77387)

(For placement of interstitial device[s] for radiation therapy guidance, see 31627, 32553, 49411, 55876)

77424   Intraoperative radiation treatment delivery, x-ray, single treatment session

77425   Intraoperative radiation treatment delivery, electrons, single treatment session

Neutron Beam Treatment Delivery

77422   High energy neutron radiation treatment delivery; single treatment area using a single port or parallel-opposed ports with no blocks or simple blocking

77423   1 or more isocenter(s) with coplanar or non-coplanar geometry with blocking and/or wedge, and/or compensator(s)

77424   Code is out of numerical sequence. See 77401-77425

77425   Code is out of numerical sequence. See 77401-77425

Radiology

Radiation Treatment Management

Radiation treatment management is reported in units of five fractions or treatment sessions, regardless of the actual time period in which the services are furnished. The services need not be furnished on consecutive days. Multiple fractions representing two or more treatment sessions furnished on the same day may be counted separately as long as there has been a distinct break in therapy sessions, and the fractions are of the character usually furnished on different days. Code 77427 is also reported if there are three or four fractions beyond a multiple of five at the end of a course of treatment; one or two fractions beyond a multiple of five at the end of a course of treatment are not reported separately.

▶Radiation treatment management requires **and includes** a minimum of one examination of the patient by the physician for medical evaluation and management (eg, assessment of the patient's response to treatment, coordination of care and treatment, review of imaging and/or lab test results with documentation) for each reporting of the radiation treatment management service. Code 77469 represents only the intraoperative session management and does not include medical evaluation and management outside of that session. The professional services furnished during treatment management typically include:

- Review of port images;
- Review of dosimetry, dose delivery, and treatment parameters;
- Review of patient treatment set-up.

Stereotactic radiosurgery (SRS-[77432]) and stereotactic body radiation treatment (SBRT-[77435]) management also include the professional component of guidance for localization of target volume for the delivery of radiation therapy (77387). *See also the Radiation Management and Treatment Table.*◀

77427 Radiation treatment management, 5 treatments

77431 Radiation therapy management with complete course of therapy consisting of 1 or 2 fractions only

(77431 is not to be used to fill in the last week of a long course of therapy)

77432 Stereotactic radiation treatment management of cranial lesion(s) (complete course of treatment consisting of 1 session)

(The same physician should not report both stereotactic radiosurgery services [61796-61800] and radiation treatment management [77432 or 77435] for cranial lesions)

(For stereotactic body radiation therapy treatment, use 77435)

(To report the technical component of guidance for localization of target volume, use 77387 with a technical component modifier [TC])

77435 Stereotactic body radiation therapy, treatment management, per treatment course, to 1 or more lesions, including image guidance, entire course not to exceed 5 fractions

(Do not report 77435 in conjunction with 77427-77432)

(The same physician should not report both stereotactic radiosurgery services [32701, 63620, 63621] and radiation treatment management [77435])

(To report the technical component of guidance for localization of target volume, use 77387 with a technical component modifier [TC])

77469 Intraoperative radiation treatment management

77470 Special treatment procedure (eg, total body irradiation, hemibody radiation, per oral or endocavitary irradiation)

(77470 assumes that the procedure is performed 1 or more times during the course of therapy, in addition to daily or weekly patient management)

(For intraoperative radiation treatment delivery and management, see 77424, 77425, 77469)

77499 Unlisted procedure, therapeutic radiology treatment management

Proton Beam Treatment Delivery

Definitions

Simple proton treatment delivery to a single treatment area utilizing a single non-tangential/oblique port, custom block with compensation (77522) and without compensation (77520).

Intermediate proton treatment delivery to one or more treatment areas utilizing two or more ports or one or more tangential/oblique ports, with custom blocks and compensators.

Complex proton treatment delivery to one or more treatment areas utilizing two or more ports per treatment area with matching or patching fields and/or multiple isocenters, with custom blocks and compensators.

77520 Proton treatment delivery; simple, without compensation

77522 simple, with compensation

77523 intermediate

77525 complex

Radiation Management and Treatment Table

Category	Code	Descriptor	IGRT TC (77387-TC) Bundled into Code?	IGRT PC (77387-PC) Bundled into Code?	Code Type (Technical / Professional)
		SRS: Stereotactic radiosurgery SBRT: Stereotactic body radiation therapy IMRT: Intensity modulated radiation therapy IGRT: Image guided radiation therapy TC: Technical component PC: Professional component (modifier 26)			
Radiation Treatment Management	77427	Treatment Management, 1-5 Treatments	N	N	Professional
	77431	Treatment Management, 1-2 Fractions	N	N	Professional
	77432	SRS Management, Cranial Lesion(s)	N	Y	Professional
	77435	SBRT Management	N	Y	Professional
SRS Treatment Delivery	77371	SRS Multisource 60 Based	Y	N	Technical
	77372	SRS Linear Based	Y	N	Technical
SBRT Treatment Delivery	77373	SBRT, 1 or More Lesions, 1-5 Fractions	Y	N	Technical
Radiation Treatment Delivery	77401	Superficial and/or Ortho Voltage	N	N	Technical
	77402	Radiation Treatment Delivery, Simple	N	N	Technical
	77407	Radiation Treatment Delivery, Intermediate	N	N	Technical
	77412	Radiation Treatment Delivery, Complex	N	N	Technical
IMRT Treatment Delivery	77385	IMRT Treatment Delivery, Simple	Y	N	Technical
	77386	IMRT Treatment Delivery, Complex	Y	N	Technical
Neutron Beam Treatment Delivery	77422	Neutron Beam Treatment, Simple	N	N	Technical
	77423	Neutron Beam Treatment, Complex	N	N	Technical
Proton Treatment Delivery	77520	Proton Treatment, Simple	N	N	Technical
	77522	Proton Treatment, Simple	N	N	Technical
	77523	Proton Treatment, Intermediate	N	N	Technical
	77525	Proton Treatment, Complex	N	N	Technical

Hyperthermia

Hyperthermia treatments as listed in this section include external (superficial and deep), interstitial, and intracavitary.

Radiation therapy when given concurrently is listed separately.

Hyperthermia is used only as an adjunct to radiation therapy or chemotherapy. It may be induced by a variety of sources (eg, microwave, ultrasound, low energy radiofrequency conduction, or by probes).

The listed treatments include management during the course of therapy and follow-up care for three months after completion.

Preliminary consultation is not included (see **Evaluation and Management** 99241-99255).

Physics planning and interstitial insertion of temperature sensors, and use of external or interstitial heat generating sources are included.

Radiology

The following descriptors are included in the treatment schedule:

⊙ **77600** Hyperthermia, externally generated; superficial (ie, heating to a depth of 4 cm or less)

⊙ **77605** deep (ie, heating to depths greater than 4 cm)

(For focused microwave thermotherapy of the breast, use 0301T)

⊙ **77610** Hyperthermia generated by interstitial probe(s); 5 or fewer interstitial applicators

⊙ **77615** more than 5 interstitial applicators

Clinical Intracavitary Hyperthermia

77620 Hyperthermia generated by intracavitary probe(s)

Clinical Brachytherapy

Clinical brachytherapy requires the use of either natural or man-made radioelements applied into or around a treatment field of interest. The supervision of radioelements and dose interpretation are performed solely by the therapeutic radiologist.

Services 77750-77799 include admission to the hospital and daily visits.

For insertion of ovoids and tandems, use 57155.

For insertion of Heyman capsules, use 58346.

Definitions

(Sources refer to intracavitary placement or permanent interstitial placement; ribbons refer to temporary interstitial placement)

A simple application has one to four sources/ribbons.

An intermediate application has five to 10 sources/ribbons.

A complex application has greater than 10 sources/ribbons.

►High dose-rate brachytherapy involves treatment with radiation sources that cannot safely be handled manually. These systems are remotely controlled and place a radionuclide source (radioelement or radioisotope) within an applicator placed in or near the target. These applicators may be placed in the body or on the skin surface.

Small electronic X-ray sources placed into an applicator within or close to the target may also be used to generate radiation at high-dose rates. This is referred to as high dose-rate electronic brachytherapy.

To report high dose-rate electronic brachytherapy, see 0394T, 0395T.◄

77750 Infusion or instillation of radioelement solution (includes 3-month follow-up care)

(For administration of radiolabeled monoclonal antibodies, use 79403)

(For non-antibody radiopharmaceutical therapy by intravenous administration only, not including 3-month follow-up care, use 79101)

77761 Intracavitary radiation source application; simple

77762 intermediate

77763 complex

►(Do not report 77761-77763 in conjunction with Category III codes 0394T, 0395T)◄

● **77767** Remote afterloading high dose rate radionuclide skin surface brachytherapy, includes basic dosimetry, when performed; lesion diameter up to 2.0 cm or 1 channel

● **77768** lesion diameter over 2.0 cm and 2 or more channels, or multiple lesions

● **77770** Remote afterloading high dose rate radionuclide interstitial or intracavitary brachytherapy, includes basic dosimetry, when performed; 1 channel

● **77771** 2-12 channels

● **77772** over 12 channels

►(Do not report 77767, 77768, 77770, 77771, 77772 in conjunction with 77300, 0394T, 0395T)◄

►(For non-brachytherapy superficial [eg, ≤200 kV] radiation treatment delivery, use 77401)◄

►(77776, 77777 have been deleted. To report, use 77799)◄

▲ **77778** Interstitial radiation source application, complex, includes supervision, handling, loading of radiation source, when performed

►(Do not report 77778 in conjunction with Category III codes 0394T, 0395T)◄

►(Do not report 77778 in conjunction with 77790)◄

►(77782-77784 have been deleted. To report, see 77767, 77768, 77770, 77771, 77772)◄

►(77785, 77786, 77787 have been deleted. To report, see 77770, 77771, 77772)◄

▲ **77789** Surface application of low dose rate radionuclide source

►(Do not report 77789 in conjunction with 77401, 77767, 77768, 0394T, 0395T)◄

77790 Supervision, handling, loading of radiation source

►(Do not report 77790 in conjunction with 77778)◄

77799 Unlisted procedure, clinical brachytherapy

Nuclear Medicine

Listed procedures may be performed independently or in the course of overall medical care. If the individual providing these services is also responsible for diagnostic workup and/or follow-up care of patient, see appropriate sections also.

Radioimmunoassay tests are found in the **Clinical Pathology** section (codes 82009-84999). These codes can be appropriately used by any specialist performing such tests in a laboratory licensed and/or certified for radioimmunoassays. The reporting of these tests is not confined to clinical pathology laboratories alone.

The services listed do not include the radiopharmaceutical or drug. To separately report supply of diagnostic and therapeutic radiopharmaceuticals and drugs, use the appropriate supply code(s), in addition to the procedure code.

Diagnostic

Endocrine System

(78000-78011 have been deleted. To report, see 78012-78014)

78012 Thyroid uptake, single or multiple quantitative measurement(s) (including stimulation, suppression, or discharge, when performed)

78013 Thyroid imaging (including vascular flow, when performed);

78014 with single or multiple uptake(s) quantitative measurement(s) (including stimulation, suppression, or discharge, when performed)

78015 Thyroid carcinoma metastases imaging; limited area (eg, neck and chest only)

78016 with additional studies (eg, urinary recovery)

78018 whole body

+ 78020 Thyroid carcinoma metastases uptake (List separately in addition to code for primary procedure)

(Use 78020 in conjunction with 78018 only)

78070 Parathyroid planar imaging (including subtraction, when performed);

78071 with tomographic (SPECT)

78072 with tomographic (SPECT), and concurrently acquired computed tomography (CT) for anatomical localization

78075 Adrenal imaging, cortex and/or medulla

78099 Unlisted endocrine procedure, diagnostic nuclear medicine

(For chemical analysis, see **Chemistry** section)

Hematopoietic, Reticuloendothelial and Lymphatic System

78102 Bone marrow imaging; limited area

78103 multiple areas

78104 whole body

78110 Plasma volume, radiopharmaceutical volume-dilution technique (separate procedure); single sampling

78111 multiple samplings

78120 Red cell volume determination (separate procedure); single sampling

78121 multiple samplings

78122 Whole blood volume determination, including separate measurement of plasma volume and red cell volume (radiopharmaceutical volume-dilution technique)

78130 Red cell survival study;

78135 differential organ/tissue kinetics (eg, splenic and/or hepatic sequestration)

78140 Labeled red cell sequestration, differential organ/tissue (eg, splenic and/or hepatic)

78185 Spleen imaging only, with or without vascular flow

(If combined with liver study, use procedures 78215 and 78216)

78190 Kinetics, study of platelet survival, with or without differential organ/tissue localization

78191 Platelet survival study

78195 Lymphatics and lymph nodes imaging

(For sentinel node identification without scintigraphy imaging, use 38792)

(For sentinel node excision, see 38500-38542)

78199 Unlisted hematopoietic, reticuloendothelial and lymphatic procedure, diagnostic nuclear medicine

(For chemical analysis, see **Chemistry** section)

Gastrointestinal System

78201 Liver imaging; static only

78202 with vascular flow

(For spleen imaging only, use 78185)

78205 Liver imaging (SPECT);

78206 with vascular flow

78215 Liver and spleen imaging; static only

78216 with vascular flow

(78220 has been deleted)

78226 Hepatobiliary system imaging, including gallbladder when present;

78227 with pharmacologic intervention, including quantitative measurement(s) when performed

78230 Salivary gland imaging;

78231 with serial images

78232 Salivary gland function study

78258 Esophageal motility

78261 Gastric mucosa imaging

78262 Gastroesophageal reflux study

Radiology

▲ **78264**   Gastric emptying imaging study (eg, solid, liquid, or both)

● **78265**   with small bowel transit

● **78266**   with small bowel and colon transit, multiple days

      ►(Report 78264, 78265, 78266 only once per imaging study)◄

78267   Urea breath test, C-14 (isotopic); acquisition for analysis

78268   analysis

     (For breath hydrogen or methane testing and analysis, use 91065)

78270   Vitamin B-12 absorption study (eg, Schilling test); without intrinsic factor

78271   with intrinsic factor

78272   Vitamin B-12 absorption studies combined, with and without intrinsic factor

78278   Acute gastrointestinal blood loss imaging

78282   Gastrointestinal protein loss

78290   Intestine imaging (eg, ectopic gastric mucosa, Meckel's localization, volvulus)

78291   Peritoneal-venous shunt patency test (eg, for LeVeen, Denver shunt)

     (For injection procedure, use 49427)

78299   Unlisted gastrointestinal procedure, diagnostic nuclear medicine

Musculoskeletal System

Bone and joint imaging can be used in the diagnosis of a variety of inflammatory processes (eg, osteomyelitis), as well as for localization of primary and/or metastatic neoplasms.

78300   Bone and/or joint imaging; limited area

78305   multiple areas

78306   whole body

78315   3 phase study

78320   tomographic (SPECT)

78350   Bone density (bone mineral content) study, 1 or more sites; single photon absorptiometry

78351   dual photon absorptiometry, 1 or more sites

78399   Unlisted musculoskeletal procedure, diagnostic nuclear medicine

Cardiovascular System

Myocardial perfusion and cardiac blood pool imaging studies may be performed at rest and/or during stress. When performed during exercise and/or pharmacologic stress, the appropriate stress testing code from the 93015-93018 series should be reported in addition to 78451-78454, 78472-78492.

78414   Determination of central c-v hemodynamics (non-imaging) (eg, ejection fraction with probe technique) with or without pharmacologic intervention or exercise, single or multiple determinations

78428   Cardiac shunt detection

78445   Non-cardiac vascular flow imaging (ie, angiography, venography)

78451   Myocardial perfusion imaging, tomographic (SPECT) (including attenuation correction, qualitative or quantitative wall motion, ejection fraction by first pass or gated technique, additional quantification, when performed); single study, at rest or stress (exercise or pharmacologic)

78452   multiple studies, at rest and/or stress (exercise or pharmacologic) and/or redistribution and/or rest reinjection

78453   Myocardial perfusion imaging, planar (including qualitative or quantitative wall motion, ejection fraction by first pass or gated technique, additional quantification, when performed); single study, at rest or stress (exercise or pharmacologic)

78454   multiple studies, at rest and/or stress (exercise or pharmacologic) and/or redistribution and/or rest reinjection

78456   Acute venous thrombosis imaging, peptide

78457   Venous thrombosis imaging, venogram; unilateral

78458   bilateral

78459   Myocardial imaging, positron emission tomography (PET), metabolic evaluation

     (For myocardial perfusion study, see 78491-78492)

     (78460-78465 have been deleted. To report, see 78451-78454)

78466   Myocardial imaging, infarct avid, planar; qualitative or quantitative

78468   with ejection fraction by first pass technique

78469   tomographic SPECT with or without quantification

     (For myocardial sympathetic innervation imaging, see 0331T, 0332T)

78472   Cardiac blood pool imaging, gated equilibrium; planar, single study at rest or stress (exercise and/or pharmacologic), wall motion study plus ejection fraction, with or without additional quantitative processing

     (For assessment of right ventricular ejection fraction by first pass technique, use 78496)

78473   multiple studies, wall motion study plus ejection fraction, at rest and stress (exercise and/or pharmacologic), with or without additional quantification

     (Do not report 78472, 78473 in conjunction with 78451-78454, 78481, 78483, 78494)

Radiology

(78478, 78480 have been deleted. To report, see 78451-78454)

78481   Cardiac blood pool imaging (planar), first pass technique; single study, at rest or with stress (exercise and/or pharmacologic), wall motion study plus ejection fraction, with or without quantification

78483   multiple studies, at rest and with stress (exercise and/or pharmacologic), wall motion study plus ejection fraction, with or without quantification

(For cerebral blood flow study, use 78610)

(Do not report 78481-78483 in conjunction with 78451-78454)

78491   Myocardial imaging, positron emission tomography (PET), perfusion; single study at rest or stress

78492   multiple studies at rest and/or stress

78494   Cardiac blood pool imaging, gated equilibrium, SPECT, at rest, wall motion study plus ejection fraction, with or without quantitative processing

+ 78496   Cardiac blood pool imaging, gated equilibrium, single study, at rest, with right ventricular ejection fraction by first pass technique (List separately in addition to code for primary procedure)

(Use 78496 in conjunction with 78472)

78499   Unlisted cardiovascular procedure, diagnostic nuclear medicine

Respiratory System

78579   Pulmonary ventilation imaging (eg, aerosol or gas)

78580   Pulmonary perfusion imaging (eg, particulate)

78582   Pulmonary ventilation (eg, aerosol or gas) and perfusion imaging

78597   Quantitative differential pulmonary perfusion, including imaging when performed

78598   Quantitative differential pulmonary perfusion and ventilation (eg, aerosol or gas), including imaging when performed

(Report 78579, 78580, 78582-78598 only once per imaging session)

(Do not report 78580, 78582-78598 in conjunction with 78451-78454)

78599   Unlisted respiratory procedure, diagnostic nuclear medicine

Nervous System

78600   Brain imaging, less than 4 static views;

78601   with vascular flow

78605   Brain imaging, minimum 4 static views;

78606   with vascular flow

78607   Brain imaging, tomographic (SPECT)

78608   Brain imaging, positron emission tomography (PET); metabolic evaluation

78609   perfusion evaluation

78610   Brain imaging, vascular flow only

78630   Cerebrospinal fluid flow, imaging (not including introduction of material); cisternography

(For injection procedure, see 61000-61070, 62270-62319)

78635   ventriculography

(For injection procedure, see 61000-61070, 62270-62294)

78645   shunt evaluation

(For injection procedure, see 61000-61070, 62270-62294)

78647   tomographic (SPECT)

78650   Cerebrospinal fluid leakage detection and localization

(For injection procedure, see 61000-61070, 62270-62294)

78660   Radiopharmaceutical dacryocystography

78699   Unlisted nervous system procedure, diagnostic nuclear medicine

Genitourinary System

78700   Kidney imaging morphology;

78701   with vascular flow

78707   with vascular flow and function, single study without pharmacological intervention

78708   with vascular flow and function, single study, with pharmacological intervention (eg, angiotensin converting enzyme inhibitor and/or diuretic)

78709   with vascular flow and function, multiple studies, with and without pharmacological intervention (eg, angiotensin converting enzyme inhibitor and/or diuretic)

▶(For introduction of radioactive substance in association with renal endoscopy, use 77778)◀

78710   tomographic (SPECT)

78725   Kidney function study, non-imaging radioisotopic study

+ 78730   Urinary bladder residual study (List separately in addition to code for primary procedure)

(Use 78730 in conjunction with 78740)

(For measurement of postvoid residual urine and/or bladder capacity by ultrasound, nonimaging, use 51798)

(For ultrasound imaging of the bladder only, with measurement of postvoid residual urine when performed, use 76857)

Radiology

78740 Ureteral reflux study (radiopharmaceutical voiding cystogram)

(Use 78740 in conjunction with 78730 for urinary bladder residual study)

(For catheterization, see 51701, 51702, 51703)

78761 Testicular imaging with vascular flow

78799 Unlisted genitourinary procedure, diagnostic nuclear medicine

(For chemical analysis, see **Chemistry** section)

Other Procedures

(For specific organ, see appropriate heading)

(For radiophosphorus tumor identification, ocular, see 78800)

78800 Radiopharmaceutical localization of tumor or distribution of radiopharmaceutical agent(s); limited area

(For specific organ, see appropriate heading)

78801 multiple areas

78802 whole body, single day imaging

78803 tomographic (SPECT)

78804 whole body, requiring 2 or more days imaging

78805 Radiopharmaceutical localization of inflammatory process; limited area

78806 whole body

78807 tomographic (SPECT)

(For imaging bone infectious or inflammatory disease with a bone imaging radiopharmaceutical, see 78300, 78305, 78306)

78808 Injection procedure for radiopharmaceutical localization by non-imaging probe study, intravenous (eg, parathyroid adenoma)

(For sentinel lymph node identification, use 38792)

(For PET of brain, see 78608, 78609)

(For PET myocardial imaging, see 78459, 78491, 78492)

78811 Positron emission tomography (PET) imaging; limited area (eg, chest, head/neck)

78812 skull base to mid-thigh

78813 whole body

78814 Positron emission tomography (PET) with concurrently acquired computed tomography (CT) for attenuation correction and anatomical localization imaging; limited area (eg, chest, head/neck)

78815 skull base to mid-thigh

78816 whole body

(Report 78811-78816 only once per imaging session)

(Computed tomography [CT] performed for other than attenuation correction and anatomical localization is reported using the appropriate site specific CT code with modifier 59)

(78890, 78891 have been deleted)

78999 Unlisted miscellaneous procedure, diagnostic nuclear medicine

Therapeutic

The oral and intravenous administration codes in this section are inclusive of the mode of administration. For intra-arterial, intra-cavitary, and intra-articular administration, also use the appropriate injection and/or procedure codes, as well as imaging guidance and radiological supervision and interpretation codes, when appropriate.

79005 Radiopharmaceutical therapy, by oral administration

(For monoclonal antibody therapy, use 79403)

79101 Radiopharmaceutical therapy, by intravenous administration

(Do not report 79101 in conjunction with 36400, 36410, 79403, 96360, 96374 or 96375, 96409)

(For radiolabeled monoclonal antibody by intravenous infusion, use 79403)

(For infusion or instillation of non-antibody radioelement solution that includes 3 months follow-up care, use 77750)

79200 Radiopharmaceutical therapy, by intracavitary administration

79300 Radiopharmaceutical therapy, by interstitial radioactive colloid administration

79403 Radiopharmaceutical therapy, radiolabeled monoclonal antibody by intravenous infusion

(For pre-treatment imaging, see 78802, 78804)

(Do not report 79403 in conjunction with 79101)

79440 Radiopharmaceutical therapy, by intra-articular administration

79445 Radiopharmaceutical therapy, by intra-arterial particulate administration

(Do not report 79445 in conjunction with 96373, 96420)

(Use appropriate procedural and radiological supervision and interpretation codes for the angiographic and interventional procedures provided prerequisite to intra-arterial radiopharmaceutical therapy)

79999 Radiopharmaceutical therapy, unlisted procedure

Pathology and Laboratory Guidelines

Guidelines to direct general reporting of services are presented in the **Introduction.** Some of the commonalities are repeated here for the convenience of those referring to this section on **Pathology and Laboratory.** Other definitions and items unique to Pathology and Laboratory are also listed.

Services in Pathology and Laboratory

Services in Pathology and Laboratory are provided by a physician or by technologists under responsible supervision of a physician.

Separate or Multiple Procedures

It is appropriate to designate multiple procedures that are rendered on the same date by separate entries.

Unlisted Service or Procedure

A service or procedure may be provided that is not listed in this edition of the CPT codebook. When reporting such a service, the appropriate "Unlisted Procedure" code may be used to indicate the service, identifying it by "Special Report" as discussed below. The "Unlisted Procedures" and accompanying codes for **Pathology and Laboratory** are as follows:

81099	Unlisted urinalysis procedure
# 81479	Unlisted molecular pathology procedure
81599	Unlisted multianalyte assay with algorithmic analysis
84999	Unlisted chemistry procedure
85999	Unlisted hematology and coagulation procedure
86486	Unlisted antigen, each
86849	Unlisted immunology procedure
86999	Unlisted transfusion medicine procedure
87999	Unlisted microbiology procedure
88099	Unlisted necropsy (autopsy) procedure
88199	Unlisted cytopathology procedure
88299	Unlisted cytogenetic study
88399	Unlisted surgical pathology procedure
88749	Unlisted in vivo (eg, transcutaneous) laboratory service
89240	Unlisted miscellaneous pathology test
89398	Unlisted reproductive medicine laboratory procedure

Special Report

A service that is rarely provided, unusual, variable, or new may require a special report. Pertinent information should include an adequate definition or description of the nature, extent, and need for the procedure; and the time, effort, and equipment necessary to provide the service.

Pathology and Laboratory

Organ or Disease-Oriented Panels

These panels were developed for coding purposes only and should not be interpreted as clinical parameters. The tests listed with each panel identify the defined components of that panel.

These panel components are not intended to limit the performance of other tests. If one performs tests in addition to those specifically indicated for a particular panel, those tests should be reported separately in addition to the panel code.

Do not report two or more panel codes that include any of the same constituent tests performed from the same patient collection. If a group of tests overlaps two or more panels, report the panel that incorporates the greater number of tests to fulfill the code definition and report the remaining tests using individual test codes (eg, do not report 80047 in conjunction with 80053).

80047   Basic metabolic panel (Calcium, ionized)

This panel must include the following:

Calcium, ionized (82330)

Carbon dioxide (bicarbonate) (82374)

Chloride (82435)

Creatinine (82565)

Glucose (82947)

Potassium (84132)

Sodium (84295)

Urea Nitrogen (BUN) (84520)

80048   Basic metabolic panel (Calcium, total)

This panel must include the following:

Calcium, total (82310)

Carbon dioxide (bicarbonate) (82374)

Chloride (82435)

Creatinine (82565)

Glucose (82947)

Potassium (84132)

Sodium (84295)

Urea nitrogen (BUN) (84520)

80050   General health panel

This panel must include the following:

Comprehensive metabolic panel (80053)

Blood count, complete (CBC), automated and automated differential WBC count (85025 or 85027 and 85004)

OR

Blood count, complete (CBC), automated (85027) and appropriate manual differential WBC count (85007 or 85009)

Thyroid stimulating hormone (TSH) (84443)

80051   Electrolyte panel

This panel must include the following:

Carbon dioxide (bicarbonate) (82374)

Chloride (82435)

Potassium (84132)

Sodium (84295)

80053   Comprehensive metabolic panel

This panel must include the following:

Albumin (82040)

Bilirubin, total (82247)

Calcium, total (82310)

Carbon dioxide (bicarbonate) (82374)

Chloride (82435)

Creatinine (82565)

Glucose (82947)

Phosphatase, alkaline (84075)

Potassium (84132)

Protein, total (84155)

Sodium (84295)

Transferase, alanine amino (ALT) (SGPT) (84460)

Transferase, aspartate amino (AST) (SGOT) (84450)

Urea nitrogen (BUN) (84520)

80055   Obstetric panel

This panel must include the following:

Blood count, complete (CBC), automated and automated differential WBC count (85025 or 85027 and 85004)

OR

Blood count, complete (CBC), automated (85027) and appropriate manual differential WBC count (85007 or 85009)

Hepatitis B surface antigen (HBsAg) (87340)

Antibody, rubella (86762)

Syphilis test, non-treponemal antibody; qualitative (eg, VDRL, RPR, ART) (86592)

Antibody screen, RBC, each serum technique (86850)

Blood typing, ABO (86900) AND

Blood typing, Rh (D) (86901)

(When syphilis screening is performed using a treponemal antibody approach [86780], do not use 80055. Use the individual codes for the tests performed in the Obstetric panel)

#● **80081**   Obstetric panel (includes HIV testing)

This panel must include the following:

Blood count, complete (CBC), and automated differential WBC count (85025 or 85027 and 85004)

OR

Blood count, complete (CBC), automated (85027) and appropriate manual differential WBC count (85007 or 85009)

Hepatitis B surface antigen (HBsAg) (87340)

HIV-1 antigen(s), with HIV-1 and HIV-2 antibodies, single result (87389)

Antibody, rubella (86762)

Syphilis test, non-treponemal antibody; qualitative (eg, VDRL, RPR, ART) (86592)

Antibody screen, RBC, each serum technique (86850)

Blood typing, ABO (86900) AND

Blood typing, Rh (D) (86901)

(When syphilis screening is performed using a treponemal antibody approach [86780], do not use 80081. Use the individual codes for the tests performed in the Obstetric panel)

80061   Lipid panel

This panel must include the following:

Cholesterol, serum, total (82465)

Lipoprotein, direct measurement, high density cholesterol (HDL cholesterol) (83718)

Triglycerides (84478)

80069   Renal function panel

This panel must include the following:

Albumin (82040)

Calcium, total (82310)

Carbon dioxide (bicarbonate) (82374)

Chloride (82435)

Creatinine (82565)

Glucose (82947)

Phosphorus inorganic (phosphate) (84100)

Potassium (84132)

Sodium (84295)

Urea nitrogen (BUN) (84520)

80074   Acute hepatitis panel

This panel must include the following:

Hepatitis A antibody (HAAb), IgM antibody (86709)

Hepatitis B core antibody (HBcAb), IgM antibody (86705)

Hepatitis B surface antigen (HBsAg) (87340)

Hepatitis C antibody (86803)

80076   Hepatic function panel

This panel must include the following:

Albumin (82040)

Bilirubin, total (82247)

Bilirubin, direct (82248)

Phosphatase, alkaline (84075)

Protein, total (84155)

Transferase, alanine amino (ALT) (SGPT) (84460)

Transferase, aspartate amino (AST) (SGOT) (84450)

80081   Code is out of numerical sequence. See 80047-80076

(80100, 80101, 80102, 80103, 80104 have been deleted. To report presumptive and/or definitive drug testing, see 80300, 80301, 80302, 80303, 80304)

Drug Assay

Drug procedures are divided into three subsections:

Therapeutic Drug Assay, **Drug Assay**, and **Chemistry**— with code selection dependent on the purpose and type of patient results obtained. Therapeutic Drug Assays are performed to monitor clinical response to a known, prescribed medication. The two major categories for drug testing in the Drug Assay subsection are:

1. **Presumptive Drug Class** procedures are used to identify possible use or non-use of a drug or drug class. A presumptive test may be followed by a definitive test in order to specifically identify drugs or metabolites.

2. **Definitive Drug Class** procedures are qualitative or quantitative test to identify possible use or non-use of a drug. These test identify specific drugs and associated metabolites, if performed. A presumptive test is not required prior to a definitive drug test.

The material for drug class procedures may be any specimen type unless otherwise specified in the code descriptor (eg, urine, blood, oral fluid, meconium, hair). Procedures can be qualitative (eg, positive/negative or present/absent), semi-quantitative, or quantitative (measured) depending on the purpose of the testing. Therapeutic drug assay (TDA) procedures are typically quantitative tests and the specimen type is whole blood, serum, plasma, or cerebrospinal fluid. *(continued on page 322)*

DEFINITIONS AND ACRONYM CONVERSION LISTING

Drug Testing Term/Acronym	Definition
6-MAM	Acronym for the heroin drug metabolite 6-monacetylmorphine
Acid	Descriptor for classifying drug/drug metabolite molecules based upon chemical ionization properties. Laboratory procedures for drug isolation and identification may include acid, base, or neutral groupings.
AM	A category of synthetic marijuana drugs discovered by and named after Alexandros Makriyannis at Northeastern University
Analog	A structural derivative of a parent chemical compound that often differs from it by a single element
Analyte	The substance or chemical constituent that is of interest in an analytical procedure
Base	Descriptor for classifying drug/drug metabolite molecules based upon chemical ionization properties. Laboratory procedures for drug isolation and identification may include acid, base, or neutral groupings.
Card(s)	Multiplexed presumptive drug class(es) immunoassay product that is read by visual observation, including instrumented when performed
Cassette(s)	Multiplexed presumptive drug class immunoassay product(s) that is read by visual observation, including instrumented when performed
CEDIA	Acronym for Cloned-Enzyme-Donor-Immuno-Assay. CEDIA immunoassay is a competitive antibody binding procedure that utilizes enzyme donor fragment-labeled antigens (drugs) to compete for antigens (drugs) contained in the patient sample. Recombination of enzyme donor fragment and enzyme acceptor fragment produces a functional enzyme. CEDIA immunoassay enzyme activity is proportional to concentration of drug(s) detected.
Chromatography	An analytical technique used to separate components of a mixture. See thin layer chromatography, gas chromatography, and high performance chromatography.
Confirmatory	Term used to describe definitive identification/quantitation procedures that are secondary to presumptive screening methods
DART	Acronym for Direct-Analysis-in-Real-Time. DART is an atmospheric pressure ionization method for mass spectrometry analysis
Definitive Drug Procedure	A procedure that provides specific identification of individual drugs and drug metabolites
DESI	Acronym for Desorption-ElectroSpray-Ionization. DESI is a combination of electrospray ionization and desorption ionization methods for mass spectrometry analysis.
Dipstick	A multiplexed presumptive drug class immunoassay product that is read by visual observation, including instrumented when performed
Drug test cup	A multiplexed presumptive drug class immunoassay product that is read by visual observation, including instrumented when performed
EDDP	Acronym for the methadone drug metabolite 2-ethylidene-1,5-dimethyl-3,3-diphenylpyrrolidine
EIA	Acronym for Enzyme-Immuno-Assay. Enzyme immunoassay is a competitive antibody binding procedure that utilizes enzyme-labeled antigens (drugs) to compete for antigens (drugs) contained in the patient sample. Enzyme immunoassay enzyme activity is proportional to concentration of drug(s) detected
ELISA	Acronym for Enzyme-Linked Immunosorbent Assay. ELISA is a competitive binding immunoassay that is design to measure antigens (drugs) or antibodies. ELISA immunoassay results are proportional to concentration of drug(s) detected.
EMIT	Acronym for Enzyme-Multiplied-Immunoassay-Test. EMIT is a trade name for a type of enzyme immunoassay (EIA).
FPIA	Acronym for Fluorescence-Polarization-Immuno-Assay. FPIA is a competitive binding immunoassay that utilizes fluorescein-labeled antigens (drugs) to compete for antigens (drugs) contained in the patient sample. The measure of polarized light emission is inversely proportional to the concentration of drug(s) detected.

Pathology and Laboratory

DEFINITIONS AND ACRONYM CONVERSION LISTING (Continued)

Drug Testing Term/Acronym	Definition
Gas chromatography	Gas chromatography is a chromatography technique in which patient sample preparations are vaporized into a gas (mobile phase) which flows through a tubular column (containing a stationary phase) and into a detector. The retention time of a drug on the column is determined by partitioning characteristics of the drug into the mobile and stationary phases. Chromatography column detectors may be non-specific (eg, flame ionization) or specific (eg, mass spectrometry). The combination of column retention time and specific detector response provides a definitive identification of the drug or drug metabolite.
GC	Acronym for gas chromatography
GC-MS	Acronym for gas chromatography mass spectrometry
GC-MS/MS	Acronym for gas chromatography mass spectrometry/mass spectrometry
High performance liquid chromatography	High performance liquid chromatography is a chromatography technique in which patient sample preparations are injected into a liquid (mobile phase) which flows through a tubular column (containing a stationary phase) and into a detector. The retention time of a drug on the column is determined by partitioning characteristics of the drug into the mobile and stationary phases. Chromatography column detectors may be non-specific (eg, ultra-violet spectrophotometry) or specific (eg, mass spectrometry). The combination of column retention time and specific detector response provides a definitive identification of the drug or drug metabolite. High performance liquid chromatography is also called high pressure liquid chromatography.
HPLC	Acronym for high performance liquid chromatography
HU	A category of synthetic marijuana drugs discovered by and named after Raphael Mechoulam at Hebrew University
IA	Acronym for immunoassay
Immunoassay	Antigen-antibody binding procedures utilized to detect antigens (eg, drugs and/or drug metabolites) in patient samples. Immunoassay designs include competitive or non-competitive with various mechanisms for detection.
Isobaric	In mass spectrometry, ions with the same mass
Isomers	Compounds that have the same molecular formula but differ in structural formula
JWH	A category of synthetic marijuana drugs discovered by and named after John W. Huffman at Clemson University.
KIMS	Acronym for kinetic interaction of microparticles in solution. KIMS immunoassay is a competitive antibody binding procedure that utilizes microparticle-labeled antigens (drugs) to compete for antigens (drugs) contained in the patient sample. Microparticle immunoassay absorbance increase is inversely proportional to concentration of drug(s) detected.
LC-MS	Acronym for liquid chromatography mass spectrometry
LC-MS/MS	Acronym for liquid chromatography mass spectrometry/mass spectrometry
LDTD	Acronym for laser diode thermal desorption. LDTD is a combination of atmospheric pressure chemical ionization and laser diode thermal desorption methods for mass spectrometry analysis.
MALDI	Acronym for matrix assisted laser desorption/Ionization mass spectrometry. MALDI is a soft ionization technique that reduces molecular fragmentation.
MDA	Acronym for the drug 3,4-methylenedioxyamphetamine. MDA is also a drug metabolite of MDMA.
MDEA	Acronym for the drug 3,4-methylenedioxy-N-ethylamphetamine
MDMA	Acronym for the drug 3,4-methylenedioxy-N-methylamphetamine
MDPV	Acronym for the drug methylenedioxypyrovalerone
MS	Acronym for mass spectrometry. MS is an identification technique that measures the charge-to-mass ratio of charged particles. There are several types of mass spectrometry instruments, such as magnetic sectoring, time of flight, quadrapole mass filter, ion traps, and Fourier transformation. Mass spectrometry is used as part of the process to assign definitive identification of drugs and drug metabolites.
MS/MS	Acronym for mass spectrometry/mass spectrometry. MS/MS instruments combine multiple units of mass spectrometry filters into a single instrument. MS/MS is also called tandem mass spectrometry.

Pathology and Laboratory

DEFINITIONS AND ACRONYM CONVERSION LISTING (Continued)

Drug Testing Term/Acronym	Definition
MS-TOF	Acronym for mass spectrometry time of flight. Time of flight is a mass spectrometry identification technique that utilizes ion velocity to determine the mass-to-charge ratio.
Multiplexed	Descriptor for a multiple component test device that simultaneously measures multiple analytes (drug classes) in a single analysis.
Neutral	Descriptor for classifying drug/drug metabolite molecules based upon chemical ionization properties. Laboratory procedures for drug isolation and identification may include acid, base, or neutral groupings.
ng/mL	Unit of measure for weight per volume calculated as nanograms per milliliter. The ng/mL unit of measure is equivalent to the ug/L unit of measure.
Optical observation	Optical observation refers to procedure results that are interpreted visually with or without instrumentation assistance.
Opiate	Medicinal category of narcotic alkaloid drugs that are natural products in the opium poppy plant *Papaver somniferum*. This immunoassay class of drugs typically includes detection of codeine, dihydrocodeine, hydrocodone, hydromorphone, and morphine.
Opioids	A category of medicinal synthetic or semi-synthetic narcotic alkaloid opioid receptor stimulating drugs including butorphanol, desomorphine, dextromethorphan, dextrorphan, levorphanol, meperidine, naloxone, naltrexone, normeperidine, and pentazocine.
Presumptive	Drug test results that indicate possible, but not definitive, presence of drugs and or drug metabolites
QTOF	Acronym for quadrapole-time of flight mass spectrometry. QTOF is a hybrid mass spectrometry identification technique that combines ion velocity with tandem quadrapole mass spectrometry (MS or MS/MS) to determine the mass-to-charge ratio.
RCS	A category of synthetic marijuana drugs that are analogs of JHW compounds. See JWH.
RIA	Acronym for radio-immuno-assay. Radioimmunoassay is a competitive antibody binding procedure that utilizes radioactive-labeled antigens (drugs) to compete for antigens (drugs) contained in the patient sample. The measure of radioactivity is inversely proportional to concentration of drug(s) detected.
Stereoisomers	Isomeric molecules that have the same molecular formula and sequence of bonded atoms (constitution), but that differ only in the three-dimensional orientations of their atoms in space
Substance	A substance is a drug that does not have an established therapeutic use as distinguished from other analytes listed in the Chemistry section (82000-84999).
TDM	Acronym for therapeutic drug monitoring
THC	Acronym for marijuana active drug ingredient tetrahydrocannabinol
Therapeutic Drug Monitoring	Analysis of blood (serum, plasma) drug concentration to monitor clinical response to therapy
Time of flight	Time of flight is a mass spectrometry technique that utilizes ion velocity to determine the mass-to-charge ratio
TLC	Acronym for thin layer chromatography
TOF	Acronym for time of flight
ug/L	Unit of measure for mass per volume calculated as micrograms per liter. The ug/L unit of measure is equivalent to the ng/mL unit of measure.

(continued from page 319)

When the same procedure(s) is performed on more than one specimen type (eg, blood and urine), the appropriate code is reported separately for each specimen type using modifier 59.

Drugs or classes of drugs may be commonly assayed first by a presumptive screening method followed by a definitive drug identification method. Presumptive methods include, but are not limited to, immunoassays (IA, EIA, ELISA, RIA, EMIT, FPIA, etc), enzymatic methods (alcohol dehydrogenase, etc), chromatographic methods without mass spectrometry (TLC, HPLC, GC, etc), or mass spectrometry without adequate drug resolution by chromatography (MS-TOF, DART, DESI, LDTD, MALDI). LC-MS, LCMS/MS, or mass spectrometry without adequate drug resolution by chromatography may also be used for presumptive testing if the chromatographic phase is not adequate to identify individual drugs and distinguish between structural isomers or isobaric compounds. All drug class immunoassays are considered presumptive, whether qualitative, semi-quantitative, or quantitative. Methods that cannot distinguish between structural isomers (such as morphine and hydromorphone or methamphetamine and phentermine) are also considered presumptive.

Definitive drug identification methods are able to identify individual drugs and distinguish between structural isomers but not necessarily stereoisomers. Definitive methods include, but are not limited to, gas chromatography with mass spectrometry (any type, single or tandem) and liquid chromatography mass spectrometry (any type, single or tandem) and excludes immunoassays (eg, IA, EIA, ELISA, RIA, EMIT, FPIA), and enzymatic methods (eg, alcohol dehydrogenase).

For chromatography, each combination of stationary and mobile phase is to be counted as one procedure.

Presumptive Drug Class Screening

Drugs or classes of drugs may be commonly assayed first by a presumptive screening method followed by a definitive drug identification method. The list of drug classes and the methodology are considered when coding presumptive procedures. If a drug class is not listed in List A or List B and it is not performed by TLC, use 80304 unless the specific analyte is listed in the Chemistry Section (82009-84830).

Drug Class List A

The following list contains drugs or classes of drugs that are commonly assayed by presumptive procedures. The methodology is typically one in which the results are capable of being read by direct optical observation, including instrument-assisted when performed (eg, dipsticks, cups, cards, cartridges), or by instrumented test systems (eg, discrete multichannel chemistry analyzers utilizing immunoassay or enzyme assay). These procedures may also be followed by a definitive procedure.

- Alcohol (Ethanol)
- Amphetamines
- Barbiturates
- Benzodiazepines
- Buprenorphine
- Cocaine metabolite
- Heroin metabolite (6-monoacetylmorphine)
- Methadone
- Methadone metabolite (EDDP)
- Methamphetamine
- Methaqualone

- Methylenedioxymethamphetamine (MDMA)
- Opiates
- Oxycodone
- Phencyclidine
- Propoxyphene
- Tetrahydrocannabinol (THC) metabolites (marijuana)
- Tricyclic Antidepressants

Drug Class List B

The following list contains drugs or classes of drugs that may be assayed by presumptive procedures. The methodology typically requires more resources than the drugs listed in Drug Class List A. The procedure may include drug class specific preanalytical sample preparation. It may be a manual process such as ELISA.

- Acetaminophen
- Carisoprodol/Meprobamate
- Ethyl Glucuronide
- Fentanyl
- Ketamine
- Meperidine
- Methylphenidate
- Nicotine/Cotinine
- Salicylate
- Synthetic Cannabinoids
- Tapentadol
- Tramadol
- Zolpidem
- Not otherwise specified

Use code 80300 to report single or multiple drug class procedures, other than TLC, using direct optical observation (eg, dipsticks, drug test cups, cassettes, and cards that are interpreted visually, with or without instrument assistance) for Class List A drug classes. Report 80300 once, irrespective of the number of direct observation drug class procedures or results on any date of service.

Use code 80301 to report single drug classes included in Drug Class List A, performed by methods other than direct optical observation or TLC, using discrete multichannel chemistry analyzers utilizing immunoassay or enzyme assay (eg, EIA, KIMS, CEDIA immunoassays) once per date of service. Use 80301 once to report single or multiple procedures performed, irrespective of the number of procedures, classes, or results on any date of service.

Use code 80302 to report presumptive, single drug classes other than those in Drug Class List A (ie, Drug Class List

B), other than direct optical observation or TLC, using immunoassays or chromatography without mass spectrometry, each drug class/procedure.

Use 80303 to report single or multiple drug procedures using thin layer chromatography (TLC), per day of service.

Use 80304 to report single or multiple drug screenings not specified elsewhere (eg, TOF, MALDI, LDTD, DESI, DART), per testing site, per date of service, each procedure.

80300   Drug screen, any number of drug classes from Drug Class List A; any number of non-TLC devices or procedures, (eg, immunoassay) capable of being read by direct optical observation, including instrumented-assisted when performed (eg, dipsticks, cups, cards, cartridges), per date of service

(Use 80303 for Drug Class List A analyte(s) performed by thin layer chromatography)

80301   single drug class method, by instrumented test systems (eg, discrete multichannel chemistry analyzers utilizing immunoassay or enzyme assay), per date of service

80302   Drug screen, presumptive, single drug class from Drug Class List B, by immunoassay (eg, ELISA) or non-TLC chromatography without mass spectrometry (eg, GC, HPLC), each procedure

(Use 80303 for Drug Class List A and List B analyte(s) performed by thin layer chromatography)

80303   Drug screen, any number of drug classes, presumptive, single or multiple drug class method; thin layer chromatography procedure(s) (TLC) (eg, acid, neutral, alkaloid plate), per date of service

80304   not otherwise specified presumptive procedure (eg, TOF, MALDI, LDTD, DESI, DART), each procedure

For example:

- To report five (5) presumptive drug classes performed using a direct optical observation device procedure (drug test cup or 5 separate dipsticks), report 80300 once per date of service.

- To report three (3) presumptive drug classes (Drug Class List A) performed using an automated chemistry analyzer, report 80301 once per facility, per date of service.

- To report thirteen (13) presumptive drug classes (Drug Class List A) performed using an automated chemistry analyzer, report 80301 once per facility, per date of service.

- To report two (2) presumptive drug classes (Drug Class List B) performed using a semi-automated analyzer, report 80302 X 2.

- To report two (2) multiple drug TLC procedures (one acid/neutral analysis for 10 drugs; one base analysis for 45 drugs), report 80303 X 1, per date of service.

- To report one (1) single drug procedure performed using TLC, report 80303 X 1, per date of service.

- To report three (3) multiple drug class procedures (one acid/neutral drug analysis; one base drug analysis; one ultra-sensitive base drug analysis) performed using time of flight (TOF) mass spectrometry (chromatography insufficient to provide definitive drug identification), report 80304 X 3.

Definitive Drug Testing

Definitive drug identification methods are able to identify individual drugs and distinguish between structural isomers but not necessarily stereoisomers. Definitive methods include, but are not limited to, gas chromatography with mass spectrometry (any type, single or tandem) and liquid chromatography mass spectrometry (any type, single or tandem) and exclude immunoassays (eg, IA, EIA, ELISA, RIA, EMIT, FPIA) and enzymatic methods (eg, alcohol dehydrogenase).

Use 80320-80377 to report definitive drug class procedures. Definitive testing may be qualitative, quantitative, or a combination of qualitative and quantitative for the same patient on the same date of service.

The **Definitive Drug Classes Listing** provides the drug classes, their associated CPT codes, and the drugs included in each class. Each category of a drug class, including metabolite(s) if performed (except stereoisomers), is reported once per date of service. Metabolites not listed in the table may be reported using the code for the parent drug. Drug class metabolite(s) is not reported separately unless the metabolite(s) is listed as a separate category in **Definitive Drug Classes Listing** (eg, heroin metabolite).

Drug classes may contain one or more codes based on the number of analytes. For example, an analysis in which five or more amphetamines and/or amphetamine metabolites would be reported with 80326. The code is based on the number of reported analytes and not the capacity of the analysis.

Definitive drug procedures that are not specified in 80320-80373 should be reported using the unlisted definitive procedure codes 80375, 80376, 80377, unless the specific analyte is listed in the **Therapeutic Drug Assays** (80150-80203) or **Chemistry** (82009-84830) sections.

See the **Definitive Drug Classes Listing** Table for a listing of the more common analytes within each drug class.

80320   Alcohols

80321   Alcohol biomarkers; 1 or 2

80322   3 or more

80323   Alkaloids, not otherwise specified

80324   Amphetamines; 1 or 2

80325   3 or 4

80326   5 or more

80327   Anabolic steroids; 1 or 2

80328   3 or more

80329   Analgesics, non-opioid; 1 or 2

80330   3-5

80331   6 or more

80332   Antidepressants, serotonergic class; 1 or 2

80333   3-5

80334   6 or more

80335   Antidepressants, tricyclic and other cyclicals; 1 or 2

80336   3-5

80337   6 or more

80338   Antidepressants, not otherwise specified

80339   Antiepileptics, not otherwise specified; 1-3

80340   4-6

80341   7 or more

(To report definitive drug testing for antihistamines, see 80375, 80376, 80377)

80342   Antipsychotics, not otherwise specified; 1-3

80343   4-6

80344   7 or more

80345   Barbiturates

80346   Benzodiazepines; 1-12

80347   13 or more

80348   Buprenorphine

80349   Cannabinoids, natural

80350   Cannabinoids, synthetic; 1-3

80351   4-6

80352   7 or more

80353   Cocaine

80354   Fentanyl

80355   Gabapentin, non-blood

(For therapeutic drug assay, use 80171)

80356   Heroin metabolite

80357   Ketamine and norketamine

80358   Methadone

80359   Methylenedioxyamphetamines (MDA, MDEA, MDMA)

80360   Methylphenidate

80361   Opiates, 1 or more

80362   Opioids and opiate analogs; 1 or 2

80363   3 or 4

80364   5 or more

80365   Oxycodone

83992   Phencyclidine (PCP)

(Phenobarbital, use 80345)

80366   Pregabalin

80367   Propoxyphene

80368   Sedative hypnotics (non-benzodiazepines)

80369   Skeletal muscle relaxants; 1 or 2

80370   3 or more

80371   Stimulants, synthetic

80372   Tapentadol

80373   Tramadol

80374   Stereoisomer (enantiomer) analysis, single drug class

(Use 80374 in conjunction with an index drug analysis, when performed)

80375   Drug(s) or substance(s), definitive, qualitative or quantitative, not otherwise specified; 1-3

80376   4-6

80377   7 or more

(To report definitive drug testing for antihistamines, see 80375, 80376, 80377)

For Example:

To report amphetamine and methamphetamine using any number of definitive procedures, report 80324 once per facility per date of service.

To report codeine, hydrocodone, hydromorphone, morphine using any number of definitive procedures, report 80361 once per facility per date of service.

To report codeine, hydrocodone, hydromorphone, morphine, oxycodone, oxymorphone, naloxone, naltrexone performed using any number of definitive procedures report 80361 X 1, 80362 X 1, and 80365 X 1 per facility per date of service.

To report benzoylecgonine, cocaine, carboxy-THC, meperidine, normeperidine using any number of definitive procedures, report 80349 X 1, 80353 X 1, and 80362 X 1 per facility per date of service.

Definitive Drug Classes Listing

Drugs and metabolites included in each definitive drug class are listed in the Definitive Drug Classes Listing table. This is not a comprehensive list. FDA classification of drugs not listed should be used where possible within the defined drug classes. Any metabolites that are not listed should be categorized with the parent drug. Drugs and metabolites not listed may be reported using codes from the Therapeutic Drug Assay (80150-80299) or Chemistry (82009-84999) sections.

Pathology and Laboratory

DEFINITIVE DRUG CLASSES LISTING

Codes	Classes	Drugs
80320	Alcohol(s)	Acetone, ethanol, ethchlorvynol, ethylene glycol, isopropanol, isopropyl alcohol, methanol
80321-80322	Alcohol Biomarkers	Ethanol conjugates (ethyl glucuronide [ETG], ethyl sulfate [ETS], fatty acid ethyl esters, phosphatidylethanol)
80323	Alkaloids, not otherwise specified	7-Hydroxymitragynine, atropine, cotinine, lysergic acid diethylamide (LSD), mescaline, mitragynine, nicotine, psilocin, psilocybin, scopolamine
80324-80326	Amphetamines	Amphetamine, ephedrinelisdexamphetamine, methamphetamine, phentermine, phenylpropanolamine, pseudoephedrine
80327-80328	Anabolic steroids	1-Androstenediol, 1-androstenedione, 1-testosterone, 4-hydroxy-testosterone, 6-oxo, 19-norandrostenedione, androstenedione, androstanolone, bolandiol, bolasterone, boldenone, boldione, calusterone, clostebol, danazol, dehydrochlormethyltestosterone, dihydrotestosterone, drostanolone, epiandrosterone, epitestosterone, fluoxymesterone, furazabol, mestanolone, mesterolone, methandienone, methandriol, methenolone, methydienolone, methyl-1-testosterone, methylnortestosterone, methyltestosterone, mibolerone, nandrolone, norbolethone, norclostebol, norethandrolone, norethindrone, oxabolone, oxandrolone, oxymesterone, oxymetholone, stanozolol, stenbolone, tibolone, trenbolone, zeranol
80329-80331	Analgesics, non-opioid	Acetaminophen, diclofenac ibuprofen, ketoprofen, naproxen, oxaprozin, salicylate
80332-80334	Antidepressants, serotonergic class	Citalopram, duloxetine, escitalopram, fluoxetine, fluvoxamine, paroxetine, sertraline
80335-80337	Antidepressants, Tricyclic and other cyclicals	Amitriptyline, amoxapine, clomipramine, demexiptiline, desipramine, doxepin, imipramine, maprotiline, mirtazpine, nortriptyline, protriptyline
80338	Antidepressants, not otherwise specified	Bupropion, desyenlafaxine, isocarboxazid, nefazodone, phenelzine, selegiline, tranylcypromine, trazodone, venlafaxine
80339-80341	Antiepileptics, not otherwise specified	Carbamazepine, clobazam, diamethadione, ethosuximide, ezogabine, lamotrigine, levetiracetam, methsuximide, oxcarbazepine, phenytoin, primidone, rufinamide, tiagabine, topiramate, trimethadione, valproic acid, zonisamide
80342-80344	Antipsychotics, not otherwise specified	Aripiprazole, chlorpromazine, clozapine, fluphenazine, haloperidol, loxapine, mesoridazine, molindone, olanzapine, paliperidone, perphenazine, phenothiazine, pimozide, prochlorperazine, quetiapine, risperidone, trifluoperazine, thiothixene, thoridazine, ziprasidone
80345	Barbiturates	Amobarbital, aprobarbital, butalbital, cyclobarbital, mephobarbital, pentobarbital, phenobarbital, secobarbital, talbutal, thiopental
80346, 80347	Benzodiazepines	Alprazolam, chlordiazepoxide, clonazepam, clorazepate, diazepam, estazolam, flunitrazepam, flurazepam, halazepamlorazepammidazolam, nitrazepam, nordazepam, oxazepam, prazepam, quazepam, temazepam
80348	Buprenorphine	Buprenorphine
80349	Cannabinoids, natural	Marijuana, dronabinol carboxy-THC
80350-80352	Cannabinoids, synthetic	CP-47,497, CP497 C8-homolog, JWH-018 and AM678, JWH-073, JWH-019, JWH-200, JWH-210, JWH-250, JWH-081, JWH-122, HWH-398, AM-2201, AM-694, SR-19 and RCS-4, SR-18 and RCS-8, JWH-203, UR-144, XLR-11, MAM-2201, AKB-48
80353	Cocaine	Benzoylecgonine, cocaethylene, cocaine, ecgonine methyl ester, norcocaine
80354	Fentanyls	Acetylfentanyl, alfentanil, fentanyl, remifentanil, sufentanil
80355	Gabapentin, non-blood	Gabapentin
80356	Heroin metabolite	6-acetylmorphine, acetylcodeine, diacetylmorphine
80368	Hypnotics, sedative (non-benzodiazepines)	See Sedative Hypnotics

DEFINITIVE DRUG CLASSES LISTING *(Continued)*

Codes	Classes	Drugs
80357	Ketamine and Norketamine	Ketamine, norketamine
80358	Methadone	Methadone and EDDP
80359	Methylenedioxyamphetamines	MDA, MDEA, MDMA
80360	Methylphenidate	Methylphenidate, ritalinic acid
80357	Norketamine	See Ketamine
80368	Non-Benzodiazepines	See Hypnotics, sedative
80361	Opiates	Codeine, dihydrocodeine, hydrocodone, hydromorphone, morphine
80362-80364	Opioids and opiate analogs	Butorphanol, desomorphine, dextromethorphan, dextrorphan, levorphanol, meperidine, naloxone, naltrexone, normeperidine, pentazocine
80365	Oxycodone	Oxycodone, oxymorphone
83992	Phencyclidine	Phencyclidine
80366	Pregabalin	Pregabalin
80367	Propoxyphene	Norpropoxyphene, propoxyphene
80368	Sedative Hypnotics (non-benzodiazepines)	Eszopiclone, zaleplon, zolpidem
80369, 80370	Skeletal muscle relaxants	Baclofen, carisoprodol, cyclobenzaprine, meprobamate, metaxalone, methocarbamol, orphenadrine, tizanidide
80371	Stimulants, synthetic	2C-B, 2C-E, 2C-I, 2C-H, 3TFMPP, 4-methylethcathinone, alpha-PVP, benzylpiperazine, bromodragonfly, cathinone, m-CPP, MDPBP, MDPPP, MDPV, mephedrone, methcathinone, methylone, phenethylamines, salvinorin, tryptamines
80372	Tapentadol	Tapentadol
80373	Tramadol	Tramadol

Therapeutic Drug Assays

Therapeutic Drug Assays are performed to monitor clinical response to a known, prescribed medication.

The material for examination is whole blood, serum, plasma, or cerebrospinal fluid. Examination is quantitative. Coding is by parent drug; measured metabolites of the drug are included in the code, if performed.

80150 Amikacin

(80152 has been deleted. To report definitive drug testing for amitryptyline, see 80335, 80336, 80337)

(80154 has been deleted. To report definitive drug testing for benzodiazepines, see 80346, 80347)

80155 Caffeine

80156 Carbamazepine; total

80157   free

80158 Cyclosporine

80159 Clozapine

(80160 has been deleted. To report definitive drug testing for desipramine, see 80335, 80336, 80337)

80162 Digoxin; total

80163   free

80164 Code is out of numerical sequence. See 80150-80299

80165 Code is out of numerical sequence. See 80150-80299

(80166 has been deleted. To report definitive drug testing for doxepin, see 80335, 80336, 80337)

80168 Ethosuximide

80169 Everolimus

 # 80171 Gabapentin, whole blood, serum, or plasma

80170 Gentamicin

80171 Code is out of numerical sequence. See 80150-80299

(80172 has been deleted. To report definitive drug testing for gold, use 80375)

80173 Haloperidol

(80174 has been deleted. To report testing for imipramine, see 80335, 80336, 80337)

80175 Lamotrigine

Pathology and Laboratory

80176	Lidocaine	80330	Code is out of numerical sequence. See 80076-80150
80177	Levetiracetam	80331	Code is out of numerical sequence. See 80076-80150
80178	Lithium	80332	Code is out of numerical sequence. See 80076-80150
80180	Mycophenolate (mycophenolic acid)	80333	Code is out of numerical sequence. See 80076-80150

(80182 has been deleted. To report definitive drug testing for nortriptyline, see 80335, 80336, 80337)

		80334	Code is out of numerical sequence. See 80076-80150
		80335	Code is out of numerical sequence. See 80076-80150
80183	Oxcarbazepine	80336	Code is out of numerical sequence. See 80076-80150
80184	Phenobarbital	80337	Code is out of numerical sequence. See 80076-80150
80185	Phenytoin; total	80338	Code is out of numerical sequence. See 80076-80150
80186	free	80339	Code is out of numerical sequence. See 80076-80150
80188	Primidone	80340	Code is out of numerical sequence. See 80076-80150
80190	Procainamide;	80341	Code is out of numerical sequence. See 80076-80150
80192	with metabolites (eg, n-acetyl procainamide)	80342	Code is out of numerical sequence. See 80076-80150
80194	Quinidine	80343	Code is out of numerical sequence. See 80076-80150
80195	Sirolimus	80344	Code is out of numerical sequence. See 80076-80150

(80196 has been deleted. To report definitive drug testing for salicylate, see 80329, 80330, 80331)

		80345	Code is out of numerical sequence. See 80076-80150
		80346	Code is out of numerical sequence. See 80076-80150
80197	Tacrolimus	80347	Code is out of numerical sequence. See 80076-80150
80198	Theophylline	80348	Code is out of numerical sequence. See 80076-80150
80199	Tiagabine	80349	Code is out of numerical sequence. See 80076-80150
80200	Tobramycin	80350	Code is out of numerical sequence. See 80076-80150
80201	Topiramate	80351	Code is out of numerical sequence. See 80076-80150
# 80164	Valproic acid (dipropylacetic acid); total	80352	Code is out of numerical sequence. See 80076-80150
# 80165	free	80353	Code is out of numerical sequence. See 80076-80150
80202	Vancomycin	80354	Code is out of numerical sequence. See 80076-80150
80203	Zonisamide	80355	Code is out of numerical sequence. See 80076-80150
80299	Quantitation of therapeutic drug, not elsewhere specified	80356	Code is out of numerical sequence. See 80076-80150
80300	Code is out of numerical sequence. See 80076-80150	80357	Code is out of numerical sequence. See 80076-80150
80301	Code is out of numerical sequence. See 80076-80150	80358	Code is out of numerical sequence. See 80076-80150
80302	Code is out of numerical sequence. See 80076-80150	80359	Code is out of numerical sequence. See 80076-80150
80303	Code is out of numerical sequence. See 80076-80150	80360	Code is out of numerical sequence. See 80076-80150
80304	Code is out of numerical sequence. See 80076-80150	80361	Code is out of numerical sequence. See 80076-80150
80320	Code is out of numerical sequence. See 80076-80150	80362	Code is out of numerical sequence. See 80076-80150
80321	Code is out of numerical sequence. See 80076-80150	80363	Code is out of numerical sequence. See 80076-80150
80322	Code is out of numerical sequence. See 80076-80150	80364	Code is out of numerical sequence. See 80076-80150
80323	Code is out of numerical sequence. See 80076-80150	80365	Code is out of numerical sequence. See 80076-80150
80324	Code is out of numerical sequence. See 80076-80150	80366	Code is out of numerical sequence. See 80076-80150
80325	Code is out of numerical sequence. See 80076-80150	80367	Code is out of numerical sequence. See 80076-80150
80326	Code is out of numerical sequence. See 80076-80150	80368	Code is out of numerical sequence. See 80076-80150
80327	Code is out of numerical sequence. See 80076-80150	80369	Code is out of numerical sequence. See 80076-80150
80328	Code is out of numerical sequence. See 80076-80150	80370	Code is out of numerical sequence. See 80076-80150
80329	Code is out of numerical sequence. See 80076-80150		

80371	Code is out of numerical sequence. See 80076-80150
80372	Code is out of numerical sequence. See 80076-80150
80373	Code is out of numerical sequence. See 80076-80150
80374	Code is out of numerical sequence. See 80076-80150
80375	Code is out of numerical sequence. See 80076-80150
80376	Code is out of numerical sequence. See 80076-80150
80377	Code is out of numerical sequence. See 80076-80150

Evocative/Suppression Testing

The following test panels involve the administration of evocative or suppressive agents and the baseline and subsequent measurement of their effects on chemical constituents. These codes are to be used for the reporting of the laboratory component of the overall testing protocol. For the administration of the evocative or suppressive agents, see Hydration, Therapeutic, Prophylactic, Diagnostic Injections and Infusions, and Chemotherapy and Other Highly Complex Drug or Highly Complex Biologic Agent Administration (eg, 96365, 96366, 96367, 96368, 96372, 96374, 96375, 96376). In the code descriptors where reference is made to a particular analyte (eg, Cortisol: 82533 x 2) the "x 2" refers to the number of times the test for that particular analyte is performed.

80400   ACTH stimulation panel; for adrenal insufficiency

This panel must include the following:

Cortisol (82533 x 2)

80402   for 21 hydroxylase deficiency

This panel must include the following:

Cortisol (82533 x 2)

17 hydroxyprogesterone (83498 x 2)

80406   for 3 beta-hydroxydehydrogenase deficiency

This panel must include the following:

Cortisol (82533 x 2)

17 hydroxypregnenolone (84143 x 2)

80408   Aldosterone suppression evaluation panel (eg, saline infusion)

This panel must include the following:

Aldosterone (82088 x 2)

Renin (84244 x 2)

80410   Calcitonin stimulation panel (eg, calcium, pentagastrin)

This panel must include the following:

Calcitonin (82308 x 3)

80412   Corticotropic releasing hormone (CRH) stimulation panel

This panel must include the following:

Cortisol (82533 x 6)

Adrenocorticotropic hormone (ACTH) (82024 x 6)

80414   Chorionic gonadotropin stimulation panel; testosterone response

This panel must include the following:

Testosterone (84403 x 2 on 3 pooled blood samples)

80415   estradiol response

This panel must include the following:

Estradiol (82670 x 2 on 3 pooled blood samples)

80416   Renal vein renin stimulation panel (eg, captopril)

This panel must include the following:

Renin (84244 x 6)

80417   Peripheral vein renin stimulation panel (eg, captopril)

This panel must include the following:

Renin (84244 x 2)

80418   Combined rapid anterior pituitary evaluation panel

This panel must include the following:

Adrenocorticotropic hormone (ACTH) (82024 x 4)

Luteinizing hormone (LH) (83002 x 4)

Follicle stimulating hormone (FSH) (83001 x 4)

Prolactin (84146 x 4)

Human growth hormone (HGH) (83003 x 4)

Cortisol (82533 x 4)

Thyroid stimulating hormone (TSH) (84443 x 4)

80420   Dexamethasone suppression panel, 48 hour

This panel must include the following:

Free cortisol, urine (82530 x 2)

Cortisol (82533 x 2)

Volume measurement for timed collection (81050 x 2)

(For single dose dexamethasone, use 82533)

80422   Glucagon tolerance panel; for insulinoma

This panel must include the following:

Glucose (82947 x 3)

Insulin (83525 x 3)

80424   for pheochromocytoma

This panel must include the following:

Catecholamines, fractionated (82384 x 2)

80426   Gonadotropin releasing hormone stimulation panel

This panel must include the following:

Follicle stimulating hormone (FSH) (83001 x 4)

Luteinizing hormone (LH) (83002 x 4)

80428   Growth hormone stimulation panel (eg, arginine infusion, l-dopa administration)

This panel must include the following:

Human growth hormone (HGH) (83003 x 4)

80430   Growth hormone suppression panel (glucose administration)

This panel must include the following:

Glucose (82947 x 3)

Human growth hormone (HGH) (83003 x 4)

80432   Insulin-induced C-peptide suppression panel

This panel must include the following:

Insulin (83525)

C-peptide (84681 x 5)

Glucose (82947 x 5)

80434   Insulin tolerance panel; for ACTH insufficiency

This panel must include the following:

Cortisol (82533 x 5)

Glucose (82947 x 5)

80435   for growth hormone deficiency

This panel must include the following:

Glucose (82947 x 5)

Human growth hormone (HGH) (83003 x 5)

80436   Metyrapone panel

This panel must include the following:

Cortisol (82533 x 2)

11 deoxycortisol (82634 x 2)

80438   Thyrotropin releasing hormone (TRH) stimulation panel; 1 hour

This panel must include the following:

Thyroid stimulating hormone (TSH) (84443 x 3)

80439   2 hour

This panel must include the following:

Thyroid stimulating hormone (TSH) (84443 x 4)

(80440 has been deleted. For prolactin, use 84146)

Consultations (Clinical Pathology)

A clinical pathology consultation is a service, including a written report, rendered by the pathologist in response to a request from a physician or qualified health care professional in relation to a test result(s) requiring additional medical interpretive judgment.

Reporting of a test result(s) without medical interpretive judgment is not considered a clinical pathology consultation.

80500   Clinical pathology consultation; limited, without review of patient's history and medical records

80502   comprehensive, for a complex diagnostic problem, with review of patient's history and medical records

(These codes may also be used for pharmacokinetic consultations)

(For consultations involving the examination and evaluation of the patient, see 99241-99255)

Urinalysis

For specific analyses, see appropriate section.

81000   Urinalysis, by dip stick or tablet reagent for bilirubin, glucose, hemoglobin, ketones, leukocytes, nitrite, pH, protein, specific gravity, urobilinogen, any number of these constituents; non-automated, with microscopy

81001   automated, with microscopy

81002   non-automated, without microscopy

81003   automated, without microscopy

81005   Urinalysis; qualitative or semiquantitative, except immunoassays

(For non-immunoassay reagent strip urinalysis, see 81000, 81002)

(For immunoassay, qualitative or semiquantitative, use 83518)

(For microalbumin, see 82043, 82044)

81007   bacteriuria screen, except by culture or dipstick

(For culture, see 87086-87088)

(For dipstick, use 81000 or 81002)

81015   microscopic only

(For sperm evaluation for retrograde ejaculation, use 89331)

81020   2 or 3 glass test

81025   Urine pregnancy test, by visual color comparison methods

81050   Volume measurement for timed collection, each

81099   Unlisted urinalysis procedure

Molecular Pathology

Molecular pathology procedures are medical laboratory procedures involving the analyses of nucleic acid to detect variants in genes that may be indicative of germline (eg, constitutional disorders) or somatic (eg, neoplasia) conditions, or to test for histocompatibility antigens (eg, HLA). Code selection is typically based on the specific gene(s) that is being analyzed. Genes are described using Human Genome Organization (HUGO) approved gene names and are italicized in the code descriptors. Gene names were taken from tables of the HUGO Gene Nomenclature Committee (HGNC) at the time the CPT codes were developed. For the most part, Human Genome Variation Society (HGVS) recommendations were followed for the names of specific molecular variants. The familiar name is used for some variants because defined criteria were not in place when the variant was first described or because HGVS recommendations were changed over time (eg, intronic variants, processed proteins). When the gene name is represented by an abbreviation, the abbreviation is listed first, followed by the full gene name italicized in parentheses (eg, "F5 *[coagulation Factor V]*"), except for the HLA series of codes. Proteins or diseases commonly associated with the genes are listed as examples in the code descriptors. The examples do not represent all conditions in which testing of the gene may be indicated.

Codes that describe tests to assess for the presence of gene variants (see definitions) use common gene variant names. Typically, all of the listed variants would be tested. However, these lists are not exclusive. If other variants are also tested in the analysis, they would be included in the procedure and not reported separately. Full gene sequencing should not be reported using codes that assess for the presence of gene variants unless specifically stated in the code descriptor.

The molecular pathology codes include all analytical services performed in the test (eg, cell lysis, nucleic acid stabilization, extraction, digestion, amplification, and detection). Any procedures required prior to cell lysis (eg, microdissection, codes 88380 and 88381) should be reported separately.

The results of the procedure may require interpretation by a physician or other qualified health care professional. When only the interpretation and report are performed, modifier 26 may be appended to the specific molecular pathology code.

All analyses are qualitative unless otherwise noted.

For microbial identification, see 87149-87153 and 87470-87801, and 87900-87904. For in situ hybridization analyses, see 88271-88275 and 88365-88368.

Molecular pathology procedures that are not specified in 81161, 81200-81383 should be reported using either the appropriate Tier 2 code (81400-81408) or the unlisted molecular pathology procedure code, 81479.

Definitions

For purposes of CPT reporting, the following definitions apply:

Abnormal allele: an alternative form of a gene that contains a disease-related variation from the normal sequence.

Breakpoint: the region at which a chromosome breaks during a translocation (defined elsewhere). These regions are often consistent for a given translocation.

Codon: a discrete unit of three nucleotides of a DNA or mRNA sequence that encodes a specific amino acid within, or signals the termination of, a polypeptide.

Common variants: variants (as defined elsewhere) that are associated with compromised gene function and are interrogated in a single round of laboratory testing (in a single, typically multiplex, assay format or using more than one assay to encompass all variants to be tested). These variants typically fit the definition of a "mutation," and are usually the predominant ones causing disease. Testing for additional uncommon variants may provide additional limited value in assessment of a patient. Often there are professional society recommendations or guidelines for which variants are most appropriate to test (eg, American College of Medical Genetics/American College of Obstetrics and Gynecology guidelines for variants used in population screening for cystic fibrosis).

Constitutional: synonymous with germline, often used in reference to the genetic code that is present at birth.

Cytogenomic: chromosome analysis using molecular techniques.

Duplication/Deletion (Dup/Del): terms that are usually used together with the "/" to refer to molecular testing, which assesses the dosage of a particular genomic region. The region tested is typically of modest to substantial size - from several dozen to several million or more nucleotides. Normal gene dosage is two copies per cell, except for the sex chromosomes (X and Y). Thus, zero or one copy represents a deletion, and three (or more) copies represent a duplication.

Dynamic mutation: polynucleotide (eg, trinucleotide) repeats that are in or associated with genes that can undergo disease-producing increases or decreases in the numbers of repeats within tissues and across generations.

Exome: DNA sequences within the human genome that code for proteins (coding regions).

Exon: typically, one of multiple nucleic acid sequences used to encode information for a gene product (polypeptide or protein). Exons are separated from each other by non-protein-coding sequences known as introns. Exons at the respective ends of a gene also contain nucleic acid sequence that does not code for the gene's protein product.

Gene: a nucleic acid sequence that typically contains information for coding a protein as well as for the regulated expression of that protein. Human genes usually contain multiple protein coding regions (exons) separated by non-protein coding regions (introns). See also *exon, intron,* and *polypeptide.*

Genome: The total (nuclear) human genetic content.

Heteroplasmy: The copy number of a variant within a cell; it is expressed as a percent. It reflects the varied distribution and dosage of mutant mitochondria in tissues and organs (mitotic segregation).

Intron: a nucleic acid sequence found between exons in human genes. An intron contains essential sequences for its proper removal (by a process known as *splicing*) to join exons together and thus facilitate production of a functional protein from a gene. An intron is sometimes referred to as an intervening sequence (IVS).

Inversion: A defect in a chromosome in which a segment breaks and reinserts in the same place but in the opposite orientation.

Loss of heterozygosity (LOH, allelic imbalance): An event that can occur in dividing cells that are heterozygous for one or more alleles, in which a daughter cell becomes hemizygous or homozygous for the allele(s) through mitotic recombination, deletion, or other chromosomal event.

Microarray: surface(s) on which multiple specific nucleic acid sequences are attached in a known arrangement. Sometimes referred to as a 'gene chip'. Examples of uses of microarrays include evaluation of a patient specimen for gains or losses of DNA sequences (copy number variants, CNVs), identification of the presence of specific nucleotide sequence variants (also known as single nucleotide polymorphisms, SNPs), mRNA expression levels, or DNA sequence analysis.

Mitochondrial DNA (mtDNA): DNA located in the mitochondria, which are cytoplasmic organelles involved with energy production. MtDNA contains 37 genes coding for oxidative phosphorylation enzymes, transfer RNAs (tRNAs) and ribosomal RNAs (rRNAs).

Mutations: typically are variants associated with altered gene function that lead to functional deficits or disease (pathogenic).

Mutation scanning: a technique (eg, single strand conformation polymorphism, temperature gradient gel electrophoresis, etc.) typically employed on multiple PCR amplicons to indicate the presence of DNA sequence variants by differences in physical properties compared to normal. Variants are then further characterized by DNA sequence analysis only in amplicons which demonstrate differences.

Nuclear DNA: DNA located in the nucleus of a cell, generally packaged in chromosomes.

Polymorphisms: typically are variants that do not compromise gene function or produce disease (benign).

Polypeptide: a sequence of amino acids covalently linked in a specified order. Polypeptides alone or in combination with other polypeptide subunits are the building blocks of proteins.

Short Tandem Repeat (STR): a region of DNA where a pattern of two or more nucleotides are repeated. The number of repeating segments can be used as genetic markers for human identity testing.

Single-nucleotide polymorphism (SNP): a DNA sequence variation existing at a significant frequency in the population, in which a single nucleotide (A, T, C, or G) differs between individuals and/or within an individual's paired chromosomes.

Somatic: synonymous with acquired, referring to genetic code alterations that develop after birth (eg, occurring in neoplastic cells).

Translocation: an abnormality resulting from the breakage of a chromosome and the relocation of a portion of that chromosome's DNA sequence to the same or another chromosome. Most common translocations involve a reciprocal exchange of DNA sequences between two differently numbered (ie, non-homologous) chromosomes, with or without a clinically significant loss of DNA.

Uniparental disomy (UPD): Abnormal inheritance of both members of a chromosome pair from one parent, with absence of the other parent's chromosome for the pair.

Variant: a nucleotide sequence difference from the "normal" (predominant) sequence for a given region. Variants are typically of two types: substitutions of one nucleotide for another, and deletions or insertions of nucleotides. Occasionally, variants reflect several nucleotide sequence changes in reasonably close proximity on the same chromosomal strand of DNA (a haplotype). These nucleotide sequence variants often result in amino acid changes in the protein made by the gene. The term *variant* does not itself carry a functional implication for those protein changes.

Variants in introns are typically described in one of two ways. The altered nucleotide(s) within a defined intervening sequence (eg, IVS3-2A>G) of a gene is listed with a "+" or "-" sign, which indicates the position relative to the first or last nucleotide of the intron. Or, the variant position is indicated relative to the last nucleotide of the preceding exon or first nucleotide of the following exon (eg, c.171+1G>A c.172-1G>T are single nucleotide changes at the first and last nucleotide of a given intron for a specific gene).

The majority of the variants described here are listed by the amino acid change using the single letter amino acid code for the original amino acid followed by the numerical position in the protein product and the amino acid substitution, eg, for *ASPA* E285A, Glutamic acid (E) at position 285 is replaced with an alanine (A). A few of the variants are described by the DNA change using the numerical position followed by the original nucleotide, a greater than sign (>) and the new nucleotide, eg, *MTHFR.* 677C>T.

A known familial variant is a specific mutation that has previously been identified within a patient's family.

Tier 1 Molecular Pathology Procedures

The following codes represent gene-specific and genomic procedures:

81161   Code is out of numerical sequence. See 81200-81383

81162   Code is out of numerical sequence. See 81170-81383

● **81170**   *ABL1 (ABL proto-oncogene 1, non-receptor tyrosine kinase)* (eg, acquired imatinib tyrosine kinase inhibitor resistance), gene analysis, variants in the kinase domain

81200   *ASPA (aspartoacylase)* (eg, Canavan disease) gene analysis, common variants (eg, E285A, Y231X)

81201   *APC (adenomatous polyposis coli)* (eg, familial adenomatosis polyposis [FAP], attenuated FAP) gene analysis; full gene sequence

81202   known familial variants

81203   duplication/deletion variants

81205   *BCKDHB (branched-chain keto acid dehydrogenase E1, beta polypeptide)* (eg, maple syrup urine disease) gene analysis, common variants (eg, R183P, G278S, E422X)

81206   *BCR/ABL1 (t(9;22))* (eg, chronic myelogenous leukemia) translocation analysis; major breakpoint, qualitative or quantitative

81207   minor breakpoint, qualitative or quantitative

81208   other breakpoint, qualitative or quantitative

81209   *BLM (Bloom syndrome, RecQ helicase-like)* (eg, Bloom syndrome) gene analysis, 2281del6ins7 variant

▲ **81210**   *BRAF (B-Raf proto-oncogene, serine/threonine kinase)* (eg, colon cancer, melanoma), gene analysis, V600 variant(s)

81211   *BRCA1, BRCA2 (breast cancer 1 and 2)* (eg, hereditary breast and ovarian cancer) gene analysis; full sequence analysis and common duplication/deletion variants in BRCA1 (ie, exon 13 del 3.835kb, exon 13 dup 6kb, exon 14-20 del 26kb, exon 22 del 510bp, exon 8-9 del 7.1kb)

▶(Do not report 81211 in conjunction with 81162)◀

#● **81162**   full sequence analysis and full duplication/deletion analysis

▶Do not report 81162 in conjunction with 81211, 81213, 81214, 81216)◀

81212   185delAG, 5385insC, 6174delT variants

81213   uncommon duplication/deletion variants

▶(Do not report 81213 in conjunction with 81162)◀

81214   *BRCA1 (breast cancer 1)* (eg, hereditary breast and ovarian cancer) gene analysis; full sequence analysis and common duplication/deletion variants (ie, exon 13 del 3.835kb, exon 13 dup 6kb, exon 14-20 del 26kb, exon 22 del 510bp, exon 8-9 del 7.1kb)

▶(When performing *BRCA1* full sequence analysis with *BRCA2* full sequence analysis, see 81162, 81211)◀

▶(Do not report 81214 in conjunction with 81162)◀

81215   known familial variant

81216   *BRCA2 (breast cancer 2)* (eg, hereditary breast and ovarian cancer) gene analysis; full sequence analysis

▶(When performing *BRCA2* full sequence analysis with *BRCA1* full sequence analysis, see 81162, 81211)◀

▶(Do not report 81216 in conjunction with 81162)◀

81217   known familial variant

● **81218**   *CEBPA (CCAAT/enhancer binding protein [C/EBP], alpha)* (eg, acute myeloid leukemia), gene analysis, full gene sequence

● **81219**   *CALR (calreticulin)* (eg, myeloproliferative disorders), gene analysis, common variants in exon 9

81220   *CFTR (cystic fibrosis transmembrane conductance regulator)* (eg, cystic fibrosis) gene analysis; common variants (eg, ACMG/ACOG guidelines)

(When Intron 8 poly-T analysis is performed in conjunction with 81220 in a R117H positive patient, do not report 81224)

81221   known familial variants

81222   duplication/deletion variants

81223   full gene sequence

81224   intron 8 poly-T analysis (eg, male infertility)

81225   *CYP2C19 (cytochrome P450, family 2, subfamily C, polypeptide 19)* (eg, drug metabolism), gene analysis, common variants (eg, *2, *3, *4, *8, *17)

81226   *CYP2D6 (cytochrome P450, family 2, subfamily D, polypeptide 6)* (eg, drug metabolism), gene analysis, common variants (eg, *2, *3, *4, *5, *6, *9, *10, *17, *19, *29, *35, *41, *1XN, *2XN, *4XN)

81227   *CYP2C9 (cytochrome P450, family 2, subfamily C, polypeptide 9)* (eg, drug metabolism), gene analysis, common variants (eg, *2, *3, *5, *6)

81228   Cytogenomic constitutional (genome-wide) microarray analysis; interrogation of genomic regions for copy number variants (eg, bacterial artificial chromosome [BAC] or oligo-based comparative genomic hybridization [CGH] microarray analysis)

81229   interrogation of genomic regions for copy number and single nucleotide polymorphism (SNP) variants for chromosomal abnormalities

(Do not report 81228 in conjunction with 81229)

(When performing cytogenomic constitutional microarray analysis that is not genome-wide [ie, regionally targeted], report the specific code for the targeted analysis if available [eg, 81405] or the unlisted molecular pathology code [81479])

Pathology and Laboratory

(Do not report analyte-specific molecular pathology procedures separately in conjunction with 81228, 81229 when the specific analytes are included as part of the microarray analysis)

(Do not report 88271 when performing cytogenomic microarray analysis)

\# **81161** *DMD (dystrophin)* (eg, Duchenne/Becker muscular dystrophy) deletion analysis, and duplication analysis, if performed

81235 *EGFR (epidermal growth factor receptor)* (eg, non-small cell lung cancer) gene analysis, common variants (eg, exon 19 LREA deletion, L858R, T790M, G719A, G719S, L861Q)

81240 *F2 (prothrombin, coagulation factor II)* (eg, hereditary hypercoagulability) gene analysis, 20210G>A variant

81241 *F5 (coagulation factor V)* (eg, hereditary hypercoagulability) gene analysis, Leiden variant

81242 *FANCC (Fanconi anemia, complementation group C)* (eg, Fanconi anemia, type C) gene analysis, common variant (eg, IVS4+4A>T)

81243 *FMR1 (fragile X mental retardation 1)* (eg, fragile X mental retardation) gene analysis; evaluation to detect abnormal (eg, expanded) alleles

(For evaluation to detect and characterize abnormal alleles, see 81243, 81244)

(For evaluation to detect and characterize abnormal alleles using a single assay [eg, PCR], use 81243)

81244 characterization of alleles (eg, expanded size and methylation status)

81245 *FLT3 (fms-related tyrosine kinase 3)* (eg, acute myeloid leukemia), gene analysis; internal tandem duplication (ITD) variants (ie, exons 14, 15)

81246 tyrosine kinase domain (TKD) variants (eg, D835, I836)

81250 *G6PC (glucose-6-phosphatase, catalytic subunit)* (eg, Glycogen storage disease, type 1a, von Gierke disease) gene analysis, common variants (eg, R83C, Q347X)

81251 *GBA (glucosidase, beta, acid)* (eg, Gaucher disease) gene analysis, common variants (eg, N370S, 84GG, L444P, IVS2+1G>A)

81252 *GJB2 (gap junction protein, beta 2, 26kDa, connexin 26)* (eg, nonsyndromic hearing loss) gene analysis; full gene sequence

81253 known familial variants

81254 *GJB6 (gap junction protein, beta 6, 30kDa, connexin 30)* (eg, nonsyndromic hearing loss) gene analysis, common variants (eg, 309kb [del(GJB6-D13S1830)] and 232kb [del(GJB6-D13S1854)])

81255 *HEXA (hexosaminidase A [alpha polypeptide])* (eg, Tay-Sachs disease) gene analysis, common variants (eg, 1278insTATC, 1421+1G>C, G269S)

81256 *HFE (hemochromatosis)* (eg, hereditary hemochromatosis) gene analysis, common variants (eg, C282Y, H63D)

81257 *HBA1/HBA2 (alpha globin 1 and alpha globin 2)* (eg, alpha thalassemia, Hb Bart hydrops fetalis syndrome, HbH disease), gene analysis, for common deletions or variant (eg, Southeast Asian, Thai, Filipino, Mediterranean, alpha3.7, alpha4.2, alpha20.5, and Constant Spring)

81260 *IKBKAP (inhibitor of kappa light polypeptide gene enhancer in B-cells, kinase complex-associated protein)* (eg, familial dysautonomia) gene analysis, common variants (eg, 2507+6T>C, R696P)

81261 *IGH@ (Immunoglobulin heavy chain locus)* (eg, leukemias and lymphomas, B-cell), gene rearrangement analysis to detect abnormal clonal population(s); amplified methodology (eg, polymerase chain reaction)

81262 direct probe methodology (eg, Southern blot)

81263 *IGH@ (Immunoglobulin heavy chain locus)* (eg, leukemia and lymphoma, B-cell), variable region somatic mutation analysis

81264 *IGK@ (Immunoglobulin kappa light chain locus)* (eg, leukemia and lymphoma, B-cell), gene rearrangement analysis, evaluation to detect abnormal clonal population(s)

(For immunoglobulin lambda gene [IGL@] rearrangement or immunoglobulin kappa deleting element, [IGKDEL] analysis, use 81479)

81265 Comparative analysis using Short Tandem Repeat (STR) markers; patient and comparative specimen (eg, pre-transplant recipient and donor germline testing, post-transplant non-hematopoietic recipient germline [eg, buccal swab or other germline tissue sample] and donor testing, twin zygosity testing, or maternal cell contamination of fetal cells)

+ 81266 each additional specimen (eg, additional cord blood donor, additional fetal samples from different cultures, or additional zygosity in multiple birth pregnancies) (List separately in addition to code for primary procedure)

(Use 81266 in conjunction with 81265)

81267 Chimerism (engraftment) analysis, post transplantation specimen (eg, hematopoietic stem cell), includes comparison to previously performed baseline analyses; without cell selection

81268 with cell selection (eg, CD3, CD33), each cell type

(If comparative STR analysis of recipient [using buccal swab or other germline tissue sample] and donor are performed after hematopoietic stem cell transplantation, report 81265, 81266 in conjunction with 81267, 81268 for chimerism testing)

81270 *JAK2 (Janus kinase 2)* (eg, myeloproliferative disorder) gene analysis, p.Val617Phe (V617F) variant

● **81272**   *KIT (v-kit Hardy-Zuckerman 4 feline sarcoma viral oncogene homolog)* (eg, gastrointestinal stromal tumor [GIST], acute myeloid leukemia, melanoma), gene analysis, targeted sequence analysis (eg, exons 8, 11, 13, 17, 18)

● **81273**   *KIT (v-kit Hardy-Zuckerman 4 feline sarcoma viral oncogene homolog)* (eg, mastocytosis), gene analysis, D816 variant(s)

▲ **81275**   *KRAS (Kirsten rat sarcoma viral oncogene homolog)* (eg, carcinoma) gene analysis; variants in exon 2 (eg, codons 12 and 13)

● **81276**   additional variant(s) (eg, codon 61, codon 146)

81280   Long QT syndrome gene analyses (eg, *KCNQ1, KCNH2, SCN5A, KCNE1, KCNE2, KCNJ2, CACNA1C, CAV3, SCN4B, AKAP, SNTA1, and ANK2)*; full sequence analysis

81281   known familial sequence variant

81282   duplication/deletion variants

81287   Code is out of numerical sequence. See 81200-81293

81288   Code is out of numerical sequence. See 81200-81293

81290   *MCOLN1 (mucolipin 1)* (eg, Mucolipidosis, type IV) gene analysis, common variants (eg, IVS3-2A>G, del6.4kb)

81287   *MGMT (O-6-methylguanine-DNA methyltransferase)* (eg, glioblastoma multiforme), methylation analysis

81291   *MTHFR (5,10-methylenetetrahydrofolate reductase)* (eg, hereditary hypercoagulability) gene analysis, common variants (eg, 677T, 1298C)

81292   *MLH1 (mutL homolog 1, colon cancer, nonpolyposis type 2)* (eg, hereditary non-polyposis colorectal cancer, Lynch syndrome) gene analysis; full sequence analysis

81288   promoter methylation analysis

81293   known familial variants

81294   duplication/deletion variants

81295   *MSH2 (mutS homolog 2, colon cancer, nonpolyposis type 1)* (eg, hereditary non-polyposis colorectal cancer, Lynch syndrome) gene analysis; full sequence analysis

81296   known familial variants

81297   duplication/deletion variants

81298   *MSH6 (mutS homolog 6 [E. coli])* (eg, hereditary non-polyposis colorectal cancer, Lynch syndrome) gene analysis; full sequence analysis

81299   known familial variants

81300   duplication/deletion variants

81301   Microsatellite instability analysis (eg, hereditary non-polyposis colorectal cancer, Lynch syndrome) of markers for mismatch repair deficiency (eg, BAT25, BAT26), includes comparison of neoplastic and normal tissue, if performed

81302   *MECP2 (methyl CpG binding protein 2)* (eg, Rett syndrome) gene analysis; full sequence analysis

81303   known familial variant

81304   duplication/deletion variants

81310   *NPM1 (nucleophosmin)* (eg, acute myeloid leukemia) gene analysis, exon 12 variants

● **81311**   *NRAS (neuroblastoma RAS viral [v-ras] oncogene homolog)* (eg, colorectal carcinoma), gene analysis, variants in exon 2 (eg, codons 12 and 13) and exon 3 (eg, codon 61)

81313   *PCA3/KLK3 (prostate cancer antigen 3 [non-protein coding]/kallikrein-related peptidase 3 [prostate specific antigen])* ratio (eg, prostate cancer)

● **81314**   *PDGFRA (platelet-derived growth factor receptor, alpha polypeptide)* (eg, gastrointestinal stromal tumor [GIST]), gene analysis, targeted sequence analysis (eg, exons 12, 18)

81315   *PML/RARalpha, (t(15;17)), (promyelocytic leukemia/ retinoic acid receptor alpha)* (eg, promyelocytic leukemia) translocation analysis; common breakpoints (eg, intron 3 and intron 6), qualitative or quantitative

81316   single breakpoint (eg, intron 3, intron 6 or exon 6), qualitative or quantitative

(For intron 3 and intron 6 [including exon 6 if performed] analysis, use 81315)

(If both intron 6 and exon 6 are analyzed, without intron 3, use one unit of 81316)

81317   *PMS2 (postmeiotic segregation increased 2 [S. cerevisiae])* (eg, hereditary non-polyposis colorectal cancer, Lynch syndrome) gene analysis; full sequence analysis

81318   known familial variants

81319   duplication/deletion variants

81321   *PTEN (phosphatase and tensin homolog)* (eg, Cowden syndrome, *PTEN* hamartoma tumor syndrome) gene analysis; full sequence analysis

81322   known familial variant

81323   duplication/deletion variant

81324   *PMP22 (peripheral myelin protein 22)* (eg, Charcot-Marie-Tooth, hereditary neuropathy with liability to pressure palsies) gene analysis; duplication/deletion analysis

81325   full sequence analysis

81326   known familial variant

81330   *SMPD1(sphingomyelin phosphodiesterase 1, acid lysosomal)* (eg, Niemann-Pick disease, Type A) gene analysis, common variants (eg, R496L, L302P, fsP330)

81331   *SNRPN/UBE3A (small nuclear ribonucleoprotein polypeptide N and ubiquitin protein ligase E3A)* (eg, Prader-Willi syndrome and/or Angelman syndrome), methylation analysis

Pathology and Laboratory

81332   *SERPINA1 (serpin peptidase inhibitor, clade A, alpha-1 antiproteinase, antitrypsin, member 1)* (eg, alpha-1-antitrypsin deficiency), gene analysis, common variants (eg, *S and *Z)

81340   *TRB@ (T cell antigen receptor, beta)* (eg, leukemia and lymphoma), gene rearrangement analysis to detect abnormal clonal population(s); using amplification methodology (eg, polymerase chain reaction)

81341   using direct probe methodology (eg, Southern blot)

81342   *TRG@ (T cell antigen receptor, gamma)* (eg, leukemia and lymphoma), gene rearrangement analysis, evaluation to detect abnormal clonal population(s)

        (For T cell antigen alpha [*TRA@*] gene rearrangement analysis, use 81479)

        (For T cell antigen delta [*TRD@*] gene rearrangement analysis, use 81402)

81350   *UGT1A1 (UDP glucuronosyltransferase 1 family, polypeptide A1)* (eg, irinotecan metabolism), gene analysis, common variants (eg, *28, *36, *37)

▲ 81355   *VKORC1 (vitamin K epoxide reductase complex, subunit 1)* (eg, warfarin metabolism), gene analysis, common variant(s) (eg, -1639G>A, c.173+1000C>T)

Human Leukocyte Antigen (HLA) typing is performed to assess compatibility of recipients and potential donors as a part of solid organ and hematopoietic stem cell pretransplant testing. HLA testing is also performed to identify HLA alleles and allele groups (antigen equivalents) associated with specific diseases and individualized responses to drug therapy (eg, HLA-B*27 and ankylosing spondylitis and HLA-B*57:01 and abacavir hypersensitivity), as well as other clinical uses. One or more HLA genes may be tested in specific clinical situations (eg, HLA-DQB1 for narcolepsy and HLA-A, -B, -C, -DRB1, and -DQB1 for kidney transplantation). Each HLA gene typically has multiple variant alleles or allele groups that can be identified by typing. For HLA result reporting, a low resolution HLA type is denoted by a two digit HLA name (eg, A*02) and intermediate resolution typing by a string of alleles or an NMDP (National Marrow Donor Program) code (eg, B*14:01/07N/08/12/14, B*39CKGN). Both low and intermediate resolutions are considered low resolution for code assignment. High resolution typing resolves the common well defined (CWD) alleles and is usually denoted by at least 4 digits (eg, A*02:02, *03:01:01:01, A*26:01:01G, and C*03:04P), however, high resolution typing may include some ambiguities for rare alleles, which may be reported as a string of alleles or an NMDP code.

If additional testing is required to resolve ambiguous allele combinations for high resolution typing, this is included in the base HLA typing codes below. The gene names have been italicized similar to the other molecular pathology codes.

        (For HLA antigen typing by non-molecular pathology techniques, see 86812-86822)

81370   HLA Class I and II typing, low resolution (eg, antigen equivalents); *HLA-A, -B, -C, -DRB1/3/4/5,* and *-DQB1*

81371   *HLA-A, -B,* and *-DRB1* (eg, verification typing)

        (When HLA typing includes a determination of the presence or absence of the DRB3/4/5 genes, that service is included in the typing and is not separately reported)

81372   HLA Class I typing, low resolution (eg, antigen equivalents); complete *(ie, HLA-A, -B,* and *-C)*

        (When performing both Class I and II low resolution *HLA typing for HLA-A,-B,-C, -DRB1/3/4/5,* and *-DQB1,* use 81370)

81373   one locus *(eg, HLA-A, -B, or -C),* each

        (When performing a complete Class I *[HLA-A,-B,* and *-C]* low resolution HLA typing, use 81372)

        (When the presence or absence of a single antigen equivalent is reported using low resolution testing, use 81374)

81374   one antigen equivalent (eg, *B*27*), each

        (When testing for presence or absence of more than 2 antigen equivalents at a locus, use 81373 for each locus tested)

81375   HLA Class II typing, low resolution (eg, antigen equivalents); *HLA-DRB1/3/4/5* and *-DQB1*

        (When performing both Class I and II low resolution HLA typing *for HLA-A,-B,-C, -DRB1/3/4/5,* and *–DQB1,* use 81370)

81376   one locus *(eg, HLA-DRB1, -DRB3/4/5, -DQB1, -DQA1, -DPB1, or -DPA1),* each

        (When low resolution typing is performed for *HLA-DRB1/3/4/5* and *-DQB1,* use 81375)

        (When HLA typing includes a determination of the presence or absence of the DRB3/4/5 genes, that service is included in the typing and is not separately reported. When low or intermediate resolution typing of any or all of the DRB3/4/5 genes is performed, treat as one locus)

81377   one antigen equivalent, each

        (When testing for presence or absence of more than 2 antigen equivalents at a locus, use 81376 for each locus)

81378   HLA Class I and II typing, high resolution (ie, alleles or allele groups), *HLA-A, -B, -C,* and *-DRB1*

81379   HLA Class I typing, high resolution (ie, alleles or allele groups); complete (ie, *HLA-A, -B,* and *-C)*

81380   one locus (eg, *HLA-A, -B,* or *-C),* each

        (When a complete Class I high resolution typing for *HLA-A,-B,* and *-C* is performed, use 81379)

        (When the presence or absence of a single allele or allele group is reported using high resolution testing, use 81381)

81381   one allele or allele group (eg, *B*57:01P*), each

(When testing for the presence or absence of more than 2 alleles or allele groups at a locus, use 81380 for each locus)

81382   HLA Class II typing, high resolution (ie, alleles or allele groups); one locus (eg, *HLA-DRB1, -DRB3/4/5, -DQB1, -DQA1, -DPB1,* or *-DPA1*), each

(When only the presence or absence of a single allele or allele group is reported using high resolution testing, use 81383)

(When high resolution typing of any or all of the DRB3/4/5 genes is performed, treat as one locus)

81383   one allele or allele group (eg, *HLA-DQB1*06:02P*), each

(When testing for the presence or absence of more than 2 alleles or allele groups at a locus, use 81382 for each locus)

Tier 2 Molecular Pathology Procedures

The following molecular pathology procedure (Tier 2) codes are used to report procedures not listed in the Tier 1 molecular pathology codes (81161, 81200-81383). They represent medically useful procedures that are generally performed in lower volumes than Tier 1 procedures (eg, the incidence of the disease being tested is rare). They are arranged by level of technical resources and interpretive work by the physician or other qualified health care professional. The individual analyses listed under each code (ie, level of procedure) utilize the definitions and coding principles as described in the introduction preceding the Tier 1 molecular pathology codes. The parenthetical examples of methodologies presented near the beginning of each code provide general guidelines used to group procedures for a given level and are not all-inclusive.

Use the appropriate molecular pathology procedure level code that includes the specific analyte listed after the code descriptor. If the analyte tested is not listed under one of the Tier 2 codes or is not represented by a Tier 1 code, use the unlisted molecular pathology procedure code, 81479.

81400   Molecular pathology procedure, Level 1 (eg, identification of single germline variant [eg, SNP] by techniques such as restriction enzyme digestion or melt curve analysis)

ACADM (acyl-CoA dehydrogenase, C-4 to C-12 straight chain, MCAD) (eg, medium chain acyl dehydrogenase deficiency), K304E variant

ACE (angiotensin converting enzyme) (eg, hereditary blood pressure regulation), insertion/deletion variant

AGTR1 (angiotensin II receptor, type 1) (eg, essential hypertension), 1166A>C variant

BCKDHA (branched chain keto acid dehydrogenase E1, alpha polypeptide) (eg, maple syrup urine disease, type 1A), Y438N variant

CCR5 (chemokine C-C motif receptor 5) (eg, HIV resistance), 32-bp deletion mutation/794 825del32 deletion

CLRN1 (clarin 1) (eg, Usher syndrome, type 3), N48K variant

DPYD (dihydropyrimidine dehydrogenase) (eg, 5-fluorouracil/5-FU and capecitabine drug metabolism), IVS14+1G>A variant

F2 (coagulation factor 2) (eg, hereditary hypercoagulability), 1199G>A variant

F5 (coagulation factor V) (eg, hereditary hypercoagulability), HR2 variant

F7 (coagulation factor VII [serum prothrombin conversion accelerator]) (eg, hereditary hypercoagulability), R353Q variant

F13B (coagulation factor XIII, B polypeptide) (eg, hereditary hypercoagulability), V34L variant

FGB (fibrinogen beta chain) (eg, hereditary ischemic heart disease), -455G>A variant

FGFR1 (fibroblast growth factor receptor 1) (eg, Pfeiffer syndrome type 1, craniosynostosis), P252R variant

FGFR3 (fibroblast growth factor receptor 3) (eg, Muenke syndrome), P250R variant

FKTN (fukutin) (eg, Fukuyama congenital muscular dystrophy), retrotransposon insertion variant

GNE (glucosamine [UDP-N-acetyl]-2-epimerase/N-acetylmannosamine kinase) (eg, inclusion body myopathy 2 [IBM2], Nonaka myopathy), M712T variant

Human Platelet Antigen 1 genotyping (HPA-1), ITGB3 (integrin, beta 3 [platelet glycoprotein IIIa], antigen CD61 [GPIIIa]) (eg, neonatal alloimmune thrombocytopenia [NAIT], post-transfusion purpura), HPA-1a/b (L33P)

Human Platelet Antigen 2 genotyping (HPA-2), GP1BA (glycoprotein Ib [platelet], alpha polypeptide [GPIba]) (eg, neonatal alloimmune thrombocytopenia [NAIT], post-transfusion purpura), HPA-2a/b (T145M)

Human Platelet Antigen 3 genotyping (HPA-3), ITGA2B (integrin, alpha 2b [platelet glycoprotein IIb of IIb/IIIa complex], antigen CD41 [GPIIb]) (eg, neonatal alloimmune thrombocytopenia [NAIT], post-transfusion purpura), HPA-3a/b (I843S)

Human Platelet Antigen 4 genotyping (HPA-4), ITGB3 (integrin, beta 3 [platelet glycoprotein IIIa], antigen CD61 [GPIIIa]) (eg, neonatal alloimmune thrombocytopenia [NAIT], post-transfusion purpura), HPA-4a/b (R143Q)

Human Platelet Antigen 5 genotyping (HPA-5), ITGA2 (integrin, alpha 2 [CD49B, alpha 2 subunit of VLA-2 receptor] [GPIa]) (eg, neonatal alloimmune thrombocytopenia [NAIT], post-transfusion purpura), HPA-5a/b (K505E)

Human Platelet Antigen 6 genotyping (HPA-6w), ITGB3 (integrin, beta 3 [platelet glycoprotein IIIa, antigen CD61] [GPIIIa]) (eg, neonatal alloimmune thrombocytopenia [NAIT], post-transfusion purpura), HPA-6a/b (R489Q)

Human Platelet Antigen 9 genotyping (HPA-9w), ITGA2B (integrin, alpha 2b [platelet glycoprotein IIb of IIb/IIIa complex, antigen CD41] [GPIIb]) (eg, neonatal alloimmune thrombocytopenia [NAIT], post-transfusion purpura), HPA-9a/b (V837M)

Human Platelet Antigen 15 genotyping (HPA-15), CD109 (CD109 molecule) (eg, neonatal alloimmune thrombocytopenia [NAIT], post-transfusion purpura), HPA-15a/b (S682Y)

IL28B (interleukin 28B [interferon, lambda 3]) (eg, drug response), rs12979860 variant

IVD (isovaleryl-CoA dehydrogenase) (eg, isovaleric acidemia), A282V variant

LCT (lactase-phlorizin hydrolase) (eg, lactose intolerance), 13910 C>T variant

NEB (nebulin) (eg, nemaline myopathy 2), exon 55 deletion variant

PCDH15 (protocadherin-related 15) (eg, Usher syndrome type 1F), R245X variant

SERPINE1 (serpine peptidase inhibitor clade E, member 1, plasminogen activator inhibitor -1, PAI-1) (eg, thrombophilia), 4G variant

SHOC2 (soc-2 suppressor of clear homolog) (eg, Noonan-like syndrome with loose anagen hair), S2G variant

SLCO1B1 (solute carrier organic anion transporter family, member 1B1) (eg, adverse drug reaction), V174A variant

SMN1 (survival of motor neuron 1, telomeric) (eg, spinal muscular atrophy), exon 7 deletion

SRY (sex determining region Y) (eg, 46,XX testicular disorder of sex development, gonadal dysgenesis), gene analysis

TOR1A (torsin family 1, member A [torsin A]) (eg, early-onset primary dystonia [DYT1]), 907_909delGAG (904_906delGAG) variant

▲ **81401** Molecular pathology procedure, Level 2 (eg, 2-10 SNPs, 1 methylated variant, or 1 somatic variant [typically using nonsequencing target variant analysis], or detection of a dynamic mutation disorder/triplet repeat)

ABCC8 (ATP-binding cassette, sub-family C [CFTR/MRP], member 8) (eg, familial hyperinsulinism), common variants (eg, c.3898-9G>A [c.3992-9G>A], F1388del)

►*ABL1 (ABL proto-oncogene 1, non-receptor tyrosine kinase) (eg, acquired imatinib resistance), T315I variant*◄

ACADM (acyl-CoA dehydrogenase, C-4 to C-12 straight chain, MCAD) (eg, medium chain acyl dehydrogenase deficiency), commons variants (eg, K304E, Y42H)

ADRB2 (adrenergic beta-2 receptor surface) (eg, drug metabolism), common variants (eg, G16R, Q27E)

AFF2 (AF4/FMR2 family, member 2 [FMR2]) (eg, fragile X mental retardation 2 [FRAXE]), evaluation to detect abnormal (eg, expanded) alleles

APOB (apolipoprotein B) (eg, familial hypercholesterolemia type B), common variants (eg, R3500Q, R3500W)

*APOE (apolipoprotein E) (eg, hyperlipoproteinemia type III, cardiovascular disease, Alzheimer disease), common variants (eg, *2, *3, *4)*

AR (androgen receptor) (eg, spinal and bulbar muscular atrophy, Kennedy disease, X chromosome inactivation), characterization of alleles (eg, expanded size or methylation status)

ATN1 (atrophin 1) (eg, dentatorubral-pallidoluysian atrophy), evaluation to detect abnormal (eg, expanded) alleles

ATXN1 (ataxin 1) (eg, spinocerebellar ataxia), evaluation to detect abnormal (eg, expanded) alleles

ATXN2 (ataxin 2) (eg, spinocerebellar ataxia), evaluation to detect abnormal (eg, expanded) alleles

ATXN3 (ataxin 3) (eg, spinocerebellar ataxia, Machado-Joseph disease), evaluation to detect abnormal (eg, expanded) alleles

ATXN7 (ataxin 7) (eg, spinocerebellar ataxia), evaluation to detect abnormal (eg, expanded) alleles

ATXN8OS (ATXN8 opposite strand [non-protein coding]) (eg, spinocerebellar ataxia), evaluation to detect abnormal (eg, expanded) alleles

ATXN10 (ataxin 10) (eg, spinocerebellar ataxia), evaluation to detect abnormal (eg, expanded) alleles

CACNA1A (calcium channel, voltage-dependent, P/Q type, alpha 1A subunit) (eg, spinocerebellar ataxia), evaluation to detect abnormal (eg, expanded) alleles

CBFB/MYH11 (inv(16)) (eg, acute myeloid leukemia), qualitative, and quantitative, if performed

CBS (cystathionine-beta-synthase) (eg, homocystinuria, cystathionine beta-synthase deficiency), common variants (eg, I278T, G307S)

CCND1/IGH (BCL1/IgH, t(11;14)) (eg, mantle cell lymphoma) translocation analysis, major breakpoint, qualitative, and quantitative, if performed

CFH/ARMS2 (complement factor H/age-related maculopathy susceptibility 2) (eg, macular degeneration), common variants (eg, Y402H [CFH], A69S [ARMS2])

CNBP (CCHC-type zinc finger, nucleic acid binding protein) (eg, myotonic dystrophy type 2), evaluation to detect abnormal (eg, expanded) alleles

CSTB (cystatin B [stefin B]) (eg, Unverricht-Lundborg disease), evaluation to detect abnormal (eg, expanded) alleles

CYP3A4 *(cytochrome P450, family 3, subfamily A, polypeptide 4)* (eg, drug metabolism), common variants (eg, *2, *3, *4, *5, *6)

CYP3A5 *(cytochrome P450, family 3, subfamily A, polypeptide 5)* (eg, drug metabolism), common variants (eg, *2, *3, *4, *5, *6)

▶DEK/NUP214 *(t(6;9))* (eg, acute myeloid leukemia), translocation analysis, qualitative, and quantitative, if performed◀

DMPK *(dystrophia myotonica-protein kinase)* (eg, myotonic dystrophy, type 1), evaluation to detect abnormal (eg, expanded) alleles

E2A/PBX1 *(t(1;19))* (eg, acute lymphocytic leukemia), translocation analysis, qualitative, and quantitative, if performed

EML4/ALK *(inv(2))* (eg, non-small cell lung cancer), translocation or inversion analysis

ETV6/NTRK3 *(t(12;15))* (eg, congenital/infantile fibrosarcoma), translocation analysis, qualitative, and quantitative, if performed

ETV6/RUNX1 *(t(12;21))* (eg, acute lymphocytic leukemia), translocation analysis, qualitative, and quantitative, if performed

EWSR1/ATF1 *(t(12;22))* (eg, clear cell sarcoma), translocation analysis, qualitative, and quantitative, if performed

EWSR1/ERG *(t(21;22))* (eg, Ewing sarcoma/peripheral neuroectodermal tumor), translocation analysis, qualitative, and quantitative, if performed

EWSR1/FLI1 *(t(11;22))* (eg, Ewing sarcoma/peripheral neuroectodermal tumor), translocation analysis, qualitative, and quantitative, if performed

EWSR1/WT1 *(t(11;22))* (eg, desmoplastic small round cell tumor), translocation analysis, qualitative, and quantitative, if performed

F11 *(coagulation factor XI)* (eg, coagulation disorder), common variants (eg, E117X [Type II], F283L [Type III], IVS14del14, and IVS14+1G>A [Type I])

FGFR3 *(fibroblast growth factor receptor 3)* (eg, achondroplasia, hypochondroplasia), common variants (eg, 1138G>A, 1138G>C, 1620C>A, 1620C>G)

FIP1L1/PDGFRA *(del(4q12))* (eg, imatinib-sensitive chronic eosinophilic leukemia), qualitative, and quantitative, if performed

FLG *(filaggrin)* (eg, icthyosis vulgaris), common variants (eg, R501X, 2282del4, R2447X, S3247X, 3702delG)

FOXO1/PAX3 *(t(2;13))* (eg, alveolar rhabdomyosarcoma), translocation analysis, qualitative, and quantitative, if performed

FOXO1/PAX7 *(t(1;13))* (eg, alveolar rhabdomyosarcoma), translocation analysis, qualitative, and quantitative, if performed

FUS/DDIT3 *(t(12;16))* (eg, myxoid liposarcoma), translocation analysis, qualitative, and quantitative, if performed

FXN *(frataxin)* (eg, Friedreich ataxia), evaluation to detect abnormal (expanded) alleles

GALC *(galactosylceramidase)* (eg, Krabbe disease), common variants (eg, c.857G>A, 30-kb deletion)

GALT *(galactose-1-phosphate uridylyltransferase)* (eg, galactosemia), common variants (eg, Q188R, S135L, K285N, T138M, L195P, Y209C, IVS2-2A>G, P171S, del5kb, N314D, L218L/N314D)

H19 *(imprinted maternally expressed transcript [non-protein coding])* (eg, Beckwith-Wiedemann syndrome), methylation analysis

HBB *(hemoglobin, beta)* (eg, sickle cell anemia, hemoglobin C, hemoglobin E), common variants (eg, HbS, HbC, HbE)

HTT *(huntingtin)* (eg, Huntington disease), evaluation to detect abnormal (eg, expanded) alleles

▶IGH@/BCL2 *(t(14;18))* (eg, follicular lymphoma), translocation analysis; single breakpoint (eg, major breakpoint region [MBR] or minor cluster region [mcr]), qualitative or quantitative◀

▶(When both MBR and mcr breakpoints are performed, use 81402)◀

KCNQ1OT1 *(KCNQ1 overlapping transcript 1 [non-protein coding])* (eg, Beckwith-Wiedemann syndrome), methylation analysis

LRRK2 *(leucine-rich repeat kinase 2)* (eg, Parkinson disease), common variants (eg, R1441G, G2019S, I2020T)

MED12 *(mediator complex subunit 12)* (eg, FG syndrome type 1, Lujan syndrome), common variants (eg, R961W, N1007S)

MEG3/DLK1 *(maternally expressed 3 [non-protein coding]/delta-like 1 homolog [Drosophila])* (eg, intrauterine growth retardation), methylation analysis

MLL/AFF1 *(t(4;11))* (eg, acute lymphoblastic leukemia), translocation analysis, qualitative, and quantitative, if performed

MLL/MLLT3 *(t(9;11))* (eg, acute myeloid leukemia), translocation analysis, qualitative, and quantitative, if performed

MT-ATP6 *(mitochondrially encoded ATP synthase 6)* (eg, neuropathy with ataxia and retinitis pigmentosa [NARP], Leigh syndrome), common variants (eg, m.8993T>G, m.8993T>C)

MT-ND4, MT-ND6 *(mitochondrially encoded NADH dehydrogenase 4, mitochondrially encoded NADH dehydrogenase 6)* (eg, Leber hereditary optic neuropathy [LHON]), common variants (eg, m.11778G>A, m.3460G>A, m.14484T>C)

MT-ND5 (mitochondrially encoded tRNA leucine 1 [UUA/G], mitochondrially encoded NADH dehydrogenase 5) (eg, mitochondrial encephalopathy with lactic acidosis and stroke-like episodes [MELAS]), common variants (eg, m.3243A>G, m.3271T>C, m.3252A>G, m.13513G>A)

MT-RNR1 (mitochondrially encoded 12S RNA) (eg, nonsyndromic hearing loss), common variants (eg, m.1555A>G, m.1494C>T)

MT-TK (mitochondrially encoded tRNA lysine) (eg, myoclonic epilepsy with ragged-red fibers [MERRF]), common variants (eg, m.8344A>G, m.8356T>C)

MT-TL1 (mitochondrially encoded tRNA leucine 1 [UUA/G]) (eg, diabetes and hearing loss), common variants (eg, m.3243A>G, m.14709 T>C) MT-TL1

MT-TS1, MT-RNR1 (mitochondrially encoded tRNA serine 1 [UCN], mitochondrially encoded 12S RNA) (eg, nonsyndromic sensorineural deafness [including aminoglycoside-induced nonsyndromic deafness]), common variants (eg, m.7445A>G, m.1555A>G)

MUTYH (mutY homolog [E. coli]) (eg, MYH-associated polyposis), common variants (eg, Y165C, G382D)

NOD2 (nucleotide-binding oligomerization domain containing 2) (eg, Crohn's disease, Blau syndrome), common variants (eg, SNP 8, SNP 12, SNP 13)

NPM1/ALK (t(2;5)) (eg, anaplastic large cell lymphoma), translocation analysis

PABPN1 (poly[A] binding protein, nuclear 1) (eg, oculopharyngeal muscular dystrophy), evaluation to detect abnormal (eg, expanded) alleles

PAX8/PPARG (t(2;3) (q13;p25)) (eg, follicular thyroid carcinoma), translocation analysis

PPP2R2B (protein phosphatase 2, regulatory subunit B, beta) (eg, spinocerebellar ataxia), evaluation to detect abnormal (eg, expanded) alleles

PRSS1 (protease, serine, 1 [trypsin 1]) (eg, hereditary pancreatitis), common variants (eg, N29I, A16V, R122H)

PYGM (phosphorylase, glycogen, muscle) (eg, glycogen storage disease type V, McArdle disease), common variants (eg, R50X, G205S)

RUNX1/RUNX1T1 (t(8;21)) (eg, acute myeloid leukemia) translocation analysis, qualitative, and quantitative, if performed

SEPT9 (septin 9) (eg, colon cancer), methylation analysis

SMN1/SMN2 (survival of motor neuron 1, telomeric/ survival of motor neuron 2, centromeric) (eg, spinal muscular atrophy), dosage analysis (eg, carrier testing)

(For duplication/deletion analysis of SMN1/SMN2, use 81401)

SS18/SSX1 (t(X;18)) (eg, synovial sarcoma), translocation analysis, qualitative, and quantitative, if performed

SS18/SSX2 (t(X;18)) (eg, synovial sarcoma), translocation analysis, qualitative, and quantitative, if performed

TBP (TATA box binding protein) (eg, spinocerebellar ataxia), evaluation to detect abnormal (eg, expanded) alleles

TPMT (thiopurine S-methyltransferase) (eg, drug metabolism), common variants (eg, *2, *3)

TYMS (thymidylate synthetase) (eg, 5-fluorouracil/5-FU drug metabolism), tandem repeat variant

VWF (von Willebrand factor) (eg, von Willebrand disease type 2N), common variants (eg, T791M, R816W, R854Q)

▲ 81402 Molecular pathology procedure, Level 3 (eg, >10 SNPs, 2-10 methylated variants, or 2-10 somatic variants [typically using non-sequencing target variant analysis], immunoglobulin and T-cell receptor gene rearrangements, duplication/deletion variants of 1 exon, loss of heterozygosity [LOH], uniparental disomy [UPD])

Chromosome 1p-/19q- (eg, glial tumors), deletion analysis

Chromosome 18q- (eg, D18S55, D18S58, D18S61, D18S64, and D18S69) (eg, colon cancer), allelic imbalance assessment (ie, loss of heterozygosity)

COL1A1/PDGFB (t(17;22)) (eg, dermatofibrosarcoma protuberans), translocation analysis, multiple breakpoints, qualitative, and quantitative, if performed

CYP21A2 (cytochrome P450, family 21, subfamily A, polypeptide 2) (eg, congenital adrenal hyperplasia, 21-hydroxylase deficiency), common variants (eg, IVS2-13G, P30L, I172N, exon 6 mutation cluster [I235N, V236E, M238K], V281L, L307FfsX6, Q318X, R356W, P453S, G110VfsX21, 30-kb deletion variant)

ESR1/PGR (receptor 1/progesterone receptor) ratio (eg, breast cancer)

IGH@/BCL2 (t(14;18)) (eg, follicular lymphoma), translocation analysis; major breakpoint region (MBR) and minor cluster region (mcr) breakpoints, qualitative or quantitative

MEFV (Mediterranean fever) (eg, familial Mediterranean fever), common variants (eg, E148Q, P369S, F479L, M680I, I692del, M694V, M694I, K695R, V726A, A744S, R761H)

MPL (myeloproliferative leukemia virus oncogene, thrombopoietin receptor, TPOR) (eg, myeloproliferative disorder), common variants (eg, W515A, W515K, W515L, W515R)

TRD@ (T cell antigen receptor, delta) (eg, leukemia and lymphoma), gene rearrangement analysis, evaluation to detect abnormal clonal population

Uniparental disomy (UPD) (eg, Russell-Silver syndrome, Prader-Willi/Angelman syndrome), short tandem repeat (STR) analysis

▲ 81403 Molecular pathology procedure, Level 4 (eg, analysis of single exon by DNA sequence analysis, analysis of >10 amplicons using multiplex PCR in 2 or more independent reactions, mutation scanning or duplication/deletion variants of 2-5 exons)

ANG (angiogenin, ribonuclease, RNase A family, 5) (eg, amyotrophic lateral sclerosis), full gene sequence

ARX (aristaless-related homeobox) (eg, X-linked lissencephaly with ambiguous genitalia, X-linked mental retardation), duplication/deletion analysis

CEL (carboxyl ester lipase [bile salt-stimulated lipase]) (eg, maturity-onset diabetes of the young [MODY]), targeted sequence analysis of exon 11 (eg, c.1785delC, c.1686delT)

CTNNB1 (catenin [cadherin-associated protein], beta 1, 88kDa) (eg, desmoid tumors), targeted sequence analysis (eg, exon 3)

DAZ/SRY (deleted in azoospermia and sex determining region Y) (eg, male infertility), common deletions (eg, AZFa, AZFb, AZFc, AZFd)

DNMT3A (DNA [cytosine-5-]-methyltransferase 3 alpha) (eg, acute myeloid leukemia), targeted sequence analysis (eg, exon 23)

EPCAM (epithelial cell adhesion molecule) (eg, Lynch syndrome), duplication/deletion analysis

F8 (coagulation factor VIII) (eg, hemophilia A), inversion analysis, intron 1 and intron 22A

F12 (coagulation factor XII [Hageman factor]) (eg, angioedema, hereditary, type III; factor XII deficiency), targeted sequence analysis of exon 9

FGFR3 (fibroblast growth factor receptor 3) (eg, isolated craniosynostosis), targeted sequence analysis (eg, exon 7)

(For targeted sequence analysis of multiple FGFR3 exons, use 81404)

GJB1 (gap junction protein, beta 1) (eg, Charcot-Marie-Tooth X-linked), full gene sequence

GNAQ (guanine nucleotide-binding protein G[q] subunit alpha) (eg, uveal melanoma), common variants (eg, R183, Q209)

HBB (hemoglobin, beta, beta-globin) (eg, beta thalassemia), duplication/deletion analysis

Human erythrocyte antigen gene analyses (eg, SLC14A1 [Kidd blood group], BCAM [Lutheran blood group], ICAM4 [Landsteiner-Wiener blood group], SLC4A1 [Diego blood group], AQP1 [Colton blood group], ERMAP [Scianna blood group], RHCE [Rh blood group, CcEe antigens], KEL [Kell blood group], DARC [Duffy blood group], GYPA, GYPB, GYPE [MNS blood group], ART4 [Dombrock blood group]) (eg, sickle-cell disease, thalassemia, hemolytic transfusion reactions, hemolytic disease of the fetus or newborn), common variants

HRAS (v-Ha-ras Harvey rat sarcoma viral oncogene homolog) (eg, Costello syndrome), exon 2 sequence

IDH1 (isocitrate dehydrogenase 1 [NADP+], soluble) (eg, glioma), common exon 4 variants (eg, R132H, R132C)

IDH2 (isocitrate dehydrogenase 2 [NADP+], mitochondrial) (eg, glioma), common exon 4 variants (eg, R140W, R172M)

JAK2 (Janus kinase 2) (eg, myeloproliferative disorder), exon 12 sequence and exon 13 sequence, if performed

KCNC3 (potassium voltage-gated channel, Shaw-related subfamily, member 3) (eg, spinocerebellar ataxia), targeted sequence analysis (eg, exon 2)

KCNJ2 (potassium inwardly-rectifying channel, subfamily J, member 2) (eg, Andersen-Tawil syndrome), full gene sequence

KCNJ11 (potassium inwardly-rectifying channel, subfamily J, member 11) (eg, familial hyperinsulinism), full gene sequence

Killer cell immunoglobulin-like receptor (KIR) gene family (eg, hematopoietic stem cell transplantation), genotyping of KIR family genes

Known familial variant not otherwise specified, for gene listed in Tier 1 or Tier 2, DNA sequence analysis, each variant exon

(For a known familial variant that is considered a common variant, use specific common variant Tier 1 or Tier 2 code)

MC4R (melanocortin 4 receptor) (eg, obesity), full gene sequence

MICA (MHC class I polypeptide-related sequence A) (eg, solid organ transplantation), common variants (eg, *001, *002)

MPL (myeloproliferative leukemia virus oncogene, thrombopoietin receptor, TPOR) (eg, myeloproliferative disorder), exon 10 sequence

MT-RNR1 (mitochondrially encoded 12S RNA) (eg, nonsyndromic hearing loss), full gene sequence

MT-TS1 (mitochondrially encoded tRNA serine 1) (eg, nonsyndromic hearing loss), full gene sequence

NDP (Norrie disease [pseudoglioma]) (eg, Norrie disease), duplication/deletion analysis

NHLRC1 (NHL repeat containing 1) (eg, progressive myoclonus epilepsy), full gene sequence

PHOX2B (paired-like homeobox 2b) (eg, congenital central hypoventilation syndrome), duplication/deletion analysis

PLN (phospholamban) (eg, dilated cardiomyopathy, hypertrophic cardiomyopathy), full gene sequence

RHD (Rh blood group, D antigen) (eg, hemolytic disease of the fetus and newborn, Rh maternal/fetal compatibility), deletion analysis (eg, exons 4, 5, and 7, pseudogene)

RHD (Rh blood group, D antigen) (eg, hemolytic disease of the fetus and newborn, Rh maternal/fetal compatibility), deletion analysis (eg, exons 4, 5, and 7, pseudogene), performed on cell-free fetal DNA in maternal blood

Pathology and Laboratory

(For human erythrocyte gene analysis of RHD, use a separate unit of 81403)

SH2D1A (SH2 domain containing 1A) (eg, X-linked lymphoproliferative syndrome), duplication/deletion analysis

SMN1 (survival of motor neuron 1, telomeric) (eg, spinal muscular atrophy), known familial sequence variant(s)

TWIST1 (twist homolog 1 [Drosophila]) (eg, Saethre-Chotzen syndrome), duplication/deletion analysis

UBA1 (ubiquitin-like modifier activating enzyme 1) (eg, spinal muscular atrophy, X-linked), targeted sequence analysis (eg, exon 15)

VHL (von Hippel-Lindau tumor suppressor) (eg, von Hippel-Lindau familial cancer syndrome), deletion/duplication analysis

VWF (von Willebrand factor) (eg, von Willebrand disease types 2A, 2B, 2M), targeted sequence analysis (eg, exon 28)

▲ **81404** Molecular pathology procedure, Level 5 (eg, analysis of 2-5 exons by DNA sequence analysis, mutation scanning or duplication/deletion variants of 6-10 exons, or characterization of a dynamic mutation disorder/triplet repeat by Southern blot analysis)

ACADS (acyl-CoA dehydrogenase, C-2 to C-3 short chain) (eg, short chain acyl-CoA dehydrogenase deficiency), targeted sequence analysis (eg, exons 5 and 6)

AFF2 (AF4/FMR2 family, member 2 [FMR2]) (eg, fragile X mental retardation 2 [FRAXE]), characterization of alleles (eg, expanded size and methylation status)

AQP2 (aquaporin 2 [collecting duct]) (eg, nephrogenic diabetes insipidus), full gene sequence

ARX (aristaless related homeobox) (eg, X-linked lissencephaly with ambiguous genitalia, X-linked mental retardation), full gene sequence

AVPR2 (arginine vasopressin receptor 2) (eg, nephrogenic diabetes insipidus), full gene sequence

BBS10 (Bardet-Biedl syndrome 10) (eg, Bardet-Biedl syndrome), full gene sequence

BTD (biotinidase) (eg, biotinidase deficiency), full gene sequence

C10orf2 (chromosome 10 open reading frame 2) (eg, mitochondrial DNA depletion syndrome), full gene sequence

CAV3 (caveolin 3) (eg, CAV3-related distal myopathy, limb-girdle muscular dystrophy type 1C), full gene sequence

CD40LG (CD40 ligand) (eg, X-linked hyper IgM syndrome), full gene sequence

CDKN2A (cyclin-dependent kinase inhibitor 2A) (eg, CDKN2A-related cutaneous malignant melanoma, familial atypical mole-malignant melanoma syndrome), full gene sequence

CLRN1 (clarin 1) (eg, Usher syndrome, type 3), full gene sequence

COX6B1 (cytochrome c oxidase subunit VIb polypeptide 1) (eg, mitochondrial respiratory chain complex IV deficiency), full gene sequence

CPT2 (carnitine palmitoyltransferase 2) (eg, carnitine palmitoyltransferase II deficiency), full gene sequence

CRX (cone-rod homeobox) (eg, cone-rod dystrophy 2, Leber congenital amaurosis), full gene sequence

CSTB (cystatin B [stefin B]) (eg, Unverricht-Lundborg disease), full gene sequence

CYP1B1 (cytochrome P450, family 1, subfamily B, polypeptide 1) (eg, primary congenital glaucoma), full gene sequence

DMPK (dystrophia myotonica-protein kinase) (eg, myotonic dystrophy type 1), characterization of abnormal (eg, expanded) alleles

EGR2 (early growth response 2) (eg, Charcot-Marie-Tooth), full gene sequence

EMD (emerin) (eg, Emery-Dreifuss muscular dystrophy), duplication/deletion analysis

EPM2A (epilepsy, progressive myoclonus type 2A, Lafora disease [laforin]) (eg, progressive myoclonus epilepsy), full gene sequence

FGF23 (fibroblast growth factor 23) (eg, hypophosphatemic rickets), full gene sequence

FGFR2 (fibroblast growth factor receptor 2) (eg, craniosynostosis, Apert syndrome, Crouzon syndrome), targeted sequence analysis (eg, exons 8, 10)

FGFR3 (fibroblast growth factor receptor 3) (eg, achondroplasia, hypochondroplasia), targeted sequence analysis (eg, exons 8, 11, 12, 13)

FHL1 (four and a half LIM domains 1) (eg, Emery-Dreifuss muscular dystrophy), full gene sequence

FKRP (fukutin related protein) (eg, congenital muscular dystrophy type 1C [MDC1C], limb-girdle muscular dystrophy [LGMD] type 2I), full gene sequence

FOXG1 (forkhead box G1) (eg, Rett syndrome), full gene sequence

FSHMD1A (facioscapulohumeral muscular dystrophy 1A) (eg, facioscapulohumeral muscular dystrophy), evaluation to detect abnormal (eg, deleted) alleles

FSHMD1A (facioscapulohumeral muscular dystrophy 1A) (eg, facioscapulohumeral muscular dystrophy), characterization of haplotype(s) (ie, chromosome 4A and 4B haplotypes)

FXN (frataxin) (eg, Friedreich ataxia), full gene sequence

GH1 (growth hormone 1) (eg, growth hormone deficiency), full gene sequence

GP1BB (glycoprotein Ib [platelet], beta polypeptide) (eg, Bernard-Soulier syndrome type B), full gene sequence

HBA1/HBA2 (alpha globin 1 and alpha globin 2) (eg, alpha thalassemia), duplication/deletion analysis

(For common deletion variants of alpha globin 1 and alpha globin 2 genes, use 81257)

HBB (hemoglobin, beta, Beta-Globin) (eg, thalassemia), full gene sequence

HNF1B (HNF1 homeobox B) (eg, maturity-onset diabetes of the young [MODY]), duplication/deletion analysis

HRAS (v-Ha-ras Harvey rat sarcoma viral oncogene homolog) (eg, Costello syndrome), full gene sequence

HSD3B2 (hydroxy-delta-5-steroid dehydrogenase, 3 beta-and steroid delta-isomerase 2) (eg, 3-beta-hydroxysteroid dehydrogenase type II deficiency), full gene sequence

HSD11B2 (hydroxysteroid [11-beta] dehydrogenase 2) (eg, mineralocorticoid excess syndrome), full gene sequence

HSPB1 (heat shock 27kDa protein 1) (eg, Charcot-Marie-Tooth disease), full gene sequence

INS (insulin) (eg, diabetes mellitus), full gene sequence

KCNJ1 (potassium inwardly-rectifying channel, subfamily J, member 1) (eg, Bartter syndrome), full gene sequence

KCNJ10 (potassium inwardly-rectifying channel, subfamily J, member 10) (eg, SeSAME syndrome, EAST syndrome, sensorineural hearing loss), full gene sequence

LITAF (lipopolysaccharide-induced TNF factor) (eg, Charcot-Marie-Tooth), full gene sequence

MEFV (Mediterranean fever) (eg, familial Mediterranean fever), full gene sequence

MEN1 (multiple endocrine neoplasia I) (eg, multiple endocrine neoplasia type 1, Wermer syndrome), duplication/deletion analysis

MMACHC (methylmalonic aciduria [cobalamin deficiency] cblC type, with homocystinuria) (eg, methylmalonic acidemia and homocystinuria), full gene sequence

MPV17 (MpV17 mitochondrial inner membrane protein) (eg, mitochondrial DNA depletion syndrome), duplication/deletion analysis

NDP (Norrie disease [pseudoglioma]) (eg, Norrie disease), full gene sequence

NDUFA1 (NADH dehydrogenase [ubiquinone] 1 alpha subcomplex, 1, 7.5kDa) (eg, Leigh syndrome, mitochondrial complex I deficiency), full gene sequence

NDUFAF2 (NADH dehydrogenase [ubiquinone] 1 alpha subcomplex, assembly factor 2) (eg, Leigh syndrome, mitochondrial complex I deficiency), full gene sequence

NDUFS4 (NADH dehydrogenase [ubiquinone] Fe-S protein 4, 18kDa [NADH-coenzyme Q reductase]) (eg, Leigh syndrome, mitochondrial complex I deficiency), full gene sequence

NIPA1 (non-imprinted in Prader-Willi/Angelman syndrome 1) (eg, spastic paraplegia), full gene sequence

NLGN4X (neuroligin 4, X-linked) (eg, autism spectrum disorders), duplication/deletion analysis

NPC2 (Niemann-Pick disease, type C2 [epididymal secretory protein E1]) (eg, Niemann-Pick disease type C2), full gene sequence

NR0B1 (nuclear receptor subfamily 0, group B, member 1) (eg, congenital adrenal hypoplasia), full gene sequence

PDX1 (pancreatic and duodenal homeobox 1) (eg, maturity-onset diabetes of the young [MODY]), full gene sequence

PHOX2B (paired-like homeobox 2b) (eg, congenital central hypoventilation syndrome), full gene sequence

PIK3CA (phosphatidylinositol-4,5-bisphosphate 3-kinase, catalytic subunit alpha) (eg, colorectal cancer), targeted sequence analysis (eg, exons 9 and 20)

PLP1 (proteolipid protein 1) (eg, Pelizaeus-Merzbacher disease, spastic paraplegia), duplication/deletion analysis

PQBP1 (polyglutamine binding protein 1) (eg, Renpenning syndrome), duplication/deletion analysis

PRNP (prion protein) (eg, genetic prion disease), full gene sequence

PROP1 (PROP paired-like homeobox 1) (eg, combined pituitary hormone deficiency), full gene sequence

PRPH2 (peripherin 2 [retinal degeneration, slow]) (eg, retinitis pigmentosa), full gene sequence

PRSS1 (protease, serine, 1 [trypsin 1]) (eg, hereditary pancreatitis), full gene sequence

RAF1 (v-raf-1 murine leukemia viral oncogene homolog 1) (eg, LEOPARD syndrome), targeted sequence analysis (eg, exons 7, 12, 14, 17)

RET (ret proto-oncogene) (eg, multiple endocrine neoplasia, type 2B and familial medullary thyroid carcinoma), common variants (eg, M918T, 2647_2648delinsTT, A883F)

RHO (rhodopsin) (eg, retinitis pigmentosa), full gene sequence

RP1 (retinitis pigmentosa 1) (eg, retinitis pigmentosa), full gene sequence

SCN1B (sodium channel, voltage-gated, type I, beta) (eg, Brugada syndrome), full gene sequence

SCO2 (SCO cytochrome oxidase deficient homolog 2 [SCO1L]) (eg, mitochondrial respiratory chain complex IV deficiency), full gene sequence

SDHC (succinate dehydrogenase complex, subunit C, integral membrane protein, 15kDa) (eg, hereditary paraganglioma-pheochromocytoma syndrome), duplication/deletion analysis

SDHD (succinate dehydrogenase complex, subunit D, integral membrane protein) (eg, hereditary paraganglioma), full gene sequence

Pathology and Laboratory

SGCG (sarcoglycan, gamma [35kDa dystrophin-associated glycoprotein]) (eg, limb-girdle muscular dystrophy), duplication/deletion analysis

SH2D1A (SH2 domain containing 1A) (eg, X-linked lymphoproliferative syndrome), full gene sequence

SLC16A2 (solute carrier family 16, member 2 [thyroid hormone transporter]) (eg, specific thyroid hormone cell transporter deficiency, Allan-Herndon-Dudley syndrome), duplication/deletion analysis

SLC25A20 (solute carrier family 25 [carnitine/ acylcarnitine translocase], member 20) (eg, carnitine-acylcarnitine translocase deficiency), duplication/deletion analysis

SLC25A4 (solute carrier family 25 [mitochondrial carrier; adenine nucleotide translocator], member 4) (eg, progressive external ophthalmoplegia), full gene sequence

SOD1 (superoxide dismutase 1, soluble) (eg, amyotrophic lateral sclerosis), full gene sequence

SPINK1 (serine peptidase inhibitor, Kazal type 1) (eg, hereditary pancreatitis), full gene sequence

STK11 (serine/threonine kinase 11) (eg, Peutz-Jeghers syndrome), duplication/deletion analysis

TACO1 (translational activator of mitochondrial encoded cytochrome c oxidase I) (eg, mitochondrial respiratory chain complex IV deficiency), full gene sequence

THAP1 (THAP domain containing, apoptosis associated protein 1) (eg, torsion dystonia), full gene sequence

TOR1A (torsin family 1, member A [torsin A]) (eg, torsion dystonia), full gene sequence

TP53 (tumor protein 53) (eg, tumor samples), targeted sequence analysis of 2-5 exons

TTPA (tocopherol [alpha] transfer protein) (eg, ataxia), full gene sequence

TTR (transthyretin) (eg, familial transthyretin amyloidosis), full gene sequence

TWIST1 (twist homolog 1 [Drosophila]) (eg, Saethre-Chotzen syndrome), full gene sequence

TYR (tyrosinase [oculocutaneous albinism IA]) (eg, oculocutaneous albinism IA), full gene sequence

USH1G (Usher syndrome 1G [autosomal recessive]) (eg, Usher syndrome, type 1), full gene sequence

VHL (von Hippel-Lindau tumor suppressor) (eg, von Hippel-Lindau familial cancer syndrome), full gene sequence

VWF (von Willebrand factor) (eg, von Willebrand disease type 1C), targeted sequence analysis (eg, exons 26, 27, 37)

ZEB2 (zinc finger E-box binding homeobox 2) (eg, Mowat-Wilson syndrome), duplication/deletion analysis

ZNF41 (zinc finger protein 41) (eg, X-linked mental retardation 89), full gene sequence

▲ 81405   Molecular pathology procedure, Level 6 (eg, analysis of 6-10 exons by DNA sequence analysis, mutation scanning or duplication/deletion variants of 11-25 exons, regionally targeted cytogenomic array analysis)

ABCD1 (ATP-binding cassette, sub-family D [ALD], member 1) (eg, adrenoleukodystrophy), full gene sequence

ACADS (acyl-CoA dehydrogenase, C-2 to C-3 short chain) (eg, short chain acyl-CoA dehydrogenase deficiency), full gene sequence

ACTA2 (actin, alpha 2, smooth muscle, aorta) (eg, thoracic aortic aneurysms and aortic dissections), full gene sequence

ACTC1 (actin, alpha, cardiac muscle 1) (eg, familial hypertrophic cardiomyopathy), full gene sequence

ANKRD1 (ankyrin repeat domain 1) (eg, dilated cardiomyopathy), full gene sequence

APTX (aprataxin) (eg, ataxia with oculomotor apraxia 1), full gene sequence

AR (androgen receptor) (eg, androgen insensitivity syndrome), full gene sequence

ARSA (arylsulfatase A) (eg, arylsulfatase A deficiency), full gene sequence

BCKDHA (branched chain keto acid dehydrogenase E1, alpha polypeptide) (eg, maple syrup urine disease, type 1A), full gene sequence

BCS1L (BCS1-like [S. cerevisiae]) (eg, Leigh syndrome, mitochondrial complex III deficiency, GRACILE syndrome), full gene sequence

BMPR2 (bone morphogenetic protein receptor, type II [serine/threonine kinase]) (eg, heritable pulmonary arterial hypertension), duplication/deletion analysis

CASQ2 (calsequestrin 2 [cardiac muscle]) (eg, catecholaminergic polymorphic ventricular tachycardia), full gene sequence

CASR (calcium-sensing receptor) (eg, hypocalcemia), full gene sequence

CDKL5 (cyclin-dependent kinase-like 5) (eg, early infantile epileptic encephalopathy), duplication/deletion analysis

CHRNA4 (cholinergic receptor, nicotinic, alpha 4) (eg, nocturnal frontal lobe epilepsy), full gene sequence

CHRNB2 (cholinergic receptor, nicotinic, beta 2 [neuronal]) (eg, nocturnal frontal lobe epilepsy), full gene sequence

COX10 (COX10 homolog, cytochrome c oxidase assembly protein) (eg, mitochondrial respiratory chain complex IV deficiency), full gene sequence

COX15 (COX15 homolog, cytochrome c oxidase assembly protein) (eg, mitochondrial respiratory chain complex IV deficiency), full gene sequence

CYP11B1 (cytochrome P450, family 11, subfamily B, polypeptide 1) (eg, congenital adrenal hyperplasia), full gene sequence

CYP17A1 (cytochrome P450, family 17, subfamily A, polypeptide 1) (eg, congenital adrenal hyperplasia), full gene sequence

CYP21A2 (cytochrome P450, family 21, subfamily A, polypeptide2) (eg, steroid 21-hydroxylase isoform, congenital adrenal hyperplasia), full gene sequence

Cytogenomic constitutional targeted microarray analysis of chromosome 22q13 by interrogation of genomic regions for copy number and single nucleotide polymorphism (SNP) variants for chromosomal abnormalities

(When performing genome-wide cytogenomic constitutional microarray analysis, see 81228, 81229)

(Do not report analyte-specific molecular pathology procedures separately when the specific analytes are included as part of the microarray analysis of chromosome 22q13)

(Do not report 88271 when performing cytogenomic microarray analysis)

DBT (dihydrolipoamide branched chain transacylase E2) (eg, maple syrup urine disease, type 2), duplication/deletion analysis

DCX (doublecortin) (eg, X-linked lissencephaly), full gene sequence

DES (desmin) (eg, myofibrillar myopathy), full gene sequence

DFNB59 (deafness, autosomal recessive 59) (eg, autosomal recessive nonsyndromic hearing impairment), full gene sequence

DGUOK (deoxyguanosine kinase) (eg, hepatocerebral mitochondrial DNA depletion syndrome), full gene sequence

DHCR7 (7-dehydrocholesterol reductase) (eg, Smith-Lemli-Opitz syndrome), full gene sequence

EIF2B2 (eukaryotic translation initiation factor 2B, subunit 2 beta, 39kDa) (eg, leukoencephalopathy with vanishing white matter), full gene sequence

EMD (emerin) (eg, Emery-Dreifuss muscular dystrophy), full gene sequence

ENG (endoglin) (eg, hereditary hemorrhagic telangiectasia, type 1), duplication/deletion analysis

EYA1 (eyes absent homolog 1 [Drosophila]) (eg, branchio-oto-renal [BOR] spectrum disorders), duplication/deletion analysis

F9 (coagulation factor IX) (eg, hemophilia B), full gene sequence

FGFR1 (fibroblast growth factor receptor 1) (eg, Kallmann syndrome 2), full gene sequence

FH (fumarate hydratase) (eg, fumarate hydratase deficiency, hereditary leiomyomatosis with renal cell cancer), full gene sequence

FKTN (fukutin) (eg, limb-girdle muscular dystrophy [LGMD] type 2M or 2L), full gene sequence

FTSJ1 (FtsJ RNA methyltransferase homolog 1 [E. coli]) (eg, X-linked mental retardation 9), duplication/deletion analysis

GABRG2 (gamma-aminobutyric acid [GABA] A receptor, gamma 2) (eg, generalized epilepsy with febrile seizures), full gene sequence

GCH1 (GTP cyclohydrolase 1) (eg, autosomal dominant dopa-responsive dystonia), full gene sequence

GDAP1 (ganglioside-induced differentiation-associated protein 1) (eg, Charcot-Marie-Tooth disease), full gene sequence

GFAP (glial fibrillary acidic protein) (eg, Alexander disease), full gene sequence

GHR (growth hormone receptor) (eg, Laron syndrome), full gene sequence

GHRHR (growth hormone releasing hormone receptor) (eg, growth hormone deficiency), full gene sequence

GLA (galactosidase, alpha) (eg, Fabry disease), full gene sequence

HBA1/HBA2 (alpha globin 1 and alpha globin 2) (eg, thalassemia), full gene sequence

HNF1A (HNF1 homeobox A) (eg, maturity-onset diabetes of the young [MODY]), full gene sequence

HNF1B (HNF1 homeobox B) (eg, maturity-onset diabetes of the young [MODY]), full gene sequence

HTRA1 (HtrA serine peptidase 1) (eg, macular degeneration), full gene sequence

IDS (iduronate 2-sulfatase) (eg, mucopolysacchridosis, type II), full gene sequence

IL2RG (interleukin 2 receptor, gamma) (eg, X-linked severe combined immunodeficiency), full gene sequence

ISPD (isoprenoid synthase domain containing) (eg, muscle-eye-brain disease, Walker-Warburg syndrome), full gene sequence

▶ *KRAS (Kirsten rat sarcoma viral oncogene homolog)* (eg, Noonan syndrome), full gene sequence◀

LAMP2 (lysosomal-associated membrane protein 2) (eg, Danon disease), full gene sequence

LDLR (low density lipoprotein receptor) (eg, familial hypercholesterolemia), duplication/deletion analysis

MEN1 (multiple endocrine neoplasia I) (eg, multiple endocrine neoplasia type 1, Wermer syndrome), full gene sequence

MMAA (methylmalonic aciduria [cobalamine deficiency] type A) (eg, MMAA-related methylmalonic acidemia), full gene sequence

Pathology and Laboratory

MMAB (methylmalonic aciduria [cobalamine deficiency] type B) (eg, MMAA-related methylmalonic acidemia), full gene sequence

MPI (mannose phosphate isomerase) (eg, congenital disorder of glycosylation 1b), full gene sequence

MPV17 (MpV17 mitochondrial inner membrane protein) (eg, mitochondrial DNA depletion syndrome), full gene sequence

MPZ (myelin protein zero) (eg, Charcot-Marie-Tooth), full gene sequence

MTM1 (myotubularin 1) (eg, X-linked centronuclear myopathy), duplication/deletion analysis

MYL2 (myosin, light chain 2, regulatory, cardiac, slow) (eg, familial hypertrophic cardiomyopathy), full gene sequence

MYL3 (myosin, light chain 3, alkali, ventricular, skeletal, slow) (eg, familial hypertrophic cardiomyopathy), full gene sequence

MYOT (myotilin) (eg, limb-girdle muscular dystrophy), full gene sequence

NDUFS7 (NADH dehydrogenase [ubiquinone] Fe-S protein 7, 20kDa [NADH-coenzyme Q reductase]) (eg, Leigh syndrome, mitochondrial complex I deficiency), full gene sequence

NDUFS8 (NADH dehydrogenase [ubiquinone] Fe-S protein 8, 23kDa [NADH-coenzyme Q reductase]) (eg, Leigh syndrome, mitochondrial complex I deficiency), full gene sequence

NDUFV1 (NADH dehydrogenase [ubiquinone] flavoprotein 1, 51kDa) (eg, Leigh syndrome, mitochondrial complex I deficiency), full gene sequence

NEFL (neurofilament, light polypeptide) (eg, Charcot-Marie-Tooth), full gene sequence

NF2 (neurofibromin 2 [merlin]) (eg, neurofibromatosis, type 2), duplication/deletion analysis

NLGN3 (neuroligin 3) (eg, autism spectrum disorders), full gene sequence

NLGN4X (neuroligin 4, X-linked) (eg, autism spectrum disorders), full gene sequence

NPHP1 (nephronophthisis 1 [juvenile]) (eg, Joubert syndrome), deletion analysis, and duplication analysis, if performed

NPHS2 (nephrosis 2, idiopathic, steroid-resistant [podocin]) (eg, steroid-resistant nephrotic syndrome), full gene sequence

NSD1 (nuclear receptor binding SET domain protein 1) (eg, Sotos syndrome), duplication/deletion analysis

OTC (ornithine carbamoyltransferase) (eg, ornithine transcarbamylase deficiency), full gene sequence

PAFAH1B1 (platelet-activating factor acetylhydrolase 1b, regulatory subunit 1 [45kDa]) (eg, lissencephaly, Miller-Dieker syndrome), duplication/deletion analysis

PARK2 (Parkinson protein 2, E3 ubiquitin protein ligase [parkin]) (eg, Parkinson disease), duplication/deletion analysis

PCCA (propionyl CoA carboxylase, alpha polypeptide) (eg, propionic acidemia, type 1), duplication/deletion analysis

PCDH19 (protocadherin 19) (eg, epileptic encephalopathy), full gene sequence

PDHA1 (pyruvate dehydrogenase [lipoamide] alpha 1) (eg, lactic acidosis), duplication/deletion analysis

PDHB (pyruvate dehydrogenase [lipoamide] beta) (eg, lactic acidosis), full gene sequence

PINK1 (PTEN induced putative kinase 1) (eg, Parkinson disease), full gene sequence

PLP1 (proteolipid protein 1) (eg, Pelizaeus-Merzbacher disease, spastic paraplegia), full gene sequence

POU1F1 (POU class 1 homeobox 1) (eg, combined pituitary hormone deficiency), full gene sequence

PRX (periaxin) (eg, Charcot-Marie-Tooth disease), full gene sequence

PQBP1 (polyglutamine binding protein 1) (eg, Renpenning syndrome), full gene sequence

PSEN1 (presenilin 1) (eg, Alzheimer disease), full gene sequence

RAB7A (RAB7A, member RAS oncogene family) (eg, Charcot-Marie-Tooth disease), full gene sequence

RAI1 (retinoic acid induced 1) (eg, Smith-Magenis syndrome), full gene sequence

REEP1 (receptor accessory protein 1) (eg, spastic paraplegia), full gene sequence

RET (ret proto-oncogene) (eg, multiple endocrine neoplasia, type 2A and familial medullary thyroid carcinoma), targeted sequence analysis (eg, exons 10, 11, 13-16)

RPS19 (ribosomal protein S19) (eg, Diamond-Blackfan anemia), full gene sequence

RRM2B (ribonucleotide reductase M2 B [TP53 inducible]) (eg, mitochondrial DNA depletion), full gene sequence

SCO1 (SCO cytochrome oxidase deficient homolog 1) (eg, mitochondrial respiratory chain complex IV deficiency), full gene sequence

SDHB (succinate dehydrogenase complex, subunit B, iron sulfur) (eg, hereditary paraganglioma), full gene sequence

SDHC (succinate dehydrogenase complex, subunit C, integral membrane protein, 15kDa) (eg, hereditary paraganglioma-pheochromocytoma syndrome), full gene sequence

SGCA (sarcoglycan, alpha [50kDa dystrophin-associated glycoprotein]) (eg, limb-girdle muscular dystrophy), full gene sequence

SGCB (sarcoglycan, beta [43kDa dystrophin-associated glycoprotein]) (eg, limb-girdle muscular dystrophy), full gene sequence

SGCD (sarcoglycan, delta [35kDa dystrophin-associated glycoprotein]) (eg, limb-girdle muscular dystrophy), full gene sequence

SGCE (sarcoglycan, epsilon) (eg, myoclonic dystonia), duplication/deletion analysis

SGCG (sarcoglycan, gamma [35kDa dystrophin-associated glycoprotein]) (eg, limb-girdle muscular dystrophy), full gene sequence

SHOC2 (soc-2 suppressor of clear homolog) (eg, Noonan-like syndrome with loose anagen hair), full gene sequence

SHOX (short stature homeobox) (eg, Langer mesomelic dysplasia), full gene sequence

SIL1 (SIL1 homolog, endoplasmic reticulum chaperone [S. cerevisiae]) (eg, ataxia), full gene sequence

SLC2A1 (solute carrier family 2 [facilitated glucose transporter], member 1) (eg, glucose transporter type 1 [GLUT 1] deficiency syndrome), full gene sequence

SLC16A2 (solute carrier family 16, member 2 [thyroid hormone transporter]) (eg, specific thyroid hormone cell transporter deficiency, Allan-Herndon-Dudley syndrome), full gene sequence

SLC22A5 (solute carrier family 22 [organic cation/carnitine transporter], member 5) (eg, systemic primary carnitine deficiency), full gene sequence

SLC25A20 (solute carrier family 25 [carnitine/acylcarnitine translocase], member 20) (eg, carnitine-acylcarnitine translocase deficiency), full gene sequence

SMAD4 (SMAD family member 4) (eg, hemorrhagic telangiectasia syndrome, juvenile polyposis), duplication/deletion analysis

SMN1 (survival of motor neuron 1, telomeric) (eg, spinal muscular atrophy), full gene sequence

SPAST (spastin) (eg, spastic paraplegia), duplication/deletion analysis

SPG7 (spastic paraplegia 7 [pure and complicated autosomal recessive]) (eg, spastic paraplegia), duplication/deletion analysis

SPRED1 (sprouty-related, EVH1 domain containing 1) (eg, Legius syndrome), full gene sequence

STAT3 (signal transducer and activator of transcription 3 [acute-phase response factor]) (eg, autosomal dominant hyper-IgE syndrome), targeted sequence analysis (eg, exons 12, 13, 14, 16, 17, 20, 21)

STK11 (serine/threonine kinase 11) (eg, Peutz-Jeghers syndrome), full gene sequence

SURF1 (surfeit 1) (eg, mitochondrial respiratory chain complex IV deficiency), full gene sequence

TARDBP (TAR DNA binding protein) (eg, amyotrophic lateral sclerosis), full gene sequence

TBX5 (T-box 5) (eg, Holt-Oram syndrome), full gene sequence

TCF4 (transcription factor 4) (eg, Pitt-Hopkins syndrome), duplication/deletion analysis

TGFBR1 (transforming growth factor, beta receptor 1) (eg, Marfan syndrome), full gene sequence

TGFBR2 (transforming growth factor, beta receptor 2) (eg, Marfan syndrome), full gene sequence

THRB (thyroid hormone receptor, beta) (eg, thyroid hormone resistance, thyroid hormone beta receptor deficiency), full gene sequence or targeted sequence analysis of >5 exons

TK2 (thymidine kinase 2, mitochondrial) (eg, mitochondrial DNA depletion syndrome), full gene sequence

TNNC1 (troponin C type 1 [slow]) (eg, hypertrophic cardiomyopathy or dilated cardiomyopathy), full gene sequence

TNNI3 (troponin I, type 3 [cardiac]) (eg, familial hypertrophic cardiomyopathy), full gene sequence

TP53 (tumor protein 53) (eg, Li-Fraumeni syndrome, tumor samples), full gene sequence or targeted sequence analysis of >5 exons

TPM1 (tropomyosin 1 [alpha]) (eg, familial hypertrophic cardiomyopathy), full gene sequence

TSC1 (tuberous sclerosis 1) (eg, tuberous sclerosis), duplication/deletion analysis

TYMP (thymidine phosphorylase) (eg, mitochondrial DNA depletion syndrome), full gene sequence

VWF (von Willebrand factor) (eg, von Willebrand disease type 2N), targeted sequence analysis (eg, exons 18-20, 23-25)

WT1 (Wilms tumor 1) (eg, Denys-Drash syndrome, familial Wilms tumor), full gene sequence

ZEB2 (zinc finger E-box binding homeobox 2) (eg, Mowat-Wilson syndrome), full gene sequence

▲ 81406   Molecular pathology procedure, Level 7 (eg, analysis of 11-25 exons by DNA sequence analysis, mutation scanning or duplication/deletion variants of 26-50 exons, cytogenomic array analysis for neoplasia)

ACADVL (acyl-CoA dehydrogenase, very long chain) (eg, very long chain acyl-coenzyme A dehydrogenase deficiency), full gene sequence

ACTN4 (actinin, alpha 4) (eg, focal segmental glomerulosclerosis), full gene sequence

AFG3L2 (AFG3 ATPase family gene 3-like 2 [S. cerevisiae]) (eg, spinocerebellar ataxia), full gene sequence

Pathology and Laboratory

AIRE (autoimmune regulator) (eg, autoimmune polyendocrinopathy syndrome type 1), full gene sequence

ALDH7A1 (aldehyde dehydrogenase 7 family, member A1) (eg, pyridoxine-dependent epilepsy), full gene sequence

ANO5 (anoctamin 5) (eg, limb-girdle muscular dystrophy), full gene sequence

APP (amyloid beta [A4] precursor protein) (eg, Alzheimer disease), full gene sequence

ASS1 (argininosuccinate synthase 1) (eg, citrullinemia type I), full gene sequence

ATL1 (atlastin GTPase 1) (eg, spastic paraplegia), full gene sequence

ATP1A2 (ATPase, Na+/K+ transporting, alpha 2 polypeptide) (eg, familial hemiplegic migraine), full gene sequence

ATP7B (ATPase, Cu++ transporting, beta polypeptide) (eg, Wilson disease), full gene sequence

BBS1 (Bardet-Biedl syndrome 1) (eg, Bardet-Biedl syndrome), full gene sequence

BBS2 (Bardet-Biedl syndrome 2) (eg, Bardet-Biedl syndrome), full gene sequence

BCKDHB (branched-chain keto acid dehydrogenase E1, beta polypeptide) (eg, maple syrup urine disease, type 1B), full gene sequence

BEST1 (bestrophin 1) (eg, vitelliform macular dystrophy), full gene sequence

BMPR2 (bone morphogenetic protein receptor, type II [serine/threonine kinase]) (eg, heritable pulmonary arterial hypertension), full gene sequence

►*BRAF (B-Raf proto-oncogene, serine/threonine kinase)* (eg, Noonan syndrome), full gene sequence◄

BSCL2 (Berardinelli-Seip congenital lipodystrophy 2 [seipin]) (eg, Berardinelli-Seip congenital lipodystrophy), full gene sequence

BTK (Bruton agammaglobulinemia tyrosine kinase) (eg, X-linked agammaglobulinemia), full gene sequence

CACNB2 (calcium channel, voltage-dependent, beta 2 subunit) (eg, Brugada syndrome), full gene sequence

CAPN3 (calpain 3) (eg, limb-girdle muscular dystrophy [LGMD] type 2A, calpainopathy), full gene sequence

CBS (cystathionine-beta-synthase) (eg, homocystinuria, cystathionine beta-synthase deficiency), full gene sequence

CDH1 (cadherin 1, type 1, E-cadherin [epithelial]) (eg, hereditary diffuse gastric cancer), full gene sequence

CDKL5 (cyclin-dependent kinase-like 5) (eg, early infantile epileptic encephalopathy), full gene sequence

CLCN1 (chloride channel 1, skeletal muscle) (eg, myotonia congenita), full gene sequence

CLCNKB (chloride channel, voltage-sensitive Kb) (eg, Bartter syndrome 3 and 4b), full gene sequence

CNTNAP2 (contactin-associated protein-like 2) (eg, Pitt-Hopkins-like syndrome 1), full gene sequence

COL6A2 (collagen, type VI, alpha 2) (eg, collagen type VI-related disorders), duplication/deletion analysis

CPT1A (carnitine palmitoyltransferase 1A [liver]) (eg, carnitine palmitoyltransferase 1A [CPT1A] deficiency), full gene sequence

CRB1 (crumbs homolog 1 [Drosophila]) (eg, Leber congenital amaurosis), full gene sequence

CREBBP (CREB binding protein) (eg, Rubinstein-Taybi syndrome), duplication/deletion analysis

Cytogenomic microarray analysis, neoplasia (eg, interrogation of copy number, and loss-of-heterozygosity via single nucleotide polymorphism [SNP]-based comparative genomic hybridization [CGH] microarray analysis)

(Do not report analyte-specific molecular pathology procedures separately when the specific analytes are included as part of the cytogenomic microarray analysis for neoplasia)

(Do not report 88271 when performing cytogenomic microarray analysis)

DBT (dihydrolipoamide branched chain transacylase E2) (eg, maple syrup urine disease, type 2), full gene sequence

DLAT (dihydrolipoamide S-acetyltransferase) (eg, pyruvate dehydrogenase E2 deficiency), full gene sequence

DLD (dihydrolipoamide dehydrogenase) (eg, maple syrup urine disease, type III), full gene sequence

DSC2 (desmocollin) (eg, arrhythmogenic right ventricular dysplasia/cardiomyopathy 11), full gene sequence

DSG2 (desmoglein 2) (eg, arrhythmogenic right ventricular dysplasia/cardiomyopathy 10), full gene sequence

DSP (desmoplakin) (eg, arrhythmogenic right ventricular dysplasia/cardiomyopathy 8), full gene sequence

EFHC1 (EF-hand domain [C-terminal] containing 1) (eg, juvenile myoclonic epilepsy), full gene sequence

EIF2B3 (eukaryotic translation initiation factor 2B, subunit 3 gamma, 58kDa) (eg, leukoencephalopathy with vanishing white matter), full gene sequence

EIF2B4 (eukaryotic translation initiation factor 2B, subunit 4 delta, 67kDa) (eg, leukoencephalopathy with vanishing white matter), full gene sequence

EIF2B5 (eukaryotic translation initiation factor 2B, subunit 5 epsilon, 82kDa) (eg, childhood ataxia with central nervous system hypomyelination/vanishing white matter), full gene sequence

⊙=Moderate sedation   ✚=Add-on code   ⇗=FDA approval pending   #=Resequenced code   ○=Recycled/reinstated code

ENG (endoglin) (eg, hereditary hemorrhagic telangiectasia, type 1), full gene sequence

EYA1 (eyes absent homolog 1 [Drosophila]) (eg, branchio-oto-renal [BOR] spectrum disorders), full gene sequence

F8 (coagulation factor VIII) (eg, hemophilia A), duplication/deletion analysis

FAH (fumarylacetoacetate hydrolase [fumarylacetoacetase]) (eg, tyrosinemia, type 1), full gene sequence

FASTKD2 (FAST kinase domains 2) (eg, mitochondrial respiratory chain complex IV deficiency), full gene sequence

FIG4 (FIG4 homolog, SAC1 lipid phosphatase domain containing [S. cerevisiae]) (eg, Charcot-Marie-Tooth disease), full gene sequence

FTSJ1 (FtsJ RNA methyltransferase homolog 1 [E. coli]) (eg, X-linked mental retardation 9), full gene sequence

FUS (fused in sarcoma) (eg, amyotrophic lateral sclerosis), full gene sequence

GAA (glucosidase, alpha; acid) (eg, glycogen storage disease type II [Pompe disease]), full gene sequence

GALC (galactosylceramidase) (eg, Krabbe disease), full gene sequence

GALT (galactose-1-phosphate uridylyltransferase) (eg, galactosemia), full gene sequence

GARS (glycyl-tRNA synthetase) (eg, Charcot-Marie-Tooth disease), full gene sequence

GCDH (glutaryl-CoA dehydrogenase) (eg, glutaricacidemia type 1), full gene sequence

GCK (glucokinase [hexokinase 4]) (eg, maturity-onset diabetes of the young [MODY]), full gene sequence

GLUD1 (glutamate dehydrogenase 1) (eg, familial hyperinsulinism), full gene sequence

GNE (glucosamine [UDP-N-acetyl]-2-epimerase/N-acetylmannosamine kinase) (eg, inclusion body myopathy 2 [IBM2], Nonaka myopathy), full gene sequence

GRN (granulin) (eg, frontotemporal dementia), full gene sequence

HADHA (hydroxyacyl-CoA dehydrogenase/3-ketoacyl-CoA thiolase/enoyl-CoA hydratase [trifunctional protein] alpha subunit) (eg, long chain acyl-coenzyme A dehydrogenase deficiency), full gene sequence

HADHB (hydroxyacyl-CoA dehydrogenase/3-ketoacyl-CoA thiolase/enoyl-CoA hydratase [trifunctional protein], beta subunit) (eg, trifunctional protein deficiency), full gene sequence

HEXA (hexosaminidase A, alpha polypeptide) (eg, Tay-Sachs disease), full gene sequence

HLCS (HLCS holocarboxylase synthetase) (eg, holocarboxylase synthetase deficiency), full gene sequence

HNF4A (hepatocyte nuclear factor 4, alpha) (eg, maturity-onset diabetes of the young [MODY]), full gene sequence

IDUA (iduronidase, alpha-L-) (eg, mucopolysaccharidosis type I), full gene sequence

INF2 (inverted formin, FH2 and WH2 domain containing) (eg, focal segmental glomerulosclerosis), full gene sequence

IVD (isovaleryl-CoA dehydrogenase) (eg, isovaleric acidemia), full gene sequence

JAG1 (jagged 1) (eg, Alagille syndrome), duplication/deletion analysis

JUP (junction plakoglobin) (eg, arrhythmogenic right ventricular dysplasia/cardiomyopathy 11), full gene sequence

KAL1 (Kallmann syndrome 1 sequence) (eg, Kallmann syndrome), full gene sequence

KCNH2 (potassium voltage-gated channel, subfamily H [eag-related], member 2) (eg, short QT syndrome, long QT syndrome), full gene sequence

(Do not report 81406 for KCNH2 full gene sequence in conjunction with 81280)

KCNQ1 (potassium voltage-gated channel, KQT-like subfamily, member 1) (eg, short QT syndrome, long QT syndrome), full gene sequence

(Do not report 81406 for KCNQ1 full gene sequence with 81280)

KCNQ2 (potassium voltage-gated channel, KQT-like subfamily, member 2) (eg, epileptic encephalopathy), full gene sequence

LDB3 (LIM domain binding 3) (eg, familial dilated cardiomyopathy, myofibrillar myopathy), full gene sequence

LDLR (low density lipoprotein receptor) (eg, familial hypercholesterolemia), full gene sequence

LEPR (leptin receptor) (eg, obesity with hypogonadism), full gene sequence

LHCGR (luteinizing hormone/choriogonadotropin receptor) (eg, precocious male puberty), full gene sequence

LMNA (lamin A/C) (eg, Emery-Dreifuss muscular dystrophy [EDMD1, 2 and 3] limb-girdle muscular dystrophy [LGMD] type 1B, dilated cardiomyopathy [CMD1A], familial partial lipodystrophy [FPLD2]), full gene sequence

LRP5 (low density lipoprotein receptor-related protein 5) (eg, osteopetrosis), full gene sequence

MAP2K1 (mitogen-activated protein kinase 1) (eg, cardiofaciocutaneous syndrome), full gene sequence

MAP2K2 (mitogen-activated protein kinase 2) (eg, cardiofaciocutaneous syndrome), full gene sequence

MAPT (microtubule-associated protein tau) (eg, frontotemporal dementia), full gene sequence

Pathology and Laboratory

MCCC1 (methylcrotonoyl-CoA carboxylase 1 [alpha]) (eg, 3-methylcrotonyl-CoA carboxylase deficiency), full gene sequence

MCCC2 (methylcrotonoyl-CoA carboxylase 2 [beta]) (eg, 3-methylcrotonyl carboxylase deficiency), full gene sequence

MFN2 (mitofusin 2) (eg, Charcot-Marie-Tooth disease), full gene sequence

MTM1 (myotubularin 1) (eg, X-linked centronuclear myopathy), full gene sequence

MUT (methylmalonyl CoA mutase) (eg, methylmalonic acidemia), full gene sequence

MUTYH (mutY homolog [E. coli]) (eg, MYH-associated polyposis), full gene sequence

NDUFS1 (NADH dehydrogenase [ubiquinone] Fe-S protein 1, 75kDa [NADH-coenzyme Q reductase]) (eg, Leigh syndrome, mitochondrial complex I deficiency), full gene sequence

NF2 (neurofibromin 2 [merlin]) (eg, neurofibromatosis, type 2), full gene sequence

NOTCH3 (notch 3) (eg, cerebral autosomal dominant arteriopathy with subcortical infarcts and leukoencephalopathy [CADASIL]), targeted sequence analysis (eg, exons 1-23)

NPC1 (Niemann-Pick disease, type C1) (eg, Niemann-Pick disease), full gene sequence

NPHP1 (nephronophthisis 1 [juvenile]) (eg, Joubert syndrome), full gene sequence

NSD1 (nuclear receptor binding SET domain protein 1) (eg, Sotos syndrome), full gene sequence

OPA1 (optic atrophy 1) (eg, optic atrophy), duplication/deletion analysis

OPTN (optineurin) (eg, amyotrophic lateral sclerosis), full gene sequence

PAFAH1B1 (platelet-activating factor acetylhydrolase 1b, regulatory subunit 1 [45kDa]) (eg, lissencephaly, Miller-Dieker syndrome), full gene sequence

PAH (phenylalanine hydroxylase) (eg, phenylketonuria), full gene sequence

PALB2 (partner and localizer of BRCA2) (eg, breast and pancreatic cancer), full gene sequence

PARK2 (Parkinson protein 2, E3 ubiquitin protein ligase [parkin]) (eg, Parkinson disease), full gene sequence

PAX2 (paired box 2) (eg, renal coloboma syndrome), full gene sequence

PC (pyruvate carboxylase) (eg, pyruvate carboxylase deficiency), full gene sequence

PCCA (propionyl CoA carboxylase, alpha polypeptide) (eg, propionic acidemia, type 1), full gene sequence

PCCB (propionyl CoA carboxylase, beta polypeptide) (eg, propionic acidemia, type 1), full gene sequence

PCDH15 (protocadherin-related 15) (eg, Usher syndrome type 1F), duplication/deletion analysis

►*PCSK9 (proprotein convertase subtilisin/kexin type 9)* (eg, familial hypercholesterolemia), full gene sequence◄

PDHA1 (pyruvate dehydrogenase [lipoamide] alpha 1) (eg, lactic acidosis), full gene sequence

PDHX (pyruvate dehydrogenase complex, component X) (eg, lactic acidosis), full gene sequence

PHEX (phosphate-regulating endopeptidase homolog, X-linked) (eg, hypophosphatemic rickets), full gene sequence

PKD2 (polycystic kidney disease 2 [autosomal dominant]) (eg, polycystic kidney disease), full gene sequence

PKP2 (plakophilin 2) (eg, arrhythmogenic right ventricular dysplasia/cardiomyopathy 9), full gene sequence

PNKD (paroxysmal nonkinesigenic dyskinesia) (eg, paroxysmal nonkinesigenic dyskinesia), full gene sequence

POLG (polymerase [DNA directed], gamma) (eg, Alpers-Huttenlocher syndrome, autosomal dominant progressive external ophthalmoplegia), full gene sequence

POMGNT1 (protein O-linked mannose beta1,2-N acetylglucosaminyltransferase) (eg, muscle-eye-brain disease, Walker-Warburg syndrome), full gene sequence

POMT1 (protein-O-mannosyltransferase 1) (eg, limb-girdle muscular dystrophy [LGMD] type 2K, Walker-Warburg syndrome), full gene sequence

POMT2 (protein-O-mannosyltransferase 2) (eg, limb-girdle muscular dystrophy [LGMD] type 2N, Walker-Warburg syndrome), full gene sequence

PRKAG2 (protein kinase, AMP-activated, gamma 2 non-catalytic subunit) (eg, familial hypertrophic cardiomyopathy with Wolff-Parkinson-White syndrome, lethal congenital glycogen storage disease of heart), full gene sequence

PRKCG (protein kinase C, gamma) (eg, spinocerebellar ataxia), full gene sequence

PSEN2 (presenilin 2 [Alzheimer disease 4]) (eg, Alzheimer disease), full gene sequence

PTPN11 (protein tyrosine phosphatase, non-receptor type 11) (eg, Noonan syndrome, LEOPARD syndrome), full gene sequence

PYGM (phosphorylase, glycogen, muscle) (eg, glycogen storage disease type V, McArdle disease), full gene sequence

RAF1 (v-raf-1 murine leukemia viral oncogene homolog 1) (eg, LEOPARD syndrome), full gene sequence

RET (ret proto-oncogene) (eg, Hirschsprung disease), full gene sequence

RPE65 (retinal pigment epithelium-specific protein 65kDa) (eg, retinitis pigmentosa, Leber congenital amaurosis), full gene sequence

⊙=Moderate sedation ✚=Add-on code ⊮=FDA approval pending #=Resequenced code ○=Recycled/reinstated code

RYR1 (ryanodine receptor 1, skeletal) (eg, malignant hyperthermia), targeted sequence analysis of exons with functionally-confirmed mutations

SCN4A (sodium channel, voltage-gated, type IV, alpha subunit) (eg, hyperkalemic periodic paralysis), full gene sequence

SCNN1A (sodium channel, nonvoltage-gated 1 alpha) (eg, pseudohypoaldosteronism), full gene sequence

SCNN1B (sodium channel, nonvoltage-gated 1, beta) (eg, Liddle syndrome, pseudohypoaldosteronism), full gene sequence

SCNN1G (sodium channel, nonvoltage-gated 1, gamma) (eg, Liddle syndrome, pseudohypoaldosteronism), full gene sequence

SDHA (succinate dehydrogenase complex, subunit A, flavoprotein [Fp]) (eg, Leigh syndrome, mitochondrial complex II deficiency), full gene sequence

SETX (senataxin) (eg, ataxia), full gene sequence

SGCE (sarcoglycan, epsilon) (eg, myoclonic dystonia), full gene sequence

SH3TC2 (SH3 domain and tetratricopeptide repeats 2) (eg, Charcot-Marie-Tooth disease), full gene sequence

SLC9A6 (solute carrier family 9 [sodium/hydrogen exchanger], member 6) (eg, Christianson syndrome), full gene sequence

SLC26A4 (solute carrier family 26, member 4) (eg, Pendred syndrome), full gene sequence

SLC37A4 (solute carrier family 37 [glucose-6-phosphate transporter], member 4) (eg, glycogen storage disease type Ib), full gene sequence

SMAD4 (SMAD family member 4) (eg, hemorrhagic telangiectasia syndrome, juvenile polyposis), full gene sequence

SOS1 (son of sevenless homolog 1) (eg, Noonan syndrome, gingival fibromatosis), full gene sequence

SPAST (spastin) (eg, spastic paraplegia), full gene sequence

SPG7 (spastic paraplegia 7 [pure and complicated autosomal recessive]) (eg, spastic paraplegia), full gene sequence

STXBP1 (syntaxin-binding protein 1) (eg, epileptic encephalopathy), full gene sequence

TAZ (tafazzin) (eg, methylglutaconic aciduria type 2, Barth syndrome), full gene sequence

TCF4 (transcription factor 4) (eg, Pitt-Hopkins syndrome), full gene sequence

TH (tyrosine hydroxylase) (eg, Segawa syndrome), full gene sequence

TMEM43 (transmembrane protein 43) (eg, arrhythmogenic right ventricular cardiomyopathy), full gene sequence

TNNT2 (troponin T, type 2 [cardiac]) (eg, familial hypertrophic cardiomyopathy), full gene sequence

TRPC6 (transient receptor potential cation channel, subfamily C, member 6) (eg, focal segmental glomerulosclerosis), full gene sequence

TSC1 (tuberous sclerosis 1) (eg, tuberous sclerosis), full gene sequence

TSC2 (tuberous sclerosis 2) (eg, tuberous sclerosis), duplication/deletion analysis

UBE3A (ubiquitin protein ligase E3A) (eg, Angelman syndrome), full gene sequence

UMOD (uromodulin) (eg, glomerulocystic kidney disease with hyperuricemia and isosthenuria), full gene sequence

VWF (von Willebrand factor) (von Willebrand disease type 2A), extended targeted sequence analysis (eg, exons 11-16, 24-26, 51, 52)

WAS (Wiskott-Aldrich syndrome [eczema-thrombocytopenia]) (eg, Wiskott-Aldrich syndrome), full gene sequence

81407   Molecular pathology procedure, Level 8 (eg, analysis of 26-50 exons by DNA sequence analysis, mutation scanning or duplication/deletion variants of >50 exons, sequence analysis of multiple genes on one platform)

ABCC8 (ATP-binding cassette, sub-family C [CFTR/MRP], member 8) (eg, familial hyperinsulinism), full gene sequence

AGL (amylo-alpha-1, 6-glucosidase, 4-alpha-glucanotransferase) (eg, glycogen storage disease type III), full gene sequence

AHI1 (Abelson helper integration site 1) (eg, Joubert syndrome), full gene sequence

ASPM (asp [abnormal spindle] homolog, microcephaly associated [Drosophila]) (eg, primary microcephaly), full gene sequence

CACNA1A (calcium channel, voltage-dependent, P/Q type, alpha 1A subunit) (eg, familial hemiplegic migraine), full gene sequence

CHD7 (chromodomain helicase DNA binding protein 7) (eg, CHARGE syndrome), full gene sequence

COL4A4 (collagen, type IV, alpha 4) (eg, Alport syndrome), full gene sequence

COL4A5 (collagen, type IV, alpha 5) (eg, Alport syndrome), duplication/deletion analysis

COL6A1 (collagen, type VI, alpha 1) (eg, collagen type VI-related disorders), full gene sequence

COL6A2 (collagen, type VI, alpha 2) (eg, collagen type VI-related disorders), full gene sequence

COL6A3 (collagen, type VI, alpha 3) (eg, collagen type VI-related disorders), full gene sequence

CREBBP (CREB binding protein) (eg, Rubinstein-Taybi syndrome), full gene sequence

F8 (coagulation factor VIII) (eg, hemophilia A), full gene sequence

JAG1 (jagged 1) (eg, Alagille syndrome), full gene sequence

KDM5C (lysine [K]-specific demethylase 5C) (eg, X-linked mental retardation), full gene sequence

KIAA0196 (KIAA0196) (eg, spastic paraplegia), full gene sequence

L1CAM (L1 cell adhesion molecule) (eg, MASA syndrome, X-linked hydrocephaly), full gene sequence

LAMB2 (laminin, beta 2 [laminin S]) (eg, Pierson syndrome), full gene sequence

MYBPC3 (myosin binding protein C, cardiac) (eg, familial hypertrophic cardiomyopathy), full gene sequence

MYH6 (myosin, heavy chain 6, cardiac muscle, alpha) (eg, familial dilated cardiomyopathy), full gene sequence

MYH7 (myosin, heavy chain 7, cardiac muscle, beta) (eg, familial hypertrophic cardiomyopathy, Liang distal myopathy), full gene sequence

MYO7A (myosin VIIA) (eg, Usher syndrome, type 1), full gene sequence

NOTCH1 (notch 1) (eg, aortic valve disease), full gene sequence

NPHS1 (nephrosis 1, congenital, Finnish type [nephrin]) (eg, congenital Finnish nephrosis), full gene sequence

OPA1 (optic atrophy 1) (eg, optic atrophy), full gene sequence

PCDH15 (protocadherin-related 15) (eg, Usher syndrome, type 1), full gene sequence

PKD1 (polycystic kidney disease 1 [autosomal dominant]) (eg, polycystic kidney disease), full gene sequence

PLCE1 (phospholipase C, epsilon 1) (eg, nephrotic syndrome type 3), full gene sequence

SCN1A (sodium channel, voltage-gated, type 1, alpha subunit) (eg, generalized epilepsy with febrile seizures), full gene sequence

SCN5A (sodium channel, voltage-gated, type V, alpha subunit) (eg, familial dilated cardiomyopathy), full gene sequence

SLC12A1 (solute carrier family 12 [sodium/potassium/chloride transporters], member 1) (eg, Bartter syndrome), full gene sequence

SLC12A3 (solute carrier family 12 [sodium/chloride transporters], member 3) (eg, Gitelman syndrome), full gene sequence

SPG11 (spastic paraplegia 11 [autosomal recessive]) (eg, spastic paraplegia), full gene sequence

SPTBN2 (spectrin, beta, non-erythrocytic 2) (eg, spinocerebellar ataxia), full gene sequence

TMEM67 (transmembrane protein 67) (eg, Joubert syndrome), full gene sequence

TSC2 (tuberous sclerosis 2) (eg, tuberous sclerosis), full gene sequence

USH1C (Usher syndrome 1C [autosomal recessive, severe]) (eg, Usher syndrome, type 1), full gene sequence

VPS13B (vacuolar protein sorting 13 homolog B [yeast]) (eg, Cohen syndrome), duplication/deletion analysis

WDR62 (WD repeat domain 62) (eg, primary autosomal recessive microcephaly), full gene sequence

81408 Molecular pathology procedure, Level 9 (eg, analysis of >50 exons in a single gene by DNA sequence analysis)

ABCA4 (ATP-binding cassette, sub-family A [ABC1], member 4) (eg, Stargardt disease, age-related macular degeneration), full gene sequence

ATM (ataxia telangiectasia mutated) (eg, ataxia telangiectasia), full gene sequence

CDH23 (cadherin-related 23) (eg, Usher syndrome, type 1), full gene sequence

CEP290 (centrosomal protein 290kDa) (eg, Joubert syndrome), full gene sequence

COL1A1 (collagen, type I, alpha 1) (eg, osteogenesis imperfecta, type I), full gene sequence

COL1A2 (collagen, type I, alpha 2) (eg, osteogenesis imperfecta, type I), full gene sequence

COL4A1 (collagen, type IV, alpha 1) (eg, brain small-vessel disease with hemorrhage), full gene sequence

COL4A3 (collagen, type IV, alpha 3 [Goodpasture antigen]) (eg, Alport syndrome), full gene sequence

COL4A5 (collagen, type IV, alpha 5) (eg, Alport syndrome), full gene sequence

DMD (dystrophin) (eg, Duchenne/Becker muscular dystrophy), full gene sequence

DYSF (dysferlin, limb girdle muscular dystrophy 2B [autosomal recessive]) (eg, limb-girdle muscular dystrophy), full gene sequence

FBN1 (fibrillin 1) (eg, Marfan syndrome), full gene sequence

ITPR1 (inositol 1,4,5-trisphosphate receptor, type 1) (eg, spinocerebellar ataxia), full gene sequence

LAMA2 (laminin, alpha 2) (eg, congenital muscular dystrophy), full gene sequence

LRRK2 (leucine-rich repeat kinase 2) (eg, Parkinson disease), full gene sequence

MYH11 (myosin, heavy chain 11, smooth muscle) (eg, thoracic aortic aneurysms and aortic dissections), full gene sequence

NEB (nebulin) (eg, nemaline myopathy 2), full gene sequence

NF1 *(neurofibromin 1)* (eg, neurofibromatosis, type 1), full gene sequence

PKHD1 *(polycystic kidney and hepatic disease 1)* (eg, autosomal recessive polycystic kidney disease), full gene sequence

RYR1 *(ryanodine receptor 1, skeletal)* (eg, malignant hyperthermia), full gene sequence

RYR2 *(ryanodine receptor 2 [cardiac])* (eg, catecholaminergic polymorphic ventricular tachycardia, arrhythmogenic right ventricular dysplasia), full gene sequence or targeted sequence analysis of > 50 exons

USH2A *(Usher syndrome 2A [autosomal recessive, mild])* (eg, Usher syndrome, type 2), full gene sequence

VPS13B *(vacuolar protein sorting 13 homolog B [yeast])* (eg, Cohen syndrome), full gene sequence

VWF *(von Willebrand factor)* (eg, von Willebrand disease types 1 and 3), full gene sequence

 # 81479   Unlisted molecular pathology procedure

Genomic Sequencing Procedures and Other Molecular Multianalyte Assays

Genomic sequencing procedures (GSPs) and other molecular multianalyte assays GSPs are DNA or RNA sequence analysis methods that simultaneously assay multiple genes or genetic regions relevant to a clinical situation. They may target specific combinations of genes or genetic material, or assay the exome or genome. The technology used for genomic sequencing is commonly referred to as next generation sequencing (NGS) or massively parallel sequencing (MPS). GSPs are performed on nucleic acids from germline or neoplastic samples. Examples of applications include aneuploidy analysis of cell-free circulating fetal DNA, gene panels for somatic alterations in neoplasms, and sequence analysis of the exome or genome to determine the cause of developmental delay. The exome and genome procedures are designed to evaluate the genetic material in totality or near totality. Although commonly used to identify sequence (base) changes, they can also be used to identify copy number, structural changes, and abnormal zygosity patterns. Another unique feature of GSPs is the ability to "re-query" or re-evaluate the sequence data (eg, complex phenotype such as developmental delay is reassessed when new genetic knowledge is attained, or for a separate unrelated clinical indication). The analyses listed below represent groups of genes that are often performed by GSPs; however, the analyses may also be performed by other molecular techniques (polymerase chain reaction [PCR] methods and microarrays). These codes should be used when the components of the descriptor(s) are fulfilled regardless of the technique used to provide the analysis, unless specifically noted in the code descriptor. When all of the components of the descriptor are not performed, use individual Tier 1 codes, Tier 2 codes, or 81479 (Unlisted molecular pathology procedure).

The assays in this section represent discrete genetic values, properties, or characteristics in which the measurement or analysis of each analyte is potentially of independent medical significance or useful in medical management. In contrast to multianalyte assays with algorithmic analyses (MAAAs), the assays in this section do not represent algorithmically combined results to obtain a risk score or other value, which in itself represents a new and distinct medical property that is of independent medical significance relative to the individual, component test results.

(For cytogenomic microarray analyses, see 81228, 81229, 81405, 81406)

(For long QT syndrome gene analyses, see 81280, 81282)

81479   Code is out of numerical sequence. See 81400-81479

81410   Aortic dysfunction or dilation (eg, Marfan syndrome, Loeys Dietz syndrome, Ehler Danlos syndrome type IV, arterial tortuosity syndrome); genomic sequence analysis panel, must include sequencing of at least 9 genes, including *FBN1, TGFBR1, TGFBR2, COL3A1, MYH11, ACTA2, SLC2A10, SMAD3,* and *MYLK*

81411   duplication/deletion analysis panel, must include analyses for *TGFBR1, TGFBR2, MYH11, and COL3A1*

● 81412   Ashkenazi Jewish associated disorders (eg, Bloom syndrome, Canavan disease, cystic fibrosis, familial dysautonomia, Fanconi anemia group C, Gaucher disease, Tay-Sachs disease), genomic sequence analysis panel, must include sequencing of at least 9 genes, including *ASPA, BLM, CFTR, FANCC, GBA, HEXA, IKBKAP, MCOLN1,* and *SMPD1*

81415   Exome (eg, unexplained constitutional or heritable disorder or syndrome); sequence analysis

+ 81416   sequence analysis, each comparator exome (eg, parents, siblings) (List separately in addition to code for primary procedure)

(Use 81416 in conjunction with 81415)

81417   re-evaluation of previously obtained exome sequence (eg, updated knowledge or unrelated condition/ syndrome)

(Do not report 81417 for incidental findings)

(For exome-wide copy number assessment by microarray, see 81228, 81229)

81420   Fetal chromosomal aneuploidy (eg, trisomy 21, monosomy X) genomic sequence analysis panel, circulating cell-free fetal DNA in maternal blood, must include analysis of chromosomes 13, 18, and 21

Pathology and Laboratory

81425   Genome (eg, unexplained constitutional or heritable disorder or syndrome); sequence analysis

+ 81426   sequence analysis, each comparator genome (eg, parents, siblings) (List separately in addition to code for primary procedure)

(Use 81426 in conjunction with 81425)

81427   re-evaluation of previously obtained genome sequence (eg, updated knowledge or unrelated condition/syndrome)

(Do not report 81427 for incidental findings)

(For genome-wide copy number assessment by microarray, see 81228, 81229)

81430   Hearing loss (eg, nonsyndromic hearing loss, Usher syndrome, Pendred syndrome); genomic sequence analysis panel, must include sequencing of at least 60 genes, including *CDH23, CLRN1, GJB2, GPR98, MTRNR1, MYO7A, MYO15A, PCDH15, OTOF, SLC26A4, TMC1, TMPRSS3, USH1C, USH1G, USH2A,* and *WFS1*

81431   duplication/deletion analysis panel, must include copy number analyses for *STRC* and *DFNB1* deletions in *GJB2* and *GJB6 genes*

● 81432   Hereditary breast cancer-related disorders (eg, hereditary breast cancer, hereditary ovarian cancer, hereditary endometrial cancer); genomic sequence analysis panel, must include sequencing of at least 14 genes, including *ATM, BRCA1, BRCA2, BRIP1, CDH1, MLH1, MSH2, MSH6, NBN, PALB2, PTEN, RAD51C, STK11,* and *TP53*

● 81433   duplication/deletion analysis panel, must include analyses for *BRCA1, BRCA2, MLH1, MSH2,* and *STK11*

● 81434   Hereditary retinal disorders (eg, retinitis pigmentosa, Leber congenital amaurosis, cone-rod dystrophy), genomic sequence analysis panel, must include sequencing of at least 15 genes, including *ABCA4, CNGA1, CRB1, EYS, PDE6A, PDE6B, PRPF31, PRPH2, RDH12, RHO, RP1, RP2, RPE65, RPGR,* and *USH2A*

▲ 81435   Hereditary colon cancer disorders (eg, Lynch syndrome, PTEN hamartoma syndrome, Cowden syndrome, familial adenomatosis polyposis); genomic sequence analysis panel, must include sequencing of at least 10 genes, including *APC, BMPR1A, CDH1, MLH1, MSH2, MSH6, MUTYH, PTEN, SMAD4,* and *STK11*

▲ 81436   duplication/deletion analysis panel, must include analysis of at least 5 genes, including *MLH1, MSH2, EPCAM, SMAD4,* and *STK11*

● 81437   Hereditary neuroendocrine tumor disorders (eg, medullary thyroid carcinoma, parathyroid carcinoma, malignant pheochromocytoma or paraganglioma); genomic sequence analysis panel, must include sequencing of at least 6 genes, including *MAX, SDHB, SDHC, SDHD, TMEM127, and VHL*

● 81438   duplication/deletion analysis panel, must include analyses for *SDHB, SDHC, SDHD,* and *VHL*

81440   Nuclear encoded mitochondrial genes (eg, neurologic or myopathic phenotypes), genomic sequence panel, must include analysis of at least 100 genes, including *BCS1L, C10orf2, COQ2, COX10, DGUOK, MPV17, OPA1, PDSS2, POLG, POLG2, RRM2B, SCO1, SCO2, SLC25A4, SUCLA2, SUCLG1, TAZ, TK2,* and *TYMP*

● 81442   Noonan spectrum disorders (eg, Noonan syndrome, cardio-facio-cutaneous syndrome, Costello syndrome, LEOPARD syndrome, Noonan-like syndrome), genomic sequence analysis panel, must include sequencing of at least 12 genes, including *BRAF, CBL, HRAS, KRAS, MAP2K1, MAP2K2, NRAS, PTPN11, RAF1, RIT1, SHOC2,* and *SOS1*

▲ 81445   Targeted genomic sequence analysis panel, solid organ neoplasm, DNA analysis, and RNA analysis when performed, 5-50 genes (eg, *ALK, BRAF, CDKN2A, EGFR, ERBB2, KIT, KRAS, NRAS, MET, PDGFRA, PDGFRB, PGR, PIK3CA, PTEN, RET*), interrogation for sequence variants and copy number variants or rearrangements, if performed

(For copy number assessment by microarray, use 81406)

▲ 81450   Targeted genomic sequence analysis panel, hematolymphoid neoplasm or disorder, DNA analysis, and RNA analysis when performed, 5-50 genes (eg, *BRAF, CEBPA, DNMT3A, EZH2, FLT3, IDH1, IDH2, JAK2, KRAS, KIT, MLL, NRAS, NPM1, NOTCH1*), interrogation for sequence variants, and copy number variants or rearrangements, or isoform expression or mRNA expression levels, if performed

(For copy number assessment by microarray, use 81406)

▲ 81455   Targeted genomic sequence analysis panel, solid organ or hematolymphoid neoplasm, DNA analysis, and RNA analysis when performed, 51 or greater genes (eg, *ALK, BRAF, CDKN2A, CEBPA, DNMT3A, EGFR, ERBB2, EZH2, FLT3, IDH1, IDH2, JAK2, KIT, KRAS, MLL, NPM1, NRAS, MET, NOTCH1, PDGFRA, PDGFRB, PGR, PIK3CA, PTEN, RET*), interrogation for sequence variants and copy number variants or rearrangements, if performed

(For copy number assessment by microarray, use 81406)

81460   Whole mitochondrial genome (eg, Leigh syndrome, mitochondrial encephalomyopathy, lactic acidosis, and stroke-like episodes [MELAS], myoclonic epilepsy with ragged-red fibers [MERFF], neuropathy, ataxia, and retinitis pigmentosa [NARP], Leber hereditary optic neuropathy [LHON]), genomic sequence, must include sequence analysis of entire mitochondrial genome with heteroplasmy detection

81465   Whole mitochondrial genome large deletion analysis panel (eg, Kearns-Sayre syndrome, chronic progressive external ophthalmoplegia), including heteroplasmy detection, if performed

81470   X-linked intellectual disability (XLID) (eg, syndromic and non-syndromic XLID); genomic sequence analysis panel, must include sequencing of at least 60 genes, including *ARX, ATRX, CDKL5, FGD1, FMR1, HUWE1, IL1RAPL, KDM5C, L1CAM, MECP2, MED12, MID1, OCRL, RPS6KA3,* and *SLC16A2*

81471   duplication/deletion gene analysis, must include analysis of at least 60 genes, including *ARX, ATRX, CDKL5, FGD1, FMR1, HUWE1, IL1RAPL, KDM5C, L1CAM, MECP2, MED12, MID1, OCRL, RPS6KA3,* and *SLC16A2*

Multianalyte Assays with Algorithmic Analyses

Multianalyte Assays with Algorithmic Analyses (MAAAs) are procedures that utilize multiple results derived from panels of analyses of various types, including molecular pathology assays, fluorescent in situ hybridization assays, and non-nucleic acid based assays (eg, proteins, polypeptides, lipids, carbohydrates). Algorithmic analysis using the results of these assays as well as other patient information (if used) is then performed and typically reported as a numeric score(s) or as a probability. MAAAs are typically unique to a single clinical laboratory or manufacturer. The results of individual component procedure(s) that are inputs to the MAAAs may be provided on the associated laboratory report; however, these assays are not separately reported using additional codes.

The format for the code descriptors of MAAAs usually include (in order):

- Disease type (eg, oncology, autoimmune, tissue rejection),
- Material(s) analyzed (eg, DNA, RNA, protein, antibody),
- Number of markers (eg, number of genes, number of proteins),
- Methodology(ies) (eg, microarray, real-time [RT]-PCR, in situ hybridization [ISH], enzyme linked immunosorbent assays [ELISA]),
- Number of functional domains (if indicated),
- Specimen type (eg, blood, fresh tissue, formalin-fixed paraffin embedded),
- Algorithm result type (eg, prognostic, diagnostic),
- Report (eg, probability index, risk score)

In contrast to GSPs and other molecular multianalyte assays, the assays in this section represent algorithmically combined results of analyses of multiple analytes to obtain a risk score or other value which in itself represents a new and distinct medical property that is of independent medical significance relative to the individual component test results in clinical context in which the assay is performed.

MAAAs, including those that do not have a Category I code, may be found in Appendix O. MAAAs that do not have a Category I code are identified in Appendix O by a four-digit number followed by the letter "M." The Category I MAAA codes that are included in this subsection are also included in Appendix O. All MAAA codes are listed in Appendix O along with the procedure's proprietary name. In order to report a MAAA code, the analysis performed must fulfill the code descriptor **and**, if proprietary, must be the test represented by the proprietary name listed in Appendix O.

When a specific MAAA procedure is not listed below or in Appendix O, the procedure must be reported using the Category I MAAA unlisted code (81599).

These codes encompass all analytical services required (eg, cell lysis, nucleic acid stabilization, extraction, digestion, amplification, hybridization, and detection) in addition to the algorithmic analysis itself. Procedures that are required prior to cell lysis (eg, microdissection, codes 88380 and 88381) should be reported separately.

● **81490**   Autoimmune (rheumatoid arthritis), analysis of 12 biomarkers using immunoassays, utilizing serum, prognostic algorithm reported as a disease activity score

     ►(Do not report 81490 in conjunction with 86140)◄

● **81493**   Coronary artery disease, mRNA, gene expression profiling by real-time RT-PCR of 23 genes, utilizing whole peripheral blood, algorithm reported as a risk score

81500   Oncology (ovarian), biochemical assays of two proteins (CA-125 and HE4), utilizing serum, with menopausal status, algorithm reported as a risk score

     (Do not report 81500 in conjunction with 86304, 86305)

81503   Oncology (ovarian), biochemical assays of five proteins (CA-125, apolipoprotein A1, beta-2 microglobulin, transferrin, and pre-albumin), utilizing serum, algorithm reported as a risk score

     (Do not report 81503 in conjunction with 82172, 82232, 83695, 83700, 84134, 84466, 86304)

81504   Oncology (tissue of origin), microarray gene expression profiling of > 2000 genes, utilizing formalin-fixed paraffin-embedded tissue, algorithm reported as tissue similarity scores

81506   Endocrinology (type 2 diabetes), biochemical assays of seven analytes (glucose, HbA1c, insulin, hs-CRP, adiponectin, ferritin, interleukin 2-receptor alpha), utilizing serum or plasma, algorithm reporting a risk score

     (Do not report 81506 in conjunction with constituent components [ie, 82728, 82947, 83036, 83525, 86141], 84999 [for adopectin], and 83520 [for interleukin 2-receptor alpha])

81507   Fetal aneuploidy (trisomy 21, 18, and 13) DNA sequence analysis of selected regions using maternal plasma, algorithm reported as a risk score for each trisomy

---

▲=Revised code   ●=New code   ►◄=Contains new or revised text   ⊘=Modifier 51 exempt

Pathology and Laboratory

81508   Fetal congenital abnormalities, biochemical assays of two proteins (PAPP-A, hCG [any form]), utilizing maternal serum, algorithm reported as a risk score

(Do not report 81508 in conjunction with 84163, 84702)

81509   Fetal congenital abnormalities, biochemical assays of three proteins (PAPP-A, hCG [any form], DIA), utilizing maternal serum, algorithm reported as a risk score

(Do not report 81509 in conjunction with 84163, 84702, 86336)

81510   Fetal congenital abnormalities, biochemical assays of three analytes (AFP, uE3, hCG [any form]), utilizing maternal serum, algorithm reported as a risk score

(Do not report 81510 in conjunction with 82105, 82677, 84702)

81511   Fetal congenital abnormalities, biochemical assays of four analytes (AFP, uE3, hCG [any form], DIA) utilizing maternal serum, algorithm reported as a risk score (may include additional results from previous biochemical testing)

(Do not report 81511 in conjunction with 82105, 82677, 84702, 86336)

81512   Fetal congenital abnormalities, biochemical assays of five analytes (AFP, uE3, total hCG, hyperglycosylated hCG, DIA) utilizing maternal serum, algorithm reported as a risk score

(Do not report 81512 in conjunction with 82105, 82677, 84702, 86336)

81519   Oncology (breast), mRNA, gene expression profiling by real-time RT-PCR of 21 genes, utilizing formalin-fixed paraffin embedded tissue, algorithm reported as recurrence score

● **81525**   Oncology (colon), mRNA, gene expression profiling by real-time RT-PCR of 12 genes (7 content and 5 housekeeping), utilizing formalin-fixed paraffin-embedded tissue, algorithm reported as a recurrence score

● **81528**   Oncology (colorectal) screening, quantitative real-time target and signal amplification of 10 DNA markers (*KRAS* mutations, promoter methylation of *NDRG4* and *BMP3*) and fecal hemoglobin, utilizing stool, algorithm reported as a positive or negative result

▶(Do not report 81528 in conjunction with 81275, 82274)◀

● **81535**   Oncology (gynecologic), live tumor cell culture and chemotherapeutic response by DAPI stain and morphology, predictive algorithm reported as a drug response score; first single drug or drug combination

+● **81536**   each additional single drug or drug combination (List separately in addition to code for primary procedure)

▶(Use 81536 in conjunction with 81535)◀

● **81538**   Oncology (lung), mass spectrometric 8-protein signature, including amyloid A, utilizing serum, prognostic and predictive algorithm reported as good versus poor overall survival

● **81540**   Oncology (tumor of unknown origin), mRNA, gene expression profiling by real-time RT-PCR of 92 genes (87 content and 5 housekeeping) to classify tumor into main cancer type and subtype, utilizing formalin-fixed paraffin-embedded tissue, algorithm reported as a probability of a predicted main cancer type and subtype

● **81545**   Oncology (thyroid), gene expression analysis of 142 genes, utilizing fine needle aspirate, algorithm reported as a categorical result (eg, benign or suspicious)

● **81595**   Cardiology (heart transplant), mRNA, gene expression profiling by real-time quantitative PCR of 20 genes (11 content and 9 housekeeping), utilizing subfraction of peripheral blood, algorithm reported as a rejection risk score

81599   Unlisted multianalyte assay with algorithmic analysis

(Do not use 81599 for multianalyte assays with algorithmic analyses listed in Appendix O)

Chemistry

The material for examination may be from any source unless otherwise specified in the code descriptor. When an analyte is measured in multiple specimens from different sources, or in specimens that are obtained at different times, the analyte is reported separately for each source and for each specimen. The examination is quantitative unless specified. To report an organ or disease oriented panel, see codes 80048-80076.

Clinical information or mathematically calculated values, which are not specifically requested by the ordering physician and are derived from the results of other ordered or performed laboratory tests, are considered part of the ordered test procedure(s) and therefore are not separately reportable service(s).

When the requested analyte result is derived using a calculation that requires values from nonrequested laboratory analyses, only the requested analyte code should be reported.

When the calculated analyte determination requires values derived from other requested and nonrequested laboratory analyses, the requested analyte codes (including those calculated) should be reported.

An exception to the above is when an analyte (eg, urinary creatinine) is performed to compensate for variations in urine concentration (eg, microalbumin, thromboxane metabolites) in random urine samples; the appropriate CPT code is reported for both the ordered analyte and the additional required analyte. When the calculated result(s) represent an algorithmically derived numeric score or probability, see the appropriate multianalyte assay with algorithmic analyses (MAAA) code or the MAAA unlisted code (81599).

(82000 has been deleted)

(82003 has been deleted. For acetaminophen, see 80329, 80330, 80331)

82009   Ketone body(s) (eg, acetone, acetoacetic acid, beta-hydroxybutyrate); qualitative

82010   quantitative

82013   Acetylcholinesterase

(For gastric acid analysis, use 82930)

(Acid phosphatase, see 84060-84066)

82016   Acylcarnitines; qualitative, each specimen

82017   quantitative, each specimen

(For carnitine, use 82379)

82024   Adrenocorticotropic hormone (ACTH)

82030   Adenosine, 5-monophosphate, cyclic (cyclic AMP)

82040   Albumin; serum, plasma or whole blood

82042   urine or other source, quantitative, each specimen

82043   urine, microalbumin, quantitative

82044   urine, microalbumin, semiquantitative (eg, reagent strip assay)

(For prealbumin, use 84134)

82045   ischemia modified

(82055 has been deleted. For alcohol, any specimen except breath, see 80320, 80321, 80322)

82075   Alcohol (ethanol), breath

82085   Aldolase

82088   Aldosterone

(Alkaline phosphatase, see 84075, 84080)

(82101 has been deleted. For alkaloids, use 80323)

(Alphaketoglutarate, see 82009, 82010)

(Alpha tocopherol [Vitamin E], use 84446)

82103   Alpha-1-antitrypsin; total

82104   phenotype

82105   Alpha-fetoprotein (AFP); serum

82106   amniotic fluid

82107   AFP-L3 fraction isoform and total AFP (including ratio)

82108   Aluminum

82120   Amines, vaginal fluid, qualitative

(For combined pH and amines test for vaginitis, use 82120 and 83986)

82127   Amino acids; single, qualitative, each specimen

82128   multiple, qualitative, each specimen

82131   single, quantitative, each specimen

82135   Aminolevulinic acid, delta (ALA)

82136   Amino acids, 2 to 5 amino acids, quantitative, each specimen

82139   Amino acids, 6 or more amino acids, quantitative, each specimen

82140   Ammonia

82143   Amniotic fluid scan (spectrophotometric)

(For L/S ratio, use 83661)

(Amobarbital, use 80345)

(82145 has been deleted. For amphetamine or methamphetamine, see 80324, 80325, 80326)

82150   Amylase

82154   Androstanediol glucuronide

82157   Androstenedione

82160   Androsterone

82163   Angiotensin II

82164   Angiotensin I - converting enzyme (ACE)

(Antidiuretic hormone (ADH), use 84588)

(Antimony, use 83015)

(Antitrypsin, alpha-1-, see 82103, 82104)

82172   Apolipoprotein, each

82175   Arsenic

(For heavy metal screening, use 83015)

82180   Ascorbic acid (Vitamin C), blood

(Aspirin, see acetylsalicylic acid, 80329, 80330, 80331)

(Atherogenic index, blood, ultracentrifugation, quantitative, use 83701)

82190   Atomic absorption spectroscopy, each analyte

(82205 has been deleted. For barbiturates not elsewhere specified, use 80345)

82232   Beta-2 microglobulin

(Bicarbonate, use 82374)

82239   Bile acids; total

82240   cholylglycine

(For bile pigments, urine, see 81000-81005)

82247   Bilirubin; total

82248   direct

82252   feces, qualitative

82261   Biotinidase, each specimen

Pathology and Laboratory

82270 Blood, occult, by peroxidase activity (eg, guaiac), qualitative; feces, consecutive collected specimens with single determination, for colorectal neoplasm screening (ie, patient was provided 3 cards or single triple card for consecutive collection)

82271 other sources

82272 Blood, occult, by peroxidase activity (eg, guaiac), qualitative, feces, 1-3 simultaneous determinations, performed for other than colorectal neoplasm screening

(Blood urea nitrogen [BUN], see 84520, 84525)

82274 Blood, occult, by fecal hemoglobin determination by immunoassay, qualitative, feces, 1-3 simultaneous determinations

82286 Bradykinin

82300 Cadmium

82306 Vitamin D; 25 hydroxy, includes fraction(s), if performed

82652 1, 25 dihydroxy, includes fraction(s), if performed

82308 Calcitonin

82310 Calcium; total

82330 ionized

82331 after calcium infusion test

82340 urine quantitative, timed specimen

82355 Calculus; qualitative analysis

82360 quantitative analysis, chemical

82365 infrared spectroscopy

82370 X-ray diffraction

(Carbamates, see individual listings)

82373 Carbohydrate deficient transferrin

82374 Carbon dioxide (bicarbonate)

(See also 82803)

82375 Carboxyhemoglobin; quantitative

82376 qualitative

(For transcutaneous measurement of carboxyhemoglobin, use 88740)

82378 Carcinoembryonic antigen (CEA)

82379 Carnitine (total and free), quantitative, each specimen

(For acylcarnitine, see 82016, 82017)

82380 Carotene

82382 Catecholamines; total urine

82383 blood

82384 fractionated

(For urine metabolites, see 83835, 84585)

82387 Cathepsin-D

82390 Ceruloplasmin

82397 Chemiluminescent assay

82415 Chloramphenicol

82435 Chloride; blood

82436 urine

82438 other source

(For sweat collection by iontophoresis, use 89230)

82441 Chlorinated hydrocarbons, screen

(Cholecalciferol [Vitamin D], use 82306)

82465 Cholesterol, serum or whole blood, total

(For high density lipoprotein [HDL], use 83718)

82480 Cholinesterase; serum

82482 RBC

82485 Chondroitin B sulfate, quantitative

(Chorionic gonadotropin, see gonadotropin, 84702, 84703)

►(82486 has been deleted. For a qualitative column chromatography procedure, use the appropriate specific analyte code, if available, or 82542)◄

►(82487, 82488 have been deleted. For a paper chromatography procedure, use the appropriate specific analyte code, if available, or 84999)◄

►(82489 has been deleted. For a thin layer chromatography procedure, use the appropriate specific analyte code, if available, or 84999)◄

►(82491 has been deleted. For a quantitative column chromatography procedure, use the appropriate specific analyte code, if available, or 82542)◄

►(82492 has been deleted. For a quantitative column chromatography procedure that detects more than one analyte, use a single specific code that represents all of the analytes, if available, or one unit of 82542 for all of the analytes)◄

82495 Chromium

82507 Citrate

(82520 has been deleted. For cocaine or metabolite, use 80353)

(Cocaine, qualitative analysis, use 80353)

(Codeine, qualitative analysis, use 80361)

(Complement, see 86160-86162)

82523 Collagen cross links, any method

82525 Copper

(Coproporphyrin, see 84119, 84120)

(Corticosteroids, use 83491)

82528 Corticosterone

82530 Cortisol; free

82533 total

(C-peptide, use 84681)

82540 Creatine

▶(82541 has been deleted. For a quantitative chromatography procedure with mass spectrometry that only detects a single specific analyte, use the appropriate specific analyte code, if applicable, or 82542)◀

▲ **82542** Column chromatography, includes mass spectrometry, if performed (eg, HPLC, LC, LC/MS, LC/MS-MS, GC, GC/MS-MS, GC/MS, HPLC/MS), non-drug analyte(s) not elsewhere specified, qualitative or quantitative, each specimen

▶(Do not report more than one unit of 82542 for each specimen)◀

▶(82543 has been deleted. For a quantitative chromatography procedure with mass spectrometry that only detects a single specific analyte, use the appropriate specific analyte code, if available, or 82542)◀

▶(82544 has been deleted. For a quantitative chromatography procedure with mass spectrometry that detects more than one analyte, use a single specific code that represents all of the analytes, if available, or one unit of 82542 for all of the analytes)◀

(For column chromatography/mass spectrometry of drugs or substances, see **Drug Assay** 80300, 80301, 80302, 80303, 80304, 80320-80377, or specific analyte code[s] in the **Chemistry** section)

82550 Creatine kinase (CK), (CPK); total

82552 isoenzymes

82553 MB fraction only

82554 isoforms

82565 Creatinine; blood

82570 other source

82575 clearance

82585 Cryofibrinogen

82595 Cryoglobulin, qualitative or semi-quantitative (eg, cryocrit)

(For quantitative, cryoglobulin, see 82784, 82785)

(Crystals, pyrophosphate vs urate, use 89060)

82600 Cyanide

82607 Cyanocobalamin (Vitamin B-12);

82608 unsaturated binding capacity

(Cyclic AMP, use 82030)

(Cyclosporine, use 80158)

82610 Cystatin C

82615 Cystine and homocystine, urine, qualitative

82626 Dehydroepiandrosterone (DHEA)

(Do not report 82626 in conjunction with 80327, 80328 to identify anabolic steroid testing for testosterone)

82627 Dehydroepiandrosterone-sulfate (DHEA-S)

(Delta-aminolevulinic acid (ALA), use 82135)

82633 Desoxycorticosterone, 11-

82634 Deoxycortisol, 11-

(Dexamethasone suppression test, use 80420)

(Diastase, urine, use 82150)

82638 Dibucaine number

(Dichloroethane, use 82441)

(Dichloromethane, use 82441)

(Diethylether, use 84600)

(82646 has been deleted. For dihydrocodeinone, use 80361)

(82649 has been deleted. For opiates, use 80361)

(82651 has been deleted. For anabolic steroids, see 80327, 80328)

82652 Code is out of numerical sequence. See 82009-84999

(82654 has been deleted. For dimethadione, see 80339, 80340, 80341)

(Dipropylacetic acid, use 80164)

(Dopamine, see 82382-82384)

(Duodenal contents, see individual enzymes; for intubation and collection, see 43756, 43757)

82656 Elastase, pancreatic (EL-1), fecal, qualitative or semi-quantitative

82657 Enzyme activity in blood cells, cultured cells, or tissue, not elsewhere specified; nonradioactive substrate, each specimen

82658 radioactive substrate, each specimen

82664 Electrophoretic technique, not elsewhere specified

(Endocrine receptor assays, see 84233-84235)

(82666 has been deleted. For epiandrosterone, see 80327, 80328)

82668 Erythropoietin

82670 Estradiol

82671 Estrogens; fractionated

82672 total

(Estrogen receptor assay, use 84233)

82677 Estriol

82679 Estrone

(Ethanol, use 80320)

(82690 has been deleted. For ethchlorvynol, ethyl alcohol, use 80320)

82693	Ethylene glycol
82696	Etiocholanolone
	(For fractionation of ketosteroids, use 83593)
82705	Fat or lipids, feces; qualitative
82710	quantitative
82715	Fat differential, feces, quantitative
82725	Fatty acids, nonesterified
82726	Very long chain fatty acids
	(For long-chain [C20-22] omega-3 fatty acids in red blood cell [RBC] membranes, use Category III code 0111T)
82728	Ferritin
	(Fetal hemoglobin, see hemoglobin 83030, 83033, and 85460)
	(Fetoprotein, alpha-1, see 82105, 82106)
82731	Fetal fibronectin, cervicovaginal secretions, semi-quantitative
82735	Fluoride
	(82742 has been deleted. For flurazepam, see 80346, 80347)
	(Foam stability test, use 83662)
82746	Folic acid; serum
82747	RBC
	(Follicle stimulating hormone [FSH], use 83001)
82757	Fructose, semen
	(Fructosamine, use 82985)
	(Fructose, TLC screen, use 84375)
82759	Galactokinase, RBC
82760	Galactose
82775	Galactose-1-phosphate uridyl transferase; quantitative
82776	screen
82777	Galectin-3
82784	Gammaglobulin (immunoglobulin); IgA, IgD, IgG, IgM, each
82785	IgE
	(For allergen specific IgE, see 86003, 86005)
82787	immunoglobulin subclasses (eg, IgG1, 2, 3, or 4), each
	(Gamma-glutamyltransferase [GGT], use 82977)
82800	Gases, blood, pH only
82803	Gases, blood, any combination of pH, pCO2, pO2, CO2, HCO3 (including calculated O2 saturation);
	(Use 82803 for 2 or more of the above listed analytes)
82805	with O2 saturation, by direct measurement, except pulse oximetry

82810	Gases, blood, O2 saturation only, by direct measurement, except pulse oximetry
	(For pulse oximetry, use 94760)
82820	Hemoglobin-oxygen affinity (pO2 for 50% hemoglobin saturation with oxygen)
	(For gastric acid analysis, use 82930)
82930	Gastric acid analysis, includes pH if performed, each specimen
82938	Gastrin after secretin stimulation
82941	Gastrin
	(Gentamicin, use 80170)
	(GGT, use 82977)
	▶(For a qualitative column chromatography procedure [eg, gas liquid chromatography], use the appropriate specific analyte code, if available, or 82542)◀
82943	Glucagon
82945	Glucose, body fluid, other than blood
82946	Glucagon tolerance test
82947	Glucose; quantitative, blood (except reagent strip)
82948	blood, reagent strip
82950	post glucose dose (includes glucose)
82951	tolerance test (GTT), 3 specimens (includes glucose)
+ 82952	tolerance test, each additional beyond 3 specimens (List separately in addition to code for primary procedure)
	(Use 82952 in conjunction with 82951)
	(82953 has been deleted)
	(For insulin tolerance test, see 80434, 80435)
	(For leucine tolerance test, use 80428)
	(For semiquantitative urine glucose, see 81000, 81002, 81005, 81099)
82955	Glucose-6-phosphate dehydrogenase (G6PD); quantitative
82960	screen
	(For glucose tolerance test with medication, use 96374 in addition)
82962	Glucose, blood by glucose monitoring device(s) cleared by the FDA specifically for home use
82963	Glucosidase, beta
82965	Glutamate dehydrogenase
	(82975 has been deleted. For glutamine [glutamic acid amide], see 82127, 82128, 82131)
82977	Glutamyltransferase, gamma (GGT)
82978	Glutathione
82979	Glutathione reductase, RBC
	(82980 has been deleted)

(Glycohemoglobin, use 83036)

82985   Glycated protein

(Gonadotropin, chorionic, see 84702, 84703)

83001   Gonadotropin; follicle stimulating hormone (FSH)

83002   luteinizing hormone (LH)

(For luteinizing releasing factor [LRH], use 83727)

83003   Growth hormone, human (HGH) (somatotropin)

(For antibody to human growth hormone, use 86277)

83006   Growth stimulation expressed gene 2 (ST2, Interleukin 1 receptor like-1)

(83008 has been deleted)

83009   Helicobacter pylori, blood test analysis for urease activity, non-radioactive isotope (eg, C-13)

(For H. pylori, breath test analysis for urease activity, see 83013, 83014)

83010   Haptoglobin; quantitative

83012   phenotypes

83013   Helicobacter pylori; breath test analysis for urease activity, non-radioactive isotope (eg, C-13)

83014   drug administration

▶(For H. pylori, stool, use 87338. For H. pylori, liquid scintillation counter, see 78267, 78268. For H. pylori, immunoassay, use 87339)◀

(For H. pylori, blood test analysis for urease activity, use 83009)

83015   Heavy metal (eg, arsenic, barium, beryllium, bismuth, antimony, mercury); screen

83018   quantitative, each

83020   Hemoglobin fractionation and quantitation; electrophoresis (eg, A2, S, C, and/or F)

83021   chromatography (eg, A2, S, C, and/or F)

(For glycosylated [A1c] hemoglobin analysis, by electrophoresis or chromatography, in the absence of an identified hemoglobin variant, use 83036)

83026   Hemoglobin; by copper sulfate method, non-automated

83030   F (fetal), chemical

83033   F (fetal), qualitative

83036   glycosylated (A1C)

(For glycosylated [A1C] hemoglobin analysis, by electrophoresis or chromatography, in the setting of an identified hemoglobin variant, see 83020, 83021)

(For fecal hemoglobin detection by immunoassay, use 82274)

83037   glycosylated (A1C) by device cleared by FDA for home use

83045   methemoglobin, qualitative

83050   methemoglobin, quantitative

(For transcutaneous quantitative methemoglobin determination, use 88741)

83051   plasma

(83055 has been deleted)

83060   sulfhemoglobin, quantitative

83065   thermolabile

83068   unstable, screen

83069   urine

83070   Hemosiderin, qualitative

(83071 has been deleted)

(HIAA, use 83497)

▶(For a qualitative column chromatography procedure [eg, high performance liquid chromatography], use the appropriate specific analyte code, if available, or 82542)◀

83080   b-Hexosaminidase, each assay

83088   Histamine

(Hollander test, see 43754, 43755)

83090   Homocysteine

83150   Homovanillic acid (HVA)

(Hormones, see individual alphabetic listings in **Chemistry** section)

(For hydrogen/methane breath test, use 91065)

83491   Hydroxycorticosteroids, 17- (17-OHCS)

(For cortisol, see 82530, 82533. For deoxycortisol, use 82634)

83497   Hydroxyindolacetic acid, 5-(HIAA)

(For urine qualitative test, use 81005)

(5-Hydroxytryptamine, use 84260)

83498   Hydroxyprogesterone, 17-d

83499   Hydroxyprogesterone, 20-

83500   Hydroxyproline; free

83505   total

83516   Immunoassay for analyte other than infectious agent antibody or infectious agent antigen; qualitative or semiquantitative, multiple step method

83518   qualitative or semiquantitative, single step method (eg, reagent strip)

83519   quantitative, by radioimmunoassay (eg, RIA)

83520   quantitative, not otherwise specified

(For immunoassays for antibodies to infectious agent antigens, see analyte and method specific codes in the **Immunology** section)

Pathology and Laboratory

(For immunoassay of tumor antigen not elsewhere specified, use 86316)

(Immunoglobulins, see 82784, 82785)

83525 Insulin; total

(For proinsulin, use 84206)

83527 free

83528 Intrinsic factor

(For intrinsic factor antibodies, use 86340)

83540 Iron

83550 Iron binding capacity

83570 Isocitric dehydrogenase (IDH)

(Isonicotinic acid hydrazide, INH, see code for specific method)

(Isopropyl alcohol, use 80320)

83582 Ketogenic steroids, fractionation

(Ketone bodies, for serum, see 82009, 82010; for urine, see 81000-81003)

83586 Ketosteroids, 17- (17-KS); total

83593 fractionation

83605 Lactate (lactic acid)

83615 Lactate dehydrogenase (LD), (LDH);

83625 isoenzymes, separation and quantitation

83630 Lactoferrin, fecal; qualitative

83631 quantitative

83632 Lactogen, human placental (HPL) human chorionic somatomammotropin

83633 Lactose, urine, qualitative

(83634 has been deleted)

(For tolerance, see 82951, 82952)

(For breath hydrogen/methane test for lactase deficiency, use 91065)

83655 Lead

83661 Fetal lung maturity assessment; lecithin sphingomyelin (L/S) ratio

83662 foam stability test

83663 fluorescence polarization

83664 lamellar body density

(For phosphatidylglycerol, use 84081)

83670 Leucine aminopeptidase (LAP)

83690 Lipase

83695 Lipoprotein (a)

83698 Lipoprotein-associated phospholipase A2 (Lp-PLA2)

83700 Lipoprotein, blood; electrophoretic separation and quantitation

83701 high resolution fractionation and quantitation of lipoproteins including lipoprotein subclasses when performed (eg, electrophoresis, ultracentrifugation)

83704 quantitation of lipoprotein particle numbers and lipoprotein particle subclasses (eg, by nuclear magnetic resonance spectroscopy)

83718 Lipoprotein, direct measurement; high density cholesterol (HDL cholesterol)

83719 VLDL cholesterol

83721 LDL cholesterol

(For fractionation by high resolution electrophoresis or ultracentrifugation, use 83701)

(For lipoprotein particle numbers and subclasses analysis by nuclear magnetic resonance spectroscopy, use 83704)

83727 Luteinizing releasing factor (LRH)

(Luteinizing hormone [LH], use 83002)

(Macroglobulins, alpha-2, use 86329)

83735 Magnesium

83775 Malate dehydrogenase

(Maltose tolerance, see 82951, 82952)

(Mammotropin, use 84146)

83785 Manganese

►(83788 has been deleted. For a qualitative mass spectrometry or tandem mass spectrometry procedure, use the specific analyte code, if available, or 83789)◄

▲ **83789** Mass spectrometry and tandem mass spectrometry (eg, MS, MS/MS, MALDI, MS-TOF, QTOF), non-drug analyte(s) not elsewhere specified, qualitative or quantitative, each specimen

►(Do not report more than one unit of 83789 for each specimen)◄

(For column chromatography/mass spectrometry of drugs or substances, see **Drug Assay** 80300, 80301, 80302, 80303, 80304, 80320-80377, or specific analyte code[s] in the **Chemistry** section)

(83805 has been deleted. For quantitative testing for meprobamate, see 80369, 80370)

83825 Mercury, quantitative

(Mercury screen, use 83015)

83835 Metanephrines

(For catecholamines, see 82382-82384)

(83840 has been deleted. For methadone, use 80358)

(Methamphetamine, see 80324, 80325, 80326)

(Methane breath test, use 91065)

83857 Methemalbumin

(Methemoglobin, see hemoglobin 83045, 83050)

(83858 has been deleted. For methsuximide, see 80339, 80340, 80341)

(Methyl alcohol, use 80320)

(Microalbumin, see 82043 for quantitative, see 82044 for semiquantitative)

83861 Microfluidic analysis utilizing an integrated collection and analysis device, tear osmolarity

(Microglobulin, beta-2, use 82232)

(For microfluidic tear osmolarity of both eyes, report 83861 twice)

83864 Mucopolysaccharides, acid, quantitative

(83866 has been deleted)

83872 Mucin, synovial fluid (Ropes test)

83873 Myelin basic protein, cerebrospinal fluid

(For oligoclonal bands, use 83916)

83874 Myoglobin

83876 Myeloperoxidase (MPO)

83880 Natriuretic peptide

83883 Nephelometry, each analyte not elsewhere specified

83885 Nickel

(83887 has been deleted. For nicotine, use 80323)

(83890-83914 have been deleted. To report, see 81161, 81200-81479)

83915 Nucleotidase 5'-

83916 Oligoclonal immune (oligoclonal bands)

83918 Organic acids; total, quantitative, each specimen

83919 qualitative, each specimen

83921 Organic acid, single, quantitative

(83925 has been deleted. For opiates, see 80361, 80362, 80363, 80364, or the specific drug [eg, fentanyls, oxycodone])

83930 Osmolality; blood

83935 urine

(For tear osmolarity using microfluidic analysis, use 83861)

83937 Osteocalcin (bone g1a protein)

83945 Oxalate

83950 Oncoprotein; HER-2/neu

(For tissue, see 88342, 88365)

83951 des-gamma-carboxy-prothrombin (DCP)

83970 Parathormone (parathyroid hormone)

(Pesticide, quantitative, see code for specific method. For screen for chlorinated hydrocarbons, use 82441)

83986 pH; body fluid, not otherwise specified

83987 exhaled breath condensate

(For blood pH, see 82800, 82803)

83992 Code is out of numerical sequence. See 80320-80374

(Phenobarbital, use 80345)

83993 Calprotectin, fecal

(84022 has been deleted. For phenothiazine, see 80342, 80343, 80344)

84030 Phenylalanine (PKU), blood

(Phenylalanine-tyrosine ratio, see 84030, 84510)

84035 Phenylketones, qualitative

84060 Phosphatase, acid; total

84061 forensic examination

84066 prostatic

84075 Phosphatase, alkaline;

84078 heat stable (total not included)

84080 isoenzymes

84081 Phosphatidylglycerol

(Phosphates inorganic, use 84100)

(Phosphates, organic, see code for specific method. For cholinesterase, see 82480, 82482)

84085 Phosphogluconate, 6-, dehydrogenase, RBC

84087 Phosphohexose isomerase

84100 Phosphorus inorganic (phosphate);

84105 urine

(Pituitary gonadotropins, see 83001-83002)

(PKU, see 84030, 84035)

84106 Porphobilinogen, urine; qualitative

84110 quantitative

84112 Evaluation of cervicovaginal fluid for specific amniotic fluid protein(s) (eg, placental alpha microglobulin-1 [PAMG-1], placental protein 12 [PP12], alpha-fetoprotein), qualitative, each specimen

84119 Porphyrins, urine; qualitative

84120 quantitation and fractionation

84126 Porphyrins, feces, quantitative

(84127 has been deleted)

(Porphyrin precursors, see 82135, 84106, 84110)

(For protoporphyrin, RBC, see 84202, 84203)

84132 Potassium; serum, plasma or whole blood

84133 urine

84134 Prealbumin

(For microalbumin, see 82043, 82044)

Pathology and Laboratory

84135	Pregnanediol
84138	Pregnanetriol
84140	Pregnenolone
84143	17-hydroxypregnenolone
84144	Progesterone

(Progesterone receptor assay, use 84234)

(For proinsulin, use 84206)

84145	Procalcitonin (PCT)
84146	Prolactin
84150	Prostaglandin, each
84152	Prostate specific antigen (PSA); complexed (direct measurement)
84153	total
84154	free
84155	Protein, total, except by refractometry; serum, plasma or whole blood
84156	urine
84157	other source (eg, synovial fluid, cerebrospinal fluid)
84160	Protein, total, by refractometry, any source

(For urine total protein by dipstick method, use 81000-81003)

84163	Pregnancy-associated plasma protein-A (PAPP-A)
84165	Protein; electrophoretic fractionation and quantitation, serum
84166	electrophoretic fractionation and quantitation, other fluids with concentration (eg, urine, CSF)
84181	Western Blot, with interpretation and report, blood or other body fluid
84182	Western Blot, with interpretation and report, blood or other body fluid, immunological probe for band identification, each

(For Western Blot tissue analysis, use 88371)

84202	Protoporphyrin, RBC; quantitative
84203	screen
84206	Proinsulin

(Pseudocholinesterase, use 82480)

84207	Pyridoxal phosphate (Vitamin B-6)
84210	Pyruvate
84220	Pyruvate kinase
84228	Quinine
84233	Receptor assay; estrogen
84234	progesterone
84235	endocrine, other than estrogen or progesterone (specify hormone)

84238	non-endocrine (specify receptor)
84244	Renin
84252	Riboflavin (Vitamin B-2)

(Salicylates, see 80329, 80330, 80331)

(Secretin test, see 99070, 43756, 43757 and appropriate analyses)

84255	Selenium
84260	Serotonin

(For urine metabolites (HIAA), use 83497)

84270	Sex hormone binding globulin (SHBG)
84275	Sialic acid

(Sickle hemoglobin, use 85660)

84285	Silica
84295	Sodium; serum, plasma or whole blood
84300	urine
84302	other source

(Somatomammotropin, use 83632)

(Somatotropin, use 83003)

84305	Somatomedin
84307	Somatostatin
84311	Spectrophotometry, analyte not elsewhere specified
84315	Specific gravity (except urine)

(For specific gravity, urine, see 81000-81003)

(Stone analysis, see 82355-82370)

(For suppression of growth stimulation expressed gene 2 [ST2] testing, use 83006)

84375	Sugars, chromatographic, TLC or paper chromatography
84376	Sugars (mono-, di-, and oligosaccharides); single qualitative, each specimen
84377	multiple qualitative, each specimen
84378	single quantitative, each specimen
84379	multiple quantitative, each specimen
84392	Sulfate, urine

(Sulfhemoglobin, use hemoglobin, 83060)

(T-3, see 84479-84481)

(T-4, see 84436-84439)

84402	Testosterone; free
84403	total

(Do not report 84402, 84403 in conjunction with 80327, 80328 to identify anabolic steroid testing for testosterone)

84425	Thiamine (Vitamin B-1)
84430	Thiocyanate

84431   Thromboxane metabolite(s), including thromboxane if performed, urine

(For concurrent urine creatinine determination, use 84431 in conjunction with 82570)

84432   Thyroglobulin

(Thyroglobulin, antibody, use 86800)

(Thyrotropin releasing hormone [TRH] test, see 80438, 80439)

84436   Thyroxine; total

84437   requiring elution (eg, neonatal)

84439   free

84442   Thyroxine binding globulin (TBG)

84443   Thyroid stimulating hormone (TSH)

84445   Thyroid stimulating immune globulins (TSI)

(Tobramycin, use 80200)

84446   Tocopherol alpha (Vitamin E)

84449   Transcortin (cortisol binding globulin)

84450   Transferase; aspartate amino (AST) (SGOT)

84460   alanine amino (ALT) (SGPT)

84466   Transferrin

(Iron binding capacity, use 83550)

84478   Triglycerides

84479   Thyroid hormone (T3 or T4) uptake or thyroid hormone binding ratio (THBR)

84480   Triiodothyronine T3; total (TT-3)

84481   free

84482   reverse

84484   Troponin, quantitative

(For troponin, qualitative assay, use 84512)

84485   Trypsin; duodenal fluid

84488   feces, qualitative

84490   feces, quantitative, 24-hour collection

84510   Tyrosine

(Urate crystal identification, use 89060)

84512   Troponin, qualitative

(For troponin, quantitative assay, use 84484)

84520   Urea nitrogen; quantitative

84525   semiquantitative (eg, reagent strip test)

84540   Urea nitrogen, urine

84545   Urea nitrogen, clearance

84550   Uric acid; blood

84560   other source

84577   Urobilinogen, feces, quantitative

84578   Urobilinogen, urine; qualitative

84580   quantitative, timed specimen

84583   semiquantitative

(Uroporphyrins, use 84120)

(Valproic acid [dipropylacetic acid], use 80164)

84585   Vanillylmandelic acid (VMA), urine

84586   Vasoactive intestinal peptide (VIP)

84588   Vasopressin (antidiuretic hormone, ADH)

84590   Vitamin A

(Vitamin B-1, use 84425)

(Vitamin B-2, use 84252)

(Vitamin B-6, use 84207)

(Vitamin B-12, use 82607)

(Vitamin B-12, absorption (Schilling), see 78270, 78271)

(Vitamin C, use 82180)

(Vitamin D, see 82306, 82652)

(Vitamin E, use 84446)

84591   Vitamin, not otherwise specified

84597   Vitamin K

(VMA, use 84585)

84600   Volatiles (eg, acetic anhydride, diethylether)

(For carbon tetrachloride, dichloroethane, dichloromethane, use 82441)

(For isopropyl alcohol and methanol, use 80320)

(Volume, blood, RISA or Cr-51, see 78110, 78111)

84620   Xylose absorption test, blood and/or urine

(For administration, use 99070)

84630   Zinc

84681   C-peptide

84702   Gonadotropin, chorionic (hCG); quantitative

84703   qualitative

(For urine pregnancy test by visual color comparison, use 81025)

84704   free beta chain

84830   Ovulation tests, by visual color comparison methods for human luteinizing hormone

84999   Unlisted chemistry procedure

(For definitive testing of a drug, not otherwise specified, see 80299, 80375, 80376, 80377)

Hematology and Coagulation

(For blood banking procedures, see **Transfusion Medicine**)

(Agglutinins, see **Immunology**)

(Antiplasmin, use 85410)

(Antithrombin III, see 85300, 85301)

85002 Bleeding time

85004 Blood count; automated differential WBC count

85007 blood smear, microscopic examination with manual differential WBC count

85008 blood smear, microscopic examination without manual differential WBC count

(For other fluids [eg, CSF], see 89050, 89051)

85009 manual differential WBC count, buffy coat

(Eosinophils, nasal smear, use 89190)

85013 spun microhematocrit

85014 hematocrit (Hct)

85018 hemoglobin (Hgb)

(For other hemoglobin determination, see 83020-83069)

(For immunoassay, hemoglobin, fecal, use 82274)

(For transcutaneous hemoglobin measurement, use 88738)

85025 complete (CBC), automated (Hgb, Hct, RBC, WBC and platelet count) and automated differential WBC count

85027 complete (CBC), automated (Hgb, Hct, RBC, WBC and platelet count)

85032 manual cell count (erythrocyte, leukocyte, or platelet) each

85041 red blood cell (RBC), automated

(Do not report code 85041 in conjunction with 85025 or 85027)

85044 reticulocyte, manual

85045 reticulocyte, automated

85046 reticulocytes, automated, including 1 or more cellular parameters (eg, reticulocyte hemoglobin content [CHr], immature reticulocyte fraction [IRF], reticulocyte volume [MRV], RNA content), direct measurement

85048 leukocyte (WBC), automated

85049 platelet, automated

85055 Reticulated platelet assay

85060 Blood smear, peripheral, interpretation by physician with written report

85097 Bone marrow, smear interpretation

(For special stains, see 88312, 88313)

(For bone biopsy, see 20220, 20225, 20240, 20245, 20250, 20251)

85130 Chromogenic substrate assay

(Circulating anti-coagulant screen [mixing studies], see 85611, 85732)

85170 Clot retraction

85175 Clot lysis time, whole blood dilution

(Clotting factor I [fibrinogen], see 85384, 85385)

85210 Clotting; factor II, prothrombin, specific

(See also 85610-85613)

85220 factor V (AcG or proaccelerin), labile factor

85230 factor VII (proconvertin, stable factor)

85240 factor VIII (AHG), 1-stage

85244 factor VIII related antigen

85245 factor VIII, VW factor, ristocetin cofactor

85246 factor VIII, VW factor antigen

85247 factor VIII, von Willebrand factor, multimetric analysis

85250 factor IX (PTC or Christmas)

85260 factor X (Stuart-Prower)

85270 factor XI (PTA)

85280 factor XII (Hageman)

85290 factor XIII (fibrin stabilizing)

85291 factor XIII (fibrin stabilizing), screen solubility

85292 prekallikrein assay (Fletcher factor assay)

85293 high molecular weight kininogen assay (Fitzgerald factor assay)

85300 Clotting inhibitors or anticoagulants; antithrombin III, activity

85301 antithrombin III, antigen assay

85302 protein C, antigen

85303 protein C, activity

85305 protein S, total

85306 protein S, free

85307 Activated Protein C (APC) resistance assay

85335 Factor inhibitor test

85337 Thrombomodulin

(For mixing studies for inhibitors, use 85732)

85345 Coagulation time; Lee and White

85347 activated

85348 other methods

(Differential count, see 85007 et seq)

(Duke bleeding time, use 85002)

(Eosinophils, nasal smear, use 89190)

85360 Euglobulin lysis

(Fetal hemoglobin, see 83030, 83033, 85460)

85362 Fibrin(ogen) degradation (split) products (FDP) (FSP); agglutination slide, semiquantitative

(Immunoelectrophoresis, use 86320)

85366   paracoagulation

85370   quantitative

85378 Fibrin degradation products, D-dimer; qualitative or semiquantitative

85379   quantitative

(For ultrasensitive and standard sensitivity quantitative D-dimer, use 85379)

85380   ultrasensitive (eg, for evaluation for venous thromboembolism), qualitative or semiquantitative

85384 Fibrinogen; activity

85385   antigen

85390 Fibrinolysins or coagulopathy screen, interpretation and report

85396 Coagulation/fibrinolysis assay, whole blood (eg, viscoelastic clot assessment), including use of any pharmacologic additive(s), as indicated, including interpretation and written report, per day

85397 Coagulation and fibrinolysis, functional activity, not otherwise specified (eg, ADAMTS-13), each analyte

85400 Fibrinolytic factors and inhibitors; plasmin

85410   alpha-2 antiplasmin

85415   plasminogen activator

85420   plasminogen, except antigenic assay

85421   plasminogen, antigenic assay

(Fragility, red blood cell, see 85547, 85555-85557)

85441 Heinz bodies; direct

85445   induced, acetyl phenylhydrazine

(Hematocrit [PCV], see 85014, 85025, 85027)

(Hemoglobin, see 83020-83068, 85018, 85025, 85027)

85460 Hemoglobin or RBCs, fetal, for fetomaternal hemorrhage; differential lysis (Kleihauer-Betke)

(See also 83030, 83033)

(Hemolysins, see 86940, 86941)

85461   rosette

85475 Hemolysin, acid

(See also 86940, 86941)

85520 Heparin assay

85525 Heparin neutralization

85530 Heparin-protamine tolerance test

85536 Iron stain, peripheral blood

(For iron stains on bone marrow or other tissues with physician evaluation, use 88313)

85540 Leukocyte alkaline phosphatase with count

85547 Mechanical fragility, RBC

85549 Muramidase

(Nitroblue tetrazolium dye test, use 86384)

85555 Osmotic fragility, RBC; unincubated

85557   incubated

(Packed cell volume, use 85013)

(Partial thromboplastin time, see 85730, 85732)

(Parasites, blood [eg, malaria smears], use 87207)

(Plasmin, use 85400)

(Plasminogen, use 85420)

(Plasminogen activator, use 85415)

85576 Platelet, aggregation (in vitro), each agent

(For thromboxane metabolite[s], including thromboxane, if performed, measurement[s] in urine, use 84431)

85597 Phospholipid neutralization; platelet

85598   hexagonal phospholipid

85610 Prothrombin time;

85611   substitution, plasma fractions, each

85612 Russell viper venom time (includes venom); undiluted

85613   diluted

(Red blood cell count, see 85025, 85027, 85041)

85635 Reptilase test

(Reticulocyte count, see 85044, 85045)

85651 Sedimentation rate, erythrocyte; non-automated

85652   automated

85660 Sickling of RBC, reduction

(Hemoglobin electrophoresis, use 83020)

(Smears [eg, for parasites, malaria], use 87207)

85670 Thrombin time; plasma

85675   titer

85705 Thromboplastin inhibition, tissue

(For individual clotting factors, see 85245-85247)

85730 Thromboplastin time, partial (PTT); plasma or whole blood

85732   substitution, plasma fractions, each

Pathology and Laboratory

85810   Viscosity

(von Willebrand factor assay, see 85245-85247)

(WBC count, see 85025, 85027, 85048, 89050)

85999   Unlisted hematology and coagulation procedure

Immunology

(Acetylcholine receptor antibody, see 83519, 86255, 86256)

(Actinomyces, antibodies to, use 86602)

(Adrenal cortex antibodies, see 86255, 86256)

86000   Agglutinins, febrile (eg, Brucella, Francisella, Murine typhus, Q fever, Rocky Mountain spotted fever, scrub typhus), each antigen

(For antibodies to infectious agents, see 86602-86804)

86001   Allergen specific IgG quantitative or semiquantitative, each allergen

(Agglutinins and autohemolysins, see 86940, 86941)

86003   Allergen specific IgE; quantitative or semiquantitative, each allergen

(For total quantitative IgE, use 82785)

86005   qualitative, multiallergen screen (dipstick, paddle, or disk)

(For total qualitative IgE, use 83518)

(Alpha-1 antitrypsin, see 82103, 82104)

(Alpha-1 feto-protein, see 82105, 82106)

(Anti-AChR [acetylcholine receptor] antibody titer, see 86255, 86256)

(Anticardiolipin antibody, use 86147)

(Anti-DNA, use 86225)

(Anti-deoxyribonuclease titer, use 86215)

86021   Antibody identification; leukocyte antibodies

86022   platelet antibodies

86023   platelet associated immunoglobulin assay

86038   Antinuclear antibodies (ANA);

86039   titer

(Antistreptococcal antibody, ie, anti-DNAse, use 86215)

(Antistreptokinase titer, use 86590)

86060   Antistreptolysin O; titer

(For antibodies to infectious agents, see 86602-86804)

86063   screen

(For antibodies to infectious agents, see 86602-86804)

(Blastomyces, antibodies to, use 86612)

86077   Blood bank physician services; difficult cross match and/or evaluation of irregular antibody(s), interpretation and written report

86078   investigation of transfusion reaction including suspicion of transmissible disease, interpretation and written report

86079   authorization for deviation from standard blood banking procedures (eg, use of outdated blood, transfusion of Rh incompatible units), with written report

(Brucella, antibodies to, use 86622)

(Candida, antibodies to, use 86628. For skin testing, use 86485)

86140   C-reactive protein;

(Candidiasis, use 86628)

86141   high sensitivity (hsCRP)

86146   Beta 2 Glycoprotein I antibody, each

86147   Cardiolipin (phospholipid) antibody, each Ig class

86152   Cell enumeration using immunologic selection and identification in fluid specimen (eg, circulating tumor cells in blood);

(For physician interpretation and report, use 86153. For cell enumeration with interpretation and report, use 86152 and 86153)

86153   physician interpretation and report, when required

(For cell enumeration, use 86152. For cell enumeration with interpretation and report, use 86152 and 86153)

(For flow cytometric immunophenotyping, see 88184-88189)

(For flow cytometric quantitation, see 86355, 86356, 86357, 86359, 86360, 86361, 86367)

86148   Anti-phosphatidylserine (phospholipid) antibody

(To report antiprothrombin [phospholipid cofactor] antibody, use 86849)

86152   Code is out of numerical sequence. See 86000-86804

86153   Code is out of numerical sequence. See 86000-86804

86155   Chemotaxis assay, specify method

(Clostridium difficile toxin, use 87230)

(Coccidioides, antibodies to, see 86635. For skin testing, use 86490)

86156   Cold agglutinin; screen

86157   titer

86160   Complement; antigen, each component

86161   functional activity, each component

86162   total hemolytic (CH50)

86171   Complement fixation tests, each antigen

(Coombs test, see 86880-86886)

86185   Counterimmunoelectrophoresis, each antigen

(Cryptococcus, antibodies to, use 86641)

86200   Cyclic citrullinated peptide (CCP), antibody

86215   Deoxyribonuclease, antibody

86225   Deoxyribonucleic acid (DNA) antibody; native or double stranded

(Echinococcus, antibodies to, see code for specific method)

(For HIV antibody tests, see 86701-86703)

86226   single stranded

(Anti D.S., DNA, IFA, eg, using C.Lucilae, see 86255 and 86256)

86235   Extractable nuclear antigen, antibody to, any method (eg, nRNP, SS-A, SS-B, Sm, RNP, Sc170, J01), each antibody

86243   Fc receptor

(Filaria, antibodies to, see code for specific method)

86255   Fluorescent noninfectious agent antibody; screen, each antibody

86256   titer, each antibody

►(Fluorescent technique for antigen identification in tissue, use 88346; for indirect fluorescence, see 88346, 88350)◄

(FTA, use 86780)

(Gel [agar] diffusion tests, use 86331)

86277   Growth hormone, human (HGH), antibody

86280   Hemagglutination inhibition test (HAI)

(For rubella, use 86762)

(For antibodies to infectious agents, see 86602-86804)

86294   Immunoassay for tumor antigen, qualitative or semiquantitative (eg, bladder tumor antigen)

(For qualitative NMP22 protein, use 86386)

86300   Immunoassay for tumor antigen, quantitative; CA 15-3 (27.29)

86301   CA 19-9

86304   CA 125

(For measurement of serum HER-2/neu oncoprotein, see 83950)

(For hepatitis delta agent, antibody, use 86692)

86305   Human epididymis protein 4 (HE4)

86308   Heterophile antibodies; screening

(For antibodies to infectious agents, see 86602-86804)

86309   titer

(For antibodies to infectious agents, see 86602-86804)

86310   titers after absorption with beef cells and guinea pig kidney

(Histoplasma, antibodies to, use 86698. For skin testing, use 86510)

(For antibodies to infectious agents, see 86602-86804)

(Human growth hormone antibody, use 86277)

86316   Immunoassay for tumor antigen, other antigen, quantitative (eg, CA 50, 72-4, 549), each

86317   Immunoassay for infectious agent antibody, quantitative, not otherwise specified

(For immunoassay techniques for antigens, see 83516, 83518, 83519, 83520, 87301-87450, 87810-87899)

(For particle agglutination procedures, use 86403)

86318   Immunoassay for infectious agent antibody, qualitative or semiquantitative, single step method (eg, reagent strip)

86320   Immunoelectrophoresis; serum

86325   other fluids (eg, urine, cerebrospinal fluid) with concentration

86327   crossed (2-dimensional assay)

86329   Immunodiffusion; not elsewhere specified

86331   gel diffusion, qualitative (Ouchterlony), each antigen or antibody

86332   Immune complex assay

86334   Immunofixation electrophoresis; serum

86335   other fluids with concentration (eg, urine, CSF)

86336   Inhibin A

86337   Insulin antibodies

86340   Intrinsic factor antibodies

(Leptospira, antibodies to, use 86720)

(Leukoagglutinins, use 86021)

86341   Islet cell antibody

86343   Leukocyte histamine release test (LHR)

86344   Leukocyte phagocytosis

86352   Cellular function assay involving stimulation (eg, mitogen or antigen) and detection of biomarker (eg, ATP)

86353   Lymphocyte transformation, mitogen (phytomitogen) or antigen induced blastogenesis

(Malaria antibodies, use 86750)

(For cellular function assay involving stimulation and detection of biomarker, use 86352)

86355   B cells, total count

86356   Mononuclear cell antigen, quantitative (eg, flow cytometry), not otherwise specified, each antigen

(Do not report 88187-88189 for interpretation of 86355, 86356, 86357, 86359, 86360, 86361, 86367)

Pathology and Laboratory

86357   Natural killer (NK) cells, total count

86359   T cells; total count

86360   absolute CD4 and CD8 count, including ratio

86361   absolute CD4 count

86367   Stem cells (ie, CD34), total count

(For flow cytometric immunophenotyping for the assessment of potential hematolymphoid neoplasia, see 88184-88189)

86376   Microsomal antibodies (eg, thyroid or liver-kidney), each

86378   Migration inhibitory factor test (MIF)

(Mitochondrial antibody, liver, see 86255, 86256)

(Mononucleosis, see 86308-86310)

86382   Neutralization test, viral

86384   Nitroblue tetrazolium dye test (NTD)

86386   Nuclear Matrix Protein 22 (NMP22), qualitative

(Ouchterlony diffusion, use 86331)

(Platelet antibodies, see 86022, 86023)

86403   Particle agglutination; screen, each antibody

86406   titer, each antibody

(Pregnancy test, see 84702, 84703)

(Rapid plasma reagin test (RPR), see 86592, 86593)

86430   Rheumatoid factor; qualitative

86431   quantitative

(Serologic test for syphilis, see 86592, 86593)

86480   Tuberculosis test, cell mediated immunity antigen response measurement; gamma interferon

86481   enumeration of gamma interferon-producing T-cells in cell suspension

86485   Skin test; candida

(For antibody, candida, use 86628)

86486   unlisted antigen, each

86490   coccidioidomycosis

86510   histoplasmosis

(For histoplasma, antibody, use 86698)

86580   tuberculosis, intradermal

(For tuberculosis test, cell mediated immunity measurement of gamma interferon antigen response, use 86480)

(For skin tests for allergy, see 95012-95199)

(Smooth muscle antibody, see 86255, 86256)

(Sporothrix, antibodies to, see code for specific method)

86590   Streptokinase, antibody

(For antibodies to infectious agents, see 86602-86804)

(Streptolysin O antibody, see antistreptolysin O, 86060, 86063)

86592   Syphilis test, non-treponemal antibody; qualitative (eg, VDRL, RPR, ART)

(For antibodies to infectious agents, see 86602-86804)

86593   quantitative

(For antibodies to infectious agents, see 86602-86804)

(Tetanus antibody, use 86774)

(Thyroglobulin antibody, use 86800)

(Thyroglobulin, use 84432)

(Thyroid microsomal antibody, use 86376)

(For toxoplasma antibody, see 86777-86778)

The following codes (86602-86804) are qualitative or semiquantitative immunoassays performed by multiple-step methods for the detection of antibodies to infectious agents. For immunoassays by single-step method (eg, reagent strips), use code 86318. Procedures for the identification of antibodies should be coded as precisely as possible. For example, an antibody to a virus could be coded with increasing specificity for virus, family, genus, species, or type. In some cases, further precision may be added to codes by specifying the class of immunoglobulin being detected. When multiple tests are done to detect antibodies to organisms classified more precisely than the specificity allowed by available codes, it is appropriate to code each as a separate service. For example, a test for antibody to an enterovirus is coded as 86658. Coxsackie viruses are enteroviruses, but there are no codes for the individual species of enterovirus. If assays are performed for antibodies to coxsackie A and B species, each assay should be separately coded. Similarly, if multiple assays are performed for antibodies of different immunoglobulin classes, each assay should be coded separately. When a coding option exists for reporting IgM specific antibodies (eg, 86632), the corresponding nonspecific code (eg, 86631) may be reported for performance of either an antibody analysis not specific for a particular immunoglobulin class or for an IgG analysis.

(For the detection of antibodies other than those to infectious agents, see specific antibody [eg, 86021-86023, 86376, 86800, 86850-86870] or specific method [eg, 83516, 86255, 86256]).

(For infectious agent/antigen detection, see 87260-87899)

86602   Antibody; actinomyces

86603   adenovirus

86606   Aspergillus

86609   bacterium, not elsewhere specified

86611   Bartonella

86612   Blastomyces

86615   Bordetella

Pathology and Laboratory

86617	Borrelia burgdorferi (Lyme disease) confirmatory test (eg, Western Blot or immunoblot)
86618	Borrelia burgdorferi (Lyme disease)
86619	Borrelia (relapsing fever)
86622	Brucella
86625	Campylobacter
86628	Candida

(For skin test, candida, use 86485)

86631	Chlamydia
86632	Chlamydia, IgM

(For chlamydia antigen, see 87270, 87320. For fluorescent antibody technique, see 86255, 86256)

86635	Coccidioides
86638	Coxiella burnetii (Q fever)
86641	Cryptococcus
86644	cytomegalovirus (CMV)
86645	cytomegalovirus (CMV), IgM
86648	Diphtheria
86651	encephalitis, California (La Crosse)
86652	encephalitis, Eastern equine
86653	encephalitis, St. Louis
86654	encephalitis, Western equine
86658	enterovirus (eg, coxsackie, echo, polio)

(Trichinella, antibodies to, use 86784)

(Trypanosoma, antibodies to, see code for specific method)

(Tuberculosis, use 86580 for skin testing)

(Viral antibodies, see code for specific method)

86663	Epstein-Barr (EB) virus, early antigen (EA)
86664	Epstein-Barr (EB) virus, nuclear antigen (EBNA)
86665	Epstein-Barr (EB) virus, viral capsid (VCA)
86666	Ehrlichia
86668	Francisella tularensis
86671	fungus, not elsewhere specified
86674	Giardia lamblia
86677	Helicobacter pylori
86682	helminth, not elsewhere specified
86684	Haemophilus influenza
86687	HTLV-I
86688	HTLV-II
86689	HTLV or HIV antibody, confirmatory test (eg, Western Blot)

86692	hepatitis, delta agent

(For hepatitis delta agent, antigen, use 87380)

86694	herpes simplex, non-specific type test
86695	herpes simplex, type 1
86696	herpes simplex, type 2
86698	histoplasma
86701	HIV-1
86702	HIV-2
86703	HIV-1 and HIV-2, single result

(For HIV-1 antigen(s) with HIV-1 and HIV-2 antibodies, single result, use 87389)

(When HIV immunoassay [HIV testing 86701-86703 or 87389] is performed using a kit or transportable instrument that wholly or in part consists of a single use, disposable analytical chamber, the service may be identified by adding modifier 92 to the usual code)

(For HIV-1 antigen, use 87390)

(For HIV-2 antigen, use 87391)

(For confirmatory test for HIV antibody (eg, Western Blot), use 86689)

86704	Hepatitis B core antibody (HBcAb); total
86705	IgM antibody
86706	Hepatitis B surface antibody (HBsAb)
86707	Hepatitis Be antibody (HBeAb)
▲ 86708	Hepatitis A antibody (HAAb)
▲ 86709	Hepatitis A antibody (HAAb), IgM antibody
86710	Antibody; influenza virus
86711	JC (John Cunningham) virus
86713	Legionella
86717	Leishmania
86720	Leptospira
86723	Listeria monocytogenes
86727	lymphocytic choriomeningitis
86729	lymphogranuloma venereum
86732	mucormycosis
86735	mumps
86738	mycoplasma
86741	Neisseria meningitidis
86744	Nocardia
86747	parvovirus
86750	Plasmodium (malaria)
86753	protozoa, not elsewhere specified
86756	respiratory syncytial virus

86757	Rickettsia
86759	rotavirus
86762	rubella
86765	rubeola
86768	Salmonella
86771	Shigella
86774	tetanus
86777	Toxoplasma
86778	Toxoplasma, IgM
86780	Treponema pallidum

(For syphilis testing by non-treponemal antibody analysis, see 86592-86593)

86784	Trichinella
86787	varicella-zoster
86788	West Nile virus, IgM
86789	West Nile virus
86790	virus, not elsewhere specified
86793	Yersinia
86800	Thyroglobulin antibody

(For thyroglobulin, use 84432)

86803	Hepatitis C antibody;
86804	confirmatory test (eg, immunoblot)

Tissue Typing

86805	Lymphocytotoxicity assay, visual crossmatch; with titration
86806	without titration
86807	Serum screening for cytotoxic percent reactive antibody (PRA); standard method
86808	quick method
86812	HLA typing; A, B, or C (eg, A10, B7, B27), single antigen
86813	A, B, or C, multiple antigens
86816	DR/DQ, single antigen
86817	DR/DQ, multiple antigens
86821	lymphocyte culture, mixed (MLC)
86822	lymphocyte culture, primed (PLC)

(For HLA typing by molecular pathology techniques, see 81370-81383)

86825	Human leukocyte antigen (HLA) crossmatch, non-cytotoxic (eg, using flow cytometry); first serum sample or dilution
+ 86826	each additional serum sample or sample dilution (List separately in addition to primary procedure)

(Use 86826 in conjunction with 86825)

(Do not report 86825, 86826 in conjunction with 86355, 86359, 88184-88189 for antibody surface markers integral to crossmatch testing)

(For autologous HLA crossmatch, see 86825, 86826)

(For lymphocytotoxicity visual crossmatch, see 86805, 86806)

86828	Antibody to human leukocyte antigens (HLA), solid phase assays (eg, microspheres or beads, ELISA, flow cytometry); qualitative assessment of the presence or absence of antibody(ies) to HLA Class I and Class II HLA antigens
86829	qualitative assessment of the presence or absence of antibody(ies) to HLA Class I or Class II HLA antigens

(If solid phase testing is performed to assess presence or absence of antibody to both HLA classes, use 86828)

86830	antibody identification by qualitative panel using complete HLA phenotypes, HLA Class I
86831	antibody identification by qualitative panel using complete HLA phenotypes, HLA Class II
86832	high definition qualitative panel for identification of antibody specificities (eg, individual antigen per bead methodology), HLA Class I
86833	high definition qualitative panel for identification of antibody specificities (eg, individual antigen per bead methodology), HLA Class II

(If solid phase testing is performed to test for HLA Class I or II antibody after treatment [eg, to remove IgM antibodies or other interfering substances], report 86828-86833 once for each panel with the untreated serum and once for each panel with the treated serum)

86834	semi-quantitative panel (eg, titer), HLA Class I
86835	semi-quantitative panel (eg, titer), HLA Class II
86849	Unlisted immunology procedure

Transfusion Medicine

(For apheresis, use 36511, 36512)

(For therapeutic phlebotomy, use 99195)

86850	Antibody screen, RBC, each serum technique
86860	Antibody elution (RBC), each elution
86870	Antibody identification, RBC antibodies, each panel for each serum technique
86880	Antihuman globulin test (Coombs test); direct, each antiserum
86885	indirect, qualitative, each reagent red cell
86886	indirect, each antibody titer

(For indirect antihuman globulin [Coombs] test for RBC antibody screening, use 86850)

(For indirect antihuman globulin [Coombs] test for RBC antibody identification using reagent red cell panels, use 86870)

86890   Autologous blood or component, collection processing and storage; predeposited

86891   intra- or postoperative salvage

86900   Blood typing, serologic; ABO

86901   Rh (D)

86902   antigen testing of donor blood using reagent serum, each antigen test

(If multiple blood units are tested for the same antigen, 86902 should be reported once for each antigen for each unit tested)

86904   antigen screening for compatible unit using patient serum, per unit screened

86905   RBC antigens, other than ABO or Rh (D), each

86906   Rh phenotyping, complete

(For human erythrocyte antigen typing by molecular pathology techniques, use 81403)

86910   Blood typing, for paternity testing, per individual; ABO, Rh and MN

86911   each additional antigen system

86920   Compatibility test each unit; immediate spin technique

86921   incubation technique

86922   antiglobulin technique

86923   electronic

(Do not use 86923 in conjunction with 86920-86922 for same unit crossmatch)

86927   Fresh frozen plasma, thawing, each unit

86930   Frozen blood, each unit; freezing (includes preparation)

86931   thawing

86932   freezing (includes preparation) and thawing

86940   Hemolysins and agglutinins; auto, screen, each

86941   incubated

86945   Irradiation of blood product, each unit

86950   Leukocyte transfusion

(For allogeneic lymphocyte infusion, use 38242)

(For leukapheresis, use 36511)

86960   Volume reduction of blood or blood product (eg, red blood cells or platelets), each unit

86965   Pooling of platelets or other blood products

(For injection(s) of platelet rich plasma, use 0232T)

86970   Pretreatment of RBCs for use in RBC antibody detection, identification, and/or compatibility testing; incubation with chemical agents or drugs, each

86971   incubation with enzymes, each

86972   by density gradient separation

86975   Pretreatment of serum for use in RBC antibody identification; incubation with drugs, each

86976   by dilution

86977   incubation with inhibitors, each

86978   by differential red cell absorption using patient RBCs or RBCs of known phenotype, each absorption

86985   Splitting of blood or blood products, each unit

86999   Unlisted transfusion medicine procedure

Microbiology

Includes bacteriology, mycology, parasitology, and virology.

Presumptive identification of microorganisms is defined as identification by colony morphology, growth on selective media, Gram stains, or up to three tests (eg, catalase, oxidase, indole, urease). Definitive identification of microorganisms is defined as an identification to the genus or species level that requires additional tests (eg, biochemical panels, slide cultures). If additional studies involve molecular probes, nucleic acid sequencing, chromatography, or immunologic techniques, these should be separately coded using 87140-87158, in addition to definitive identification codes. The molecular diagnostic codes (eg, 81161, 81200-81408) are not to be used in combination with or instead of the procedures represented by 87140-87158. For multiple specimens/sites use modifier 59. For repeat laboratory tests performed on the same day, use modifier 91.

(87001 has been deleted)

87003   Animal inoculation, small animal, with observation and dissection

87015   Concentration (any type), for infectious agents

(Do not report 87015 in conjunction with 87177)

87040   Culture, bacterial; blood, aerobic, with isolation and presumptive identification of isolates (includes anaerobic culture, if appropriate)

87045   stool, aerobic, with isolation and preliminary examination (eg, KIA, LIA), Salmonella and Shigella species

87046   stool, aerobic, additional pathogens, isolation and presumptive identification of isolates, each plate

87070   any other source except urine, blood or stool, aerobic, with isolation and presumptive identification of isolates

(For urine, use 87088)

87071 quantitative, aerobic with isolation and presumptive identification of isolates, any source except urine, blood or stool

(For urine, use 87088)

87073 quantitative, anaerobic with isolation and presumptive identification of isolates, any source except urine, blood or stool

(For definitive identification of isolates, use 87076 or 87077. For typing of isolates see 87140-87158)

87075 any source, except blood, anaerobic with isolation and presumptive identification of isolates

87076 anaerobic isolate, additional methods required for definitive identification, each isolate

87077 aerobic isolate, additional methods required for definitive identification, each isolate

87081 Culture, presumptive, pathogenic organisms, screening only;

87084 with colony estimation from density chart

87086 Culture, bacterial; quantitative colony count, urine

87088 with isolation and presumptive identification of each isolate, urine

87101 Culture, fungi (mold or yeast) isolation, with presumptive identification of isolates; skin, hair, or nail

87102 other source (except blood)

87103 blood

87106 Culture, fungi, definitive identification, each organism; yeast

87107 mold

87109 Culture, mycoplasma, any source

87110 Culture, chlamydia, any source

(For immunofluorescence staining of shell vials, use 87140)

87116 Culture, tubercle or other acid-fast bacilli (eg, TB, AFB, mycobacteria) any source, with isolation and presumptive identification of isolates

(For concentration, use 87015)

87118 Culture, mycobacterial, definitive identification, each isolate

87140 Culture, typing; immunofluorescent method, each antiserum

87143 gas liquid chromatography (GLC) or high pressure liquid chromatography (HPLC) method

87147 immunologic method, other than immunofluoresence (eg, agglutination grouping), per antiserum

87149 identification by nucleic acid (DNA or RNA) probe, direct probe technique, per culture or isolate, each organism probed

(Do not report 87149 in conjunction with 81161, 81200-81408)

87150 identification by nucleic acid (DNA or RNA) probe, amplified probe technique, per culture or isolate, each organism probed

(Do not report 87150 in conjunction with 81161, 81200-81408)

87152 identification by pulse field gel typing

(Do not report 87152 in conjunction with 81161, 81200-81408)

87153 identification by nucleic acid sequencing method, each isolate (eg, sequencing of the 16S rRNA gene)

87158 other methods

87164 Dark field examination, any source (eg, penile, vaginal, oral, skin); includes specimen collection

87166 without collection

87168 Macroscopic examination; arthropod

87169 parasite

87172 Pinworm exam (eg, cellophane tape prep)

87176 Homogenization, tissue, for culture

87177 Ova and parasites, direct smears, concentration and identification

(Do not report 87177 in conjunction with 87015)

(For direct smears from a primary source, use 87207)

(For coccidia or microsporidia exam, use 87207)

(For complex special stain (trichrome, iron hematoxylin), use 87209)

(For nucleic acid probes in cytologic material, use 88365)

87181 Susceptibility studies, antimicrobial agent; agar dilution method, per agent (eg, antibiotic gradient strip)

87184 disk method, per plate (12 or fewer agents)

87185 enzyme detection (eg, beta lactamase), per enzyme

87186 microdilution or agar dilution (minimum inhibitory concentration [MIC] or breakpoint), each multi-antimicrobial, per plate

+ 87187 microdilution or agar dilution, minimum lethal concentration (MLC), each plate (List separately in addition to code for primary procedure)

(Use 87187 in conjunction with 87186 or 87188)

87188 macrobroth dilution method, each agent

87190 mycobacteria, proportion method, each agent

(For other mycobacterial susceptibility studies, see 87181, 87184, 87186, or 87188)

87197 Serum bactericidal titer (Schlicter test)

87205 Smear, primary source with interpretation; Gram or Giemsa stain for bacteria, fungi, or cell types

87206 fluorescent and/or acid fast stain for bacteria, fungi, parasites, viruses or cell types

87207   special stain for inclusion bodies or parasites (eg, malaria, coccidia, microsporidia, trypanosomes, herpes viruses)

(For direct smears with concentration and identification, use 87177)

(For thick smear preparation, use 87015)

(For fat, meat, fibers, nasal eosinophils, and starch, see miscellaneous section)

87209   complex special stain (eg, trichrome, iron hemotoxylin) for ova and parasites

87210   wet mount for infectious agents (eg, saline, India ink, KOH preps)

(For KOH examination of skin, hair or nails, see 87220)

87220   Tissue examination by KOH slide of samples from skin, hair, or nails for fungi or ectoparasite ova or mites (eg, scabies)

87230   Toxin or antitoxin assay, tissue culture (eg, Clostridium difficile toxin)

87250   Virus isolation; inoculation of embryonated eggs, or small animal, includes observation and dissection

87252   tissue culture inoculation, observation, and presumptive identification by cytopathic effect

87253   tissue culture, additional studies or definitive identification (eg, hemabsorption, neutralization, immunofluoresence stain), each isolate

(Electron microscopy, use 88348)

(Inclusion bodies in tissue sections, see 88304-88309; in smears, see 87207-87210; in fluids, use 88106)

87254   centrifuge enhanced (shell vial) technique, includes identification with immunofluorescence stain, each virus

(Report 87254 in addition to 87252 as appropriate)

87255   including identification by non-immunologic method, other than by cytopathic effect (eg, virus specific enzymatic activity)

These codes are intended for primary source only. For similar studies on culture material, refer to codes 87140-87158. Infectious agents by antigen detection, immunofluorescence microscopy, or nucleic acid probe techniques should be reported as precisely as possible. The molecular pathology procedures codes (81161, 81200-81408) are not to be used in combination with or instead of the procedures represented by 87470-87801. The most specific code possible should be reported. If there is no specific agent code, the general methodology code (eg, 87299, 87449, 87450, 87797, 87798, 87799, 87899) should be used. For identification of antibodies to many of the listed infectious agents, see 86602-86804. When separate results are reported for different species or strain of organisms, each result should be coded separately. Use modifier 59 when separate results are reported for different species or strains that are described by the same code.

87260   Infectious agent antigen detection by immunofluorescent technique; adenovirus

87265   Bordetella pertussis/parapertussis

87267   Enterovirus, direct fluorescent antibody (DFA)

87269   giardia

87270   Chlamydia trachomatis

87271   Cytomegalovirus, direct fluorescent antibody (DFA)

87272   cryptosporidium

87273   Herpes simplex virus type 2

87274   Herpes simplex virus type 1

87275   influenza B virus

87276   influenza A virus

87277   Legionella micdadei

87278   Legionella pneumophila

87279   Parainfluenza virus, each type

87280   respiratory syncytial virus

87281   Pneumocystis carinii

87283   Rubeola

87285   Treponema pallidum

87290   Varicella zoster virus

87299   not otherwise specified, each organism

87300   Infectious agent antigen detection by immunofluorescent technique, polyvalent for multiple organisms, each polyvalent antiserum

(For physician evaluation of infectious disease agents by immunofluorescence, use 88346)

▲ **87301**   Infectious agent antigen detection by immunoassay technique, (eg, enzyme immunoassay [EIA], enzyme-linked immunosorbent assay [ELISA], immunochemiluminometric assay [IMCA]) qualitative or semiquantitative, multiple-step method; adenovirus enteric types 40/41

▲ **87305**   Aspergillus

▲ **87320**   Chlamydia trachomatis

▲ **87324**   Clostridium difficile toxin(s)

▲ **87327**   Cryptococcus neoformans

(For Cryptococcus latex agglutination, use 86403)

▲ **87328**   cryptosporidium

▲ **87329**   giardia

▲ **87332**   cytomegalovirus

▲ **87335**   Escherichia coli 0157

(For giardia antigen, use 87329)

▲ **87336**   Entamoeba histolytica dispar group

▲ **87337**   Entamoeba histolytica group

Pathology and Laboratory

▲ 87338   Helicobacter pylori, stool

▲ 87339   Helicobacter pylori

(For H. pylori, stool, use 87338. For H. pylori, breath and blood by mass spectrometry, see 83013, 83014. For H. pylori, liquid scintillation counter, see 78267, 78268)

▲ 87340   hepatitis B surface antigen (HBsAg)

▲ 87341   hepatitis B surface antigen (HBsAg) neutralization

▲ 87350   hepatitis Be antigen (HBeAg)

▲ 87380   hepatitis, delta agent

▲ 87385   Histoplasma capsulatum

▲ 87389   HIV-1 antigen(s), with HIV-1 and HIV-2 antibodies, single result

▲ 87390   HIV-1

▲ 87391   HIV-2

▲ 87400   Influenza, A or B, each

▲ 87420   respiratory syncytial virus

▲ 87425   rotavirus

▲ 87427   Shiga-like toxin

▲ 87430   Streptococcus, group A

▲ 87449   Infectious agent antigen detection by immunoassay technique, (eg, enzyme immunoassay [EIA], enzyme-linked immunosorbent assay [ELISA], immunochemiluminometric assay [IMCA]), qualitative or semiquantitative; multiple-step method, not otherwise specified, each organism

▲ 87450   single step method, not otherwise specified, each organism

▲ 87451   multiple step method, polyvalent for multiple organisms, each polyvalent antiserum

87470   Infectious agent detection by nucleic acid (DNA or RNA); Bartonella henselae and Bartonella quintana, direct probe technique

87471   Bartonella henselae and Bartonella quintana, amplified probe technique

87472   Bartonella henselae and Bartonella quintana, quantification

87475   Borrelia burgdorferi, direct probe technique

87476   Borrelia burgdorferi, amplified probe technique

87477   Borrelia burgdorferi, quantification

87480   Candida species, direct probe technique

87481   Candida species, amplified probe technique

87482   Candida species, quantification

87485   Chlamydia pneumoniae, direct probe technique

87486   Chlamydia pneumoniae, amplified probe technique

87487   Chlamydia pneumoniae, quantification

87490   Chlamydia trachomatis, direct probe technique

87491   Chlamydia trachomatis, amplified probe technique

87492   Chlamydia trachomatis, quantification

87493   Clostridium difficile, toxin gene(s), amplified probe technique

87495   cytomegalovirus, direct probe technique

87496   cytomegalovirus, amplified probe technique

87497   cytomegalovirus, quantification

87498   enterovirus, amplified probe technique, includes reverse transcription when performed

87500   vancomycin resistance (eg, enterococcus species van A, van B), amplified probe technique

87501   influenza virus, includes reverse transcription, when performed, and amplified probe technique, each type or subtype

▲ 87502   influenza virus, for multiple types or sub-types, includes multiplex reverse transcription, when performed, and multiplex amplified probe technique, first 2 types or sub-types

+▲ 87503   influenza virus, for multiple types or sub-types, includes multiplex reverse transcription, when performed, and multiplex amplified probe technique, each additional influenza virus type or sub-type beyond 2 (List separately in addition to code for primary procedure)

(Use 87503 in conjunction with 87502)

87505   gastrointestinal pathogen (eg, Clostridium difficile, E. coli, Salmonella, Shigella, norovirus, Giardia), includes multiplex reverse transcription, when performed, and multiplex amplified probe technique, multiple types or subtypes, 3-5 targets

87506   gastrointestinal pathogen (eg, Clostridium difficile, E. coli, Salmonella, Shigella, norovirus, Giardia), includes multiplex reverse transcription, when performed, and multiplex amplified probe technique, multiple types or subtypes, 6-11 targets

87507   gastrointestinal pathogen (eg, Clostridium difficile, E. coli, Salmonella, Shigella, norovirus, Giardia), includes multiplex reverse transcription, when performed, and multiplex amplified probe technique, multiple types or subtypes, 12-25 targets

87510   Gardnerella vaginalis, direct probe technique

87511   Gardnerella vaginalis, amplified probe technique

87512   Gardnerella vaginalis, quantification

87515   hepatitis B virus, direct probe technique

87516   hepatitis B virus, amplified probe technique

87517   hepatitis B virus, quantification

87520   hepatitis C, direct probe technique

87521   hepatitis C, amplified probe technique, includes reverse transcription when performed

87522	hepatitis C, quantification, includes reverse transcription when performed
87525	hepatitis G, direct probe technique
87526	hepatitis G, amplified probe technique
87527	hepatitis G, quantification
87528	Herpes simplex virus, direct probe technique
87529	Herpes simplex virus, amplified probe technique
87530	Herpes simplex virus, quantification
87531	Herpes virus-6, direct probe technique
87532	Herpes virus-6, amplified probe technique
87533	Herpes virus-6, quantification
87534	HIV-1, direct probe technique
87535	HIV-1, amplified probe technique, includes reverse transcription when performed
87536	HIV-1, quantification, includes reverse transcription when performed
87537	HIV-2, direct probe technique
87538	HIV-2, amplified probe technique, includes reverse transcription when performed
87539	HIV-2, quantification, includes reverse transcription when performed
# 87623	Human Papillomavirus (HPV), low-risk types (eg, 6, 11, 42, 43, 44)
# 87624	Human Papillomavirus (HPV), high-risk types (eg, 16, 18, 31, 33, 35, 39, 45, 51, 52, 56, 58, 59, 68)
	(When both low-risk and high-risk HPV types are performed in a single assay, use only 87624)
# 87625	Human Papillomavirus (HPV), types 16 and 18 only, includes type 45, if performed
87540	Legionella pneumophila, direct probe technique
87541	Legionella pneumophila, amplified probe technique
87542	Legionella pneumophila, quantification
87550	Mycobacteria species, direct probe technique
87551	Mycobacteria species, amplified probe technique
87552	Mycobacteria species, quantification
87555	Mycobacteria tuberculosis, direct probe technique
87556	Mycobacteria tuberculosis, amplified probe technique
87557	Mycobacteria tuberculosis, quantification
87560	Mycobacteria avium-intracellulare, direct probe technique
87561	Mycobacteria avium-intracellulare, amplified probe technique
87562	Mycobacteria avium-intracellulare, quantification
87580	Mycoplasma pneumoniae, direct probe technique
87581	Mycoplasma pneumoniae, amplified probe technique

87582	Mycoplasma pneumoniae, quantification
87590	Neisseria gonorrhoeae, direct probe technique
87591	Neisseria gonorrhoeae, amplified probe technique
87592	Neisseria gonorrhoeae, quantification
	(87620 has been deleted. To report, see 87623, 87624, 87625)
	(87621 has been deleted. To report, see 87623, 87624, 87625)
	(87622 has been deleted. To report, see 87623, 87624, 87625)
87623	Code is out of numerical sequence. See 87003-87999
87624	Code is out of numerical sequence. See 87003-87999
87625	Code is out of numerical sequence. See 87003-87999
87631	respiratory virus (eg, adenovirus, influenza virus, coronavirus, metapneumovirus, parainfluenza virus, respiratory syncytial virus, rhinovirus), includes multiplex reverse transcription, when performed, and multiplex amplified probe technique, multiple types or subtypes, 3-5 targets
87632	respiratory virus (eg, adenovirus, influenza virus, coronavirus, metapneumovirus, parainfluenza virus, respiratory syncytial virus, rhinovirus), includes multiplex reverse transcription, when performed, and multiplex amplified probe technique, multiple types or subtypes, 6-11 targets
87633	respiratory virus (eg, adenovirus, influenza virus, coronavirus, metapneumovirus, parainfluenza virus, respiratory syncytial virus, rhinovirus), includes multiplex reverse transcription, when performed, and multiplex amplified probe technique, multiple types or subtypes, 12-25 targets
	(Use 87631-87633 for nucleic acid assays which detect multiple respiratory viruses in a multiplex reaction [ie, single procedure with multiple results])
	(For assays that are used to type or subtype influenza viruses only, see 87501-87503)
	(For assays that include influenza viruses with additional respiratory viruses, see 87631-87633)
	(For detection of multiple infectious agents not otherwise specified which report a single result, see 87800, 87801)
87640	Staphylococcus aureus, amplified probe technique
87641	Staphylococcus aureus, methicillin resistant, amplified probe technique
	(For assays that detect methicillin resistance and identify Staphylococcus aureus using a single nucleic acid sequence, use 87641)
87650	Streptococcus, group A, direct probe technique
87651	Streptococcus, group A, amplified probe technique
87652	Streptococcus, group A, quantification
87653	Streptococcus, group B, amplified probe technique

Pathology and Laboratory

87660   Trichomonas vaginalis, direct probe technique

87661   Trichomonas vaginalis, amplified probe technique

87797   Infectious agent detection by nucleic acid (DNA or RNA), not otherwise specified; direct probe technique, each organism

87798   amplified probe technique, each organism

87799   quantification, each organism

87800   Infectious agent detection by nucleic acid (DNA or RNA), multiple organisms; direct probe(s) technique

87801   amplified probe(s) technique

(For each specific organism nucleic acid detection from a primary source, see 87470-87660. For detection of specific infectious agents not otherwise specified, see 87797, 87798, or 87799 1 time for each agent)

(For detection of multiple infectious agents not otherwise specified which report a single result, see 87800, 87801)

(Do not use 87801 for nucleic acid assays that detect multiple respiratory viruses in a multiplex reaction [ie, single procedure with multiple results], see 87631-87633)

87802   Infectious agent antigen detection by immunoassay with direct optical observation; Streptococcus, group B

87803   Clostridium difficile toxin A

87806   HIV-1 antigen(s), with HIV-1 and HIV-2 antibodies

87804   Influenza

87806   Code is out of numerical sequence. See 87003-87999

87807   respiratory syncytial virus

87808   Trichomonas vaginalis

87809   adenovirus

87810   Chlamydia trachomatis

87850   Neisseria gonorrhoeae

87880   Streptococcus, group A

87899   not otherwise specified

87900   Infectious agent drug susceptibility phenotype prediction using regularly updated genotypic bioinformatics

87910   Infectious agent genotype analysis by nucleic acid (DNA or RNA); cytomegalovirus

87901   HIV-1, reverse transcriptase and protease regions

87906   HIV-1, other region (eg, integrase, fusion)

(For infectious agent drug susceptibility phenotype prediction for HIV-1, use 87900)

87912   Hepatitis B virus

87902   Hepatitis C virus

87903   Infectious agent phenotype analysis by nucleic acid (DNA or RNA) with drug resistance tissue culture analysis, HIV 1; first through 10 drugs tested

+ 87904   each additional drug tested (List separately in addition to code for primary procedure)

(Use 87904 in conjunction with 87903)

87905   Infectious agent enzymatic activity other than virus (eg, sialidase activity in vaginal fluid)

(For virus isolation including identification by non-immunologic method, other than by cytopathic effect, use 87255)

87906   Code is out of numerical sequence. See 87003-87999

87910   Code is out of numerical sequence. See 87003-87999

87912   Code is out of numerical sequence. See 87003-87999

87999   Unlisted microbiology procedure

Anatomic Pathology

Postmortem Examination

Procedures 88000 through 88099 represent physician services only. Use modifier 90 for outside laboratory services.

88000   Necropsy (autopsy), gross examination only; without CNS

88005   with brain

88007   with brain and spinal cord

88012   infant with brain

88014   stillborn or newborn with brain

88016   macerated stillborn

88020   Necropsy (autopsy), gross and microscopic; without CNS

88025   with brain

88027   with brain and spinal cord

88028   infant with brain

88029   stillborn or newborn with brain

88036   Necropsy (autopsy), limited, gross and/or microscopic; regional

88037   single organ

88040   Necropsy (autopsy); forensic examination

88045   coroner's call

88099   Unlisted necropsy (autopsy) procedure

Cytopathology

88104   Cytopathology, fluids, washings or brushings, except cervical or vaginal; smears with interpretation

88106   simple filter method with interpretation

(Do not report 88106 in conjunction with 88104)

(For nongynecological selective cellular enhancement including filter transfer techniques, use 88112)

88108   Cytopathology, concentration technique, smears and interpretation (eg, Saccomanno technique)

(For cervical or vaginal smears, see 88150-88155)

(For gastric intubation with lavage, see 43754, 43755)

(For x-ray localization, use 74340)

88112   Cytopathology, selective cellular enhancement technique with interpretation (eg, liquid based slide preparation method), except cervical or vaginal

(Do not report 88112 with 88108)

88120   Cytopathology, in situ hybridization (eg, FISH), urinary tract specimen with morphometric analysis, 3-5 molecular probes, each specimen; manual

88121   using computer-assisted technology

(For morphometric in situ hybridization on cytologic specimens other than urinary tract, see 88367, 88368)

(For more than 5 probes, use 88399)

88125   Cytopathology, forensic (eg, sperm)

88130   Sex chromatin identification; Barr bodies

88140   peripheral blood smear, polymorphonuclear drumsticks

(For Guard stain, use 88313)

Codes 88141-88155, 88164-88167, 88174-88175 are used to report cervical or vaginal screening by various methods and to report physician interpretation services. Use codes 88150-88154 to report conventional Pap smears that are examined using non-Bethesda reporting. Use codes 88164-88167 to report conventional Pap smears that are examined using the Bethesda System of reporting. Use codes 88142-88143 to report liquid-based specimens processed as thin-layer preparations that are examined using any system of reporting (Bethesda or non-Bethesda). Use codes 88174-88175 to report automated screening of liquid-based specimens that are examined using any system of reporting (Bethesda or non-Bethesda). Within each of these three code families choose the one code that describes the screening method(s) used. Codes 88141 and 88155 should be reported in addition to the screening code chosen when the additional services are provided. Manual rescreening requires a complete visual reassessment of the entire slide initially screened by either an automated or manual process. Manual review represents an assessment of selected cells or regions of a slide identified by initial automated review.

88141   Cytopathology, cervical or vaginal (any reporting system), requiring interpretation by physician

(Use 88141 in conjunction with 88142-88154, 88164-88167, 88174-88175)

88142   Cytopathology, cervical or vaginal (any reporting system), collected in preservative fluid, automated thin layer preparation; manual screening under physician supervision

88143   with manual screening and rescreening under physician supervision

(For automated screening of automated thin layer preparation, see 88174, 88175)

88147   Cytopathology smears, cervical or vaginal; screening by automated system under physician supervision

88148   screening by automated system with manual rescreening under physician supervision

88150   Cytopathology, slides, cervical or vaginal; manual screening under physician supervision

88152   with manual screening and computer-assisted rescreening under physician supervision

88153   with manual screening and rescreening under physician supervision

88154   with manual screening and computer-assisted rescreening using cell selection and review under physician supervision

+ **88155**   Cytopathology, slides, cervical or vaginal, definitive hormonal evaluation (eg, maturation index, karyopyknotic index, estrogenic index) (List separately in addition to code[s] for other technical and interpretation services)

(Use 88155 in conjunction with 88142-88154, 88164-88167, 88174-88175)

88160   Cytopathology, smears, any other source; screening and interpretation

88161   preparation, screening and interpretation

88162   extended study involving over 5 slides and/or multiple stains

(For aerosol collection of sputum, use 89220)

(For special stains, see 88312-88314)

88164   Cytopathology, slides, cervical or vaginal (the Bethesda System); manual screening under physician supervision

88165   with manual screening and rescreening under physician supervision

88166   with manual screening and computer-assisted rescreening under physician supervision

88167   with manual screening and computer-assisted rescreening using cell selection and review under physician supervision

(To report collection of specimen via fine needle aspiration, see 10021, 10022)

88172   Cytopathology, evaluation of fine needle aspirate; immediate cytohistologic study to determine adequacy for diagnosis, first evaluation episode, each site

(The evaluation episode represents a complete set of cytologic material submitted for evaluation and is independent of the number of needle passes or slides prepared. A separate evaluation episode occurs if the proceduralist provider obtains additional material from the same site, based on the prior immediate adequacy assessment, or a separate lesion is aspirated)

Pathology and Laboratory

88173   interpretation and report

(Report one unit of 88173 for the interpretation and report from each anatomic site, regardless of the number of passes or evaluation episodes performed during the aspiration procedure)

(For fine needle aspirate, see 10021, 10022)

(Do not report 88172, 88173 in conjunction with 88333 and 88334 for the same specimen)

#+ 88177   immediate cytohistologic study to determine adequacy for diagnosis, each separate additional evaluation episode, same site (List separately in addition to code for primary procedure)

(When repeat immediate evaluation episode(s) is required on subsequent cytologic material from the same site, eg, following determination the prior sampling that was not adequate for diagnosis, use 1 unit of 88177 for each additional evaluation episode)

(Use 88177 in conjunction with 88172)

88174   Cytopathology, cervical or vaginal (any reporting system), collected in preservative fluid, automated thin layer preparation; screening by automated system, under physician supervision

88175   with screening by automated system and manual rescreening or review, under physician supervision

(For manual screening, see 88142, 88143)

88177   Code is out of numerical sequence. See 88104-88199

88182   Flow cytometry, cell cycle or DNA analysis

(For DNA ploidy analysis by morphometric technique, use 88358)

88184   Flow cytometry, cell surface, cytoplasmic, or nuclear marker, technical component only; first marker

+ 88185   each additional marker (List separately in addition to code for first marker)

(Report 88185 in conjunction with 88184)

88187   Flow cytometry, interpretation; 2 to 8 markers

88188   9 to 15 markers

88189   16 or more markers

(Do not report 88187-88189 for interpretation of 86355, 86356, 86357, 86359, 86360, 86361, 86367)

(For assessment of circulating antibodies by flow cytometric techniques, see analyte and method-specific codes in the Chemistry section [83516-83520] or Immunology section [86000-86849])

(For cell enumeration using immunologic selection and identification in fluid specimen [eg, circulating tumor cells in blood], see 86152, 86153)

88199   Unlisted cytopathology procedure

(For electron microscopy, use 88348)

Cytogenetic Studies

Molecular pathology procedures should be reported using the appropriate code from Tier 1 (81161, 81200-81383), Tier 2 (81400-81408), Genomic Sequencing Procedures and Other Molecular Multianalyte Assays (81410-81471), or Multianalyte Assays with Algorithmic Analyses (81500-81512) sections. If no specific code exists, one of the unlisted codes (81479 or 81599) should be used.

(For acetylcholinesterase, use 82013)

(For alpha-fetoprotein, serum or amniotic fluid, see 82105, 82106)

(For laser microdissection of cells from tissue sample, see 88380)

88230   Tissue culture for non-neoplastic disorders; lymphocyte

88233   skin or other solid tissue biopsy

88235   amniotic fluid or chorionic villus cells

88237   Tissue culture for neoplastic disorders; bone marrow, blood cells

88239   solid tumor

88240   Cryopreservation, freezing and storage of cells, each cell line

(For therapeutic cryopreservation and storage, use 38207)

88241   Thawing and expansion of frozen cells, each aliquot

(For therapeutic thawing of previous harvest, use 38208)

88245   Chromosome analysis for breakage syndromes; baseline Sister Chromatid Exchange (SCE), 20-25 cells

88248   baseline breakage, score 50-100 cells, count 20 cells, 2 karyotypes (eg, for ataxia telangiectasia, Fanconi anemia, fragile X)

88249   score 100 cells, clastogen stress (eg, diepoxybutane, mitomycin C, ionizing radiation, UV radiation)

88261   Chromosome analysis; count 5 cells, 1 karyotype, with banding

88262   count 15-20 cells, 2 karyotypes, with banding

88263   count 45 cells for mosaicism, 2 karyotypes, with banding

88264   analyze 20-25 cells

88267   Chromosome analysis, amniotic fluid or chorionic villus, count 15 cells, 1 karyotype, with banding

88269   Chromosome analysis, in situ for amniotic fluid cells, count cells from 6-12 colonies, 1 karyotype, with banding

88271   Molecular cytogenetics; DNA probe, each (eg, FISH)

(For cytogenomic microarray analysis, see 81228, 81229, 81405, 81406, 81479)

88272   chromosomal in situ hybridization, analyze 3-5 cells (eg, for derivatives and markers)

88273	chromosomal in situ hybridization, analyze 10-30 cells (eg, for microdeletions)
88274	interphase in situ hybridization, analyze 25-99 cells
88275	interphase in situ hybridization, analyze 100-300 cells
88280	Chromosome analysis; additional karyotypes, each study
88283	additional specialized banding technique (eg, NOR, C-banding)
88285	additional cells counted, each study
88289	additional high resolution study
88291	Cytogenetics and molecular cytogenetics, interpretation and report
88299	Unlisted cytogenetic study

Surgical Pathology

Services 88300 through 88309 include accession, examination, and reporting. They do not include the services designated in codes 88311 through 88365 and 88399, which are coded in addition when provided.

The unit of service for codes 88300 through 88309 is the specimen.

A specimen is defined as tissue or tissues that is (are) submitted for individual and separate attention, requiring individual examination and pathologic diagnosis. Two or more such specimens from the same patient (eg, separately identified endoscopic biopsies, skin lesions) are each appropriately assigned an individual code reflective of its proper level of service.

Service code 88300 is used for any specimen that in the opinion of the examining pathologist can be accurately diagnosed without microscopic examination. Service code 88302 is used when gross and microscopic examination is performed on a specimen to confirm identification and the absence of disease. Service codes 88304 through 88309 describe all other specimens requiring gross and microscopic examination, and represent additional ascending levels of physician work. Levels 88302 through 88309 are specifically defined by the assigned specimens.

Any unlisted specimen should be assigned to the code which most closely reflects the physician work involved when compared to other specimens assigned to that code.

(Do not report 88302-88309 on the same specimen as part of Mohs surgery)

| 88300 | **Level I** - Surgical pathology, gross examination only |
| 88302 | **Level II** - Surgical pathology, gross and microscopic examination |

Appendix, incidental

Fallopian tube, sterilization

Fingers/toes, amputation, traumatic

Foreskin, newborn

Hernia sac, any location

Hydrocele sac

Nerve

Skin, plastic repair

Sympathetic ganglion

Testis, castration

Vaginal mucosa, incidental

Vas deferens, sterilization

| 88304 | **Level III** - Surgical pathology, gross and microscopic examination |

Abortion, induced

Abscess

Aneurysm - arterial/ventricular

Anus, tag

Appendix, other than incidental

Artery, atheromatous plaque

Bartholin's gland cyst

Bone fragment(s), other than pathologic fracture

Bursa/synovial cyst

Carpal tunnel tissue

Cartilage, shavings

Cholesteatoma

Colon, colostomy stoma

Conjunctiva - biopsy/pterygium

Cornea

Diverticulum - esophagus/small intestine

Dupuytren's contracture tissue

Femoral head, other than fracture

Fissure/fistula

Foreskin, other than newborn

Gallbladder

Ganglion cyst

Hematoma

Hemorrhoids

Hydatid of Morgagni

Intervertebral disc

Joint, loose body

Meniscus

Mucocele, salivary

Neuroma - Morton's/traumatic

Pilonidal cyst/sinus

Pathology and Laboratory

Polyps, inflammatory - nasal/sinusoidal

Skin - cyst/tag/debridement

Soft tissue, debridement

Soft tissue, lipoma

Spermatocele

Tendon/tendon sheath

Testicular appendage

Thrombus or embolus

Tonsil and/or adenoids

Varicocele

Vas deferens, other than sterilization

Vein, varicosity

88305   **Level IV** - Surgical pathology, gross and microscopic examination

Abortion - spontaneous/missed

Artery, biopsy

Bone marrow, biopsy

Bone exostosis

Brain/meninges, other than for tumor resection

Breast, biopsy, not requiring microscopic evaluation of surgical margins

Breast, reduction mammoplasty

Bronchus, biopsy

Cell block, any source

Cervix, biopsy

Colon, biopsy

Duodenum, biopsy

Endocervix, curettings/biopsy

Endometrium, curettings/biopsy

Esophagus, biopsy

Extremity, amputation, traumatic

Fallopian tube, biopsy

Fallopian tube, ectopic pregnancy

Femoral head, fracture

Fingers/toes, amputation, non-traumatic

Gingiva/oral mucosa, biopsy

Heart valve

Joint, resection

Kidney, biopsy

Larynx, biopsy

Leiomyoma(s), uterine myomectomy - without uterus

Lip, biopsy/wedge resection

Lung, transbronchial biopsy

Lymph node, biopsy

Muscle, biopsy

Nasal mucosa, biopsy

Nasopharynx/oropharynx, biopsy

Nerve, biopsy

Odontogenic/dental cyst

Omentum, biopsy

Ovary with or without tube, non-neoplastic

Ovary, biopsy/wedge resection

Parathyroid gland

Peritoneum, biopsy

Pituitary tumor

Placenta, other than third trimester

Pleura/pericardium - biopsy/tissue

Polyp, cervical/endometrial

Polyp, colorectal

Polyp, stomach/small intestine

Prostate, needle biopsy

Prostate, TUR

Salivary gland, biopsy

Sinus, paranasal biopsy

Skin, other than cyst/tag/debridement/plastic repair

Small intestine, biopsy

Soft tissue, other than tumor/mass/lipoma/debridement

Spleen

Stomach, biopsy

Synovium

Testis, other than tumor/biopsy/castration

Thyroglossal duct/brachial cleft cyst

Tongue, biopsy

Tonsil, biopsy

Trachea, biopsy

Ureter, biopsy

Urethra, biopsy

Urinary bladder, biopsy

Uterus, with or without tubes and ovaries, for prolapse

Vagina, biopsy

Vulva/labia, biopsy

88307   **Level V** - Surgical pathology, gross and microscopic examination

Adrenal, resection

   ⊙=Moderate sedation   ✚=Add-on code   ✗=FDA approval pending   #=Resequenced code   ○=Recycled/reinstated code

Bone - biopsy/curettings

Bone fragment(s), pathologic fracture

Brain, biopsy

Brain/meninges, tumor resection

Breast, excision of lesion, requiring microscopic evaluation of surgical margins

Breast, mastectomy - partial/simple

Cervix, conization

Colon, segmental resection, other than for tumor

Extremity, amputation, non-traumatic

Eye, enucleation

Kidney, partial/total nephrectomy

Larynx, partial/total resection

Liver, biopsy - needle/wedge

Liver, partial resection

Lung, wedge biopsy

Lymph nodes, regional resection

Mediastinum, mass

Myocardium, biopsy

Odontogenic tumor

Ovary with or without tube, neoplastic

Pancreas, biopsy

Placenta, third trimester

Prostate, except radical resection

Salivary gland

Sentinel lymph node

Small intestine, resection, other than for tumor

Soft tissue mass (except lipoma) - biopsy/simple excision

Stomach - subtotal/total resection, other than for tumor

Testis, biopsy

Thymus, tumor

Thyroid, total/lobe

Ureter, resection

Urinary bladder, TUR

Uterus, with or without tubes and ovaries, other than neoplastic/prolapse

88309   **Level VI** - Surgical pathology, gross and microscopic examination

Bone resection

Breast, mastectomy - with regional lymph nodes

Colon, segmental resection for tumor

Colon, total resection

Esophagus, partial/total resection

Extremity, disarticulation

Fetus, with dissection

Larynx, partial/total resection - with regional lymph nodes

Lung - total/lobe/segment resection

Pancreas, total/subtotal resection

Prostate, radical resection

Small intestine, resection for tumor

Soft tissue tumor, extensive resection

Stomach - subtotal/total resection for tumor

Testis, tumor

Tongue/tonsil -resection for tumor

Urinary bladder, partial/total resection

Uterus, with or without tubes and ovaries, neoplastic

Vulva, total/subtotal resection

(For fine needle aspiration, see 10021, 10022)

(For evaluation of fine needle aspirate, see 88172-88173)

(Do not report 88302-88309 on the same specimen as part of Mohs surgery)

+ 88311   Decalcification procedure (List separately in addition to code for surgical pathology examination)

88312   Special stain including interpretation and report; Group I for microorganisms (eg, acid fast, methenamine silver)

(Report one unit of 88312 for each special stain, on each surgical pathology block, cytologic specimen, or hematologic smear)

88313   Group II, all other (eg, iron, trichrome), except stain for microorganisms, stains for enzyme constituents, or immunocytochemistry and immunohistochemistry

(Report one unit of 88313 for each special stain, on each surgical pathology block, cytologic specimen, or hematologic smear)

(For immunocytochemistry and immunohistochemistry, use 88342)

+ 88314   histochemical stain on frozen tissue block (List separately in addition to code for primary procedure)

(Use 88314 in conjunction with 17311-17315, 88302-88309, 88331, 88332)

(Do not report 88314 with 17311-17315 for routine frozen section stain [eg, hematoxylin and eosin, toluidine blue], performed during Mohs surgery. When a nonroutine histochemical stain on frozen tissue during Mohs surgery is utilized, report 88314 with modifier 59)

(Report one unit of 88314 for each special stain on each frozen surgical pathology block)

Pathology and Laboratory

(For a special stain performed on frozen tissue section material to identify enzyme constituents, use 88319)

(For determinative histochemistry to identify chemical components, use 88313)

88319   Group III, for enzyme constituents

(For each stain on each surgical pathology block, cytologic specimen, or hematologic smear, use one unit of 88319)

(For detection of enzyme constituents by immunohistochemical or immunocytochemical technique, use 88342)

88321 Consultation and report on referred slides prepared elsewhere

88323 Consultation and report on referred material requiring preparation of slides

88325 Consultation, comprehensive, with review of records and specimens, with report on referred material

88329 Pathology consultation during surgery;

88331   first tissue block, with frozen section(s), single specimen

+ 88332   each additional tissue block with frozen section(s) (List separately in addition to code for primary procedure)

(Use 88332 in conjunction with 88331)

88333   cytologic examination (eg, touch prep, squash prep), initial site

+ 88334   cytologic examination (eg, touch prep, squash prep), each additional site (List separately in addition to code for primary procedure)

(Use 88334 in conjunction with 88331, 88333)

(For intraoperative consultation on a specimen requiring both frozen section and cytologic evaluation, use 88331 and 88334)

(For percutaneous needle biopsy requiring intraprocedural cytologic examination, use 88333)

(Do not report 88333 and 88334 for non-intraoperative cytologic examination, see 88160-88162)

(Do not report 88333 and 88334 for intraprocedural cytologic evaluation of fine needle aspirate, see 88172)

88341 Code is out of numerical sequence. See 88300-88399

88342 Immunohistochemistry or immunocytochemistry, per specimen; initial single antibody stain procedure

(For quantitative or semiquantitative immunohistochemistry, see 88360, 88361)

(88343 has been deleted. For multiplex antibody stain procedure, use 88344)

#+ 88341   each additional single antibody stain procedure (List separately in addition to code for primary procedure)

(Use 88341 in conjunction with 88342)

(For multiplex antibody stain procedure, use 88344)

88344   each multiplex antibody stain procedure

(Do not use more than one unit of 88341, 88342, or 88344 for the same separately identifiable antibody per specimen)

(Do not report 88341, 88342, 88344 in conjunction with 88360, 88361 unless each procedure is for a different antibody)

(When multiple separately identifiable antibodies are applied to the same specimen [ie, multiplex antibody stain procedure], use one unit of 88344)

(When multiple antibodies are applied to the same slide that are not separately identifiable, [eg, antibody cocktails], use 88342, unless an additional separately identifiable antibody is also used, then use 88344)

▲ **88346** Immunofluorescence, per specimen; initial single antibody stain procedure

►(88347 has been deleted. To report, see 88346, 88350)◄

#+● 88350   each additional single antibody stain procedure (List separately in addition to code for primary procedure)

►(Report 88350 in conjunction with 88346)◄

►(Do not report 88346 and 88350 for fluorescent in situ hybridization studies, see 88364, 88365, 88366, 88367, 88368, 88369, 88373, 88374, and 88377)◄

►(Do not report 88346 and 88350 for multiplex immunofluorescence analysis, use 88399)◄

88348 Electron microscopy, diagnostic

(88349 has been deleted. To report, use 88348)

88350 Code is out of numerical sequence. See 88300-88399

88355 Morphometric analysis; skeletal muscle

88356   nerve

88358   tumor (eg, DNA ploidy)

(Do not report 88358 with 88313 unless each procedure is for a different special stain)

88360 Morphometric analysis, tumor immunohistochemistry (eg, Her-2/neu, estrogen receptor/progesterone receptor), quantitative or semiquantitative, per specimen, each single antibody stain procedure; manual

88361   using computer-assisted technology

(Do not report 88360, 88361 in conjunction with 88341, 88342, or 88344 unless each procedure is for a different antibody)

(Morphometric analysis of a multiplex antibody stain should be reported with one unit of 88360 or 88361, per specimen)

(For morphometric analysis using in situ hybridization techniques, see 88367, 88368)

(When semi-thin plastic-embedded sections are performed in conjunction with morphometric analysis, only the morphometric analysis should be reported; if performed as an independent procedure, see codes 88300-88309 for surgical pathology.)

88362   Nerve teasing preparations

88363   Examination and selection of retrieved archival (ie, previously diagnosed) tissue(s) for molecular analysis (eg, KRAS mutational analysis)

88364   Code is out of numerical sequence. See 88300-88399

88365   In situ hybridization (eg, FISH), per specimen; initial single probe stain procedure

#+ 88364   each additional single probe stain procedure (List separately in addition to code for primary procedure)

(Use 88364 in conjunction with 88365)

88366   each multiplex probe stain procedure

(Do not report 88365, 88366 in conjunction with 88367, 88368, 88374, 88377 for the same probe)

88367   Morphometric analysis, in situ hybridization (quantitative or semi-quantitative), using computer-assisted technology, per specimen; initial single probe stain procedure

#+ 88373   each additional single probe stain procedure (List separately in addition to code for primary procedure)

(Use 88373 in conjunction with 88367)

 # 88374   each multiplex probe stain procedure

(Do not report 88367, 88374 in conjunction with 88365, 88366, 88368, 88377 for the same probe)

88368   Morphometric analysis, in situ hybridization (quantitative or semi-quantitative), manual, per specimen; initial single probe stain procedure

+ 88369   each additional single probe stain procedure (List separately in addition to code for primary procedure)

(Use 88369 in conjunction with 88368)

 # 88377   each multiplex probe stain procedure

(Do not report 88368 or 88377 in conjunction with 88365, 88366, 88367, 88374 for the same probe)

(For morphometric in situ hybridization evaluation of urinary tract cytologic specimens, see 88120, 88121)

88371   Protein analysis of tissue by Western Blot, with interpretation and report;

88372   immunological probe for band identification, each

88373   Code is out of numerical sequence. See 88300-88399

88374   Code is out of numerical sequence. See 88300-88399

88375   Optical endomicroscopic image(s), interpretation and report, real-time or referred, each endoscopic session

►(Do not report 88375 in conjunction with 43206, 43252, 0397T)◄

88377   Code is out of numerical sequence. See 88300-88399

88380   Microdissection (ie, sample preparation of microscopically identified target); laser capture

88381   manual

(Do not report 88380 in conjunction with 88381)

(88384-88386 have been deleted. To report, see 81161, 81200-81479)

88387   Macroscopic examination, dissection, and preparation of tissue for non-microscopic analytical studies (eg, nucleic acid-based molecular studies); each tissue preparation (eg, a single lymph node)

(Do not report 88387 for tissue preparation for microbiologic cultures or flow cytometric studies)

(Do not report 88387 in conjunction with 88388, 88329-88334)

+ 88388   in conjunction with a touch imprint, intraoperative consultation, or frozen section, each tissue preparation (eg, a single lymph node) (List separately in addition to code for primary procedure)

(Use 88388 in conjunction with 88329-88334)

(Do not report 88387 or 88388 for tissue preparation for microbiologic cultures or flow cytometric studies)

88399   Unlisted surgical pathology procedure

In Vivo (eg, Transcutaneous) Laboratory Procedures

(For all in vivo measurements not specifically listed, use 88749)

►(For wavelength fluorescent spectroscopy of advanced glycation end products [skin], use 88749)◄

(For transcutaneous oxyhemoglobin measurement in a lower extremity wound by near infrared spectroscopy, use 0286T)

88720   Bilirubin, total, transcutaneous

(For transdermal oxygen saturation, see 94760-94762)

88738   Hemoglobin (Hgb), quantitative, transcutaneous

(For in vitro hemoglobin measurement, use 85018)

88740   Hemoglobin, quantitative, transcutaneous, per day; carboxyhemoglobin

(For in vitro carboxyhemoglobin measurement, use 82375)

88741   methemoglobin

(For in vitro quantitative methemoglobin determination, use 83050)

88749   Unlisted in vivo (eg, transcutaneous) laboratory service

Pathology and Laboratory

Other Procedures

89049   Caffeine halothane contracture test (CHCT) for malignant hyperthermia susceptibility, including interpretation and report

89050   Cell count, miscellaneous body fluids (eg, cerebrospinal fluid, joint fluid), except blood;

89051   with differential count

89055   Leukocyte assessment, fecal, qualitative or semiquantitative

89060   Crystal identification by light microscopy with or without polarizing lens analysis, tissue or any body fluid (except urine)

(Do not report 89060 for crystal identification on paraffin-embedded tissue)

89125   Fat stain, feces, urine, or respiratory secretions

89160   Meat fibers, feces

89190   Nasal smear for eosinophils

(Occult blood, feces, use 82270)

(Paternity tests, use 86910)

89220   Sputum, obtaining specimen, aerosol induced technique (separate procedure)

(89225 has been deleted)

89230   Sweat collection by iontophoresis

(89235 has been deleted)

89240   Unlisted miscellaneous pathology test

Reproductive Medicine Procedures

89250   Culture of oocyte(s)/embryo(s), less than 4 days;

89251   with co-culture of oocyte(s)/embryos

(For extended culture of oocyte[s]/embryo[s], see 89272)

89253   Assisted embryo hatching, microtechniques (any method)

89254   Oocyte identification from follicular fluid

89255   Preparation of embryo for transfer (any method)

89257   Sperm identification from aspiration (other than seminal fluid)

(For semen analysis, see 89300-89320)

(For sperm identification from testis tissue, use 89264)

89258   Cryopreservation; embryo(s)

89259   sperm

(For cryopreservation of reproductive tissue, testicular, use 89335)

89260   Sperm isolation; simple prep (eg, sperm wash and swim-up) for insemination or diagnosis with semen analysis

89261   complex prep (eg, Percoll gradient, albumin gradient) for insemination or diagnosis with semen analysis

(For semen analysis without sperm wash or swim-up, use 89320)

89264   Sperm identification from testis tissue, fresh or cryopreserved

(For biopsy of testis, see 54500, 54505)

(For sperm identification from aspiration, use 89257)

(For semen analysis, see 89300-89320)

89268   Insemination of oocytes

89272   Extended culture of oocyte(s)/embryo(s), 4-7 days

89280   Assisted oocyte fertilization, microtechnique; less than or equal to 10 oocytes

89281   greater than 10 oocytes

89290   Biopsy, oocyte polar body or embryo blastomere, microtechnique (for pre-implantation genetic diagnosis); less than or equal to 5 embryos

89291   greater than 5 embryos

89300   Semen analysis; presence and/or motility of sperm including Huhner test (post coital)

89310   motility and count (not including Huhner test)

89320   volume, count, motility, and differential

(Skin tests, see 86485-86580 and 95012-95199)

89321   sperm presence and motility of sperm, if performed

(To report Hyaluronan binding assay [HBA], use 89398)

89322   volume, count, motility, and differential using strict morphologic criteria (eg, Kruger)

89325   Sperm antibodies

(For medicolegal identification of sperm, use 88125)

89329   Sperm evaluation; hamster penetration test

89330   cervical mucus penetration test, with or without spinnbarkeit test

89331   Sperm evaluation, for retrograde ejaculation, urine (sperm concentration, motility, and morphology, as indicated)

(For semen analysis on concurrent semen specimen, see 89300-89322 in conjunction with 89331)

(For detection of sperm in urine, use 81015)

89335   Cryopreservation, reproductive tissue, testicular

(For cryopreservation of embryo[s], use 89258. For cryopreservation of sperm, use 89259)

(For cryopreservation, ovarian tissue, oocytes, use 0058T; for mature oocytes, use 89337; for immature oocytes, use 0357T)

89337   Cryopreservation, mature oocyte(s)

(For cryopreservation of immature oocyte[s], use 0357T)

89342   Storage (per year); embryo(s)

89343   sperm/semen

89344   reproductive tissue, testicular/ovarian

89346   oocyte(s)

89352   Thawing of cryopreserved; embryo(s)

89353   sperm/semen, each aliquot

89354   reproductive tissue, testicular/ovarian

89356   oocytes, each aliquot

89398   Unlisted reproductive medicine laboratory procedure

Pathology and Laboratory

Notes

⊙=Moderate sedation ✦=Add-on code ✗=FDA approval pending #=Resequenced code ○=Recycled/reinstated code

Pathology and Laboratory

Medicine Guidelines

In addition to the definitions and commonly used terms presented in the **Introduction**, several other items unique to this section on **Medicine** are defined or identified here.

Add-on Codes

Some of the listed procedures are commonly carried out in addition to the primary procedure performed. All add-on codes found in the CPT codebook are exempt from the multiple procedure concept. They are exempt from the use of modifier 51, as these procedures are not reported as stand-alone codes. These additional or supplemental procedures are designated as "add-on" codes. Add-on codes in the CPT codebook can be readily identified by specific descriptor nomenclature which includes phrases such as "each additional" or "(List separately in addition to primary procedure)."

Separate Procedures

Some of the procedures or services listed in the CPT codebook that are commonly carried out as an integral component of a total service or procedure have been identified by the inclusion of the term "separate procedure." The codes designated as "separate procedure" should not be reported in addition to the code for the total procedure or service of which it is considered an integral component.

However, when a procedure or service that is designated as a "separate procedure" is carried out independently or considered to be unrelated or distinct from other procedures/services provided at that time, it may be reported by itself, or in addition to other procedures/services by appending modifier 59 to the specific "separate procedure" code to indicate that the procedure is not considered to be a component of another procedure, but is a distinct, independent procedure. This may represent a different session or patient encounter, different procedure or surgery, different site or organ system, separate incision/excision, separate lesion, or separate injury (or area of injury in extensive injuries).

Unlisted Service or Procedure

A service or procedure may be provided that is not listed in this edition of the CPT codebook. When reporting such a service, the appropriate "Unlisted Procedure" code may be used to indicate the service, identifying it by "Special Report" as discussed on the following page. The "Unlisted Procedures" and accompanying codes for **Medicine** are as follows:

90399	Unlisted immune globulin
90749	Unlisted vaccine/toxoid
90899	Unlisted psychiatric service or procedure
90999	Unlisted dialysis procedure, inpatient or outpatient
91299	Unlisted diagnostic gastroenterology procedure
92499	Unlisted ophthalmological service or procedure
92700	Unlisted otorhinolaryngological service or procedure
93799	Unlisted cardiovascular service or procedure
93998	Unlisted noninvasive vascular diagnostic study
94799	Unlisted pulmonary service or procedure
95199	Unlisted allergy/clinical immunologic service or procedure
95999	Unlisted neurological or neuromuscular diagnostic procedure
96379	Unlisted therapeutic, prophylactic, or diagnostic intravenous or intra-arterial injection or infusion
96549	Unlisted chemotherapy procedure
96999	Unlisted special dermatological service or procedure
97039	Unlisted modality (specify type and time if constant attendance)
97139	Unlisted therapeutic procedure (specify)
97799	Unlisted physical medicine/rehabilitation service or procedure
99199	Unlisted special service, procedure or report
99600	Unlisted home visit service or procedure

Medicine

Special Report

A service that is rarely provided, unusual, variable, or new may require a special report. Pertinent information should include an adequate definition or description of the nature, extent, and need for the procedure; and the time, effort, and equipment necessary to provide the service.

►Imaging Guidance◄

►When imaging guidance or imaging supervision and interpretation is included in a procedure, guidelines for image documentation and report, included in the guidelines for Radiology (Including Nuclear Medicine and Diagnostic Ultrasound) will apply.◄

Supplied Materials

Supplies and materials (eg, trays, drug supplies, and materials) over and above those usually included with the procedure(s) rendered are reported separately using code 99070 or a specific supply code.

Medicine

Immune Globulins, Serum or Recombinant Products

►Codes 90281-90399 identify the serum globulins, extracted from human blood; or recombinant immune globulin products created in a laboratory through genetic modification of human and/or animal proteins. Both are reported in addition to the administration codes 96365, 96366, 96367, 96368, 96369, 96370, 96371, 96372, 96374, 96375, as appropriate. Modifier 51 should not be reported with this section of products codes when performed with another procedure. The serum or recombinant globulin products listed here include broad-spectrum anti-infective immune globulins, antitoxins, various isoantibodies, and monoclonal antibodies.◄

90281	Immune globulin (Ig), human, for intramuscular use
90283	Immune globulin (IgIV), human, for intravenous use
90284	Immune globulin (SCIg), human, for use in subcutaneous infusions, 100 mg, each
90287	Botulinum antitoxin, equine, any route
90288	Botulism immune globulin, human, for intravenous use
90291	Cytomegalovirus immune globulin (CMV-IgIV), human, for intravenous use
90296	Diphtheria antitoxin, equine, any route
90371	Hepatitis B immune globulin (HBIg), human, for intramuscular use
90375	Rabies immune globulin (RIg), human, for intramuscular and/or subcutaneous use
90376	Rabies immune globulin, heat-treated (RIg-HT), human, for intramuscular and/or subcutaneous use
90378	Respiratory syncytial virus, monoclonal antibody, recombinant, for intramuscular use, 50 mg, each
90384	Rho(D) immune globulin (RhIg), human, full-dose, for intramuscular use
90385	Rho(D) immune globulin (RhIg), human, mini-dose, for intramuscular use
90386	Rho(D) immune globulin (RhIgIV), human, for intravenous use
90389	Tetanus immune globulin (TIg), human, for intramuscular use
90393	Vaccinia immune globulin, human, for intramuscular use
90396	Varicella-zoster immune globulin, human, for intramuscular use
90399	Unlisted immune globulin

Immunization Administration for Vaccines/Toxoids

Report vaccine immunization administration codes 90460, 90461, 90471-90474 in addition to the vaccine and toxoid code(s) 90476-90749.

Report codes 90460 and 90461 only when the physician or qualified health care professional provides face-to-face counseling of the patient/family during the administration of a vaccine. For immunization administration of any vaccine that is not accompanied by face-to-face physician or qualified health care professional counseling to the patient/family or for administration of vaccines to patients over 18 years of age, report codes 90471-90474. (See also **Instructions for Use of the CPT Codebook** for definition of reporting qualifications.)

If a significant separately identifiable Evaluation and Management service (eg, new or established patient office or other outpatient services [99201-99215], office or other outpatient consultations [99241-99245], emergency department services [99281-99285], preventive medicine services [99381-99429]) is performed, the appropriate E/M service code should be reported in addition to the vaccine and toxoid administration codes.

A component refers to all antigens in a vaccine that prevent disease(s) caused by one organism (90460 and 90461). Multi-valent antigens or multiple serotypes of antigens against a single organism are considered a single component of vaccines. Combination vaccines are those vaccines that contain multiple vaccine components. Conjugates or adjuvants contained in vaccines are not considered to be component parts of the vaccine as defined above.

(For allergy testing, see 95004 et seq)

(For skin testing of bacterial, viral, fungal extracts, see 86485-86580)

(For therapeutic or diagnostic injections, see 96372-96379)

90460	Immunization administration through 18 years of age via any route of administration, with counseling by physician or other qualified health care professional; first or only component of each vaccine or toxoid administered

Medicine

+ 90461   each additional vaccine or toxoid component administered (List separately in addition to code for primary procedure)

(Use 90460 for each vaccine administered. For vaccines with multiple components [combination vaccines], report 90460 in conjunction with 90461 for each additional component in a given vaccine)

(90465-90468 have been deleted. To report, see 90460, 90461, 90471-90474)

90471   Immunization administration (includes percutaneous, intradermal, subcutaneous, or intramuscular injections); 1 vaccine (single or combination vaccine/toxoid)

(Do not report 90471 in conjunction with 90473)

+ 90472   each additional vaccine (single or combination vaccine/toxoid) (List separately in addition to code for primary procedure)

(Use 90472 in conjunction with 90460, 90471, 90473)

▶(For immune globulins, see 90281-90399. For administration of immune globulins, see 96365, 96366, 96367, 96368, 96369, 96370, 96371, 96374)◀

(For intravesical administration of BCG vaccine, see 51720, 90586)

90473   Immunization administration by intranasal or oral route; 1 vaccine (single or combination vaccine/toxoid)

(Do not report 90473 in conjunction with 90471)

+ 90474   each additional vaccine (single or combination vaccine/toxoid) (List separately in addition to code for primary procedure)

(Use 90474 in conjunction with 90460, 90471, 90473)

Vaccines, Toxoids

To assist users to report the most recent new or revised vaccine product codes, the American Medical Association (AMA) currently uses the CPT website, which features updates of CPT Editorial Panel actions regarding these products. Once approved by the CPT Editorial Panel, these codes will be made available for release on a semi-annual (twice a year: July 1 and January 1) basis. As part of the electronic distribution, there is a six-month implementation period from the initial release date (ie, codes released on January 1 are eligible for use on July 1 and codes released on July 1 are eligible for use January 1).

The CPT Editorial Panel, in recognition of the public health interest in vaccine products, has chosen to publish new vaccine product codes prior to approval by the US Food and Drug Administration (FDA). These codes are indicated with the ⁄ symbol and will be tracked by the AMA to monitor FDA approval status. Once the FDA status changes to approval, the ⁄ symbol will be removed. CPT users should refer to the AMA CPT website (www.ama-assn.org/go/cpt-vaccine) for the most up-to-date information on codes with the ⁄ symbol.

Codes 90476-90749 identify the vaccine product **only**. To report the administration of a vaccine/toxoid, the vaccine/toxoid product codes 90476-90749 must be used in addition to an immunization administration code(s) 90460, 90461, 90471, 90472, 90473, 90474. Modifier 51 should not be reported with vaccine/toxoid codes 90476-90749, when reported in conjunction with administration codes 90460, 90461, 90471, 90472, 90473, 90474.

If a significantly separately identifiable Evaluation and Management (E/M) service (eg, office or other outpatient services, preventive medicine services) is performed, the appropriate E/M service code should be reported in addition to the vaccine and toxoid administration codes.

To meet the reporting requirements of immunization registries, vaccine distribution programs, and reporting systems (eg, Vaccine Adverse Event Reporting System) the exact vaccine product administered needs to be reported. Multiple codes for a particular vaccine are provided in the CPT codebook when the schedule (number of doses or timing) differs for two or more products of the same vaccine type (eg, hepatitis A, Hib) or the vaccine product is available in more than one chemical formulation, dosage, or route of administration.

The "when administered to" age descriptions included in CPT vaccine codes are not intended to identify a product's licensed age indication. The term "preservative free" includes use for vaccines that contain no preservative and vaccines that contain trace amounts of preservative agents that are not present in a sufficient concentration for the purpose of preserving the final vaccine formulation. The absence of a designation regarding a preservative does not necessarily indicate the presence or absence of preservative in the vaccine. Refer to the product's prescribing information (PI) for the licensed age indication before administering vaccine to a patient.

Separate codes are available for combination vaccines (eg, Hib-HepB, DTap-IPV/Hib). It is inappropriate to code each component of a combination vaccine separately. If a specific vaccine code is not available, the unlisted procedure code should be reported, until a new code becomes available.

The vaccine/toxoid abbreviations listed in codes 90476-90748 reflect the most recent US vaccine abbreviations references used in the Advisory Committee on Immunization Practices (ACIP) recommendations at the time of CPT code set publication. Interim updates to vaccine code descriptors will be made following abbreviation approval by the ACIP on a timely basis via the AMA CPT website (www.ama-assn.org/go/cpt-vaccine). The accuracy of the ACIP vaccine abbreviation designations in the CPT code set does not affect the validity of the vaccine code and its reporting function.

▶(For immune globulins, see 90281-90399. For administration of immune globulins, see 96365-96375)◀

Medicine

90476　Adenovirus vaccine, type 4, live, for oral use

90477　Adenovirus vaccine, type 7, live, for oral use

90581　Anthrax vaccine, for subcutaneous or intramuscular use

90585　Bacillus Calmette-Guerin vaccine (BCG) for tuberculosis, live, for percutaneous use

90586　Bacillus Calmette-Guerin vaccine (BCG) for bladder cancer, live, for intravesical use

90620　Code is out of numerical sequence. See 90476-90749

90621　Code is out of numerical sequence. See 90476-90749

90625　Code is out of numerical sequence. See 90476-90749

90630　Code is out of numerical sequence. See 90476-90749

▲ 90632　Hepatitis A vaccine (HepA), adult dosage, for intramuscular use

▲ 90633　Hepatitis A vaccine (HepA), pediatric/adolescent dosage-2 dose schedule, for intramuscular use

▲ 90634　Hepatitis A vaccine (HepA), pediatric/adolescent dosage-3 dose schedule, for intramuscular use

90636　Hepatitis A and hepatitis B vaccine (HepA-HepB), adult dosage, for intramuscular use

90644　Code is out of numerical sequence. See 90476-90749

►(90645 has been deleted)◄

►(90646 has been deleted)◄

▲ 90647　Haemophilus influenzae type b vaccine (Hib), PRP-OMP conjugate, 3 dose schedule, for intramuscular use

▲ 90648　Haemophilus influenzae type b vaccine (Hib), PRP-T conjugate, 4 dose schedule, for intramuscular use

▲ 90649　Human Papillomavirus vaccine, types 6, 11, 16, 18, quadrivalent (4vHPV), 3 dose schedule, for intramuscular use

▲ 90650　Human Papillomavirus vaccine, types 16, 18, bivalent (2vHPV), 3 dose schedule, for intramuscular use

▲ 90651　Human Papillomavirus vaccine types 6, 11, 16, 18, 31, 33, 45, 52, 58, nonavalent (9vHPV), 3 dose schedule, for intramuscular use

✎▲ 90653　Influenza vaccine, inactivated (IIV), subunit, adjuvanted, for intramuscular use

90654　Influenza virus vaccine, trivalent (IIV3), split virus, preservative-free, for intradermal use

90630　Influenza virus vaccine, quadrivalent (IIV4), split virus, preservative free, for intradermal use

▲ 90655　Influenza virus vaccine, trivalent (IIV3), split virus, preservative free, when administered to children 6-35 months of age, for intramuscular use

▲ 90656　Influenza virus vaccine, trivalent (IIV3), split virus, preservative free, when administered to individuals 3 years and older, for intramuscular use

▲ 90657　Influenza virus vaccine, trivalent (IIV3), split virus, when administered to children 6-35 months of age, for intramuscular use

▲ 90658　Influenza virus vaccine, trivalent (IIV3), split virus, when administered to individuals 3 years of age and older, for intramuscular use

▲ 90660　Influenza virus vaccine, trivalent, live (LAIV3), for intranasal use

#▲ 90672　Influenza virus vaccine, quadrivalent, live (LAIV4), for intranasal use

▲ 90661　Influenza virus vaccine (ccIIV3), derived from cell cultures, subunit, preservative and antibiotic free, for intramuscular use

#▲ 90673　Influenza virus vaccine, trivalent (RIV3), derived from recombinant DNA, hemagglutinin (HA) protein only, preservative and antibiotic free, for intramuscular use

▲ 90662　Influenza virus vaccine (IIV), split virus, preservative free, enhanced immunogenicity via increased antigen content, for intramuscular use

▲ 90664　Influenza virus vaccine, live (LAIV), pandemic formulation, for intranasal use

(90665 has been deleted)

✎▲ 90666　Influenza virus vaccine (IIV), pandemic formulation, split virus, preservative free, for intramuscular use

✎▲ 90667　Influenza virus vaccine (IIV), pandemic formulation, split virus, adjuvanted, for intramuscular use

✎▲ 90668　Influenza virus vaccine (IIV), pandemic formulation, split virus, for intramuscular use

►(90669 has been deleted)◄

▲ 90670　Pneumococcal conjugate vaccine, 13 valent (PCV13), for intramuscular use

90672　Code is out of numerical sequence. See 90476-90749

90673　Code is out of numerical sequence. See 90476-90749

90675　Rabies vaccine, for intramuscular use

90676　Rabies vaccine, for intradermal use

▲ 90680　Rotavirus vaccine, pentavalent (RV5), 3 dose schedule, live, for oral use

▲ 90681　Rotavirus vaccine, human, attenuated (RV1), 2 dose schedule, live, for oral use

▲ 90685　Influenza virus vaccine, quadrivalent (IIV4), split virus, preservative free, when administered to children 6-35 months of age, for intramuscular use

▲ 90686　Influenza virus vaccine, quadrivalent (IIV4), split virus, preservative free, when administered to individuals 3 years of age and older, for intramuscular use

▲ 90687　Influenza virus vaccine, quadrivalent (IIV4), split virus, when administered to children 6-35 months of age, for intramuscular use

Medicine

▲ 90688 Influenza virus vaccine, quadrivalent (IIV4), split virus, when administered to individuals 3 years of age and older, for intramuscular use

90690 Typhoid vaccine, live, oral

90691 Typhoid vaccine, Vi capsular polysaccharide (ViCPs), for intramuscular use

►(90692 has been deleted)◄

►(90693 has been deleted)◄

▲ 90696 Diphtheria, tetanus toxoids, acellular pertussis vaccine and inactivated poliovirus vaccine (DTaP-IPV), when administered to children 4 through 6 years of age, for intramuscular use

✗● 90697 Diphtheria, tetanus toxoids, acellular pertussis vaccine, inactivated poliovirus vaccine, Haemophilus influenzae type b PRP-OMP conjugate vaccine, and hepatitis B vaccine (DTaP-IPV-Hib--HepB), for intramuscular use

▲ 90698 Diphtheria, tetanus toxoids, acellular pertussis vaccine, Haemophilus influenzae type b, and inactivated poliovirus vaccine, (DTap-IPV/Hib), for intramuscular use

90700 Diphtheria, tetanus toxoids, and acellular pertussis vaccine (DTaP), when administered to individuals younger than 7 years, for intramuscular use

(90701 has been deleted)

▲ 90702 Diphtheria and tetanus toxoids adsorbed (DT) when administered to individuals younger than 7 years, for intramuscular use

►(90703 has been deleted)◄

►(90704 has been deleted)◄

►(90705 has been deleted)◄

►(90706 has been deleted)◄

90707 Measles, mumps and rubella virus vaccine (MMR), live, for subcutaneous use

►(90708 has been deleted)◄

90710 Measles, mumps, rubella, and varicella vaccine (MMRV), live, for subcutaneous use

►(90712 has been deleted)◄

90713 Poliovirus vaccine, inactivated (IPV), for subcutaneous or intramuscular use

▲ 90714 Tetanus and diphtheria toxoids adsorbed (Td), preservative free, when administered to individuals 7 years or older, for intramuscular use

90715 Tetanus, diphtheria toxoids and acellular pertussis vaccine (Tdap), when administered to individuals 7 years or older, for intramuscular use

▲ 90716 Varicella virus vaccine (VAR), live, for subcutaneous use

90717 Yellow fever vaccine, live, for subcutaneous use

(90718 has been deleted)

►(90719 has been deleted)◄

►(90720 has been deleted)◄

►(90721 has been deleted)◄

90723 Diphtheria, tetanus toxoids, acellular pertussis vaccine, hepatitis B, and inactivated poliovirus vaccine (DTaP-HepB-IPV), for intramuscular use

►(90725 has been deleted)◄

#✗● 90625 Cholera vaccine, live, adult dosage, 1 dose schedule, for oral use

►(90727 has been deleted)◄

▲ 90732 Pneumococcal polysaccharide vaccine, 23-valent (PPSV23), adult or immunosuppressed patient dosage, when administered to individuals 2 years or older, for subcutaneous or intramuscular use

#▲ 90644 Meningococcal conjugate vaccine, serogroups C & Y and Haemophilus influenzae type b vaccine (Hib-MenCY), 4 dose schedule, when administered to children 2-18 months of age, for intramuscular use

▲ 90733 Meningococcal polysaccharide vaccine, serogroups A, C, Y, W-135, quadrivalent (MPSV4), for subcutaneous use

▲ 90734 Meningococcal conjugate vaccine, serogroups A, C, Y and W-135, quadrivalent (MenACWY), for intramuscular use

#● 90620 Meningococcal recombinant protein and outer membrane vesicle vaccine, serogroup B (MenB), 2 dose schedule, for intramuscular use

#● 90621 Meningococcal recombinant lipoprotein vaccine, serogroup B (MenB), 3 dose schedule, for intramuscular use

►(90735 has been deleted)◄

▲ 90736 Zoster (shingles) vaccine (HZV), live, for subcutaneous injection

90738 Japanese encephalitis virus vaccine, inactivated, for intramuscular use

✗▲ 90739 Hepatitis B vaccine (HepB), adult dosage, 2 dose schedule, for intramuscular use

▲ 90740 Hepatitis B vaccine (HepB), dialysis or immunosuppressed patient dosage, 3 dose schedule, for intramuscular use

▲ 90743 Hepatitis B vaccine (HepB), adolescent, 2 dose schedule, for intramuscular use

▲ 90744 Hepatitis B vaccine (HepB), pediatric/adolescent dosage, 3 dose schedule, for intramuscular use

▲ 90746 Hepatitis B vaccine (HepB), adult dosage, 3 dose schedule, for intramuscular use

▲ 90747 Hepatitis B vaccine (HepB), dialysis or immunosuppressed patient dosage, 4 dose schedule, for intramuscular use

▲ 90748 Hepatitis B and Haemophilus influenzae type b vaccine (Hib-HepB), for intramuscular use

90749 Unlisted vaccine/toxoid

Medicine

Psychiatry

Psychiatry services include diagnostic services, psychotherapy, and other services to an individual, family, or group. Patient condition, characteristics, or situational factors may require services described as being with interactive complexity. Services may be provided to a patient in crisis. Services are provided in all settings of care and psychiatry services codes are reported without regard to setting. Services may be provided by a physician or other qualified health care professional. Some psychiatry services may be reported with **Evaluation and Management Services** (99201-99255, 99281-99285, 99304-99337, 99341-99350) or other services when performed. **Evaluation and Management Services** (99201-99285, 99304-99337, 99341-99350) may be reported for treatment of psychiatric conditions, rather than using **Psychiatry Services** codes, when appropriate.

Hospital care in treating a psychiatric inpatient or partial hospitalization may be initial or subsequent in nature (see 99221-99233).

Some patients receive hospital evaluation and management services only and others receive hospital evaluation and management services and other procedures. If other procedures such as electroconvulsive therapy or psychotherapy are rendered in addition to hospital evaluation and management services, these may be listed separately (eg, hospital care services [99221-99223, 99231-99233] plus electroconvulsive therapy [90870]), or when psychotherapy is done, with appropriate code(s) defining psychotherapy services.

Consultation for psychiatric evaluation of a patient includes examination of a patient and exchange of information with the primary physician and other informants such as nurses or family members, and preparation of a report. These services may be reported using consultation codes (see **Consultations**).

(Do not report 90785-90899 in conjunction with 90839, 90840, 0364T, 0365T, 0366T, 0367T, 0373T, 0374T)

Interactive Complexity

Code 90785 is an add-on code for interactive complexity to be reported in conjunction with codes for diagnostic psychiatric evaluation (90791, 90792), psychotherapy (90832, 90834, 90837), psychotherapy when performed with an evaluation and management service (90833, 90836, 90838, 99201-99255, 99304-99337, 99341-99350), and group psychotherapy (90853).

Interactive complexity refers to specific communication factors that complicate the delivery of a psychiatric procedure. Common factors include more difficult communication with discordant or emotional family members and engagement of young and verbally undeveloped or impaired patients. Typical patients are those who have third parties, such as parents, guardians, other family members, interpreters, language translators, agencies, court officers, or schools involved in their psychiatric care.

These factors are typically present with patients who:

- Have other individuals legally responsible for their care, such as minors or adults with guardians, or

- Request others to be involved in their care during the visit, such as adults accompanied by one or more participating family members or interpreter or language translator, or

- Require the involvement of other third parties, such as child welfare agencies, parole or probation officers, or schools.

Psychiatric procedures may be reported "with interactive complexity" when at least one of the following is present:

1. The need to manage maladaptive communication (related to, eg, high anxiety, high reactivity, repeated questions, or disagreement) among participants that complicates delivery of care.

2. Caregiver emotions or behavior that interferes with the caregiver's understanding and ability to assist in the implementation of the treatment plan.

3. Evidence or disclosure of a sentinel event and mandated report to third party (eg, abuse or neglect with report to state agency) with initiation of discussion of the sentinel event and/or report with patient and other visit participants.

4. Use of play equipment, other physical devices, interpreter, or translator to communicate with the patient to overcome barriers to therapeutic or diagnostic interaction between the physician or other qualified health care professional and a patient who:

- Is not fluent in the same language as the physician or other qualified health care professional, or

- Has not developed, or has lost, either the expressive language communication skills to explain his/her symptoms and response to treatment, or the receptive communication skills to understand the physician or other qualified health care professional if he/she were to use typical language for communication.

When provided in conjunction with the psychotherapy services (90832-90838), the amount of time spent by a physician or other qualified health care professional providing interactive complexity services should be reflected in the timed service code for psychotherapy (90832, 90834, 90837) or the psychotherapy add-on code performed with an evaluation and management service (90833, 90836, 90838) and must relate to the psychotherapy service only. Interactive complexity is not a factor for evaluation and management services selection (99201-99255, 99281-99285, 99304-99337, 99341-99350), except as it directly affects key components as defined in the Evaluation and Management Services Guidelines (ie, history, examination, and medical decision making).

Medicine

+ 90785 Interactive complexity (List separately in addition to the code for primary procedure)

> (Use 90785 in conjunction with codes for diagnostic psychiatric evaluation [90791, 90792], psychotherapy [90832, 90834, 90837], psychotherapy when performed with an evaluation and management service [90833, 90836, 90838, 99201-99255, 99304-99337, 99341-99350], and group psychotherapy [90853])

> (Do not report 90785 in conjunction with 90839, 90840, or in conjunction with E/M services when no psychotherapy service is also reported)

> (Do not report 90785 in conjunction with 90839, 90840, 0364T, 0365T, 0366T, 0367T, 0373T, 0374T)

Psychiatric Diagnostic Procedures

Psychiatric diagnostic evaluation is an integrated biopsychosocial assessment, including history, mental status, and recommendations. The evaluation may include communication with family or other sources and review and ordering of diagnostic studies.

Psychiatric diagnostic evaluation with medical services is an integrated biopsychosocial and medical assessment, including history, mental status, other physical examination elements as indicated, and recommendations. The evaluation may include communication with family or other sources, prescription of medications, and review and ordering of laboratory or other diagnostic studies.

In certain circumstances one or more other informants (family members, guardians, or significant others) may be seen in lieu of the patient. Codes 90791, 90792 may be reported more than once for the patient when separate diagnostic evaluations are conducted with the patient and other informants. Report services as being provided to the patient and not the informant or other party in such circumstances. Codes 90791, 90792 may be reported once per day and not on the same day as an evaluation and management service performed by the same individual for the same patient.

The psychiatric diagnostic evaluation may include interactive complexity services when factors exist that complicate the delivery of the psychiatric procedure. These services should be reported with add-on code 90785 used in conjunction with the diagnostic psychiatric evaluation codes 90791, 90792.

Codes 90791, 90792 are used for the diagnostic assessment(s) or reassessment(s), if required, and do not include psychotherapeutic services. Psychotherapy services, including for crisis, may not be reported on the same day.

> (Do not report 90791-90899 in conjunction with 90839, 90840, 0364T, 0365T, 0366T, 0367T, 0373T, 0374T)

90791 Psychiatric diagnostic evaluation

90792 Psychiatric diagnostic evaluation with medical services

> (Do not report 90791 or 90792 in conjunction with 99201-99337, 99341-99350, 99366-99368, 99401-99444, 0368T, 0369T, 0370T, 0371T)

> (Use 90785 in conjunction with 90791, 90792 when the diagnostic evaluation includes interactive complexity services)

> (90801 and 90802 have been deleted. To report diagnostic evaluations, see 90791, 90792)

> (90804, 90805, 90806, 90807, 90808, 90809 have been deleted. To report, see psychotherapy codes 90832, 90834, 90837 or psychotherapy add-on codes when performed with an evaluation and management service [90833, 90836, 90838, 99201-99255, 99304-99337, 99341-99350])

> (90810, 90811, 90812, 90813, 90814, 90815 have been deleted. To report interactive psychotherapy, report 90785 in conjunction with psychotherapy codes 90832, 90834, 90837 or psychotherapy add-on codes when performed with an evaluation and management service [90833, 90836, 90838, 99201-99255, 99304-99337, 99341-99350])

> (90816, 90817, 90818, 90819, 90821, 90822 have been deleted. To report, see psychotherapy codes 90832, 90834, 90837 or psychotherapy add-on codes when performed with an evaluation and management service [90833, 90836, 90838, 99201-99255, 99304-99337, 99341-99350])

> (90823, 90824, 90826, 90827, 90828, 90829 have been deleted. To report interactive psychotherapy, report 90785 in conjunction with psychotherapy codes 90832, 90834, 90837 or psychotherapy add-on codes when performed with an evaluation and management service [90833, 90836, 90838, 99201-99255, 99304-99337, 99341-99350])

Psychotherapy

Psychotherapy is the treatment of mental illness and behavioral disturbances in which the physician or other qualified health care professional, through definitive therapeutic communication, attempts to alleviate the emotional disturbances, reverse or change maladaptive patterns of behavior, and encourage personality growth and development.

The psychotherapy service codes 90832-90838 include ongoing assessment and adjustment of psychotherapeutic interventions, and may include involvement of family member(s) or others in the treatment process.

Psychotherapy times are for face-to-face services with patient and/or family member. The patient must be present for all or some of the service. For family psychotherapy without the patient present, use 90846. In reporting, choose the code closest to the actual time (ie, 16-37 minutes for 90832 and 90833, 38-52 minutes for

⊙=Moderate sedation ✚=Add-on code ✗=FDA approval pending #=Resequenced code ○=Recycled/reinstated code

90834 and 90836, and 53 or more minutes for 90837 and 90838). Do not report psychotherapy of less than 16 minutes duration. (See instructions for the usage of time in the Introduction of the CPT code set.)

Psychotherapy provided to a patient in a crisis state is reported with codes 90839 and 90840 and cannot be reported in addition to the psychotherapy codes 90832-90838. For psychotherapy for crisis, see "Other Psychotherapy."

Code 90785 is an add-on code to report interactive complexity services when provided in conjunction with the psychotherapy codes 90832-90838. The amount of time spent by a physician or other qualified health care professional providing interactive complexity services should be reflected in the timed service code for psychotherapy (90832, 90834, 90837) or the psychotherapy add-on code performed with an evaluation and management service (90833, 90836, 90838).

Some psychiatric patients receive a medical evaluation and management (E/M) service on the same day as a psychotherapy service by the same physician or other qualified health care professional. To report both E/M and psychotherapy, the two services must be significant and separately identifiable. These services are reported by using codes specific for psychotherapy when performed with evaluation and management services (90833, 90836, 90838) as add-on codes to the evaluation and management service.

Medical symptoms and disorders inform treatment choices of psychotherapeutic interventions, and data from therapeutic communication are used to evaluate the presence, type, and severity of medical symptoms and disorders. For the purposes of reporting, the medical and psychotherapeutic components of the service may be separately identified as follows:

1. The type and level of E/M service is selected first based upon the key components of history, examination, and medical decision-making.

2. Time associated with activities used to meet criteria for the E/M service is not included in the time used for reporting the psychotherapy service (ie, time spent on history, examination and medical decision making **when used for the E/M service** is not psychotherapy time). Time may not be used as the basis of E/M code selection and Prolonged Services may not be reported when psychotherapy with E/M (90833, 90836, 90838) are reported.

3. A separate diagnosis is not required for the reporting of E/M and psychotherapy on the same date of service.

90832   Psychotherapy, 30 minutes with patient and/or family member

+ **90833**   Psychotherapy, 30 minutes with patient and/or family member when performed with an evaluation and management service (List separately in addition to the code for primary procedure)

(Use 90833 in conjunction with 99201-99255, 99304-99337, 99341-99350)

90834   Psychotherapy, 45 minutes with patient and/or family member

+ **90836**   Psychotherapy, 45 minutes with patient and/or family member when performed with an evaluation and management service (List separately in addition to the code for primary procedure)

(Use 90836 in conjunction with 99201-99255, 99304-99337, 99341-99350)

90837   Psychotherapy, 60 minutes with patient and/or family member

(Use the appropriate prolonged services code [99354, 99355, 99356, 99357] for psychotherapy services not performed with an E/M service of 90 minutes or longer face-to-face with the patient)

+ **90838**   Psychotherapy, 60 minutes with patient and/or family member when performed with an evaluation and management service (List separately in addition to the code for primary procedure)

(Use 90838 in conjunction with 99201-99255, 99304-99337, 99341-99350)

(Use 90785 in conjunction with 90832, 90833, 90834, 90836, 90837, 90838 when psychotherapy includes interactive complexity services)

Psychotherapy for Crisis

Psychotherapy for crisis is an urgent assessment and history of a crisis state, a mental status exam, and a disposition. The treatment includes psychotherapy, mobilization of resources to defuse the crisis and restore safety, and implementation of psychotherapeutic interventions to minimize the potential for psychological trauma. The presenting problem is typically life threatening or complex and requires immediate attention to a patient in high distress.

Codes 90839, 90840 are used to report the total duration of time face-to-face with the patient and/or family spent by the physician or other qualified health care professional providing psychotherapy for crisis, even if the time spent on that date is not continuous. For any given period of time spent providing psychotherapy for crisis state, the physician or other qualified health care professional must devote his or her full attention to the patient and, therefore, cannot provide services to any other patient during the same time period. The patient must be present for all or some of the service. Do not report with 90791 or 90792.

Medicine

Code 90839 is used to report the first 30-74 minutes of psychotherapy for crisis on a given date. It should be used only once per date even if the time spent by the physician or other health care professional is not continuous on that date. Psychotherapy for crisis of less than 30 minutes total duration on a given date should be reported with 90832 or 90833 (when provided with evaluation and management services).

Code 90840 is used to report additional block(s) of time, of up to 30 minutes each beyond the first 74 minutes.

90839 Psychotherapy for crisis; first 60 minutes

+ 90840 each additional 30 minutes (List separately in addition to code for primary service)

(Use 90840 in conjunction with 90839)

(Do not report 90839, 90840 in conjunction with 90791, 90792, psychotherapy codes 90832-90838 or other psychiatric services, or 90785-90899)

Other Psychotherapy

90845 Psychoanalysis

90846 Family psychotherapy (without the patient present)

90847 Family psychotherapy (conjoint psychotherapy) (with patient present)

(Do not report 90846, 90847 in conjunction with 0368T, 0369T, 0370T, 0371T)

90849 Multiple-family group psychotherapy

90853 Group psychotherapy (other than of a multiple-family group)

(Use 90853 in conjunction with 90785 for the specified patient when group psychotherapy includes interactive complexity)

(Do not report 90853 in conjunction with 0372T)

(90857 has been deleted. To report, use 90785 in conjunction with 90853)

Other Psychiatric Services or Procedures

(For analysis/programming of neurostimulators used for vagus nerve stimulation therapy, see 95970, 95974, 95975)

(90862 has been deleted. To report, see 90863 or Evaluation and Management services codes 99201-99255, 99281-99285, 99304-99337, 99341-99350)

+ 90863 Pharmacologic management, including prescription and review of medication, when performed with psychotherapy services (List separately in addition to the code for primary procedure)

(Use 90863 in conjunction with 90832, 90834, 90837)

(For pharmacologic management with psychotherapy services performed by a physician or other qualified health care professional who may report evaluation and management codes, use the appropriate evaluation and management codes 99201-99255, 99281-99285, 99304-99337, 99341-99350 and the appropriate psychotherapy with evaluation and management service 90833, 90836, 90838)

(Do not count time spent on providing pharmacologic management services in the time used for selection of the psychotherapy service)

90865 Narcosynthesis for psychiatric diagnostic and therapeutic purposes (eg, sodium amobarbital (Amytal) interview)

90867 Therapeutic repetitive transcranial magnetic stimulation (TMS) treatment; initial, including cortical mapping, motor threshold determination, delivery and management

(Report only once per course of treatment)

(Do not report 90867 in conjunction with 90868, 90869, 95860, 95870, 95928, 95929, 95939)

90868 subsequent delivery and management, per session

90869 subsequent motor threshold re-determination with delivery and management

(Do not report 90869 in conjunction with 90867, 90868, 95860-95870, 95928, 95929, 95939)

(If a significant, separately identifiable evaluation and management, medication management, or psychotherapy service is performed, the appropriate E/M or psychotherapy code may be reported in addition to 90867-90869. Evaluation and management activities directly related to cortical mapping, motor threshold determination, delivery and management of TMS are not separately reported)

(For transcranial magnetic stimulation motor function mapping for therapeutic planning other than for repetitive transcranial magnetic stimulation, use 0310T)

90870 Electroconvulsive therapy (includes necessary monitoring)

90875 Individual psychophysiological therapy incorporating biofeedback training by any modality (face-to-face with the patient), with psychotherapy (eg, insight oriented, behavior modifying or supportive psychotherapy); 30 minutes

90876 45 minutes

90880 Hypnotherapy

90882 Environmental intervention for medical management purposes on a psychiatric patient's behalf with agencies, employers, or institutions

90885 Psychiatric evaluation of hospital records, other psychiatric reports, psychometric and/or projective tests, and other accumulated data for medical diagnostic purposes

Medicine

90887   Interpretation or explanation of results of psychiatric, other medical examinations and procedures, or other accumulated data to family or other responsible persons, or advising them how to assist patient

(Do not report 90887 in conjunction with 0368T, 0369T, 0370T, 0371T)

90889   Preparation of report of patient's psychiatric status, history, treatment, or progress (other than for legal or consultative purposes) for other individuals, agencies, or insurance carriers

90899   Unlisted psychiatric service or procedure

Biofeedback

(For psychophysiological therapy incorporating biofeedback training, see 90875, 90876)

90901   Biofeedback training by any modality

90911   Biofeedback training, perineal muscles, anorectal or urethral sphincter, including EMG and/or manometry

(For testing of rectal sensation, tone and compliance, use 91120)

(For incontinence treatment by pulsed magnetic neuromodulation, use 53899)

Dialysis

(90918, 90922 have been deleted. To report ESRD-related services for patients younger than 2 years of age, see 90951-90953, 90963, 90967)

(90919, 90923 have been deleted. To report ESRD-related services for patients between 2 and 11 years of age, see 90954-90956, 90964, 90968)

(90920, 90924 have been deleted. To report ESRD-related services for patients between 12 and 19 years of age, see 90957-90959, 90965, 90969)

(90921, 90925 have been deleted. To report ESRD-related services for patients 20 years of age and older, see 90960-90962, 90966, 90970)

Hemodialysis

Codes 90935, 90937 are reported to describe the hemodialysis procedure with all evaluation and management services related to the patient's renal disease on the day of the hemodialysis procedure. These codes are used for inpatient ESRD and non-ESRD procedures or for outpatient non-ESRD dialysis services. Code 90935 is reported if only one evaluation of the patient is required related to that hemodialysis procedure. Code 90937 is reported when patient re-evaluation(s) is required during a hemodialysis procedure. Use modifier 25 with evaluation and management codes including new or established patient office or other outpatient services

(99201-99215), office or other outpatient consultations (99241-99245), observation care (99217-99220, 99224-99226), observation or inpatient care including admission and discharge (99234-99236), initial hospital care (99221-99226, 99231-99239), new or established patient emergency department services (99281-99285), critical care services (99291, 99292), inpatient neonatal intensive care services and pediatric and neonatal critical care services (99466-99480), nursing facility services (99304-99318), domiciliary, rest home services, or custodial care (99324-99337), and home services (99341-99350), for separately identifiable services unrelated to the dialysis procedure or renal failure which cannot be rendered during the dialysis session.

(For home visit hemodialysis services performed by a non-physician health care professional, use 99512)

(For cannula declotting, see 36831, 36833, 36860, 36861)

(For declotting of implanted vascular access device or catheter by thrombolytic agent, use 36593)

(For collection of blood specimen from a partially or completely implantable venous access device, use 36591)

(For prolonged attendance by a physician or other qualified health care professional, see 99354-99360)

90935   Hemodialysis procedure with single evaluation by a physician or other qualified health care professional

90937   Hemodialysis procedure requiring repeated evaluation(s) with or without substantial revision of dialysis prescription

90940   Hemodialysis access flow study to determine blood flow in grafts and arteriovenous fistulae by an indicator method

(For duplex scan of hemodialysis access, use 93990)

Miscellaneous Dialysis Procedures

Codes 90945, 90947 describe dialysis procedures other than hemodialysis (eg, peritoneal dialysis, hemofiltration or continuous renal replacement therapies), and all evaluation and management services related to the patient's renal disease on the day of the procedure. Code 90945 is reported if only one evaluation of the patient is required related to that procedure. Code 90947 is reported when patient re-evaluation(s) is required during a procedure. Use modifier 25 with Evaluation and Management codes including office or other outpatient services (99201-99215), office or other outpatient consultations (99241-99245), observation care (99217-99220, 99224-99226), observation or inpatient care including admission and discharge (99234-99239), hospital care (99221-99226, 99231-99239), new or established patient emergency department services (99281-99285), critical care services (99291, 99292), inpatient neonatal intensive care services and pediatric and neonatal critical care services (99466-99480), nursing facility services (99304-99318), domiciliary, rest home, or custodial care services (99324-99337), and home services

Medicine

(99341-99350) for separately identifiable services unrelated to the procedure or the renal failure which cannot be rendered during the dialysis session.

(For percutaneous insertion of intraperitoneal tunneled catheter, use 49418. For open insertion of tunneled intraperitoneal catheter, use 49421)

(For prolonged attendance by a physician or other qualified health care professional, see 99354-99360)

90945   Dialysis procedure other than hemodialysis (eg, peritoneal dialysis, hemofiltration, or other continuous renal replacement therapies), with single evaluation by a physician or other qualified health care professional

(For home infusion of peritoneal dialysis, use 99601, 99602)

90947   Dialysis procedure other than hemodialysis (eg, peritoneal dialysis, hemofiltration, or other continuous renal replacement therapies) requiring repeated evaluations by a physician or other qualified health care professional, with or without substantial revision of dialysis prescription

End-Stage Renal Disease Services

Codes 90951-90962 are reported **once** per month to distinguish age-specific services related to the patient's end-stage renal disease (ESRD) performed in an outpatient setting with three levels of service based on the number of face-to-face visits. ESRD-related services by a physician or other qualified health care professional include establishment of a dialyzing cycle, outpatient evaluation and management of the dialysis visits, telephone calls, and patient management during the dialysis provided during a full month. In the circumstances in which the patient has had a complete assessment visit during the month and services are provided over a period of less than a month, 90951-90962 may be used according to the number of visits performed.

Codes 90963-90966 are reported once per month for a full month of service to distinguish age-specific services for end-stage renal disease (ESRD) services for home dialysis patients.

For ESRD and non-ESRD dialysis services performed in an inpatient setting, and for non-ESRD dialysis services performed in an outpatient setting, see 90935-90937 and 90945-90947.

Evaluation and management services unrelated to ESRD services that cannot be performed during the dialysis session may be reported separately.

Codes 90967-90970 are reported to distinguish age-specific services for end-stage renal disease (ESRD) services for less than a full month of service, per day, for services provided under the following circumstances: home dialysis patients less than a full month, transient patients, partial month where there was one or more face-to-face visits without the complete assessment, the patient

was hospitalized before a complete assessment was furnished, dialysis was stopped due to recovery or death, or the patient received a kidney transplant. For reporting purposes, each month is considered 30 days.

Examples:

ESRD-related services:

ESRD-related services are initiated on July 1 for a 57-year-old male. On July 11, he is admitted to the hospital as an inpatient and is discharged on July 27. He has had a complete assessment and the physician or other qualified health care professional has performed two face-to-face visits prior to admission. Another face-to-face visit occurs after discharge during the month.

In this example, 90961 is reported for the three face-to-face outpatient visits. Report inpatient E/M services as appropriate. Dialysis procedures rendered during the hospitalization (July 11-27) should be reported as appropriate (90935-90937, 90945-90947).

If the patient did not have a complete assessment during the month or was a transient or dialysis was stopped due to recovery or death, 90970 would be used to report each day outside the inpatient hospitalization as described in the home dialysis example below.

ESRD-related services for the home dialysis patient:

Home ESRD-related services are initiated on July 1 for a 57-year-old male. On July 11, he is admitted to the hospital as an inpatient and is discharged on July 27.

In this example, 90970 should be reported for each day outside of the inpatient hospitalization (30 days/month less 17 days/hospitalization = 13 days). Report inpatient E/M services as appropriate. Dialysis procedures rendered during the hospitalization (July 11-27) should be reported as appropriate (90935-90937, 90945-90947).

(Do not report 90951-90970 during the same month in conjunction with 99487-99489)

(Do not report 90951-90970 during the service time of 99495-99496)

90951   End-stage renal disease (ESRD) related services monthly, for patients younger than 2 years of age to include monitoring for the adequacy of nutrition, assessment of growth and development, and counseling of parents; with 4 or more face-to-face visits by a physician or other qualified health care professional per month

90952   with 2-3 face-to-face visits by a physician or other qualified health care professional per month

90953   with 1 face-to-face visit by a physician or other qualified health care professional per month

90954   End-stage renal disease (ESRD) related services monthly, for patients 2-11 years of age to include monitoring for the adequacy of nutrition, assessment of growth and development, and counseling of parents; with 4 or more face-to-face visits by a physician or other qualified health care professional per month

90955   with 2-3 face-to-face visits by a physician or other qualified health care professional per month

90956   with 1 face-to-face visit by a physician or other qualified health care professional per month

90957   End-stage renal disease (ESRD) related services monthly, for patients 12-19 years of age to include monitoring for the adequacy of nutrition, assessment of growth and development, and counseling of parents; with 4 or more face-to-face visits by a physician or other qualified health care professional per month

90958   with 2-3 face-to-face visits by a physician or other qualified health care professional per month

90959   with 1 face-to-face visit by a physician or other qualified health care professional per month

90960   End-stage renal disease (ESRD) related services monthly, for patients 20 years of age and older; with 4 or more face-to-face visits by a physician or other qualified health care professional per month

90961   with 2-3 face-to-face visits by a physician or other qualified health care professional per month

90962   with 1 face-to-face visit by a physician or other qualified health care professional per month

90963   End-stage renal disease (ESRD) related services for home dialysis per full month, for patients younger than 2 years of age to include monitoring for the adequacy of nutrition, assessment of growth and development, and counseling of parents

90964   End-stage renal disease (ESRD) related services for home dialysis per full month, for patients 2-11 years of age to include monitoring for the adequacy of nutrition, assessment of growth and development, and counseling of parents

90965   End-stage renal disease (ESRD) related services for home dialysis per full month, for patients 12-19 years of age to include monitoring for the adequacy of nutrition, assessment of growth and development, and counseling of parents

90966   End-stage renal disease (ESRD) related services for home dialysis per full month, for patients 20 years of age and older

90967   End-stage renal disease (ESRD) related services for dialysis less than a full month of service, per day; for patients younger than 2 years of age

90968   for patients 2-11 years of age

90969   for patients 12-19 years of age

90970   for patients 20 years of age and older

Other Dialysis Procedures

90989   Dialysis training, patient, including helper where applicable, any mode, completed course

90993   Dialysis training, patient, including helper where applicable, any mode, course not completed, per training session

90997   Hemoperfusion (eg, with activated charcoal or resin)

90999   Unlisted dialysis procedure, inpatient or outpatient

Gastroenterology

(91000 has been deleted)

91010   Esophageal motility (manometric study of the esophagus and/or gastroesophageal junction) study with interpretation and report;

(91011, 91012 have been deleted)

+ 91013   with stimulation or perfusion (eg, stimulant, acid or alkali perfusion) (List separately in addition to code for primary procedure)

(Use 91013 in conjunction with 91010)

(Do not report 91013 more than once per session)

►(To report esophageal motility studies with high resolution esophageal pressure topography, use 91299)◄

91020   Gastric motility (manometric) studies

91022   Duodenal motility (manometric) study

(If gastrointestinal endoscopy is performed, use 43235)

(If fluoroscopy is performed, use 76000)

(If gastric motility study is performed, use 91020)

(Do not report 91020, 91022 in conjunction with 91112)

91030   Esophagus, acid perfusion (Bernstein) test for esophagitis

91034   Esophagus, gastroesophageal reflux test; with nasal catheter pH electrode(s) placement, recording, analysis and interpretation

91035   with mucosal attached telemetry pH electrode placement, recording, analysis and interpretation

91037   Esophageal function test, gastroesophageal reflux test with nasal catheter intraluminal impedance electrode(s) placement, recording, analysis and interpretation;

91038   prolonged (greater than 1 hour, up to 24 hours)

▲ **91040**   Esophageal balloon distension study, diagnostic, with provocation when performed

►(Do not report 91040 more than once per session)◄

91065   Breath hydrogen or methane test (eg, for detection of lactase deficiency, fructose intolerance, bacterial overgrowth, or oro-cecal gastrointestinal transit)

(Report 91065 once for each administered challenge)

(For H. pylori breath test analysis, use 83013 for non-radioactive (C-13) isotope or 78268 for radioactive (C-14) isotope)

(To report placement of an esophageal tamponade tube for management of variceal bleeding, use 43460. To report placement of a long intestinal Miller-Abbott tube, use 44500)

Medicine

(For abdominal paracentesis, see 49082, 49083, 49084; with instillation of medication, see 96440, 96446)

(For peritoneoscopy, use 49320; with biopsy, use 49321)

(For splenoportography, see 38200, 75810)

91110 Gastrointestinal tract imaging, intraluminal (eg, capsule endoscopy), esophagus through ileum, with interpretation and report

(Do not report 91110 in conjunction with 91111, 0355T)

(Visualization of the colon is not reported separately)

(Append modifier 52 if the ileum is not visualized)

91111 Gastrointestinal tract imaging, intraluminal (eg, capsule endoscopy), esophagus with interpretation and report

(Do not report 91111 in conjunction with 91110, 0355T)

(For measurement of gastrointestinal tract transit times or pressure using wireless capsule, use 91112)

91112 Gastrointestinal transit and pressure measurement, stomach through colon, wireless capsule, with interpretation and report

(Do not report 91112 in conjunction with 83986, 91020, 91022, 91117)

91117 Colon motility (manometric) study, minimum 6 hours continuous recording (including provocation tests, eg, meal, intracolonic balloon distension, pharmacologic agents, if performed), with interpretation and report

(For wireless capsule pressure measurements, use 91112)

(Do not report 91117 in conjunction with 91120, 91122)

91120 Rectal sensation, tone, and compliance test (ie, response to graded balloon distention)

(For biofeedback training, use 90911)

(For anorectal manometry, use 91122)

91122 Anorectal manometry

(Do not report 91120, 91122 in conjunction with 91117)

Gastric Physiology

91132 Electrogastrography, diagnostic, transcutaneous;

91133 with provocative testing

Other Procedures

91200 Liver elastography, mechanically induced shear wave (eg, vibration), without imaging, with interpretation and report

91299 Unlisted diagnostic gastroenterology procedure

Ophthalmology

(For surgical procedures, see **Surgery**, Eye and Ocular Adnexa, 65091 et seq)

Definitions

Intermediate ophthalmological services describes an evaluation of a new or existing condition complicated with a new diagnostic or management problem not necessarily relating to the primary diagnosis, including history, general medical observation, external ocular and adnexal examination and other diagnostic procedures as indicated; may include the use of mydriasis for ophthalmoscopy.

For example:

a. Review of history, external examination, ophthalmoscopy, biomicroscopy for an acute complicated condition (eg, iritis) not requiring comprehensive ophthalmological services.

b. Review of interval history, external examination, ophthalmoscopy, biomicroscopy and tonometry in established patient with known cataract not requiring comprehensive ophthalmological services.

Comprehensive ophthalmological services describes a general evaluation of the complete visual system. The comprehensive services constitute a single service entity but need not be performed at one session. The service includes history, general medical observation, external and ophthalmoscopic examinations, gross visual fields and basic sensorimotor examination. It often includes, as indicated: biomicroscopy, examination with cycloplegia or mydriasis and tonometry. It always includes initiation of diagnostic and treatment programs.

Intermediate and comprehensive ophthalmological services constitute integrated services in which medical decision making cannot be separated from the examining techniques used. Itemization of service components, such as slit lamp examination, keratometry, routine ophthalmoscopy, retinoscopy, tonometry, or motor evaluation is not applicable.

For example:

The comprehensive services required for diagnosis and treatment of a patient with symptoms indicating possible disease of the visual system, such as glaucoma, cataract or retinal disease, or to rule out disease of the visual system, new or established patient.

Initiation of diagnostic and treatment program includes the prescription of medication, and arranging for special ophthalmological diagnostic or treatment services, consultations, laboratory procedures and radiological services.

Special ophthalmological services describes services in which a special evaluation of part of the visual system is

Medicine

made, which goes beyond the services included under general ophthalmological services, or in which special treatment is given. Special ophthalmological services may be reported in addition to the general ophthalmological services or evaluation and management services.

For example:

Fluorescein angioscopy, quantitative visual field examination, refraction or extended color vision examination (such as Nagel's anomaloscope) should be separately reported.

Prescription of lenses, when required, is included in 92015. It includes specification of lens type (monofocal, bifocal, other), lens power, axis, prism, absorptive factor, impact resistance, and other factors.

Interpretation and report by the physician or other qualified health care professional is an integral part of special ophthalmological services where indicated. Technical procedures (which may or may not be performed personally) are often part of the service, but should not be mistaken to constitute the service itself.

General Ophthalmological Services

New Patient

(For distinguishing between new and established patients, see **Evaluation and Management** guidelines)

92002   Ophthalmological services: medical examination and evaluation with initiation of diagnostic and treatment program; intermediate, new patient

►(Do not report 92002 in conjunction with 99173, 99174, 99177)◄

92004   comprehensive, new patient, 1 or more visits

►(Do not report 92004 in conjunction with 99173, 99174, 99177)◄

Established Patient

(For distinguishing between new and established patients, see **Evaluation and Management** guidelines)

92012   Ophthalmological services: medical examination and evaluation, with initiation or continuation of diagnostic and treatment program; intermediate, established patient

►(Do not report 92012 in conjunction with 99173, 99174, 99177)◄

92014   comprehensive, established patient, 1 or more visits

►(Do not report 92014 in conjunction with 99173, 99174, 99177)◄

(For surgical procedures, see **Surgery**, Eye and Ocular Adnexa, 65091 et seq)

Special Ophthalmological Services

92015   Determination of refractive state

►(Do not report 92015 in conjunction with 99173, 99174, 99177)◄

►(For instrument-based ocular screening, use 99174, 99177)◄

92018   Ophthalmological examination and evaluation, under general anesthesia, with or without manipulation of globe for passive range of motion or other manipulation to facilitate diagnostic examination; complete

92019   limited

92020   Gonioscopy (separate procedure)

(For gonioscopy under general anesthesia, use 92018)

92025   Computerized corneal topography, unilateral or bilateral, with interpretation and report

(Do not report 92025 in conjunction with 65710-65771)

(92025 is not used for manual keratoscopy, which is part of a single system Evaluation and Management or ophthalmological service)

92060   Sensorimotor examination with multiple measurements of ocular deviation (eg, restrictive or paretic muscle with diplopia) with interpretation and report (separate procedure)

92065   Orthoptic and/or pleoptic training, with continuing medical direction and evaluation

92071   Fitting of contact lens for treatment of ocular surface disease

(Do not report 92071 in conjunction with 92072)

(Report supply of lens separately with 99070 or appropriate supply code)

92072   Fitting of contact lens for management of keratoconus, initial fitting

(For subsequent fittings, report using evaluation and management services or general ophthalmological services)

(Do not report 92072 in conjunction with 92071)

(Report supply of lens separately with 99070 or appropriate supply code)

92081   Visual field examination, unilateral or bilateral, with interpretation and report; limited examination (eg, tangent screen, Autoplot, arc perimeter, or single stimulus level automated test, such as Octopus 3 or 7 equivalent)

92082   intermediate examination (eg, at least 2 isopters on Goldmann perimeter, or semiquantitative, automated suprathreshold screening program, Humphrey suprathreshold automatic diagnostic test, Octopus program 33)

Medicine

92083 extended examination (eg, Goldmann visual fields with at least 3 isopters plotted and static determination within the central 30°, or quantitative, automated threshold perimetry, Octopus program G-1, 32 or 42, Humphrey visual field analyzer full threshold programs 30-2, 24-2, or 30/60-2)

(Gross visual field testing (eg, confrontation testing) is a part of general ophthalmological services and is not reported separately)

(For visual field assessment by patient activitated data transmission to a remote surveillance center, see 0378T, 0379T)

92100 Serial tonometry (separate procedure) with multiple measurements of intraocular pressure over an extended time period with interpretation and report, same day (eg, diurnal curve or medical treatment of acute elevation of intraocular pressure)

(For monitoring of intraocular pressure for 24 hours or longer, use 0329T)

(Ocular blood flow measurements are reported with 0198T. Single-episode tonometry is a component of general ophthalmological service or E/M service)

92132 Scanning computerized ophthalmic diagnostic imaging, anterior segment, with interpretation and report, unilateral or bilateral

(For specular microscopy and endothelial cell analysis, use 92286)

(For tear film imaging, use 0330T)

92133 Scanning computerized ophthalmic diagnostic imaging, posterior segment, with interpretation and report, unilateral or bilateral; optic nerve

92134 retina

(Do not report 92133 and 92134 at the same patient encounter)

(92135 has been deleted)

(For scanning computerized ophthalmic diagnostic imaging of the optic nerve and retina, see 92133, 92134)

92136 Ophthalmic biometry by partial coherence interferometry with intraocular lens power calculation

(For tear film imaging, use 0330T)

92140 Provocative tests for glaucoma, with interpretation and report, without tonography

92145 Corneal hysteresis determination, by air impulse stimulation, unilateral or bilateral, with interpretation and report

Ophthalmoscopy

Routine ophthalmoscopy is part of general and special ophthalmologic services whenever indicated. It is a non-itemized service and is not reported separately.

92225 Ophthalmoscopy, extended, with retinal drawing (eg, for retinal detachment, melanoma), with interpretation and report; initial

92226 subsequent

92227 Remote imaging for detection of retinal disease (eg, retinopathy in a patient with diabetes) with analysis and report under physician supervision, unilateral or bilateral

(Do not report 92227 in conjunction with 92002-92014, 92133, 92134, 92250, 92228 or with the evaluation and management of the single organ system, the eye, 99201-99350)

92228 Remote imaging for monitoring and management of active retinal disease (eg, diabetic retinopathy) with physician review, interpretation and report, unilateral or bilateral

(Do not report 92228 in conjunction with 92002-92014, 92133, 92134, 92250, 92227 or with the evaluation and management of the single organ system, the eye, 99201-99350)

92230 Fluorescein angioscopy with interpretation and report

92235 Fluorescein angiography (includes multiframe imaging) with interpretation and report

92240 Indocyanine-green angiography (includes multiframe imaging) with interpretation and report

92250 Fundus photography with interpretation and report

92260 Ophthalmodynamometry

(For ophthalmoscopy under general anesthesia, use 92018)

Other Specialized Services

For prescription, fitting, and/or medical supervision of ocular prosthetic (artificial eye) adaptation by a physician, see evaluation and management services including office or other outpatient services (99201-99215), office or other outpatient consultations (99241-99245) or general ophthalmological service codes 92002-92014.

92265 Needle oculoelectromyography, 1 or more extraocular muscles, 1 or both eyes, with interpretation and report

92270 Electro-oculography with interpretation and report

▶(For vestibular function tests with recording, see 92537, 92538, 92540, 92541, 92542, 92544, 92545, 92546, 92547, 92548)◄

▶(Do not report 92270 in conjunction with 92537, 92538, 92540, 92541, 92542, 92544, 92545, 92546, 92547, 92548)◄

(To report saccadic eye movement testing with recording, use 92700)

92275 Electroretinography with interpretation and report

(For electronystagmography for vestibular function studies, see 92541 et seq)

⊙=Moderate sedation ✛=Add-on code ✗=FDA approval pending #=Resequenced code ○=Recycled/reinstated code

(For ophthalmic echography (diagnostic ultrasound), see 76511-76529)

92283   Color vision examination, extended, eg, anomaloscope or equivalent

(Color vision testing with pseudoisochromatic plates [such as HRR or Ishihara] is not reported separately. It is included in the appropriate general or ophthalmological service, or 99172)

92284   Dark adaptation examination with interpretation and report

92285   External ocular photography with interpretation and report for documentation of medical progress (eg, close-up photography, slit lamp photography, goniophotography, stereo-photography)

(For tear film imaging, use 0330T)

92286   Anterior segment imaging with interpretation and report; with specular microscopy and endothelial cell analysis

92287   with fluorescein angiography

Contact Lens Services

The prescription of contact lens includes specification of optical and physical characteristics (such as power, size, curvature, flexibility, gas-permeability). It is **not** a part of the general ophthalmological services.

The fitting of contact lens includes instruction and training of the wearer and incidental revision of the lens during the training period.

Follow-up of successfully fitted extended wear lenses is reported as part of a general ophthalmological service (92012 et seq).

The supply of contact lenses may be reported as part of the service of fitting. It may also be reported separately by using the appropriate supply codes.

(For therapeutic or surgical use of contact lens, see 68340, 92071, 92072)

92310   Prescription of optical and physical characteristics of and fitting of contact lens, with medical supervision of adaptation; corneal lens, both eyes, except for aphakia

(For prescription and fitting of 1 eye, add modifier 52)

92311   corneal lens for aphakia, 1 eye

92312   corneal lens for aphakia, both eyes

92313   corneoscleral lens

92314   Prescription of optical and physical characteristics of contact lens, with medical supervision of adaptation and direction of fitting by independent technician; corneal lens, both eyes except for aphakia

(For prescription and fitting of 1 eye, add modifier 52)

92315   corneal lens for aphakia, 1 eye

92316   corneal lens for aphakia, both eyes

92317   corneoscleral lens

92325   Modification of contact lens (separate procedure), with medical supervision of adaptation

92326   Replacement of contact lens

Spectacle Services (Including Prosthesis for Aphakia)

Prescription of lenses, when required, is included in 92015 Determination of refractive state. It includes specification of lens type (monofocal, bifocal, other), lens power, axis, prism, absorptive factor, impact resistance, and other factors.

When provided, fitting of spectacles is a separate service and is reported as indicated by 92340-92371.

Fitting includes measurement of anatomical facial characteristics, the writing of laboratory specifications, and the final adjustment of the spectacles to the visual axes and anatomical topography. Presence of the physician or other qualified health care professional is not required.

Supply of materials is a separate service component; it is not part of the service of fitting spectacles.

92340   Fitting of spectacles, except for aphakia; monofocal

92341   bifocal

92342   multifocal, other than bifocal

92352   Fitting of spectacle prosthesis for aphakia; monofocal

92353   multifocal

92354   Fitting of spectacle mounted low vision aid; single element system

92355   telescopic or other compound lens system

92358   Prosthesis service for aphakia, temporary (disposable or loan, including materials)

92370   Repair and refitting spectacles; except for aphakia

92371   spectacle prosthesis for aphakia

Other Procedures

92499   Unlisted ophthalmological service or procedure

Special Otorhinolaryngologic Services

Diagnostic or treatment procedures that are reported as evaluation and management services (eg, otoscopy, anterior rhinoscopy, tuning fork test, removal of non-impacted cerumen) are not reported separately.

Special otorhinolaryngologic services are those diagnostic and treatment services not included in an evaluation and management service, including office or other outpatient

Medicine

services (99201-99215), or office or other outpatient consultations (99241-99245).

►Codes 92507, 92508, 92520, 92521, 92522, 92523, 92524, and 92526 are used to report evaluation and treatment of speech sound production, receptive language, and expressive language abilities, voice and resonance production, speech fluency, and swallowing. Evaluations may include examination of speech sound production, articulatory movements of oral musculature, oral-pharyngeal swallowing function, qualitative analysis of voice and resonance, and measures of frequency, type, and duration of stuttering. Evaluations may also include the patient's ability to understand the meaning and intent of written and verbal expressions, as well as the appropriate formulation and utterance of expressive thought. In contrast, 92626 and 92627 are reported for an evaluation of auditory rehabilitation status determining the patient's ability to use residual hearing in order to identify the acoustic characteristics of sounds associated with speech communication.◄

(For laryngoscopy with stroboscopy, use 31579)

92502   Otolaryngologic examination under general anesthesia

92504   Binocular microscopy (separate diagnostic procedure)

(92506 has been deleted. To report, see 92521, 92522, 92523, 92524)

92507   Treatment of speech, language, voice, communication, and/or auditory processing disorder; individual

(Do not report 92507 in conjunction with 0364T, 0365T, 0368T, 0369T)

92508   group, 2 or more individuals

(Do not report 92508 in conjunction with 0366T, 0367T, 0372T)

(For auditory rehabilitation, prelingual hearing loss, use 92630)

(For auditory rehabilitation, postlingual hearing loss, use 92633)

(For cochlear implant programming, see 92601-92604)

92511   Nasopharyngoscopy with endoscope (separate procedure)

(Do not report 92511 in conjunction with 43197, 43198)

92512   Nasal function studies (eg, rhinomanometry)

92516   Facial nerve function studies (eg, electroneuronography)

92520   Laryngeal function studies (ie, aerodynamic testing and acoustic testing)

(For performance of a single test, use modifier 52)

(To report flexible fiberoptic laryngeal evaluation of swallowing and laryngeal sensory testing, see 92611-92617)

(To report other testing of laryngeal function (eg, electroglottography), use 92700)

92521   Evaluation of speech fluency (eg, stuttering, cluttering)

92522   Evaluation of speech sound production (eg, articulation, phonological process, apraxia, dysarthria)

92523   with evaluation of language comprehension and expression (eg, receptive and expressive language)

92524   Behavioral and qualitative analysis of voice and resonance

92526   Treatment of swallowing dysfunction and/or oral function for feeding

Vestibular Function Tests, Without Electrical Recording

92531   Spontaneous nystagmus, including gaze

92532   Positional nystagmus test

(Do not report 92531, 92532 with evaluation and management services including office or other outpatient services [99201-99215], observation care [99218-99220, 99224-99226], observation or inpatient care including admission and discharge [99234-99236], hospital care [99221-99223, 99231-99233], office or other outpatient consultations [99241-99245], nursing facility services [99304-99318], and domiciliary, rest home, or custodial care services [99324-99337])

92533   Caloric vestibular test, each irrigation (binaural, bithermal stimulation constitutes 4 tests)

92534   Optokinetic nystagmus test

Vestibular Function Tests, With Recording (eg, ENG)

● **92537**   Caloric vestibular test with recording, bilateral; bithermal (ie, one warm and one cool irrigation in each ear for a total of four irrigations)

►(Do not report 92537 in conjunction with 92270, 92538)◄

►(For three irrigations, use modifier 52)◄

►(For monothermal caloric vestibular testing, use 92538)◄

● **92538**   monothermal (ie, one irrigation in each ear for a total of two irrigations)

►(Do not report 92538 in conjunction with 92270, 92537)◄

►(For one irrigation, use modifier 52)◄

►(For bilateral, bithermal caloric vestibular testing, use 92537)◄

92540   Basic vestibular evaluation, includes spontaneous nystagmus test with eccentric gaze fixation nystagmus, with recording, positional nystagmus test, minimum of 4 positions, with recording, optokinetic nystagmus test, bidirectional foveal and peripheral stimulation, with recording, and oscillating tracking test, with recording

Medicine

(Do not report 92540 in conjunction with 92270, 92541, 92542, 92544, 92545)

92541 Spontaneous nystagmus test, including gaze and fixation nystagmus, with recording

(Do not report 92541 in conjunction with 92270, 92540 or the set of 92542, 92544, and 92545)

92542 Positional nystagmus test, minimum of 4 positions, with recording

(Do not report 92542 in conjunction with 92270, 92540 or the set of 92541, 92544, and 92545)

►(92543 has been deleted. To report caloric vestibular testing, see 92537, 92538)◄

92544 Optokinetic nystagmus test, bidirectional, foveal or peripheral stimulation, with recording

(Do not report 92544 in conjunction with 92270, 92540 or the set of 92541, 92542, and 92545)

92545 Oscillating tracking test, with recording

(Do not report 92545 in conjunction with 92270, 92540 or the set of 92541, 92542, and 92544)

92546 Sinusoidal vertical axis rotational testing

(Do not report 92546 in conjunction with 92270)

+ 92547 Use of vertical electrodes (List separately in addition to code for primary procedure)

(Use 92547 in conjunction with 92540-92546)

(For unlisted vestibular tests, use 92700)

(Do not report 92547 in conjunction with 92270)

92548 Computerized dynamic posturography

(Do not report 92548 in conjunction with 92270)

Audiologic Function Tests

The audiometric tests listed below require the use of calibrated electronic equipment, recording of results and a report with interpretation. Hearing tests (such as whispered voice, tuning fork) that are otorhinolaryngologic Evaluation and Management services are not reported separately. All services include testing of both ears. Use modifier 52 if a test is applied to one ear instead of two ears. All codes (except 92559) apply to testing of individuals. For testing of groups, use 92559 and specify test(s) used.

(For evaluation of speech, language, and/or hearing problems through observation and assessment of performance, see 92521, 92522, 92523, 92524)

92550 Tympanometry and reflex threshold measurements

(Do not report 92550 in conjunction with 92567, 92568)

92551 Screening test, pure tone, air only

92552 Pure tone audiometry (threshold); air only

92553   air and bone

92555 Speech audiometry threshold;

92556   with speech recognition

92557 Comprehensive audiometry threshold evaluation and speech recognition (92553 and 92556 combined)

(For hearing aid evaluation and selection, see 92590-92595)

(For automated audiometry, see 0208T-0212T)

92558 Code is out of numerical sequence. See 92550-92597

92559 Audiometric testing of groups

92560 Bekesy audiometry; screening

92561   diagnostic

92562 Loudness balance test, alternate binaural or monaural

92563 Tone decay test

92564 Short increment sensitivity index (SISI)

92565 Stenger test, pure tone

92567 Tympanometry (impedance testing)

92568 Acoustic reflex testing, threshold

92570 Acoustic immittance testing, includes tympanometry (impedance testing), acoustic reflex threshold testing, and acoustic reflex decay testing

(Do not report 92570 in conjunction with 92567, 92568)

92571 Filtered speech test

92572 Staggered spondaic word test

92575 Sensorineural acuity level test

92576 Synthetic sentence identification test

92577 Stenger test, speech

92579 Visual reinforcement audiometry (VRA)

92582 Conditioning play audiometry

92583 Select picture audiometry

92584 Electrocochleography

92585 Auditory evoked potentials for evoked response audiometry and/or testing of the central nervous system; comprehensive

92586   limited

 # 92558 Evoked otoacoustic emissions, screening (qualitative measurement of distortion product or transient evoked otoacoustic emissions), automated analysis

92587 Distortion product evoked otoacoustic emissions; limited evaluation (to confirm the presence or absence of hearing disorder, 3-6 frequencies) or transient evoked otoacoustic emissions, with interpretation and report

92588   comprehensive diagnostic evaluation (quantitative analysis of outer hair cell function by cochlear mapping, minimum of 12 frequencies), with interpretation and report

(For central auditory function evaluation, see 92620, 92621)

Medicine

92590 Hearing aid examination and selection; monaural

92591   binaural

92592 Hearing aid check; monaural

92593   binaural

92594 Electroacoustic evaluation for hearing aid; monaural

92595   binaural

92596 Ear protector attenuation measurements

92597 Code is out of numerical sequence. See 92601-92633

Evaluative and Therapeutic Services

Codes 92601 and 92603 describe post-operative analysis and fitting of previously placed external devices, connection to the cochlear implant, and programming of the stimulator. Codes 92602 and 92604 describe subsequent sessions for measurements and adjustment of the external transmitter and re-programming of the internal stimulator.

(For placement of cochlear implant, use 69930)

92601 Diagnostic analysis of cochlear implant, patient younger than 7 years of age; with programming

92602   subsequent reprogramming

(Do not report 92602 in addition to 92601)

(For aural rehabilitation services following cochlear implant, including evaluation of rehabilitation status, see 92626-92627, 92630-92633)

92603 Diagnostic analysis of cochlear implant, age 7 years or older; with programming

92604   subsequent reprogramming

(Do not report 92604 in addition to 92603)

 # 92597 Evaluation for use and/or fitting of voice prosthetic device to supplement oral speech

▶(To report augmentative and alternative communication device services, see 92605, 92607, 92608, 92618)◀

92605 Evaluation for prescription of non-speech-generating augmentative and alternative communication device, face-to-face with the patient; first hour

▶(To report evaluation for use and/or fitting of voice prosthetic device, use 92597)◀

#✚ 92618   each additional 30 minutes (List separately in addition to code for primary procedure)

(Use 92618 in conjunction with 92605)

92606 Therapeutic service(s) for the use of non-speech-generating device, including programming and modification

92607 Evaluation for prescription for speech-generating augmentative and alternative communication device, face-to-face with the patient; first hour

▶(To report evaluation for use and/or fitting of voice prosthetic device, use 92597)◀

(For evaluation for prescription of a non-speech-generating device, use 92605)

✚ 92608   each additional 30 minutes (List separately in addition to code for primary procedure)

(Use 92608 in conjunction with 92607)

92609 Therapeutic services for the use of speech-generating device, including programming and modification

(For therapeutic service(s) for the use of a non-speech-generating device, use 92606)

92610 Evaluation of oral and pharyngeal swallowing function

(For motion fluoroscopic evaluation of swallowing function, use 92611)

(For flexible endoscopic examination, use 92612-92617)

92611 Motion fluoroscopic evaluation of swallowing function by cine or video recording

(For radiological supervision and interpretation, use 74230)

(For evaluation of oral and pharyngeal swallowing function, use 92610)

(For flexible fiberoptic diagnostic laryngoscopy, use 31575. Do not report 31575 in conjunction with 92612-92617)

92612 Flexible fiberoptic endoscopic evaluation of swallowing by cine or video recording;

(If flexible fiberoptic or endoscopic evaluation of swallowing is performed without cine or video recording, use 92700)

92613   interpretation and report only

(To report an evaluation of oral and pharyngeal swallowing function, use 92610)

(To report motion fluoroscopic evaluation of swallowing function, use 92611)

92614 Flexible fiberoptic endoscopic evaluation, laryngeal sensory testing by cine or video recording;

(If flexible fiberoptic or endoscopic evaluation of swallowing is performed without cine or video recording, use 92700)

92615   interpretation and report only

92616 Flexible fiberoptic endoscopic evaluation of swallowing and laryngeal sensory testing by cine or video recording;

(If flexible fiberoptic or endoscopic evaluation of swallowing is performed without cine or video recording, use 92700)

92617   interpretation and report only

92618 Code is out of numerical sequence. See 92601-92633

92620 Evaluation of central auditory function, with report; initial 60 minutes

+ 92621 each additional 15 minutes (List separately in addition to code for primary procedure)

(Use 92621 in conjunction with 92620)

(Do not report 92620, 92621 in conjunction with 92521, 92522, 92523, 92524)

92625 Assessment of tinnitus (includes pitch, loudness matching, and masking)

(Do not report 92625 in conjunction with 92562)

(For unilateral assessment, use modifier 52)

92626 Evaluation of auditory rehabilitation status; first hour

+ 92627 each additional 15 minutes (List separately in addition to code for primary procedure)

(Use 92627 in conjunction with 92626)

(When reporting 92626, 92627, use the face-to-face time with the patient or family)

92630 Auditory rehabilitation; prelingual hearing loss

92633 postlingual hearing loss

Special Diagnostic Procedures

92640 Diagnostic analysis with programming of auditory brainstem implant, per hour

(Report nonprogramming services separately [eg, cardiac monitoring])

Other Procedures

92700 Unlisted otorhinolaryngological service or procedure

Cardiovascular

Therapeutic Services and Procedures

92920 Code is out of numerical sequence. See 92998-93000

92921 Code is out of numerical sequence. See 92998-93000

92924 Code is out of numerical sequence. See 92998-93000

92925 Code is out of numerical sequence. See 92998-93000

92928 Code is out of numerical sequence. See 92998-93000

92929 Code is out of numerical sequence. See 92998-93000

92933 Code is out of numerical sequence. See 92998-93000

92934 Code is out of numerical sequence. See 92998-93000

92937 Code is out of numerical sequence. See 92998-93000

92938 Code is out of numerical sequence. See 92998-93000

92941 Code is out of numerical sequence. See 92998-93000

92943 Code is out of numerical sequence. See 92998-93000

92944 Code is out of numerical sequence. See 92998-93000

Other Therapeutic Services and Procedures

92950 Cardiopulmonary resuscitation (eg, in cardiac arrest)

(See also critical care services, 99291, 99292)

⊙ **92953** Temporary transcutaneous pacing

(For direction of ambulance or rescue personnel outside the hospital by a physician or other qualified health care professional, use 99288)

⊙ **92960** Cardioversion, elective, electrical conversion of arrhythmia; external

⊙ **92961** internal (separate procedure)

(Do not report 92961 in conjunction with 93282-93284, 93287, 93289, 93295, 93296, 93618-93624, 93631, 93640-93642, 93650, 93653-93657, 93662)

92970 Cardioassist-method of circulatory assist; internal

92971 external

(For balloon atrial-septostomy, use 92992)

(For placement of catheters for use in circulatory assist devices such as intra-aortic balloon pump, use 33970)

92973 Code is out of numerical sequence. See 92998-93000

92974 Code is out of numerical sequence. See 92998-93000

92975 Code is out of numerical sequence. See 92998-93000

92977 Code is out of numerical sequence. See 92998-93000

92978 Code is out of numerical sequence. See 92998-93000

92979 Code is out of numerical sequence. See 92998-93000

(92980, 92981, 92982, 92984 have been deleted. To report, see 92920-92944)

⊙ **92986** Percutaneous balloon valvuloplasty; aortic valve

⊙ **92987** mitral valve

92990 pulmonary valve

92992 Atrial septectomy or septostomy; transvenous method, balloon (eg, Rashkind type) (includes cardiac catheterization)

92993 blade method (Park septostomy) (includes cardiac catheterization)

(92995, 92996 have been deleted. To report, see 92924, 92925, 92933-92944)

92997 Percutaneous transluminal pulmonary artery balloon angioplasty; single vessel

+ 92998 each additional vessel (List separately in addition to code for primary procedure)

(Use 92998 in conjunction with 92997)

Medicine

Coronary Therapeutic Services and Procedures

Codes 92920-92944 describe percutaneous revascularization services performed for occlusive disease of the coronary vessels (major coronary arteries, coronary artery branches, or coronary artery bypass grafts). These percutaneous coronary intervention (PCI) codes are built on progressive hierarchies with more intensive services inclusive of lesser intensive services. These PCI codes all include the work of accessing and selectively catheterizing the vessel, traversing the lesion, radiological supervision and interpretation directly related to the intervention(s) performed, closure of the arteriotomy when performed through the access sheath, and imaging performed to document completion of the intervention in addition to the intervention(s) performed. These codes include angioplasty (eg, balloon, cutting balloon, wired balloons, cryoplasty), atherectomy (eg, directional, rotational, laser), and stenting (eg, balloon expandable, self-expanding, bare metal, drug eluting, covered). Each code in this family includes balloon angioplasty, when performed. Diagnostic coronary angiography may be reported separately under specific circumstances.

Diagnostic coronary angiography codes (93454-93461) and injection procedure codes (93563-93564) should not be used with percutaneous coronary revascularization services (92920-92944) to report:

1. Contrast injections, angiography, roadmapping, and/or fluoroscopic guidance for the coronary intervention,

2. Vessel measurement for the coronary intervention, **or**

3. Post-coronary angioplasty/stent/atherectomy angiography, as this work is captured in the percutaneous coronary revascularization services codes (92920-92944).

Diagnostic angiography performed at the time of a coronary interventional procedure may be separately reportable if:

1. No prior catheter-based coronary angiography study is available, and a full diagnostic study is performed, and a decision to intervene is based on the diagnostic angiography, **or**

2. A prior study is available, but as documented in the medical record:

   a. The patient's condition with respect to the clinical indication has changed since the prior study, **or**

   b. There is inadequate visualization of the anatomy and/or pathology, **or**

   c. There is a clinical change during the procedure that requires new evaluation outside the target area of intervention.

Diagnostic coronary angiography performed at a separate session from an interventional procedure is separately reportable.

Major coronary arteries: The major coronary arteries are the left main, left anterior descending, left circumflex, right, and ramus intermedius arteries. All PCI procedures performed in all segments (proximal, mid, distal) of a single major coronary artery through the native coronary circulation are reported with one code. When one segment of a major coronary artery is treated through the native circulation and treatment of another segment of the same artery requires access through a coronary artery bypass graft, the intervention through the bypass graft is reported separately.

Coronary artery branches: Up to two coronary artery branches of the left anterior descending (diagonals), left circumflex (marginals), and right (posterior descending, posterolaterals) coronary arteries are recognized. The left main and ramus intermedius coronary arteries do not have recognized branches for reporting purposes. All PCI(s) performed in any segment (proximal, mid, distal) of a coronary artery branch is reported with one code. PCI is reported for up to two branches of a major coronary artery. Additional PCI in a third branch of the same major coronary artery is not separately reportable.

Coronary artery bypass grafts: Each coronary artery bypass graft represents a coronary vessel. A sequential bypass graft with more than one distal anastomosis represents only one graft. A branching bypass graft (eg, Y graft) represents a coronary vessel for the main graft, and each branch off the main graft constitutes an additional coronary vessel. PCI performed on major coronary arteries or coronary artery branches by access through a bypass graft is reported using the bypass graft PCI codes. All bypass graft PCI codes include the use of coronary artery embolic protection devices when performed.

Only one base code from this family may be reported for revascularization of a major coronary artery and its recognized branches. Only one base code should be reported for revascularization of a coronary artery bypass graft, its subtended coronary artery, and recognized branches of the subtended coronary artery. If one segment of a major coronary artery and its recognized branches is treated through the native circulation, and treatment of another segment of the same vessel requires access through a coronary artery bypass graft, an additional base code is reported to describe the intervention performed through the bypass graft. The PCI base codes are 92920, 92924, 92928, 92933, 92937, 92941, and 92943. The PCI base code that includes the most intensive service provided for the target vessel should be reported. The hierarchy of these services is built on an intensity of service ranked from highest to lowest as 92943 = 92941 = 92933 > 92924 > 92937 = 92928 > 92920.

PCI performed during the same session in additional recognized branches of the target vessel should be reported using the applicable add-on code(s). The add-on codes are 92921, 92925, 92928, 92934, 92938, and 92944 and follow the same principle in regard to reporting the most intensive service provided. The intensity of service is ranked from highest to lowest as 92944 = 92938 > 92934 > 92925 > 92929 > 92921.

PCI performed during the same session in additional major coronary or in additional coronary artery bypass grafts should be reported using the applicable additional base code(s). PCI performed during the same session in additional coronary artery branches should be reported using the applicable additional add-on code(s).

If a single lesion extends from one target vessel (major coronary artery, coronary artery bypass graft, or coronary artery branch) into another target vessel, but can be revascularized with a single intervention bridging the two vessels, this PCI should be reported with a single code despite treating more than one vessel. For example, if a left main coronary lesion extends into the proximal left circumflex coronary artery and a single stent is placed to treat the entire lesion, this PCI should be reported as a single vessel stent (92928). In this example, a code for additional vessel treatment (92929) would not be additionally reported.

When bifurcation lesions are treated, PCI is reported for both vessels treated. For example, when a bifurcation lesion involving the left anterior descending artery and the first diagonal artery is treated by stenting both vessels, 92928 and 92929 are both reported.

Target vessel PCI for acute myocardial infarction is inclusive of all balloon angioplasty, atherectomy, stenting, manual aspiration thrombectomy, distal protection, and intracoronary rheolytic agent administration performed. Mechanical thrombectomy is reported separately.

Chronic total occlusion of a coronary vessel is present when there is no antegrade flow through the true lumen, accompanied by suggestive angiographic and clinical criteria (eg, antegrade "bridging" collaterals present, calcification at the occlusion site, no current presentation with ST elevation or Q wave acute myocardial infarction attributable to the occluded target lesion). Current presentation with ST elevation or Q wave acute myocardial infarction attributable to the occluded target lesion, subtotal occlusion, and occlusion with dye staining at the site consistent with fresh thrombus are not considered chronic total occlusion.

Codes 92973 (percutaneous transluminal coronary thrombectomy, mechanical), 92974 (coronary brachytherapy), 92978 and 92979 (intravascular ultrasound), and 93571 and 93572 (intravascular Doppler velocity and/or pressure [fractional flow reserve (FFR) or coronary flow reserve (CFR)]) are add-on codes for reporting procedures performed in addition to coronary and bypass graft diagnostic and interventional services, unless included in the base code. Non-mechanical, aspiration thrombectomy is not reported with 92973, and is included in the PCI code for acute myocardial infarction (92941), when performed.

(To report transcatheter placement of radiation delivery device for coronary intravascular brachytherapy, use 92974)

►(For intravascular radioelement application, see 77770, 77771, 77772)◄

(For nonsurgical septal reduction therapy [eg, alcohol ablation], use 93799)

#⊙ **92920** Percutaneous transluminal coronary angioplasty; single major coronary artery or branch

#⊙+ **92921**   each additional branch of a major coronary artery (List separately in addition to code for primary procedure)

(Use 92921 in conjunction with 92920, 92924, 92928, 92933, 92937, 92941, 92943)

#⊙ **92924** Percutaneous transluminal coronary atherectomy, with coronary angioplasty when performed; single major coronary artery or branch

#⊙+ **92925**   each additional branch of a major coronary artery (List separately in addition to code for primary procedure)

(Use 92925 in conjunction with 92924, 92928, 92933, 92937, 92941, 92943)

#⊙ **92928** Percutaneous transcatheter placement of intracoronary stent(s), with coronary angioplasty when performed; single major coronary artery or branch

#⊙+ **92929**   each additional branch of a major coronary artery (List separately in addition to code for primary procedure)

(Use 92929 in conjunction with 92928, 92933, 92937, 92941, 92943)

#⊙ **92933** Percutaneous transluminal coronary atherectomy, with intracoronary stent, with coronary angioplasty when performed; single major coronary artery or branch

#⊙+ **92934**   each additional branch of a major coronary artery (List separately in addition to code for primary procedure)

(Use 92934 in conjunction with 92933, 92937, 92941, 92943)

#⊙ **92937** Percutaneous transluminal revascularization of or through coronary artery bypass graft (internal mammary, free arterial, venous), any combination of intracoronary stent, atherectomy and angioplasty, including distal protection when performed; single vessel

#⊙+ **92938**   each additional branch subtended by the bypass graft (List separately in addition to code for primary procedure)

(Use 92938 in conjunction with 92937)

Medicine

▲=Revised code   ●=New code   ►◄=Contains new or revised text   ⊘=Modifier 51 exempt

#⊙ **92941**   Percutaneous transluminal revascularization of acute total/subtotal occlusion during acute myocardial infarction, coronary artery or coronary artery bypass graft, any combination of intracoronary stent, atherectomy and angioplasty, including aspiration thrombectomy when performed, single vessel

(For additional vessels treated, see 92920-92938, 92943, 92944)

#⊙ **92943**   Percutaneous transluminal revascularization of chronic total occlusion, coronary artery, coronary artery branch, or coronary artery bypass graft, any combination of intracoronary stent, atherectomy and angioplasty; single vessel

#⊙+ **92944**   each additional coronary artery, coronary artery branch, or bypass graft (List separately in addition to code for primary procedure)

(Use 92944 in conjunction with 92924, 92928, 92933, 92937, 92941, 92943)

(To report transcatheter placement of radiation delivery device for coronary intravascular brachytherapy, use 92974)

▶(For intravascular radioelement application, see 77770, 77771, 77772)◀

#⊙+ **92973**   Percutaneous transluminal coronary thrombectomy mechanical (List separately in addition to code for primary procedure)

(Use 92973 in conjunction with 92920, 92924, 92928, 92933, 92937, 92941, 92943, 92975, 93454-93461, 93563, 93564)

(Do not report 92973 for aspiration thrombectomy)

#⊙+ **92974**   Transcatheter placement of radiation delivery device for subsequent coronary intravascular brachytherapy (List separately in addition to code for primary procedure)

(Use 92974 in conjunction with 92920, 92924, 92928, 92933, 92937, 92941, 92943, 93454-93461)

▶(For intravascular radioelement application, see 77770, 77771, 77772)◀

#⊙ **92975**   Thrombolysis, coronary; by intracoronary infusion, including selective coronary angiography

92977   by intravenous infusion

(For thrombolysis of vessels other than coronary, see 37211-37214)

(For cerebral thrombolysis, use 37195)

#⊙+ **92978**   Intravascular ultrasound (coronary vessel or graft) during diagnostic evaluation and/or therapeutic intervention including imaging supervision, interpretation and report; initial vessel (List separately in addition to code for primary procedure)

(Use 92978 in conjunction with 92975, 92920, 92924, 92928, 92933, 92937, 92941, 92943, 93454-93461, 93563, 93564)

#⊙+ **92979**   each additional vessel (List separately in addition to code for primary procedure)

(Use 92979 in conjunction with 92978)

(Intravascular ultrasound services include all transducer manipulations and repositioning within the specific vessel being examined, both before and after therapeutic intervention [eg, stent placement])

(For intravascular spectroscopy, use 0205T)

(For intravascular optical coherence tomography, see 0291T, 0292T)

Cardiography

Codes 93040-93042 are appropriate when an order for the test is triggered by an event, the rhythm strip is used to help diagnose the presence or absence of an arrhythmia, and a report is generated. There must be a specific order for an electrocardiogram or rhythm strip followed by a separate, signed, written, and retrievable report. It is not appropriate to use these codes for reviewing the telemetry monitor strips taken from a monitoring system. The need for an electrocardiogram or rhythm strip should be supported by documentation in the patient medical record.

(For echocardiography, see 93303-93350)

(For electrocardiogram, 64 leads or greater, with graphic presentation and analysis, see 0178T-0180T)

▶(For acoustic cardiography services, use 93799)◀

93000   Electrocardiogram, routine ECG with at least 12 leads; with interpretation and report

93005   tracing only, without interpretation and report

93010   interpretation and report only

(For ECG monitoring, see 99354-99360)

93015   Cardiovascular stress test using maximal or submaximal treadmill or bicycle exercise, continuous electrocardiographic monitoring, and/or pharmacological stress; with supervision, interpretation and report

93016   supervision only, without interpretation and report

93017   tracing only, without interpretation and report

93018   interpretation and report only

93024   Ergonovine provocation test

93025   Microvolt T-wave alternans for assessment of ventricular arrhythmias

93040   Rhythm ECG, 1-3 leads; with interpretation and report

93041   tracing only without interpretation and report

93042   interpretation and report only

● **93050**   Arterial pressure waveform analysis for assessment of central arterial pressures, includes obtaining waveform(s), digitization and application of nonlinear mathematical transformations to determine central arterial pressures and augmentation index, with interpretation and report, upper extremity artery, non-invasive

▶(Do not report 93050 in conjunction with diagnostic or interventional intra-arterial procedures)◀

Cardiovascular Monitoring Services

Cardiovascular monitoring services are diagnostic medical procedures using in-person and remote technology to assess cardiovascular rhythm (ECG) data. Holter monitors (93224-93227) include up to 48 hours of continuous recording. Mobile cardiac telemetry monitors (93228, 93229) have the capability of transmitting a tracing at any time, always have internal ECG analysis algorithms designed to detect major arrhythmias, and transmit to an attended surveillance center. Event monitors (93268-93272) record segments of ECGs with recording initiation triggered either by patient activation or by an internal automatic, pre-programmed detection algorithm (or both) and transmit the recorded electrocardiographic data when requested (but cannot transmit immediately based upon the patient or algorithmic activation rhythm) and require attended surveillance.

Attended surveillance: is the immediate availability of a remote technician to respond to rhythm or device alert transmissions from a patient, either from an implanted or wearable monitoring or therapy device, as they are generated and transmitted to the remote surveillance location or center.

Electrocardiographic rhythm derived elements: elements derived from recordings of the electrical activation of the heart including, but not limited to heart rhythm, rate, ST analysis, heart rate variability, T-wave alternans.

Mobile cardiovascular telemetry (MCT): continuously records the electrocardiographic rhythm from external electrodes placed on the patient's body. Segments of the ECG data are automatically (without patient intervention) transmitted to a remote surveillance location by cellular or landline telephone signal. The segments of the rhythm, selected for transmission, are triggered automatically (MCT device algorithm) by rapid and slow heart rates or by the patient during a symptomatic episode. There is continuous real time data analysis by preprogrammed algorithms in the device and attended surveillance of the transmitted rhythm segments by a surveillance center technician to evaluate any arrhythmias and to determine signal quality. The surveillance center technician reviews the data and

notifies the physician or other qualified health care professional depending on the prescribed criteria.

ECG rhythm derived elements are distinct from physiologic data, even when the same device is capable of producing both. Implantable cardiovascular monitor (ICM) device services are always separately reported from implantable cardioverter-defibrillator (ICD) service.

93224   External electrocardiographic recording up to 48 hours by continuous rhythm recording and storage; includes recording, scanning analysis with report, review and interpretation by a physician or other qualified health care professional

93225   recording (includes connection, recording, and disconnection)

93226   scanning analysis with report

93227   review and interpretation by a physician or other qualified health care professional

(For less than 12 hours of continuous recording, use modifier 52)

(For greater than 48 hours of monitoring, see Category III codes 0295T-0298T)

93228   External mobile cardiovascular telemetry with electrocardiographic recording, concurrent computerized real time data analysis and greater than 24 hours of accessible ECG data storage (retrievable with query) with ECG triggered and patient selected events transmitted to a remote attended surveillance center for up to 30 days; review and interpretation with report by a physician or other qualified health care professional

(Report 93228 only once per 30 days)

(Do not report 93228 in conjunction with 93224, 93227)

93229   technical support for connection and patient instructions for use, attended surveillance, analysis and transmission of daily and emergent data reports as prescribed by a physician or other qualified health care professional

(Report 93229 only once per 30 days)

(Do not report 93229 in conjunction with 93224, 93226)

(For external cardiovascular monitors that do not perform automatic ECG triggered transmissions to an attended surveillance center, see 93224-93227, 93268-93272)

93260   Code is out of numerical sequence. See 93279-93299

93261   Code is out of numerical sequence. See 93279-93299

93268   External patient and, when performed, auto activated electrocardiographic rhythm derived event recording with symptom-related memory loop with remote download capability up to 30 days, 24-hour attended monitoring; includes transmission, review and interpretation by a physician or other qualified health care professional

93270   recording (includes connection, recording, and disconnection)

Medicine

93271   transmission and analysis

93272   review and interpretation by a physician or other qualified health care professional

(For implanted patient activated cardiac event recording, see 33282, 93285, 93291, 93298)

93278   Signal-averaged electrocardiography (SAECG), with or without ECG

(For interpretation and report only, use 93278 with modifier 26)

(For unlisted cardiographic procedure, use 93799)

Implantable and Wearable Cardiac Device Evaluations

Cardiac device evaluation services are diagnostic medical procedures using in-person and remote technology to assess device therapy and cardiovascular physiologic data. Codes 93260, 93261, 93279-93299 describe this technology and technical/professional and service center practice. Codes 93260, 93261, 93279-93292 are reported per procedure. Codes 93293, 93294, 93295, 93296 are reported no more than **once** every 90 days. Do not report 93293, 93294, 93295, 93296, if the monitoring period is less than 30 days. Codes 93297, 93298 are reported no more than **once** up to every 30 days. Do not report 93297-93299, if the monitoring period is less than 10 days.

A service center may report 93296 or 93299 during a period in which a physician or other qualified health care professional performs an in-person interrogation device evaluation. The same individual may not report an in-person and remote interrogation of the same device during the same period. Report only remote services when an in-person interrogation device evaluation is performed during a period of remote interrogation device evaluation. A period is established by the initiation of the remote monitoring or the 91st day of a pacemaker or implantable defibrillator monitoring or the 31st day of an implantable loop recorder (ILR) or implantable cardiovascular monitor (ICM) monitoring, and extends for the subsequent 90 or 30 days respectively, for which remote monitoring is occurring. Programming device evaluations and in-person interrogation device evaluations may not be reported on the same date by the same individual. Programming device evaluations and remote interrogation device evaluations may both be reported during the remote interrogation device evaluation period.

For monitoring by wearable devices, see 93224-93272.

ECG rhythm derived elements are distinct from physiologic data, even when the same device is capable of producing both. ICM device services are always separately reported from implantable defibrillator services. When ILR data is derived from an implantable defibrillator or pacemaker, do not report ILR services with pacemaker or implantable defibrillator services.

Do not report 93268-93272 when performing 93260, 93261, 93279-93289, 93291-93296, or 93298-93299. Do not report 93040, 93041, 93042 when performing 93260, 93261, 93279-93289, 93291-93296, or 93298-93299.

The pacemaker and implantable defibrillator interrogation device evaluations, peri-procedural device evaluations and programming, and programming device evaluations may not be reported in conjunction with pacemaker or implantable defibrillator device and/or lead insertion or revision services by the same individual.

The following definitions and instructions apply to codes 93260, 93261, 93279-93299.

Attended surveillance: the immediate availability of a remote technician to respond to rhythm or device alert transmissions from a patient, either from an implanted or wearable monitoring or therapy device, as they are generated and transmitted to the remote surveillance location or center.

Device, single lead: a pacemaker or implantable defibrillator with pacing and sensing function in only one chamber of the heart or a subcutaneous electrode.

Device, dual lead: a pacemaker or implantable defibrillator with pacing and sensing function in only two chambers of the heart.

Device, multiple lead: a pacemaker or implantable defibrillator with pacing and sensing function in three or more chambers of the heart.

Electrocardiographic rhythm derived elements: elements derived from recordings of the electrical activation of the heart including, but not limited to heart rhythm, rate, ST analysis, heart rate variability, T-wave alternans.

Implantable cardiovascular monitor (ICM): an implantable cardiovascular device used to assist the physician in the management of non-rhythm related cardiac conditions such as heart failure. The device collects longitudinal physiologic cardiovascular data elements from one or more internal sensors (such as right ventricular pressure, left atrial pressure, or an index of lung water) and/or external sensors (such as blood pressure or body weight) for patient assessment and management. The data are stored and transmitted by either local telemetry or remotely to an Internet-based file server or surveillance technician. The function of the ICM may be an additional function of an implantable cardiac device (eg, implantable defibrillator) or a function of a stand-alone device. When ICM functionality is included in an implantable defibrillator device or pacemaker, the ICM data and the implantable defibrillator or pacemaker, heart rhythm data such as sensing, pacing, and tachycardia detection therapy are distinct and, therefore, the monitoring processes are distinct.

Implantable defibrillator: two general categories of implantable defibrillators exist: transvenous implantable pacing cardioverter-defibrillator (ICD) and subcutaneous implantable defibrillator (SICD). An implantable pacing cardioverter-defibrillator device provides high-energy and low-energy stimulation to one or more chambers of the heart to terminate rapid heart rhythms called tachycardia or fibrillation. Implantable pacing cardioverter-defibrillators also have pacemaker functions to treat slow heart rhythms called bradycardia. In addition to the tachycardia and bradycardia functions, the implantable pacing cardioverter-defibrillator may or may not include the functionality of an implantable cardiovascular monitor or an implantable loop recorder. The subcutaneous implantable defibrillator uses a single subcutaneous electrode to treat ventricular tachyarrhythmias. Subcutaneous implantable defibrillators differ from transvenous implantable pacing cardioverter-defibrillators in that subcutaneous implantable defibrillators do not provide antitachycardia pacing or chronic pacing. For subcutaneous implantable defibrillator device evaluation, see 93260, 93261.

Implantable loop recorder (ILR): an implantable device that continuously records the electrocardiographic rhythm triggered automatically by rapid and slow heart rates or by the patient during a symptomatic episode. The ILR function may be the only function of the device or it may be part of a pacemaker or implantable defibrillator device. The data are stored and transmitted by either local telemetry or remotely to an Internet-based file server or surveillance technician. Extraction of data and compilation or report for physician or qualified health care professional interpretation is usually performed in the office setting.

Interrogation device evaluation: an evaluation of an implantable device such as a cardiac pacemaker, implantable defibrillator, implantable cardiovascular monitor, or implantable loop recorder. Using an office, hospital, or emergency room instrument or via a remote interrogation system, stored and measured information about the lead(s) when present, sensor(s) when present, battery and the implanted device function, as well as data collected about the patient's heart rhythm and heart rate is retrieved. The retrieved information is evaluated to determine the current programming of the device and to evaluate certain aspects of the device function such as battery voltage, lead impedance, tachycardia detection settings, and rhythm treatment settings.

The components that must be evaluated for the various types of implantable cardiac devices are listed below. (The required components for both remote and in-person interrogations are the same.)

   Pacemaker: Programmed parameters, lead(s), battery, capture and sensing function and heart rhythm.

   Implantable defibrillator: programmed parameters, lead(s), battery, capture and sensing function, presence or absence of therapy for ventricular tachyarrhythmias and underlying heart rhythm.

   Implantable cardiovascular monitor: Programmed parameters and analysis of at least one recorded physiologic cardiovascular data element from either internal or external sensors.

   Implantable loop recorder: Programmed parameters and the heart rate and rhythm during recorded episodes from both patient initiated and device algorithm detected events, when present.

Interrogation device evaluation (remote): a procedure performed for patients with pacemakers, implantable defibrillators, or implantable loop recorders using data obtained remotely. All device functions, including the programmed parameters, lead(s), battery, capture and sensing function, presence or absence of therapy for ventricular tachyarrhythmias (for implantable defibrillators) and underlying heart rhythm are evaluated.

The components that must be evaluated for the various types of implantable cardiac devices are listed below. (The required components for both remote and in person interrogations are the same.)

   Pacemaker: Programmed parameters, lead(s), battery, capture and sensing function, and heart rhythm.

   Implantable defibrillator: Programmed parameters, lead(s), battery, capture and sensing function, presence or absence of therapy for ventricular tachyarrhythmias, and underlying heart rhythm.

   Implantable cardiovascular monitor: Programmed parameters and analysis of at least one recorded physiologic cardiovascular data element from either internal or external sensors.

   Implantable loop recorder: Programmed parameters and the heart rate and rhythm during recorded episodes from both patient-initiated and device algorithm detected events, when present.

Pacemaker: an implantable device that provides low energy localized stimulation to one or more chambers of the heart to initiate contraction in that chamber.

Peri-procedural device evaluation and programming: an evaluation of an implantable device system (either a pacemaker or implantable defibrillator) to adjust the device to settings appropriate for the patient prior to a surgery, procedure, or test. The device system data are interrogated to evaluate the lead(s), sensor(s), and battery in addition to review of stored information, including patient and system measurements. The device is programmed to settings appropriate for the surgery, procedure, or test, as required. A second evaluation and programming are performed after the surgery, procedure, or test to provide settings appropriate to the post procedural situation, as required. If one performs both the pre- and post-evaluation and programming service, the appropriate code, either 93286 or 93287, would be reported two times. If one performs the pre-surgical

Medicine

service and a separate individual performs the post-surgical service, each reports either 93286 or 93287 only one time.

Physiologic cardiovascular data elements: data elements from one or more internal sensors (such as right ventricular pressure, left atrial pressure or an index of lung water) and/or external sensors (such as blood pressure or body weight) for patient assessement and management. It does not include ECG rhythm derived data elements.

Programming device evaluation (in person): a procedure performed for patients with a pacemaker, implantable defibrillator, or implantable loop recorder. All device functions, including the battery, programmable settings and lead(s), when present, are evaluated. To assess capture thresholds, iterative adjustments (eg, progressive changes in pacing output of a pacing lead) of the programmable parameters are conducted. The iterative adjustments provide information that permits the operator to assess and select the most appropriate final program parameters to provide for consistent delivery of the appropriate therapy and to verify the function of the device. The final program parameters may or may not change after evaluation.

The programming device evaluation includes all of the components of the interrogation device evaluation (remote) or the interrogation device evaluation (in person), and it includes the selection of patient specific programmed parameters depending on the type of device.

The components that must be evaluated for the various types of programming device evaluations are listed below. (See also required interrogation device evaluation [remote and in person] components above.)

Pacemaker: Programmed parameters, lead(s), battery, capture and sensing function, and heart rhythm. Often, but not always, the sensor rate response, lower and upper heart rates, AV intervals, pacing voltage and pulse duration, sensing value, and diagnostics will be adjusted during a programming evaluation.

Implantable defibrillator: Programmed parameters, lead(s), battery, capture and sensing function, presence or absence of therapy for ventricular tachyarrhythmias and underlying heart rhythm. Often, but not always, the sensor rate response, lower and upper heart rates, AV intervals, pacing voltage and pulse duration, sensing value, and diagnostics will be adjusted during a programming evaluation. In addition, ventricular tachycardia detection and therapies are sometimes altered depending on the interrogated data, patient's rhythm, symptoms, and condition.

Implantable loop recorder: Programmed parameters and the heart rhythm during recorded episodes from both patient initiated and device algorithm detected events. Often, but not always, the tachycardia and bradycardia detection criteria will be adjusted during a programming evaluation.

Transtelephonic rhythm strip pacemaker evaluation: service of transmission of an electrocardiographic rhythm strip over the telephone by the patient using a transmitter and recorded by a receiving location using a receiver/recorder (also commonly known as transtelephonic pacemaker monitoring). The electrocardiographic rhythm strip is recorded both with and without a magnet applied over the pacemaker. The rhythm strip is evaluated for heart rate and rhythm, atrial and ventricular capture (if observed) and atrial and ventricular sensing (if observed). In addition, the battery status of the pacemaker is determined by measurement of the paced rate on the electrocardiographic rhythm strip recorded with the magnet applied.

93279   Programming device evaluation (in person) with iterative adjustment of the implantable device to test the function of the device and select optimal permanent programmed values with analysis, review and report by a physician or other qualified health care professional; single lead pacemaker system

(Do not report 93279 in conjunction with 93286, 93288)

93280   dual lead pacemaker system

(Do not report 93280 in conjunction with 93286, 93288)

93281   multiple lead pacemaker system

(Do not report 93281 in conjunction with 93286, 93288)

93282   single lead transvenous implantable defibrillator system

(Do not report 93282 in conjunction with 93260, 93287, 93289, 93745)

93283   dual lead transvenous implantable defibrillator system

(Do not report 93283 in conjunction with 93287, 93289)

93284   multiple lead transvenous implantable defibrillator system

(Do not report 93284 in conjunction with 93287, 93289)

 # 93260   implantable subcutaneous lead defibrillator system

(Do not report 93260 in conjunction with 93261, 93282, 93287)

(Do not report 93260 in conjunction with pulse generator and lead insertion or repositioning codes 33240, 33241, 33262, 33270, 33271, 33272, 33273)

93285   implantable loop recorder system

(Do not report 93285 in conjunction with 33282, 93279-93284, 93291)

93286   Peri-procedural device evaluation (in person) and programming of device system parameters before or after a surgery, procedure, or test with analysis, review and report by a physician or other qualified health care professional; single, dual, or multiple lead pacemaker system

(Report 93286 once before and once after surgery, procedure, or test, when device evaluation and programming is performed before and after surgery, procedure, or test)

(Do not report 93286 in conjunction with 93279-93281, 93288)

93287   single, dual, or multiple lead implantable defibrillator system

(Report 93287 once before and once after surgery, procedure, or test, when device evaluation and programming is performed before and after surgery, procedure, or test)

(Do not report 93287 in conjunction with 93260, 93261, 93282, 93283, 93284, 93289)

93288   Interrogation device evaluation (in person) with analysis, review and report by a physician or other qualified health care professional, includes connection, recording and disconnection per patient encounter; single, dual, or multiple lead pacemaker system

(Do not report 93288 in conjunction with 93279-93281, 93286, 93294, 93296)

93289   single, dual, or multiple lead transvenous implantable defibrillator system, including analysis of heart rhythm derived data elements

(For monitoring physiologic cardiovascular data elements derived from an implantable defibrillator, use 93290)

(Do not report 93289 in conjunction with 93261, 93282, 93283, 93284, 93287, 93295, 93296)

 # 93261   implantable subcutaneous lead defibrillator system

(Do not report 93261 in conjunction with 93260, 93287, 93289)

(Do not report 93261 in conjunction with pulse generator and lead insertion or repositioning codes 33240, 33241, 33262, 33270, 33271, 33272, 33273)

93290   implantable cardiovascular monitor system, including analysis of 1 or more recorded physiologic cardiovascular data elements from all internal and external sensors

(For heart rhythm derived data elements, use 93289)

(Do not report 93290 in conjunction with 93297, 93299)

93291   implantable loop recorder system, including heart rhythm derived data analysis

(Do not report 93291 in conjunction with 33282, 93288-93290, 93298, 93299)

93292   wearable defibrillator system

(Do not report 93292 in conjunction with 93745)

93293   Transtelephonic rhythm strip pacemaker evaluation(s) single, dual, or multiple lead pacemaker system, includes recording with and without magnet application with analysis, review and report(s) by a physician or other qualified health care professional, up to 90 days

(Do not report 93293 in conjunction with 93294)

(For in person evaluation, see 93040, 93041, 93042)

(Report 93293 only once per 90 days)

93294   Interrogation device evaluation(s) (remote), up to 90 days; single, dual, or multiple lead pacemaker system with interim analysis, review(s) and report(s) by a physician or other qualified health care professional

(Do not report 93294 in conjunction with 93288, 93293)

(Report 93294 only once per 90 days)

93295   single, dual, or multiple lead implantable defibrillator system with interim analysis, review(s) and report(s) by a physician or other qualified health care professional

(For remote monitoring of physiologic cardiovascular data elements derived from an ICD, use 93297)

(Do not report 93295 in conjunction with 93289)

(Report 93295 only once per 90 days)

93296   single, dual, or multiple lead pacemaker system or implantable defibrillator system, remote data acquisition(s), receipt of transmissions and technician review, technical support and distribution of results

(Do not report 93296 in conjunction with 93288, 93289, 93299)

(Report 93296 only once per 90 days)

93297   Interrogation device evaluation(s), (remote) up to 30 days; implantable cardiovascular monitor system, including analysis of 1 or more recorded physiologic cardiovascular data elements from all internal and external sensors, analysis, review(s) and report(s) by a physician or other qualified health care professional

(For heart rhythm derived data elements, use 93295)

(Do not report 93297 in conjunction with 93290, 93298)

(Report 93297 only once per 30 days)

93298   implantable loop recorder system, including analysis of recorded heart rhythm data, analysis, review(s) and report(s) by a physician or other qualified health care professional

(Do not report 93298 in conjunction with 33282, 93291, 93297)

(Report 93298 only once per 30 days)

93299   implantable cardiovascular monitor system or implantable loop recorder system, remote data acquisition(s), receipt of transmissions and technician review, technical support and distribution of results

(Do not report 93299 in conjunction with 93290, 93291, 93296)

(Report 93299 only once per 30 days)

Medicine

Echocardiography

Echocardiography includes obtaining ultrasonic signals from the heart and great vessels, with real time image and/or Doppler ultrasonic signal documentation, with interpretation and report. When interpretation is performed separately, use modifier 26.

A complete transthoracic echocardiogram without spectral or color flow Doppler (93307) is a comprehensive procedure that includes 2-dimensional and, when performed, selected M-mode examination of the left and right atria, left and right ventricles, the aortic, mitral, and tricuspid valves, the pericardium, and adjacent portions of the aorta. Multiple views are required to obtain a complete functional and anatomic evaluation, and appropriate measurements are obtained and recorded. Despite significant effort, identification and measurement of some structures may not always be possible. In such instances, the reason that an element could not be visualized must be documented. Additional structures that may be visualized (eg, pulmonary veins, pulmonary artery, pulmonic valve, inferior vena cava) would be included as part of the service.

A complete transthoracic echocardiogram with spectral and color flow Doppler (93306) is a comprehensive procedure that includes spectral Doppler and color flow Doppler in addition to the 2-dimensional and selected M-mode examinations, when performed. Spectral Doppler (93320, 93321) and color flow Doppler (93325) provide information regarding intracardiac blood flow and hemodynamics.

A follow-up or limited echocardiographic study (93308) is an examination that does not evaluate or document the attempt to evaluate all the structures that comprise the complete echocardiographic exam. This is typically limited to, or performed in follow-up of a focused clinical concern.

In stress echocardiography, echocardiographic images are recorded from multiple cardiac windows before, after, and in some protocols, during stress. The stress is achieved by (1) walking on a treadmill; (2) using a bicycle (supine or upright); or (3) the administration of pharmacological agents that either simulate exercise (by increasing heart rate, blood pressure, or myocardial contractility) or alter coronary flow (vasodilation). The patient's ECG, heart rate, and blood pressure are monitored at baseline, throughout the procedure and during recovery. Reports are prepared to evaluate (1) the duration of stress, the reason for stopping, and the hemodynamic response to stress; (2) the electrocardiographic response to stress; and (3) the echocardiographic response to stress.

When a stress echocardiogram is performed with a complete cardiovascular stress test (continuous electrocardiographic monitoring, supervision, interpretation and report by a physician or other qualified health care professional), use 93351. When only the professional components of a complete stress test and a stress echocardiogram are provided (eg, in a facility setting) by the same physician, use 93351 with modifier 26. When all professional services of a stress test are not performed by the same physician performing the stress echocardiogram, use 93350 in conjunction with the appropriate codes (93016-93018) for the components of the cardiovascular stress test that are provided.

When left ventricular endocardial borders cannot be adequately identified by standard echocardiographic imaging, echocardiographic contrast may be infused intravenously both at rest and with stress to achieve that purpose. Code 93352 is used to report the administration of echocardiographic contrast agent in conjunction with the stress echocardiography codes (93350 or 93351). Supply of contrast agent and/or drugs used for pharmacological stress is reported separately in addition to the procedure code.

Code 93355 is used to report transesophageal echocardiography (TEE) services during transcatheter intracardiac therapies. Code 93355 is reported once per intervention and only by an individual who is not performing the interventional procedure. Code 93355 includes the work of passing the endoscopic ultrasound transducer through the mouth into the esophagus, when performed by the individual performing the TEE, diagnostic transesophageal echocardiography and ongoing manipulation of the transducer to guide sizing and/or placement of implants, determination of adequacy of the intervention, and assessment for potential complications. Real-time image acquisition, measurements, and interpretation of image(s), documentation of completion of the intervention, and final written report are included in this code.

A range of intracardiac therapies may be performed with TEE guidance. Code 93355 describes TEE during advanced transcatheter structural heart procedures (eg, transcatheter aortic valve replacement [TAVR], left atrial appendage closure [LAA], or percutaneous mitral valve repair).

See 93313 for separate reporting of the probe insertion by a physician other than the physician performing the TEE.

Report of an echocardiographic study, whether complete or limited, includes an interpretation of all obtained information, documentation of all clinically relevant findings including quantitative measurements obtained, plus a description of any recognized abnormalities. Pertinent images, videotape, and/or digital data are archived for permanent storage and are available for subsequent review. Use of echocardiography not meeting these criteria is not separately reportable.

Use of ultrasound, without thorough evaluation of organ(s) or anatomic region, image documentation and final, written report, is not separately reportable.

(For fetal echocardiography, see 76825-76828)

93303   Transthoracic echocardiography for congenital cardiac anomalies; complete

93304   follow-up or limited study

93306   Echocardiography, transthoracic, real-time with image documentation (2D), includes M-mode recording, when performed, complete, with spectral Doppler echocardiography, and with color flow Doppler echocardiography

(For transthoracic echocardiography without spectral and color Doppler, use 93307)

93307   Echocardiography, transthoracic, real-time with image documentation (2D), includes M-mode recording, when performed, complete, without spectral or color Doppler echocardiography

(Do not report 93307 in conjunction with 93320, 93321, 93325)

93308   Echocardiography, transthoracic, real-time with image documentation (2D), includes M-mode recording, when performed, follow-up or limited study

⊙ **93312**   Echocardiography, transesophageal, real-time with image documentation (2D) (with or without M-mode recording); including probe placement, image acquisition, interpretation and report

(Do not report 93312 in conjunction with 93355)

⊙ **93313**   placement of transesophageal probe only

(The same individual may not report 93313 in conjunction with 93355)

⊙ **93314**   image acquisition, interpretation and report only

(Do not report 93314 in conjunction with 93355)

⊙ **93315**   Transesophageal echocardiography for congenital cardiac anomalies; including probe placement, image acquisition, interpretation and report

(Do not report 93315 in conjunction with 93355)

⊙ **93316**   placement of transesophageal probe only

(Do not report 93316 in conjunction with 93355)

⊙ **93317**   image acquisition, interpretation and report only

(Do not report 93317 in conjunction with 93355)

⊙ **93318**   Echocardiography, transesophageal (TEE) for monitoring purposes, including probe placement, real time 2-dimensional image acquisition and interpretation leading to ongoing (continuous) assessment of (dynamically changing) cardiac pumping function and to therapeutic measures on an immediate time basis

(Do not report 93318 in conjunction with 93355)

+ **93320**   Doppler echocardiography, pulsed wave and/or continuous wave with spectral display (List separately in addition to codes for echocardiographic imaging); complete

(Use 93320 in conjunction with 93303, 93304, 93312, 93314, 93315, 93317, 93350, 93351)

(Do not report 93320 in conjunction with 93355)

+ **93321**   follow-up or limited study (List separately in addition to codes for echocardiographic imaging)

(Use 93321 in conjunction with 93303, 93304, 93308, 93312, 93314, 93315, 93317, 93350, 93351)

(Do not report 93321 in conjunction with 93355)

+ **93325**   Doppler echocardiography color flow velocity mapping (List separately in addition to codes for echocardiography)

(Use 93325 in conjunction with 76825, 76826, 76827, 76828, 93303, 93304, 93308, 93312, 93314, 93315, 93317, 93350, 93351)

(Do not report 93325 in conjunction with 93355)

93350   Echocardiography, transthoracic, real-time with image documentation (2D), includes M-mode recording, when performed, during rest and cardiovascular stress test using treadmill, bicycle exercise and/or pharmacologically induced stress, with interpretation and report;

(Stress testing codes 93016-93018 should be reported, when appropriate, in conjunction with 93350 to capture the cardiovascular stress portion of the study)

(Do not report 93350 in conjunction with 93015)

93351   including performance of continuous electrocardiographic monitoring, with supervision by a physician or other qualified health care professional

(Do not report 93351 in conjunction with 93015-93018, 93350. Do not report 93351-26 in conjunction with 93016, 93018, 93350-26)

+ **93352**   Use of echocardiographic contrast agent during stress echocardiography (List separately in addition to code for primary procedure)

(Do not report 93352 more than once per stress echocardiogram)

(Use 93352 in conjunction with 93350, 93351)

93355   Echocardiography, transesophageal (TEE) for guidance of a transcatheter intracardiac or great vessel(s) structural intervention(s) (eg, TAVR, transcathether pulmonary valve replacement, mitral valve repair, paravalvular regurgitation repair, left atrial appendage occlusion/closure, ventricular septal defect closure) (peri-and intra-procedural), real-time image acquisition and documentation, guidance with quantitative measurements, probe manipulation, interpretation, and report, including diagnostic transesophageal echocardiography and, when performed, administration of ultrasound contrast, Doppler, color flow, and 3D

(To report placement of transesophageal probe by separate physician, use 93313)

(Do not report 93355 in conjunction with 76376, 76377, 93312, 93313, 93314, 93315, 93316, 93317, 93318, 93320, 93321, 93325)

Medicine

Cardiac Catheterization

Cardiac catheterization is a diagnostic medical procedure which includes introduction, positioning and repositioning, when necessary, of catheter(s), within the vascular system, recording of intracardiac and/or intravascular pressure(s), and final evaluation and report of procedure. There are two code families for cardiac catheterization: one for congenital heart disease and one for all other conditions. Anomalous coronary arteries, patent foramen ovale, mitral valve prolapse, and bicuspid aortic valve are to be reported with 93451-93464, 93566-93568.

Right heart catheterization includes catheter placement in one or more right-sided cardiac chamber(s) or structures (ie, the right atrium, right ventricle, pulmonary artery, pulmonary wedge), obtaining blood samples for measurement of blood gases, and cardiac output measurements (Fick or other method), when performed. Left heart catheterization involves catheter placement in a left-sided (systemic) cardiac chamber(s) (left ventricle or left atrium) and includes left ventricular injection(s) when performed. Do not report 93503 in conjunction with other diagnostic cardiac catheterization codes. When right heart catheterization is performed in conjunction with other cardiac catheterization services, report 93453, 93456, 93457, 93460, or 93461. For placement of a flow directed catheter (eg, Swan-Ganz) performed for hemodynamic monitoring purposes not in conjunction with other catheterization services, use 93503. Right heart catheterization does not include right ventricular or right atrial angiography (93566). When left heart catheterization is performed using either transapical puncture of the left ventricle or transseptal puncture of an intact septum, report 93462 in conjunction with 93452, 93453, 93458-93461, 93653, 93654. Catheter placement(s) in coronary artery(ies) involves selective engagement of the origins of the native coronary artery(ies) for the purpose of coronary angiography. Catheter placement(s) in bypass graft(s) (venous, internal mammary, free arterial graft[s]) involve selective engagement of the origins of the graft(s) for the purpose of bypass angiography. It is typically performed only in conjunction with coronary angiography of native vessels.

The cardiac catheterization codes (93452-93461), other than those for congenital heart disease, include contrast injection(s), imaging supervision, interpretation, and report for imaging typically performed. Codes for left heart catheterization (93452, 93453, 93458-93461), other than those for congenital heart disease, include intraprocedural injection(s) for left ventricular/left atrial angiography, imaging supervision, and interpretation, when performed. Codes for coronary catheter placement(s) (93454-93461), other than those for congenital heart disease, include intraprocedural injection(s) for coronary angiography, imaging

supervision, and interpretation. Codes for catheter placement(s) in bypass graft(s) (93455, 93457, 93459, 93461), other than those for congenital heart disease, include intraprocedural injection(s) for bypass graft angiography, imaging supervision, and interpretation. Do not report 93563-93565 in conjunction with 93452-93461.

For cardiac catheterization for congenital cardiac anomalies, see 93530-93533. When contrast injection(s) are performed in conjunction with cardiac catheterization for congenital anomalies, see 93563-93568.

Cardiac catheterization (93451-93461) includes all roadmapping angiography in order to place the catheters, including any injections and imaging supervision, interpretation, and report. It does not include contrast injection(s) and imaging supervision, interpretation, and report for imaging that is separately identified by specific procedure code(s). For right ventricular or right atrial angiography performed in conjunction with cardiac catheterization for congenital or noncongenital heart disease (93451-93461, 93530-93533), use 93566. For aortography, use 93567. For pulmonary angiography, use 93568. For angiography of noncoronary arteries and veins, performed as a distinct service, use appropriate codes from the Radiology section and the Vascular Injection Procedures section.

When cardiac catheterization is combined with pharmacologic agent administration with the specific purpose of repeating hemodynamic measurements to evaluate hemodynamic response, use 93463 in conjunction with 93451-93453 and 93456-93461. Do not report 93463 for intracoronary administration of pharmacologic agents during percutaneous coronary interventional procedures, during intracoronary assessment of coronary pressure, flow or resistance, or during intracoronary imaging procedures. Do not report 93463 in conjunction with 92920-92944, 92975, 92977.

When cardiac catheterization is combined with exercise (eg, walking or arm or leg ergometry protocol) with the specific purpose of repeating hemodynamic measurements to evaluate hemodynamic response, report 93464 in conjunction with 93451-93453, 93456-93461, and 93530-93533.

Contrast injection to image the access site(s) for the specific purpose of placing a closure device is inherent to the catheterization procedure and not separately reportable. Closure device placement at the vascular access site is inherent to the catheterization procedure and not separately reportable.

Modifier 51 should not be appended to 93451, 93456, 93503.

Please see the cardiac catheterization table located following 93571.

⊙⊘ **93451**   Right heart catheterization including measurement(s) of oxygen saturation and cardiac output, when performed

(Do not report 93451 in conjunction with 93453, 93456, 93457, 93460, 93461)

(Do not report 93451 in conjunction with 0345T for diagnostic left and right heart catheterization procedures intrinsic to the valve repair procedure)

⊙ **93452**   Left heart catheterization including intraprocedural injection(s) for left ventriculography, imaging supervision and interpretation, when performed

(Do not report 93452 in conjunction with 93453, 93458-93461)

⊙ **93453**   Combined right and left heart catheterization including intraprocedural injection(s) for left ventriculography, imaging supervision and interpretation, when performed

(Do not report 93453 in conjunction with 93451, 93452, 93456-93461)

(Do not report 93453 in conjunction with 0345T for diagnostic left and right heart catheterization procedures intrinsic to the valve repair procedure)

⊙ **93454**   Catheter placement in coronary artery(s) for coronary angiography, including intraprocedural injection(s) for coronary angiography, imaging supervision and interpretation;

(Do not report 93453, 93454 in conjunction with 0345T for coronary angiography intrinsic to the valve repair procedure)

⊙ **93455**   with catheter placement(s) in bypass graft(s) (internal mammary, free arterial, venous grafts) including intraprocedural injection(s) for bypass graft angiography

⊙⊘ **93456**   with right heart catheterization

(Do not report 93456 in conjunction with 0345T for diagnostic left and right heart catheterization procedures intrinsic to the valve repair procedure)

⊙ **93457**   with catheter placement(s) in bypass graft(s) (internal mammary, free arterial, venous grafts) including intraprocedural injection(s) for bypass graft angiography and right heart catheterization

⊙ **93458**   with left heart catheterization including intraprocedural injection(s) for left ventriculography, when performed

⊙ **93459**   with left heart catheterization including intraprocedural injection(s) for left ventriculography, when performed, catheter placement(s) in bypass graft(s) (internal mammary, free arterial, venous grafts) with bypass graft angiography

⊙ **93460**   with right and left heart catheterization including intraprocedural injection(s) for left ventriculography, when performed

⊙ **93461**   with right and left heart catheterization including intraprocedural injection(s) for left ventriculography, when performed, catheter placement(s) in bypass graft(s) (internal mammary, free arterial, venous grafts) with bypass graft angiography

(Do not report 93461 in conjunction with 0345T for diagnostic left and right heart catheterization procedures intrinsic to the valve repair procedure)

⊙+ **93462**   Left heart catheterization by transseptal puncture through intact septum or by transapical puncture (List separately in addition to code for primary procedure)

▶(Use 93462 in conjunction with 33477, 93452, 93453, 93458, 93459, 93460, 93461, 93582, 93653, 93654)◀

(Do not report 93462 in conjunction with 93656)

(Do not report 93462 in conjunction with 0345T unless transapical puncture is performed)

⊙+ **93463**   Pharmacologic agent administration (eg, inhaled nitric oxide, intravenous infusion of nitroprusside, dobutamine, milrinone, or other agent) including assessing hemodynamic measurements before, during, after and repeat pharmacologic agent administration, when performed (List separately in addition to code for primary procedure)

▶(Use 93463 in conjunction with 33477, 93451-93453, 93456-93461, 93530, 93531, 93532, 93533, 93580, 93581)◀

(Report 93463 only once per catheterization procedure)

(Do not report 93463 for pharmacologic agent administration in conjunction with coronary interventional procedure 92920-92944, 92975, 92977)

⊙+ **93464**   Physiologic exercise study (eg, bicycle or arm ergometry) including assessing hemodynamic measurements before and after (List separately in addition to code for primary procedure)

▶(Use 93464 in conjunction with 33477, 93451-93453, 93456-93461, 93530-93533)◀

(Report 93464 only once per catheterization procedure)

(For pharmacologic agent administration, use 93463)

(For bundle of His recording, use 93600)

⊘ **93503**   Insertion and placement of flow directed catheter (eg, Swan-Ganz) for monitoring purposes

(For subsequent monitoring, see 99356-99357)

⊙ **93505**   Endomyocardial biopsy

(To report transcatheter placement of radiation delivery device for coronary intravascular brachytherapy, use 92974)

▶(For intravascular radioelement application, see 77770, 77771, 77772)◀

Medicine

⊙ **93530** Right heart catheterization, for congenital cardiac anomalies

93531 Combined right heart catheterization and retrograde left heart catheterization, for congenital cardiac anomalies

93532 Combined right heart catheterization and transseptal left heart catheterization through intact septum with or without retrograde left heart catheterization, for congenital cardiac anomalies

93533 Combined right heart catheterization and transseptal left heart catheterization through existing septal opening, with or without retrograde left heart catheterization, for congenital cardiac anomalies

Injection Procedures

All injection codes include radiological supervision, interpretation, and report. Cardiac catheterization codes (93452-93461), other than those for congenital heart disease, include contrast injection(s) for imaging typically performed during these procedures (see Cardiac Catheterization above). Do not report 93563-93565 in conjunction with 93452-93461. When injection procedures for right ventricular, right atrial, aortic, or pulmonary angiography are performed in conjunction with cardiac catheterization, these services are reported separately (93566-93568). When right ventricular or right atrial angiography is performed at the time of heart catheterization, use 93566 with the appropriate catheterization code (93451, 93453, 93456, 93457, 93460, or 93461). Use 93567 when supravalvular ascending aortography is performed at the time of heart catheterization. Use 93568 with the appropriate right heart catheterization code when pulmonary angiography is performed. Separately reported injection procedures do not include introduction of catheters but do include repositioning of catheters when necessary and use of automatic power injectors, when performed.

When contrast injection(s) are performed in conjunction with cardiac catheterization for congenital cardiac anomalies (93530-93533), see 93563-93568. Injection procedure codes 93563-93568 include imaging supervision, interpretation, and report.

▶Injection procedures 93563-93568 represent separate identifiable services and may be coded in conjunction with one another when appropriate. The technical details of angiography, supervision of imaging and processing, interpretation, and report are included.◀

⊙ **93561** Indicator dilution studies such as dye or thermodilution, including arterial and/or venous catheterization; with cardiac output measurement (separate procedure)

⊙ **93562** subsequent measurement of cardiac output

(Do not report 93561, 93562 in conjunction with 93451-93462, 93582)

(For radioisotope method of cardiac output, see 78472, 78473, or 78481)

⊙✚ **93563** Injection procedure during cardiac catheterization including imaging supervision, interpretation, and report; for selective coronary angiography during congenital heart catheterization (List separately in addition to code for primary procedure)

⊙✚ **93564** for selective opacification of aortocoronary venous or arterial bypass graft(s) (eg, aortocoronary saphenous vein, free radial artery, or free mammary artery graft) to one or more coronary arteries and in situ arterial conduits (eg, internal mammary), whether native or used for bypass to one or more coronary arteries during congenital heart catheterization, when performed (List separately in addition to code for primary procedure)

(Do not report 93563, 93564 in conjunction with 0345T for coronary angiography intrinsic to the valve repair procedure)

⊙✚ **93565** for selective left ventricular or left atrial angiography (List separately in addition to code for primary procedure)

(Do not report 93563-93565 in conjunction with 93452-93461)

(Use 93563-93565 in conjunction with 93530-93533)

⊙✚ **93566** for selective right ventricular or right atrial angiography (List separately in addition to code for primary procedure)

(Use 93566 in conjunction with 93451, 93453, 93456, 93457, 93460, 93461, 93530-93533)

▶(Do not report 93566 in conjunction with 0387T for right ventriculography performed during leadless pacemaker insertion)◀

⊙✚ **93567** for supravalvular aortography (List separately in addition to code for primary procedure)

(Use 93567 in conjunction with 93451-93461, 93530-93533)

(For non-supravalvular thoracic aortography or abdominal aortography performed at the time of cardiac catheterization, use the appropriate radiological supervision and interpretation codes [36221, 75600-75630])

⊙✚ **93568** for pulmonary angiography (List separately in addition to code for primary procedure)

(Use 93568 in conjunction with 93451, 93453, 93456, 93457, 93460, 93461, 93530-93533)

⊙✚ **93571** Intravascular Doppler velocity and/or pressure derived coronary flow reserve measurement (coronary vessel or graft) during coronary angiography including pharmacologically induced stress; initial vessel (List separately in addition to code for primary procedure)

(Use 93571 in conjunction with 92920, 92924, 92928, 92933, 92937, 92941, 92943, 92975, 93454-93461, 93563, 93564)

Medicine

⊙**+ 93572**   each additional vessel (List separately in addition to code for primary procedure)

(Use 93572 in conjunction with 93571)

(Intravascular distal coronary blood flow velocity measurements include all Doppler transducer manipulations and repositioning within the specific vessel being examined, during coronary angiography or therapeutic intervention [eg, angioplasty])

(For unlisted cardiac catheterization procedure, use 93799)

Repair of Structural Heart Defect

93580   Percutaneous transcatheter closure of congenital interatrial communication (ie, Fontan fenestration, atrial septal defect) with implant

(Percutaneous transcatheter closure of atrial septal defect includes a right heart catheterization procedure. Code 93580 includes injection of contrast for atrial and ventricular angiograms. Codes 93451-93453, 93455-93461, 93530-93533, 93564-93566 should not be reported separately in addition to code 93580)

93581   Percutaneous transcatheter closure of a congenital ventricular septal defect with implant

(Percutaneous transcatheter closure of ventricular septal defect includes a right heart catheterization procedure. Code 93581 includes injection of contrast for atrial and ventricular angiograms. Codes 93451-93453, 93455-93461, 93530-93533, 93564-93566 should not be reported separately in addition to code 93581)

(For echocardiographic services performed in addition to 93580, 93581, see 93303-93317, 93662 as appropriate)

⊙ **93582**   Percutaneous transcatheter closure of patent ductus arteriosus

(93582 includes congenital right and left heart catheterization, catheter placement in the aorta, and aortic arch angiography, when performed)

(Do not report 93582 in conjunction with 36013, 36014, 36200, 75600, 75605, 93451-93461, 93530, 93531, 93532, 93533, 93567)

(For other cardiac angiographic procedures performed at the time of transcatheter PDA closure, see 93563, 93564, 93565, 93566, 93568 as appropriate)

(For left heart catheterization by transseptal puncture through intact septum or by transapical puncture performed at the time of transcatheter PDA closure, use 93462)

(For repair of patent ductus arteriosus by ligation, see 33820, 33822, 33824)

(For intracardiac echocardiographic services performed at the time of transcatheter PDA closure, use 93662. Other echocardiographic services provided by a separate individual are reported using the appropriate echocardiography service codes, 93315, 93316, 93317)

⊙ **93583**   Percutaneous transcatheter septal reduction therapy (eg, alcohol septal ablation) including temporary pacemaker insertion when performed

(93583 includes insertion of temporary pacemaker, when performed, and left heart catheterization)

(Do not report 93583 in conjunction with 33210, 93452, 93453, 93458, 93459, 93460, 93461, 93531, 93532, 93533, 93565)

(93583 includes left anterior descending coronary angiography for the purpose of roadmapping to guide the intervention. Do not report 93454, 93455, 93456, 93457, 93458, 93459, 93460, 93461, 93563 for coronary angiography performed during alcohol septal ablation for the purpose of roadmapping, guidance of the intervention, vessel measurement, and completion angiography)

(Diagnostic cardiac catheterization procedures may be separately reportable when no prior catheter-based diagnostic study of the treatment zone is available, the prior diagnostic study is inadequate, or the patient's condition with respect to the clinical indication has changed since the prior study or during the intervention. Use the appropriate codes from 93451, 93454, 93455, 93456, 93457, 93530, 93563, 93564, 93566, 93567, 93568)

(Do not report 93583 in conjunction with 33210, 33211)

(Do not report 93463 for the injection of alcohol for this procedure)

(For intracardiac echocardiographic services performed at the time of alcohol septal ablation, use 93662)

(Other echocardiographic services provided by a separate physician are reported using the appropriate echocardiography services codes, 93312, 93313, 93314, 93315, 93316, 93317)

(For surgical ventriculomyotomy [-myectomy] for idiopathic hypertrophic subaortic stenosis, use 33416)

Medicine

Cardiac Catheterization Codes

CPT Code	Code Descriptor	Catheter Placement Type				Add-on Procedures (Can Be Reported Separately)					
		RHC	LHC	Coronary Artery Placement	Bypass Graft(s)	With Transseptal or Transapical Puncture (93462)	With Pharmacological Study (93463)	With Exercise Study (93464)	Injection Procedure for Selective Right Ventricular or Right Atrial Angiography (93566)	Injection Procedure for Supravalvular Aortography (93567)	Injection Procedure for Pulmonary Angiography (93568)
93451	Right heart catheterization including measurement(s) of oxygen saturation and cardiac output, when performed	X					X	X	X		X
93452	Left heart catheterization including intraprocedural injection(s) for left ventriculography, imaging supervision and interpretation, when performed		X			X	X	X		X	
93453	Combined right and left heart catheterization including intraprocedural injection(s) for left ventriculography, imaging supervision and interpretation, when performed	X	X			X	X	X	X	X	X
93454	Catheter placement in coronary artery(s) for coronary angiography, including intraprocedural injection(s) for coronary angiography, imaging supervision and interpretation;			X						X	
93455	Catheter placement in coronary artery(s) for coronary angiography, including intraprocedural injection(s) for coronary angiography, imaging supervision and interpretation; **with catheter placement(s) in bypass graft(s), (internal mammary, free arterial, venous grafts) including intraprocedural injection(s) for bypass graft angiography**			X	X					X	

⊙ = Moderate sedation   ✚ = Add-on code   ✗ = FDA approval pending   # = Resequenced code   ○ = Recycled/reinstated code

Medicine

Cardiac Catheterization Codes, *continued*

CPT Code	Code Descriptor	Catheter Placement Type				Add-on Procedures (Can Be Reported Separately)					
		RHC	LHC	Coronary Artery Placement	Bypass Graft(s)	With Transseptal or Transapical Puncture (93462)	With Pharmacological Study (93463)	With Exercise Study (93464)	Injection Procedure for Selective Right Ventricular or Right Atrial Angiography (93566)	Injection Procedure for Supravalvular Aortography (93567)	Injection Procedure for Pulmonary Angiography (93568)
93456	Catheter placement in coronary artery(s) for coronary angiography, including intraprocedural injection(s) for coronary angiography, imaging supervision and interpretation; **with right heart catheterization**	X		X			X	X	X	X	X
93457	Catheter placement in coronary artery(s) for coronary angiography, including intraprocedural injection(s) for coronary angiography, imaging supervision and interpretation; **with catheter placement(s) in bypass graft(s) (internal mammary, free arterial, venous grafts) including intraprocedural injection(s) for bypass graft angiography and right heart catheterization**	X		X	X		X	X	X	X	X
93458	Catheter placement in coronary artery(s) for coronary angiography, including intraprocedural injection(s) for coronary angiography, imaging supervision and interpretation; **with left heart catheterization including intraprocedural injection(s) for left ventriculography, when performed**		X	X		X	X	X		X	

Medicine

Medicine

Cardiac Catheterization Codes, *continued*

CPT Code	Code Descriptor	Catheter Placement Type				Add-on Procedures (Can Be Reported Separately)					
		RHC	LHC	Coronary Artery Placement	Bypass Graft(s)	With Transseptal or Transapical Puncture 93462	With Pharmacological Study 93463	With Exercise Study 93464	Injection Procedure for Selective Right Ventricular or Right Atrial Angiography 93566	Injection Procedure for Supravalvular Aortography 93567	Injection Procedure for Pulmonary Angiography 93568
93459	Catheter placement in coronary artery(s) for coronary angiography, including intraprocedural injection(s) for coronary angiography, imaging supervision and interpretation; **with left heart catheterization including intraprocedural injection(s) for left ventriculography, when performed, catheter placement(s) in bypass graft(s) (internal mammary, free arterial, venous grafts) with bypass graft angiography**		X	X	X	X	X	X		X	
93460	Catheter placement in coronary artery(s) for coronary angiography, including intraprocedural injection(s) for coronary angiography, imaging supervision and interpretation; **with right and left heart catheterization including intraprocedural injection(s) for left ventriculography, when performed**	X	X	X		X	X	X	X	X	X
93461	Catheter placement in coronary artery(s) for coronary angiography, including intraprocedural injection(s) for coronary angiography, imaging supervision and interpretation; **with right and left heart catheterization including intraprocedural injection(s) for left ventriculography, when performed, catheter placement(s) in bypass graft(s) (internal mammary, free arterial, venous grafts) with bypass graft angiography**	X	X	X	X	X	X	X	X	X	X

Intracardiac Electrophysiological Procedures/Studies

Intracardiac electrophysiologic studies (EPS) are invasive diagnostic medical procedures which include the insertion and repositioning of electrode catheters, recording of electrograms before and during pacing, programmed stimulation of multiple locations in the heart, analysis of recorded information, and report of the procedure. In many circumstances, patients with arrhythmias are evaluated and treated at the same encounter. In this situation, a diagnostic *electrophysiologic study* is performed, induced tachycardia(s) are *mapped*, and on the basis of the diagnostic and mapping information, the tissue is *ablated*.

Definitions

Arrhythmia Induction: In most electrophysiologic studies, an attempt is made to induce arrhythmia(s) from single or multiple sites within the heart. Arrhythmia induction may be achieved by multiple techniques, eg, by performing pacing at different rates or programmed stimulation (introduction of critically timed electrical impulses). Because arrhythmia induction occurs via the same catheter(s) inserted for the electrophysiologic study(ies), catheter insertion and temporary pacemaker codes are not additionally reported. Codes 93600-93603, 93610, 93612, and 93618 are used to describe unusual situations where there may be recording, pacing, or an attempt at arrhythmia induction from only one site in the heart. Code 93619 describes only evaluation of the sinus node, atrioventricular node, and His-Purkinje conduction system, without arrhythmia induction. Codes 93620-93624, 93640-93642, 93653, 93654, and 93656 all include recording, pacing, and attempted arrhythmia induction from one or more site(s) in the heart.

Mapping: When a tachycardia is induced, the site of tachycardia origination or its electrical path through the heart is often defined by mapping. Mapping creates a multidimensional depiction of a tachycardia by recording multiple electrograms obtained sequentially or simultaneously from multiple catheter sites in the heart. Depending upon the technique, certain types of mapping catheters may be repositioned from point-to-point within the heart, allowing sequential recording from the various sites to construct maps. Other types of mapping catheters allow mapping without a point-to-point technique by allowing simultaneous recording from many electrodes on the same catheter and computer-assisted three-dimensional reconstruction of the tachycardia activation sequence.

Mapping is a distinct procedure performed in addition to a diagnostic electrophysiologic study or ablation procedure and may be separately reported using 93609 or 93613. Do not report standard mapping (93609) in addition to 3-dimensional mapping (93613).

Ablation: Once the part of the heart involved in the tachycardia is localized, the tachycardia may be treated by ablation (the delivery of a radiofrequency or cryo-energy to the area to selectively destroy cardiac tissue). Ablation procedures (93653-93657) are performed at the same session as electrophysiology studies and therefore represent a combined code description. When reporting ablation therapy codes (93653-93657), the single site electrophysiology studies (93600-93603, 93610, 93612, 93618) and the comprehensive electrophysiology studies (93619, 93620) may not be reported separately. Code 93622 may be reported separately with 93653 and 93656. Code 93623 may be reported separately with 93653, 93654, and 93656. However, 93621 for left atrial pacing and recording from coronary sinus or left atrium should not be reported in conjunction with 93656, as this procedure is a component of 93656. Codes 93653 and 93654 include right ventricular pacing and recording and His bundle recording when clinically indicated. When performance of one or more components is not possible or indicated, document the reason for not performing. Code 93656 includes each of left atrial pacing/recording, right ventricular pacing/recording, and His bundle recording when clinically indicated. When performance of one or more components is not possible or indicated, document the reason for not performing.

The differences in the techniques involved for ablation of supraventricular arrhythmias, ventricular arrhythmias, and atrial fibrillation are reflected within the descriptions for 93653-93657. Code 93653 is a primary code for catheter ablation for treatment of supraventricular tachycardia caused by dual atrioventricular nodal pathways, accessory atrioventricular connections, or other atrial foci. Code 93654 describes catheter ablation for treatment of ventricular tachycardia or focus of ventricular ectopy. Code 93656 is a primary code for reporting treatment of atrial fibrillation by ablation to achieve complete pulmonary vein electrical isolation. Codes 93653, 93654, and 93656 are distinct primary procedure codes and may not be reported together.

Codes 93655 and 93657 are add-on codes listed in addition to the primary ablation code to report ablation of sites distinct from the primary ablation site. After ablation of the primary target site, post-ablation electrophysiologic evaluation is performed as part of those ablation services (93653, 93654, 93656) and additional mechanisms of tachycardia may be identified. For example, if the primary tachycardia ablated was atrioventricular nodal reentrant tachycardia and during post-ablation testing an atrial tachycardia, atrial flutter, or accessory pathway with orthodromic reentry tachycardia was identified, this would be considered a separate mechanism of tachycardia. Pacing maneuvers are performed to define the mechanism(s) of the new tachycardia(s). Catheter ablation of this distinct mechanism of tachycardia is then performed at the newly discovered atrial or ventricular origin. Appropriate post-

Medicine

---

ablation attempts at re-induction and observation are again performed. Code 93655 is listed in conjunction with 93653 when repeat ablation is for treatment of an additional supraventricular tachycardia mechanism and with 93654 when the repeat ablation is for treatment of an additional ventricular tachycardia mechanism. Code 93655 may be reported with 93656 when an additional non-atrial fibrillation tachycardia is separately diagnosed after pulmonary vein isolation. Code 93657 is reported in conjunction with 93656 when successful pulmonary vein isolation is achieved, attempts at re-induction of atrial fibrillation identify an additional left or right atrial focus for atrial fibrillation, and further ablation of this new focus is performed.

In certain circumstances, depending on the chamber of origin, a catheter or catheters may be maneuvered into the left ventricle to facilitate arrhythmia diagnosis. This may be accomplished via a retrograde aortic approach by means of the arterial access or through a transseptal puncture. For ablation treatment of supraventricular tachycardia (93653) and ventricular tachycardia (93654), the left heart catheterization by transseptal puncture through intact septum (93462) may be reported separately as an add-on code. However, for ablation treatment of atrial fibrillation (93656), the transseptal puncture (93462) is a standard component of the procedure and may not be reported separately. Do not report 93462 in conjunction with 93656.

Modifier 51 should not be appended to 93600-93603, 93610, 93612, 93615-93618, 93631.

⊘ **93600**   Bundle of His recording

(Do not report 93600 in conjunction with 93619, 93620, 93653, 93654, 93656)

⊘ **93602**   Intra-atrial recording

(Do not report 93602 in conjunction with 93619, 93620, 93653, 93654, 93656)

⊘ **93603**   Right ventricular recording

(Do not report 93603 in conjunction with 93619, 93620, 93653, 93654, 93656)

⊙✚ **93609**   Intraventricular and/or intra-atrial mapping of tachycardia site(s) with catheter manipulation to record from multiple sites to identify origin of tachycardia (List separately in addition to code for primary procedure)

(Use 93609 in conjunction with 93620, 93653, 93656)

(Do not report 93609 in conjunction with 93613, 93654)

⊘ **93610**   Intra-atrial pacing

(Do not report 93610 in conjunction with 93619, 93620, 93653, 93654, 93656)

⊘ **93612**   Intraventricular pacing

(Do not report 93612 in conjunction with 93619, 93620, 93621, 93622, 93653, 93654, 93656)

⊙✚ **93613**   Intracardiac electrophysiologic 3-dimensional mapping (List separately in addition to code for primary procedure)

(Use 93613 in conjunction with 93620, 93653, 93656)

(Do not report 93613 in conjunction with 93609, 93654)

⊙⊘ **93615**   Esophageal recording of atrial electrogram with or without ventricular electrogram(s);

⊙⊘ **93616**   with pacing

⊙⊘ **93618**   Induction of arrhythmia by electrical pacing

(Do not report 93618 in conjunction with 93619, 93620, 93621, 93622, 93653, 93654, 93656)

(For intracardiac phonocardiogram, use 93799)

⊙ **93619**   Comprehensive electrophysiologic evaluation with right atrial pacing and recording, right ventricular pacing and recording, His bundle recording, including insertion and repositioning of multiple electrode catheters, without induction or attempted induction of arrhythmia

(Do not report 93619 in conjunction with 93600, 93602, 93603, 93610, 93612, 93618, 93620, 93621, 93622, 93653, 93654, 93655, 93656, 93657)

⊙ **93620**   Comprehensive electrophysiologic evaluation including insertion and repositioning of multiple electrode catheters with induction or attempted induction of arrhythmia; with right atrial pacing and recording, right ventricular pacing and recording, His bundle recording

(Do not report 93620 in conjunction with 93600, 93602, 93603, 93610, 93612, 93618, 93619, 93653, 93654, 93655, 93656, 93657)

⊙✚ **93621**   with left atrial pacing and recording from coronary sinus or left atrium (List separately in addition to code for primary procedure)

(Use 93621 in conjunction with 93620, 93653, 93654)

(Do not report 93621 in conjunction with 93656)

⊙✚ **93622**   with left ventricular pacing and recording (List separately in addition to code for primary procedure)

(Use 93622 in conjunction with 93620, 93653, 93656)

(Do not report 93622 in conjunction with 93654)

✚ **93623**   Programmed stimulation and pacing after intravenous drug infusion (List separately in addition to code for primary procedure)

(Use 93623 in conjunction with 93610, 93612, 93619, 93620, 93653, 93654, 93656)

⊙ **93624**   Electrophysiologic follow-up study with pacing and recording to test effectiveness of therapy, including induction or attempted induction of arrhythmia

⊘ **93631**   Intra-operative epicardial and endocardial pacing and mapping to localize the site of tachycardia or zone of slow conduction for surgical correction

(For operative ablation of an arrhythmogenic focus or pathway by a separate individual, see 33250-33261)

⊙ **93640** Electrophysiologic evaluation of single or dual chamber pacing cardioverter-defibrillator leads including defibrillation threshold evaluation (induction of arrhythmia, evaluation of sensing and pacing for arrhythmia termination) at time of initial implantation or replacement;

⊙ **93641** with testing of single or dual chamber pacing cardioverter-defibrillator pulse generator

(For subsequent or periodic electronic analysis and/or reprogramming of single or dual chamber pacing cardioverter-defibrillators, see 93282, 93283, 93289, 93292, 93295, 93642)

⊙ **93642** Electrophysiologic evaluation of single or dual chamber transvenous pacing cardioverter-defibrillator (includes defibrillation threshold evaluation, induction of arrhythmia, evaluation of sensing and pacing for arrhythmia termination, and programming or reprogramming of sensing or therapeutic parameters)

⊙ **93644** Electrophysiologic evaluation of subcutaneous implantable defibrillator (includes defibrillation threshold evaluation, induction of arrhythmia, evaluation of sensing for arrhythmia termination, and programming or reprogramming of sensing or therapeutic parameters)

(Do not report 93644 in conjunction with 33270 at the time of subcutaneous implantable defibrillator device insertion)

(For subsequent or periodic electrophysiologic evaluation of a subcutaneous implantable defibrillator device, see 93260, 93261)

⊙ **93650** Intracardiac catheter ablation of atrioventricular node function, atrioventricular conduction for creation of complete heart block, with or without temporary pacemaker placement

(93651, 93652 have been deleted. To report, see 93653-93657)

⊙ **93653** Comprehensive electrophysiologic evaluation including insertion and repositioning of multiple electrode catheters with induction or attempted induction of an arrhythmia with right atrial pacing and recording, right ventricular pacing and recording (when necessary), and His bundle recording (when necessary) with intracardiac catheter ablation of arrhythmogenic focus; with treatment of supraventricular tachycardia by ablation of fast or slow atrioventricular pathway, accessory atrioventricular connection, cavo-tricuspid isthmus or other single atrial focus or source of atrial re-entry

(Do not report 93653 in conjunction with 93600-93603, 93610, 93612, 93618-93620, 93642, 93654, 93656)

⊙ **93654** with treatment of ventricular tachycardia or focus of ventricular ectopy including intracardiac electrophysiologic 3D mapping, when performed, and left ventricular pacing and recording, when performed

(Do not report 93654 in conjunction with 93279-93284, 93286-93289, 93600-93603, 93609, 93610, 93612, 93613, 93618-93620, 93622, 93642, 93653, 93656)

⊙➕ **93655** Intracardiac catheter ablation of a discrete mechanism of arrhythmia which is distinct from the primary ablated mechanism, including repeat diagnostic maneuvers, to treat a spontaneous or induced arrhythmia (List separately in addition to code for primary procedure)

(Use 93655 in conjunction with 93653, 93654, 93656)

⊙ **93656** Comprehensive electrophysiologic evaluation including transseptal catheterizations, insertion and repositioning of multiple electrode catheters with induction or attempted induction of an arrhythmia including left or right atrial pacing/recording when necessary, right ventricular pacing/recording when necessary, and His bundle recording when necessary with intracardiac catheter ablation of atrial fibrillation by pulmonary vein isolation

(Do not report 93656 in conjunction with 93279-93284, 93286-93289, 93462, 93600, 93602, 93603, 93610, 93612, 93618, 93619, 93620, 93621, 93653, 93654)

⊙➕ **93657** Additional linear or focal intracardiac catheter ablation of the left or right atrium for treatment of atrial fibrillation remaining after completion of pulmonary vein isolation (List separately in addition to code for primary procedure)

(Use 93657 in conjunction with 93656)

93660 Evaluation of cardiovascular function with tilt table evaluation, with continuous ECG monitoring and intermittent blood pressure monitoring, with or without pharmacological intervention

(For testing of autonomic nervous system function, see 95921, 95924, 95943)

➕ **93662** Intracardiac echocardiography during therapeutic/diagnostic intervention, including imaging supervision and interpretation (List separately in addition to code for primary procedure)

(Use 93662 in conjunction with 92987, 93453, 93460-93462, 93532, 93580, 93581, 93620, 93621, 93622, 93653, 93654, 93656 as appropriate)

(Do not report 92961 in addition to 93662)

Peripheral Arterial Disease Rehabilitation

Peripheral arterial disease (PAD) rehabilitative physical exercise consists of a series of sessions, lasting 45-60 minutes per session, involving use of either a motorized treadmill or a track to permit each patient to achieve symptom-limited claudication. Each session is supervised by an exercise physiologist or nurse. The supervising provider monitors the individual patient's claudication threshold and other cardiovascular limitations for adjustment of workload. During this supervised rehabilitation program, the development of new arrhythmias, symptoms that might suggest angina or the continued inability of the patient to progress to an adequate level of exercise may require review and examination of the patient by a physician or other qualified health care professional. These services would be

Medicine

separately reported with an appropriate level E/M service code including office or other outpatient services (99201-99215), initial hospital care (99221-99223), subsequent hospital care (99231-99233), critical care services (99291-99292).

93668 Peripheral arterial disease (PAD) rehabilitation, per session

Noninvasive Physiologic Studies and Procedures

(For arterial cannulization and recording of direct arterial pressure, use 36620)

(For radiographic injection procedures, see 36000-36299)

(For vascular cannulization for hemodialysis, see 36800-36821)

(For chemotherapy for malignant disease, see 96409-96549)

(For penile plethysmography, use 54240)

93701 Bioimpedance-derived physiologic cardiovascular analysis

(For bioelectrical impedance analysis whole body composition, use 0358T. For left ventricular filling pressure indirect measurement by computerized calibration of the arterial waveform response to Valsalva, use 93799)

93702 Bioimpedance spectroscopy (BIS), extracellular fluid analysis for lymphedema assessment(s)

(For bioelectrical impedance analysis whole body composition, use 0358T)

(For bioimpedance-derived physiological cardiovascular analysis, use 93701)

93724 Electronic analysis of antitachycardia pacemaker system (includes electrocardiographic recording, programming of device, induction and termination of tachycardia via implanted pacemaker, and interpretation of recordings)

(93731, 93732 have been deleted. For interrogation of dual lead pacemaker, see 93288, 93294. For programming of dual chamber pacemaker, use 93280)

(93734, 93735 have been deleted. For interrogation of single lead pacemaker, see 93288, 93294. For programming of single lead pacemaker, use 93279)

93740 Temperature gradient studies

(93741, 93742 have been deleted. For interrogation of single implantable cardioverter-defibrillator [ICD], see 93289, 93295. For programming of single ICD, use 93282. For interrogation of wearable cardioverter-defibrillator, use 93292)

(93743, 93744 have been deleted. For interrogation of dual implantable cardioverter-defibrillator [ICD], see 93289, 93295. For programming of dual ICD, use 93283)

93745 Initial set-up and programming by a physician or other qualified health care professional of wearable cardioverter-defibrillator includes initial programming of system, establishing baseline electronic ECG, transmission of data to data repository, patient instruction in wearing system and patient reporting of problems or events

(Do not report 93745 in conjunction with 93282, 93292)

93750 Interrogation of ventricular assist device (VAD), in person, with physician or other qualified health care professional analysis of device parameters (eg, drivelines, alarms, power surges), review of device function (eg, flow and volume status, septum status, recovery), with programming, if performed, and report

(Do not report 93750 in conjunction with 33975, 33976, 33979, 33981-33983)

(93760, 93762 have been deleted)

93770 Determination of venous pressure

(For central venous cannulization see 36555-36556, 36500)

93784 Ambulatory blood pressure monitoring, utilizing a system such as magnetic tape and/or computer disk, for 24 hours or longer; including recording, scanning analysis, interpretation and report

93786 recording only

93788 scanning analysis with report

93790 review with interpretation and report

Other Procedures

93797 Physician or other qualified health care professional services for outpatient cardiac rehabilitation; without continuous ECG monitoring (per session)

93798 with continuous ECG monitoring (per session)

93799 Unlisted cardiovascular service or procedure

Noninvasive Vascular Diagnostic Studies

Vascular studies include patient care required to perform the studies, supervision of the studies and interpretation of study results with copies for patient records of hard copy output with analysis of all data, including bidirectional vascular flow or imaging when provided.

The use of a simple hand-held or other Doppler device that does not produce hard copy output, or that produces a record that does not permit analysis of bidirectional vascular flow, is considered to be part of the physical examination of the vascular system and is not separately reported. The Ankle-Brachial Index (or ABI) is reportable with 93922 or 93923 as long as simultaneous Doppler recording and analysis of bidirectional blood flow, volume

Medicine

plethysmography, or transcutaneous oxygen tension measurements are also performed.

Duplex scan (eg, 93880, 93882) describes an ultrasonic scanning procedure for characterizing the pattern and direction of blood flow in arteries or veins with the production of real-time images integrating B-mode two-dimensional vascular structure, Doppler spectral analysis, and color flow Doppler imaging.

Physiologic studies Noninvasive physiologic studies are performed using equipment separate and distinct from the duplex ultrasound imager. Codes 93922, 93923, 93924, and 93965 describe the evaluation of non-imaging physiologic recordings of pressures with Doppler analysis of bi-directional blood flow, plethysmography, and/or oxygen tension measurements appropriate for the anatomic area studied.

Limited studies for lower extremity require either:

(1) ankle/brachial indices at distal posterior tibial and anterior tibial/dorsalis pedis arteries plus bidirectional Doppler waveform recording and analysis at 1-2 levels; or (2) ankle/brachial indices at distal posterior tibial and anterior tibial/dorsalis pedis arteries plus volume plethysmography at 1-2 levels; or (3) ankle/brachial indices at distal posterior tibial and anterior tibial/dorsalis pedis arteries with transcutaneous oxygen tension measurements at 1-2 levels. Potential levels include high thigh, low thigh, calf, ankle, metatarsal and toes.

Limited studies for upper extremity require either:

(1) Doppler-determined systolic pressures and bidirectional Doppler waveform recording and analysis at 1-2 levels; or (2) Doppler-determined systolic pressures and volume plethysmography at 1-2 levels; or (3) Doppler-determined systolic pressures and transcutaneous oxygen tension measurements at 1-2 levels. Potential levels include arm, forearm, wrist, and digits.

Complete studies for lower extremity require either:

(1) ankle/brachial indices at distal posterior tibial and anterior tibial/dorsalis pedis arteries plus bidirectional Doppler waveform recording and analysis at 3 or more levels; or (2) ankle/brachial indices at distal posterior tibial and anterior tibial/dorsalis pedis arteries plus volume plethysmography at 3 or more levels; or (3) ankle/brachial indices at distal posterior tibial and anterior tibial/dorsalis pedis arteries with transcutaneous oxygen tension measurements at 3 or more levels. Alternatively, a complete study may be reported with measurements at a single level if provocative functional maneuvers (eg, measurements with postural provocative tests, or measurements with reactive hyperemia) are performed.

Complete studies for upper extremity require either:

(1) Doppler-determined systolic pressures and bidirectional Doppler waveform recording and analysis at 3 or more levels; or (2) Doppler-determined systolic pressures and volume plethysmography at 3 or more

levels; or (3) Doppler-determined systolic pressures and transcutaneous oxygen tension measurements at 3 or more levels. Potential levels include arm, forearm, wrist, and digits. Alternatively, a complete study may be reported with measurements at a single level if provocative functional maneuvers (eg, measurements with postural provocative tests, or measurements with cold stress) are performed.

Cerebrovascular Arterial Studies

A complete transcranial Doppler (TCD) study (93886) includes ultrasound evaluation of the right and left anterior circulation territories and the posterior circulation territory (to include vertebral arteries and basilar artery). In a limited TCD study (93888) there is ultrasound evaluation of two or fewer of these territories. For TCD, ultrasound evaluation is a reasonable and concerted attempt to identify arterial signals through an acoustic window.

Code 93895 includes the acquisition and storage of images of the common carotid arteries, carotid bulbs, and internal carotid arteries bilaterally with quantification of intima media thickness (common carotid artery mean and maximal values) and determination of presence of atherosclerotic plaque. When any of these elements are not obtained, use 0126T.

(93875 has been deleted)

93880   Duplex scan of extracranial arteries; complete bilateral study

(Do not report 93880 in conjunction with 93895, 0126T)

93882   unilateral or limited study

(Do not report 93882 in conjunction with 93895, 0126T)

(To report common carotid intima-media thickness (IMT) study for evaluation of atherosclerotic burden or coronary heart disease risk factor assessment, use Category III code 0126T)

93886   Transcranial Doppler study of the intracranial arteries; complete study

93888   limited study

93890   vasoreactivity study

93892   emboli detection without intravenous microbubble injection

93893   emboli detection with intravenous microbubble injection

93895   Quantitative carotid intima media thickness and carotid atheroma evaluation, bilateral

(Do not report 93895 in conjunction with 93880, 93882, 0126T)

(Do not report 93890-93893 in conjunction with 93888)

Medicine

Extremity Arterial Studies (Including Digits)

93922 Limited bilateral noninvasive physiologic studies of upper or lower extremity arteries, (eg, for lower extremity: ankle/brachial indices at distal posterior tibial and anterior tibial/dorsalis pedis arteries plus bidirectional, Doppler waveform recording and analysis at 1-2 levels, or ankle/brachial indices at distal posterior tibial and anterior tibial/dorsalis pedis arteries plus volume plethysmography at 1-2 levels, or ankle/brachial indices at distal posterior tibial and anterior tibial/dorsalis pedis arteries with, transcutaneous oxygen tension measurement at 1-2 levels)

(When only 1 arm or leg is available for study, report 93922 with modifier 52 for a unilateral study when recording 1-2 levels. Report 93922 when recording 3 or more levels or performing provocative functional maneuvers)

(Report 93922 only once in the upper extremity(s) and/or once in the lower extremity(s). When both the upper and lower extremities are evaluated in the same setting, 93922 may be reported twice by adding modifier 59 to the second procedure)

(For transcutaneous oxyhemoglobin measurement in a lower extremity wound by near infrared spectroscopy, use 0286T)

(Do not report 93922 in conjunction with 0337T)

93923 Complete bilateral noninvasive physiologic studies of upper or lower extremity arteries, 3 or more levels (eg, for lower extremity: ankle/brachial indices at distal posterior tibial and anterior tibial/dorsalis pedis arteries plus segmental blood pressure measurements with bidirectional Doppler waveform recording and analysis, at 3 or more levels, or ankle/brachial indices at distal posterior tibial and anterior tibial/dorsalis pedis arteries plus segmental volume plethysmography at 3 or more levels, or ankle/brachial indices at distal posterior tibial and anterior tibial/dorsalis pedis arteries plus segmental transcutaneous oxygen tension measurements at 3 or more levels), or single level study with provocative functional maneuvers (eg, measurements with postural provocative tests, or measurements with reactive hyperemia)

(When only 1 arm or leg is available for study, report 93922 for a unilateral study when recording 3 or more levels or when performing provocative functional maneuvers)

(Report 93923 only once in the upper extremity(s) and/or once in the lower extremity(s). When both the upper and lower extremities are evaluated in the same setting, 93923 may be reported twice by adding modifier 59 to the second procedure)

(For transcutaneous oxyhemoglobin measurement in a lower extremity wound by near infrared spectroscopy, use 0286T)

(Do not report 93923 in conjunction with 0337T)

93924 Noninvasive physiologic studies of lower extremity arteries, at rest and following treadmill stress testing, (ie, bidirectional Doppler waveform or volume plethysmography recording and analysis at rest with ankle/brachial indices immediately after and at timed intervals following performance of a standardized protocol on a motorized treadmill plus recording of time of onset of claudication or other symptoms, maximal walking time, and time to recovery) complete bilateral study

(Do not report 93924 in conjunction with 93922, 93923)

93925 Duplex scan of lower extremity arteries or arterial bypass grafts; complete bilateral study

93926   unilateral or limited study

93930 Duplex scan of upper extremity arteries or arterial bypass grafts; complete bilateral study

93931   unilateral or limited study

Extremity Venous Studies (Including Digits)

93965 Noninvasive physiologic studies of extremity veins, complete bilateral study (eg, Doppler waveform analysis with responses to compression and other maneuvers, phleborheography, impedance plethysmography)

93970 Duplex scan of extremity veins including responses to compression and other maneuvers; complete bilateral study

93971   unilateral or limited study

(Do not report 93970, 93971 in conjunction with 36475, 36476, 36478, 36479)

Visceral and Penile Vascular Studies

93975 Duplex scan of arterial inflow and venous outflow of abdominal, pelvic, scrotal contents and/or retroperitoneal organs; complete study

93976   limited study

93978 Duplex scan of aorta, inferior vena cava, iliac vasculature, or bypass grafts; complete study

93979   unilateral or limited study

93980 Duplex scan of arterial inflow and venous outflow of penile vessels; complete study

93981   follow-up or limited study

93982 Noninvasive physiologic study of implanted wireless pressure sensor in aneurysmal sac following endovascular repair, complete study including recording, analysis of pressure and waveform tracings, interpretation and report

(Do not report 93982 in conjunction with 34806)

Extremity Arterial-Venous Studies

93990   Duplex scan of hemodialysis access (including arterial inflow, body of access and venous outflow)

(For measurement of hemodialysis access flow using indicator dilution methods, use 90940)

Other Noninvasive Vascular Diagnostic Studies

93998   Unlisted noninvasive vascular diagnostic study

Pulmonary

Ventilator Management

94002   Ventilation assist and management, initiation of pressure or volume preset ventilators for assisted or controlled breathing; hospital inpatient/observation, initial day

94003   hospital inpatient/observation, each subsequent day

94004   nursing facility, per day

(Do not report 94002-94004 in conjunction with Evaluation and Management services 99201-99499)

94005   Home ventilator management care plan oversight of a patient (patient not present) in home, domiciliary or rest home (eg, assisted living) requiring review of status, review of laboratories and other studies and revision of orders and respiratory care plan (as appropriate), within a calendar month, 30 minutes or more

(Do not report 94005 in conjunction with 99339, 99340, 99374-99378)

(Ventilator management care plan oversight is reported separately from home or domiciliary, rest home [eg, assisted living] services. A physician or other qualified health care professional may report 94005, when performed, including when a different individual reports 99339, 99340, 99374-99378 for the same 30 days)

Pulmonary Diagnostic Testing and Therapies

Codes 94010-94799 include laboratory procedure(s) and interpretation of test results. If a separate identifiable evaluation and management service is performed, the appropriate E/M service code including new or established patient office or other outpatient services (99201-99215), office or other outpatient consultations (99241-99245), emergency department services (99281-99285), nursing facility services (99304-99318), domiciliary, rest home, or custodial care services (99324-99337), and home services (99341-99350) may be reported in addition to 94010-94799.

Spirometry (94010) measures expiratory airflow and volumes and forms the basis of most pulmonary function testing. When spirometry is performed before and after administration of a bronchodilator, report 94060. Measurement of vital capacity (94150) is a component of spirometry and is only reported when performed alone. The flow-volume loop (94375) is used to identify patterns of inspiratory and/or expiratory obstruction in central or peripheral airways. Spirometry (94010, 94060) includes maximal breathing capacity (94200) and flow-volume loop (94375), when performed.

Measurement of lung volumes may be performed using plethysmography, helium dilution or nitrogen washout. Plethysmography (94726) is utilized to determine total lung capacity, residual volume, functional residual capacity, and airway resistance. Nitrogen washout or helium dilution (94727) may be used to measure lung volumes, distribution of ventilation and closing volume. Impulse oscillometry (94728) assesses airway resistance and may be reported in addition to gas dilution techniques. Spirometry (94010, 94060) and bronchial provocation (94070) are not included in 94726 and 94727 and may be reported separately.

Diffusing capacity (94729) is most commonly performed in conjunction with lung volumes or spirometry and is an add-on code to 94726-94728, 94010, 94060, 94070, and 94375.

Pulmonary function tests (94011-94013) are reported for measurements in infants and young children through 2 years of age.

Pulmonary function testing measurements are reported as actual values and as a percent of predicted values by age, gender, height, and race.

Chest wall manipulation for the mobilization of secretions and improvement in lung function can be performed using manual (94667, 94668) or mechanical (94669) methods. Manual techniques include cupping, percussing, and use of a hand-held vibration device. A mechanical technique is the application of an external vest or wrap that delivers mechanical oscillation.

94010   Spirometry, including graphic record, total and timed vital capacity, expiratory flow rate measurement(s), with or without maximal voluntary ventilation

(Do not report 94010 in conjunction with 94150, 94200, 94375, 94728)

⊙ **94011**   Measurement of spirometric forced expiratory flows in an infant or child through 2 years of age

⊙ **94012**   Measurement of spirometric forced expiratory flows, before and after bronchodilator, in an infant or child through 2 years of age

⊙ **94013**   Measurement of lung volumes (ie, functional residual capacity [FRC], forced vital capacity [FVC], and expiratory reserve volume [ERV]) in an infant or child through 2 years of age

Medicine

94014 Patient-initiated spirometric recording per 30-day period of time; includes reinforced education, transmission of spirometric tracing, data capture, analysis of transmitted data, periodic recalibration and review and interpretation by a physician or other qualified health care professional

94015 recording (includes hook-up, reinforced education, data transmission, data capture, trend analysis, and periodic recalibration)

94016 review and interpretation only by a physician or other qualified health care professional

94060 Bronchodilation responsiveness, spirometry as in 94010, pre- and post-bronchodilator administration

►(Do not report 94060 in conjunction with 94150, 94200, 94375, 94640, 94728)◄

(Report bronchodilator supply separately with 99070 or appropriate supply code)

(For prolonged exercise test for bronchospasm with pre- and post-spirometry, use 94620)

94070 Bronchospasm provocation evaluation, multiple spirometric determinations as in 94010, with administered agents (eg, antigen[s], cold air, methacholine)

►(Do not report 94070 in conjunction with 94640)◄

(Report antigen[s] administration separately with 99070 or appropriate supply code)

94150 Vital capacity, total (separate procedure)

(Do not report 94150 in conjunction with 94010, 94060, 94728. To report thoracic gas volumes, see 94726, 94727)

94200 Maximum breathing capacity, maximal voluntary ventilation

(Do not report 94200 in conjunction with 94010, 94060)

(94240 has been deleted. To report thoracic gas volumes, see 94726, 94727)

94250 Expired gas collection, quantitative, single procedure (separate procedure)

94375 Respiratory flow volume loop

(Do not report 94375 in conjunction with 94010, 94060, 94728)

94400 Breathing response to CO2 (CO2 response curve)

►(Do not report 94400 in conjunction with 94640)◄

94450 Breathing response to hypoxia (hypoxia response curve)

(For high altitude simulation test [HAST], see 94452, 94453)

94452 High altitude simulation test (HAST), with interpretation and report by a physician or other qualified health care professional;

(For obtaining arterial blood gases, use 36600)

(Do not report 94452 in conjunction with 94453, 94760, 94761)

94453 with supplemental oxygen titration

(For obtaining arterial blood gases, use 36600)

(Do not report 94453 in conjunction with 94452, 94760, 94761)

⊘ **94610** Intrapulmonary surfactant administration by a physician or other qualified health care professional through endotracheal tube

(Do not report 94610 in conjunction with 99468-99472)

(For endotracheal intubation, use 31500)

(Report 94610 once per dosing episode)

94620 Pulmonary stress testing; simple (eg, 6-minute walk test, prolonged exercise test for bronchospasm with pre- and post-spirometry and oximetry)

94621 complex (including measurements of CO_2 production, O_2 uptake, and electrocardiographic recordings)

▲ **94640** Pressurized or nonpressurized inhalation treatment for acute airway obstruction for therapeutic purposes and/or for diagnostic purposes such as sputum induction with an aerosol generator, nebulizer, metered dose inhaler or intermittent positive pressure breathing (IPPB) device

►(Do not report 94640 in conjunction with 94060, 94070, or 94400)◄

(For more than 1 inhalation treatment performed on the same date, append modifier 76)

(For continuous inhalation treatment of 1 hour or more, see 94644, 94645)

94642 Aerosol inhalation of pentamidine for pneumocystis carinii pneumonia treatment or prophylaxis

94644 Continuous inhalation treatment with aerosol medication for acute airway obstruction; first hour

(For services of less than 1 hour, use 94640)

+ **94645** each additional hour (List separately in addition to code for primary procedure)

(Use 94645 in conjunction with 94644)

94660 Continuous positive airway pressure ventilation (CPAP), initiation and management

94662 Continuous negative pressure ventilation (CNP), initiation and management

94664 Demonstration and/or evaluation of patient utilization of an aerosol generator, nebulizer, metered dose inhaler or IPPB device

(94664 can be reported 1 time only per day of service)

94667 Manipulation chest wall, such as cupping, percussing, and vibration to facilitate lung function; initial demonstration and/or evaluation

94668 subsequent

94669 Mechanical chest wall oscillation to facilitate lung function, per session

94680 Oxygen uptake, expired gas analysis; rest and exercise, direct, simple

94681   including CO$_2$ output, percentage oxygen extracted

94690   rest, indirect (separate procedure)

(For single arterial puncture, use 36600)

94726 Plethysmography for determination of lung volumes and, when performed, airway resistance

(Do not report 94726 in conjunction with 94727, 94728)

94727 Gas dilution or washout for determination of lung volumes and, when performed, distribution of ventilation and closing volumes

(Do not report 94727 in conjunction with 94726)

94728 Airway resistance by impulse oscillometry

(Do not report 94728 in conjunction with 94010, 94060, 94070, 94375, 94726)

+ 94729 Diffusing capacity (eg, carbon monoxide, membrane) (List separately in addition to code for primary procedure)

(Report 94729 in conjunction with 94010, 94060, 94070, 94375, 94726-94728)

94750 Pulmonary compliance study (eg, plethysmography, volume and pressure measurements)

94760 Noninvasive ear or pulse oximetry for oxygen saturation; single determination

(For blood gases, see 82803-82810)

94761   multiple determinations (eg, during exercise)

94762   by continuous overnight monitoring (separate procedure)

(For other in vivo laboratory procedures, see 88720-88741)

94770 Carbon dioxide, expired gas determination by infrared analyzer

(For bronchoscopy, see 31622-31646)

(For placement of flow directed catheter, use 93503)

(For venipuncture, use 36410)

(For central venous catheter placement, see 36555-36556)

(For arterial puncture, use 36600)

(For arterial catheterization, use 36620)

(For thoracentesis, use 32554, 32555)

(For phlebotomy, therapeutic, use 99195)

(For lung biopsy, needle, use 32405)

(For intubation, orotracheal or nasotracheal, use 31500)

94772 Circadian respiratory pattern recording (pediatric pneumogram), 12-24 hour continuous recording, infant

(Separate procedure codes for electromyograms, EEG, ECG, and recordings of respiration are excluded when 94772 is reported)

94774 Pediatric home apnea monitoring event recording including respiratory rate, pattern and heart rate per 30-day period of time; includes monitor attachment, download of data, review, interpretation, and preparation of a report by a physician or other qualified health care professional

(Do not report 94774 in conjunction with 94775-94777 during the same reporting period)

94775   monitor attachment only (includes hook-up, initiation of recording and disconnection)

94776   monitoring, download of information, receipt of transmission(s) and analyses by computer only

94777   review, interpretation and preparation of report only by a physician or other qualified health care professional

(When oxygen saturation monitoring is used in addition to heart rate and respiratory monitoring, it is not reported separately)

(Do not report 94774-94777 in conjunction with 93224-93272)

(Do not report apnea recording device separately)

(For sleep study, see 95805-95811)

94780 Car seat/bed testing for airway integrity, neonate, with continual nursing observation and continuous recording of pulse oximetry, heart rate and respiratory rate, with interpretation and report; 60 minutes

(Do not report 94780 for less than 60 minutes)

(Do not report 94780 in conjunction with 93040-93042, 94760, 94761, 99468-99472, 99477-99480)

+ 94781   each additional full 30 minutes (List separately in addition to code for primary procedure)

(Use 94781 in conjunction with 94780)

94799 Unlisted pulmonary service or procedure

Allergy and Clinical Immunology

Definitions

Immunotherapy (desensitization, hyposensitization): is the parenteral administration of allergenic extracts as antigens at periodic intervals, usually on an increasing dosage scale to a dosage which is maintained as maintenance therapy. Indications for immunotherapy are determined by appropriate diagnostic procedures coordinated with clinical judgment and knowledge of the natural history of allergic diseases.

Medicine

Other therapy: for medical conferences on the use of mechanical and electronic devices (precipitators, air conditioners, air filters, humidifiers, dehumidifiers), climatotherapy, physical therapy, occupational and recreational therapy, see Evaluation and Management services.

Do not report Evaluation and Management (E/M) services for test interpretation and report. If a significant separately identifiable E/M service is performed, the appropriate E/M service code, which may include new or established patient office or other outpatient services (99201-99215), hospital observation services (99217-99220, 99224-99226), hospital care (99221-99223, 99231-99233), consultations (99241-99255), emergency department services (99281-99285), nursing facility services (99304-99318), domiciliary, rest home, or custodial care services (99324-99337), home services (99341-99350), or preventive medicine services (99381-99429), should be reported using modifier 25.

Allergy Testing

(For allergy laboratory tests, see 86000-86999)

(For administration of medications [eg, epinephrine, steroidal agents, antihistamines] for therapy for severe or intractable allergic reaction, use 96372)

95004   Percutaneous tests (scratch, puncture, prick) with allergenic extracts, immediate type reaction, including test interpretation and report, specify number of tests

95012   Nitric oxide expired gas determination

(95010 and 95015 have been deleted. To report, see 95017 and 95018)

95017   Allergy testing, any combination of percutaneous (scratch, puncture, prick) and intracutaneous (intradermal), sequential and incremental, with venoms, immediate type reaction, including test interpretation and report, specify number of tests

95018   Allergy testing, any combination of percutaneous (scratch, puncture, prick) and intracutaneous (intradermal), sequential and incremental, with drugs or biologicals, immediate type reaction, including test interpretation and report, specify number of tests

95024   Intracutaneous (intradermal) tests with allergenic extracts, immediate type reaction, including test interpretation and report, specify number of tests

95027   Intracutaneous (intradermal) tests, sequential and incremental, with allergenic extracts for airborne allergens, immediate type reaction, including test interpretation and report, specify number of tests

95028   Intracutaneous (intradermal) tests with allergenic extracts, delayed type reaction, including reading, specify number of tests

95044   Patch or application test(s) (specify number of tests)

95052   Photo patch test(s) (specify number of tests)

95056   Photo tests

95060   Ophthalmic mucous membrane tests

95065   Direct nasal mucous membrane test

95070   Inhalation bronchial challenge testing (not including necessary pulmonary function tests); with histamine, methacholine, or similar compounds

95071   with antigens or gases, specify

(For pulmonary function tests, see 94060, 94070)

(95075 has been deleted. For ingestion challenge testing, see 95076, 95079)

Ingestion Challenge Testing

Codes 95076 and 95079 are used to report ingestion challenge testing. Report 95076 for initial 120 minutes of testing time (ie, not physician face-to-face time). Report 95079 for each additional 60 minutes of testing time (ie, not physician face-to-face time). For total testing time less than 61 minutes (eg, positive challenge resulting in cessation of testing), report an evaluation and management service, if appropriate. Patient assessment/monitoring activities for allergic reaction (eg, blood pressure testing, peak flow meter testing) are not separately reported. Intervention therapy (eg, injection of steroid or epinephrine) may be reported separately as appropriate.

For purposes of reporting testing times, if an evaluation and management service is required, then testing time ends.

95076   Ingestion challenge test (sequential and incremental ingestion of test items, eg, food, drug or other substance); initial 120 minutes of testing

+ 95079   each additional 60 minutes of testing (List separately in addition to code for primary procedure)

(Use 95079 in conjunction with 95076)

Allergen Immunotherapy

Codes 95115-95199 include the professional services necessary for allergen immunotherapy. Office visit codes may be used in addition to allergen immunotherapy if other identifiable services are provided at that time.

95115   Professional services for allergen immunotherapy not including provision of allergenic extracts; single injection

95117   2 or more injections

95120   Professional services for allergen immunotherapy in the office or institution of the prescribing physician or other qualified health care professional, including provision of allergenic extract; single injection

95125   2 or more injections

95130   single stinging insect venom

95131   2 stinging insect venoms

95132   3 stinging insect venoms

95133	4 stinging insect venoms
95134	5 stinging insect venoms
95144	Professional services for the supervision of preparation and provision of antigens for allergen immunotherapy, single dose vial(s) (specify number of vials)

(A single dose vial contains a single dose of antigen administered in 1 injection)

95145	Professional services for the supervision of preparation and provision of antigens for allergen immunotherapy (specify number of doses); single stinging insect venom
95146	2 single stinging insect venoms
95147	3 single stinging insect venoms
95148	4 single stinging insect venoms
95149	5 single stinging insect venoms
95165	Professional services for the supervision of preparation and provision of antigens for allergen immunotherapy; single or multiple antigens (specify number of doses)
95170	whole body extract of biting insect or other arthropod (specify number of doses)

(For allergy immunotherapy reporting, a dose is the amount of antigen[s] administered in a single injection from a multiple dose vial)

95180	Rapid desensitization procedure, each hour (eg, insulin, penicillin, equine serum)
95199	Unlisted allergy/clinical immunologic service or procedure

(For skin testing of bacterial, viral, fungal extracts, see 86485-86580, 95028)

(For special reports on allergy patients, use 99080)

(For testing procedures such as radioallergosorbent testing [RAST], rat mast cell technique [RMCT], mast cell degranulation test [MCDT], lymphocytic transformation test [LTT], leukocyte histamine release [LHR], migration inhibitory factor test [MIF], transfer factor test [TFT], nitroblue tetrazolium dye test [NTD], see Immunology section in **Pathology** or use 95199)

Endocrinology

95250	Ambulatory continuous glucose monitoring of interstitial tissue fluid via a subcutaneous sensor for a minimum of 72 hours; sensor placement, hook-up, calibration of monitor, patient training, removal of sensor, and printout of recording

(Do not report 95250 more than once per month)

(Do not report 95250 in conjunction with 99091)

95251	interpretation and report

(Do not report 95251 more than once per month)

(Do not report 95251 in conjunction with 99091)

Neurology and Neuromuscular Procedures

Neurologic services are typically consultative, and any of the levels of consultation (99241-99255) may be appropriate.

In addition, services and skills outlined under **Evaluation and Management** levels of service appropriate to neurologic illnesses should be reported similarly.

The EEG, autonomic function, evoked potential, reflex tests, EMG, NCV, and MEG services (95812-95829 and 95860-95967) include recording, interpretation, and report by a physician or other qualified health care professional. For interpretation only, use modifier 26. For EMG guidance, see 95873, 95874.

Codes 95812-95822, 95950-95953 and 95956 use recording time as a basis for code use. Recording time is when the recording is underway and data is being collected. Recording time excludes set up and take down time. Codes 95961-95962 use physician or other qualified health care professional attendance time as a basis for code use.

(Do not report codes 95860-95875 in addition to 96000-96004)

Sleep Medicine Testing

Sleep medicine services include procedures that evaluate adult and pediatric patients for a variety of sleep disorders. Sleep medicine testing services are diagnostic procedures using in-laboratory and portable technology to assess physiologic data and therapy.

All sleep services (95800-95811) include recording, interpretation, and report. (Report with modifier 52 if less than 6 hours of recording for 95800, 95801 and 95806, 95807, 95810, 95811; if less than 7 hours of recording for 95782, 95783, or if less than four nap opportunities are recorded for 95805).

Definitions

For purposes of CPT reporting of sleep medicine testing services, the following definitions apply:

Actigraphy: the use of a portable, non-invasive, device that continuously records gross motor movement over an extended period of time. The periods of activity and rest are indirect parameters for estimates of the periods of wakefulness and sleep of an individual.

Attended: a technologist or qualified health care professional is physically present (ie, sufficient proximity such that the qualified health care professional can physically respond to emergencies, to other appropriate patient needs or to technical problems at the bedside) throughout the recording session.

Electrooculogram (EOG): a recording of electrical activity indicative of eye movement.

Medicine

Maintenance of wakefulness test (MWT): a standardized objective test used to determine a person's ability to stay awake. MWT requires sleep staging of the trials that are performed at defined intervals and is attended by a qualified health care professional.

Multiple sleep latency test (MSLT): a standardized objective test of the tendency to fall asleep. MSLT requires sleep staging of the nap opportunities that are performed at defined intervals and is attended by a technologist or qualified health care professional.

Peripheral arterial tonometry (PAT): a plethysmography technique that continuously measures pulsatile volume changes in a digit. This reflects the relative change of blood volume as an indirect measure of sympathetic nervous system activity which is used in respiratory analysis.

Physiological measurements of sleep as used in 95805: the parameters measured are a frontal, central and occipital lead of EEG (3 leads), submental EMG lead and a left and right EOG. These parameters are used together for staging sleep.

Polysomnography: a sleep test involving the continuous, simultaneous, recording of physiological parameters for a period of at least 6 hours that is performed in a sleep laboratory and attended by a technologist or qualified health care professional. The parameters measured are a frontal, central and occipital lead of EEG (3 leads), submental EMG lead and a left and right EOG, (from which sleep is staged), plus four or more additional parameters. The additional parameters typically required in polysomnography are listed below:

    a. Electrocardiogram (ECG)

    b. Nasal and/or oral airflow

    c. Respiratory effort

    d. Oxyhemoglobin saturation, SpO_2

    e. Bilateral anterior tibialis EMG

Positive airway pressure (PAP): a device used to treat sleep-related breathing disorders with the use of non-invasive delivery of positive pressure to the airway. Examples include but are not limited to: CPAP (continuous positive airway pressure), bilevel PAP, AutoPAP (autotitrating or adjusting PAP), ASV (adaptive-servo ventilation).

Remote: the site of service is distant from the monitoring center. Neither a technologist nor a qualified health care professional is physically present at the testing site.

Respiratory airflow (ventilation): the movement of air during inhaled and exhaled breaths. This is typically assessed using thermistor and nasal pressure sensors.

Respiratory analysis: generation of derived parameters that describe components of respiration obtained by using direct or indirect parameters, eg, by airflow or peripheral arterial tone.

Respiratory effort: contraction of the diaphragmatic and/or intercostal muscles to cause (or attempt to cause) respiratory airflow. This is typically measured using transducers that estimate motion of the thorax and abdomen such as respiratory inductive plethysmography, transducers that estimate pressures generated by breathing muscles such as esophageal monometry, or by contraction of breathing muscles, such as diaphragmatic/intercostal EMG.

Respiratory (thoracoabdominal) movement: movement of the chest and abdomen during respiratory effort.

Sleep latency: the length of time it takes to transition from wakefulness to sleep. In the sleep laboratory it is the time from "lights out" to the first epoch scored as any stage of sleep.

Sleep staging: the delineation of the distinct sleep levels through the simultaneous evaluation of physiologic measures including a frontal, central and occipital lead of EEG (3 leads), submental EMG lead and a left and right EOG.

Sleep testing (or sleep study): the continuous, simultaneous monitoring of physiological parameters during sleep (eg, polysomnography, EEG).

Total sleep time: a derived parameter obtained by sleep staging or may be estimated indirectly using actigraphy or other methods.

Unattended: a technologist or qualified health care professional is not physically present with the patient during the recording session.

    (Report with modifier 52 if less than 6 hours of recording or in other cases of reduced services as appropriate)

    (For unattended sleep study, use 95806)

95782   Code is out of numerical sequence. See 95803-95783

95783   Code is out of numerical sequence. See 95803-95783

95800   Code is out of numerical sequence. See 95803-95811

95801   Code is out of numerical sequence. See 95800-95811

95803   Actigraphy testing, recording, analysis, interpretation, and report (minimum of 72 hours to 14 consecutive days of recording)

    (Do not report 95803 more than once in any 14 day period)

    (Do not report 95803 in conjunction with 95806-95811)

95805   Multiple sleep latency or maintenance of wakefulness testing, recording, analysis and interpretation of physiological measurements of sleep during multiple trials to assess sleepiness

95806   Sleep study, unattended, simultaneous recording of, heart rate, oxygen saturation, respiratory airflow, and respiratory effort (eg, thoracoabdominal movement)

    (Do not report 95806 in conjunction with 93041-93227, 93228, 93229, 93268-93272, 95800, 95801)

Medicine

(For unattended sleep study that measures heart rate, oxygen saturation, respiratory analysis, and sleep time, use 95800)

(For unattended sleep study that measures a minimum heart rate, oxygen saturation, and respiratory analysis, use 95801)

 # 95800   Sleep study, unattended, simultaneous recording; heart rate, oxygen saturation, respiratory analysis (eg, by airflow or peripheral arterial tone), and sleep time

(Do not report 95800 in conjunction with 93041-93227, 93228, 93229, 93268-93272, 95801, 95803, 95806)

(For unattended sleep study that measures a minimum of heart rate, oxygen saturation, and respiratory analysis, use 95801)

 # 95801   minimum of heart rate, oxygen saturation, and respiratory analysis (eg, by airflow or peripheral arterial tone)

(Do not report 95801 in conjunction with 93041-93227, 93228, 93229, 93268-93272, 95800, 95806)

(For unattended sleep study that measures heart rate, oxygen saturation, respiratory analysis and sleep time, use 95800)

95807   Sleep study, simultaneous recording of ventilation, respiratory effort, ECG or heart rate, and oxygen saturation, attended by a technologist

95808   Polysomnography; any age, sleep staging with 1-3 additional parameters of sleep, attended by a technologist

95810   age 6 years or older, sleep staging with 4 or more additional parameters of sleep, attended by a technologist

95811   age 6 years or older, sleep staging with 4 or more additional parameters of sleep, with initiation of continuous positive airway pressure therapy or bilevel ventilation, attended by a technologist

 # 95782   younger than 6 years, sleep staging with 4 or more additional parameters of sleep, attended by a technologist

 # 95783   younger than 6 years, sleep staging with 4 or more additional parameters of sleep, with initiation of continuous positive airway pressure therapy or bi-level ventilation, attended by a technologist

Routine Electroencephalography (EEG)

EEG codes 95812-95822 include hyperventilation and/or photic stimulation when appropriate. Routine EEG codes 95816-95822 include 20 to 40 minutes of recording. Extended EEG codes 95812-95813 include reporting times longer than 40 minutes.

95812   Electroencephalogram (EEG) extended monitoring; 41-60 minutes

95813   greater than 1 hour

95816   Electroencephalogram (EEG); including recording awake and drowsy

95819   including recording awake and asleep

95822   recording in coma or sleep only

95824   cerebral death evaluation only

95827   all night recording

(For 24-hour EEG monitoring, see 95950-95953 or 95956)

(For EEG during nonintracranial surgery, use 95955)

(For Wada test, use 95958)

(For digital analysis of EEG, use 95957)

95829   Electrocorticogram at surgery (separate procedure)

95830   Insertion by physician or other qualified health care professional of sphenoidal electrodes for electroencephalographic (EEG) recording

Muscle and Range of Motion Testing

95831   Muscle testing, manual (separate procedure) with report; extremity (excluding hand) or trunk

95832   hand, with or without comparison with normal side

95833   total evaluation of body, excluding hands

95834   total evaluation of body, including hands

95851   Range of motion measurements and report (separate procedure); each extremity (excluding hand) or each trunk section (spine)

95852   hand, with or without comparison with normal side

95857   Cholinesterase inhibitor challenge test for myasthenia gravis

Electromyography

Needle electromyographic (EMG) procedures include the interpretation of electrical waveforms measured by equipment that produces both visible and audible components of electrical signals recorded from the muscle(s) studied by the needle electrode.

Use 95870 or 95885 when four or fewer muscles are tested in an extremity. Use 95860-95864 or 95886 when five or more muscles are tested in an extremity.

Use EMG codes (95860-95864 and 95867-95870) when no nerve conduction studies (95907-95913) are performed on that day. Use 95885, 95886, and 95887 for EMG services when nerve conduction studies (95907-95913) are performed in conjunction with EMG on the same day.

Report either 95885 or 95886 once per extremity. Codes 95885 and 95886 can be reported together up to a combined total of four units of service per patient when all four extremities are tested.

Report 95887 once per anatomic site (ie, cervical paraspinal muscle[s], thoracic paraspinal muscle[s],

Medicine

lumbar paraspinal muscle[s], chest wall muscle[s], and abdominal wall muscle[s]). Use 95887 for a unilateral study of the cranial nerve innervated muscles (excluding extra-ocular and larynx); when performed bilaterally, 95887 may be reported twice.

Use 95887 when a study of the cervical paraspinal muscle(s), or the lumbar paraspinal muscle(s) is performed with no corresponding limb study (95885 or 95886) on the same day.

(For needle electromyography of anal or urethral sphincter, use 51785)

(For non-needle electromyography of anal or urethral sphincter, use 51784)

(For needle electromyography of larynx, use 95865)

(For needle electromyography of hemidiaphragm, use 95866)

(For needle electromyography of extra-ocular muscles, use 92265)

95860   Needle electromyography; 1 extremity with or without related paraspinal areas

95861   2 extremities with or without related paraspinal areas

(For dynamic electromyography performed during motion analysis studies, see 96002-96003)

95863   3 extremities with or without related paraspinal areas

95864   4 extremities with or without related paraspinal areas

95865   larynx

(Do not report modifier 50 in conjunction with 95865)

(For unilateral procedure, report modifier 52 in conjunction with 95865)

95866   hemidiaphragm

95867   cranial nerve supplied muscle(s), unilateral

95868   cranial nerve supplied muscles, bilateral

95869   thoracic paraspinal muscles (excluding T1 or T12)

95870   limited study of muscles in 1 extremity or non-limb (axial) muscles (unilateral or bilateral), other than thoracic paraspinal, cranial nerve supplied muscles, or sphincters

(To report a complete study of the extremities, see 95860-95864)

(For anal or urethral sphincter, detrusor, urethra, perineum musculature, see 51785-51792)

(For eye muscles, use 92265)

95872   Needle electromyography using single fiber electrode, with quantitative measurement of jitter, blocking and/or fiber density, any/all sites of each muscle studied

#✚ **95885**   Needle electromyography, each extremity, with related paraspinal areas, when performed, done with nerve conduction, amplitude and latency/velocity study; limited (List separately in addition to code for primary procedure)

#✚ **95886**   complete, five or more muscles studied, innervated by three or more nerves or four or more spinal levels (List separately in addition to code for primary procedure)

(Use 95885, 95886 in conjunction with 95907-95913)

(Do not report 95885, 95886 in conjunction with 95860-95864, 95870, 95905)

#✚ **95887**   Needle electromyography, non-extremity (cranial nerve supplied or axial) muscle(s) done with nerve conduction, amplitude and latency/velocity study (List separately in addition to code for primary procedure)

(Use 95887 in conjunction with 95907-95913)

(Do not report 95887 in conjunction with 95867-95870, 95905)

Ischemic Muscle Testing and Guidance for Chemodenervation

✚ **95873**   Electrical stimulation for guidance in conjunction with chemodenervation (List separately in addition to code for primary procedure)

(Do not report 95873 in conjunction with 64617, 95860-95870, 95874)

✚ **95874**   Needle electromyography for guidance in conjunction with chemodenervation (List separately in addition to code for primary procedure)

(Use 95873, 95874 in conjunction with 64612, 64615, 64616, 64642, 64643, 64644, 64645, 64646, 64647)

(Do not report more than one guidance code for each corresponding chemodenervation code)

(Do not report 95874 in conjunction with 64617, 95860-95870, 95873)

95875   Ischemic limb exercise test with serial specimen(s) acquisition for muscle(s) metabolite(s)

(For listing of nerves considered for separate study, see **Appendix J**)

95885   Code is out of numerical sequence. See 95860-95887

95886   Code is out of numerical sequence. See 95860-95887

95887   Code is out of numerical sequence. See 95860-95887

Nerve Conduction Tests

The following applies to nerve conduction tests (95907-95913): Codes 95907-95913 describe nerve conduction tests when performed with individually placed stimulating, recording, and ground electrodes. The stimulating, recording, and ground electrode placement and the test design must be individualized to the patient's unique anatomy. Nerves tested must be limited to the specific nerves and conduction studies needed for the particular clinical question being investigated. The stimulating electrode must be placed directly over the nerve to be tested, and stimulation parameters properly adjusted to avoid stimulating other nerves or nerve branches. In most motor nerve conduction studies, and in some sensory and mixed nerve conduction studies, both proximal and distal stimulation will be used. Motor nerve conduction study recordings must be made from electrodes placed directly over the motor point of the specific muscle to be tested. Sensory nerve conduction study recordings must be made from electrodes placed directly over the specific nerve to be tested. Waveforms must be reviewed on site in real time, and the technique (stimulus site, recording site, ground site, filter settings) must be adjusted, as appropriate, as the test proceeds in order to minimize artifact, and to minimize the chances of unintended stimulation of adjacent nerves and the unintended recording from adjacent muscles or nerves. Reports must be prepared on site by the examiner, and consist of the work product of the interpretation of numerous test results, using well-established techniques to assess the amplitude, latency, and configuration of waveforms elicited by stimulation at each site of each nerve tested. This includes the calculation of nerve conduction velocities, sometimes including specialized F-wave indices, along with comparison to normal values, summarization of clinical and electrodiagnostic data, and physician or other qualified health care professional interpretation. Codes 95907-95913 describe one or more nerve conduction studies. For the purposes of coding, a single conduction study is defined as a sensory conduction test, a motor conduction test with or without an F wave test, or an H-reflex test. Each type of study (sensory, motor with or without F wave, H-reflex) for each nerve includes all orthodromic and antidromic impulses associated with that nerve and constitutes a distinct study when determining the number of studies in each grouping (eg, 1-2 or 3-4 nerve conduction studies). Each type of nerve conduction study is counted only once when multiple sites on the same nerve are stimulated or recorded. The numbers of these separate tests should be added to determine which code to use. For a list of nerves, see Appendix J. Use 95885-95887 in conjunction with 95907-95913 when performing electromyography with nerve conduction studies.

Code 95905 describes nerve conduction tests when performed with preconfigured electrodes customized to a specific anatomic site.

(95900, 95903, 95904 have been deleted. For nerve conduction studies, see 95907-95913)

⊘ **95905**　　Motor and/or sensory nerve conduction, using preconfigured electrode array(s), amplitude and latency/velocity study, each limb, includes F-wave study when performed, with interpretation and report;

(Report 95905 only once per limb studied)

(Do not report 95905 in conjunction with 95885, 95886, 95907-95913)

95907　　Nerve conduction studies; 1-2 studies

95908　　　　3-4 studies

95909　　　　5-6 studies

95910　　　　7-8 studies

95911　　　　9-10 studies

95912　　　　11-12 studies

95913　　　　13 or more studies

Intraoperative Neurophysiology

Codes 95940, 95941 describe ongoing neurophysiologic monitoring, testing, and data interpretation distinct from performance of specific type(s) of baseline neurophysiologic study(s) performed during surgical procedures. When the service is performed by the surgeon or anesthesiologist, the professional services are included in the surgeon's or anesthesiologist's primary service code(s) for the procedure and are not reported separately. Do not report these codes for automated monitoring devices that do not require continuous attendance by a professional qualified to interpret the testing and monitoring.

Recording and testing are performed either personally or by a technologist who is physically present with the patient during the service. Supervision is performed either in the operating room or by real time connection outside the operating room. The monitoring professional must be solely dedicated to performing the intraoperative neurophysiologic monitoring and must be available to intervene at all times during the service as necessary, for the reported time period(s). For any given period of time spent providing these services, the service takes full attention and, therefore, other clinical activities beyond providing and interpreting of monitoring cannot be provided during the same period of time.

Throughout the monitoring, there must be provisions for continuous and immediate communication directly with the operating room team in the surgical suite. One or more simultaneous cases may be reported (95941). When monitoring more than one procedure, there must be the immediate ability to transfer patient monitoring to another monitoring professional during the surgical procedure should that individual's exclusive attention be required for another procedure. Report 95941 for all remote or non-one-on-one monitoring time connected to each case regardless of overlap with other cases.

Codes 95940, 95941 include only the ongoing neurophysiologic monitoring time distinct from performance of specific type(s) of baseline neurophysiologic study(s), or other services such as intraoperative functional cortical or subcortical mapping. Codes 95940 and 95941 are reported based upon the time spent monitoring only, and not the number of baseline tests performed or parameters monitored. The time spent performing or interpreting the baseline neurophysiologic study(ies) should not be counted as intraoperative monitoring, but represents separately reportable procedures. When reporting 95940 and 95941, the same neurophysiologic study(ies) performed at baseline should be reported not more than once per

Medicine

operative session. Baseline study reporting is based upon the total unique studies performed. For example, if during the course of baseline testing and one-on-one monitoring, two separate nerves have motor testing performed in conjunction with limited single extremity EMG, then 95885 and 95907 would be reported in addition to 95940. Time spent monitoring (95940, 95941) excludes time to set up, record, and interpret the baseline studies, and to remove electrodes at the end of the procedure. To report time spent waiting on standby for a case to start, use 99360. For procedures that last beyond midnight, report services using the day on which the monitoring began and using the total time monitored.

Code 95940 is reported per 15 minutes of service. Code 95940 requires reporting only the portion of time the monitoring professional was physically present in the operating room providing one-on-one patient monitoring, and no other cases may be monitored at the same time. Time spent in the operating room is cumulative. To determine units of service of 95940, use the total minutes monitoring in the operating room one-on-one. Monitoring may begin prior to incision (eg, when positioning on the table is a time of risk). Report continuous intraoperative neurophysiologic monitoring in the operating room (95940) in addition to the services related to monitoring from outside the operating room (95941).

Code 95941 should be used once per hour even if multiple methods of neurophysiologic monitoring are used during the time. Code 95941 requires the monitoring of neurophysiological data that is collected from the operating room continuously on-line in real time via a secure data link. When reporting 95941, real-time ability must be available through sufficient data bandwidth transfer rates to view and interrogate the neurophysiologic data contemporaneously.

Report 95941 for all cases in which there was no physical presence by the monitoring professional in the operating room during the monitoring time or when monitoring more than one case in an operating room. It is also used to report the time of monitoring physically performed outside of the operating room in those cases where monitoring occurred both within and outside the operating room. Do not report 95941 if the monitoring lasts 30 minutes or less.

Intraoperative neurophysiology monitoring codes 95940 and 95941 are each used to report the total duration of respective time spent providing each service, even if that time is not in a single continuous block.

(95920 has been deleted. To report, see 95940, 95941)

#+ **95940**　Continuous intraoperative neurophysiology monitoring in the operating room, one on one monitoring requiring personal attendance, each 15 minutes (List separately in addition to code for primary procedure)

(Use 95940 in conjunction with the study performed, 92585, 95822, 95860-95870, 95907-95913, 95925, 95926, 95927, 95928, 95929, 95930-95937, 95938, 95939)

#+ **95941**　Continuous intraoperative neurophysiology monitoring, from outside the operating room (remote or nearby) or for monitoring of more than one case while in the operating room, per hour (List separately in addition to code for primary procedure)

(Use 95941 in conjunction with the study performed, 92585, 95822, 95860-95870, 95907-95913, 95925, 95926, 95927, 95928, 95929, 95930-95937, 95938, 95939)

(For time spent waiting on standby before monitoring, use 99360)

(For electrocorticography, use 95829)

(For intraoperative EEG during nonintracranial surgery, use 95955)

(For intraoperative functional cortical or subcortical mapping, see 95961-95962)

(For intraoperative neurostimulator programming and analysis, see 95970-95975)

Autonomic Function Tests

The purpose of autonomic nervous system function testing is to determine the presence of autonomic dysfunction, the site of autonomic dysfunction, and the various autonomic subsystems that may be disordered.

Code 95921 should be reported only when electrocardiographic monitoring of heart rate derived from the time elapsing between two consecutive R waves in the electrocardiogram, or the R-R interval, is displayed on a monitor and stored for subsequent analysis of waveforms. Testing is typically performed in the prone position. A tilt table may be used, but is not required equipment for testing of the parasympathetic function. At least two of the following components need to be included in testing:

1. Heart rate response to deep breathing derived from a visual quantitative analysis of recordings with subject breathing at a rate of 5-6 breaths per minute.

2. Valsalva ratio determined by dividing the maximum heart rate by the lowest heart rate. The initial heart rate responses to sustained oral pressure (blowing into a tube with an open glottis) consist of tachycardia followed by a bradycardia at 15-45 seconds after the Valsalva pressure has been released. A minimum of two Valsalva maneuvers are to be performed. The initial cardioacceleration is an exercise reflex while the subsequent tachycardia and bradycardia are baroreflex-mediated.

3. A 30:15 ratio (R-R interval at beat 30)/(R-R interval at beat 15) used as an index of cardiovascular function.

Code 95922 should be reported only when all of the following components are included in testing:

1. Continuous recording of beat-to-beat BP and heart rate. The heart rate needs to be derived from an electrocardiogram (ECG) unit such that an accurate quantitative graphical measurement of the R-R interval is obtained.

2. A period of supine rest of at least 20 minutes prior to testing.

3. The performance and recording of beat-to-beat blood pressure and heart rate during a minimum of two (2) Valsalva maneuvers.

4. The performance of passive head-up tilt with continuous recording of beat-to-beat blood pressure and heart rate for a minimum of five minutes, followed by passive tilt-back to the supine position. This must be performed using a tilt table.

Code 95924 should be reported only when both the parasympathetic function and the adrenergic function are tested together with the use of a tilt table.

(To report autonomic function testing that does not include beat-to-beat recording or for testing without use of a tilt table, use 95943)

95921 Testing of autonomic nervous system function; cardiovagal innervation (parasympathetic function), including 2 or more of the following: heart rate response to deep breathing with recorded R-R interval, Valsalva ratio, and 30:15 ratio

95922 vasomotor adrenergic innervation (sympathetic adrenergic function), including beat-to-beat blood pressure and R-R interval changes during Valsalva maneuver and at least 5 minutes of passive tilt

(Do not report 95922 in conjunction with 95921)

95923 sudomotor, including 1 or more of the following: quantitative sudomotor axon reflex test (QSART), silastic sweat imprint, thermoregulatory sweat test, and changes in sympathetic skin potential

95924 combined parasympathetic and sympathetic adrenergic function testing with at least 5 minutes of passive tilt

(Do not report 95924 in conjunction with 95921 or 95922)

 # 95943 Simultaneous, independent, quantitative measures of both parasympathetic function and sympathetic function, based on time-frequency analysis of heart rate variability concurrent with time-frequency analysis of continuous respiratory activity, with mean heart rate and blood pressure measures, during rest, paced (deep) breathing, Valsalva maneuvers, and head-up postural change

(Do not report 95943 in conjunction with 93040, 95921, 95922, 95924)

Evoked Potentials and Reflex Tests

95925 Short-latency somatosensory evoked potential study, stimulation of any/all peripheral nerves or skin sites, recording from the central nervous system; in upper limbs

(Do not report 95925 in conjunction with 95926)

95926 in lower limbs

(Do not report 95926 in conjunction with 95925)

 # 95938 in upper and lower limbs

(Do not report 95938 in conjunction with 95925, 95926)

95927 in the trunk or head

(To report a unilateral study, use modifier 52)

(For auditory evoked potentials, use 92585)

95928 Central motor evoked potential study (transcranial motor stimulation); upper limbs

(Do not report 95928 in conjunction with 95929)

95929 lower limbs

(Do not report 95929 in conjunction with 95928)

 # 95939 in upper and lower limbs

(Do not report 95939 in conjunction with 95928, 95929)

95930 Visual evoked potential (VEP) testing central nervous system, checkerboard or flash

(For screening of visual acuity using automated visual evoked potential devices, use 0333T)

95933 Orbicularis oculi (blink) reflex, by electrodiagnostic testing

(95934, 95936 have been deleted. To report H-reflex testing, see 95907-95913)

95937 Neuromuscular junction testing (repetitive stimulation, paired stimuli), each nerve, any 1 method

95938 Code is out of numerical sequence. See 95925-95939

95939 Code is out of numerical sequence. See 95925-95939

95940 Code is out of numerical sequence. See 95921-95943

95941 Code is out of numerical sequence. See 95921-95943

95943 Code is out of numerical sequence. See 95921-95943

Special EEG Tests

Codes 95950-95953 and 95956 are used per 24 hours of recording. For recording more than 12 hours, do not use modifier 52. For recording 12 hours or less, use modifier 52. Codes 95951 and 95956 are used for recordings in which interpretations can be made throughout the recording time, with interventions to alter or end the recording or to alter the patient care during the recordings as needed.

Medicine

Codes 95961 and 95962 use physician or other qualified health care professional time as a basis for unit of service. Report 95961 for the first hour of attendance. Use modifier 52 with 95961 for 30 minutes or less. Report 95962 for each additional hour of attendance.

95950 Monitoring for identification and lateralization of cerebral seizure focus, electroencephalographic (eg, 8 channel EEG) recording and interpretation, each 24 hours

95951 Monitoring for localization of cerebral seizure focus by cable or radio, 16 or more channel telemetry, combined electroencephalographic (EEG) and video recording and interpretation (eg, for presurgical localization), each 24 hours

95953 Monitoring for localization of cerebral seizure focus by computerized portable 16 or more channel EEG, electroencephalographic (EEG) recording and interpretation, each 24 hours, unattended

95954 Pharmacological or physical activation requiring physician or other qualified health care professional attendance during EEG recording of activation phase (eg, thiopental activation test)

95955 Electroencephalogram (EEG) during nonintracranial surgery (eg, carotid surgery)

95956 Monitoring for localization of cerebral seizure focus by cable or radio, 16 or more channel telemetry, electroencephalographic (EEG) recording and interpretation, each 24 hours, attended by a technologist or nurse

95957 Digital analysis of electroencephalogram (EEG) (eg, for epileptic spike analysis)

95958 Wada activation test for hemispheric function, including electroencephalographic (EEG) monitoring

95961 Functional cortical and subcortical mapping by stimulation and/or recording of electrodes on brain surface, or of depth electrodes, to provoke seizures or identify vital brain structures; initial hour of attendance by a physician or other qualified health care professional

+ 95962 each additional hour of attendance by a physician or other qualified health care professional (List separately in addition to code for primary procedure)

(Use 95962 in conjunction with 95961)

95965 Magnetoencephalography (MEG), recording and analysis; for spontaneous brain magnetic activity (eg, epileptic cerebral cortex localization)

95966 for evoked magnetic fields, single modality (eg, sensory, motor, language, or visual cortex localization)

+ 95967 for evoked magnetic fields, each additional modality (eg, sensory, motor, language, or visual cortex localization) (List separately in addition to code for primary procedure)

(Use 95967 in conjunction with 95966)

(For electroencephalography performed in addition to magnetoencephalography, see 95812-95827)

(For somatosensory evoked potentials, auditory evoked potentials, and visual evoked potentials performed in addition to magnetic evoked field responses, see 92585, 95925, 95926, and/or 95930)

(For computerized tomography performed in addition to magnetoencephalography, see 70450-70470, 70496)

(For magnetic resonance imaging performed in addition to magnetoencephalography, see 70551-70553)

Neurostimulators, Analysis-Programming

Simple intraoperative or subsequent programming of the neurostimulator pulse generator/transmitter (95971) includes changes to three or fewer of the following parameters: rate, pulse amplitude, pulse duration, pulse frequency, eight or more electrode contacts, cycling, stimulation train duration, train spacing, number of programs, number of channels, alternating electrode polarities, dose time (stimulation parameters changing in time periods of minutes including dose lockout times), more than one clinical feature (eg, rigidity, dyskinesia, tremor). Complex intraoperative or subsequent programming (95972-95979) includes changes to more than three of the above.

►Code 95970 describes subsequent electronic analysis of a previously implanted simple or complex brain, spinal cord, or peripheral neurostimulator pulse generator system, without reprogramming. Code 95971 describes intraoperative or subsequent electronic analysis of an implanted simple spinal cord, or peripheral (ie, peripheral nerve, autonomic nerve, neuromuscular) neurostimulator pulse generator system, with programming. Code 95972 describes intraoperative (at initial insertion/revision) or subsequent electronic analysis of an implanted complex spinal cord or peripheral (except cranial nerve) neurostimulator pulse generator system, with programming. Codes 95974 and 95975 describe intraoperative (at initial insertion/revision) or subsequent electronic analysis of an implanted complex cranial nerve neurostimulator pulse generator system, with programming. Codes 95978 and 95979 describe initial or subsequent electronic analysis of an implanted brain neurostimulator pulse generator system, with programming.◄

Code 95980 describes intraoperative electronic analysis of an implanted gastric neurostimulator pulse generator system, with programming; code 95981 describes subsequent analysis of the device; code 95982 describes subsequent analysis and reprogramming. For electronic analysis and reprogramming of gastric neurostimulator, lesser curvature, see 95980-95982.

►For 95974 and 95978, use modifier 52 if less than 31 minutes in duration.◄

(For electronic analysis and reprogramming of a peripheral subcutaneous field stimulation pulse generator, use 0285T)

(For insertion of neurostimulator pulse generator, see 61885, 63685, 64590)

(For revision or removal of neurostimulator pulse generator or receiver, see 61888, 63688, 64595)

(For implantation of neurostimulator electrodes, see 43647, 43881, 61850-61870, 63650-63655, 64553-64580. For revision or removal of neurostimulator electrodes, see 43648, 43882, 61880, 63661-63664, 64585)

95970   Electronic analysis of implanted neurostimulator pulse generator system (eg, rate, pulse amplitude, pulse duration, configuration of wave form, battery status, electrode selectability, output modulation, cycling, impedance and patient compliance measurements); simple or complex brain, spinal cord, or peripheral (ie, cranial nerve, peripheral nerve, sacral nerve, neuromuscular) neurostimulator pulse generator/transmitter, without reprogramming

95971   simple spinal cord, or peripheral (ie, peripheral nerve, sacral nerve, neuromuscular) neurostimulator pulse generator/transmitter, with intraoperative or subsequent programming

▲ **95972**   complex spinal cord, or peripheral (ie, peripheral nerve, sacral nerve, neuromuscular) (except cranial nerve) neurostimulator pulse generator/transmitter, with intraoperative or subsequent programming

►(95973 has been deleted)◄

95974   complex cranial nerve neurostimulator pulse generator/transmitter, with intraoperative or subsequent programming, with or without nerve interface testing, first hour

+ **95975**   complex cranial nerve neurostimulator pulse generator/transmitter, with intraoperative or subsequent programming, each additional 30 minutes after first hour (List separately in addition to code for primary procedure)

(Use 95975 in conjunction with 95974)

95978   Electronic analysis of implanted neurostimulator pulse generator system (eg, rate, pulse amplitude and duration, battery status, electrode selectability and polarity, impedance and patient compliance measurements), complex deep brain neurostimulator pulse generator/transmitter, with initial or subsequent programming; first hour

+ **95979**   each additional 30 minutes after first hour (List separately in addition to code for primary procedure)

(Use 95979 in conjunction with 95978)

95980   Electronic analysis of implanted neurostimulator pulse generator system (eg, rate, pulse amplitude and duration, configuration of wave form, battery status, electrode selectability, output modulation, cycling, impedance and patient measurements) gastric neurostimulator pulse generator/transmitter; intraoperative, with programming

95981   subsequent, without reprogramming

95982   subsequent, with reprogramming

(For intraoperative or subsequent analysis, with programming, when performed, of vagus nerve trunk stimulator used for blocking therapy [morbid obesity], see 0312T, 0317T)

Other Procedures

95990   Refilling and maintenance of implantable pump or reservoir for drug delivery, spinal (intrathecal, epidural) or brain (intraventricular), includes electronic analysis of pump, when performed;

95991   requiring skill of a physician or other qualified health care professional

(Do not report 95990, 95991 in conjunction with 62367-62370. For analysis and/or reprogramming of implantable infusion pump, see 62367-62370)

(For refill and maintenance of implanted infusion pump or reservoir for systemic drug therapy [eg, chemotherapy], use 96522)

⊘ **95992**   Canalith repositioning procedure(s) (eg, Epley maneuver, Semont maneuver), per day

(Do not report 95992 in conjunction with 92531, 92532)

95999   Unlisted neurological or neuromuscular diagnostic procedure

Motion Analysis

Codes 96000-96004 describe services performed as part of a major therapeutic or diagnostic decision making process. Motion analysis is performed in a dedicated motion analysis laboratory (ie, a facility capable of performing videotaping from the front, back and both sides, computerized 3D kinematics, 3D kinetics, and dynamic electromyography). Code 96000 may include 3D kinetics and stride characteristics. Codes 96002-96003 describe dynamic electromyography.

Code 96004 should only be reported once regardless of the number of study(ies) reviewed/interpreted.

(For performance of needle electromyography procedures, see 95860-95870, 95872, 95885-95887)

(For gait training, use 97116)

96000   Comprehensive computer-based motion analysis by video-taping and 3D kinematics;

96001   with dynamic plantar pressure measurements during walking

Medicine

96002   Dynamic surface electromyography, during walking or other functional activities, 1-12 muscles

96003   Dynamic fine wire electromyography, during walking or other functional activities, 1 muscle

         (Do not report 96002, 96003 in conjunction with 95860-95866, 95869-95872, 95885-95887)

96004   Review and interpretation by physician or other qualified health care professional of comprehensive computer-based motion analysis, dynamic plantar pressure measurements, dynamic surface electromyography during walking or other functional activities, and dynamic fine wire electromyography, with written report

Functional Brain Mapping

Code 96020 includes selection and administration of testing of language, memory, cognition, movement, sensation, and other neurological functions when conducted in association with functional neuroimaging, monitoring of performance of this testing, and determination of validity of neurofunctional testing relative to separately interpreted functional magnetic resonance images.

96020   Neurofunctional testing selection and administration during noninvasive imaging functional brain mapping, with test administered entirely by a physician or other qualified health care professional (ie, psychologist), with review of test results and report

         (For functional magnetic resonance imaging [fMRI], brain, use 70555)

         (Do not report 96020 in conjunction with 96101-96103, 96116-96120)

         (Do not report 96020 in conjunction with 70554)

         (Evaluation and Management services codes should not be reported on the same day as 96020)

Medical Genetics and Genetic Counseling Services

These services are provided by trained genetic counselors and may include obtaining a structured family genetic history, pedigree construction, analysis for genetic risk assessment, and counseling of the patient and family. These activities may be provided during one or more sessions and may include review of medical data and family information, face-to-face interviews, and counseling services.

Code 96040 is reported for each 30-minute increment of face-to-face time. Do not report 96040 for 15 minutes or less of face-to-face time. Report 96040 once for 16 to 30 minutes of face-to-face time.

96040   Medical genetics and genetic counseling services, each 30 minutes face-to-face with patient/family

         (For genetic counseling and education provided to an individual by a physician or other qualified health care professional who may report evaluation and management services, see the appropriate Evaluation and Management codes)

         (For genetic counseling and education to a group by a physician or other qualified health care professional, use 99078)

         (For education regarding genetic risks by a nonphysician to a group, see 98961, 98962)

         (For genetic counseling and/or risk factor reduction intervention provided to patient(s) without symptoms or established disease, by a physician or other qualified health care professional who may report evaluation and management services, see 99401-99412)

Central Nervous System Assessments/Tests (eg, Neuro-Cognitive, Mental Status, Speech Testing)

The following codes are used to report the services provided during testing of the cognitive function of the central nervous system. The testing of cognitive processes, visual motor responses, and abstractive abilities is accomplished by the combination of several types of testing procedures. It is expected that the administration of these tests will generate material that will be formulated into a report. A minimum of 31 minutes must be provided to report any per hour code. Services 96101, 96116, 96118 and 96125 report time as face-to-face time with the patient and the time spent interpreting and preparing the report.

         (For development of cognitive skills, see 97532, 97533)

         (For mini-mental status examination performed by a physician, see **Evaluation and Management** services codes)

         (Do not report 96101-96125 in conjunction with 0364T, 0365T, 0366T, 0367T, 0373T, 0374T)

96101   Psychological testing (includes psychodiagnostic assessment of emotionality, intellectual abilities, personality and psychopathology, eg, MMPI, Rorschach, WAIS), per hour of the psychologist's or physician's time, both face-to-face time administering tests to the patient and time interpreting these test results and preparing the report

         (96101 is also used in those circumstances when additional time is necessary to integrate other sources of clinical data, including previously completed and reported technician- and computer-administered tests)

         (Do not report 96101 for the interpretation and report of 96102, 96103)

96102   Psychological testing (includes psychodiagnostic assessment of emotionality, intellectual abilities, personality and psychopathology, eg, MMPI and WAIS), with qualified health care professional interpretation and report, administered by technician, per hour of technician time, face-to-face

96103   Psychological testing (includes psychodiagnostic assessment of emotionality, intellectual abilities, personality and psychopathology, eg, MMPI), administered by a computer, with qualified health care professional interpretation and report

96105   Assessment of aphasia (includes assessment of expressive and receptive speech and language function, language comprehension, speech production ability, reading, spelling, writing, eg, by Boston Diagnostic Aphasia Examination) with interpretation and report, per hour

96110   Developmental screening (eg, developmental milestone survey, speech and language delay screen), with scoring and documentation, per standardized instrument

(For an emotional/behavioral assessment, use 96127)

96111   Developmental testing, (includes assessment of motor, language, social, adaptive, and/or cognitive functioning by standardized developmental instruments) with interpretation and report

96116   Neurobehavioral status exam (clinical assessment of thinking, reasoning and judgment, eg, acquired knowledge, attention, language, memory, planning and problem solving, and visual spatial abilities), per hour of the psychologist's or physician's time, both face-to-face time with the patient and time interpreting test results and preparing the report

96118   Neuropsychological testing (eg, Halstead-Reitan Neuropsychological Battery, Wechsler Memory Scales and Wisconsin Card Sorting Test), per hour of the psychologist's or physician's time, both face-to-face time administering tests to the patient and time interpreting these test results and preparing the report

(96118 is also used in those circumstances when additional time is necessary to integrate other sources of clinical data, including previously completed and reported technician- and computer-administered tests)

(Do not report 96118 for the interpretation and report of 96119 or 96120)

96119   Neuropsychological testing (eg, Halstead-Reitan Neuropsychological Battery, Wechsler Memory Scales and Wisconsin Card Sorting Test), with qualified health care professional interpretation and report, administered by technician, per hour of technician time, face-to-face

96120   Neuropsychological testing (eg, Wisconsin Card Sorting Test), administered by a computer, with qualified health care professional interpretation and report

96125   Standardized cognitive performance testing (eg, Ross Information Processing Assessment) per hour of a qualified health care professional's time, both face-to-face time administering tests to the patient and time interpreting these test results and preparing the report

(For psychological and neuropsychological testing by a physician or psychologist, see 96101-96103, 96118-96120)

96127   Brief emotional/behavioral assessment (eg, depression inventory, attention-deficit/hyperactivity disorder [ADHD] scale), with scoring and documentation, per standardized instrument

(For developmental screening, use 96110)

Health and Behavior Assessment/Intervention

Health and behavior assessment procedures are used to identify the psychological, behavioral, emotional, cognitive, and social factors important to the prevention, treatment, or management of physical health problems.

The focus of the assessment is not on mental health but on the biopsychosocial factors important to physical health problems and treatments. The focus of the intervention is to improve the patient's health and well-being utilizing cognitive, behavioral, social, and/or psychophysiological procedures designed to ameliorate specific disease-related problems.

Codes 96150-96155 describe services offered to patients who present with primary physical illnesses, diagnoses, or symptoms and may benefit from assessments and interventions that focus on the biopsychosocial factors related to the patient's health status. These services do not represent preventive medicine counseling and risk factor reduction interventions.

For patients that require psychiatric services (90785-90899) as well as health and behavior assessment/intervention (96150-96155), report the predominant service performed. Do not report 96150-96155 in conjunction with 90785-90899 on the same date.

Evaluation and Management services codes (including Counseling Risk Factor Reduction and Behavior Change Intervention [99401-99412]), should not be reported on the same day.

(For health and behavior assessment and/or intervention performed by a physician or other qualified health care professional who may report evaluation and management services, see **Evaluation and Management** or **Preventive Medicine** services codes)

(Do not report 96150, 96151, 96152, 96153, 96154, 96155 in conjunction with 0364T, 0365T, 0366T, 0367T, 0373T, 0374T)

Medicine

96150 Health and behavior assessment (eg, health-focused clinical interview, behavioral observations, psychophysiological monitoring, health-oriented questionnaires), each 15 minutes face-to-face with the patient; initial assessment

96151 re-assessment

96152 Health and behavior intervention, each 15 minutes, face-to-face; individual

96153 group (2 or more patients)

96154 family (with the patient present)

96155 family (without the patient present)

Hydration, Therapeutic, Prophylactic, Diagnostic Injections and Infusions, and Chemotherapy and Other Highly Complex Drug or Highly Complex Biologic Agent Administration

Physician or other qualified health care professional work related to hydration, injection, and infusion services predominantly involves affirmation of treatment plan and direct supervision of staff.

Codes 96360-96379, 96401, 96402, 96409-96425, 96521-96523 are not intended to be reported by the physician in the facility setting. If a significant, separately identifiable office or other outpatient Evaluation and Management service is performed, the appropriate E/M service (99201-99215, 99241-99245, 99354-99355) should be reported using modifier 25 in addition to 96360-96549. For same day E/M service, a different diagnosis is not required.

If performed to facilitate the infusion or injection, the following services are included and are not reported separately:

a. Use of local anesthesia

b. IV start

c. Access to indwelling IV, subcutaneous catheter or port

d. Flush at conclusion of infusion

e. Standard tubing, syringes, and supplies

> (For declotting a catheter or port, use 36593)

When multiple drugs are administered, report the service(s) and the specific materials or drugs for each.

When administering multiple infusions, injections or combinations, only one "initial" service code should be reported for a given date, unless protocol requires that two separate IV sites must be used. Do not report a second initial service on the same date due to an intravenous line requiring a re-start, an IV rate not being able to be reached without two lines, or for accessing a port of a multi-lumen catheter. If an injection or infusion is of a subsequent or concurrent nature, even if it is the first such service within that group of services, then a subsequent or concurrent code from the appropriate section should be reported (eg, the first IV push given subsequent to an initial one-hour infusion is reported using a subsequent IV push code).

Initial infusion: For physician or other qualified health care professional reporting, an initial infusion is the *key or primary reason for the encounter* reported irrespective of the temporal order in which the infusion(s) or injection(s) are administered. For facility reporting, an initial infusion is based using the hierarchy. For both physician or other qualified health care professional and facility reporting, only one *initial* service code (eg, 96365) should be reported unless the protocol or patient condition requires that two separate IV sites must be utilized. The difference in time and effort in providing this second IV site access is also reported using the *initial* service code with modifier 59 appended (eg, 96365, 96365-59).

Sequential infusion: A sequential infusion is an infusion or IV push of a new substance or drug following a primary or initial service. All sequential services require that there be a new substance or drug, except that facilities may report a sequential intravenous push of the same drug using 96376.

Concurrent infusion: A concurrent infusion is an infusion of a new substance or drug infused at the same time as another substance or drug. A concurrent infusion service is not time based and is only reported once per day regardless of whether an additional new drug or substance is administered concurrently. Hydration may not be reported concurrently with any other service. A separate subsequent concurrent administration of another new drug or substance (the third substance or drug) is not reported.

In order to determine which service should be reported as the initial service when there is more than one type of service, hierarchies have been created. These vary by whether the physician or other qualified health care professional or a facility is reporting. The order of selection for reporting is based upon the physician's or other qualified health care professional's knowledge of the clinical condition(s) and treatment(s). The hierarchy that facilities are to use is based upon a structural algorithm. When these codes are reported by the physician or other qualified health care professional, the "initial" code that best describes the key or primary reason for the encounter should always be reported irrespective of the order in which the infusions or injections occur.

When these codes are reported *by the facility*, the following instructions apply. The initial code should be selected using a hierarchy whereby chemotherapy services are primary to therapeutic, prophylactic, and diagnostic services which are primary to hydration services. Infusions are primary to pushes, which are primary to injections. This hierarchy is to be followed by facilities and supersedes parenthetical instructions for add-on codes that suggest an add-on of a higher hierarchical position may be reported in conjunction with a base code of a lower position. (For example, the hierarchy would not permit reporting 96376 with 96360, as 96376 is a higher order code. IV push is primary to hydration.)

When reporting multiple infusions of the same drug/substance on the same date of service, the initial code should be selected. The second and subsequent infusion(s) should be reported based on the individual time(s) of each additional infusion(s) of the same drug/substance using the appropriate add-on code.

Example: In the outpatient observation setting, a patient receives one-hour intravenous infusions of the same antibiotic every 8 hours on the same date of service through the same IV access. The hierarchy for facility reporting permits the reporting of code 96365 for the first one-hour dose administered. Add-on 96366 would be reported twice (once for the second and third one-hour infusions of the same drug).

When reporting codes for which infusion time is a factor, use the actual time over which the infusion is administered. Intravenous or intra-arterial push is defined as: (a) an injection in which the individual who administers the drug/substance is continuously present to administer the injection and observe the patient, or (b) an infusion of 15 minutes or less. If intravenous hydration (96360, 96361) is given from 11 PM to 2 AM, 96360 would be reported once and 96361 twice. For continuous services that last beyond midnight, use the date in which the service began and report the total units of time provided continuously. However, if instead of a continuous infusion, a medication was given by intravenous push at 10 PM and 2 AM, as the service was not continuous, the two administrations would be reported as an initial service (96374) and sequential (96376) as: (1) no other infusion services were performed; and (2) the push of the same drug was performed more than 30 minutes beyond the initial administration. A "keep open" infusion of any type is not separately reported.

Hydration

Codes 96360-96361 are intended to report a hydration IV infusion to consist of a pre-packaged fluid and electrolytes (eg, normal saline, D5-1/2 normal saline+30mEq KCl/liter), but are not used to report infusion of drugs or other substances. Hydration IV infusions typically require direct supervision for purposes of consent, safety oversight, or intraservice supervision of staff. Typically such infusions require little special handling to prepare or dispose of, and staff that administer these do not typically require advanced

practice training. After initial set-up, infusion typically entails little patient risk and thus little monitoring. These codes are not intended to be reported by the physician or other qualified health care professional in the facility setting.

Some chemotherapeutic agents and other therapeutic agents require pre- and/or post-hydration to be given in order to avoid specific toxicities. A minimum time duration of 31 minutes of hydration infusion is required to report the service. However, the hydration codes 96360 or 96361 are not used when the purpose of the intravenous fluid is to "keep open" an IV line prior or subsequent to a therapeutic infusion, or as a free-flowing IV during chemotherapy or other therapeutic infusion.

96360 Intravenous infusion, hydration; initial, 31 minutes to 1 hour

(Do not report 96360 if performed as a concurrent infusion service)

(Do not report intravenous infusion for hydration of 30 minutes or less)

+ 96361 each additional hour (List separately in addition to code for primary procedure)

(Use 96361 in conjunction with 96360)

(Report 96361 for hydration infusion intervals of greater than 30 minutes beyond 1 hour increments)

(Report 96361 to identify hydration if provided as a secondary or subsequent service after a different initial service [96360, 96365, 96374, 96409, 96413] is administered through the same IV access)

Therapeutic, Prophylactic, and Diagnostic Injections and Infusions (Excludes Chemotherapy and Other Highly Complex Drug or Highly Complex Biologic Agent Administration)

A therapeutic, prophylactic, or diagnostic IV infusion or injection (other than hydration) is for the administration of substances/drugs. When fluids are used to administer the drug(s), the administration of the fluid is considered incidental hydration and is not separately reportable. These services typically require direct supervision for any or all purposes of patient assessment, provision of consent, safety oversight, and intra-service supervision of staff. Typically, such infusions require special consideration to prepare, dose or dispose of, require practice training and competency for staff who administer the infusions, and require periodic patient assessment with vital sign monitoring during the infusion. These codes are not intended to be reported by the physician or other qualified health care professional in the facility setting.

Medicine

See codes 96401-96549 for the administration of chemotherapy or other highly complex drug or highly complex biologic agent services. These highly complex services require advanced practice training and competency for staff who provide these services; special considerations for preparation, dosage or disposal; and commonly, these services entail significant patient risk and frequent monitoring. Examples are frequent changes in the infusion rate, prolonged presence of nurse administering the solution for patient monitoring and infusion adjustments, and frequent conferring with the physician or other qualified health care professional about these issues.

(Do not report 96365-96379 with codes for which IV push or infusion is an inherent part of the procedure [eg, administration of contrast material for a diagnostic imaging study])

96365   Intravenous infusion, for therapy, prophylaxis, or diagnosis (specify substance or drug); initial, up to 1 hour

+ 96366   each additional hour (List separately in addition to code for primary procedure)

(Report 96366 in conjunction with 96365, 96367)

(Report 96366 for additional hour[s] of sequential infusion)

(Report 96366 for infusion intervals of greater than 30 minutes beyond 1 hour increments)

(Report 96366 in conjunction with 96365 to identify each second and subsequent infusions of the same drug/substance)

+ 96367   additional sequential infusion of a new drug/substance, up to 1 hour (List separately in addition to code for primary procedure)

(Report 96367 in conjunction with 96365, 96374, 96409, 96413 to identify the infusion of a new drug/substance provided as a secondary or subsequent service after a different initial service is administered through the same IV access. Report 96367 only once per sequential infusion of same infusate mix)

+ 96368   concurrent infusion (List separately in addition to code for primary procedure)

(Report 96368 only once per date of service)

(Report 96368 in conjunction with 96365, 96366, 96413, 96415, 96416)

96369   Subcutaneous infusion for therapy or prophylaxis (specify substance or drug); initial, up to 1 hour, including pump set-up and establishment of subcutaneous infusion site(s)

(For infusions of 15 minutes or less, use 96372)

+ 96370   each additional hour (List separately in addition to code for primary procedure)

(Use 96370 in conjunction with 96369)

(Use 96370 for infusion intervals of greater than 30 minutes beyond 1 hour increments)

+ 96371   additional pump set-up with establishment of new subcutaneous infusion site(s) (List separately in addition to code for primary procedure)

(Use 96371 in conjunction with 96369)

(Use 96369, 96371 only once per encounter)

96372   Therapeutic, prophylactic, or diagnostic injection (specify substance or drug); subcutaneous or intramuscular

(For administration of vaccines/toxoids, see 90460, 90461, 90471, 90472)

(Report 96372 for non-antineoplastic hormonal therapy injections)

(Report 96401 for anti-neoplastic nonhormonal injection therapy)

(Report 96402 for anti-neoplastic hormonal injection therapy)

(Do not report 96372 for injections given without direct physician or other qualified health care professional supervision. To report, use 99211. Hospitals may report 96372 when the physician or other qualified health care professional is not present)

(96372 does not include injections for allergen immunotherapy. For allergen immunotherapy injections, see 95115-95117)

96373   intra-arterial

96374   intravenous push, single or initial substance/drug

+ 96375   each additional sequential intravenous push of a new substance/drug (List separately in addition to code for primary procedure)

(Use 96375 in conjunction with 96365, 96374, 96409, 96413)

(Report 96375 to identify intravenous push of a new substance/drug if provided as a secondary or subsequent service after a different initial service is administered through the same IV access)

+ 96376   each additional sequential intravenous push of the same substance/drug provided in a facility (List separately in addition to code for primary procedure)

(Do not report 96376 for a push performed within 30 minutes of a reported push of the same substance or drug)

(96376 may be reported by facilities only)

(Report 96376 in conjunction with 96365, 96374, 96409, 96413)

96379   Unlisted therapeutic, prophylactic, or diagnostic intravenous or intra-arterial injection or infusion

(For allergy immunology, see 95004 et seq)

Chemotherapy and Other Highly Complex Drug or Highly Complex Biologic Agent Administration

Chemotherapy administration codes 96401-96549 apply to parenteral administration of non-radionuclide anti-neoplastic drugs; and also to anti-neoplastic agents provided for treatment of noncancer diagnoses (eg, cyclophosphamide for auto-immune conditions) or to substances such as certain monoclonal antibody agents, and other biologic response modifiers. The highly complex infusion of chemotherapy or other drug or biologic agents requires physician or other qualified health care professional work and/or clinical staff monitoring well beyond that of therapeutic drug agents (96360-96379) because the incidence of severe adverse patient reactions are typically greater. These services can be provided by any physician or other qualified health care professional. Chemotherapy services are typically highly complex and require direct supervision for any or all purposes of patient assessment, provision of consent, safety oversight, and intraservice supervision of staff. Typically, such chemotherapy services require advanced practice training and competency for staff who provide these services; special considerations for preparation, dosage, or disposal; and commonly, these services entail significant patient risk and frequent monitoring. Examples are frequent changes in the infusion rate, prolonged presence of the nurse administering the solution for patient monitoring and infusion adjustments, and frequent conferring with the physician or other qualified health care professional about these issues. When performed to facilitate the infusion of injection, preparation of chemotherapy agent(s), highly complex agent(s), or other highly complex drugs is included and is not reported separately. To report infusions that do not require this level of complexity, see 96360-96379. Codes 96401-96402, 96409-96425, 96521-96523 are not intended to be reported by the individual physician or other qualified health care professional in the facility setting.

The term "chemotherapy" in 96401-96549 includes other highly complex drugs or highly complex biologic agents.

Report separate codes for each parenteral method of administration employed when chemotherapy is administered by different techniques. The administration of medications (eg, antibiotics, steroidal agents, antiemetics, narcotics, analgesics) administered independently or sequentially as supportive management of chemotherapy administration, should be separately reported using 96360, 96361, 96365, 96379 as appropriate.

Report both the specific service as well as code(s) for the specific substance(s) or drug(s) provided. The fluid used to administer the drug(s) is considered incidental hydration and is not separately reportable.

Regional (isolation) chemotherapy perfusion should be reported using the codes for arterial infusion (96420-96425). Placement of the intra-arterial catheter should be reported using the appropriate code from the **Cardiovascular Surgery** section. Placement of arterial and venous cannula(s) for extracorporeal circulation via a membrane oxygenator perfusion pump should be reported using 36823. Code 36823 includes dose calculation and administration of the chemotherapy agent by injection into the perfusate. Do not report 96409-96425 in conjunction with 36823.

(For home infusion services, see 99601-99602)

Injection and Intravenous Infusion Chemotherapy and Other Highly Complex Drug or Highly Complex Biologic Agent Administration

Intravenous or intra-arterial push is defined as: (a) an injection in which the healthcare professional who administers the substance/drug is continuously present to administer the injection and observe the patient, or (b) an infusion of 15 minutes or less.

96401 Chemotherapy administration, subcutaneous or intramuscular; non-hormonal anti-neoplastic

96402 hormonal anti-neoplastic

96405 Chemotherapy administration; intralesional, up to and including 7 lesions

96406 intralesional, more than 7 lesions

96409 intravenous, push technique, single or initial substance/drug

+ 96411 intravenous, push technique, each additional substance/drug (List separately in addition to code for primary procedure)

(Use 96411 in conjunction with 96409, 96413)

96413 Chemotherapy administration, intravenous infusion technique; up to 1 hour, single or initial substance/drug

(Report 96361 to identify hydration if administered as a secondary or subsequent service in association with 96413 through the same IV access)

(Report 96366, 96367, 96375 to identify therapeutic, prophylactic, or diagnostic drug infusion or injection, if administered as a secondary or subsequent service in association with 96413 through the same IV access)

+ 96415 each additional hour (List separately in addition to code for primary procedure)

(Use 96415 in conjunction with 96413)

(Report 96415 for infusion intervals of greater than 30 minutes beyond 1-hour increments)

96416 initiation of prolonged chemotherapy infusion (more than 8 hours), requiring use of a portable or implantable pump

Medicine

(For refilling and maintenance of a portable pump or an implantable infusion pump or reservoir for drug delivery, see 96521-96523)

+ 96417   each additional sequential infusion (different substance/drug), up to 1 hour (List separately in addition to code for primary procedure)

(Use 96417 in conjunction with 96413)

(Report only once per sequential infusion. Report 96415 for additional hour(s) of sequential infusion)

Intra-Arterial Chemotherapy and Other Highly Complex Drug or Highly Complex Biologic Agent Administration

96420   Chemotherapy administration, intra-arterial; push technique

96422   infusion technique, up to 1 hour

+ 96423   infusion technique, each additional hour (List separately in addition to code for primary procedure)

(Use 96423 in conjunction with 96422)

(Report 96423 for infusion intervals of greater than 30 minutes beyond 1-hour increments)

(For regional chemotherapy perfusion via membrane oxygenator perfusion pump to an extremity, use 36823)

96425   infusion technique, initiation of prolonged infusion (more than 8 hours), requiring the use of a portable or implantable pump

(For refilling and maintenance of a portable pump or an implantable infusion pump or reservoir for drug delivery, see 96521-96523)

Other Injection and Infusion Services

Code 96523 does not require direct supervision. Codes 96521-96523 may be reported when these devices are used for therapeutic drugs other than chemotherapy.

(For collection of blood specimen from a completely implantable venous access device, use 36591)

96440   Chemotherapy administration into pleural cavity, requiring and including thoracentesis

96446   Chemotherapy administration into the peritoneal cavity via indwelling port or catheter

96450   Chemotherapy administration, into CNS (eg, intrathecal), requiring and including spinal puncture

(For intravesical (bladder) chemotherapy administration, use 51720)

(For insertion of subarachnoid catheter and reservoir for infusion of drug, see 62350, 62351, 62360-62362; for insertion of intraventricular catheter and reservoir, see 61210, 61215)

96521   Refilling and maintenance of portable pump

96522   Refilling and maintenance of implantable pump or reservoir for drug delivery, systemic (eg, intravenous, intra-arterial)

(For refilling and maintenance of an implantable infusion pump for spinal or brain drug infusion, use 95990-95991)

96523   Irrigation of implanted venous access device for drug delivery systems

(Do not report 96523 in conjunction with other services. To report collection of blood specimen, use 36591)

96542   Chemotherapy injection, subarachnoid or intraventricular via subcutaneous reservoir, single or multiple agents

(For radioactive isotope therapy, use 79005)

96549   Unlisted chemotherapy procedure

Photodynamic Therapy

(To report ocular photodynamic therapy, use 67221)

96567   Photodynamic therapy by external application of light to destroy premalignant and/or malignant lesions of the skin and adjacent mucosa (eg, lip) by activation of photosensitive drug(s), each phototherapy exposure session

+ 96570   Photodynamic therapy by endoscopic application of light to ablate abnormal tissue via activation of photosensitive drug(s); first 30 minutes (List separately in addition to code for endoscopy or bronchoscopy procedures of lung and gastrointestinal tract)

(Report 96570 with modifier 52 for service of less than 23 minutes with report)

+ 96571   each additional 15 minutes (List separately in addition to code for endoscopy or bronchoscopy procedures of lung and gastrointestinal tract)

(For 23-37 minutes of service, use 96570. For 38-52 minutes of service, use 96570 in conjunction with 96571)

(96570, 96571 are to be used in addition to bronchoscopy, endoscopy codes)

(Use 96570, 96571 in conjunction with 31641, 43229 as appropriate)

Special Dermatological Procedures

See the **Evaluation and Management coding guidelines** for further instructions on reporting that is appropriate for management of dermatologic illnesses.

(For intralesional injections, see 11900, 11901)

(For Tzanck smear, see 88160-88161)

96900   Actinotherapy (ultraviolet light)

(For rhinophototherapy, intranasal application of ultraviolet and visible light, use 30999)

Medicine

96902 Microscopic examination of hairs plucked or clipped by the examiner (excluding hair collected by the patient) to determine telogen and anagen counts, or structural hair shaft abnormality

96904 Whole body integumentary photography, for monitoring of high risk patients with dysplastic nevus syndrome or a history of dysplastic nevi, or patients with a personal or familial history of melanoma

96910 Photochemotherapy; tar and ultraviolet B (Goeckerman treatment) or petrolatum and ultraviolet B

96912   psoralens and ultraviolet A (PUVA)

96913 Photochemotherapy (Goeckerman and/or PUVA) for severe photoresponsive dermatoses requiring at least 4-8 hours of care under direct supervision of the physician (includes application of medication and dressings)

96920 Laser treatment for inflammatory skin disease (psoriasis); total area less than 250 sq cm

96921   250 sq cm to 500 sq cm

96922   over 500 sq cm

(For laser destruction of premalignant lesions, see 17000-17004)

(For laser destruction of cutaneous vascular proliferative lesions, see 17106-17108)

(For laser destruction of benign lesions, see 17110-17111)

(For laser destruction of malignant lesions, see 17260-17286)

● **96931** Reflectance confocal microscopy (RCM) for cellular and sub-cellular imaging of skin; image acquisition and interpretation and report, first lesion

● **96932**   image acquisition only, first lesion

● **96933**   interpretation and report only, first lesion

+● **96934**   image acquisition and interpretation and report, each additional lesion (List separately in addition to code for primary procedure)

►(Use 96934 in conjunction with 96931)◄

+● **96935**   image acquisition only, each additional lesion (List separately in addition to code for primary procedure)

►(Use 96935 in conjunction with 96932)◄

+● **96936**   interpretation and report only, each additional lesion (List separately in addition to code for primary procedure)

►(Use 96936 in conjunction with 96933)◄

96999 Unlisted special dermatological service or procedure

Physical Medicine and Rehabilitation

Codes 97001-97755 should be used to report each distinct procedure performed. Do not append modifier 51 to 97001-97755.

The work of the physician or other qualified health care professional consists of face-to-face time with the patient (and caregiver, if applicable) delivering skilled services. For the purpose of determining the total time of a service, incremental intervals of treatment at the same visit may be accumulated.

(For muscle testing, range of joint motion, electromyography, see 95831 et seq)

(For biofeedback training by EMG, use 90901)

(For transcutaneous nerve stimulation (TNS), use 64550)

97001 Physical therapy evaluation

97002 Physical therapy re-evaluation

97003 Occupational therapy evaluation

97004 Occupational therapy re-evaluation

97005 Athletic training evaluation

97006 Athletic training re-evaluation

Modalities

Any physical agent applied to produce therapeutic changes to biologic tissue; includes but not limited to thermal, acoustic, light, mechanical, or electric energy.

Supervised

The application of a modality that does not require direct (one-on-one) patient contact.

97010 Application of a modality to 1 or more areas; hot or cold packs

97012   traction, mechanical

97014   electrical stimulation (unattended)

(For acupuncture with electrical stimulation, see 97813, 97814)

97016   vasopneumatic devices

97018   paraffin bath

97022   whirlpool

97024   diathermy (eg, microwave)

97026   infrared

97028   ultraviolet

Medicine

Constant Attendance

The application of a modality that requires direct (one-on-one) patient contact.

97032 Application of a modality to 1 or more areas; electrical stimulation (manual), each 15 minutes

(For transcutaneous electrical modulation pain reprocessing [TEMPR/scrambler therapy], use 0278T)

97033 iontophoresis, each 15 minutes

97034 contrast baths, each 15 minutes

97035 ultrasound, each 15 minutes

97036 Hubbard tank, each 15 minutes

97039 Unlisted modality (specify type and time if constant attendance)

Therapeutic Procedures

A manner of effecting change through the application of clinical skills and/or services that attempt to improve function.

Physician or other qualified health care professional (ie, therapist) required to have direct (one-on-one) patient contact.

97110 Therapeutic procedure, 1 or more areas, each 15 minutes; therapeutic exercises to develop strength and endurance, range of motion and flexibility

97112 neuromuscular reeducation of movement, balance, coordination, kinesthetic sense, posture, and/or proprioception for sitting and/or standing activities

97113 aquatic therapy with therapeutic exercises

97116 gait training (includes stair climbing)

(Use 96000-96003 to report comprehensive gait and motion analysis procedures)

97124 massage, including effleurage, petrissage and/or tapotement (stroking, compression, percussion)

(For myofascial release, use 97140)

97139 Unlisted therapeutic procedure (specify)

97140 Manual therapy techniques (eg, mobilization/manipulation, manual lymphatic drainage, manual traction), 1 or more regions, each 15 minutes

97150 Therapeutic procedure(s), group (2 or more individuals)

(Report 97150 for each member of group)

(Group therapy procedures involve constant attendance of the physician or other qualified health care professional [ie, therapist], but by definition do not require one-on-one patient contact by the same physician or other qualified health care professional)

(For manipulation under general anesthesia, see appropriate anatomic section in **Musculoskeletal System**)

(For osteopathic manipulative treatment [OMT], see 98925-98929)

(Do not report 97150 in conjunction with 0366T, 0367T, 0372T)

97530 Therapeutic activities, direct (one-on-one) patient contact (use of dynamic activities to improve functional performance), each 15 minutes

97532 Development of cognitive skills to improve attention, memory, problem solving (includes compensatory training), direct (one-on-one) patient contact, each 15 minutes

(Do not report 97532 in conjunction with 0364T, 0365T, 0368T, 0369T)

97533 Sensory integrative techniques to enhance sensory processing and promote adaptive responses to environmental demands, direct (one-on-one) patient contact, each 15 minutes

97535 Self-care/home management training (eg, activities of daily living (ADL) and compensatory training, meal preparation, safety procedures, and instructions in use of assistive technology devices/adaptive equipment) direct one-on-one contact, each 15 minutes

97537 Community/work reintegration training (eg, shopping, transportation, money management, avocational activities and/or work environment/modification analysis, work task analysis, use of assistive technology device/adaptive equipment), direct one-on-one contact, each 15 minutes

(For wheelchair management/propulsion training, use 97542)

97542 Wheelchair management (eg, assessment, fitting, training), each 15 minutes

97545 Work hardening/conditioning; initial 2 hours

+ 97546 each additional hour (List separately in addition to code for primary procedure)

(Use 97546 in conjunction with 97545)

Active Wound Care Management

Active wound care procedures are performed to remove devitalized and/or necrotic tissue and promote healing. Services require direct (one-on-one) contact with the patient.

(Do not report 97597-97602 in conjunction with 11042-11047 for the same wound)

(For debridement of burn wounds, see 16020-16030)

97597 Debridement (eg, high pressure waterjet with/without suction, sharp selective debridement with scissors, scalpel and forceps), open wound, (eg, fibrin, devitalized epidermis and/or dermis, exudate, debris, biofilm), including topical application(s), wound assessment, use of a whirlpool, when performed and instruction(s) for ongoing care, per session, total wound(s) surface area; first 20 sq cm or less

Medicine

+ 97598   each additional 20 sq cm, or part thereof (List separately in addition to code for primary procedure)

(Use 97598 in conjunction with 97597)

97602   Removal of devitalized tissue from wound(s), non-selective debridement, without anesthesia (eg, wet-to-moist dressings, enzymatic, abrasion), including topical application(s), wound assessment, and instruction(s) for ongoing care, per session

97605   Negative pressure wound therapy (eg, vacuum assisted drainage collection), utilizing durable medical equipment (DME), including topical application(s), wound assessment, and instruction(s) for ongoing care, per session; total wound(s) surface area less than or equal to 50 square centimeters

97606   total wound(s) surface area greater than 50 square centimeters

97607   Negative pressure wound therapy, (eg, vacuum assisted drainage collection), utilizing disposable, non-durable medical equipment including provision of exudate management collection system, topical application(s), wound assessment, and instructions for ongoing care, per session; total wound(s) surface area less than or equal to 50 square centimeters

97608   total wound(s) surface area greater than 50 square centimeters

(Do not report 97607, 97608 in conjunction with 97605, 97606)

97610   Low frequency, non-contact, non-thermal ultrasound, including topical application(s), when performed, wound assessment, and instruction(s) for ongoing care, per day

Tests and Measurements

Requires direct one-on-one patient contact.

(For muscle testing, manual or electrical, joint range of motion, electromyography, or nerve velocity determination, see 95831-95857, 95860-95872, 95885-95887, 95907-95913)

97750   Physical performance test or measurement (eg, musculoskeletal, functional capacity), with written report, each 15 minutes

97755   Assistive technology assessment (eg, to restore, augment or compensate for existing function, optimize functional tasks and/or maximize environmental accessibility), direct one-on-one contact, with written report, each 15 minutes

(To report augmentative and alternative communication devices, see 92605, 92607)

Orthotic Management and Prosthetic Management

97760   Orthotic(s) management and training (including assessment and fitting when not otherwise reported), upper extremity(s), lower extremity(s) and/or trunk, each 15 minutes

(Code 97760 should not be reported with 97116 for the same extremity)

97761   Prosthetic training, upper and/or lower extremity(s), each 15 minutes

97762   Checkout for orthotic/prosthetic use, established patient, each 15 minutes

Other Procedures

(For extracorporeal shock wave musculoskeletal therapy, see Category III codes 0019T, 0101T, 0102T)

97799   Unlisted physical medicine/rehabilitation service or procedure

Medical Nutrition Therapy

97802   Medical nutrition therapy; initial assessment and intervention, individual, face-to-face with the patient, each 15 minutes

97803   re-assessment and intervention, individual, face-to-face with the patient, each 15 minutes

97804   group (2 or more individual(s)), each 30 minutes

(Physicians and other qualified health care professionals who may report evaluation and management services should use the appropriate evaluation and management codes)

Acupuncture

Acupuncture is reported based on 15-minute increments of personal (face-to-face) contact with the patient, not the duration of acupuncture needle(s) placement.

If no electrical stimulation is used during a 15-minute increment, use 97810, 97811. If electrical stimulation of any needle is used during a 15-minute increment, use 97813, 97814.

Only one code may be reported for each 15-minute increment. Use either 97810 or 97813 for the initial 15-minute increment. Only one initial code is reported per day.

Evaluation and management services may be reported in addition to acupuncture procedures when performed by physicians or other health care professionals, who may report evaluation and management services, including new or established patient office or other outpatient services (99201-99215), hospital observation care

Medicine

(99217-99220, 99224-99226), hospital care (99221-99223, 99231-99233), office or other outpatient consultations (99241-99245), inpatient consultations (99251-99255), critical care services (99291, 99292), inpatient neonatal intensive care services and pediatric and neonatal critical care services (99466-99480), emergency department services (99281-99285), nursing facility services (99304-99318), domiciliary, rest home, or custodial care services (99324-99337), and home services (99341-99350) may be reported separately using modifier 25 if the patient's condition requires a significant, separately identifiable E/M service above and beyond the usual preservice and postservice work associated with the acupuncture services. The time of the E/M service is not included in the time of the acupuncture service.

97810 Acupuncture, 1 or more needles; without electrical stimulation, initial 15 minutes of personal one-on-one contact with the patient

(Do not report 97810 in conjunction with 97813)

+ 97811 without electrical stimulation, each additional 15 minutes of personal one-on-one contact with the patient, with re-insertion of needle(s) (List separately in addition to code for primary procedure)

(Use 97811 in conjunction with 97810, 97813)

97813 with electrical stimulation, initial 15 minutes of personal one-on-one contact with the patient

(Do not report 97813 in conjunction with 97810)

+ 97814 with electrical stimulation, each additional 15 minutes of personal one-on-one contact with the patient, with re-insertion of needle(s) (List separately in addition to code for primary procedure)

(Use 97814 in conjunction with 97810, 97813)

Osteopathic Manipulative Treatment

Osteopathic manipulative treatment (OMT) is a form of manual treatment applied by a physician or other qualified health care professional to eliminate or alleviate somatic dysfunction and related disorders. This treatment may be accomplished by a variety of techniques.

Evaluation and Management services including new or established patient office or other outpatient services (99201-99215), hospital observation care (99217-99220, 99224-99226), hospital care (99221-99223, 99231-99233), critical care services (99291, 99292), observation or inpatient care services (99234-99236), office or other outpatient consultations (99241-99245), emergency department services (99281-99285), nursing facility services (99304-99318), domiciliary, rest home, or custodial care services (99324-99337), and home services (99341-99350) may be reported separately using modifier 25 if the patient's condition requires a significant,

separately identifiable E/M service above and beyond the usual preservice and postservice work associated with the procedure. The E/M service may be caused or prompted by the same symptoms or condition for which the OMT service was provided. As such, different diagnoses are not required for the reporting of the OMT and E/M service on the same date.

Body regions referred to are: head region; cervical region; thoracic region; lumbar region; sacral region; pelvic region; lower extremities; upper extremities; rib cage region; abdomen and viscera region.

98925 Osteopathic manipulative treatment (OMT); 1-2 body regions involved

98926 3-4 body regions involved

98927 5-6 body regions involved

98928 7-8 body regions involved

98929 9-10 body regions involved

Chiropractic Manipulative Treatment

Chiropractic manipulative treatment (CMT) is a form of manual treatment to influence joint and neurophysiological function. This treatment may be accomplished using a variety of techniques.

The chiropractic manipulative treatment codes include a pre-manipulation patient assessment. Additional evaluation and management services including office or other outpatient services (99201-99215), subsequent observation care (99224-99226), subsequent hospital care (99231-99233), office or other outpatient consultations (99241-99245), subsequent nursing facility services (99307-99310), domiciliary, rest home, or custodial care services (99324-99337), and home services (99341-99350) may be reported separately using modifier 25 if the patient's condition requires a significant, separately identifiable E/M service above and beyond the usual preservice and postservice work associated with the procedure. The E/M service may be caused or prompted by the same symptoms or condition for which the CMT service was provided. As such, different diagnoses are not required for the reporting of the CMT and E/M service on the same date.

For purposes of CMT, the five spinal regions referred to are: cervical region (includes atlanto-occipital joint); thoracic region (includes costovertebral and costotransverse joints); lumbar region; sacral region; and pelvic (sacro-iliac joint) region. The five extraspinal regions referred to are: head (including temporomandibular joint, excluding atlanto-occipital) region; lower extremities; upper extremities; rib cage (excluding costotransverse and costovertebral joints) and abdomen.

⊙=Moderate sedation ✦=Add-on code ✒=FDA approval pending #=Resequenced code ○=Recycled/reinstated code

Medicine

98940	Chiropractic manipulative treatment (CMT); spinal, 1-2 regions
98941	spinal, 3-4 regions
98942	spinal, 5 regions
98943	extraspinal, 1 or more regions

Education and Training for Patient Self-Management

The following codes are used to report educational and training services prescribed by a physician or other qualified health care professional and provided by a qualified, nonphysician health care professional using a standardized curriculum to an individual or a group of patients for the treatment of established illness(s)/disease(s) or to delay comorbidity(s). Education and training for patient self-management may be reported with these codes only when using a standardized curriculum as described below. This curriculum may be modified as necessary for the clinical needs, cultural norms and health literacy of the individual patient(s).

The purpose of the educational and training services is to teach the patient (may include caregiver[s]) how to effectively self-manage the patient's illness(s)/disease(s) or delay disease comorbidity(s) in conjunction with the patient's professional healthcare team. Education and training related to subsequent reinforcement or due to changes in the patient's condition or treatment plan are reported in the same manner as the original education and training. The type of education and training provided for the patient's clinical condition will be identified by the appropriate diagnosis code(s) reported.

The qualifications of the nonphysician healthcare professionals and the content of the educational and training program must be consistent with guidelines or standards established or recognized by a physician society, nonphysician healthcare professional society/association, or other appropriate source.

(For counseling and education provided by a physician to an individual, see the appropriate evaluation and management codes including office or other outpatient services [99201-99215], hospital observation care [99217-99220, 99224-99226], hospital care [99221-99223, 99231-99233], new or established patient office or other outpatient consultations [99241-99245], inpatient consultations [99251-99255], emergency department services [99281-99285], nursing facility services [99304-99318], domiciliary, rest home, or custodial care services [99324-99337], home services [99341-99350], and counseling risk factor reduction and behavior change intervention [99401-99429]. See also **Instructions for Use of the CPT Codebook** for definition of reporting qualifications)

(For counseling and education provided by a physician to a group, use 99078)

(For counseling and/or risk factor reduction intervention provided by a physician to patient[s] without symptoms or established disease, see 99401-99412)

(For medical nutrition therapy, see 97802-97804)

(For health and behavior assessment/intervention that is not part of a standardized curriculum, see 96150-96155)

(For education provided as genetic counseling services, use 96040. For education to a group regarding genetic risks, see 98961, 98962)

98960	Education and training for patient self-management by a qualified, nonphysician health care professional using a standardized curriculum, face-to-face with the patient (could include caregiver/family) each 30 minutes; individual patient
98961	2-4 patients
98962	5-8 patients

Non-Face-to-Face Nonphysician Services

Telephone Services

Telephone services are non-face-to-face assessment and management services provided by a qualified health care professional to a patient using the telephone. These codes are used to report episodes of care by the qualified health care professional initiated by an established patient or guardian of an established patient. If the telephone service ends with a decision to see the patient within 24 hours or the next available urgent visit appointment, the code is not reported; rather the encounter is considered part of the preservice work of the subsequent assessment and management service, procedure, and visit. Likewise, if the telephone call refers to a service performed and reported by the qualified health care professional within the previous seven days (either qualified health care professional requested or unsolicited patient follow-up) or within the postoperative period of the previously completed procedure, then the service(s) are considered part of that previous service or procedure. (Do not report 98966-98969 if reporting 98966-98969 performed in the previous seven days.)

(For telephone services provided by a physician, see 99441-99443)

Medicine

98966   Telephone assessment and management service provided by a qualified nonphysician health care professional to an established patient, parent, or guardian not originating from a related assessment and management service provided within the previous 7 days nor leading to an assessment and management service or procedure within the next 24 hours or soonest available appointment; 5-10 minutes of medical discussion

98967   11-20 minutes of medical discussion

98968   21-30 minutes of medical discussion

(Do not report 98966-98968 during the same month with 99487-99489)

(Do not report 98966-98968 when performed during the service time of codes 99495, 99496)

On-line Medical Evaluation

An on-line electronic medical evaluation is a non-face-to-face assessment and management service by a qualified health care professional to a patient using Internet resources in response to a patient's on-line inquiry. Reportable services involve the qualified health care professional's personal timely response to the patient's inquiry and must involve permanent storage (electronic or hard copy) of the encounter. This service is reported only once for the same episode of care during a seven-day period, although multiple qualified health care professionals could report their exchange with the same patient. If the on-line medical evaluation refers to an assessment and management service previously performed and reported by the qualified health care professional within the previous seven days (either qualified health care professional requested or unsolicited patient follow-up) or within the postoperative period of the previously completed procedure, then the service(s) are considered covered by the previous assessment and management office service or procedure. A reportable service encompasses the sum of communication (eg, related telephone calls, prescription provision, laboratory orders) pertaining to the on-line patient encounter.

(For an on-line medical evaluation provided by a physician, use 99444)

98969   Online assessment and management service provided by a qualified nonphysician health care professional to an established patient or guardian, not originating from a related assessment and management service provided within the previous 7 days, using the Internet or similar electronic communications network

(Do not report 98969 when using 99339-99340, 99374-99380 for the same communication[s])

(Do not report 98969 for anticoagulation management when reporting 99363, 99364)

(Do not report 98969 during the same month with 99487-99489)

(Do not report 98969 when performed during the service time of codes 99495, 99496)

Special Services, Procedures and Reports

The procedures with code numbers 99000 through 99091 provide the reporting physician or other qualified health care professional with the means of identifying the completion of special reports and services that are an adjunct to the basic services rendered. The specific number assigned indicates the special circumstances under which a basic procedure is performed.

Code 99091 should be reported no more than once in a 30-day period to include the physician or other qualified health care professional time involved with data accession, review and interpretation, modification of care plan as necessary (including communication to patient and/or caregiver), and associated documentation.

If the services described by 99091 are provided on the same day the patient presents for an E/M service, these services should be considered part of the E/M service and not separately reported.

Do not report 99091 if it occurs within 30 days of care plan oversight services 99374-99380. Do not report 99091 if other more specific CPT codes exist (eg, 93227, 93272 for cardiographic services; 95250 for continuous glucose monitoring). Do not report 99091 for transfer and interpretation of data from hospital or clinical laboratory computers.

Codes 99050-99060 are reported in addition to an associated basic service. Do not append modifier 51 to 99050-99060. Typically only a single adjunct code from among 99050-99060 would be reported per patient encounter. However, there may be circumstances in which reporting multiple adjunct codes per patient encounter may be appropriate.

Miscellaneous Services

99000   Handling and/or conveyance of specimen for transfer from the office to a laboratory

99001   Handling and/or conveyance of specimen for transfer from the patient in other than an office to a laboratory (distance may be indicated)

99002   Handling, conveyance, and/or any other service in connection with the implementation of an order involving devices (eg, designing, fitting, packaging, handling, delivery or mailing) when devices such as orthotics, protectives, prosthetics are fabricated by an outside laboratory or shop but which items have been designed, and are to be fitted and adjusted by the attending physician or other qualified health care professional

(For routine collection of venous blood, use 36415)

99024   Postoperative follow-up visit, normally included in the surgical package, to indicate that an evaluation and management service was performed during a postoperative period for a reason(s) related to the original procedure

Medicine

(As a component of a surgical "package," see **Surgery Guidelines**)

99026   Hospital mandated on call service; in-hospital, each hour

99027   out-of-hospital, each hour

(For standby services requiring prolonged attendance, use 99360, as appropriate. Time spent performing separately reportable procedure(s) or service(s) should not be included in the time reported as mandated on-call service)

99050   Services provided in the office at times other than regularly scheduled office hours, or days when the office is normally closed (eg, holidays, Saturday or Sunday), in addition to basic service

99051   Service(s) provided in the office during regularly scheduled evening, weekend, or holiday office hours, in addition to basic service

99053   Service(s) provided between 10:00 PM and 8:00 AM at 24-hour facility, in addition to basic service

99056   Service(s) typically provided in the office, provided out of the office at request of patient, in addition to basic service

99058   Service(s) provided on an emergency basis in the office, which disrupts other scheduled office services, in addition to basic service

99060   Service(s) provided on an emergency basis, out of the office, which disrupts other scheduled office services, in addition to basic service

99070   Supplies and materials (except spectacles), provided by the physician or other qualified health care professional over and above those usually included with the office visit or other services rendered (list drugs, trays, supplies, or materials provided)

(For supply of spectacles, use the appropriate supply codes)

99071   Educational supplies, such as books, tapes, and pamphlets, for the patient's education at cost to physician or other qualified health care professional

99075   Medical testimony

99078   Physician or other qualified health care professional qualified by education, training, licensure/regulation (when applicable) educational services rendered to patients in a group setting (eg, prenatal, obesity, or diabetic instructions)

99080   Special reports such as insurance forms, more than the information conveyed in the usual medical communications or standard reporting form

(Do not report 99080 in conjunction with 99455, 99456 for the completion of Workmen's Compensation forms)

99082   Unusual travel (eg, transportation and escort of patient)

99090   Analysis of clinical data stored in computers (eg, ECGs, blood pressures, hematologic data)

(For physician/or other qualified health care professional qualified by education, training, licensure/regulation [when applicable] collection and interpretation of physiologic data stored/transmitted by patient/caregiver, see 99091)

(Do not report 99090 if other more specific CPT codes exist, eg, 93227, 93272, 0206T for cardiographic services; 95250 for continuous glucose monitoring; 97750 for musculoskeletal function testing)

99091   Collection and interpretation of physiologic data (eg, ECG, blood pressure, glucose monitoring) digitally stored and/or transmitted by the patient and/or caregiver to the physician or other qualified health care professional, qualified by education, training, licensure/regulation (when applicable) requiring a minimum of 30 minutes of time

Qualifying Circumstances for Anesthesia

(For explanation of these services, see **Anesthesia Guidelines**)

+ 99100   Anesthesia for patient of extreme age, younger than 1 year and older than 70 (List separately in addition to code for primary anesthesia procedure)

(For procedure performed on infants younger than 1 year of age at time of surgery, see 00326, 00561, 00834, 00836)

+ 99116   Anesthesia complicated by utilization of total body hypothermia (List separately in addition to code for primary anesthesia procedure)

+ 99135   Anesthesia complicated by utilization of controlled hypotension (List separately in addition to code for primary anesthesia procedure)

+ 99140   Anesthesia complicated by emergency conditions (specify) (List separately in addition to code for primary anesthesia procedure)

(An emergency is defined as existing when delay in treatment of the patient would lead to a significant increase in the threat to life or body part)

Moderate (Conscious) Sedation

Moderate (conscious) sedation is a drug induced depression of consciousness during which patients respond purposefully to verbal commands, either alone or accompanied by light tactile stimulation. No interventions are required to maintain a patent airway, and spontaneous ventilation is adequate. Cardiovascular function is usually maintained.

Medicine

Moderate sedation does not include minimal sedation (anxiolysis), deep sedation or monitored anesthesia care (00100-01999).

When providing moderate sedation, the following services are included and **not** reported separately:

- Assessment of the patient (not included in intraservice time);

- Establishment of IV access and fluids to maintain patency, when performed;

- Administration of agent(s);

- Maintenance of sedation;

- Monitoring of oxygen saturation, heart rate and blood pressure; and

- Recovery (not included in intraservice time).

Intraservice time starts with the administration of the sedation agent(s), requires continuous face-to-face attendance, and ends at the conclusion of personal contact by the physician providing the sedation.

Do not report 99143-99150 in conjunction with 94760-94762.

Do not report 99143-99145 in conjunction with codes listed in Appendix G. Do not report 99148-99150 in conjunction with codes listed in Appendix G when performed in the nonfacility setting.

When a second physician or other qualified health care professional other than the health care professional performing the diagnostic or therapeutic services provides moderate sedation in the facility setting (eg, hospital, outpatient hospital/ambulatory surgery center, skilled nursing facility) for the procedures listed in Appendix G, the second physician or other qualified health care professional reports 99148-99150. However, for the circumstance in which these services are performed by the second physician or other qualified health care professional in the nonfacility setting (eg, office, freestanding imaging center), codes 99148-99150 are not reported. See also **Instructions for Use of the CPT Codebook** for definition of reporting qualifications.

⊘ **99143** Moderate sedation services (other than those services described by codes 00100-01999) provided by the same physician or other qualified health care professional performing the diagnostic or therapeutic service that the sedation supports, requiring the presence of an independent trained observer to assist in the monitoring of the patient's level of consciousness and physiological status; younger than 5 years of age, first 30 minutes intra-service time

⊘ **99144** age 5 years or older, first 30 minutes intra-service time

+ **99145** each additional 15 minutes intra-service time (List separately in addition to code for primary service)

(Use 99145 in conjunction with 99143, 99144)

99148 Moderate sedation services (other than those services described by codes 00100-01999), provided by a physician or other qualified health care professional other than the health care professional performing the diagnostic or therapeutic service that the sedation supports; younger than 5 years of age, first 30 minutes intra-service time

99149 age 5 years or older, first 30 minutes intra-service time

+ **99150** each additional 15 minutes intra-service time (List separately in addition to code for primary service)

(Use 99150 in conjunction with 99148, 99149)

Other Services and Procedures

99170 Anogenital examination, magnified, in childhood for suspected trauma, including image recording when performed

(For moderate sedation, use 99143-99150)

99172 Visual function screening, automated or semi-automated bilateral quantitative determination of visual acuity, ocular alignment, color vision by pseudoisochromatic plates, and field of vision (may include all or some screening of the determination[s] for contrast sensitivity, vision under glare)

(This service must employ graduated visual acuity stimuli that allow a quantitative determination of visual acuity [eg, Snellen chart]. This service may not be used in addition to a general ophthalmological service or an E/M service)

►(Do not report 99172 in conjunction with 99173, 99174, 99177)◄

99173 Screening test of visual acuity, quantitative, bilateral

(The screening test used must employ graduated visual acuity stimuli that allow a quantitative estimate of visual acuity [eg, Snellen chart]. Other identifiable services unrelated to this screening test provided at the same time may be reported separately [eg, preventive medicine services]. When acuity is measured as part of a general ophthalmological service or of an E/M service of the eye, it is a diagnostic examination and not a screening test.)

►(Do not report 99173 in conjunction with 99172, 99174, 99177)◄

▲ **99174** Instrument-based ocular screening (eg, photoscreening, automated-refraction), bilateral; with remote analysis and report

►(Do not report 99174 in conjunction with 92002-92014, 99172, 99173, 99177)◄

#● **99177**   with on-site analysis

▶(Do not report 99177 in conjunction with 92002-92014, 99172, 99173, 99174)◀

99175   Ipecac or similar administration for individual emesis and continued observation until stomach adequately emptied of poison

(For diagnostic intubation, see 43754, 43755)

(For gastric lavage for diagnostic purposes, see 43754, 43755)

99177   Code is out of numerical sequence. See 99170-99199

99183   Physician or other qualified health care professional attendance and supervision of hyperbaric oxygen therapy, per session

(Evaluation and Management services and/or procedures [eg, wound debridement] provided in a hyperbaric oxygen treatment facility in conjunction with a hyperbaric oxygen therapy session should be reported separately)

99184   Initiation of selective head or total body hypothermia in the critically ill neonate, includes appropriate patient selection by review of clinical, imaging and laboratory data, confirmation of esophageal temperature probe location, evaluation of amplitude EEG, supervision of controlled hypothermia, and assessment of patient tolerance of cooling

(Do not report 99184 more than once per hospital stay)

(99185, 99186 have been deleted)

99188   Application of topical fluoride varnish by a physician or other qualified health care professional

99190   Assembly and operation of pump with oxygenator or heat exchanger (with or without ECG and/or pressure monitoring); each hour

99191   45 minutes

99192   30 minutes

99195   Phlebotomy, therapeutic (separate procedure)

99199   Unlisted special service, procedure or report

Home Health Procedures/ Services

These codes are used by non-physician health care professionals. Physicians should utilize the home visit codes 99341-99350 and utilize CPT codes other than 99500-99600 for any additional procedure/service provided to a patient living in a residence.

The following codes are used to report services provided in a patient's residence (including assisted living apartments, group homes, nontraditional private homes, custodial care facilities, or schools).

Health care professionals who are authorized to use Evaluation and Management (E/M) Home Visit codes (99341-99350) may report 99500-99600 in addition to 99341-99350 if both services are performed. E/M services may be reported separately, using modifier 25, if the patient's condition requires a significant separately identifiable E/M service, above and beyond the home health service(s)/procedure(s) codes 99500-99600.

99500   Home visit for prenatal monitoring and assessment to include fetal heart rate, non-stress test, uterine monitoring, and gestational diabetes monitoring

99501   Home visit for postnatal assessment and follow-up care

99502   Home visit for newborn care and assessment

99503   Home visit for respiratory therapy care (eg, bronchodilator, oxygen therapy, respiratory assessment, apnea evaluation)

99504   Home visit for mechanical ventilation care

99505   Home visit for stoma care and maintenance including colostomy and cystostomy

99506   Home visit for intramuscular injections

99507   Home visit for care and maintenance of catheter(s) (eg, urinary, drainage, and enteral)

99509   Home visit for assistance with activities of daily living and personal care

(To report self-care/home management training, see 97535)

(To report home medical nutrition assessment and intervention services, see 97802-97804)

(To report home speech therapy services, see 92507-92508)

99510   Home visit for individual, family, or marriage counseling

99511   Home visit for fecal impaction management and enema administration

99512   Home visit for hemodialysis

(For home infusion of peritoneal dialysis, use 99601, 99602)

99600   Unlisted home visit service or procedure

Home Infusion Procedures/Services

99601   Home infusion/specialty drug administration, per visit (up to 2 hours);

+ **99602**   each additional hour (List separately in addition to code for primary procedure)

(Use 99602 in conjunction with 99601)

Medicine

Medication Therapy Management Services

Medication therapy management service(s) (MTMS) describe face-to-face patient assessment and intervention as appropriate, by a pharmacist, upon request. MTMS is provided to optimize the response to medications or to manage treatment-related medication interactions or complications.

MTMS includes the following documented elements: review of the pertinent patient history, medication profile (prescription and nonprescription), and recommendations for improving health outcomes and treatment compliance. These codes are not to be used to describe the provision of product-specific information at the point of dispensing or any other routine dispensing-related activities.

99605 Medication therapy management service(s) provided by a pharmacist, individual, face-to-face with patient, with assessment and intervention if provided; initial 15 minutes, new patient

99606 initial 15 minutes, established patient

+ 99607 each additional 15 minutes (List separately in addition to code for primary service)

(Use 99607 in conjunction with 99605, 99606)

Medicine

Category II Codes

The following section of *Current Procedural Terminology* (CPT) contains a set of supplemental tracking codes that can be used for performance measurement. It is anticipated that the use of Category II codes for performance measurement will decrease the need for record abstraction and chart review, and thereby minimize administrative burden on physicians, other health care professionals, hospitals, and entities seeking to measure the quality of patient care. These codes are intended to facilitate data collection about the quality of care rendered by coding certain services and test results that support nationally established performance measures and that have an evidence base as contributing to quality patient care.

The use of these codes is optional. The codes are not required for correct coding and may not be used as a substitute for Category I codes.

These codes describe clinical components that may be typically included in evaluation and management services or clinical services and, therefore, do not have a relative value associated with them. Category II codes may also describe results from clinical laboratory or radiology tests and other procedures, identified processes intended to address patient safety practices, or services reflecting compliance with state or federal law.

Category II codes described in this section make use of alphabetical characters as the 5th character in the string (ie, 4 digits followed by the letter **F**). These digits are not intended to reflect the placement of the code in the regular (Category I) part of the CPT code set. To promote understanding of these codes and their associated measures, users are referred to the Alphabetical Clinical Topics Listing, which contains information about performance measurement exclusion modifiers, measures, and the measure's source.

Cross-references to the measures associated with each Category II code and their source are included for reference in the Alphabetical Clinical Topics Listing. In addition, acronyms for the related diseases or clinical condition(s) have been added at the end of each code descriptor to identify the topic or clinical category in which that code is included. A complete listing of the diseases/clinical conditions, and their acronyms are provided in alphabetical order in the Alphabetical Clinical Topics Listing. The Alphabetical Clinical Topics Listing can be accessed on the website at www.ama-assn.org, under the Category II link. Users should review the complete measure(s) associated with each code prior to implementation.

Category II codes are reviewed by the Performance Measures Advisory Group (PMAG), an advisory body to the CPT Editorial Panel and the CPT/HCPAC Advisory Committee. The PMAG is comprised of performance measurement experts representing the Agency for Healthcare Research and Quality (AHRQ), the American Medical Association (AMA), the Centers for Medicare and Medicaid Services (CMS), The Joint Commission (TJC), and the Physician Consortium for Performance Improvement® (PCPI). The PMAG may seek additional expertise and/or input from other national health care organizations, as necessary, for the development of tracking codes. These may include national medical specialty societies, other national health care professional associations, accrediting bodies, and federal regulatory agencies.

The most current listing of Category II codes, including guidelines, Code Change Proposal forms, and release and implementation dates for Category II codes may be accessed at www.ama-assn.org/go/cpt.

The superscripted numbers included at the end of each code descriptor direct users to the footnotes. The following information identifies the name and Web address of the measure developers that are associated with these footnotes:

Footnotes

[1] Physician Consortium for Performance Improvement®(PCPI), www.physicianconsortium.org.

[2] National Committee on Quality Assurance (NCQA), Health Employer Data Information Set (HEDIS®), www.ncqa.org.

[3] The Joint Commission (TJC), ORYX Initiative Performance Measures, www.jointcommission.org/performancemeasurement/aspx.

[4] National Diabetes Quality Improvement Alliance (NDQIA),www.nationaldiabetesalliance.org.

[5] Joint measure from The Physician Consortium for Performance Improvement, www.physicianconsortium.org, and National Committee on Quality Assurance (NCQA), www.ncqa.org.

[6] The Society of Thoracic Surgeons at www.sts.org and National Quality Forum, www.qualityforum.org.

[7] Optum, www.optum.com.

[8] American Academy of Neurology, www.aan.com/go/practice/quality/measurements or quality@aan.com.

[9] College of American Pathologists (CAP), www.cap.org/apps/docs/advocacy/pathology performance measurement.pdf.

[10] American Gastroenterological Association (AGA), www.gastro.org/quality.

[11] American Society of Anesthesiologists (ASA), www.asahq.org.

[12] American College of Gastroenterology (ACG), www.gi.org; American Gastroenterological Association (AGA), www.gastro.org; and American Society for Gastrointestinal Endoscopy (ASGE), www.asge.org.

Modifiers

The following performance measurement modifiers may be used for Category II codes to indicate that a service specified in the associated measure(s) was considered but, due to either medical, patient, or system circumstance(s) documented in the medical record, the service was not provided. These modifiers serve as denominator exclusions from the performance measure. The user should note that not all listed measures provide for exclusions (see Alphabetical Clinical Topics Listing for more discussion regarding exclusion criteria).

Category II modifiers should only be reported with Category II codes—they should not be reported with Category I or Category III codes. In addition, the modifiers in the Category II section should only be used where specified in the guidelines, reporting instructions, parenthetic notes, or code descriptor language listed in the Category II section (code listing and the Alphabetical Clinical Topics Listing).

1P Performance Measure Exclusion Modifier due to Medical Reasons

Reasons include:

- Not indicated (absence of organ/limb, already received/performed, other)

- Contraindicated (patient allergic history, potential adverse drug interaction, other)

- Other medical reasons

2P Performance Measure Exclusion Modifier due to Patient Reasons

Reasons include:

- Patient declined

- Economic, social, or religious reasons

- Other patient reasons

3P Performance Measure Exclusion Modifier due to System Reasons

Reasons include:

- Resources to perform the services not available

- Insurance coverage/payor-related limitations

- Other reasons attributable to health care delivery system

Modifier 8P is intended to be used as a "reporting modifier" to allow the reporting of circumstances when an action described in a measure's numerator is not performed and the reason is not otherwise specified.

8P Performance measure reporting modifier—action not performed, reason not otherwise specified

Composite Codes

Composite codes combine several measures grouped within a single code descriptor to facilitate reporting for a clinical condition when all components are met. If only some of the components are met or if services are provided in addition to those included in the composite code, they may be reported individually using the corresponding CPT Category II codes for those services.

0001F Heart failure assessed (includes assessment of all the following components) (CAD)[1]:

Blood pressure measured (2000F)[1]

Level of activity assessed (1003F)[1]

Clinical symptoms of volume overload (excess) assessed (1004F)[1]

Weight, recorded (2001F)[1]

Clinical signs of volume overload (excess) assessed (2002F)[1]

(To report blood pressure measured, use 2000F)

0005F Osteoarthritis assessed (OA)[1]

Includes assessment of all the following components:

Osteoarthritis symptoms and functional status assessed (1006F)[1]

Use of anti-inflammatory or over-the-counter (OTC) analgesic medications assessed (1007F)[1]

Initial examination of the involved joint(s) (includes visual inspection, palpation, range of motion) (2004F)[1]

(To report tobacco use cessation intervention, use 4001F)

0012F Community-acquired bacterial pneumonia assessment (includes all of the following components) (CAP)[1]:

Co-morbid conditions assessed (1026F)[1]

Vital signs recorded (2010F)[1]

Mental status assessed (2014F)[1]

Hydration status assessed (2018F)[1]

0014F Comprehensive preoperative assessment performed for cataract surgery with intraocular lens (IOL) placement (includes assessment of all of the following components) (EC)[5]:

Dilated fundus evaluation performed within 12 months prior to cataract surgery (2020F)[5]

Pre-surgical (cataract) axial length, corneal power measurement and method of intraocular lens power calculation documented (must be performed within 12 months prior to surgery) (3073F)[5]

Preoperative assessment of functional or medical indication(s) for surgery prior to the cataract surgery with intraocular lens placement (must be performed within 12 months prior to cataract surgery) (3325F)[5]

Category II

0015F   Melanoma follow up completed (includes assessment of all of the following components) (ML)[5]:

    History obtained regarding new or changing moles (1050F)[5]

    Complete physical skin exam performed (2029F)[5]

    Patient counseled to perform a monthly self skin examination (5005F)[5]

Patient Management

Patient management codes describe utilization measures or measures of patient care provided for specific clinical purposes (eg, prenatal care, pre- and post-surgical care).

0500F   Initial prenatal care visit (report at first prenatal encounter with health care professional providing obstetrical care. Report also date of visit and, in a separate field, the date of the last menstrual period [LMP]) (Prenatal)[2]

0501F   Prenatal flow sheet documented in medical record by first prenatal visit (documentation includes at minimum blood pressure, weight, urine protein, uterine size, fetal heart tones, and estimated date of delivery). Report also: date of visit and, in a separate field, the date of the last menstrual period [LMP] (Note: If reporting 0501F Prenatal flow sheet, it is not necessary to report 0500F Initial prenatal care visit) (Prenatal)[1]

0502F   Subsequent prenatal care visit (Prenatal)[2]

    [Excludes: patients who are seen for a condition unrelated to pregnancy or prenatal care (eg, an upper respiratory infection; patients seen for consultation only, not for continuing care)]

0503F   Postpartum care visit (Prenatal)[2]

0505F   Hemodialysis plan of care documented (ESRD, P-ESRD)[1]

0507F   Peritoneal dialysis plan of care documented (ESRD)[1]

0509F   Urinary incontinence plan of care documented (GER)[5]

0513F   Elevated blood pressure plan of care documented (CKD)[1]

0514F   Plan of care for elevated hemoglobin level documented for patient receiving Erythropoiesis-Stimulating Agent therapy (ESA) (CKD)[1]

0516F   Anemia plan of care documented (ESRD)[1]

0517F   Glaucoma plan of care documented (EC)[5]

0518F   Falls plan of care documented (GER)[5]

0519F   Planned chemotherapy regimen, including at a minimum: drug(s) prescribed, dose, and duration, documented prior to initiation of a new treatment regimen (ONC)[1]

0520F   Radiation dose limits to normal tissues established prior to the initiation of a course of 3D conformal radiation for a minimum of 2 tissue/organ (ONC)[1]

0521F   Plan of care to address pain documented (COA)[2] (ONC)[1]

0525F   Initial visit for episode (BkP)[2]

0526F   Subsequent visit for episode (BkP)[2]

0528F   Recommended follow-up interval for repeat colonoscopy of at least 10 years documented in colonoscopy report (End/Polyp)[5]

0529F   Interval of 3 or more years since patient's last colonoscopy, documented (End/Polyp)[5]

0535F   Dyspnea management plan of care, documented (Pall Cr)[5]

0540F   Glucorticoid Management Plan Documented (RA)[5]

0545F   Plan for follow-up care for major depressive disorder, documented (MDD ADOL)[1]

0550F   Cytopathology report on routine nongynecologic specimen finalized within two working days of accession date (PATH)[9]

0551F   Cytopathology report on nongynecologic specimen with documentation that the specimen was non-routine (PATH)[9]

0555F   Symptom management plan of care documented (HF)[1]

0556F   Plan of care to achieve lipid control documented (CAD)[1]

0557F   Plan of care to manage anginal symptoms documented (CAD)[1]

0575F   HIV RNA control plan of care, documented (HIV)[5]

0580F   Multidisciplinary care plan developed or updated (ALS)[8]

0581F   Patient transferred directly from anesthetizing location to critical care unit (Peri2)[11]

0582F   Patient not transferred directly from anesthetizing location to critical care unit (Peri2)[11]

0583F   Transfer of care checklist used (Peri2)[11]

0584F   Transfer of care checklist not used (Peri2)[11]

Patient History

Patient history codes describe measures for select aspects of patient history or review of systems.

1000F   Tobacco use assessed (CAD, CAP, COPD, PV)[1] (DM)[4]

1002F   Anginal symptoms and level of activity assessed (NMA–No Measure Associated)

1003F   Level of activity assessed (NMA–No Measure Associated)

1004F   Clinical symptoms of volume overload (excess) assessed (NMA–No Measure Associated)

1005F   Asthma symptoms evaluated (includes documentation of numeric frequency of symptoms or patient completion of an asthma assessment tool/survey/questionnaire) (NMA–No Measure Associated)

Category II

1006F   Osteoarthritis symptoms and functional status assessed (may include the use of a standardized scale or the completion of an assessment questionnaire, such as the SF-36, AAOS Hip & Knee Questionnaire) (OA)[1]

[Instructions: Report when osteoarthritis is addressed during the patient encounter]

1007F   Use of anti-inflammatory or analgesic over-the-counter (OTC) medications for symptom relief assessed (OA)[1]

1008F   Gastrointestinal and renal risk factors assessed for patients on prescribed or OTC non-steroidal anti-inflammatory drug (NSAID) (OA)[1]

1010F   Severity of angina assessed by level of activity (CAD)[1]

1011F   Angina present (CAD)[1]

1012F   Angina absent (CAD)[1]

1015F   Chronic obstructive pulmonary disease (COPD) symptoms assessed (Includes assessment of at least 1 of the following: dyspnea, cough/sputum, wheezing), or respiratory symptom assessment tool completed (COPD)[1]

1018F   Dyspnea assessed, not present (COPD)[1]

1019F   Dyspnea assessed, present (COPD)[1]

1022F   Pneumococcus immunization status assessed (CAP, COPD)[1]

1026F   Co-morbid conditions assessed (eg, includes assessment for presence or absence of: malignancy, liver disease, congestive heart failure, cerebrovascular disease, renal disease, chronic obstructive pulmonary disease, asthma, diabetes, other co-morbid conditions) (CAP)[1]

1030F   Influenza immunization status assessed (CAP)[1]

1031F   Smoking status and exposure to second hand smoke in the home assessed (Asthma)[1]

1032F   Current tobacco smoker **or** currently exposed to secondhand smoke (Asthma)[1]

1033F   Current tobacco non-smoker **and** not currently exposed to secondhand smoke (Asthma)[1]

1034F   Current tobacco smoker (CAD, CAP, COPD, PV)[1] (DM)[4]

1035F   Current smokeless tobacco user (eg, chew, snuff) (PV)[1]

1036F   Current tobacco non-user (CAD, CAP, COPD, PV)[1] (DM)[4] (IBD)[10]

1038F   Persistent asthma (mild, moderate or severe) (Asthma)[1]

1039F   Intermittent asthma (Asthma)[1]

1040F   DSM-5 criteria for major depressive disorder documented at the initial evaluation (MDD, MDD ADOL)[1]

1050F   History obtained regarding new or changing moles (ML)[5]

1052F   Type, anatomic location, and activity all assessed (IBD)[10]

1055F   Visual functional status assessed (EC)[5]

1060F   Documentation of permanent **or** persistent **or** paroxysmal atrial fibrillation (STR)[5]

1061F   Documentation of absence of permanent **and** persistent **and** paroxysmal atrial fibrillation (STR)[5]

1065F   Ischemic stroke symptom onset of less than 3 hours prior to arrival (STR)[5]

1066F   Ischemic stroke symptom onset greater than or equal to 3 hours prior to arrival (STR)[5]

1070F   Alarm symptoms (involuntary weight loss, dysphagia, or gastrointestinal bleeding) assessed; none present (GERD)[5]

1071F   1 or more present (GERD)[5]

(1080F has been deleted. To report Surrogate decision maker or advance care plan documented in the medical record, report code 1123F or 1124F.)

1090F   Presence or absence of urinary incontinence assessed (GER)[5]

1091F   Urinary incontinence characterized (eg, frequency, volume, timing, type of symptoms, how bothersome) (GER)[5]

1100F   Patient screened for future fall risk; documentation of 2 or more falls in the past year or any fall with injury in the past year (GER)[5]

1101F   documentation of no falls in the past year or only 1 fall without injury in the past year (GER)[5]

1110F   Patient discharged from an inpatient facility (eg, hospital, skilled nursing facility, or rehabilitation facility) within the last 60 days (GER)[5]

1111F   Discharge medications reconciled with the current medication list in outpatient medical record (COA)[2] (GER)[5]

1116F   Auricular or periauricular pain assessed (AOE)[1]

1118F   GERD symptoms assessed after 12 months of therapy (GERD)[5]

1119F   Initial evaluation for condition (HEP C)[1](EPI, DSP)[8]

1121F   Subsequent evaluation for condition (HEP C)[1](EPI)[8]

1123F   Advance Care Planning discussed and documented advance care plan or surrogate decision maker documented in the medical record (DEM)[1] (GER, Pall Cr)[5]

1124F   Advance Care Planning discussed and documented in the medical record, patient did not wish or was not able to name a surrogate decision maker or provide an advance care plan (DEM)[1] (GER, Pall Cr)[5]

1125F   Pain severity quantified; pain present (COA)[2] (ONC)[1]

1126F   no pain present (COA)[2] (ONC)[1]

1127F   New episode for condition (NMA–No Measure Associated)

1128F   Subsequent episode for condition (NMA–No Measure Associated)

1130F   Back pain and function assessed, including all of the following: Pain assessment **and** functional status **and** patient history, including notation of presence or absence of "red flags" (warning signs) **and** assessment of prior treatment and response, **and** employment status (BkP)[2]

1134F   Episode of back pain lasting 6 weeks or less (BkP)[2]

Category II

1135F   Episode of back pain lasting longer than 6 weeks (BkP)[2]

1136F   Episode of back pain lasting 12 weeks or less (BkP)[2]

1137F   Episode of back pain lasting longer than 12 weeks (BkP)[2]

1150F   Documentation that a patient has a substantial risk of death within 1 year (Pall Cr)[5]

1151F   Documentation that a patient does not have a substantial risk of death within one year (Pall Cr)[5]

1152F   Documentation of advanced disease diagnosis, goals of care prioritize comfort (Pall Cr)[5]

1153F   Documentation of advanced disease diagnosis, goals of care do not prioritize comfort (Pall Cr)[5]

1157F   Advance care plan or similar legal document present in the medical record (COA)[2]

1158F   Advance care planning discussion documented in the medical record (COA)[2]

1159F   Medication list documented in medical record (COA)[2]

1160F   Review of all medications by a prescribing practitioner or clinical pharmacist (such as, prescriptions, OTCs, herbal therapies and supplements) documented in the medical record (COA)[2]

1170F   Functional status assessed (COA)[2] (RA)[5]

1175F   Functional status for dementia assessed and results reviewed (DEM)[1]

1180F   All specified thromboembolic risk factors assessed (AFIB)[1]

1181F   Neuropsychiatric symptoms assessed and results reviewed (DEM)[1]

1182F   Neuropsychiatric symptoms, one or more present (DEM)[1]

1183F   Neuropsychiatric symptoms, absent (DEM)[1]

1200F   Seizure type(s) and current seizure frequency(ies) documented (EPI)[8]

1205F   Etiology of epilepsy or epilepsy syndrome(s) reviewed and documented (EPI)[8]

1220F   Patient screened for depression (SUD)[5]

1400F   Parkinson's disease diagnosis reviewed (Prkns)[8]

1450F   Symptoms improved or remained consistent with treatment goals since last assessment (HF)[1]

1451F   Symptoms demonstrated clinically important deterioration since last assessment (HF)[1]

1460F   Qualifying cardiac event/diagnosis in previous 12 months (CAD)[1]

1461F   No qualifying cardiac event/diagnosis in previous 12 months (CAD)[1]

1490F   Dementia severity classified, mild (DEM)[1]

1491F   Dementia severity classified, moderate (DEM)[1]

1493F   Dementia severity classified, severe (DEM)[1]

1494F   Cognition assessed and reviewed (DEM)[1]

1500F   Symptoms and signs of distal symmetric polyneuropathy reviewed and documented (DSP)[8]

1501F   Not initial evaluation for condition (DSP)[8]

1502F   Patient queried about pain and pain interference with function using a valid and reliable instrument (DSP)[8]

1503F   Patient queried about symptoms of respiratory insufficiency (ALS)[8]

1504F   Patient has respiratory insufficiency (ALS)[8]

1505F   Patient does not have respiratory insufficiency (ALS)[8]

Physical Examination

Physical examination codes describe aspects of physical examination or clinical assessment.

2000F   Blood pressure measured (CKD)[1](DM)[2,4]

2001F   Weight recorded (PAG)[1]

2002F   Clinical signs of volume overload (excess) assessed (NMA–No Measure Associated)

2004F   Initial examination of the involved joint(s) (includes visual inspection, palpation, range of motion) (OA)[1]

       [Instructions: Report only for initial osteoarthritis visit or for visits for new joint involvement]

2010F   Vital signs (temperature, pulse, respiratory rate, and blood pressure) documented and reviewed (CAP)[1] (EM)[5]

2014F   Mental status assessed (CAP)[1] (EM)[5]

2015F   Asthma impairment assessed (Asthma)[1]

2016F   Asthma risk assessed (Asthma)[1]

2018F   Hydration status assessed (normal/mildly dehydrated/severely dehydrated) (CAP)[1]

2019F   Dilated macular exam performed, including documentation of the presence or absence of macular thickening or hemorrhage **and** the level of macular degeneration severity (EC)[5]

2020F   Dilated fundus evaluation performed within 12 months prior to cataract surgery (EC)[5]

2021F   Dilated macular or fundus exam performed, including documentation of the presence or absence of macular edema **and** level of severity of retinopathy (EC)[5]

2022F   Dilated retinal eye exam with interpretation by an ophthalmologist or optometrist documented and reviewed (DM)[2,4]

2024F   7 standard field stereoscopic photos with interpretation by an ophthalmologist or optometrist documented and reviewed (DM)[2,4]

2026F   Eye imaging validated to match diagnosis from 7 standard field stereoscopic photos results documented and reviewed (DM)[2,4]

2027F   Optic nerve head evaluation performed (EC)[5]

Category II

2028F Foot examination performed (includes examination through visual inspection, sensory exam with monofilament, and pulse exam – report when any of the 3 components are completed) (DM)[4]

2029F Complete physical skin exam performed (ML)[5]

2030F Hydration status documented, normally hydrated (PAG)[1]

2031F Hydration status documented, dehydrated (PAG)[1]

2035F Tympanic membrane mobility assessed with pneumatic otoscopy or tympanometry (OME)[1]

2040F Physical examination on the date of the initial visit for low back pain performed, in accordance with specifications (BkP)[2]

2044F Documentation of mental health assessment prior to intervention (back surgery or epidural steroid injection) or for back pain episode lasting longer than 6 weeks (BkP)[2]

2050F Wound characteristics including size **and** nature of wound base tissue **and** amount of drainage prior to debridement documented (CWC)[5]

2060F Patient interviewed directly on or before date of diagnosis of major depressive disorder (MDD ADOL)[1]

Diagnostic/Screening Processes or Results

Diagnostic/screening processes or results codes describe results of tests ordered (clinical laboratory tests, radiological or other procedural examinations, and conclusions of medical decision-making).

3006F Chest X-ray results documented and reviewed (CAP)[1]

3008F Body Mass Index (BMI), documented (PV)[1]

3011F Lipid panel results documented and reviewed (must include total cholesterol, HDL-C, triglycerides and calculated LDL-C) (CAD)[1]

3014F Screening mammography results documented and reviewed (PV)[1,2]

3015F Cervical cancer screening results documented and reviewed (PV)[1]

3016F Patient screened for unhealthy alcohol use using a systematic screening method (PV)[1] (DSP)[8]

3017F Colorectal cancer screening results documented and reviewed (PV)[12]

3018F Pre-procedure risk assessment **and** depth of insertion **and** quality of the bowel prep **and** complete description of polyp(s) found, including location of each polyp, size, number and gross morphology **and** recommendations for follow-up in final colonoscopy report documented (End/Polyp)[5]

3019F Left ventricular ejection fraction (LVEF) assessment planned post discharge (HF)[1]

3020F Left ventricular function (LVF) assessment (eg, echocardiography, nuclear test, or ventriculography) documented in the medical record (Includes quantitative or qualitative assessment results) (NMA–No Measure Associated)

3021F Left ventricular ejection fraction (LVEF) less than 40% or documentation of moderately or severely depressed left ventricular systolic function (CAD, HF)[1]

3022F Left ventricular ejection fraction (LVEF) greater than or equal to 40% or documentation as normal or mildly depressed left ventricular systolic function (CAD, HF)[1]

3023F Spirometry results documented and reviewed (COPD)[1]

3025F Spirometry test results demonstrate FEV_1/FVC less than 70% with COPD symptoms (eg, dyspnea, cough/sputum, wheezing) (CAP, COPD)[1]

3027F Spirometry test results demonstrate FEV_1/FVC greater than or equal to 70% or patient does not have COPD symptoms (COPD)[1]

3028F Oxygen saturation results documented and reviewed (includes assessment through pulse oximetry or arterial blood gas measurement) (CAP, COPD)[1] (EM)[5]

3035F Oxygen saturation less than or equal to 88% or a PaO_2 less than or equal to 55 mm Hg (COPD)[1]

3037F Oxygen saturation greater than 88% or PaO_2 greater than 55 mm Hg (COPD)[1]

3038F Pulmonary function test performed within 12 months prior to surgery (Lung/Esop Cx)[6]

3040F Functional expiratory volume (FEV_1) less than 40% of predicted value (COPD)[1]

3042F Functional expiratory volume (FEV_1) greater than or equal to 40% of predicted value (COPD)[1]

3044F Most recent hemoglobin A1c (HbA1c) level less than 7.0% (DM)[2,4]

3045F Most recent hemoglobin A1c (HbA1c) level 7.0–9.0% (DM)[2,4]

3046F Most recent hemoglobin A1c level greater than 9.0% (DM)[4]

(To report most recent hemoglobin A1c level less than or equal to 9.0%, see codes 3044F-3045F)

3048F Most recent LDL-C less than 100 mg/dL (CAD)[1] (DM)[4]

3049F Most recent LDL-C 100-129 mg/dL (CAD)[1] (DM)[4]

3050F Most recent LDL-C greater than or equal to 130 mg/dL (CAD)[1] (DM)[4]

3055F Left ventricular ejection fraction (LVEF) less than or equal to 35% (HF)[1]

3056F Left ventricular ejection fraction (LVEF) greater than 35% or no LVEF result available (HF)[1]

3060F Positive microalbuminuria test result documented and reviewed (DM)[2,4]

Category II

3061F Negative microalbuminuria test result documented and reviewed (DM)[2,4]

3062F Positive macroalbuminuria test result documented and reviewed (DM)[2,4]

3066F Documentation of treatment for nephropathy (eg, patient receiving dialysis, patient being treated for ESRD, CRF, ARF, or renal insufficiency, any visit to a nephrologist) (DM)[2,4]

3072F Low risk for retinopathy (no evidence of retinopathy in the prior year) (DM)[2,4]

3073F Pre-surgical (cataract) axial length, corneal power measurement and method of intraocular lens power calculation documented within 12 months prior to surgery (EC)[5]

3074F Most recent systolic blood pressure less than 130 mm Hg (DM)[2,4] (HTN, CKD, CAD)[1]

3075F Most recent systolic blood pressure 130 - 139 mm Hg (DM)[2,4](HTN, CKD, CAD)[1]

(To report most recent systolic blood pressure less than 140 mm Hg, see codes 3074F-3075F)

3077F Most recent systolic blood pressure greater than or equal to 140 mm Hg (HTN, CKD, CAD)[1] (DM)[2,4]

3078F Most recent diastolic blood pressure less than 80 mm Hg (HTN, CKD, CAD)[1] (DM)[2,4]

3079F Most recent diastolic blood pressure 80-89 mm Hg (HTN, CKD, CAD)[1] (DM)[2,4]

3080F Most recent diastolic blood pressure greater than or equal to 90 mm Hg (HTN, CKD, CAD)[1] (DM)[2,4]

3082F Kt/V less than 1.2 (Clearance of urea [Kt]/volume [V]) (ESRD, P-ESRD)[1]

3083F Kt/V equal to or greater than 1.2 and less than 1.7 (Clearance of urea [Kt]/volume [V]) (ESRD, P-ESRD)[1]

3084F Kt/V greater than or equal to 1.7 (Clearance of urea [Kt]/volume [V]) (ESRD, P-ESRD)[1]

3085F Suicide risk assessed (MDD, MDD ADOL)[1]

3088F Major depressive disorder, mild (MDD)[1]

3089F Major depressive disorder, moderate (MDD)[1]

3090F Major depressive disorder, severe without psychotic features (MDD)[1]

3091F Major depressive disorder, severe with psychotic features (MDD)[1]

3092F Major depressive disorder, in remission (MDD)[1]

3093F Documentation of new diagnosis of initial or recurrent episode of major depressive disorder (MDD)[1]

3095F Central dual-energy X-ray absorptiometry (DXA) results documented (OP)[5](IBD)[10]

3096F Central dual-energy X-ray absorptiometry (DXA) ordered (OP)[5](IBD)[10]

3100F Carotid imaging study report (includes direct or indirect reference to measurements of distal internal carotid diameter as the denominator for stenosis measurement) (STR, RAD)[5]

3110F Documentation in final CT or MRI report of presence or absence of hemorrhage and mass lesion and acute infarction (STR)[5]

3111F CT or MRI of the brain performed in the hospital within 24 hours of arrival **or** performed in an outpatient imaging center, to confirm initial diagnosis of stroke, TIA or intracranial hemorrhage (STR)[5]

3112F CT or MRI of the brain performed greater than 24 hours after arrival to the hospital **or** performed in an outpatient imaging center for purpose other than confirmation of initial diagnosis of stroke, TIA, or intracranial hemorrhage (STR)[5]

3115F Quantitative results of an evaluation of current level of activity and clinical symptoms (HF)[1]

3117F Heart failure disease specific structured assessment tool completed (HF)[1]

3118F New York Heart Association (NYHA) Class documented (HF)[1]

3119F No evaluation of level of activity or clinical symptoms (HF)[1]

3120F 12-Lead ECG Performed (EM)[5]

(3125F has been deleted)

3126F Esophageal biopsy report with a statement about dysplasia (present, absent, or indefinite, and if present, contains appropriate grading) (PATH)[9]

3130F Upper gastrointestinal endoscopy performed (GERD)[5]

3132F Documentation of referral for upper gastrointestinal endoscopy (GERD)[5]

3140F Upper gastrointestinal endoscopy report indicates suspicion of Barrett's esophagus (GERD)[5]

3141F Upper gastrointestinal endoscopy report indicates no suspicion of Barrett's esophagus (GERD)[5]

3142F Barium swallow test ordered (GERD)[1]

(To report documentation of barium swallow study, use 3142F)

3150F Forceps esophageal biopsy performed (GERD)[5]

3155F Cytogenetic testing performed on bone marrow at time of diagnosis or prior to initiating treatment (HEM)[1]

3160F Documentation of iron stores prior to initiating erythropoietin therapy (HEM)[1]

3170F Flow cytometry studies performed at time of diagnosis or prior to initiating treatment (HEM)[1]

3200F Barium swallow test not ordered (GERD)[5]

3210F Group A Strep Test Performed (PHAR)[2]

Category II

3215F Patient has documented immunity to Hepatitis A (HEP-C)[1]

3216F Patient has documented immunity to Hepatitis B (HEP-C)[1](IBD)[10]

3218F RNA testing for Hepatitis C documented as performed within 6 months prior to initiation of antiviral treatment for Hepatitis C (HEP-C)[1]

3220F Hepatitis C quantitative RNA testing documented as performed at 12 weeks from initiation of antiviral treatment (HEP-C)[1]

3230F Documentation that hearing test was performed within 6 months prior to tympanostomy tube insertion (OME)[1]

3250F Specimen site other than anatomic location of primary tumor (PATH)[1]

3260F pT category (primary tumor), pN category (regional lymph nodes), and histologic grade documented in pathology report (PATH)[1]

3265F Ribonucleic acid (RNA) testing for Hepatitis C viremia ordered or results documented (HEP C)[1]

3266F Hepatitis C genotype testing documented as performed prior to initiation of antiviral treatment for Hepatitis C (HEP C)[1]

3267F Pathology report includes pT category, pN category, Gleason score, and statement about margin status (PATH)[9]

3268F Prostate-specific antigen (PSA), **and** primary tumor (T) stage, **and** Gleason score documented prior to initiation of treatment (PRCA)[1]

3269F Bone scan performed prior to initiation of treatment or at any time since diagnosis of prostate cancer (PRCA)[1]

3270F Bone scan not performed prior to initiation of treatment nor at any time since diagnosis of prostate cancer (PRCA)[1]

3271F Low risk of recurrence, prostate cancer (PRCA)[1]

3272F Intermediate risk of recurrence, prostate cancer (PRCA)[1]

3273F High risk of recurrence, prostate cancer (PRCA)[1]

3274F Prostate cancer risk of recurrence not determined or neither low, intermediate nor high (PRCA)[1]

3278F Serum levels of calcium, phosphorus, intact Parathyroid Hormone (PTH) and lipid profile ordered (CKD)[1]

3279F Hemoglobin level greater than or equal to 13 g/dL (CKD, ESRD)[1]

3280F Hemoglobin level 11 g/dL to 12.9 g/dL (CKD, ESRD)[1]

3281F Hemoglobin level less than 11 g/dL (CKD, ESRD)[1]

3284F Intraocular pressure (IOP) reduced by a value of greater than or equal to 15% from the pre-intervention level (EC)[5]

3285F Intraocular pressure (IOP) reduced by a value less than 15% from the pre-intervention level (EC)[5]

3288F Falls risk assessment documented (GER)[5]

3290F Patient is D (Rh) negative and unsensitized (Pre-Cr)[1]

3291F Patient is D (Rh) positive or sensitized (Pre-Cr)[1]

3292F HIV testing ordered or documented and reviewed during the first or second prenatal visit (Pre-Cr)[1]

3293F ABO and Rh blood typing documented as performed (Pre-Cr)[7]

3294F Group B Streptococcus (GBS) screening documented as performed during week 35-37 gestation (Pre-Cr)[7]

3300F American Joint Committee on Cancer (AJCC) stage documented and reviewed (ONC)[1]

3301F Cancer stage documented in medical record as metastatic and reviewed (ONC)[1]

(Codes 3302F-3312F have been deleted)

(To report measures for cancer staging, see 3321F-3390F)

3315F Estrogen receptor (ER) or progesterone receptor (PR) positive breast cancer (ONC)[1]

3316F Estrogen receptor (ER) and progesterone receptor (PR) negative breast cancer (ONC)[1]

3317F Pathology report confirming malignancy documented in the medical record and reviewed prior to the initiation of chemotherapy (ONC)[1]

3318F Pathology report confirming malignancy documented in the medical record and reviewed prior to the initiation of radiation therapy (ONC)[1]

3319F 1 of the following diagnostic imaging studies ordered: chest x-ray, CT, Ultrasound, MRI, PET, or nuclear medicine scans (ML)[5]

3320F None of the following diagnostic imaging studies ordered: chest X-ray, CT, Ultrasound, MRI, PET, or nuclear medicine scans (ML)[5]

3321F AJCC Cancer Stage 0 or IA Melanoma, documented (ML)[5]

3322F Melanoma greater than AJCC Stage 0 or IA (ML)[5]

3323F Clinical tumor, node and metastases (TNM) staging documented and reviewed prior to surgery (Lung/Esop Cx)[6]

3324F MRI or CT scan ordered, reviewed or requested (EPI)[8]

3325F Preoperative assessment of functional or medical indication(s) for surgery prior to the cataract surgery with intraocular lens placement (must be performed within 12 months prior to cataract surgery) (EC)[5]

3328F Performance status documented and reviewed within 2 weeks prior to surgery (Lung/Esop Cx)[6]

3330F Imaging study ordered (BkP)[2]

3331F Imaging study not ordered (BkP)[2]

3340F Mammogram assessment category of "incomplete: need additional imaging evaluation" documented (RAD)[5]

3341F Mammogram assessment category of "negative," documented (RAD)[5]

3342F Mammogram assessment category of "benign," documented (RAD)[5]

Category II

3343F Mammogram assessment category of "probably benign," documented (RAD)[5]

3344F Mammogram assessment category of "suspicious," documented (RAD)[5]

3345F Mammogram assessment category of "highly suggestive of malignancy," documented (RAD)[5]

3350F Mammogram assessment category of "known biopsy proven malignancy," documented (RAD)[5]

3351F Negative screen for depressive symptoms as categorized by using a standardized depression screening/assessment tool (MDD)[2]

3352F No significant depressive symptoms as categorized by using a standardized depression assessment tool (MDD)[2]

3353F Mild to moderate depressive symptoms as categorized by using a standardized depression screening/assessment tool (MDD)[2]

3354F Clinically significant depressive symptoms as categorized by using a standardized depression screening/assessment tool (MDD)[2]

3370F AJCC Breast Cancer Stage 0 documented (ONC)[1]

3372F AJCC Breast Cancer Stage I: T1mic, T1a or T1b (tumor size ≤ 1 cm) documented (ONC)[1]

3374F AJCC Breast Cancer Stage I: T1c (tumor size > 1 cm to 2 cm) documented (ONC)[1]

3376F AJCC Breast Cancer Stage II documented (ONC)[1]

3378F AJCC Breast Cancer Stage III documented (ONC)[1]

3380F AJCC Breast Cancer Stage IV documented (ONC)[1]

3382F AJCC colon cancer, Stage 0 documented (ONC)[1]

3384F AJCC colon cancer, Stage I documented (ONC)[1]

3386F AJCC colon cancer, Stage II documented (ONC)[1]

3388F AJCC colon cancer, Stage III documented (ONC)[1]

3390F AJCC colon cancer, Stage IV documented (ONC)[1]

3394F Quantitative HER2 immunohistochemistry (IHC) evaluation of breast cancer consistent with the scoring system defined in the ASCO/CAP guidelines (PATH)[9]

3395F Quantitative non-HER2 immunohistochemistry (IHC) evaluation of breast cancer (eg, testing for estrogen or progesterone receptors [ER/PR]) performed (PATH)[9]

3450F Dyspnea screened, no dyspnea or mild dyspnea (Pall Cr)[5]

3451F Dyspnea screened, moderate or severe dyspnea (Pall Cr)[5]

3452F Dyspnea not screened (Pall Cr)[5]

3455F TB screening performed and results interpreted within six months prior to initiation of first-time biologic disease modifying anti-rheumatic drug therapy for RA (RA)[5]

3470F Rheumatoid arthritis (RA) disease activity, low (RA)[5]

3471F Rheumatoid arthritis (RA) disease activity, moderate (RA)[5]

3472F Rheumatoid arthritis (RA) disease activity, high (RA)[5]

3475F Disease prognosis for rheumatoid arthritis assessed, poor prognosis documented (RA)[5]

3476F Disease prognosis for rheumatoid arthritis assessed, good prognosis documented (RA)[5]

3490F History of AIDS-defining condition (HIV)[5]

3491F HIV indeterminate (infants of undetermined HIV status born of HIV-infected mothers) (HIV)[5]

3492F History of nadir CD4+ cell count <350 cells/mm^3 (HIV)[5]

3493F No history of nadir CD4+ cell count <350 cells/mm^3 **and** no history of AIDS-defining condition (HIV)[5]

3494F CD4+ cell count <200 cells/mm^3 (HIV)[5]

3495F CD4+ cell count 200 – 499 cells/mm^3 (HIV)[5]

3496F CD4+ cell count ≥500 cells/mm^3 (HIV)[5]

3497F CD4+ cell percentage <15% (HIV)[5]

3498F CD4+ cell percentage ≥15% (HIV)[5]

3500F CD4+ cell count or CD4+ cell percentage documented as performed (HIV)[5]

3502F HIV RNA viral load below limits of quantification (HIV)[5]

3503F HIV RNA viral load not below limits of quantification (HIV)[5]

3510F Documentation that tuberculosis (TB) screening test performed and results interpreted (HIV)[5] (IBD)[10]

3511F Chlamydia and gonorrhea screenings documented as performed (HIV)[5]

3512F Syphilis screening documented as performed (HIV)[5]

3513F Hepatitis B screening documented as performed (HIV)[5]

3514F Hepatitis C screening documented as performed (HIV)[5]

3515F Patient has documented immunity to Hepatitis C (HIV)[5]

3517F Hepatitis B Virus (HBV) status assessed and results interpreted within one year prior to receiving a first course of anti-TNF (tumor necrosis factor) therapy (IBD)[10]

3520F Clostridium difficile testing performed (IBD)[10]

3550F Low risk for thromboembolism (AFIB)[1]

3551F Intermediate risk for thromboembolism (AFIB)[1]

3552F High risk for thromboembolism (AFIB)[1]

3555F Patient had International Normalized Ratio (INR) measurement performed (AFIB)[1]

3570F Final report for bone scintigraphy study includes correlation with existing relevant imaging studies (eg, x-ray, MRI, CT) corresponding to the same anatomical region in question (NUC_MED)[1]

3572F Patient considered to be potentially at risk for fracture in a weight-bearing site (NUC_MED)[1]

3573F Patient not considered to be potentially at risk for fracture in a weight-bearing site (NUC_MED)[1]

3650F Electroencephalogram (EEG) ordered, reviewed or requested (EPI)[8]

3700F Psychiatric disorders or disturbances assessed (Prkns)[8]

3720F Cognitive impairment or dysfunction assessed (Prkns)[8]

3725F Screening for depression performed (DEM)[1]

3750F Patient not receiving dose of corticosteroids greater than or equal to 10mg/day for 60 or greater consecutive days (IBD)[10]

3751F Electrodiagnostic studies for distal symmetric polyneuropathy conducted (or requested), documented, and reviewed within 6 months of initial evaluation for condition (DSP)[8]

3752F Electrodiagnostic studies for distal symmetric polyneuropathy **not** conducted (or requested), documented, or reviewed within 6 months of initial evaluation for condition (DSP)[8]

3753F Patient has clear clinical symptoms and signs that are highly suggestive of neuropathy AND cannot be attributed to another condition, AND has an obvious cause for the neuropathy (DSP)[8]

3754F Screening tests for diabetes mellitus reviewed, requested, or ordered (DSP)[8]

3755F Cognitive and behavioral impairment screening performed (ALS)[8]

3756F Patient has pseudobulbar affect, sialorrhea, or ALS-related symptoms (ALS)[8]

3757F Patient does not have pseudobulbar affect, sialorrhea, or ALS-related symptoms (ALS)[8]

3758F Patient referred for pulmonary function testing or peak cough expiratory flow (ALS)[8]

3759F Patient screened for dysphagia, weight loss, and impaired nutrition, and results documented (ALS)[8]

3760F Patient exhibits dysphagia, weight loss, or impaired nutrition (ALS)[8]

3761F Patient does not exhibit dysphagia, weight loss, or impaired nutrition (ALS)[8]

3762F Patient is dysarthric (ALS)[8]

3763F Patient is not dysarthric (ALS)[8]

3775F Adenoma(s) or other neoplasm detected during screening colonoscopy (SCADR)[12]

3776F Adenoma(s) or other neoplasm not detected during screening colonoscopy (SCADR)[12]

Therapeutic, Preventive, or Other Interventions

Therapeutic, preventive, or other interventions codes describe pharmacologic, procedural, or behavioral therapies, including preventive services such as patient education and counseling.

4000F Tobacco use cessation intervention, counseling (COPD, CAP, CAD, Asthma)[1] (DM)[4] (PV)[2]

4001F Tobacco use cessation intervention, pharmacologic therapy (COPD, CAD, CAP, PV, Asthma)[1] (DM)[4] (PV)[2]

4003F Patient education, written/oral, appropriate for patients with heart failure, performed (NMA–No Measure Associated)[1]

4004F Patient screened for tobacco use **and** received tobacco cessation intervention (counseling, pharmacotherapy, or both), if identified as a tobacco user (PV, CAD)[1]

4005F Pharmacologic therapy (other than minerals/vitamins) for osteoporosis prescribed (OP)[5] (IBD)[10]

(4007F has been deleted. To report age related eye disease study (AREDS) formulation prescribed or recommended, use code 4177F)

4008F Beta-blocker therapy prescribed or currently being taken (CAD,HF)[1]

(4009F has been deleted. To report angiotensin converting enzyme [ACE] inhibitor or angiotensin receptor blocker [ARB] therapy, use 4010F)

4010F Angiotensin Converting Enzyme (ACE) Inhibitor or Angiotensin Receptor Blocker (ARB) therapy prescribed or currently being taken (CAD, CKD, HF)[1] (DM)[2]

4011F Oral antiplatelet therapy prescribed (CAD)[1]

4012F Warfarin therapy prescribed (NMA–No Measure Associated)

4013F Statin therapy prescribed or currently being taken (CAD)[1]

4014F Written discharge instructions provided to heart failure patients discharged home (Instructions include all of the following components: activity level, diet, discharge medications, follow-up appointment, weight monitoring, what to do if symptoms worsen) (NMA–No Measure Associated)

4015F Persistent asthma, preferred long term control medication or an acceptable alternative treatment, prescribed (NMA–No Measure Associated)

(Note: There are no medical exclusion criteria)

(Do not report modifier 1P with 4015F)

(To report patient reasons for not prescribing, use modifier 2P)

4016F Anti-inflammatory/analgesic agent prescribed (OA)[1]

(Use for prescribed or continued medication[s], including over-the-counter medication[s])

4017F Gastrointestinal prophylaxis for NSAID use prescribed (OA)[1]

4018F Therapeutic exercise for the involved joint(s) instructed or physical or occupational therapy prescribed (OA)[1]

4019F Documentation of receipt of counseling on exercise **and** either both calcium and vitamin D use or counseling regarding both calcium and vitamin D use (OP)[5]

4025F Inhaled bronchodilator prescribed (COPD)[1]

4030F Long-term oxygen therapy prescribed (more than 15 hours per day) (COPD)[1]

4033F Pulmonary rehabilitation exercise training recommended (COPD)[1]

(Report 4033F with 1019F)

4035F Influenza immunization recommended (COPD)[1] (IBD)[10]

4037F Influenza immunization ordered or administered (COPD, PV, CKD, ESRD)[1](IBD)[10]

4040F Pneumococcal vaccine administered or previously received (COPD)[1] (PV)[1,2] (IBD)[10]

4041F Documentation of order for cefazolin OR cefuroxime for antimicrobial prophylaxis (PERI 2)[5]

4042F Documentation that prophylactic antibiotics were neither given within 4 hours prior to surgical incision nor given intraoperatively (PERI 2)[5]

4043F Documentation that an order was given to discontinue prophylactic antibiotics within 48 hours of surgical end time, cardiac procedures (PERI 2)[5]

4044F Documentation that an order was given for venous thromboembolism (VTE) prophylaxis to be given within 24 hours prior to incision time or 24 hours after surgery end time (PERI 2)[5]

4045F Appropriate empiric antibiotic prescribed (CAP)[1], (EM)[5]

4046F Documentation that prophylactic antibiotics were given within 4 hours prior to surgical incision or given intraoperatively (PERI 2)[5]

4047F Documentation of order for prophylactic parenteral antibiotics to be given within 1 hour (if fluoroquinolone or vancomycin, 2 hours) prior to surgical incision (or start of procedure when no incision is required) (PERI 2)[5]

4048F Documentation that administration of prophylactic parenteral antibiotic was initiated within 1 hour (if fluoroquinolone or vancomycin, 2 hours) prior to surgical incision (or start of procedure when no incision is required) as ordered (PERI 2)[5]

4049F Documentation that order was given to discontinue prophylactic antibiotics within 24 hours of surgical end time, non-cardiac procedure (PERI 2)[5]

4050F Hypertension plan of care documented as appropriate (NMA-No Measure Associated)[1]

4051F Referred for an arteriovenous (AV) fistula (ESRD, CKD)[1]

4052F Hemodialysis via functioning arteriovenous (AV) fistula (ESRD)[1]

4053F Hemodialysis via functioning arteriovenous (AV) graft (ESRD)[1]

4054F Hemodialysis via catheter (ESRD)[1]

4055F Patient receiving peritoneal dialysis (ESRD)[1]

4056F Appropriate oral rehydration solution recommended (PAG)[1]

4058F Pediatric gastroenteritis education provided to caregiver (PAG)[1]

4060F Psychotherapy services provided (MDD, MDD ADOL)[1]

4062F Patient referral for psychotherapy documented (MDD, MDD ADOL)[1]

4063F Antidepressant pharmacotherapy considered and not prescribed (MDD ADOL)[1]

4064F Antidepressant pharmacotherapy prescribed (MDD, MDD ADOL)[1]

4065F Antipsychotic pharmacotherapy prescribed (MDD)[1]

4066F Electroconvulsive therapy (ECT) provided (MDD)[1]

4067F Patient referral for electroconvulsive therapy (ECT) documented (MDD)[1]

4069F Venous thromboembolism (VTE) prophylaxis received (IBD)[10]

4070F Deep vein thrombosis (DVT) prophylaxis received by end of hospital day 2 (STR)[5]

4073F Oral antiplatelet therapy prescribed at discharge (STR)[5]

4075F Anticoagulant therapy prescribed at discharge (STR)[5]

4077F Documentation that tissue plasminogen activator (t-PA) administration was considered (STR)[5]

4079F Documentation that rehabilitation services were considered (STR)[5]

4084F Aspirin received within 24 hours before emergency department arrival or during emergency department stay (EM)[5]

4086F Aspirin or clopidogrel prescribed or currently being taken (CAD)[1]

4090F Patient receiving erythropoietin therapy (HEM)[1]

4095F Patient not receiving erythropoietin therapy (HEM)[1]

4100F Bisphosphonate therapy, intravenous, ordered or received (HEM)[1]

4110F Internal mammary artery graft performed for primary, isolated coronary artery bypass graft procedure (CABG)[6]

4115F Beta blocker administered within 24 hours prior to surgical incision (CABG)[6]

4120F Antibiotic prescribed or dispensed (URI, PHAR)[2], (A-BRONCH)[2]

4124F Antibiotic neither prescribed nor dispensed (URI, PHAR)[2], (A-BRONCH)[2]

4130F Topical preparations (including OTC) prescribed for acute otitis externa (AOE)[1]

4131F Systemic antimicrobial therapy prescribed (AOE)[1]

4132F Systemic antimicrobial therapy not prescribed (AOE)[1]

4133F Antihistamines or decongestants prescribed or recommended (OME)[1]

4134F Antihistamines or decongestants neither prescribed nor recommended (OME)[1]

Category II

4135F Systemic corticosteroids prescribed (OME)[1]

4136F Systemic corticosteroids not prescribed (OME)[1]

4140F Inhaled corticosteroids prescribed (Asthma)[1]

4142F Corticosteroid sparing therapy prescribed (IBD)[10]

4144F Alternative long-term control medication prescribed (Asthma)[1]

4145F Two or more anti-hypertensive agents prescribed or currently being taken (CAD, HTN)[1]

4148F Hepatitis A vaccine injection administered or previously received (HEP-C)[1]

4149F Hepatitis B vaccine injection administered or previously received (HEP-C, HIV)[1] (IBD)[10]

4150F Patient receiving antiviral treatment for Hepatitis C (HEP-C)[1]

4151F Patient not receiving antiviral treatment for Hepatitis C (HEP-C)[1]

4153F Combination peginterferon and ribavirin therapy prescribed (HEP-C)[1]

4155F Hepatitis A vaccine series previously received (HEP-C)[1]

4157F Hepatitis B vaccine series previously received (HEP-C)[1]

4158F Patient counseled about risks of alcohol use (HEP-C)[1]

4159F Counseling regarding contraception received prior to initiation of antiviral treatment (HEP-C)[1]

4163F Patient counseling at a minimum on all of the following treatment options for clinically localized prostate cancer: active surveillance, **and** interstitial prostate brachytherapy, **and** external beam radiotherapy, **and** radical prostatectomy, provided prior to initiation of treatment (PRCA)[1]

4164F Adjuvant (ie, in combination with external beam radiotherapy to the prostate for prostate cancer) hormonal therapy (gonadotropin-releasing hormone [GnRH] agonist or antagonist) prescribed/administered (PRCA)[1]

4165F 3-dimensional conformal radiotherapy (3D-CRT) or intensity modulated radiation therapy (IMRT) received (PRCA)[1]

4167F Head of bed elevation (30-45 degrees) on first ventilator day ordered (CRIT)[1]

4168F Patient receiving care in the intensive care unit (ICU) and receiving mechanical ventilation, 24 hours or less (CRIT)[1]

4169F Patient either not receiving care in the intensive care unit (ICU) OR not receiving mechanical ventilation OR receiving mechanical ventilation greater than 24 hours (CRIT)[1]

4171F Patient receiving erythropoiesis-stimulating agents (ESA) therapy (CKD)[1]

4172F Patient not receiving erythropoiesis-stimulating agents (ESA) therapy (CKD)[1]

4174F Counseling about the potential impact of glaucoma on visual functioning and quality of life, and importance of treatment adherence provided to patient and/or caregiver(s) (EC)[5]

4175F Best-corrected visual acuity of 20/40 or better (distance or near) achieved within the 90 days following cataract surgery (EC)[5]

4176F Counseling about value of protection from UV light and lack of proven efficacy of nutritional supplements in prevention or progression of cataract development provided to patient and/or caregiver(s) (NMA-No Measure Associated)

4177F Counseling about the benefits and/or risks of the Age-Related Eye Disease Study (AREDS) formulation for preventing progression of age-related macular degeneration (AMD) provided to patient and/or caregiver(s) (EC)[5]

4178F Anti-D immune globulin received between 26 and 30 weeks gestation (Pre-Cr)[1]

4179F Tamoxifen or aromatase inhibitor (AI) prescribed (ONC)[1]

4180F Adjuvant chemotherapy referred, prescribed, or previously received for Stage III colon cancer (ONC)[1]

4181F Conformal radiation therapy received (NMA—No Measure Associated)

4182F Conformal radiation therapy not received (NMA—No Measure Associated)

4185F Continuous (12-months) therapy with proton pump inhibitor (PPI) or histamine H2 receptor antagonist (H2RA) received (GERD)[5]

4186F No continuous (12-months) therapy with either proton pump inhibitor (PPI) or histamine H2 receptor antagonist (H2RA) received (GERD)[5]

4187F Disease modifying anti-rheumatic drug therapy prescribed or dispensed (RA)[2]

4188F Appropriate angiotensin converting enzyme (ACE)/ angiotensin receptor blockers (ARB) therapeutic monitoring test ordered or performed (AM)[2]

4189F Appropriate digoxin therapeutic monitoring test ordered or performed (AM)[2]

4190F Appropriate diuretic therapeutic monitoring test ordered or performed (AM)[2]

4191F Appropriate anticonvulsant therapeutic monitoring test ordered or performed (AM)[2]

4192F Patient not receiving glucocorticoid therapy (RA)[5]

4193F Patient receiving <10 mg daily prednisone (or equivalent), or RA activity is worsening, or glucocorticoid use is for less than 6 months (RA)[5]

4194F Patient receiving ≥10 mg daily prednisone (or equivalent) for longer than 6 months, and improvement or no change in disease activity (RA)[5]

4195F Patient receiving first-time biologic disease modifying anti-rheumatic drug therapy for rheumatoid arthritis (RA)[5]

⊙=Moderate sedation ✚=Add-on code ⌁=FDA approval pending #=Resequenced code ○=Recycled/reinstated code

Category II

4196F Patient not receiving first-time biologic disease modifying anti-rheumatic drug therapy for rheumatoid arthritis (RA)[5]

4200F External beam radiotherapy as primary therapy to prostate with or without nodal irradiation (PRCA)[1]

4201F External beam radiotherapy with or without nodal irradiation as adjuvant or salvage therapy for prostate cancer patient (PRCA)[1]

4210F Angiotensin converting enzyme (ACE) or angiotensin receptor blockers (ARB) medication therapy for 6 months or more (MM)[2]

4220F Digoxin medication therapy for 6 months or more (MM)[2]

4221F Diuretic medication therapy for 6 months or more (MM)[2]

4230F Anticonvulsant medication therapy for 6 months or more (MM)[2]

4240F Instruction in therapeutic exercise with follow-up provided to patients during episode of back pain lasting longer than 12 weeks (BkP)[2]

4242F Counseling for supervised exercise program provided to patients during episode of back pain lasting longer than 12 weeks (BkP)[2]

4245F Patient counseled during the initial visit to maintain or resume normal activities (BkP)[2]

4248F Patient counseled during the initial visit for an episode of back pain against bed rest lasting 4 days or longer (BkP)[2]

4250F Active warming used intraoperatively for the purpose of maintaining normothermia, **or** at least 1 body temperature equal to or greater than 36 degrees Centigrade (or 96.8 degrees Fahrenheit) recorded within the 30 minutes immediately before or the 15 minutes immediately after anesthesia end time (CRIT)[1]

4255F Duration of general or neuraxial anesthesia 60 minutes or longer, as documented in the anesthesia record (CRIT)[5] (Peri2)[11]

4256F Duration of general or neuraxial anesthesia less than 60 minutes, as documented in the anesthesia record (CRIT)[5] (Peri2)[11]

4260F Wound surface culture technique used (CWC)[5]

4261F Technique other than surface culture of the wound exudate used (eg, Levine/deep swab technique, semi-quantitative or quantitative swab technique) **or** wound surface culture technique not used (CWC)[5]

4265F Use of wet to dry dressings prescribed or recommended (CWC)[5]

4266F Use of wet to dry dressings neither prescribed nor recommended (CWC)[5]

4267F Compression therapy prescribed (CWC)[5]

4268F Patient education regarding the need for long term compression therapy including interval replacement of compression stockings received (CWC)[5]

4269F Appropriate method of offloading (pressure relief) prescribed (CWC)[5]

4270F Patient receiving potent antiretroviral therapy for 6 months or longer (HIV)[5]

4271F Patient receiving potent antiretroviral therapy for less than 6 months or not receiving potent antiretroviral therapy (HIV)[5]

4274F Influenza immunization administered or previously received (HIV)[5] (P-ESRD)[1]

4276F Potent antiretroviral therapy prescribed (HIV)[5]

4279F Pneumocystis jiroveci pneumonia prophylaxis prescribed (HIV)[5]

4280F Pneumocystis jiroveci pneumonia prophylaxis prescribed within 3 months of low CD4+ cell count or percentage (HIV)[5]

4290F Patient screened for injection drug use (HIV)[5]

4293F Patient screened for high-risk sexual behavior (HIV)[5]

4300F Patient receiving warfarin therapy for nonvalvular atrial fibrillation or atrial flutter (AFIB)[1]

4301F Patient not receiving warfarin therapy for nonvalvular atrial fibrillation or atrial flutter (AFIB)[1]

4305F Patient education regarding appropriate foot care **and** daily inspection of the feet received (CWC)[5]

4306F Patient counseled regarding psychosocial **and** pharmacologic treatment options for opioid addiction (SUD)[1]

4320F Patient counseled regarding psychosocial **and** pharmacologic treatment options for alcohol dependence (SUD)[5]

4322F Caregiver provided with education and referred to additional resources for support (DEM)[1]

4324F Patient (or caregiver) queried about Parkinson's disease medication related motor complications (Prkns)[8]

4325F Medical and surgical treatment options reviewed with patient (or caregiver) (Prkns)[8]

4326F Patient (or caregiver) queried about symptoms of autonomic dysfunction (Prkns)[8]

4328F Patient (or caregiver) queried about sleep disturbances (Prkns)[8]

4330F Counseling about epilepsy specific safety issues provided to patient (or caregiver(s)) (EPI)[8]

4340F Counseling for women of childbearing potential with epilepsy (EPI)[8]

4350F Counseling provided on symptom management, end of life decisions, and palliation (DEM)[1]

4400F Rehabilitative therapy options discussed with patient (or caregiver) (Prkns)[8]

Category II

4450F Self-care education provided to patient (HF)[1]

4470F Implantable cardioverter-defibrillator (ICD) counseling provided (HF)[1]

4480F Patient receiving ACE inhibitor/ARB therapy and beta-blocker therapy for 3 months or longer (HF)[1]

4481F Patient receiving ACE inhibitor/ARB therapy and beta-blocker therapy for less than 3 months or patient not receiving ACE inhibitor/ARB therapy and beta-blocker therapy (HF)[1]

4500F Referred to an outpatient cardiac rehabilitation program (CAD)[1]

4510F Previous cardiac rehabilitation for qualifying cardiac event completed (CAD)[1]

4525F Neuropsychiatric intervention ordered (DEM)[1]

4526F Neuropsychiatric intervention received (DEM)[1]

4540F Disease modifying pharmacotherapy discussed (ALS)[8]

4541F Patient offered treatment for pseudobulbar affect, sialorrhea, or ALS-related symptoms (ALS)[8]

4550F Options for noninvasive respiratory support discussed with patient (ALS)[8]

4551F Nutritional support offered (ALS)[8]

4552F Patient offered referral to a speech language pathologist (ALS)[8]

4553F Patient offered assistance in planning for end of life issues (ALS)[8]

4554F Patient received inhalational anesthetic agent (Peri2)[11]

4555F Patient did not receive inhalational anesthetic agent (Peri2)[11]

4556F Patient exhibits 3 or more risk factors for post-operative nausea and vomiting (Peri2)[11]

4557F Patient does not exhibit 3 or more risk factors for post-operative nausea and vomiting (Peri2)[11]

4558F Patient received at least 2 prophylactic pharmacologic anti-emetic agents of different classes preoperatively and intraoperatively (Peri2)[11]

4559F At least 1 body temperature measurement equal to or greater than 35.5 degrees Celsius (or 95.9 degrees Fahrenheit) recorded within the 30 minutes immediately before or the 15 minutes immediately after anesthesia end time (Peri2)[11]

4560F Anesthesia technique did not involve general or neuraxial anesthesia (Peri2)[11]

4561F Patient has a coronary artery stent (Peri2)[11]

4562F Patient does not have a coronary artery stent (Peri2)[11]

4563F Patient received aspirin within 24 hours prior to anesthesia start time (Peri2)[11]

Follow-up or Other Outcomes

Follow-up or other outcomes codes describe review and communication of test results to patients, patient satisfaction or experience with care, patient functional status, and patient morbidity and mortality.

5005F Patient counseled on self-examination for new or changing moles (ML)[5]

5010F Findings of dilated macular or fundus exam communicated to the physician or other qualified health care professional managing the diabetes care (EC)[5]

5015F Documentation of communication that a fracture occurred and that the patient was or should be tested or treated for osteoporosis (OP)[5]

5020F Treatment summary report communicated to physician(s) or other qualified health care professional(s) managing continuing care and to the patient within 1 month of completing treatment (ONC)[1]

5050F Treatment plan communicated to provider(s) managing continuing care within 1 month of diagnosis (ML)[5]

5060F Findings from diagnostic mammogram communicated to practice managing patient's on-going care within 3 business days of exam interpretation (RAD)[5]

5062F Findings from diagnostic mammogram communicated to the patient within 5 days of exam interpretation (RAD)[5]

5100F Potential risk for fracture communicated to the referring physician or other qualified health care professional within 24 hours of completion of the imaging study (NUC_MED)[1]

5200F Consideration of referral for a neurological evaluation of appropriateness for surgical therapy for intractable epilepsy within the past 3 years (EPI)[8]

5250F Asthma discharge plan provided to patient (Asthma)[1]

Patient Safety

Patient safety codes that describe patient safety practices.

6005F Rationale (eg, severity of illness and safety) for level of care (eg, home, hospital) documented (CAP)[1]

6010F Dysphagia screening conducted prior to order for or receipt of any foods, fluids, or medication by mouth (STR)[5]

6015F Patient receiving or eligible to receive foods, fluids, or medication by mouth (STR)[5]

6020F NPO (nothing by mouth) ordered (STR)[5]

▲ **6030F** All elements of maximal sterile barrier technique, hand hygiene, skin preparation and, if ultrasound is used, sterile ultrasound techniques followed (CRIT)[1]

6040F Use of appropriate radiation dose reduction devices OR manual techniques for appropriate moderation of exposure, documented (RAD)[5]

6045F	Radiation exposure or exposure time in final report for procedure using fluoroscopy, documented (RAD)[5]
6070F	Patient queried and counseled about anti-epileptic drug (AED) side effects (EPI)[8]
6080F	Patient (or caregiver) queried about falls (Prkns, DSP)[8]
6090F	Patient (or caregiver) counseled about safety issues appropriate to patient's stage of disease (Prkns)[8]
6100F	Timeout to verify correct patient, correct site, and correct procedure, documented (PATH)[9]
6101F	Safety counseling for dementia provided (DEM)[1]
6102F	Safety counseling for dementia ordered (DEM)[1]
6110F	Counseling provided regarding risks of driving and the alternatives to driving (DEM)[1]
6150F	Patient not receiving a first course of anti-TNF (tumor necrosis factor) therapy (IBD)[10]

Structural Measures

Structural measures codes are used to identify measures that address the setting or system of the delivered care. These codes also address aspects of the capabilities of the organization or health care professional providing the care.

7010F	Patient information entered into a recall system that includes: target date for the next exam specified **and** a process to follow up with patients regarding missed or unscheduled appointments (ML)[5]
7020F	Mammogram assessment category (eg, Mammography Quality Standards Act [MQSA], Breast Imaging Reporting and Data System [BI-RADS®], or FDA approved equivalent categories) entered into an internal database to allow for analysis of abnormal interpretation (recall) rate (RAD)[5]
7025F	Patient information entered into a reminder system with a target due date for the next mammogram (RAD)[5]

Nonmeasure Code Listing

The following codes are included for reporting of certain aspects of care. These factors are not represented by measures developed by existing measures organizations or recognized measures-development processes at the time they are placed in the CPT code set, but may ultimately be associated with measures approved by an appropriate quality improvement organization.

9001F	Aortic aneurysm less than 5.0 cm maximum diameter on centerline formatted CT or minor diameter on axial formatted CT (NMA–No Measure Associated)
9002F	Aortic aneurysm 5.0 - 5.4 cm maximum diameter on centerline formatted CT or minor diameter on axial formatted CT (NMA–No Measure Associated)
9003F	Aortic aneurysm 5.5 - 5.9 cm maximum diameter on centerline formatted CT or minor diameter on axial formatted CT (NMA–No Measure Associated)
9004F	Aortic aneurysm 6.0 cm or greater maximum diameter on centerline formatted CT or minor diameter on axial formatted CT (NMA–No Measure Associated)
9005F	Asymptomatic carotid stenosis: No history of any transient ischemic attack or stroke in any carotid or vertebrobasilar territory (NMA–No Measure Associated)
9006F	Symptomatic carotid stenosis: Ipsilateral carotid territory TIA or stroke less than 120 days prior to procedure (NMA–No Measure Associated)
9007F	Other carotid stenosis: Ipsilateral TIA or stroke 120 days or greater prior to procedure or any prior contralateral carotid territory or vertebrobasilar TIA or stroke (NMA–No Measure Associated)

Notes

⊙=Moderate sedation ✚=Add-on code ✗=FDA approval pending #=Resequenced code ○=Recycled/reinstated code

Category III Codes

The following section contains a set of temporary codes for emerging technology, services, and procedures. Category III codes allow data collection for these services/procedures. Use of unlisted codes does not offer the opportunity for the collection of specific data. If a Category III code is available, this code must be reported instead of a Category I unlisted code. This is an activity that is critically important in the evaluation of health care delivery and the formation of public and private policy. The use of the codes in this section allow physicians and other qualified health care professionals, insurers, health services researchers, and health policy experts to identify emerging technology, services, and procedures for clinical efficacy, utilization and outcomes.

►The inclusion of a service or procedure in this section does not constitute a finding of support, or lack thereof, with regard to clinical efficacy, safety, applicability to clinical practice, or payer coverage. The codes in this section may not conform to the usual requirements for CPT Category I codes established by the Editorial Panel. For Category I codes, the Panel requires that the service/procedure be performed by many health care professionals in clinical practice in multiple locations and that FDA approval, as appropriate, has already been received. The nature of emerging technology, services, and procedures is such that these requirements may not be met. For these reasons, temporary codes for emerging technology, services, and procedures have been placed in a separate section of the CPT code set and the codes are differentiated from Category I CPT codes by the use of alphanumeric characters.◄

Services and procedures described in this section make use of alphanumeric characters. These codes have an alpha character as the 5th character in the string (ie, four digits followed by the letter T). The digits are not intended to reflect the placement of the code in the Category I section of CPT nomenclature. Codes in this section may or may not eventually receive a Category I CPT code. In either case, in general, a given Category III code will be archived five years from the date of initial publication or extension unless a modification of the archival date is specifically noted at the time of a revision or change to a code (eg, addition of parenthetical instructions, reinstatement). Services and procedures described by Category III codes which have been archived after five years, without conversion, must be reported using the Category I unlisted code unless another specific cross-reference is established at the time of archiving. New codes or revised codes in this section are released semi-annually via the AMA CPT website, to expedite dissemination for reporting. The full set of temporary

codes for emerging technology, services, and procedures are published annually in the CPT code set. Go to www.ama-assn.org/go/cpt for the most current listing.

(For destruction of localized lesion of choroid by transpupillary thermotherapy, use 67299)

(For destruction of macular drusen, photocoagulation, use 67299)

0019T Extracorporeal shock wave involving musculoskeletal system, not otherwise specified, low energy
Sunset January 2017

(For application of high energy extracorporeal shock wave involving musculoskeletal system not otherwise specified, use 0101T)

(For application of high energy extracorporeal shock wave involving lateral humeral epicondyle, use 0102T)

(For non-surgical septal reduction therapy, use 93799)

(For lipoprotein, direct measurement, intermediate density lipoproteins [IDL] [remnant lipoprotein], use 84999)

(For endoscopic lysis of epidural adhesions with direct visualization using mechanical means or solution injection [eg, normal saline], use 64999)

(For dual energy x-ray absorptiometry [DXA] body composition study, use 76499)

(For pulsed magnetic neuromodulation incontinence treatment, use 53899)

(0030T has been deleted)

(To report antiprothrombin [phospholipid cofactor] antibody, use 86849)

(0031T, 0032T have been deleted)

(For speculoscopy, including sampling, use 58999)

(For urinalysis infectious agent detection, semi-quantitative analysis of volatile compounds, use 81099)

0042T Cerebral perfusion analysis using computed tomography with contrast administration, including post-processing of parametric maps with determination of cerebral blood flow, cerebral blood volume, and mean transit time
Sunset January 2019

(For carbon monoxide, expired gas analysis [eg, ETCO$_c$/hemolysis breath test], use 84999)

(0046T, 0047T have been deleted)

(For mammary duct[s] catheter lavage, use 19499)

(0048T has been deleted. To report, use 33991)

(0050T has been deleted. To report, see 33990-33993)

Category III

0051T Implantation of a total replacement heart system (artificial heart) with recipient cardiectomy
Sunset January 2019

(For implantation of heart assist or ventricular assist device, see 33975, 33976)

0052T Replacement or repair of thoracic unit of a total replacement heart system (artificial heart)
Sunset January 2019

(For replacement or repair of other implantable components in a total replacement heart system (artificial heart), use 0053T)

0053T Replacement or repair of implantable component or components of total replacement heart system (artificial heart), excluding thoracic unit
Sunset January 2019

(For replacement or repair of a thoracic unit of a total replacement heart system (artificial heart), use 0052T)

+ 0054T Computer-assisted musculoskeletal surgical navigational orthopedic procedure, with image-guidance based on fluoroscopic images (List separately in addition to code for primary procedure)
Sunset January 2019

+ 0055T Computer-assisted musculoskeletal surgical navigational orthopedic procedure, with image-guidance based on CT/MRI images (List separately in addition to code for primary procedure)
Sunset January 2019

(When CT and MRI are both performed, report 0055T only once)

0058T Cryopreservation; reproductive tissue, ovarian
Sunset January 2021

(0059T has been deleted)

(For cryopreservation of mature oocyte(s), use 89337. For cryopreservation of immature oocyte(s), use 0357T)

 # 0357T immature oocyte(s)
Sunset January 2020

(For cryopreservation of mature oocyte(s), use 89337)

(For cryopreservation of embryo(s), sperm and testicular reproductive tissue, see 89258, 89259, 89335)

(For electrical impedance breast scan, use 76499)

(For destruction/reduction of malignant breast tumor, microwave phased array thermotherapy, use 19499)

(0062T, 0063T have been deleted)

(For percutaneous intradiscal annuloplasty, any method other than electrothermal, use 22899)

(For intradiscal electrothermal annuloplasty, see 22526, 22527)

(To report CT colon, screening, use 74263)

(To report CT colon, diagnostic, see 74261-74262)

(0068T-0070T have been deleted)

(For acoustic heart sound recording and computer analysis, use 93799)

0071T Focused ultrasound ablation of uterine leiomyomata, including MR guidance; total leiomyomata volume less than 200 cc of tissue
Sunset January 2020

0072T total leiomyomata volume greater or equal to 200 cc of tissue
Sunset January 2020

(Do not report 0071T, 0072T in conjunction with 51702 or 77022)

(0073T has been deleted. To report, use 77385)

0075T Transcatheter placement of extracranial vertebral artery stent(s), including radiologic supervision and interpretation, open or percutaneous; initial vessel
Sunset January 2020

+ 0076T each additional vessel (List separately in addition to code for primary procedure)
Sunset January 2020

(Use 0076T in conjunction with 0075T)

(When the ipsilateral extracranial vertebral arteriogram (including imaging and selective catheterization) confirms the need for stenting, then 0075T and 0076T include all ipsilateral extracranial vertebral catheterization, all diagnostic imaging for ipsilateral extracranial vertebral artery stenting, and all related radiologic supervision and interpretation. If stenting is not indicated, then the appropriate codes for selective catheterization and imaging should be reported in lieu of 0075T or 0076T)

(0078T-0081T have been deleted. To report, see 34841-34848)

0085T Breath test for heart transplant rejection
Sunset January 2021

(To report total disc lumbar arthroplasty, use 22857)

(0092T has been deleted)

(For cervical arthroplasty procedure on three or more levels, use 0375T)

+ 0095T Removal of total disc arthroplasty (artificial disc), anterior approach, each additional interspace, cervical (List separately in addition to code for primary procedure)
Sunset January 2019

(Use 0095T in conjunction with 22864)

(To report revision of total disc lumbar arthroplasty, use 22862)

+ 0098T Revision including replacement of total disc arthroplasty (artificial disc), anterior approach, each additional interspace, cervical (List separately in addition to code for primary procedure)
Sunset January 2019

(Use 0098T in conjunction with 22861)

(Do not report 0098T in conjunction with 0095T)

(Do not report 0098T in conjunction with 22851 when performed at the same level)

(For decompression, see 63001-63048)

►(0099T has been deleted. To report, use 65785)◄

0100T Placement of a subconjunctival retinal prosthesis receiver and pulse generator, and implantation of intra-ocular retinal electrode array, with vitrectomy
Sunset January 2021

0101T Extracorporeal shock wave involving musculoskeletal system, not otherwise specified, high energy
Sunset January 2021

(For application of low energy musculoskeletal system extracorporeal shock wave, use 0019T)

(For extracorporeal shock wave therapy involving integumentary system not otherwise specified, see 0299T, 0300T)

(Do not report 0101T in conjunction with 0299T, 0300T when treating same area)

0102T Extracorporeal shock wave, high energy, performed by a physician, requiring anesthesia other than local, involving lateral humeral epicondyle
Sunset January 2021

(For application of low energy musculoskeletal system extracorporeal shock wave, use 0019T)

►(0103T has been deleted)◄

►(For holotranscobalamin, quantitative, use 84999)◄

(For inert gas rebreathing for cardiac output measurement during rest, use 93799)

(For inert gas rebreathing for cardiac output measurement during exercise, use 93799)

0106T Quantitative sensory testing (QST), testing and interpretation per extremity; using touch pressure stimuli to assess large diameter sensation
Sunset January 2021

0107T using vibration stimuli to assess large diameter fiber sensation
Sunset January 2021

0108T using cooling stimuli to assess small nerve fiber sensation and hyperalgesia
Sunset January 2021

0109T using heat-pain stimuli to assess small nerve fiber sensation and hyperalgesia
Sunset January 2021

0110T using other stimuli to assess sensation
Sunset January 2021

0111T Long-chain (C20-22) omega-3 fatty acids in red blood cell (RBC) membranes
Sunset January 2021

(For very long chain fatty acids, use 82726)

►(0123T has been deleted)◄

►(For fistulization of sclera for glaucoma, through ciliary body, use 66999)◄

(0124T has been deleted)

(For conjunctival incision with posterior extrascleral placement of pharmacological agent, use 68399)

0126T Common carotid intima-media thickness (IMT) study for evaluation of atherosclerotic burden or coronary heart disease risk factor assessment
Sunset January 2021

(Do not report 0126T in conjunction with 93880, 93882, 93895)

(For bilateral quantitative carotid intima media thickness and carotid atheroma evaluation that includes all required elements, use 93895)

(0130T has been deleted)

(For validated, statistically reliable, randomized, controlled, single-patient clinical investigation of FDA approved chronic care drugs, provided by a pharmacist, interpretation and report to the prescribing health care professional, use 99199)

(0141T-0143T have been deleted)

(To report pancreatic islet cell transplantation, use 48999)

(0144T-0151T have been deleted. To report, see 75571-75574)

(For laparoscopic implantation, replacement, revision, or removal of gastric stimulation electrodes, lesser curvature, use 43659)

(For open implantation, replacement, revision, or removal of gastric stimulation electrodes, lesser curvature, use 43999)

+ 0159T Computer-aided detection, including computer algorithm analysis of MRI image data for lesion detection/characterization, pharmacokinetic analysis, with further physician review for interpretation, breast MRI (List separately in addition to code for primary procedure)
Sunset January 2017

(Use 0159T in conjunction with 77058, 77059)

(Do not report 0159T in conjunction with 76376, 76377)

(0160T, 0161T have been deleted. To report, see 90867, 90869)

+ 0163T Total disc arthroplasty (artificial disc), anterior approach, including discectomy to prepare interspace (other than for decompression), each additional interspace, lumbar (List separately in addition to code for primary procedure)
Sunset January 2019

(Use 0163T in conjunction with 22857)

Category III

+ 0164T   Removal of total disc arthroplasty, (artificial disc), anterior approach, each additional interspace, lumbar (List separately in addition to code for primary procedure)
Sunset January 2019

(Use 0164T in conjunction with 22865)

+ 0165T   Revision including replacement of total disc arthroplasty (artificial disc), anterior approach, each additional interspace, lumbar (List separately in addition to code for primary procedure)
Sunset January 2019

(Use 0165T in conjunction with 22862)

(Do not report 0163T-0165T in conjunction with 22851, 49010, when performed at the same level)

(For decompression, see 63001-63048)

(For transmyocardial transcatheter closure of ventricular septal defect, with implant, including cardiopulmonary bypass if performed, use 33999)

(For rhinophototherapy, intranasal application of ultraviolet and visible light, use 30999)

0169T   Stereotactic placement of infusion catheter(s) in the brain for delivery of therapeutic agent(s), including computerized stereotactic planning and burr hole(s)
Sunset January 2017

(Do not report code 0169T in conjunction with 20660, 61107, 61781, 61782, 61783)

0171T   Insertion of posterior spinous process distraction device (including necessary removal of bone or ligament for insertion and imaging guidance), lumbar; single level
Sunset January 2017

+ 0172T   each additional level (List separately in addition to code for primary procedure)
Sunset January 2017

(Use 0172T in conjunction with 0171T)

(0173T has been deleted)

+ 0174T   Computer-aided detection (CAD) (computer algorithm analysis of digital image data for lesion detection) with further physician review for interpretation and report, with or without digitization of film radiographic images, chest radiograph(s), performed concurrent with primary interpretation (List separately in addition to code for primary procedure)
Sunset January 2017

(Use 0174T in conjunction with 71010, 71020, 71021, 71022, 71030)

0175T   Computer-aided detection (CAD) (computer algorithm analysis of digital image data for lesion detection) with further physician review for interpretation and report, with or without digitization of film radiographic images, chest radiograph(s), performed remote from primary interpretation
Sunset January 2017

(Do not report 0175T in conjunction with 71010, 71020, 71021, 71022, 71030)

0178T   Electrocardiogram, 64 leads or greater, with graphic presentation and analysis; with interpretation and report
Sunset January 2018

0179T   tracing and graphics only, without interpretation and report
Sunset January 2018

0180T   interpretation and report only
Sunset January 2018

(For electrocardiogram routine, with at least 12 leads separately performed, see 93000-93010)

(0181T has been deleted. To report, use 92145)

►(0182T has been deleted, To report, see 0394T, 0395T)◄

(0183T has been deleted. To report, use 97610)

0184T   Excision of rectal tumor, transanal endoscopic microsurgical approach (ie, TEMS), including muscularis propria (ie, full thickness)
Sunset January 2019

(For non-endoscopic excision of rectal tumor, see 45160, 45171, 45172)

(Do not report 0184T in conjunction with 45300-45327, 69990)

(0185T has been deleted)

(For multivariate analysis of patient-specific findings with quantifiable computer probability assessment, including report, use 99199)

(0186T has been deleted)

(For suprachoroidal delivery of pharmacologic agent, use 67299)

Remote Real-Time Interactive Video-conferenced Critical Care Services

Remote real-time interactive video-conferenced critical care is the direct delivery by a physician(s) or other qualified health care professional(s) of medical care for a critically ill or critically injured patient from an off-site location. Remote real-time interactive video-conferenced critical care is intended to supplement on-site critical care services at times when a critically ill or injured patient requires additional critical care resources than are available on-site. (For definitions of critical illness or injury and critical care services, see **Critical Care Services** section.)

In order to report remote real-time interactive video-conferenced critical care, the physician(s) or other qualified health care professional(s) in the remote location must have real-time access to the patient's medical record including progress notes, nursing notes, current medications, vital signs, clinical laboratory test results, other diagnostic test results, and radiographic images.

The remote physician or other qualified health care professional must have real-time capability to enter electronic orders; document the remote care services provided in the hospital medical record; video conference with the on-site health care team in the patient room; assess patients in their individual rooms, using high fidelity audio and video capabilities, including clear observation of the patient, monitors, ventilators, and infusion pumps; and speak to patients and family members.

The review and/or interpretation of all diagnostic information is included in reporting remote real-time interactive video-conferenced critical care when performed during the critical period by the individual(s) providing remote real-time interactive video-conferenced critical care and should not be reported separately.

The remote real-time interactive video-conferenced critical care codes 0188T and 0189T are used to report the total duration of time spent by the individual providing remote real-time interactive video-conferenced critical care services to a critically ill or critically injured patient, even if the time spent by the individual on that date is not continuous. For any given period of time spent providing remote real-time interactive video-conferenced critical care services, the physician or other qualified health care professional must devote his or her full attention to the patient and, therefore, cannot provide services to any other patient during the same period of time.

Time spent with the individual patient should be recorded in the patient's record. The time that can be reported as remote real-time interactive video-conferenced critical care is the time spent engaged in work directly related to the individual patient's care. For example, time spent reviewing test results or imaging studies, discussing the critically ill patient's care with other medical staff or documenting remote real-time interactive video-conferenced critical care services in the medical record would be reported as remote real-time interactive video-conferenced critical care, even though it does not occur at the bedside. Also, when the patient is unable or lacks capacity to participate in discussions, time spent from the remote site with family members or surrogate decision makers obtaining a medical history, reviewing the patient's condition or prognosis, or discussing treatment or limitation(s) of treatment may be reported as remote real-time interactive video-conferenced critical care, provided that the conversation bears directly on the management of the patient.

Time spent in activities that occur away from the bedside when the individual does not have the real-time capabilities described above may not be reported as remote real-time interactive video-conferenced critical care because the individual is not immediately available to the patient. Time spent in activities that do not directly contribute to the treatment of the patient may not be reported as remote real-time interactive video-conferenced critical care, even if they are performed in the remote site (eg, participation in administrative meetings or telephone calls to discuss other patients). Only one physician or other qualified health care professional may report either critical care services (99291, 99292) or remote real-time interactive video-conferenced critical care for the same period of time. Do not report remote real-time interactive video-conferenced critical care if another individual reports pediatric or neonatal critical care or intensive care services (99468-99476).

Code 0188T is used to report the first 30 to 74 minutes of remote real-time interactive video-conferenced, critical care on a given date. It should be used only once per date even if the time spent by the physician or other qualified health care professional is not continuous on that date. Remote real-time interactive video-conferenced, critical care of less than 30 minutes total duration on a given date should not be reported.

Code 0189T is used to report additional block(s) of time, of up to 30 minutes each, beyond the first 74 minutes (see table below).

The following examples illustrate the correct reporting of remote critical care services:

Total Duration of Critical Care	Codes
less than 30 minutes (less than 1/2 hour)	do not report
30-74 minutes (1/2 hr. - 1 hr. 14 min.)	0188T X 1
75-104 minutes (1 hr. 15 min. - 1 hr. 44 min.)	0188T X 1 AND 0189T X 1
105-134 minutes (1 hr. 45 min. - 2 hr. 14 min.)	0188T X 1 AND 0189T X 2

0188T   Remote real-time interactive video-conferenced critical care, evaluation and management of the critically ill or critically injured patient; first 30-74 minutes
Sunset January 2019

+ 0189T   each additional 30 minutes (List separately in addition to code for primary service)
Sunset January 2019

(Use 0189T in conjunction with 0188T)

+ 0190T   Placement of intraocular radiation source applicator (List separately in addition to primary procedure)
Sunset January 2019

(Use 0190T in conjunction with 67036)

(For application of the source by radiation oncologist, see Clinical Brachytherapy section)

Category III

0191T Insertion of anterior segment aqueous drainage device, without extraocular reservoir, internal approach, into the trabecular meshwork; initial insertion
Sunset January 2019

#+ 0376T each additional device insertion (List separately in addition to code for primary procedure)
Sunset January 2020

(Use 0376T in conjunction with 0191T)

 # 0253T Insertion of anterior segment aqueous drainage device, without extraocular reservoir, internal approach, into the suprachoroidal space
Sunset January 2019

(0192T has been deleted)

(To report insertion of drainage device by external approach, use 66183)

0195T Arthrodesis, pre-sacral interbody technique, disc space preparation, discectomy, without instrumentation, with image guidance, includes bone graft when performed; L5-S1 interspace
Sunset January 2019

+ 0196T L4-L5 interspace (List separately in addition to code for primary procedure)
Sunset January 2019

(Use 0196T in conjunction with 0195T)

(Do not report 0195T, 0196T in conjunction with 20930-20938, 22558, 22840, 22845, 22848, 22851, 72275, 76000, 76380, 76496, 76497, 77002, 77003, 77011, 77012)

(0197T has been deleted. To report, use 77387)

0198T Measurement of ocular blood flow by repetitive intraocular pressure sampling, with interpretation and report
Sunset January 2020

(0199T has been deleted)

(For tremor measurement with accelerometer(s) and/or gyroscope(s), use 95999)

⊙ 0200T Percutaneous sacral augmentation (sacroplasty), unilateral injection(s), including the use of a balloon or mechanical device, when used, 1 or more needles, includes imaging guidance and bone biopsy, when performed
Sunset January 2020

⊙ 0201T Percutaneous sacral augmentation (sacroplasty), bilateral injections, including the use of a balloon or mechanical device, when used, 2 or more needles, includes imaging guidance and bone biopsy, when performed
Sunset January 2020

(Do not report 0200T, 0201T in conjunction with 20225 when performed at the same level)

0202T Posterior vertebral joint(s) arthroplasty (eg, facet joint[s] replacement), including facetectomy, laminectomy, foraminotomy, and vertebral column fixation, injection of bone cement, when performed, including fluoroscopy, single level, lumbar spine
Sunset January 2020

(Do not report 0202T in conjunction with 22511, 22514, 22840, 22851, 22857, 63005, 63012, 63017, 63030, 63042, 63047, 63056 at the same level)

+ 0205T Intravascular catheter-based coronary vessel or graft spectroscopy (eg, infrared) during diagnostic evaluation and/or therapeutic intervention including imaging supervision, interpretation, and report, each vessel (List separately in addition to code for primary procedure)
Sunset January 2020

(Use 0205T in conjunction with 92920, 92924, 92928, 92933, 92937, 92941, 92943, 92975, 93454-93461, 93563, 93564)

0206T Computerized database analysis of multiple cycles of digitized cardiac electrical data from two or more ECG leads, including transmission to a remote center, application of multiple nonlinear mathematical transformations, with coronary artery obstruction severity assessment
Sunset January 2020

(When a 12-lead ECG is performed, 93000-93010 may be reported, as appropriate)

0207T Evacuation of meibomian glands, automated, using heat and intermittent pressure, unilateral
Sunset January 2020

0208T Pure tone audiometry (threshold), automated; air only
Sunset January 2021

0209T air and bone
Sunset January 2021

0210T Speech audiometry threshold, automated;
Sunset January 2021

0211T with speech recognition
Sunset January 2021

0212T Comprehensive audiometry threshold evaluation and speech recognition (0209T, 0211T combined), automated
Sunset January 2021

(For audiometric testing using audiometers performed manually by a qualified health care professional, see 92551-92557)

0213T Injection(s), diagnostic or therapeutic agent, paravertebral facet (zygapophyseal) joint (or nerves innervating that joint) with ultrasound guidance, cervical or thoracic; single level
Sunset January 2021

(To report bilateral procedure, use 0213T with modifier 50)

+ 0214T   second level (List separately in addition to code for primary procedure)
Sunset January 2021

(Use 0214T in conjunction with 0213T)

(To report bilateral procedure, use 0214T with modifier 50)

+ 0215T   third and any additional level(s) (List separately in addition to code for primary procedure)
Sunset January 2021

(Do not report 0215T more than once per day)

(Use 0215T in conjunction with 0213T, 0214T)

(To report bilateral procedure, use 0215T with modifier 50)

0216T   Injection(s), diagnostic or therapeutic agent, paravertebral facet (zygapophyseal) joint (or nerves innervating that joint) with ultrasound guidance, lumbar or sacral; single level
Sunset January 2021

(To report bilateral procedure, use 0216T with modifier 50)

+ 0217T   second level (List separately in addition to code for primary procedure)
Sunset January 2021

(Use 0217T in conjunction with 0216T)

(To report bilateral procedure, use 0217T with modifier 50)

+ 0218T   third and any additional level(s) (List separately in addition to code for primary procedure)
Sunset January 2021

(Do not report 0218T more than once per day)

(Use 0218T in conjunction with 0216T, 0217T)

(If injection(s) are performed using fluoroscopy or CT, see 64490-64495)

(To report bilateral procedure, use 0218T with modifier 50)

0219T   Placement of a posterior intrafacet implant(s), unilateral or bilateral, including imaging and placement of bone graft(s) or synthetic device(s), single level; cervical
Sunset January 2021

0220T   thoracic
Sunset January 2021

0221T   lumbar
Sunset January 2021

(Do not report 0219T-0221T in conjunction with any radiological service)

(Do not report 0219T-0221T in conjunction with 20930, 20931, 22600-22614, 22840, 22851 at the same level)

+ 0222T   each additional vertebral segment (List separately in addition to code for primary procedure)
Sunset January 2021

(Use 0222T in conjunction with 0219T-0221T)

(For posterior or posterolateral arthrodesis technique, see 22600-22614)

▶(0223T, 0224T, 0225T have been deleted. To report acoustic cardiography, use 93799)◀

(0226T has been deleted. To report, use 46601)

(0227T has been deleted. To report, use 46607)

0228T   Injection(s), anesthetic agent and/or steroid, transforaminal epidural, with ultrasound guidance, cervical or thoracic; single level
Sunset January 2021

+ 0229T   each additional level (List separately in addition to code for primary procedure)
Sunset January 2021

(Use 0229T in conjunction with 0228T)

0230T   Injection(s), anesthetic agent and/or steroid, transforaminal epidural, with ultrasound guidance, lumbar or sacral; single level
Sunset January 2021

+ 0231T   each additional level (List separately in addition to code for primary procedure)
Sunset January 2021

(Use 0231T in conjunction with 0230T)

(For transforaminal epidural injections performed under fluoroscopy or CT, see 64479–64484)

(Do not report 0228T-0231T in conjunction with 76942, 76998, 76999)

0232T   Injection(s), platelet rich plasma, any site, including image guidance, harvesting and preparation when performed
Sunset January 2017

(Do not report 0232T in conjunction with 20550, 20551, 20600-20610, 20926, 76942, 77002, 77012, 77021, 86965)

(Do not report 38220-38230 for bone marrow aspiration for platelet rich stem cell injection. For bone marrow aspiration for platelet rich stem cell injection, use 0232T)

▶(0233T has been deleted. To report skin advanced glycation endproducts measurement by multi-wavelength fluorescent spectroscopy, use 88749)◀

Category III

Atherectomy (Open or Percutaneous) for Supra-Inguinal Arteries

Codes 0234T-0238T describe atherectomy performed by any method (eg, directional, rotational, laser) in arteries above the inguinal ligaments. These codes are structured differently than the codes describing atherectomy performed below the inguinal ligaments (37225, 37227, 37229, 37231, 37233, 37235).

These supra-inguinal atherectomy codes all include the surgical work of performing the atherectomy plus the radiological supervision and interpretation of the atherectomy. Unlike the atherectomy codes for infra-inguinal arteries, this set of Category III codes does not include accessing and selectively catheterizing the vessel, traversing the lesion, embolic protection if used, other intervention used to treat the same or other vessels, or closure of the arteriotomy by any method. These codes describe endovascular procedures performed percutaneously and/or through an open surgical exposure.

0234T Transluminal peripheral atherectomy, open or percutaneous, including radiological supervision and interpretation; renal artery
Sunset January 2021

0235T visceral artery (except renal), each vessel
Sunset January 2021

0236T abdominal aorta
Sunset January 2021

0237T brachiocephalic trunk and branches, each vessel
Sunset January 2021

0238T iliac artery, each vessel
Sunset January 2021

(0239T has been deleted. To report, use 93702)

▶(0240T, 0241T have been deleted)◀

(To report esophageal motility studies without high resolution esophageal pressure topography, use 91010 and with stimulant or perfusion, use 91013)

(0242T has been deleted. To report, use 91112)

▶(0243T, 0244T have been deleted. To report intermittent measurement of wheeze rate for bronchodilator or bronchial challenge diagnostic evaluation, use 94799)◀

(0245T, 0246T, 0247T, 0248T have been deleted. To report, see 21811, 21812, 21813)

0249T Ligation, hemorrhoidal vascular bundle(s), including ultrasound guidance
Sunset January 2021

(Do not report 0249T in conjunction with 46020, 46221, 46250-46262, 46600, 46945, 46946, 76872, 76942, 76998)

(0250T-0252T have been deleted. For airway sizing and insertion and removal of bronchial valve[s], see 31647-31649)

0253T Code is out of numerical sequence. See 0188T-0254T

0254T Endovascular repair of iliac artery bifurcation (eg, aneurysm, pseudoaneurysm, arteriovenous malformation, trauma) using bifurcated endoprosthesis from the common iliac artery into both the external and internal iliac artery, unilateral;
Sunset January 2021

0255T radiological supervision and interpretation
Sunset January 2021

(0256T has been deleted. To report, see 33361, 33362, 33363, 33364)

(0257T has been deleted. To report, see 33365, 33366)

(0258T has been deleted. To report, see 33365, 33366)

(0259T has been deleted. To report, see 33365, 33367, 33368, 33369)

(0260T, 0261T have been deleted. To report, use 99184)

▶(0262T has been deleted. To report transcatheter pulmonary valve implantation, use 33477)◀

0263T Intramuscular autologous bone marrow cell therapy, with preparation of harvested cells, multiple injections, one leg, including ultrasound guidance, if performed; complete procedure including unilateral or bilateral bone marrow harvest
Sunset January 2017

(Do not report 0263T in conjunction with 38204-38242, 76942, 93925, 93926)

0264T complete procedure excluding bone marrow harvest
Sunset January 2017

(Do not report 0264T in conjunction with 38204-38242, 76942, 93925, 93926, 0265T)

0265T unilateral or bilateral bone marrow harvest only for intramuscular autologous bone marrow cell therapy
Sunset January 2017

(Do not report 0265T in conjunction with 38204-38242, 0264T. For complete procedure, use 0263T)

0266T Implantation or replacement of carotid sinus baroreflex activation device; total system (includes generator placement, unilateral or bilateral lead placement, intra-operative interrogation, programming, and repositioning, when performed)
Sunset January 2017

0267T lead only, unilateral (includes intra-operative interrogation, programming, and repositioning, when performed)
Sunset January 2017

(For bilateral lead implantation or replacement, use 0267T with modifier 50)

0268T pulse generator only (includes intra-operative interrogation, programming, and repositioning, when performed)
Sunset January 2017

(Do not report 0267T, 0268T in conjunction with 0266T, 0269T-0273T)

0269T Revision or removal of carotid sinus baroreflex activation device; total system (includes generator placement, unilateral or bilateral lead placement, intra-operative interrogation, programming, and repositioning, when performed)
Sunset January 2017

(Do not report 0269T in conjunction with 0266T-0268T, 0270T-0273T)

0270T lead only, unilateral (includes intra-operative interrogation, programming, and repositioning, when performed)
Sunset January 2017

(Do not report 0270T in conjunction with 0266T-0269T, 0271T-0273T)

(For bilateral lead removal, use 0270T with modifier 50)

(For removal of total carotid sinus baroreflex activation device, use 0269T)

0271T pulse generator only (includes intra-operative interrogation, programming, and repositioning, when performed)
Sunset January 2017

(Do not report 0271T in conjunction with 0266T-0270T, 0272T, 0273T)

(For removal and replacement, see 0266T, 0267T, 0268T)

0272T Interrogation device evaluation (in person), carotid sinus baroreflex activation system, including telemetric iterative communication with the implantable device to monitor device diagnostics and programmed therapy values, with interpretation and report (eg, battery status, lead impedance, pulse amplitude, pulse width, therapy frequency, pathway mode, burst mode, therapy start/stop times each day);
Sunset January 2017

(Do not report 0272T in conjunction with 0266T-0271T, 0273T)

0273T with programming
Sunset January 2017

(Do not report 0273T in conjunction with 0266T-0272T)

0274T Percutaneous laminotomy/laminectomy (interlaminar approach) for decompression of neural elements, (with or without ligamentous resection, discectomy, facetectomy and/or foraminotomy), any method, under indirect image guidance (eg, fluoroscopic, CT), with or without the use of an endoscope, single or multiple levels, unilateral or bilateral; cervical or thoracic
Sunset January 2017

0275T lumbar
Sunset January 2017

(For laminotomy/hemilaminectomy performed using an open and endoscopically-assisted approach, see 63020-63035)

(For percutaneous decompression of the nucleus pulposus of intervertebral disc utilizing needle based technique, use 62287)

(0276T, 0277T have been deleted. To report, see 31660, 31661)

0278T Transcutaneous electrical modulation pain reprocessing (eg, scrambler therapy), each treatment session (includes placement of electrodes)
Sunset January 2017

(0279T, 0280T have been deleted. To report, see 86152, 86153)

0281T Percutaneous transcatheter closure of the left atrial appendage with implant, including fluoroscopy, transseptal puncture, catheter placement(s), left atrial angiography, left atrial appendage angiography, radiological supervision and interpretation
Sunset January 2017

(Do not report 0281T in conjunction with 93462 [left heart catheterization by transseptal puncture])

(Report cardiac catheterization procedures [93451-93461, 93530-93533] separately for indications distinct from the left atrial appendage closure procedure)

(For left ventriculography performed by transseptal approach for indications distinct from the left atrial appendage closure procedure, use 93565)

(Do not report 0281T in conjunction with 93452, 93453, 93458-93461, 93531-93533 unless catheterization of the left ventricle is performed by a non-transseptal approach for indications distinct from the left atrial appendage closure procedure)

(Do not report 0281T in conjunction with 93451, 93453, 93456, 93460, 93461, 93530-93533 unless complete right heart catheterization is performed for indications distinct from the left atrial appendage closure procedure)

⊙ **0282T** Percutaneous or open implantation of neurostimulator electrode array(s), subcutaneous (peripheral subcutaneous field stimulation), including imaging guidance, when performed, cervical, thoracic or lumbar; for trial, including removal at the conclusion of trial period
Sunset January 2017

⊙ **0283T** permanent, with implantation of a pulse generator
Sunset January 2017

⊙ **0284T** Revision or removal of pulse generator or electrodes, including imaging guidance, when performed, including addition of new electrodes, when performed
Sunset January 2017

0285T Electronic analysis of implanted peripheral subcutaneous field stimulation pulse generator, with reprogramming when performed
Sunset January 2017

►(Do not report 0282T, 0283T, 0284T, 0285T in conjunction with 64550-64595, 77002, 77003, 95970, 95971, 95972)◄

Category III

0286T   Near-infrared spectroscopy studies of lower extremity wounds (eg, for oxyhemoglobin measurement)
Sunset January 2017

0287T   Near-infrared guidance for vascular access requiring real-time digital visualization of subcutaneous vasculature for evaluation of potential access sites and vessel patency
Sunset January 2017

0288T   Anoscopy, with delivery of thermal energy to the muscle of the anal canal (eg, for fecal incontinence)
Sunset January 2017

(Do not report 0288T in conjunction with 46600-46615)

+ 0289T   Corneal incisions in the donor cornea created using a laser, in preparation for penetrating or lamellar keratoplasty (List separately in addition to code for primary procedure)
Sunset January 2017

(Use 0289T in conjunction with 65710, 65730, 65750, 65755)

+ 0290T   Corneal incisions in the recipient cornea created using a laser, in preparation for penetrating or lamellar keratoplasty (List separately in addition to code for primary procedure)
Sunset January 2017

(Use 0290T in conjunction with 65710, 65730, 65750, 65755)

⊙+ 0291T   Intravascular optical coherence tomography (coronary native vessel or graft) during diagnostic evaluation and/or therapeutic intervention, including imaging supervision, interpretation, and report; initial vessel (List separately in addition to primary procedure)
Sunset January 2018

(Use 0291T in conjunction with cardiac catheterization codes 92920, 92924, 92928, 92933, 92937, 92941, 92943, 92975, 93454-93461, 93563, 93564)

(Intravascular optical coherence tomography services include all transducer manipulations and repositioning within the specific vessel being examined, both before and after therapeutic intervention [eg, stent placement])

⊙+ 0292T   each additional vessel (List separately in addition to primary procedure)
Sunset January 2018

(Use 0292T in conjunction with 0291T)

(For intravascular spectroscopy, use 0205T)

⊙ 0293T   Insertion of left atrial hemodynamic monitor; complete system, includes implanted communication module and pressure sensor lead in left atrium including transseptal access, radiological supervision and interpretation, and associated injection procedures, when performed
Sunset January 2018

(Do not report 0293T in conjunction with 93462, 93662)

⊙+ 0294T   pressure sensor lead at time of insertion of pacing cardioverter-defibrillator pulse generator including radiological supervision and interpretation and associated injection procedures, when performed (List separately in addition to code for primary procedure)
Sunset January 2018

(Use 0294T in conjunction with 33230, 33231, 33240, 33262-33264, 33249)

(Do not report 0294T in conjunction with 93462, 93662)

(Do not report 0293T or 0294T in conjunction with 33202-33249, 93451-93453 unless performed for separate and distinct clinical indication other than for placement or calibration of left atrial hemodynamic monitoring system)

0295T   External electrocardiographic recording for more than 48 hours up to 21 days by continuous rhythm recording and storage; includes recording, scanning analysis with report, review and interpretation
Sunset January 2018

0296T   recording (includes connection and initial recording)
Sunset January 2018

0297T   scanning analysis with report
Sunset January 2018

0298T   review and interpretation
Sunset January 2018

(Do not report 0295T-0298T in conjunction with 93224-93272 for same monitoring period)

0299T   Extracorporeal shock wave for integumentary wound healing, high energy, including topical application and dressing care; initial wound
Sunset January 2018

+ 0300T   each additional wound (List separately in addition to code for primary procedure)
Sunset January 2018

(Use 0300T in conjunction with 0299T)

(Do not report 0300T in conjunction with 28890, 0101T, 0102T when treating same area)

⊙ 0301T   Destruction/reduction of malignant breast tumor with externally applied focused microwave, including interstitial placement of disposable catheter with combined temperature monitoring probe and microwave focusing sensocatheter under ultrasound thermotherapy guidance
Sunset January 2018

(Do not report 0301T in conjunction with 76641, 76642, 76942, 76998, 77600, 77605, 77610, 77615)

Category III

⊙ **0302T**   Insertion or removal and replacement of intracardiac ischemia monitoring system including imaging supervision and interpretation when performed and intra-operative interrogation and programming when performed; complete system (includes device and electrode)
Sunset January 2018

⊙ **0303T**   electrode only
Sunset January 2018

⊙ **0304T**   device only
Sunset January 2018

(Do not report 0302T-0304T in conjunction with 93000-93010)

0305T   Programming device evaluation (in person) of intracardiac ischemia monitoring system with iterative adjustment of programmed values, with analysis, review, and report
Sunset January 2018

(Do not report 0305T in conjunction with 93000-93010, 0302T-0304T, 0306T)

0306T   Interrogation device evaluation (in person) of intracardiac ischemia monitoring system with analysis, review, and report
Sunset January 2018

(Do not report 0306T in conjunction with 93000-93010, 0302T-0305T)

⊙ **0307T**   Removal of intracardiac ischemia monitoring device
Sunset January 2018

⊙▲ **0308T**   Insertion of ocular telescope prosthesis including removal of crystalline lens or intraocular lens prosthesis
Sunset January 2021

(Do not report 0308T in conjunction with 65800-65815, 66020, 66030, 66600-66635, 66761, 66825, 66982-66986, 69990)

+ **0309T**   Arthrodesis, pre-sacral interbody technique, including disc space preparation, discectomy, with posterior instrumentation, with image guidance, includes bone graft, when performed, lumbar, L4-L5 interspace (List separately in addition to code for primary procedure)
Sunset January 2018

(Use 0309T in conjunction with 22586)

(Do not report 0309T in conjunction with 20930-20938, 22840, 22848, 72275, 77002, 77003, 77011, 77012)

0310T   Motor function mapping using non-invasive navigated transcranial magnetic stimulation (nTMS) for therapeutic treatment planning, upper and lower extremity
Sunset January 2018

(Do not report 0310T in conjunction with 95860-95870, 95928, 95929, 95939)

▶(0311T has been deleted. To report, use 93050)◀

0312T   Vagus nerve blocking therapy (morbid obesity); laparoscopic implantation of neurostimulator electrode array, anterior and posterior vagal trunks adjacent to esophagogastric junction (EGJ), with implantation of pulse generator, includes programming
Sunset January 2018

0313T   laparoscopic revision or replacement of vagal trunk neurostimulator electrode array, including connection to existing pulse generator
Sunset January 2018

0314T   laparoscopic removal of vagal trunk neurostimulator electrode array and pulse generator
Sunset January 2018

0315T   removal of pulse generator
Sunset January 2018

0316T   replacement of pulse generator
Sunset January 2018

(Do not report 0315T in conjunction with 0316T)

0317T   neurostimulator pulse generator electronic analysis, includes reprogramming when performed
Sunset January 2018

(For implantation, revision, replacement, and/or removal of vagus [cranial] nerve neurostimulator electrode array and/or pulse generator for vagus nerve stimulation performed other than at the EGJ [eg, epilepsy], see 64568-64570)

(For analysis and/or [re]programming for vagus nerve stimulator, see 95970, 95974, 95975)

(0318T has been deleted. To report, use 33366)

Subcutaneous Implantable Defibrillator System

(0319T, 0320T, 0321T, 0322T, 0323T, 0324T, 0325T, 0326T, 0327T, 0328T have been deleted. To report, see 33240, 33241, 33262, 33270, 33271, 33272, 33273, 93260, 93261, 93644)

0329T   Monitoring of intraocular pressure for 24 hours or longer, unilateral or bilateral, with interpretation and report
Sunset January 2019

0330T   Tear film imaging, unilateral or bilateral, with interpretation and report
Sunset January 2019

0331T   Myocardial sympathetic innervation imaging, planar qualitative and quantitative assessment
Sunset January 2019

0332T   with tomographic SPECT
Sunset January 2019

(For myocardial infarct avid imaging, see 78466, 78468, 78469)

Category III

0333T   Visual evoked potential, screening of visual acuity,
automated
Sunset January 2019

(0334T has been deleted)

(To report percutaneous/minimally invasive [indirect
visualization] arthrodesis of the sacroiliac joint with
image guidance, use 27279)

⊙ **0335T**   Extra-osseous subtalar joint implant for talotarsal
stabilization
Sunset January 2019

0336T   Laparoscopy, surgical, ablation of uterine fibroid(s),
including intraoperative ultrasound guidance and
monitoring, radiofrequency
Sunset January 2019

(Do not report 0336T in conjunction with 76998, 0071T)

0337T   Endothelial function assessment, using peripheral
vascular response to reactive hyperemia, non-invasive
(eg, brachial artery ultrasound, peripheral artery
tonometry), unilateral or bilateral
Sunset January 2019

(Do not report 0337T in conjunction with 93922, 93923)

0338T   Transcatheter renal sympathetic denervation,
percutaneous approach including arterial puncture,
selective catheter placement(s) renal artery(ies),
fluoroscopy, contrast injection(s), intraprocedural
roadmapping and radiological supervision and
interpretation, including pressure gradient
measurements, flush aortogram and diagnostic renal
angiography when performed; unilateral
Sunset January 2019

0339T   bilateral
Sunset January 2019

(Do not report 0338T, 0339T in conjunction with 36251,
36252, 36253, 36254)

⊙ **0340T**   Ablation, pulmonary tumor(s), including pleura or chest
wall when involved by tumor extension, percutaneous,
cryoablation, unilateral, includes imaging guidance
Sunset January 2019

(Do not report 0340T in conjunction with 76940, 77013,
77022)

0341T   Quantitative pupillometry with interpretation and report,
unilateral or bilateral
Sunset January 2020

0342T   Therapeutic apheresis with selective HDL delipidation
and plasma reinfusion
Sunset January 2020

Fluoroscopy (76000, 76001) and radiologic supervision
and interpretation are inherent to the transcatheter mitral
valve repair (TMVR) procedure and are not separately
reportable. Diagnostic cardiac catheterization (93451,
93452, 93453, 93454, 93455, 93456, 93457, 93458,
93459, 93460, 93461, 93530, 93531, 93532, 93533)
should **not** be reported with transcatheter mitral valve
repair 0345T for:

- Contrast injections, angiography, roadmapping, and/or
fluoroscopic guidance for the transcatheter mitral valve
repair (TMVR),

- Left ventricular angiography to assess mitral
regurgitation, for guidance of TMVR, or

- Right and left heart catheterization for hemodynamic
measurements before, during, and after TMVR for
guidance of TMVR.

Diagnostic right and left heart catheterization (93451,
93452, 93453, 93456, 93457, 93458, 93459, 93460,
93461, 93530, 93531, 93532, 93533), and diagnostic
coronary angiography (93454, 93455, 93456, 93457,
93458, 93459, 93460, 93461, 93563, 93564) not
inherent to the TMVR, may be reported with 0345T,
appended with modifier 59 if:

1. No prior study is available and a full diagnostic
study is performed, or

2. A prior study is available, but as documented in the
medical record:

   a. There is inadequate visualization of the anatomy
   and/or pathology, or

   b. The patient's condition with respect to the clinical
   indication has changed since the prior study, or

   c. There is a clinical change during the procedure
   that requires new evaluation.

Percutaneous coronary interventional procedures may be
reported separately, when performed.

Other cardiac catheterization services may be reported
separately, when performed for diagnostic purposes not
intrinsic to the TMVR.

When transcatheter ventricular support is required, the
appropriate code may be reported with the appropriate
ventricular assist device (VAD) procedure (33990, 33991,
33992, 33993) or balloon pump insertion (33967,
33970, 33973).

(0343T has been deleted. To report, use 33418)

(0344T has been deleted. To report, use 33419)

0345T   Transcatheter mitral valve repair percutaneous approach
via the coronary sinus
Sunset January 2020

(For transcatheter mitral valve repair percutaneous approach including transseptal puncture when performed, see 33418, 33419)

(Do not report 0345T in conjunction with 93451, 93452, 93453, 93456, 93457, 93458, 93459, 93460, 93461 for diagnostic left and right heart catheterization procedures intrinsic to the valve repair procedure)

(Do not report 0345T in conjunction with 93453, 93454, 93563, 93564 for coronary angiography intrinsic to the valve repair procedure)

+ 0346T Ultrasound, elastography (List separately in addition to code for primary procedure)
Sunset January 2020

(Use 0346T in conjunction with 76536, 76604, 76641, 76642, 76700, 76705, 76770, 76775, 76830, 76856, 76857, 76870, 76872, 76881, 76882)

0347T Placement of interstitial device(s) in bone for radiostereometric analysis (RSA)
Sunset January 2020

0348T Radiologic examination, radiostereometric analysis (RSA); spine, (includes cervical, thoracic and lumbosacral, when performed)
Sunset January 2020

0349T upper extremity(ies), (includes shoulder, elbow, and wrist, when performed)
Sunset January 2020

0350T lower extremity(ies), (includes hip, proximal femur, knee, and ankle, when performed)
Sunset January 2020

0351T Optical coherence tomography of breast or axillary lymph node, excised tissue, each specimen; real-time intraoperative
Sunset January 2020

0352T interpretation and report, real-time or referred
Sunset January 2020

(Do not report 0352T in conjunction with 0351T, when performed by the same physician)

0353T Optical coherence tomography of breast, surgical cavity; real-time intraoperative
Sunset January 2020

(Report 0353T once per session)

0354T interpretation and report, real-time or referred
Sunset January 2020

(Do not report 0354T in conjunction with 0353T, when performed by the same physician)

0355T Gastrointestinal tract imaging, intraluminal (eg, capsule endoscopy), colon, with interpretation and report
Sunset January 2020

(Use 0355T for imaging of distal ileum, when performed)

(Do not report 0355T in conjunction with 91110, 91111)

0356T Insertion of drug-eluting implant (including punctal dilation and implant removal when performed) into lacrimal canaliculus, each
Sunset January 2020

0357T Code is out of numerical sequence. See 0019T-0359T

▲ 0358T Bioelectrical impedance analysis whole body composition assessment, with interpretation and report
Sunset January 2020

(For bioimpedance-derived physiological cardiovascular analysis, use 93701)

(For bioimpedance spectroscopy (BIS), use 93702)

Adaptive Behavior Assessments

Behavior identification assessment (0359T) conducted by the physician or other qualified health care professional includes a detailed behavioral history, patient observation, administration of standardized and non-standardized tests, and structured guardian/caregiver interview to identify and describe deficient adaptive or maladaptive behaviors (eg, impaired social skills and communication deficits, destructive behaviors, and additional functional limitations secondary to maladaptive behaviors). Code 0359T also includes the physician's or other qualified health care professional's interpretation of results and development of plan of care, which may include further observational or exposure behavioral follow-up assessment(s) (0360T, 0361T, 0362T, 0363T), discussion of findings and recommendations with the primary guardian(s)/caregiver(s), and preparation of report.

Observational behavioral follow-up assessment (0360T, 0361T) is administered by a technician under the direction of a physician or other qualified health care professional. The physician or other qualified health care professional may or may not be on site during the face-to-face assessment process. Codes 0360T and 0361T include the physician's or other qualified health care professional's interpretation of results, discussion of findings and recommendations with the primary caregiver(s), and preparation of report.

Codes 0360T and 0361T describe services provided to patients who present with specific destructive behavior(s) (eg, self-injurious behavior, aggression, property destruction) or behavioral problems secondary to repetitive behaviors or deficits in communication or social relatedness. These assessments include use of structured observation and/or standardized and non-standardized tests to determine levels of adaptive behavior. Areas assessed may include cooperation, motivation, visual understanding, receptive and expressive language, imitation, requests, labeling, play and leisure, and social interactions. Specific destructive behavior(s) assessments include structured observational testing to examine events, cues, responses, and consequences associated with the behavior(s).

Category III

Exposure behavioral follow-up assessment (0362T, 0363T) is administered by the physician or other qualified health care professional with the assistance of one or more technicians. Codes 0362T and 0363T include the physician's or other qualified health care professional's interpretation of results, discussion of findings and recommendations with the primary caregiver(s), and preparation of report.

The typical patients for 0362T and 0363T include patients with one or more specific severe destructive behavior(s) (eg, self-injurious behavior, aggression, property destruction). Specific severe destructive behavior(s) are assessed using structured testing to examine events, cues, responses, and consequences associated with the behavior(s).

Codes 0362T and 0363T include exposing the patient to a series of social and environmental conditions associated with the destructive behavior(s). Assessment methods include using testing methods designed to examine triggers, events, cues, responses, and consequences associated with the aforementioned maladaptive behavior(s). This assessment is completed in a structured, safe environment.

Codes 0360T, 0361T, 0362T, and 0363T are reported following 0359T based on the time that the patient is face-to-face with one or more technician(s). Only count the time of one technician when two or more are present. Codes 0360T, 0361T, 0362T, and 0363T are reported per the CPT Time–Rule (eg, a unit of time is attained when the mid-point is passed). See CPT Time-Rule for Face-to-Face Technician Time Table. The time reported with 0360T, 0361T, 0362T, and 0363T is over a single day and is not cumulative over a longer period.

(Do not report 0359T, 0360T, 0361T, 0362T, 0363T in conjunction with 90785-90899, 96101-96125, 96150, 96151, 96152, 96153, 96154, 96155 on the same date)

(For psychiatric diagnostic evaluation, see 90791, 90792)

(For speech evaluations, see 92521, 92522, 92523, 92524)

(For occupational therapy evaluation, see 97003, 97004)

(For medical team conference, see 99366, 99367, 99368)

(For health and behavior assessment/intervention, see 96150, 96151, 96152, 96153, 96154, 96155)

(For neurobehavioral status exam, use 96116)

(For neuropsychological testing, use 96118)

CPT Time–Rule for Face-to-Face Technician Time: Codes 0360T, 0361T, 0362T, 0363T

Time	CPT Code(s)
Less than 16 min	Not reportable
16-45 min	0360T or 0362T
46-75 min	0360T and 0361T or 0362T and 0363T
Each additional increment up to 30 min	Additional 0361T or 0363T

0359T **Behavior identification assessment,** by the physician or other qualified health care professional, face-to-face with patient and caregiver(s), includes administration of standardized and non-standardized tests, detailed behavioral history, patient observation and caregiver interview, interpretation of test results, discussion of findings and recommendations with the primary guardian(s)/caregiver(s), and preparation of report
Sunset January 2020

0360T **Observational behavioral follow-up assessment,** includes physician or other qualified health care professional direction with interpretation and report, administered by one technician; first 30 minutes of technician time, face-to-face with the patient
Sunset January 2020

+ **0361T** each additional 30 minutes of technician time, face-to-face with the patient (List separately in addition to code for primary service)
Sunset January 2020

(Use 0361T in conjunction with 0360T)

0362T **Exposure behavioral follow-up assessment,** includes physician or other qualified health care professional direction with interpretation and report, administered by physician or other qualified health care professional with the assistance of one or more technicians; first 30 minutes of technician(s) time, face-to-face with the patient
Sunset January 2020

+ **0363T** each additional 30 minutes of technician(s) time, face-to-face with the patient (List separately in addition to code for primary procedure)
Sunset January 2020

(Use 0363T in conjunction with 0362T)

(0362T, 0363T are reported based on a single technician's face-to-face time with the patient and not the combined time of multiple technicians)

(Do not report 0359T, 0360T, 0361T, 0362T, 0363T in conjunction with 90785-90899, 96101-96125, 96150, 96151, 96152, 96153, 96154, 96155)

Adaptive Behavior Treatment

Adaptive behavior treatment codes 0364T, 0365T, 0366T, 0367T, 0368T, 0369T, 0370T, 0371T, 0372T, 0373T, 0374T describe services provided to patients who present with deficient adaptive or maladaptive behaviors (eg, impaired social skills and communication, destructive behaviors, or additional functional limitations secondary to maladaptive behaviors). Specific target problems and treatment goals are based on results of previous assessments (see 0359T, 0360T, 0361T, 0362T, 0363T).

Adaptive behavior treatment by protocol and group adaptive behavior treatment by protocol are administered by a technician face-to-face with one patient (0364T, 0365T), or two or more patients (0366T, 0367T) under the direction of a physician or other qualified health care professional, utilizing a behavioral intervention protocol designed in advance by the physician or other qualified health care professional, who may or may not provide direct supervision during the face-to-face therapy. Do not report 0366T, 0367T if the group is larger than eight patients.

Adaptive behavior treatment with protocol modification (0368T, 0369T) is administered by a physician or other qualified health care professional face-to-face with a single patient. The physician or other qualified health care professional resolves one or more problems with the protocol and may simultaneously instruct a technician and/or guardian(s)/caregiver(s) in administering the modified protocol. Physician or other qualified health care professional instruction to the technician without the patient present is not reported separately.

Family adaptive behavior treatment guidance and multiple-family group adaptive behavior treatment guidance are administered by a physician or other qualified health care professional face-to-face with guardian(s)/caregiver(s), without the presence of a patient, and involve identifying problem behaviors and deficits and teaching guardian(s)/caregiver(s) of one patient (0370T) or multiple patients (0371T) to utilize treatment protocols designed to reduce maladaptive behaviors and/or skill deficits. Do not report 0371T if the group is larger than eight patients.

Adaptive behavior treatment social skills group (0372T) is administered by a physician or other qualified health care professional face-to-face with multiple patients, focusing on social skills training and identifying and targeting individual patient social deficits and problem behaviors. The physician or other qualified health care professional monitors the needs of individual patients and adjusts the therapeutic techniques during the group, as needed. Services to increase target social skills may include modeling, rehearsing, corrective feedback, and homework assignments. In contrast to adaptive behavior treatment by protocol techniques (0364T, 0365T, 0366T, 0367T), adjustments required in social skills group setting are made in real time rather than for a subsequent service. Do not report 0372T if the group is larger than eight patients.

Codes 0364T, 0365T, 0366T, 0367T, 0368T, 0369T, 0372T may include services involving patient interaction with other individuals, including other patients. Report group services (0366T, 0367T, 0372T) only for patients who are participating in the interaction in order to meet their own individual treatment goals.

0364T   Adaptive behavior treatment by protocol, administered by technician, face-to-face with one patient; first 30 minutes of technician time
Sunset January 2020

+ 0365T   each additional 30 minutes of technician time (List separately in addition to code for primary procedure)
Sunset January 2020

(Use 0365T in conjunction with 0364T)

(Do not report 0364T, 0365T in conjunction with 90785-90899, 92507, 96101-96155, 97532)

0366T   Group adaptive behavior treatment by protocol, administered by technician, face-to-face with two or more patients; first 30 minutes of technician time
Sunset January 2020

+ 0367T   each additional 30 minutes of technician time (List separately in addition to code for primary procedure)
Sunset January 2020

(Use 0367T in conjunction with 0366T)

(Do not report 0366T, 0367T if the group is larger than eight patients)

(Do not report 0366T, 0367T in conjunction with 90785-90899, 92508, 96101-96155, 97150)

0368T   Adaptive behavior treatment with protocol modification administered by physician or other qualified health care professional with one patient; first 30 minutes of patient face-to-face time
Sunset January 2020

+ 0369T   each additional 30 minutes of patient face-to-face time (List separately in addition to code for primary procedure)
Sunset January 2020

(Use 0369T in conjunction with 0368T)

(Do not report 0368T, 0369T in conjunction with 90791, 90792, 90846, 90847, 90887, 92507, 97532)

0370T   Family adaptive behavior treatment guidance, administered by physician or other qualified health care professional (without the patient present)
Sunset January 2020

Category III

0371T Multiple-family group adaptive behavior treatment guidance, administered by physician or other qualified health care professional (without the patient present)
Sunset January 2020

(Do not report 0371T when the families of more than eight patients are participants)

(Do not report 0370T, 0371T in conjunction with 90791, 90792, 90846, 90847, 90887)

0372T Adaptive behavior treatment social skills group, administered by physician or other qualified health care professional face-to-face with multiple patients
Sunset January 2020

(Do not report 0372T if the group is larger than eight patients)

(Do not report 0372T in conjunction with 90853, 92508, 97150)

Exposure Adaptive Behavior Treatment With Protocol Modification

Codes 0373T and 0374T describe services provided to patients with one or more specific severe destructive behaviors (eg, self-injurious behavior, aggression, property destruction), with direct supervision by a physician or other qualified health care professional that requires two or more technicians face-to-face with the patient for safe treatment. Technicians elicit behavioral effects of exposing the patient to specific environmental conditions and treatments. Technicians record all occurrences of targeted behaviors. The physician or other qualified health care professional reviews and analyzes data and refines the therapy using single-case designs; ineffective components are modified or replaced until discharge goals are achieved (eg, reducing destructive behavior by at least 90%, generalizing the treatment effects across caregivers and settings, or maintaining the treatment effects over time). The therapy is conducted in a structured, safe environment. Precautions may include environmental modifications and/or protective equipment for the safety of the patient or the technicians.

0373T Exposure adaptive behavior treatment with protocol modification requiring two or more technicians for severe maladaptive behavior(s); first 60 minutes of technicians' time, face-to-face with patient
Sunset January 2020

+ **0374T** each additional 30 minutes of technicians' time face-to-face with patient (List separately in addition to code for primary procedure)
Sunset January 2020

(Use 0374T in conjunction with 0373T)

(0373T, 0374T are reported based on a single technician's face-to-face time with the patient and not the combined time of multiple technicians)

(Do not report 0373T, 0374T in conjunction with 90785-90899, 96101-96155)

0375T Total disc arthroplasty (artificial disc), anterior approach, including discectomy with end plate preparation (includes osteophytectomy for nerve root or spinal cord decompression and microdissection), cervical, three or more levels
Sunset January 2020

(Do not report 0375T in conjunction with 22851, 22856, 22858 when performed at the same level)

0376T Code is out of numerical sequence. See 0019T-0375T

0377T Anoscopy with directed submucosal injection of bulking agent for fecal incontinence
Sunset January 2020

(Do not report 0377T in conjunction with 46600)

0378T Visual field assessment, with concurrent real time data analysis and accessible data storage with patient initiated data transmitted to a remote surveillance center for up to 30 days; review and interpretation with report by a physician or other qualified health care professional
Sunset January 2020

0379T technical support and patient instructions, surveillance, analysis, and transmission of daily and emergent data reports as prescribed by a physician or other qualified health care professional
Sunset January 2020

0380T Computer-aided animation and analysis of time series retinal images for the monitoring of disease progression, unilateral or bilateral, with interpretation and report
Sunset January 2020

● **0381T** External heart rate and 3-axis accelerometer data recording up to 14 days to assess changes in heart rate and to monitor motion analysis for the purposes of diagnosing nocturnal epilepsy seizure events; includes report, scanning analysis with report, review and interpretation by a physician or other qualified health care professional
Sunset January 2021

● **0382T** review and interpretation only
Sunset January 2021

►(Do not report 0381T, 0382T in conjunction with 0383T, 0384T, 0385T, 0386T)◄

● **0383T** External heart rate and 3-axis accelerometer data recording from 15 to 30 days to assess changes in heart rate and to monitor motion analysis for the purposes of diagnosing nocturnal epilepsy seizure events; includes report, scanning analysis with report, review and interpretation by a physician or other qualified health care professional
Sunset January 2021

● **0384T** review and interpretation only
Sunset January 2021

►(Do not report 0383T, 0384T in conjunction with 0381T, 0382T, 0385T, 0386T)◄

● **0385T**   External heart rate and 3-axis accelerometer data recording more than 30 days to assess changes in heart rate and to monitor motion analysis for the purposes of diagnosing nocturnal epilepsy seizure events; includes report, scanning analysis with report, review and interpretation by a physician or other qualified health care professional
Sunset January 2021

● **0386T**   review and interpretation only
Sunset January 2021

►(Do not report 0385T, 0386T in conjunction with 0381T, 0382T, 0383T, 0384T)◄

►Pacemaker—Leadless and Pocketless System◄

►A leadless cardiac pacemaker system is a pulse generator with built-in battery and electrode for implantation in a cardiac chamber via a transfemoral catheter approach. For these services, see 0387T, 0388T, 0389T, 0390T, 0391T. Codes 0387T, 0388T include fluoroscopy (76000), right ventriculography (93566), and femoral venography (75820) intrinsic to procedure, when performed.◄

● **0387T**   Transcatheter insertion or replacement of permanent leadless pacemaker, ventricular
Sunset January 2021

►(For insertion, repositioning, or replacement of pacemaker systems with lead[s], use the appropriate epicardial [33202, 33203] or transvenous codes [33206-33222, 33224, 33225, 33226])◄

►(Do not report 0387T in conjunction with 0388T, 0389T, 0390T, 0391T)◄

►(Do not report 0387T in conjunction with 93566 for right ventriculography performed during leadless pacemaker insertion)◄

● **0388T**   Transcatheter removal of permanent leadless pacemaker, ventricular
Sunset January 2021

►(For removal of pacemaker systems with lead[s], see the appropriate transvenous [33227, 33228, 33229, 33233, 33234, 33235] or thoracotomy codes [33236, 33237, 33238])◄

►(Do not report 0388T in conjunction with 0387T)◄

● **0389T**   Programming device evaluation (in person) with iterative adjustment of the implantable device to test the function of the device and select optimal permanent programmed values with analysis, review and report, leadless pacemaker system
Sunset January 2021

►(Do not report 0389T in conjunction with 0387T, 0390T, 0391T)◄

►(For programming device evaluations of pacemaker systems with lead[s], see 93279, 93280, 93281)◄

● **0390T**   Peri-procedural device evaluation (in person) and programming of device system parameters before or after a surgery, procedure or test with analysis, review and report, leadless pacemaker system
Sunset January 2021

►(Do not report 0390T in conjunction with 0387T, 0389T, 0391T)◄

►(For peri-procedural device evaluation of systems with lead[s], see 93286, 93287)◄

● **0391T**   Interrogation device evaluation (in person) with analysis, review and report, includes connection, recording and disconnection per patient encounter, leadless pacemaker system
Sunset January 2021

►(Do not report 0391T in conjunction with 0387T, 0389T, 0390T)◄

►(For interrogation device evaluation of systems with lead[s], see 93288, 93289)◄

● **0392T**   Laparoscopy, surgical, esophageal sphincter augmentation procedure, placement of sphincter augmentation device (ie, magnetic band)
Sunset January 2021

● **0393T**   Removal of esophageal sphincter augmentation device
Sunset January 2021

►(Do not report 0393T in conjunction with 43279, 43280, 43281, 43282)◄

►(Electronic brachytherapy is a form of radiation therapy in which an electrically generated X-ray source of ionizing radiation is placed inside or in close proximity to the tumor or target tissue to deliver therapeutic radiation dosage)◄

● **0394T**   High dose rate electronic brachytherapy, skin surface application, per fraction, includes basic dosimetry, when performed
Sunset January 2021

►(Do not report 0394T in conjunction with 77261, 77262, 77263, 77300, 77306, 77307, 77316, 77317, 77318, 77332, 77333, 77334, 77336, 77427, 77431, 77432, 77435, 77469, 77470, 77499, 77761, 77762, 77763, 77767, 77768, 77770, 77771, 77772, 77778, 77789)◄

►(For high dose rate radionuclide surface brachytherapy, see 77767, 77768)◄

►(For non-brachytherapy superficial [eg, ≤200 kV] radiation treatment delivery, use 77401)◄

Category III

● **0395T** High dose rate electronic brachytherapy, interstitial or intracavitary treatment, per fraction, includes basic dosimetry, when performed
Sunset January 2021

►(Do not report 0395T in conjunction with 77261, 77262, 77263, 77300, 77306, 77307, 77316, 77317, 77318, 77332, 77333, 77334, 77336, 77427, 77431, 77432, 77435, 77469, 77470, 77499, 77761, 77762, 77763, 77767, 77768, 77770, 77771, 77772, 77778, 77789)◄

►(For skin surface application of high dose rate electronic brachytherapy, use 0394T)◄

+● **0396T** Intra-operative use of kinetic balance sensor for implant stability during knee replacement arthroplasty (List separately in addition to code for primary procedure)
Sunset January 2021

►(Use 0396T in conjunction with 27445, 27446, 27447, 27486, 27487, 27488)◄

⊙+● **0397T** Endoscopic retrograde cholangiopancreatography (ERCP), with optical endomicroscopy (List separately in addition to code for primary procedure)
Sunset January 2021

►(Use 0397T in conjunction with 43260, 43261, 43262, 43263, 43264, 43265, 43274, 43275, 43276, 43277, 43278)◄

►(Do not report 0397T in conjunction with 88375)◄

►(Do not report optical endomicroscopy more than once per session)◄

● **0398T** Magnetic resonance image guided high intensity focused ultrasound (MRgFUS), stereotactic ablation lesion, intracranial for movement disorder including stereotactic navigation and frame placement when performed
Sunset January 2021

►(Do not report 0398T in conjunction with 61781, 61800)◄

+● **0399T** Myocardial strain imaging (quantitative assessment of myocardial mechanics using image-based analysis of local myocardial dynamics) (List separately in addition to code for primary procedure)
Sunset January 2021

►(Use 0399T in conjunction with 93303, 93304, 93306, 93307, 93308, 93312, 93314, 93315, 93317, 93350, 93351, 93355)◄

►(Report 0399T once per session)◄

● **0400T** Multi-spectral digital skin lesion analysis of clinically atypical cutaneous pigmented lesions for detection of melanomas and high risk melanocytic atypia; one to five lesions
Sunset January 2021

● **0401T** six or more lesions
Sunset January 2021

►(Do not report 0401T in conjunction with 0400T)◄

● **0402T** Collagen cross-linking of cornea (including removal of the corneal epithelium and intraoperative pachymetry when performed)
Sunset January 2021

►(Do not report 0402T in conjunction with 65435, 69990, 76514)◄

● **0403T** Preventive behavior change, intensive program of prevention of diabetes using a standardized diabetes prevention program curriculum, provided to individuals in a group setting, minimum 60 minutes, per day
Sunset January 2021

● **0404T** Transcervical uterine fibroid(s) ablation with ultrasound guidance, radiofrequency
Sunset January 2021

● **0405T** Oversight of the care of an extracorporeal liver assist system patient requiring review of status, review of laboratories and other studies, and revision of orders and liver assist care plan (as appropriate), within a calendar month, 30 minutes or more of non-face-to-face time
Sunset January 2021

● **0406T** Nasal endoscopy, surgical, ethmoid sinus, placement of drug eluting implant;
Sunset January 2021

● **0407T** with biopsy, polypectomy or debridement
Sunset January 2021

►(Do not report 0406T, 0407T in conjunction with 31200, 31201, 31205, 31231, 31237, 31240, 31254, 31255, 31288, 31290 when performed on the same side)◄

►(Do not report 0407T in conjunction with 0406T if performed on the same side)◄

Category III

Appendix A

Modifiers

This list includes all of the modifiers applicable to CPT 2016 codes.

A modifier provides the means to report or indicate that a service or procedure that has been performed has been altered by some specific circumstance but not changed in its definition or code. Modifiers also enable health care professionals to effectively respond to payment policy requirements established by other entities.

22 **Increased Procedural Services:** When the work required to provide a service is substantially greater than typically required, it may be identified by adding modifier 22 to the usual procedure code. Documentation must support the substantial additional work and the reason for the additional work (ie, increased intensity, time, technical difficulty of procedure, severity of patient's condition, physical and mental effort required). **Note:** This modifier should not be appended to an E/M service.

23 **Unusual Anesthesia:** Occasionally, a procedure, which usually requires either no anesthesia or local anesthesia, because of unusual circumstances must be done under general anesthesia. This circumstance may be reported by adding modifier 23 to the procedure code of the basic service.

24 **Unrelated Evaluation and Management Service by the Same Physician or Other Qualified Health Care Professional During a Postoperative Period:** The physician or other qualified health care professional may need to indicate that an evaluation and management service was performed during a postoperative period for a reason(s) unrelated to the original procedure. This circumstance may be reported by adding modifier 24 to the appropriate level of E/M service.

25 **Significant, Separately Identifiable Evaluation and Management Service by the Same Physician or Other Qualified Health Care Professional on the Same Day of the Procedure or Other Service:** It may be necessary to indicate that on the day a procedure or service identified by a CPT code was performed, the patient's condition required a significant, separately identifiable E/M service above and beyond the other service provided or beyond the usual preoperative and postoperative care associated with the procedure that was performed. A significant, separately identifiable E/M service is defined or substantiated by documentation that satisfies the relevant criteria for the respective E/M service to be reported (see **Evaluation and Management Services Guidelines** for instructions on determining level of E/M service). The E/M service may be prompted by the symptom or condition for which the procedure and/or service was provided. As such, different diagnoses are not required for reporting of the E/M services on the same date. This circumstance may be reported by adding modifier 25 to the appropriate level of E/M service.

Note: This modifier is not used to report an E/M service that resulted in a decision to perform surgery. See modifier 57. For significant, separately identifiable non-E/M services, see modifier 59.

26 **Professional Component:** Certain procedures are a combination of a physician or other qualified health care professional component and a technical component. When the physician or other qualified health care professional component is reported separately, the service may be identified by adding modifier 26 to the usual procedure number.

32 **Mandated Services:** Services related to *mandated* consultation and/or related services (eg, third party payer, governmental, legislative or regulatory requirement) may be identified by adding modifier 32 to the basic procedure.

33 **Preventive Services:** When the primary purpose of the service is the delivery of an evidence based service in accordance with a US Preventive Services Task Force A or B rating in effect and other preventive services identified in preventive services mandates (legislative or regulatory), the service may be identified by adding 33 to the procedure. For separately reported services specifically identified as preventive, the modifier should not be used.

47 **Anesthesia by Surgeon:** Regional or general anesthesia provided by the surgeon may be reported by adding modifier 47 to the basic service. (This does not include local anesthesia.) **Note:** Modifier 47 would not be used as a modifier for the anesthesia procedures.

50 **Bilateral Procedure:** Unless otherwise identified in the listings, bilateral procedures that are performed at the same session, should be identified by adding modifier 50 to the appropriate 5 digit code.

51 **Multiple Procedures:** When multiple procedures, other than E/M services, Physical Medicine and Rehabilitation services or provision of supplies (eg, vaccines), are performed at the same session by the same individual, the primary procedure or service may be reported as listed. The additional procedure(s) or service(s) may be identified by appending modifier 51 to the additional procedure or service code(s). **Note:** This modifier should not be appended to designated "add-on" codes (see Appendix D).

52 **Reduced Services:** Under certain circumstances a service or procedure is partially reduced or eliminated at the discretion of the physician or other qualified health care professional. Under these circumstances the service provided can be identified by its usual procedure number and the addition of modifier 52, signifying that the service is reduced. This provides a means of reporting reduced services without disturbing the identification of the basic service. **Note:** For hospital outpatient reporting of a previously scheduled procedure/service that is partially reduced or cancelled as a result of extenuating

Appendix A

circumstances or those that threaten the well-being of the patient prior to or after administration of anesthesia, see modifiers 73 and 74 (see modifiers approved for ASC hospital outpatient use).

53 **Discontinued Procedure:** Under certain circumstances, the physician or other qualified health care professional may elect to terminate a surgical or diagnostic procedure. Due to extenuating circumstances or those that threaten the well being of the patient, it may be necessary to indicate that a surgical or diagnostic procedure was started but discontinued. This circumstance may be reported by adding modifier 53 to the code reported by the individual for the discontinued procedure. **Note:** This modifier is not used to report the elective cancellation of a procedure prior to the patient's anesthesia induction and/or surgical preparation in the operating suite. For outpatient hospital/ambulatory surgery center (ASC) reporting of a previously scheduled procedure/service that is partially reduced or cancelled as a result of extenuating circumstances or those that threaten the well being of the patient prior to or after administration of anesthesia, see modifiers 73 and 74 (see modifiers approved for ASC hospital outpatient use).

54 **Surgical Care Only:** When 1 physician or other qualified health care professional performs a surgical procedure and another provides preoperative and/or postoperative management, surgical services may be identified by adding modifier 54 to the usual procedure number.

55 **Postoperative Management Only:** When 1 physician or other qualified health care professional performed the postoperative management and another performed the surgical procedure, the postoperative component may be identified by adding modifier 55 to the usual procedure number.

56 **Preoperative Management Only:** When 1 physician or other qualified health care professional performed the preoperative care and evaluation and another performed the surgical procedure, the preoperative component may be identified by adding modifier 56 to the usual procedure number.

57 **Decision for Surgery:** An evaluation and management service that resulted in the initial decision to perform the surgery may be identified by adding modifier 57 to the appropriate level of E/M service.

58 **Staged or Related Procedure or Service by the Same Physician or Other Qualified Health Care Professional During the Postoperative Period:** It may be necessary to indicate that the performance of a procedure or service during the postoperative period was: (a) planned or anticipated (staged); (b) more extensive than the original procedure; or (c) for therapy following a surgical procedure. This circumstance may be reported by adding modifier 58 to the staged or related procedure. **Note:** For treatment of a problem that requires a return to the operating/procedure room (eg, unanticipated clinical condition), see modifier 78.

59 **Distinct Procedural Service:** Under certain circumstances, it may be necessary to indicate that a procedure or service was distinct or independent from other non-E/M services performed on the same day. Modifier 59 is used to identify procedures/services, other than E/M services, that are not normally reported together, but are appropriate under the circumstances. Documentation must support a different session, different procedure or surgery, different site or organ system, separate incision/excision, separate lesion, or separate injury (or area of injury in extensive injuries) not ordinarily encountered or performed on the same day by the same individual. However, when another already established modifier is appropriate it should be used rather than modifier 59. Only if no more descriptive modifier is available, and the use of modifier 59 best explains the circumstances, should modifier 59 be used. **Note:** Modifier 59 should not be appended to an E/M service. To report a separate and distinct E/M service with a non-E/M service performed on the same date, see modifier 25. See also page 502, Level II (HCPCS/National) Modifiers listing.

62 **Two Surgeons:** When 2 surgeons work together as primary surgeons performing distinct part(s) of a procedure, each surgeon should report his/her distinct operative work by adding modifier 62 to the procedure code and any associated add-on code(s) for that procedure as long as both surgeons continue to work together as primary surgeons. Each surgeon should report the co-surgery once using the same procedure code. If additional procedure(s) (including add-on procedure(s) are performed during the same surgical session, separate code(s) may also be reported with modifier 62 added. **Note:** If a co-surgeon acts as an assistant in the performance of additional procedure(s), other than those reported with the modifier 62, during the same surgical session, those services may be reported using separate procedure code(s) with modifier 80 or modifier 82 added, as appropriate.

63 **Procedure Performed on Infants less than 4 kg:** Procedures performed on neonates and infants up to a present body weight of 4 kg may involve significantly increased complexity and physician or other qualified health care professional work commonly associated with these patients. This circumstance may be reported by adding modifier 63 to the procedure number. **Note:** Unless otherwise designated, this modifier may only be appended to procedures/services listed in the 20005-69990 code series. Modifier 63 should not be appended to any CPT codes listed in the **Evaluation and Management Services, Anesthesia, Radiology, Pathology/Laboratory, or Medicine** sections.

66 **Surgical Team:** Under some circumstances, highly complex procedures (requiring the concomitant services of several physicians or other qualified health care professionals, often of different specialties, plus other highly skilled, specially trained personnel, various types of complex equipment) are carried out under the "surgical team" concept. Such circumstances may be identified by each participating individual with the addition of modifier 66 to the basic procedure number used for reporting services.

76 Repeat Procedure or Service by Same Physician or Other Qualified Health Care Professional: It may be necessary to indicate that a procedure or service was repeated by the same physician or other qualified health care professional subsequent to the original procedure or service. This circumstance may be reported by adding modifier 76 to the repeated procedure or service. **Note:** This modifier should not be appended to an E/M service.

77 Repeat Procedure by Another Physician or Other Qualified Health Care Professional: It may be necessary to indicate that a basic procedure or service was repeated by another physician or other qualified health care professional subsequent to the original procedure or service. This circumstance may be reported by adding modifier 77 to the repeated procedure or service. **Note:** This modifier should not be appended to an E/M service.

78 Unplanned Return to the Operating/Procedure Room by the Same Physician or Other Qualified Health Care Professional Following Initial Procedure for a Related Procedure During the Postoperative Period: It may be necessary to indicate that another procedure was performed during the postoperative period of the initial procedure (unplanned procedure following initial procedure). When this procedure is related to the first, and requires the use of an operating/procedure room, it may be reported by adding modifier 78 to the related procedure. (For repeat procedures, see modifier 76.)

79 Unrelated Procedure or Service by the Same Physician or Other Qualified Health Care Professional During the Postoperative Period: The individual may need to indicate that the performance of a procedure or service during the postoperative period was unrelated to the original procedure. This circumstance may be reported by using modifier 79. (For repeat procedures on the same day, see modifier 76.)

80 Assistant Surgeon: Surgical assistant services may be identified by adding modifier 80 to the usual procedure number(s).

81 Minimum Assistant Surgeon: Minimum surgical assistant services are identified by adding modifier 81 to the usual procedure number.

82 Assistant Surgeon (when qualified resident surgeon not available): The unavailability of a qualified resident surgeon is a prerequisite for use of modifier 82 appended to the usual procedure code number(s).

90 Reference (Outside) Laboratory: When laboratory procedures are performed by a party other than the treating or reporting physician or other qualified health care professional, the procedure may be identified by adding modifier 90 to the usual procedure number.

91 Repeat Clinical Diagnostic Laboratory Test: In the course of treatment of the patient, it may be necessary to repeat the same laboratory test on the same day to obtain subsequent (multiple) test results. Under these circumstances, the laboratory test performed can be identified by its usual procedure number and the addition of modifier 91. **Note:** This modifier may not be used when tests are rerun to confirm initial results; due to testing problems with specimens or equipment; or for any other reason when a normal, one-time, reportable result is all that is required. This modifier may not be used when other code(s) describe a series of test results (eg, glucose tolerance tests, evocative/suppression testing). This modifier may only be used for laboratory test(s) performed more than once on the same day on the same patient.

92 Alternative Laboratory Platform Testing: When laboratory testing is being performed using a kit or transportable instrument that wholly or in part consists of a single use, disposable analytical chamber, the service may be identified by adding modifier 92 to the usual laboratory procedure code (HIV testing 86701-86703, and 87389). The test does not require permanent dedicated space, hence by its design may be hand carried or transported to the vicinity of the patient for immediate testing at that site, although location of the testing is not in itself determinative of the use of this modifier.

99 Multiple Modifiers: Under certain circumstances 2 or more modifiers may be necessary to completely delineate a service. In such situations modifier 99 should be added to the basic procedure, and other applicable modifiers may be listed as part of the description of the service.

Anesthesia Physical Status Modifiers

The Physical Status modifiers are consistent with the American Society of Anesthesiologists ranking of patient physical status, and distinguishing various levels of complexity of the anesthesia service provided. All anesthesia services are reported by use of the anesthesia five-digit procedure code (00100-01999) with the appropriate physical status modifier appended.

Example: 00100-P1

Under certain circumstances, when another established modifier(s) is appropriate, it should be used in addition to the physical status modifier.

Example: 00100-P4-53

Physical Status Modifier P1: A normal healthy patient

Physical Status Modifier P2: A patient with mild systemic disease

Physical Status Modifier P3: A patient with severe systemic disease

Physical Status Modifier P4: A patient with severe systemic disease that is a constant threat to life

Physical Status Modifier P5: A moribund patient who is not expected to survive without the operation

Physical Status Modifier P6: A declared brain-dead patient whose organs are being removed for donor purposes

Modifiers Approved for Ambulatory Surgery Center (ASC) Hospital Outpatient Use

CPT Level I Modifiers

25 **Significant, Separately Identifiable Evaluation and Management Service by the Same Physician or Other Qualified Health Care Professional on the Same Day of the Procedure or Other Service:** It may be necessary to indicate that on the day a procedure or service identified by a CPT code was performed, the patient's condition required a significant, separately identifiable E/M service above and beyond the other service provided or beyond the usual preoperative and postoperative care associated with the procedure that was performed. A significant, separately identifiable E/M service is defined or substantiated by documentation that satisfies the relevant criteria for the respective E/M service to be reported (see **Evaluation and Management Services Guidelines** for instructions on determining level of E/M service). The E/M service may be prompted by the symptom or condition for which the procedure and/or service was provided. As such, different diagnoses are not required for reporting of the E/M services on the same date. This circumstance may be reported by adding modifier 25 to the appropriate level of E/M service. **Note:** This modifier is not used to report an E/M service that resulted in a decision to perform surgery. See modifier 57. For significant, separately identifiable non-E/M services, see modifier 59.

27 **Multiple Outpatient Hospital E/M Encounters on the Same Date:** For hospital outpatient reporting purposes, utilization of hospital resources related to separate and distinct E/M encounters performed in multiple outpatient hospital settings on the same date may be reported by adding modifier 27 to each appropriate level outpatient and/or emergency department E/M code(s). This modifier provides a means of reporting circumstances involving evaluation and management services provided by physician(s) in more than one (multiple) outpatient hospital setting(s) (eg, hospital emergency department, clinic). **Note:** This modifier is not to be used for physician reporting of multiple E/M services performed by the same physician on the same date. For physician reporting of all outpatient evaluation and management services provided by the same physician on the same date and performed in multiple outpatient setting(s) (eg, hospital emergency department, clinic), see **Evaluation and Management, Emergency Department, or Preventive Medicine Services** codes.

50 **Bilateral Procedure:** Unless otherwise identified in the listings, bilateral procedures that are performed at the same session, should be identified by adding modifier 50 to the appropriate 5 digit code.

52 **Reduced Services:** Under certain circumstances a service or procedure is partially reduced or eliminated at the discretion of the physician or other qualified health care professional. Under these circumstances the service provided can be identified by its usual procedure number and the addition of modifier 52, signifying that the service is reduced. This provides a means of reporting reduced services without disturbing the identification of the basic service. **Note:** For hospital outpatient reporting of a previously scheduled procedure/service that is partially reduced or cancelled as a result of extenuating circumstances or those that threaten the well-being of the patient prior to or after administration of anesthesia, see modifiers 73 and 74 (see modifiers approved for ASC hospital outpatient use).

58 **Staged or Related Procedure or Service by the Same Physician or Other Qualified Health Care Professional During the Postoperative Period:** It may be necessary to indicate that the performance of a procedure or service during the postoperative period was: (a) planned or anticipated (staged); (b) more extensive than the original procedure; or (c) for therapy following a surgical procedure. This circumstance may be reported by adding modifier 58 to the staged or related procedure. **Note:** For treatment of a problem that requires a return to the operating/procedure room (eg, unanticipated clinical condition), see modifier 78.

59 **Distinct Procedural Service:** Under certain circumstances, it may be necessary to indicate that a procedure or service was distinct or independent from other non-E/M services performed on the same day. Modifier 59 is used to identify procedures/services, other than E/M services, that are not normally reported together, but are appropriate under the circumstances. Documentation must support a different session, different procedure or surgery, different site or organ system, separate incision/excision, separate lesion, or separate injury (or area of injury in extensive injuries) not ordinarily encountered or performed on the same day by the same individual. However, when another already established modifier is appropriate it should be used rather than modifier 59. Only if no more descriptive modifier is available, and the use of modifier 59 best explains the circumstances, should modifier 59 be used. **Note:** Modifier 59 should not be appended to an E/M service. To report a separate and distinct E/M service with a non-E/M service performed on the same date, see modifier 25. See also page 502, Level II (HCPCS/National) Modifiers listing.

73 **Discontinued Out-Patient Hospital/Ambulatory Surgery Center (ASC) Procedure Prior to the Administration of Anesthesia:** Due to extenuating circumstances or those that threaten the well being of the patient, the physician may cancel a surgical or diagnostic procedure subsequent to the patient's surgical preparation (including sedation when provided, and being taken to the room where the procedure is to be performed), but prior to the administration of anesthesia (local, regional block(s) or general). Under these circumstances, the intended service that is prepared for but cancelled can be reported by its usual procedure number and the addition of modifier 73. **Note:** The elective cancellation of a service prior to the administration of anesthesia and/or surgical preparation of the patient should not be reported. For physician reporting of a discontinued procedure, see modifier 53.

74 Discontinued Out-Patient Hospital/Ambulatory Surgery Center (ASC) Procedure After Administration of Anesthesia: Due to extenuating circumstances or those that threaten the well being of the patient, the physician may terminate a surgical or diagnostic procedure after the administration of anesthesia (local, regional block(s), general) or after the procedure was started (incision made, intubation started, scope inserted, etc). Under these circumstances, the procedure started but terminated can be reported by its usual procedure number and the addition of modifier 74. **Note:** The elective cancellation of a service prior to the administration of anesthesia and/or surgical preparation of the patient should not be reported. For physician reporting of a discontinued procedure, see modifier 53.

76 Repeat Procedure or Service by Same Physician or Other Qualified Health Care Professional: It may be necessary to indicate that a procedure or service was repeated by the same physician or other qualified health care professional subsequent to the original procedure or service. This circumstance may be reported by adding modifier 76 to the repeated procedure or service. **Note:** This modifier should not be appended to an E/M service.

77 Repeat Procedure by Another Physician or Other Qualified Health Care Professional: It may be necessary to indicate that a basic procedure or service was repeated by another physician or other qualified health care professional subsequent to the original procedure or service. This circumstance may be reported by adding modifier 77 to the repeated procedure or service. **Note:** This modifier should not be appended to an E/M service.

78 Unplanned Return to the Operating/Procedure Room by the Same Physician or Other Qualified Health Care Professional Following Initial Procedure for a Related Procedure During the Postoperative Period: It may be necessary to indicate that another procedure was performed during the postoperative period of the initial procedure (unplanned procedure following initial procedure). When this procedure is related to the first, and requires the use of an operating/procedure room, it may be reported by adding modifier 78 to the related procedure. (For repeat procedures, see modifier 76.)

79 Unrelated Procedure or Service by the Same Physician or Other Qualified Health Care Professional During the Postoperative Period: The individual may need to indicate that the performance of a procedure or service during the postoperative period was unrelated to the original procedure. This circumstance may be reported by using modifier 79. (For repeat procedures on the same day, see modifier 76.)

91 Repeat Clinical Diagnostic Laboratory Test: In the course of treatment of the patient, it may be necessary to repeat the same laboratory test on the same day to obtain subsequent (multiple) test results. Under these circumstances, the laboratory test performed can be identified by its usual procedure number and the addition of modifier 91. **Note:** This modifier may not be used when tests are rerun to confirm initial results; due to testing problems with specimens or equipment; or for any other reason when a normal, one-time, reportable result is all that is required. This modifier may not be used when other code(s) describe a series of test results (eg, glucose tolerance tests, evocative/suppression testing). This modifier may only be used for laboratory test(s) performed more than once on the same day on the same patient.

Level II (HCPCS/National) Modifiers

E1 Upper left, eyelid

E2 Lower left, eyelid

E3 Upper right, eyelid

E4 Lower right, eyelid

F1 Left hand, second digit

F2 Left hand, third digit

F3 Left hand, fourth digit

F4 Left hand, fifth digit

F5 Right hand, thumb

F6 Right hand, second digit

F7 Right hand, third digit

F8 Right hand, fourth digit

F9 Right hand, fifth digit

FA Left hand, thumb

GG Performance and payment of a screening mammogram and diagnostic mammogram on the same patient, same day

GH Diagnostic mammogram converted from screening mammogram on same day

LC Left circumflex coronary artery

LD Left anterior descending coronary artery

LM Left main coronary artery

LT Left side (used to identify procedures performed on the left side of the body)

QM Ambulance service provided under arrangement by a provider of services

QN Ambulance service furnished directly by a provider of services

RC Right coronary artery

RI Ramus intermedius coronary artery

RT Right side (used to identify procedures performed on the right side of the body)

T1 Left foot, second digit

T2 Left foot, third digit

T3 Left foot, fourth digit

T4 Left foot, fifth digit

T5 Right foot, great toe

T6 Right foot, second digit

T7 Right foot, third digit

T8 Right foot, fourth digit

T9 Right foot, fifth digit

TA Left foot, great toe

XE Separate Encounter *

XS Separate Structure *

XP Separate Practitioner *

XU Unusual Non-Overlapping Service *

(*HCPCS modifiers for selective identification of subsets of
Distinct Procedural Services [-59 modifier])

Appendix B

Summary of Additions, Deletions, and Revisions

Appendix B shows the actual changes that were made to the code descriptors. New codes appear with a bullet (●) and are indicated as "Code Added." Revised codes are preceded with a triangle (▲). Within revised codes, the deleted language appears with a ~~strikethrough~~, while new text appears <u>underlined</u>. Codes with which moderate sedation would not be separately reported when performed at the same session by the same individual are denoted with the bullseye (⊙). The symbol ⟋ is used to identify codes for vaccines that are pending FDA approval (see **Appendix K**). The symbol # is used to identify codes that have been resequenced (see **Appendix N**). CPT add-on codes are annotated by the symbol ✚ (see **Appendix D**). The symbol ⊘ is used to identify codes that are exempt from the use of modifier 51 (see **Appendix E**).

Evaluation and Management

✚▲ 99354 Prolonged <u>evaluation and management or pscyhotherapy service(s) (beyond the typical</u> service <u>time of the primary procedure)</u> in the office or other outpatient setting requiring direct patient contact beyond the usual service; first hour (List separately in addition to code for office or other outpatient **Evaluation and Management** <u>or psychotherapy</u> service)

✚▲ 99355 each additional 30 minutes (List separately in addition to code for prolonged service)

#✚● 99415 Code added

#✚● 99416 Code added

Surgery

● 10035 Code added

✚● 10036 Code added

~~21805~~ ~~Open treatment of rib fracture without fixation, each~~

~~31620~~ ~~Endobronchial ultrasound (EBUS) during bronchoscopic diagnostic or therapeutic intervention(s) (List separately in addition to code for primary procedure[s])~~

⊙✚▲ 31632 with transbronchial lung biopsy(s), each additional lobe (List separately in addition to code for primary procedure)

⊙✚▲ 31633 with transbronchial needle aspiration biopsy(s), each additional lobe (List separately in addition to code for primary procedure)

⊙● 31652 Code added

⊙● 31653 Code added

⊙✚● 31654 Code added

● 33477 · Code added

⊙▲ 37184 Primary percutaneous transluminal mechanical thrombectomy, noncoronary, <u>non-intracranial,</u> arterial or arterial bypass graft, including fluoroscopic guidance and intraprocedural pharmacological thrombolytic injection(s); initial vessel

⊙✚▲ 37185 second and all subsequent vessel(s) within the same vascular family (List separately in addition to code for primary mechanical thrombectomy procedure)

⊙✚▲ 37186 Secondary percutaneous transluminal thrombectomy (eg, nonprimary mechanical, snare basket, suction technique), noncoronary, <u>non-intracranial,</u> arterial or arterial bypass graft, including fluoroscopic guidance and intraprocedural pharmacological thrombolytic injections, provided in conjunction with another percutaneous intervention other than primary mechanical thrombectomy (List separately in addition to code for primary procedure)

~~37202~~ ~~Transcatheter therapy, infusion other than for thrombolysis, any type (eg, spasmolytic, vasoconstrictive)~~

#⊙▲ 37211 Transcatheter therapy, arterial infusion for thrombolysis other than coronary, <u>intracranial,</u> any method, including radiological supervision and interpretation, initial treatment day

~~37250~~ ~~Intravascular ultrasound (non-coronary vessel) during diagnostic evaluation and/or therapeutic intervention; initial vessel (List separately in addition to code for primary procedure)~~

~~37251~~ ~~each additional vessel (List separately in addition to code for primary procedure)~~

⊙✚● 37252 Code added

⊙✚● 37253 Code added

~~39400~~ ~~Mediastinoscopy, includes biopsy(ies), when performed~~

● 39401 Code added

● 39402 Code added

#● **43210**   Code added

47136   ~~heterotopic, partial or whole, from cadaver or living donor, any age~~

47500   ~~Injection procedure for percutaneous transhepatic cholangiography~~

47505   ~~Injection procedure for cholangiography through an existing catheter (eg, percutaneous transhepatic or T-tube)~~

47510   ~~Introduction of percutaneous transhepatic catheter for biliary drainage~~

47511   ~~Introduction of percutaneous transhepatic stent for internal and external biliary drainage~~

47525   ~~Change of percutaneous biliary drainage catheter~~

47530   ~~Revision and/or reinsertion of transhepatic tube~~

● **47531**   Code added

⊙● **47532**   Code added

⊙● **47533**   Code added

⊙● **47534**   Code added

⊙● **47535**   Code added

⊙● **47536**   Code added

● **47537**   Code added

⊙● **47538**   Code added

⊙● **47539**   Code added

⊙● **47540**   Code added

⊙● **47541**   Code added

⊙+● **47542**   Code added

⊙+● **47543**   Code added

⊙+● **47544**   Code added

47560   ~~Laparoscopy, surgical; with guided transhepatic cholangiography, without biopsy~~

47561   ~~with guided transhepatic cholangiography with biopsy~~

47630   ~~Biliary duct stone extraction, percutaneous via T-tube tract, basket, or snare (eg, Burhenne technique)~~

● **49185**   Code added

⊙▲ **50387**   Removal and replacement of externally accessible ~~transnephric ureteral stent~~nephroureteral catheter (eg, external/internal stent) requiring fluoroscopic guidance, including radiological supervision and interpretation

50392   ~~Introduction of intracatheter or catheter into renal pelvis for drainage and/or injection, percutaneous~~

50393   ~~Introduction of ureteral catheter or stent into ureter through renal pelvis for drainage and/or injection, percutaneous~~

50394   ~~Injection procedure for pyelography (as nephrostogram, pyelostogram, antegrade pyeloureterograms) through nephrostomy or pyelostomy tube, or indwelling ureteral catheter~~

50398   ~~Change of nephrostomy or pyelostomy tube~~

#⊙● **50430**   Code added

#● **50431**   Code added

#⊙● **50432**   Code added

#⊙● **50433**   Code added

#⊙● **50434**   Code added

#● **50435**   Code added

⊙+● **50606**   Code added

⊙● **50693**   Code added

⊙● **50694**   Code added

⊙● **50695**   Code added

⊙+● **50705**   Code added

⊙+● **50706**   Code added

● **54437**   Code added

● **54438**   Code added

● **61645**   Code added

● **61650**   Code added

+● **61651**   Code added

64412   ~~spinal accessory nerve~~

#● **64461**   Code added

#+● **64462**   Code added

#● **64463**   Code added

● **65785**   Code added

▲ **65855**   Trabeculoplasty by laser surgery~~, 1 or more sessions (defined treatment series)~~

▲ **67101**   Repair of retinal detachment, 1 or more sessions; cryotherapy or diathermy, ~~with or without~~including drainage of subretinal fluid, when performed

▲ **67105**   photocoagulation, ~~with or without~~including drainage of subretinal fluid, when performed

▲ **67107**   Repair of retinal detachment; scleral buckling (such as lamellar scleral dissection, imbrication or encircling procedure), ~~with or without~~including, when performed, implant, ~~with or without~~ cryotherapy, photocoagulation, and drainage of subretinal fluid

▲ **67108**   with vitrectomy, any method, ~~with or without~~including, when performed, air or gas tamponade, focal endolaser photocoagulation, cryotherapy, drainage of subretinal fluid, scleral buckling, and/or removal of lens by same technique

67112   ~~by scleral buckling or vitrectomy, on patient having previous ipsilateral retinal detachment repair(s) using scleral buckling or vitrectomy techniques~~

▲ **67113**   Repair of complex retinal detachment (eg, proliferative vitreoretinopathy, stage C-1 or greater, diabetic traction retinal detachment, retinopathy of prematurity, retinal tear of greater than 90 degrees), with vitrectomy and membrane peeling, including, ~~may include~~when performed, air, gas, or silicone oil tamponade, cryotherapy, endolaser photocoagulation, drainage of subretinal fluid, scleral buckling, and/or removal of lens

▲ **67227**   Destruction of extensive or progressive retinopathy (eg, diabetic retinopathy)~~, 1 or more sessions~~, cryotherapy, diathermy

▲ **67228**   Treatment of extensive or progressive retinopathy (eg, ~~1 or more sessions~~diabetic retinopathy), photocoagulation~~; (eg, diabetic retinopathy), photocoagulation~~

● **69209**   Code added

Radiology

70373   ~~Laryngography, contrast, radiological supervision and interpretation~~

72010   ~~Radiologic examination, spine, entire, survey study, anteroposterior and lateral~~

72069   ~~Radiologic examination, spine, thoracolumbar, standing (scoliosis)~~

▲ 72080   thoracolumbar junction, minimum of 2 views

● 72081   Code added

● 72082   Code added

● 72083   Code added

● 72084   Code added

~~72090~~   ~~scoliosis study, including supine and erect studies~~

~~73500~~   ~~Radiologic examination, hip, unilateral; 1 view~~

● 73501   Code added

● 73502   Code added

● 73503   Code added

~~73510~~   ~~complete, minimum of 2 views~~

~~73520~~   ~~Radiologic examination, hips, bilateral, minimum of 2 views of each hip, including anteroposterior view of pelvis~~

● 73521   Code added

● 73522   Code added

● 73523   Code added

~~73530~~   ~~Radiologic examination, hip, during operative procedure~~

~~73540~~   ~~Radiologic examination, pelvis and hips, infant or child, minimum of 2 views~~

~~73550~~   ~~Radiologic examination, femur, 2 views~~

● 73551   Code added

● 73552   Code added

▲ 74240   Radiologic examination, gastrointestinal tract, upper; with or without delayed ~~films~~images, without KUB

▲ 74241   with or without delayed ~~films~~images, with KUB

▲ 74245   with small intestine, includes multiple serial ~~films~~images

▲ 74246   Radiological examination, gastrointestinal tract, upper, air contrast, with specific high density barium, effervescent agent, with or without glucagon; with or without delayed ~~films~~images, without KUB

▲ 74247   with or without delayed ~~films~~images, with KUB

▲ 74250   Radiologic examination, small intestine, includes multiple serial ~~films~~images:

▲ 74251   via enteroclysis tube

~~74305~~   ~~through existing catheter, radiological supervision and interpretation~~

~~74320~~   ~~Cholangiography, percutaneous, transhepatic, radiological supervision and interpretation~~

~~74327~~   ~~Postoperative biliary duct calculus removal, percutaneous via T-tube tract, basket, or snare (eg, Burhenne technique), radiological supervision and interpretation~~

▲ 74340   Introduction of long gastrointestinal tube (eg, Miller-Abbott), including multiple fluoroscopies and ~~films~~images, radiological supervision and interpretation

~~74475~~   ~~Introduction of intracatheter or catheter into renal pelvis for drainage and/or injection, percutaneous, radiological supervision and interpretation~~

~~74480~~   ~~Introduction of ureteral catheter or stent into ureter through renal pelvis for drainage and/or injection, percutaneous, radiological supervision and interpretation~~

● 74712   Code added

+● 74713   Code added

~~75896~~   ~~Transcatheter therapy, infusion, other than for thrombolysis, radiological supervision and interpretation~~

~~75945~~   ~~Intravascular ultrasound (non-coronary vessel), radiological supervision and interpretation; initial vessel~~

~~75946~~   ~~each additional non-coronary vessel (List separately in addition to code for primary procedure)~~

~~75980~~   ~~Percutaneous transhepatic biliary drainage with contrast monitoring, radiological supervision and interpretation~~

~~75982~~   ~~Percutaneous placement of drainage catheter for combined internal and external biliary drainage or of a drainage stent for internal biliary drainage in patients with an inoperable mechanical biliary obstruction, radiological supervision and interpretation~~

▲ 77057   Screening mammography, bilateral (2-view ~~film~~ study of each breast)

▲ 77417   Therapeutic radiology port ~~film~~image(s)

● 77767   Code added

● 77768   Code added

● 77770   Code added

● 77771   Code added

● 77772   Code added

~~77776~~   ~~Interstitial radiation source application; simple~~

~~77777~~   ~~intermediate~~

▲ 77778   Interstitial radiation source application, complex, includes supervision, handling, loading of radiation source, when performed~~; complex~~

~~77785~~   ~~Remote afterloading high dose rate radionuclide brachytherapy; 1 channel~~

~~77786~~   ~~2-12 channels~~

~~77787~~   ~~over 12 channels~~

▲ 77789   Surface application of ~~radiation~~low dose rate radionuclide source

▲ 78264   Gastric emptying imaging study (eg, solid, liquid, or both):

● 78265   Code added

● 78266   Code added

Pathology and Laboratory

#● 80081   Code added

● 81170   Code added

▲ 81210   BRAF (~~vB raf murine sarcoma viral~~ Raf proto-oncogene ~~homolog B1, serine/threonine kinase~~) (eg, colon cancer, melanoma), gene analysis, V600E variant(s);

#● 81162   Code added

● 81218   Code added

● 81219   Code added

● 81272   Code added

● 81273   Code added

▲ 81275   KRAS (~~v-Ki-ras2~~ Kirsten rat sarcoma viral oncogene homolog) (eg, carcinoma) gene analysis,~~variants in codons 12 and 13~~; variants in exon 2 (eg, codons 12 and 13)

● 81276   Code added

● 81311   Code added

● 81314   Code added

▲ 81355   *VKORC1 (vitamin K epoxide reductase complex, subunit 1)* (eg, warfarin metabolism), gene analysis, common variants(s) (eg, -1639/3673 1639G>A, c.173+1000C>T)

▲ 81401   Molecular pathology procedure, Level 2 (eg, 2-10 SNPs, 1 methylated variant, or 1 somatic variant [typically using nonsequencing target variant analysis], or detection of a dynamic mutation disorder/triplet repeat)

   ABL1 (ABL (eproto-abl oncogene 1, non-receptor tyrosine kinase) (eg, acquired imatinib resistance), T315l variant

   DEK/NUP214 (t(6;9)) (eg, acute myeloid leukemia), translocation analysis, qualitative, and quantitative, if performed

   IGH@/BCL2 (t(14;18)) (eg, follicular lymphoma), translocation analysis; single breakpoint (eg, major breakpoint region [MBR] or minor cluster region [mcr]), qualitative or quantitative

   (When both MBR and mcr breakpoints are performed use 81402)

▲ 81402   Molecular pathology procedure, Level 3 (eg, >10 SNPs, 2-10 methylated variants, or 2-10 somatic variants [typically using non-sequencing target variant analysis], immunoglobulin and T-cell receptor gene rearrangements, duplication/deletion variants of 1 exon, loss of heterozygosity [LOH], uniparental disomy [UPD])

   KIT (v-kit Hardy-Zuckerman 4 feline sarcoma viral oncogene homolog) (eg, mastocytosis), common variants (eg, D816V, D816Y, D816F)

▲ 81403   Molecular pathology procedure, Level 4 (eg, analysis of single exon by DNA sequence analysis, analysis of >10 amplicons using multiplex PCR in 2 or more independent reactions, mutation scanning or duplication/deletion variants of 2-5 exons)

   ABL1 (c-abl oncogene 1, receptor tyrosine kinase) (eg, acquired imatinib tyrosine kinase inhibitor resistance), variants in the kinase domain

   CEBPA (CCAAT/enhancer binding protein [C/EBP], alpha) (eg, acute myeloid leukemia), full gene sequence

   KRAS (v-Ki-ras2 Kirsten rat sarcoma viral oncogene) (eg, carcinoma), gene analysis, variant(s) in exon 3 (eg, codon 61)

▲ 81404   Molecular pathology procedure, Level 5 (eg, analysis of 2-5 exons by DNA sequence analysis, mutation scanning or duplication/deletion variants of 6-10 exons, or characterization of a dynamic mutation disorder/triplet repeat by Southern blot analysis)

   KIT (C-kit) (v-kit Hardy-Zuckerman 4 feline sarcoma viral oncogene homolog) (eg, GIST, acute myeloid leukemia, melanoma), targeted gene analysis (eg, exons 8, 11, 13, 17, 18)

   NRAS (neuroblastoma RAS viral oncogene homolog) (eg, colorectal carcinoma), exon 1 and exon 2 sequences

   PDGFRA (platelet-derived growth factor receptor alpha polypeptide) (eg, gastrointestinal stromal tumor), targeted sequence analysis (eg, exons 12, 18)

▲ 81405   Molecular pathology procedure, Level 6 (eg, analysis of 6-10 exons by DNA sequence analysis, mutation scanning or duplication/deletion variants of 11-25 exons, regionally targeted cytogenomic array analysis)

   KRAS (v-Ki-ras2 Kirsten rat sarcoma viral oncogene homolog) (eg, Noonan syndrome), full gene sequence

▲ 81406   Molecular pathology procedure, Level 7 (eg, analysis of 11-25 exons by DNA sequence analysis, mutation scanning or duplication/deletion variants of 26-50 exons, cytogenomic array analysis for neoplasia)

   BRAF (vB-raf murine sarcoma viral Raf proto-oncogene homolog B1, serine/threonine kinase) (eg, Noonan syndrome), full gene sequence

   PCSK9 (proprotein convertase subtilisin/kexin type 9) (eg, familial hypercholesterolemia), full gene sequence

● 81412   Code added

● 81432   Code added

● 81433   Code added

● 81434   Code added

▲ 81435   Hereditary colon cancer syndromes disorders (eg, Lynch syndrome, PTEN hamartoma syndrome, Cowden syndrome, familial adenomatosis polyposis); genomic sequence analysis panel, must include analysis sequencing of at least 7 10 genes, including APC, BMPR1A, CHEK2 CDH1, MLH1, MSH2, MSH6, MUTYH, PTEN, SMAD4, and PMS2 STK11

▲ 81436   duplication/deletion gene analysis panel, must include analysis of at least 8 5 genes, including APC, MLH1, MSH2, MSH6, PMS2, EPCAM, CHEK2 SMAD4, and MUTYH STK11

● 81437   Code added

● 81438   Code added

● 81442   Code added

▲ 81445   Targeted genomic sequence analysis panel, solid organ neoplasm, DNA analysis, and RNA analysis when performed, 5-50 genes (eg, ALK, BRAF, CDKN2A, EGFR, ERBB2, KIT, KRAS, NRAS, MET, PDGFRA, PDGFRB, PGR, PIK3CA, PTEN, RET), interrogation for sequence variants and copy number variants or rearrangements, if performed

▲ 81450   Targeted genomic sequence analysis panel, hematolymphoid neoplasm or disorder, DNA analysis, and RNA analysis when performed, 5-50 genes (eg, BRAF, CEBPA, DNMT3A, EZH2, FLT3, IDH1, IDH2, JAK2, KRAS, KIT, MLL, NRAS, NPM1, NOTCH1), interrogation for sequence variants, and copy number variants or rearrangements, or isoform expression or mRNA expression levels, if performed

▲ 81455   Targeted genomic sequence analysis panel, solid organ or hematolymphoid neoplasm, DNA analysis, and RNA analysis when performed, 51 or greater genes (eg, ALK, BRAF, CDKN2A, CEBPA, DNMT3A, EGFR, ERBB2, EZH2, FLT3, IDH1, IDH2, JAK2, KIT, KRAS, MLL, NPM1, NRAS, MET, NOTCH1, PDGFRA, PDGFRB, PGR, PIK3CA, PTEN, RET), interrogation for sequence variants and copy number variants or rearrangements, if performed

● 81490   Code added

● 81493   Code added

● 81525   Code added

● 81528   Code added

● 81535   Code added

+● 81536   Code added

● 81538   Code added

● 81540   Code added

● 81545   Code added

● 81595   Code added

82486   Chromatography, qualitative; column (eg, gas liquid or HPLC), analyte not elsewhere specified

82487   paper, 1-dimensional, analyte not elsewhere specified

82488   paper, 2-dimensional, analyte not elsewhere specified

82489   thin layer, analyte not elsewhere specified

82491 ~~Chromatography, quantitative, column (eg, gas liquid or HPLC); single analyte not elsewhere specified, single stationary and mobile phase~~

82492 ~~multiple analytes, single stationary and mobile phase~~

82541 ~~Column chromatography/mass spectrometry (eg, GC/MS, or HPLC/MS), non-drug analyte not elsewhere specified; qualitative, single stationary and mobile phase~~

▲ 82542 Column chromatography/, includes mass spectrometry, if performed (eg, HPLC, LC, LC/MS, LC/MS-MS, GC, GC/MS-MS, orGC/MS, HPLC/MS), non-drug analyte(s) not elsewhere specified, qualitative or quantitative, each specimen; quantitative, single stationary and mobile phase

82543 ~~stable isotope dilution, single analyte, quantitative, single stationary and mobile phase~~

82544 ~~stable isotope dilution, multiple analytes, quantitative, single stationary and mobile phase~~

83788 ~~Mass spectrometry and tandem mass spectrometry (MS, MS/MS), analyte not elsewhere specified; qualitative, each specimen~~

▲ 83789 Mass spectrometry and tandem mass spectrometry (eg, MS, MS/MS, MALDI, MS-TOF, QTOF), non-drug analyte(s) not elsewhere specified, qualitative or quantitative, each specimen; quantitative, each specimen

▲ 86708 Hepatitis A antibody (HAAb); total

▲ 86709 Hepatitis A antibody (HAAb), IgM antibody; IgM antibody

▲ 87301 Infectious agent antigen detection by immunoassay technique, (eg, enzyme immunoassay technique[EIA], enzyme-linked immunosorbent assay [ELISA], immunochemiluminometric assay [IMCA]) qualitative or semiquantitative, multiple-step method; adenovirus enteric types 40/41

▲ 87305 Aspergillus

▲ 87320 Chlamydia trachomatis

▲ 87324 Clostridium difficile toxin(s)

▲ 87327 Cryptococcus neoformans

▲ 87328 cryptosporidium

▲ 87329 giardia

▲ 87332 cytomegalovirus

▲ 87335 Escherichia coli 0157

▲ 87336 Entamoeba histolytica dispar group

▲ 87337 Entamoeba histolytica group

▲ 87338 Helicobacter pylori, stool

▲ 87339 Helicobacter pylori

▲ 87340 hepatitis B surface antigen (HBsAg)

▲ 87341 hepatitis B surface antigen (HBsAg) neutralization

▲ 87350 hepatitis Be antigen (HBeAg)

▲ 87380 hepatitis, delta agent

▲ 87385 Histoplasma capsulatum

▲ 87389 HIV-1 antigen(s), with HIV-1 and HIV-2 antibodies, single result

▲ 87390 HIV-1

▲ 87391 HIV-2

▲ 87400 Influenza, A or B, each

▲ 87420 respiratory syncytial virus

▲ 87425 rotavirus

▲ 87427 Shiga-like toxin

▲ 87430 Streptococcus, group A

▲ 87449 Infectious agent antigen detection by immunoassay technique, (eg, enzyme immunoassay technique[EIA, enzyme-linked immunosorbent assay [ELISA], immunochemiluminometric assay [IMCA]), qualitative or semiquantitative; multiple-step method, not otherwise specified, each organism

▲ 87450 single step method, not otherwise specified, each organism

▲ 87451 multiple step method, polyvalent for multiple organisms, each polyvalent antiserum

▲ 87502 influenza virus, for multiple types or sub-types, includes multiplex reverse transcription, when performed, and multiplex amplified probe technique, first 2 types or sub-types

+▲ 87503 influenza virus, for multiple types or sub-types, includes multiplex reverse transcription, when performed, and multiplex amplified probe technique, each additional influenza virus type or sub-type beyond 2 (List separately in addition to code for primary procedure)

▲ 88346 Immunofluorescent studyImmunofluorescence, each antibodyper specimen; direct methodinitial single antibody stain procedure

88347 ~~indirect method~~

#+● 88350 Code added

Medicine

▲ 90632 Hepatitis A vaccine (HepA), adult dosage, for intramuscular use

▲ 90633 Hepatitis A vaccine (HepA), pediatric/adolescent dosage-2 dose schedule, for intramuscular use

▲ 90634 Hepatitis A vaccine (HepA), pediatric/adolescent dosage-3 dose schedule, for intramuscular use

90645 ~~Hemophilus influenza b vaccine (Hib), HbOC conjugate (4 dose schedule), for intramuscular use~~

90646 ~~Hemophilus influenza b vaccine (Hib), PRP-D conjugate, for booster use only, intramuscular use~~

▲ 90647 Hemophilus influenzaHaemophilus influenzae type b vaccine (Hib), PRP-OMP conjugate (, 3 dose schedule), for intramuscular use

▲ 90648 Hemophilus influenzaHaemophilus influenzae type b vaccine (Hib), PRP-T conjugate (, 4 dose schedule), for intramuscular use

▲ 90649 Human Papilloma virus (HPV)Papillomavirus vaccine, types 6, 11, 16, 18 (quadrivalent), quadrivalent (4vHPV), 3 dose schedule, for intramuscular use

▲ 90650 Human Papilloma virus (HPV)Papillomavirus vaccine, types 16, 18, bivalent (2vHPV), 3 dose schedule, for intramuscular use

▲ 90651 Human Papillomavirus vaccine types 6, 11, 16, 18, 31, 33, 45, 52, 58, nonavalent (HPV)(9vHPV), 3 dose schedule, for intramuscular use

✗ ▲ 90653 Influenza vaccine, inactivated (IIV), subunit, adjuvanted, for intramuscular use

▲ 90655 Influenza virus vaccine, trivalent (IIV3), split virus, preservative free, when administered to children 6-35 months of age, for intramuscular use

▲ 90656 Influenza virus vaccine, trivalent (IIV3), split virus, preservative free, when administered to individuals 3 years and older, for intramuscular use

▲ 90657 Influenza virus vaccine, trivalent (IIV3), split virus, when administered to children 6-35 months of age, for intramuscular use

▲ 90658   Influenza virus vaccine, trivalent (IIV3), split virus, when administered to individuals 3 years of age and older, for intramuscular use

▲ 90660   Influenza virus vaccine, trivalent, live (LAIV3), for intranasal use

#▲ 90672   Influenza virus vaccine, quadrivalent, live (LAIV4), for intranasal use

▲ 90661   Influenza virus vaccine (ccIIV3), derived from cell cultures, subunit, preservative and antibiotic free, for intramuscular use

#▲ 90673   Influenza virus vaccine, trivalent (RIV3), derived from recombinant DNA, hemagglutinin (HA) protein only, preservative and antibiotic free, for intramuscular use

▲ 90662   Influenza virus vaccine (IIV), split virus, preservative free, enhanced immunogenicity via increased antigen content, for intramuscular use

▲ 90664   Influenza virus vaccine, live (LAIV), pandemic formulation, live, for intranasal use

✎▲ 90666   Influenza virus vaccine (IIV), pandemic formulation, split virus, preservative free, for intramuscular use

✎▲ 90667   Influenza virus vaccine (IIV), pandemic formulation, split virus, adjuvanted, for intramuscular use

✎▲ 90668   Influenza virus vaccine (IIV), pandemic formulation, split virus, for intramuscular use

90669   ~~Pneumococcal conjugate vaccine, 7 valent (PCV7), for intramuscular use~~

▲ 90670   Pneumococcal conjugate vaccine, 13 valent (PCV13), for intramuscular use

▲ 90680   Rotavirus vaccine, pentavalent (RV5), 3 dose schedule, live, for oral use

▲ 90681   Rotavirus vaccine, human, attenuated (RV1), 2 dose schedule, live, for oral use

▲ 90685   Influenza virus vaccine, quadrivalent (IIV4), split virus, preservative free, when administered to children 6-35 months of age, for intramuscular use

▲ 90686   Influenza virus vaccine, quadrivalent (IIV4), split virus, preservative free, when administered to individuals 3 years of age and older, for intramuscular use

▲ 90687   Influenza virus vaccine, quadrivalent (IIV4), split virus, when administered to children 6-35 months of age, for intramuscular use;

▲ 90688   Influenza virus vaccine, quadrivalent (IIV4), split virus, when administered to individuals 3 years of age and older, for intramuscular use

90692   ~~Typhoid vaccine, heat- and phenol-inactivated (H-P), for subcutaneous or intradermal use~~

90693   ~~Typhoid vaccine, acetone-killed, dried (AKD), for subcutaneous use (U.S. military)~~

▲ 90696   Diphtheria, tetanus toxoids, acellular pertussis vaccine and inactivated poliovirus vaccine, inactivated (DTaP-IPV), when administered to children 4 through 6 years of age, for intramuscular use

✎● 90697   Code added

▲ 90698   Diphtheria, tetanus toxoids, acellular pertussis vaccine, hHaemophilus influenza Type Binfluenzae type b, and inactivated poliovirus vaccine (DTap-IPV/Hib), for intramuscular use

▲ 90702   Diphtheria and tetanus toxoids adsorbed (DT) adsorbed when administered to individuals younger than 7 years, for intramuscular use

90703   ~~Tetanus toxoid adsorbed, for intramuscular use~~

90704   ~~Mumps virus vaccine, live, for subcutaneous use~~

90705   ~~Measles virus vaccine, live, for subcutaneous use~~

90706   ~~Rubella virus vaccine, live, for subcutaneous use~~

90708   ~~Measles and rubella virus vaccine, live, for subcutaneous use~~

90712   ~~Poliovirus vaccine, (any type[s]) (OPV), live, for oral use~~

▲ 90714   Tetanus and diphtheria toxoids adsorbed (Td) adsorbed, preservative free, when administered to individuals 7 years or older, for intramuscular use

▲ 90716   Varicella virus vaccine (VAR), live, for subcutaneous use

90719   ~~Diphtheria toxoid, for intramuscular use~~

90720   ~~Diphtheria, tetanus toxoids, and whole cell pertussis vaccine and Haemophilus influenzae b vaccine (DTwP-Hib), for intramuscular use~~

90721   ~~Diphtheria, tetanus toxoids, and acellular pertussis vaccine and Haemophilus influenzae b vaccine (DTaP/Hib), for intramuscular use~~

90725   ~~Cholera vaccine for injectable use~~

#✎● 90625   Code added

90727   ~~Plague vaccine, for intramuscular use~~

▲ 90732   Pneumococcal polysaccharide vaccine, 23-valent (PPSV23), adult or immunosuppressed patient dosage, when administered to individuals 2 years or older, for subcutaneous or intramuscular use

#▲ 90644   Meningococcal conjugate vaccine, serogroups C & Y and Hemophilus influenza BHaemophilus influenzae type b vaccine (Hib-MenCY), 4 dose schedule, when administered to children 2-1518 months of age, for intramuscular use

▲ 90733   Meningococcal polysaccharide vaccine (any group[s]), serogroups A, C, Y, W-135, quadrivalent (MPSV4), for subcutaneous use

▲ 90734   Meningococcal conjugate vaccine, serogroups A, C, Y and W-135, quadrivalent (MenACWY), for intramuscular use

#● 90620   Code added

#● 90621   Code added

90735   ~~Japanese encephalitis virus vaccine, for subcutaneous use~~

▲ 90736   Zoster (shingles) vaccine (HZV), live, for subcutaneous injection

✎▲ 90739   Hepatitis B vaccine (HepB), adult dosage, 2 dose schedule, for intramuscular use

▲ 90740   Hepatitis B vaccine (HepB), dialysis or immunosuppressed patient dosage (, 3 dose schedule), for intramuscular use

▲ 90743   Hepatitis B vaccine (HepB), adolescent (, 2 dose schedule), for intramuscular use

▲ 90744   Hepatitis B vaccine (HepB), pediatric/adolescent dosage (, 3 dose schedule), for intramuscular use

▲ 90746   Hepatitis B vaccine (HepB), adult dosage (, 3 dose schedule), for intramuscular use

▲ 90747   Hepatitis B vaccine (HepB), dialysis or immunosuppressed patient dosage (, 4 dose schedule), for intramuscular use

▲ 90748   Hepatitis B and Hemophilus influenzaHaemophilus influenzae type b vaccine (HepB-Hib)(Hib-HepB), for intramuscular use

▲ 91040   Esophageal balloon distension study, diagnostic, with provocation studywhen performed

● 92537   Code added

● 92538   Code added

92543   ~~Caloric vestibular test, each irrigation (binaural, bithermal stimulation constitutes 4 tests), with recording~~

● 93050   Code added

▲ 94640   Pressurized or nonpressurized inhalation treatment for acute airway obstruction ~~or for sputum induction~~therapeutic purposes and/or for diagnostic purposes ~~(eg,~~such as sputum induction with an aerosol generator, nebulizer, metered dose inhaler or intermittent positive pressure breathing ~~(IPPB)~~(IPPB) device)

▲ 95972   complex spinal cord, or peripheral (ie, peripheral nerve, sacral nerve, neuromuscular) (except cranial nerve) neurostimulator pulse generator/transmitter, with intraoperative or subsequent programming~~, up to 1 hour~~

95973   ~~complex spinal cord, or peripheral (ie, peripheral nerve, sacral nerve, neuromuscular) (except cranial nerve) neurostimulator pulse generator/transmitter, with intraoperative or subsequent programming, each additional 30 minutes after first hour (List separately in addition to code for primary procedure)~~

● 96931   Code added

● 96932   Code added

● 96933   Code added

+● 96934   Code added

+● 96935   Code added

+● 96936   Code added

▲ 99174   Instrument-based ocular screening (eg, photoscreening, automated-refraction), bilateral; with remote analysis and report

#● 99177   Code added

Category II Codes

▲ 6030F   All elements of maximal sterile barrier technique, ~~followed including:~~ cap **and** mask **and** ~~sterile gown **and** sterile gloves **and**~~ a large sterile sheet **and** hand hygiene, skin preparation and, if ultrasound is used, sterile ultrasound techniques followed **and** 2% chlorhexidine for cutaneous antisepsis (or acceptable alternative antiseptics, per current guideline) (CRIT)[1]

Category III Codes

~~0099T~~   ~~Implantation of intrastromal corneal ring segments~~

~~0103T~~   ~~Holotranscobalamin, quantitative~~

~~0123T~~   ~~Fistulization of sclera for glaucoma, through ciliary body~~

~~0182T~~   ~~High dose rate electronic brachytherapy, per fraction~~

~~0223T~~   ~~Acoustic cardiography, including automated analysis of combined acoustic and electrical intervals; single, with interpretation and report~~

~~0224T~~   ~~multiple, including serial trended analysis and limited reprogramming of device parameter, AV or VV delays only, with interpretation and report~~

~~0225T~~   ~~multiple, including serial trended analysis and limited reprogramming of device parameter, AV and VV delays, with interpretation and report~~

~~0233T~~   ~~Skin advanced glycation endproducts (AGE) measurement by multi-wavelength fluorescent spectroscopy~~

~~0240T~~   ~~Esophageal motility (manometric study of the esophagus and/or gastroesophageal junction) study with interpretation and report; with high resolution esophageal pressure topography~~

~~0241T~~   ~~with stimulation or perfusion during high resolution esophageal pressure topography study (eg, stimulant, acid or alkali perfusion) (List separately in addition to code for primary procedure)~~

~~0243T~~   ~~Intermittent measurement of wheeze rate for bronchodilator or bronchial-challenge diagnostic evaluation(s), with interpretation and report~~

~~0244T~~   ~~Continuous measurement of wheeze rate during treatment assessment or during sleep for documentation of nocturnal wheeze and cough for diagnostic evaluation 3 to 24 hours, with interpretation and report~~

~~0262T~~   ~~Implantation of catheter-delivered prosthetic pulmonary valve, endovascular approach~~

⊙▲ 0308T   Insertion of ocular telescope prosthesis including removal of crystalline lens or intraocular lens prosthesis

~~0311T~~   ~~Non-invasive calculation and analysis of central arterial pressure waveforms with interpretation and report~~

▲ 0358T   Bioelectrical impedance analysis whole body composition assessment~~, supine position~~, with interpretation and report

● 0381T   Code added

● 0382T   Code added

● 0383T   Code added

● 0384T   Code added

● 0385T   Code added

● 0386T   Code added

● 0387T   Code added

● 0388T   Code added

● 0389T   Code added

● 0390T   Code added

● 0391T   Code added

● 0392T   Code added

● 0393T   Code added

● 0394T   Code added

● 0395T   Code added

+● 0396T   Code added

⊙+● 0397T   Code added

● 0398T   Code added

+● 0399T   Code added

● 0400T   Code added

● 0401T   Code added

● 0402T   Code added

● 0403T   Code added

● 0404T   Code added

● 0405T   Code added

● 0406T   Code added

● 0407T   Code added

Appendix C

Clinical Examples

As described in the CPT 2016 code set, clinical examples of the CPT codes for Evaluation and Management (E/M) services are intended to be an important element of the coding system. The clinical examples, when used with the E/M descriptors contained in the full text of the CPT code set, provide a useful tool and guidance for individuals to report the services provided to their patients. Clinical examples of the codes for E/M services are provided to assist physicians in understanding the meaning of the descriptors and selecting the correct code. Each example was developed by physicians in the specialties shown.

The same problem, when seen by physicians in different specialties, may involve different amounts of work. Therefore, the appropriate level of encounter should be reported using the descriptors rather than the examples.

The American Medical Association is pleased to provide you with these clinical examples for the CPT 2016 code set. The clinical examples that are provided in this supplement are limited to Office or Other Outpatient Services, Hospital Inpatient Services, Consultations, Critical Care, Prolonged Services, and Care Plan Oversight.

These clinical examples are used to describe presenting problems that are frequently encountered in a given specialty. Typical patients with such problems may commonly require the listed Evaluation and Management (E/M) service. Therefore, these examples are **not** appropriately used for any review of correct coding or estimating physician or qualified health care professional work. These clinical examples do not encompass the entire scope of medical practice. Inclusion or exclusion of any particular specialty group does not infer any judgment of importance or lack thereof; nor does it limit the applicability of the example to any particular specialty. We present these examples to provide additional educational context when used in conjunction with the E/M descriptors and guidelines.

Of utmost importance is that these clinical examples are just that: examples. A particular patient encounter, depending on the specific circumstances, must be judged by the services provided by the physician or other qualified health care professional for that particular patient. Simply because the patient's complaints, symptoms, or diagnoses match those of a particular clinical example does not automatically assign that patient encounter to that particular level of service. Moreover, simply because the patient's complaints, symptoms, or diagnoses **do not** match those of a particular clinical example does not automatically **exclude** that patient encounter from a particular level of service. The three components (history, examination, and medical decision making) must be met, consistent with the Nature of Presenting Problem, and documented in the medical record to report a particular level of service.

Office or Other Outpatient Service

New Patient

99201   Initial office visit for a 50-year-old male from out-of-town who needs a prescription refill for a nonsteroidal anti-inflammatory drug. (Anesthesiology)

Initial office visit for a 40-year-old female, new patient, requesting information about local pain clinics. (Anesthesiology/Pain Medicine)

Initial office visit for a 10-year-old female for determination of visual acuity as part of a summer camp physical (does not include determination of refractive error). (Ophthalmology)

Initial office visit for an out-of-town patient requiring topical refill. (Dermatology/Podiatry Surgery)

Initial office visit for a 65-year-old male for reassurance about an isolated seborrheic keratosis on upper back. (Dermatology)

Initial office visit for an out-of-state visitor who needs refill of topical steroid to treat lichen planus. (Dermatology)

Initial office visit for an 86-year-old male, out-of-town visitor, who needs prescription refilled for an anal skin preparation that he forgot. (Colon & Rectal Surgery)

Initial office visit for a patient following surgery in another OMS practice. Timing and symptoms suggest diagnosis of alveolar osteitis for which packing will be indicated. (Oral & Maxillofacial Surgery)

Initial office visit for a patient with a pedunculated lesion of the neck which is unsightly. (Dermatology)

Initial office visit for a 10-year-old male, for limited subungual hematoma not requiring drainage. (Podiatry Surgery)

Initial office visit with a 9-month-old female with diaper rash. (Pediatrics)

Initial office visit with a 5-year-old female to remove sutures from simple wound placed by another physician. (Dermatology)

Initial office visit for a patient with a small area of sunburn requiring first aid. (Dermatology)

Initial office visit for the evaluation and management of a contusion of a finger. (Orthopaedic Surgery)

Initial office visit for a 22-year-old male with a small area of sunburn requiring first aid. (Family Medicine/Internal Medicine)

Initial office visit for a 25-year-old female, presents with complaints of skin tags on her neck. (Plastic Surgery)

Initial office visit for an 86-year-old male with a 2 cm lipoma on back that he is concerned is infected. (General Surgery)

Initial office visit with a 5-year-old female who had absorbable sutures, in for a wound check with no complications. (Plastic Surgery)

Initial office visit for an 85-year-old patient with a history of cigarette smoking now with an asymmetrical neck mass, referred by primary care physician for fine-needle aspiration. (Pathology)

Initial office visit for a 25-year-old patient with brief history of cigarette smoking now with a symmetrical neck enlargement, referred by primary care physician for fine-needle aspiration. (Pathology)

Initial office visit for a 55-year-old male, out-of-town visitor, with treated sleep apnea who requests a prescription for a replacement CPAP interface. (Sleep Medicine)

99202 Initial office visit for a 13-year-old patient with comedopapular acne of the face unresponsive to over-the-counter medications. (Family Medicine)

Initial office visit for a patient with a clinically benign lesion or nodule of the lower leg that has been present for many years. (Dermatology)

Initial office visit for a patient with a circumscribed patch of dermatitis of the leg. (Dermatology)

Initial office visit for a patient with papulosquamous eruption of elbows. (Dermatology)

Initial office visit for a 9-year-old patient with erythematous grouped, vesicular eruption of the lip of three days' duration. (Pediatrics)

Initial office visit for an 18-year-old male referred by an orthodontist for advice regarding removal of four wisdom teeth. (Oral & Maxillofacial Surgery)

Initial office visit for a 14-year-old male, who was referred by his orthodontist, for advice on the exposure of impacted maxillary cuspids. (Oral & Maxillofacial Surgery)

Initial office visit for a patient presenting with itching patches on the wrists and ankles. (Dermatology)

Initial office visit for a 30-year-old male with a two-week-old burn of the hand, now healed but patient concerned with redness and swelling. (Plastic Surgery)

Initial evaluation and management of recurrent urinary infection in female. (Internal Medicine)

Initial office visit with a 10-year-old female with history of chronic otitis media and a draining ear. (Pediatrics)

Initial office visit for a 10-year-old female with acute maxillary sinusitis. (Family Medicine)

Initial office visit for a patient with papulopustular and comedonal acne. (Dermatology)

Initial office visit for a patient with recurring episodes of herpes simplex who has developed a clustering of vesicles on the upper lip. (Internal Medicine)

Initial office visit with a 10-year-old male with severe rash and itching for the past 24 hours, positive history for contact with poison oak 48 hours prior to the visit. (Family Medicine)

Initial office visit for a 65-year-old female with low hemoglobin level, no evidence of clinical bleeding, who was referred by her internist for possible bone marrow aspiration. (Pathology)

Initial office visit for a 55-year-old patient with a history of cigarette smoking now with an asymmetrical neck mass, referred by primary care physician for fine-needle aspiration. (Pathology)

Initial office visit for a 45-year-old male with known sleep apnea and an inability to tolerate CPAP due to dry mouth. (Sleep Medicine)

Initial office visit for an 18-year-old male with cellulitis around a superficial puncture wound of the skin. (General Surgery)

Initial office visit for a 61-year-old male with a macerated, itching rash between the toes that has been present for three weeks. (Podiatry Surgery)

Initial office visit for a healthy 16-year-old male with an ingrown nail with paronychia. (Podiatry Surgery)

99203 Initial office visit of a 76-year-old male with a stasis ulcer of three months' duration. (Dermatology)

Initial office visit for a 30-year-old female with pain in the lateral aspect of the forearm. (Physical Medicine & Rehabilitation)

Initial office visit for a patient with cystic acne of the face, chest, and back. Discussion of use of systemic medication. (Dermatology)

Initial office visit for a patient with a patchy, scaly erythematous eruption of the extremities. (Dermatology)

Initial office visit for a 57-year-old female who complains of painful parotid swelling of one week's duration. (Oral & Maxillofacial Surgery)

Initial office visit for a diffusely photodamaged patient with multiple crusted lesions. (Dermatology)

Initial office visit for a patient with dermatitis of the antecubital and popliteal fossae. (Dermatology)

Initial office visit for a 22-year-old female with irregular menses. (Family Medicine)

Initial office visit for a 50-year-old female with dyspepsia and nausea. (Family Medicine)

Initial office visit for a 53-year-old laborer with degenerative joint disease of the knee with no prior treatment. (Orthopaedic Surgery)

Initial office visit for a 60-year-old male with Dupuytren's contracture of one hand with multiple digit involvement. (Orthopaedic Surgery)

Initial office visit for a 33-year-old male with painless gross hematuria without cystoscopy. (Internal Medicine)

Initial office visit for a 55-year-old female with chronic blepharitis. There is a history of use of many medications. (Ophthalmology)

Initial office visit for an 18-year-old female with a two-day history of acute conjunctivitis. Extensive history of possible exposures, prior normal ocular history, and medication use is obtained. (Ophthalmology)

Initial office visit for a 14-year-old male with unilateral anterior knee pain. (Physical Medicine & Rehabilitation)

Initial office visit of an adult who presents with symtoms of an upper-respiratory infection that has progressed to unilateral purulent nasal discharge and discomfort in the right maxillary teeth. (Otolaryngology/Head & Neck Surgery)

Initial office visit of a 65-year-old with long-standing nasal stuffiness on multiple medications and continuous positive airway pressure (CPAP) for obstructive sleep apnea syndrome (OSAS). (Otolaryngology/Head & Neck Surgery)

Initial office visit for a 35-year-old female with postprandial right upper quadrant abdominal pain. (General Surgery)

Initial office visit with couple for counseling concerning voluntary vasectomy for sterility. Spent 30 minutes discussing procedure, risks and benefits, and answering questions. (Urology)

Initial office visit for evaluation, diagnosis, and management of painless gross hematuria in a new patient, without cystoscopy. (Internal Medicine)

Initial office visit for evaluation of a 13-year-old female with progressive scoliosis. (Physical Medicine & Rehabilitation)

Initial office visit for a 21-year-old female desiring counseling and evaluation of initiation of contraception. (Family Practice/Internal Medicine/Obstetrics & Gynecology)

Initial office visit for a 49-year-old male presenting with painless blood per rectum associated with bowel movement. (Colon & Rectal Surgery)

Initial office visit for a 19-year-old football player with three-day-old acute knee injury; now with swelling and pain. (Orthopaedic Surgery)

Initial office visit of a 49-year-old male with nasal obstruction. Detailed exam with topical anesthesia. (Plastic Surgery)

Initial office evaluation for gradual symmetric hearing loss, without other otologic symptoms or history, 58-year-old male, history and physical examination, with interpretation of complete audiogram, air bone, etc. (Otolaryngology)

25-year-old male with back pain of six weeks' duration. (Neurology)

Initial office visit for a 61-year-old female whose husband reports loud disruptive snoring that interferes with his sleep. (Sleep Medicine)

Initial office evaluation of a 58-year-old male, gradual symmetric hearing loss, without other otologic symptoms or history. (Otolaryngology)

Initial office visit for a 45-year-old hypertensive female with a two-month history of plantar heel pain. (Podiatry Surgery)

Initial office visit for a 12-year-old male athlete with retrocalcaneal pain and swelling with no prior treatment. (Podiatry Surgery)

99204 Initial office visit for a 13-year-old female with progressive scoliosis. (Orthopaedic Surgery)

Initial office visit for a 34-year-old female with primary infertility for evaluation and counseling. (Obstetrics & Gynecology)

Initial office visit for a patient with a personal history of multiple non-melanoma skin cancers who presents with a rapidly enlarging 2 cm nodule located on the left temple along with associated tingling in the area and fullness of the subcutaneous tissue in the left prearuricular region. (Dermatology)

Initial office visit for an adolescent who was referred by school counselor because of repeated skipping school and declining grades. (Psychiatry)

Initial office visit for a 50-year-old machinist with a generalized eruption. (Dermatology)

Initial office visit for a 45-year-old female who has been abstinent from alcohol and benzodiazepines for three months but complains of headaches, insomnia, and anxiety. (Psychiatry)

Initial office visit for a 60-year-old male with recent change in bowel habits, weight loss, and abdominal pain. (Abdominal Surgery/Colon & Rectal Surgery)

Initial office visit for a 50-year-old male with an aortic aneurysm who is considering surgery. (General Surgery)

Initial office visit for a 17-year-old female with depression. (Internal Medicine)

Initial office visit of a 40-year-old with chronic draining ear, progressive hearing loss and imbalance, with findings consistent with chronic otitis media and cholesteatoma. (Otolaryngology/Head & Neck Surgery)

Initial office visit for initial evaluation of a 63-year-old male with chest pain on exertion. (Cardiology/Internal Medicine)

Initial office visit for evaluation of a 70-year-old patient with recent onset of episodic confusion. (Internal Medicine)

Initial office visit for a 7-year-old female with juvenile diabetes mellitus, new to area, past history of hospitalization times three. (Pediatrics)

Initial office visit of a 50-year-old female with progressive solid food dysphagia. (Gastroenterology)

Initial office visit for a 34-year-old patient with primary infertility, including counseling. (Obstetrics & Gynecology)

Initial office visit for evaluation of a 70-year-old female with polyarthralgia. (Rheumatology)

Initial office visit for a patient with papulosquamous eruption involving 60 percent of the cutaneous surface with joint pain. Combinations of topical and systemic treatments discussed. (Dermatology)

Initial office visit of a 40-year-old female with symptoms of atopic allergies including eye and sinus congestion, often associated with infections. She would like to be tested for allergies. (Otolaryngology/Head & Neck Surgery)

An 8-year-old healthy male with attention problems in school. (Neurology)

Initial office visit for a 67-year-old male with nocturnal choking, witnessed apneas, and excessive daytime sleepiness. (Sleep Medicine)

Initial office visit for a 42-year-old female with Charcot-Marie-Tooth disease, pes cavus, and worsening painful hammer toes. (Podiatry Surgery)

Initial office visit for a 55-year-old-male with progressive rheumatoid arthritis and deformity of the ankle secondary to previous injury. (Podiatry Surgery)

99205 Initial office visit for a patient with disseminated lupus erythematosus with kidney disease, edema, purpura, and scarring lesions on the extremities plus cardiac symptoms. (Dermatology/Internal Medicine)

Initial office visit for a 25-year-old female with systemic lupus erythematosus, fever, seizures, and profound thrombocytopenia. (Rheumatology)

Initial office visit for an adult with multiple cutaneous blisters, denuded secondarily infected ulcerations, oral lesions, weight loss, and increasing weakness refractory to high dose corticosteroid. Initiation of new immunosuppressive therapy. (Dermatology)

Initial office visit for a 28-year-old male with systemic vasculitis and compromised circulation to the limbs. (Rheumatology)

Initial office visit for a 41-year-old female new to the area requesting rheumatologic care, on disability due to scleroderma and recent hospitalization for malignant hypertension. (Rheumatology)

Initial office visit for a 52-year-old female with acute four extemity weakness and shortness of breath one week post-flu vaccination. (Physical Medicine & Rehabilitation)

Initial office visit for a 60-year-old male with previous back surgery; now presents with back and pelvic pain, two-month history of bilateral progressive calf and thigh tightness and weakness when walking, causing several falls. (Orthopaedic Surgery)

Initial office visit for an adolescent referred from emergency department after taking a near-lethal overdose that required hospitalization. (Psychiatry)

Initial office visit for a 49-year-old female with a history of headaches and dependence on opioids. She reports weight loss, progressive headache, and depression. (Psychiatry)

Initial office visit for a 34-year-old uremic Type I diabetic patient referred for ESRD modality assessment and planning. (Nephrology)

Initial office visit for a 75-year-old female with neck and bilateral shoulder pain, brisk deep tendon reflexes, and stress incontinence. (Physical Medicine & Rehabilitation)

Initial office visit for an 8-year-old male with cerebral palsy and spastic quadriparesis. (Physical Medicine & Rehabilitation)

Initial office visit for a 73-year-old male with known prostate malignancy, who presents with severe back pain and a recent onset of lower extremity weakness. (Physical Medicine & Rehabilitation)

Initial office visit for a 38-year-old male with paranoid delusions and a history of alcohol abuse. (Psychiatry)

Initial office visit for a 12-week-old with bilateral hip dislocations and bilateral club feet. (Orthopaedic Surgery)

Initial office visit for a 29-year-old female with acute orbital congestion, eyelid retraction, and bilateral visual loss from optic neuropathy. (Ophthalmology)

Initial office visit for a 70-year-old diabetic patient with progressive visual field loss, advanced optic disc cupping, and neovascularization of retina. (Ophthalmology)

Initial office visit for a newly diagnosed Type I diabetic patient. (Endocrinology)

Initial office evaluation of a 65-year-old female with exertional chest pain, intermittent claudication, syncope, and a murmur of aortic stenosis. (Cardiology)

Initial office visit for a 73-year-old male with an unexplained 20 lb weight loss. (Hematology/Oncology)

Initial office evaluaton and management of patient with systemic vasculitis and compromised circulation to the limbs. (Rheumatology)

Initial office visit for a 24-year-old with risk factors for HIV infection who has a fever, cough, and shortness of breath. (Infectious Disease)

Initial outpatient evaluation of a 69-year-old male with severe chronic obstructive pulmonary disease, congestive heart failure, and hypertension. (Family Medicine)

Initial office visit for a 17-year-old female who is having school problems and has told a friend that she is considering suicide. She has recently cut herself. The patient and her family are consulted in regard to treatment options. (Psychiatry)

Initial office visit for a female with severe hirsutism, amenorrhea, weight loss, and a desire to have children. (Obstetrics & Gynecology)

Initial office visit for a 42-year-old male on hypertensive medication, newly arrived to the area, with diastolic blood pressure of 110, history of recurrent calculi, episodic headaches, intermittent chest pain, and orthopnea. (Internal Medicine)

Initial office visit for 70-year-old female with hypertension, diabetes, morbid obesity and recurrent incisional hernia that has become increasingly painful. (General Surgery)

57-year-old man with new-onset dementia. (Neurology)

Initial office visit for a 25-year-old female with a history of depression who presents with complaints of difficulty maintaining sleep, excessive daytime somnolence, and fatigue. She also complains of episodes of muscle weakness. (Sleep Medicine)

Initial office visit for a 75-year-old febrile female with an infected posterior heel ulceration penetrating to bone with comorbidities of diabetes and peripheral vascular disease. (Podiatry Surgery)

Initial office visit for a 36-year-old hypertensive laborer with inability to bear weight due to multiple metatarsal fractures and forefoot compartment syndrome stemming from a crush injury suffered two days prior. (Podiatry Surgery)

Initial office visit for a child with a long history of bipolar disorder, ADHD, anxiety, and school problems, relatively stable and recently moved from another state. (Psychiatry)

Initial office visit for 61-year-old male with depression and a history of diabetes mellitus, arthritis, hypertension, and coronary artery disease. (Psychiatry)

Initial office visit of a 40-year-old with chronic draining ear, progressive hearing loss, and imbalance, with findings consistent with chronic otitis media and cholesteatoma. (Head & Neck Surgery/Otolaryngology)

Established Patient

99211 Office visit for an 82-year-old female, established patient, for a monthly B12 injection with documented Vitamin B12 deficiency. (Geriatrics/Internal Medicine/Family Medicine)

Office visit for a 50-year-old male, established patient, for removal of uncomplicated facial sutures. (Plastic Surgery)

Office visit for an established patient who lost prescription for lichen planus. Returned for new copy. (Dermatology)

Office visit for an established patient undergoing orthodontics who complains of a wire and is irritating his/her cheek and asks you to check it. (Oral & Maxillofacial Surgery)

Office visit for a 50-year-old female, established patient, seen for her gold injection by the nurse. (Rheumatology)

Office visit for a 73-year-old female, established patient, with pernicious anemia for weekly B12 injection. (Gastroenterology)

Office visit for an established patient for dressing change on a skin biopsy. (Dermatology/Podiatry Surgery)

Office visit for a 19-year-old, established patient, three days postirrigation and drainage of an infected sebaceous cyst, for removal of packing. (Plastic Surgery)

Office visit of a 20-year-old female, established patient, who receives an allergy vaccine injection and is observed for a reaction by the nurse. (Otolaryngology/Head & Neck Surgery)

Office visit for a 45-year-old male, established patient, with chronic renal failure for the administration of erythropoietin. (Nephrology)

Office visit for an established patient, a Peace Corps enlistee, who requests documentation that third molars have been removed. (Oral & Maxillofacial Surgery)

Office visit for a 45-year-old female, established patient, three weeks post simple repair of scalp laceration, noted a retained suture in healed wound, removed by nurse. (Plastic Surgery)

Office visit for a 9-year-old, established patient, successfully treated for impetigo, requiring release to return to school. (Dermatology/Pediatrics)

Office visit for an established patient requesting a return-to-work certificate for resolving contact dermatitis. (Dermatology)

Office visit for an established patient who is performing glucose monitoring and wants to check accuracy of machine with lab blood glucose by technician who checks accuracy and function of patient machine. (Endocrinology)

Follow-up office visit for a 65-year-old female with a chronic indwelling percutaneous nephrostomy catheter seen for routine pericatheter skin care and dressing change. (Interventional Radiology)

Outpatient visit with 19-year-old male, established patient, for supervised drug screen. (Addiction Medicine)

Office visit with 12-year-old male, established patient, for cursory check of hematoma one day after venipuncture. (Internal Medicine)

Office visit with 31-year-old female, established patient, for return to work certificate. (Anesthesiology)

Office visit for 14-year-old, established patient, to re-dress an abrasion. (Orthopaedic Surgery)

Office visit for a 45-year-old female, established patient, for a blood pressure check. (Obstetrics & Gynecology)

Office visit for prescription refill for a 35-year-old female, established patient, with schizophrenia who is stable but has run out of neuroleptic and is scheduled to be seen in a week. (Psychiatry)

Office visit with a nurse for a 6-year-old asthmatic patient who brings his nebulizer to learn how to use it with the new medicine he was prescribed. (Allergy & Immunology)

Office visit for a 38-year-old male, established patient, for evaluation of resolving nasal erythema from use of CPAP interface. (Sleep Medicine)

Office visit for a 58-year-old male presenting for nursing examination of wound. Patient had incsion and drainage of abscess in ER. (General Surgery)

Office visit for a patient treated four months ago. He presents as scheduled for examination of final healing of an intraoral incision at a bone graft site. (Oral & Maxillofacial Surgery)

99212 Office visit for an 11-year-old, established patient, seen in follow-up for mild comedonal acne of the cheeks on topical desquamating agents. (Dermatology/Family Medicine/Pediatrics)

Office visit for a 10-year-old female, established patient, who has been swimming in a lake, now presents with a one-day history of left ear pain with purulent drainage. (Family Medicine)

Office visit for an established patient seen in follow-up of clearing patch of localized contact dermatitis. (Family Medicine/Dermatology)

Office visit for an established patient returning for evaluation of response to treatment of lichen planus on wrists and ankles. (Dermatology)

Office visit for an established patient with tinea pedis being treated with topical therapy. (Dermatology)

Office visit for an established patient with localized erythematous plaque of psoriasis with topical hydration. (Dermatology)

Office visit for a 23-year-old healthy female fully recovered from Bell's palsy, seen one week after onset and initial visit. (Neurology)

Office visit for an established patient with recurring episodes of herpes simplex who has developed a clustering of vesicles on the upper lip. (Oral & Maxillofacial Surgery)

Evaluation of a 50-year-old male, established patient, who has experienced a recurrence of knee pain after he discontinued NSAID. (Anesthesiology/Pain Medicine)

Office visit for an established patient with an irritated skin tag for reassurance. (Dermatology)

Office visit for a 33-year-old, established patient, for contusion and abrasion of lower extremity. (Orthopaedic Surgery)

Office visit for a 22-year-old male, established patient, one month after incision and drainage of sebacious cyst. (Plastic Surgery)

Office visit for a 21-year-old, established patient, who is seen in follow-up after antibiotic therapy for acute bacterial tonsillitis with resolution of symptoms. (Otolaryngology/Head & Neck Surgery)

Office visit, established patient, 6-year-old with sore throat and headache. (Family Medicine/Pediatrics)

Office evaluation for possible purulent bacterial conjunctivitis with one- to two-day history of redness and discharge, 16-year-old female, established patient. (Pediatrics/Internal Medicine/Family Medicine)

Office visit for a 65-year-old female, established patient, returns for three-week follow-up for resolving severe ankle sprain. (Orthopaedic Surgery)

Office visit, sore throat, fever, and fatigue in a 19-year-old college student, established patient. (Internal Medicine)

Office visit for 66-year-old male, with sebaceous cyst on shoulder. (General Surgery)

Office visit with a 36-year-old male, established patient, for follow-up on effectiveness of medicine management of oral candidiasis. (Oral & Maxillofacial Surgery)

Office visit for a 27-year-old female, established patient, with complaints of vaginal itching. (Obstetrics & Gynecology)

Office visit with a 36-year-old male, established patient, for follow-up on effectiveness of medicine management of oral candidiasis, with improvement in symptoms. (Oral & Maxillofacial Surgery)

Office visit for a 32-year-old patient who has allergic rhinitis that is controlled with intranasal steroids but now is having eye symptoms. (Allergy & Immunology)

Office visit for a 45-year-old asthmatic patient who is seen for renewal of inhaler prescription. She is noted to have wheezing on exam and the dose of medication is increased. (Allergy & Immunology)

Office visit for a 65-year-old, established patient, for CPAP compliance data review. (Sleep Medicine)

Office visit for 66-year-old male with sebaceous cyst on shoulder. (General Surgery)

Office visit for an established patient returning for evaluation of response to medication prescribed for plantar warts. (Podiatry Surgery)

Office visit for an established patient with tinea pedis being treated with topical therapy. (Dermatology/Podiatry Surgery)

Office visit for a 65-year-old female, established patient, returns for three-week follow-up for resolving severe ankle sprain. (Orthopaedic Surgery/Podiatry Surgery)

99213 Office visit for a child, established patient, with chronic secretory otitis media history and physical exam, with interpretation of audiogram. (Otolaryngology/Head & Neck Surgery)

Office visit, established patient, for evaluation and treatment of an acutely draining ear in a 5-year-old with tympanotomy tubes. (Otolaryngology/Head & Neck Surgery)

Office visit for an established patient with new lesions of lichen planus in spite of topical therapies. (Dermatology)

Office visit for a 13-year-old, established patient, with comedopapular acne of the face that has shown poor response to topical medication. Discussion of use of systemic medication. (Dermatology)

Office visit for a 62-year-old female, established patient, for follow-up for stable cirrhosis of the liver. (Internal Medicine/Family Medicine)

Office visit for an 80-year-old female, established patient, to evaluate medical management of osteoarthritis of the temporomandibular joint. (Rheumatology)

Office visit for a healthy 45-year-old female, established patient. Presents with suspicious lesion on the back. (Plastic Surgery)

Office visit for a 68-year-old female, established patient, with polymyalgia rheumatic, maintained on chronic low-dose corticosteroid, with no new complaints. (Rheumatology)

Office visit for a 3-year-old female, established patient, for earache and dyshidrosis of feet. (Pediatrics/Family Medicine)

Office visit for an established patient for 18-months post-operative follow-up of TMJ repair. (Oral & Maxillofacial Surgery)

Office visit for a 45-year-old male, established patient, being re-evaluated for recurrent acute prostatitis. (Urology)

Office visit for a 43-year-old male, established patient, with known reflex sympathetic dystrophy. (Anesthesiology)

Office visit for an established patient with an evenly pigmented superficial nodule of leg that is symptomatic. (Dermatology)

Office visit for an established patient with psoriasis involvement of the elbows, pitting of the nails, and itchy scalp. (Dermatology)

Office visit for a 27-year-old male, established patient, with deep follicular and perifollicular inflammation unable to tolerate systemic antibiotics due to GI upset, requires change of systemic medication. (Dermatology)

Office visit for a 60-year-old, established patient, with chronic essential hypertension on multiple drug regimen, for blood pressure check. (Family Medicine)

Office visit for a 20-year-old male, established patient, for removal of sutures in hand. (Family Medicine)

Office visit for a 58-year-old female, established patient, with unilateral painful bunion. (Orthopaedic Surgery)

Office visit for a 45-year-old female, established patient, with known osteoarthritis and painful swollen knees. (Rheumatology)

Office visit for a 25-year-old female, established patient, complaining of bleeding and heavy menses. (Obstetrics & Gynecology)

Office visit for a 55-year-old male, established patient, with hypertension managed by a beta blocker/thiazide regime; now experiencing mild fatigue. (Nephrology)

Office visit for a 65-year-old female, established patient, with primary glaucoma for interval determination of intraocular pressure and possible adjustment of medication. (Ophthalmology)

Office visit for a 56-year-old male, established patient, with stable exertional angina who complains of new onset of calf pain while walking. (Cardiology)

Office visit for a 63-year-old female, established patient, with rheumatoid arthritis on auranofin and ibuprofen, seen for routine follow-up visit. (Rheumatology)

Office visit for an established patient with Graves' disease, three months post I-131 therapy, who presents with lassitude and malaise. (Endocrinology)

Office visit for the quarterly follow-up of a 63-year-old male, established patient, with chronic myofascial pain syndrome, effectively managed by doxepin, who presents with new onset urinary hesitancy. (Pain Medicine)

Office visit for the biannual follow-up of an established patient with migraine variant having infrequent, intermittent, moderate to severe headaches with nausea and vomiting, which are sometimes effectively managed by ergotamine tartrate and an antiemetic, but occasionally requiring visits to an emergency department. (Pain Medicine)

Office visit for an established patient after discharge from a pain rehabilitation program to review and adjust medication dosage. (Pain Medicine)

Office visit with 55-year-old male, established patient, for management of hypertension, mild fatigue, on beta blocker/thiazide regimen. (Family Medicine/Internal Medicine)

Outpatient visit for a 35-year-old female who had plastic surgery in Mexico two weeks before, presents for wound evaluation and suture removal. (General Surgery)

Office visit for a 70-year-old diabetic hypertensive established patient with recent change in insulin requirement. (Internal Medicine/Nephrology)

Office visit with 80-year-old female, established patient, for follow-up osteoporosis, status-post compression fractures. (Rheumatology)

Office visit for an established patient with stable cirrhosis of the liver. (Gastroenterology)

Routine, follow-up office evaluation at a three-month interval for a 77-year-old female, established patient, with nodular small cleaved-cell lymphoma. (Hematology/Oncology)

Quarterly follow-up office visit for a 45-year-old male, established patient, with stable chronic asthma, on steroid and bronchodilator therapy. (Pulmonary Medicine)

Office visit for a 50-year-old female, established patient, with insulin-dependent diabetes mellitus and stable coronary artery disease, for monitoring. (Family Medicine/Internal Medicine)

Office visit for a patient followed for a diagnosis of allergic rhinitis who recently acquired a cat. Oral nasal medicines are no longer controlling symptoms. Head congestion and yellow drainage are constant. (Allergy & Immunology)

Office visit for a 60-year-old asthmatic who recently developed high blood pressure and is now on BP medicine is seen for worsening asthma and found to have reduced pulmonary function tests compared to last year. (Allergy & Immunology)

Office visit for a 40-year-old female with well-controlled migraine who desires to remain on the same medication. (Neurology)

Office visit for a 25-year-old male, established patient, for periodic follow-up of narcolepsy, stable on stimulant medication. (Sleep Medicine)

Office visit for an established patient with photodamage and a new onset of a bleeding papulonodule on the leg. (Dermatology)

Quarterly follow-up office visit for a 45-year-old male, established patient, with stable chronic asthma, on steroid and bronchodilator therapy. (Pulmonary Medicine)

Office visit for an established diabetic patient, reevaluation of a worsening plantar fasciitis requiring a change in therapy. (Podiatry Surgery)

Office visit for a 58-year-old female, established patient, with unilateral painful bunion. (Orthopaedic Surgery/Podiatry Surgery)

Office visit for a 9-year-old male, established patient, with ADHD. Mild symptoms and minimal medication side effects. (Psychiatry)

Office visit for a 27-year-old female, established patient, with stable depression and anxiety. Intermittent moderate stress. (Psychiatry)

Office visit for a 16-year-old female, established patient, with intermittent moderate depression. (Psychiatry)

99214 Office visit, established patient, presenting with a new onset of a generalized pruritic to painful eruption and mouth sores. (Dermatology)

Office visit for a 32-year-old female, established patient, with new onset right lower quadrant pain. (Family Medicine)

Office visit for reassessment and reassurance/counseling of a 40-year-old female, established patient, who is experiencing increased symptoms while on a pain management treatment program. (Pain Medicine)

Office visit for a 30-year-old, established patient, under management for intractable low back pain, who now presents with new onset right posterior thigh pain. (Pain Medicine)

Office visit for an established patient with frequent intermittent, moderate to severe headaches requiring beta blocker or tricyclic antidepressant prophylaxis, as well as four symptomatic treatments, but who is still experiencing headaches at a frequency of several times a month that are unresponsive to treatment. (Pain Medicine)

Office visit for an established patient with psoriasis with extensive involvement of scalp, trunk, palms, and soles with joint pain. Combinations of topical and systemic treatments discussed and instituted. (Dermatology)

Office visit for a 55-year-old male, established patient, with increasing night pain, limp, and progressive varus of both knees. (Orthopaedic Surgery)

Follow-up visit for a 15-year-old withdrawn patient with four-year history of papulocystic acne of the face, chest, and back with early scarring and poor response to past treatment. Discussion of use of systemic medication. (Dermatology)

Office visit for a 28-year-old male, established patient, with regional enteritis, diarrhea, and low-grade fever. (Internal Medicine)

Office visit for a 25-year-old female, established patient, following recent arthrogram and MR imaging for TMJ pain. (Oral & Maxillofacial Surgery)

Office visit for a 32-year-old female, established patient, with large obstructing stone in left mid-ureter, to discuss management options including urethroscopy with extraction or ESWL. (Urology)

Evaluation for a 28-year-old male, established patient, with new onset of low back pain. (Anesthesiology/Pain Medicine)

Office visit for a 28-year-old female, established patient, with right lower quadrant abdominal pain, fever, and anorexia. (Internal Medicine/Family Medicine)

Office visit for a 45-year-old male, established patient, four months follow-up of L4-5 diskectomy, with persistent incapacitating low back and leg pain. (Orthopaedic Surgery)

Outpatient visit for a 77-year-old male, established patient, with hypertension, presenting with a three-month history of episodic substernal chest pain on exertion. (Cardiology)

Office visit for a 25-year-old female, established patient, for evaluation of progressive saddle nose deformity of unknown etiology. (Plastic Surgery)

Office visit for a 65-year-old male, established patient, with BPH and severe bladder outlet obstruction, to discuss management options such as TURP. (Urology)

Office visit for an established patient with lichen planus and 60% of the cutaneous surface involved, not responsive to systemic steroids, as well as developing symptoms of progressive heartburn and paranoid ideation. (Dermatology)

Office visit for a 52-year-old male, established patient, with a 12-year history of bipolar disorder responding to lithium carbonate and brief psychotherapy. Psychotherapy and prescription provided. (Psychiatry)

Office visit for a 63-year-old female, established patient, with a history of familial polyposis, status post-colectomy with sphincter sparing procedure, who now presents with rectal bleeding and increase in stooling frequency. (General Surgery)

Office visit for a 68-year-old male, established patient, with the sudden onset of multiple flashes and floaters in the right eye due to a posterior vitreous detachment. (Ophthalmology)

Office visit for a 55-year-old female, established patient, on cyclosporin for treatment of resistant, small vessel vasculitis. (Rheumatology)

Follow-up office visit for a 55-year-old male, two months after iliac angioplasty with new onset of contralateral extremity claudication. (Interventional Radiology)

Office visit for a 68-year-old male, established patient, with stable angina, two months post myocardial infarction, who is not tolerating one of his medications. (Cardiology)

Weekly office visit for 5FU therapy for an ambulatory established patient with metastatic colon cancer and increasing shortness of breath. (Hematology/Oncology)

Office visit for a 65-year-old male with Parkinson disease, on medication with sleep disturbance after medication increase. (Neurology)

Office visit for a 32-year-old female with obesity and diabetes. presents with new onset right lower quadrant pain. (Urology/General Surgery/Internal Medicine/Family Medicine)

Office evaluation of 28-year-old, established patient, with regional enteritis, diarrhea, and low-grade fever. (Family Medicine/Internal Medicine)

Office visit with 50-year-old female, established patient, diabetic, blood sugar controlled by diet. She now complains of frequency of urination and weight loss, blood sugar of 320 and negative ketones on dipstick. (Internal Medicine)

Follow-up office visit for a 45-year-old, established patient, with rheumatoid arthritis on gold, methotrexate, or immunosuppressive therapy. (Rheumatology)

Office visit for a 60-year-old male, established patient, two years post-removal of intracranial meningioma, now with new headaches and visual disturbance. (Neurosurgery)

Office visit for a 68-year-old female, established patient, for routine review and follow-up of non-insulin dependent diabetes, obesity, hypertension, and congestive heart failure. Complains of vision difficulties and admits dietary noncompliance. Patient is counseled concerning diet and current medications adjusted. (Family Medicine)

Office visit for an established patient who presents with severe dysphagia, oynophagia, and trismus and is found on physical exam to have a peritonsilar abscess. (Otolaryngology/Head & Neck Surgery)

Office visit for a 65-year-old male with hypertension, BPH, and allergic rhinitis seen because he cannot sleep due to nasal congestion. He was told by his PCP not to use decongestant pills so he uses a nasal decongestant spray regularly to breathe. He has been using the spray daily for the past six months. (Allergy & Immunology)

Office visit for an asthmatic patient who has missed three days of work due to asthma exacerbation and is found to have acute maxillary sinusitis and nocturnal asthma requiring treatment of both the sinusitis and altering the medication regimen. (Allergy & Immunology)

Office visit for an established diabetic patient with peripheral vascular disease with a new noninfected deep plantar ulceration. (Podiatry Surgery)

Office visit for a 48-year-old male, established patient, with bipolar disorder, marital problems, chronic insomnia, and several medical conditions. Mild psychiatric symptoms and minimal medication side effects. (Psychiatry)

Office visit for 7-year-old female, established patient, with ADHD. The patient has been disruptive in school, resulting in daily phone calls to parents over the last two weeks. Low appetite from the medication has been improving. (Psychiatry)

Office visit for a 13-year-old male, established patient, with depression, anxiety, and anger outbursts. (Psychiatry)

Office visit for a 22-year-old female, established patient, with bipolar disorder and obesity. The patient wants to stop the medication because of resulting weight gain. (Psychiatry)

Office visit for a 70-year-old male, established patient, with stable depression and recent mild forgetfulness. (Psychiatry)

Quarterly follow-up office visit for a 45-year-old male, established patient, with chronic asthma, on steroid and bronchodilator therapy. (Pulmonary Medicine)

Office visit for a 70-year-old female, established patient with sleep apnea and diabetes, who continues to have difficulty staying awake during the day despite treatment. (Sleep Medicine)

99215 Office visit for an adult diabetic established patient with a past history of recurrent sinusitis who presents with a one-week history of double vision and CT scan consistent with periorbital abscess. (Otolaryngology/Head & Neck Surgery)

Office visit for an established patient with disseminated lupus erythematosus, extensive edema of extremities, kidney disease, and weakness requiring monitored course on azathioprene and corticosteroid and complicated by acute depression. (Internal Medicine/Rheumatology)

Office visit for a patient with history of metastatic melanoma presenting with clinical lymphadenopathy distant to the primary tumor and subcutaneous nodules requiring a detailed discussion of treatment alternatives. (Dermatology)

Office visit for an established male patient with dermatomyositis, accelerated weakness, recent onset of fever, diffuse skin rash, nasal speech, and dysphagia with burning retrosternal pain. (Dermatology)

Office visit for an established adolescent patient with history of bipolar disorder treated with lithium; seen on urgent basis at family's request because of severe depressive symptoms. (Psychiatry)

Office visit for an established patient having acute migraine with new onset neurological symptoms and whose headaches are unresponsive to previous attempts at management with a combination of preventive and abortive medication. (Pain Medicine)

Office visit for an established patient with exfoliative lichen planus with daily fever spikes, disorientation, and shortness of breath. (Dermatology)

Office visit for a 25-year-old, established patient, two years post-burn with bilateral ectropion, hypertrophic facial burn scars, near absence of left breast, and burn syndactyly of both hands. Discussion of treatment options following examination. (Plastic Surgery)

Office visit for a 36-year-old, established patient, three-month status post-transplant, with new onset of peripheral edema, increased blood pressure, and progressive fatigue. (Nephrology)

Office visit for a 27-year-old female, established patient, with bipolar disorder who was stable on lithium carbonate and monthly supportive psychotherapy but now has developed symptoms of hypomania. (Psychiatry)

Office visit for a 25-year-old male, established patient with a history of schizophrenia who has been seen bi-monthly but is complaining of auditory hallucinations. (Psychiatry)

Office visit for a 62-year-old male, established patient, three years postoperative abdominal perineal resection, now with a rising carcinoembryonic antigen, weight loss, and pelvic pain. (Abdominal Surgery)

Office visit for a 42-year-old male, established patient, nine months postoperative emergency vena cava shunt for variceal bleeding, now presents with complaints of one episode of "dark" bowel movement, weight gain, tightness in abdomen, whites of eyes seem yellow, and occasional drowsiness after eating hamburgers. (Abdominal Surgery)

Office visit for a 68-year-old male with biopsy-proven rectal carcinoma, for evaluation and discussion of treatment options. (General Surgery)

Office visit for a 60-year-old, established patient, with diabetic nephropathy with increasing edema and dyspnea. (Endocrinology)

Office visit with 30-year-old male, established patient for three-month history of fatigue, weight loss, intermittent fever, and presenting with diffuse adenopathy and splenomegaly. (Family Medicine)

Office visit for restaging of an established patient with new lymphadenopathy one year post-therapy for lymphoma. (Hematology/Oncology)

Office visit for evaluation of recent onset syncopal attacks in a 70-year-old female, established patient. (Internal Medicine)

Follow-up visit, 40-year-old female mother of three, established patient, with acute rheumatoid arthritis, anatomical Stage 3, ARA function Class 3 rheumatoid arthritis, and deteriorating function. (Rheumatology)

Follow-up office visit for a 65-year-old male with a fever of recent onset while on outpatient antibiotic therapy for endocarditis. (Infectious Disease)

Office visit for a healthy 16-year-old male who suffered a concussion a week ago, now fully recovered, needing an evaluation to return to playing football. (Neurology)

Office visit for a 70-year-old female, established patient, with diabetes mellitus and hypertension, presenting with a two-month history of increasing confusion, agitation, and short-term memory loss. (Family Medicine/Internal Medicine)

Office visit for a 28-year-old female, established patient, who is abstinent from previous cocaine dependence but reports progressive panic attacks and chest pains. (Psychiatry)

Office visit for a 10-year-old asthmatic who has been to the emergency room for severe persistent asthma and is on combination therapy and oral steroids but has not stopped wheezing or coughing at night. (Allergy & Immunology)

Office visit, established patient, female with systemic lupus erythematosus and renal disease requiring combination systemic immunosuppressive therapy presents with a new onset of peripheral edema, diffuse skin rash, weakness, and acute depression. (Dermatology)

Office visit for a 53-year-old female, established patient, with sleep apnea and new-onset heart failure, who presents with a recent weight gain as well as recurrence of symptoms of daytime sleepiness and frequent nocturnal awakenings. (Sleep Medicine)

Office visit for an established diabetic patient with a cellulitic deep plantar abscess and history of previous forefoot amputation on the contralateral side. (Podiatry Surgery)

Hospital Inpatient Services

Initial Hospital Care

New or Established Patient

99221   Initial hospital visit following admission for a 42-year-old male for observation following institution of IV antibiotics for a cellulitis of the forearm. (Plastic Surgery/Oral & Maxillofacial Surgery)

Initial hospital visit for a 40-year-old patient with a thrombosed synthetic arteriovenous conduit. (Nephrology)

Initial hospital visit for a healthy 24-year-old male with an acute onset of low back pain following a lifting injury. (Internal Medicine/Anesthesiology/Pain Medicine)

Initial hospital visit for a 69-year-old female with controlled hypertension, scheduled for surgery. (Internal Medicine/Cardiology)

Initial hospital visit for a 24-year-old healthy female with benign tumor of palate. (Oral & Maxillofacial Surgery)

Initial hospital visit for a 14-year-old female with infectious mononucleosis and dehydration. (Internal Medicine)

Initial hospital visit for a 62-year-old female with stable rheumatoid arthritis, admitted for total joint replacement. (Rheumatology)

Initial hospital visit for a 6-month-old infant admitted for observation for apnea after craniofacial CT scan with sedation. (Plastic Surgery)

Initial hospital visit for a 69-year-old female with controlled hypertension, scheduled for surgery. (Cardiology)

Hospital admission, examination, and initiation of treatment program for a 67-year-old male with uncomplicated pneumonia who requires IV antibiotic therapy. (Internal Medicine)

Hospital admission for a 12-year-old with a laceration of the upper eyelid involving the lid margin admitted prior to surgery for IV antibiotic therapy. (Ophthalmology)

Hospital admission for a 32-year-old female with severe flank pain, hematuria, and presumed diagnosis of ureteral calculus as determined by Emergency Department physician. (Urology)

Initial hospital visit for a patient with several large venous stasis ulcers not responding to outpatient therapy. (Dermatology)

Initial hospital visit for 21-year-old pregnant patient (nine-weeks gestation) with hyperemesis gravidarum. (Obstetrics & Gynecology)

Initial hospital visit for a 73-year-old female with acute pyelonephritis who is otherwise generally healthy. (Geriatrics)

Initial hospital visit for 62-year-old patient with cellulitis of the foot requiring bedrest and intravenous antibiotics. (Orthopaedic Surgery)

Initial hospital visit for a 55-year-old female admitted to the hospital with nausea and vomiting, has a benign exam and a nonspecific bowel gas pattern on X ray. (General Surgery)

99222   Hospital admission for an 18-month-old with 10% dehydration. (Pediatrics)

Initial hospital visit for a 65-year-old female with right upper quadrant pain, mild jaundice, and gallstones. (General Surgery/Abdominal Surgery/Colon & Rectal Surgery)

Initial hospital visit for airway management, due to a benign laryngeal mass. (Otolaryngology/Head & Neck Surgery)

Initial hospital visit for a 66-year-old female with an L-2 vertebral compression fracture with acute onset of paralytic ileus; seen in the office two days previously. (Orthopaedic Surgery)

Initial hospital visit and evaluation of a 15-year-old male admitted with peritonsillar abscess or cellulitis requiring intravenous antibiotic therapy. (Otolaryngology/Head & Neck Surgery)

Initial hospital visit for a 42-year-old male with vertebral compression fracture following a motor vehicle accident. (Orthopaedic Surgery)

Initial hospital evaluation of a patient with a diffuse erythematous maculopapular eruption of new onset. Patient has multiple medical problems requiring various medications. (Dermatology)

Initial hospital visit for a 3-year-old patient with high temperature, limp, and painful hip motion of 18 hours' duration. (Pediatrics/Orthopaedic Surgery)

Initial hospital visit for an 18-year-old male who has suppurative sialoadenitis and dehydration. (Oral & Maxillofacial Surgery)

Initial hospital visit for a 65-year-old female for acute onset of thrombotic cerebrovascular accident with contralateral paralysis and aphasia. (Neurology)

Initial hospital visit for a 50-year-old male chronic paraplegic patient with pain and spasm below the lesion. (Anesthesiology)

Partial hospital admission for an adolescent patient from chaotic blended family, transferred from inpatient setting, for continued treatment to maintain symptomatic control of hostility and depression. (Psychiatry)

Initial hospital visit for a 61-year-old male with history of previous myocardial infarction, who now complains of chest pain. (Internal Medicine)

Initial hospital visit of a 15-year-old on medications for a sore throat over the last two weeks. The sore throat has worsened and patient now has dysphagia. The exam shows large necrotic tonsils with an adequate airway and small palpable nodes. The initial mono test was negative. (Otolaryngology/Head & Neck Surgery)

Initial hospital evaluation of a 23-year-old allergy patient admitted with eyelid edema and pain on fifth day of oral antibiotic therapy. (Otolaryngology/Head & Neck Surgery)

Hospital admission for a 30-year-old female with epilepsy, not compliant with medication, admitted after three seizures. (Neurology)

Hospital admission, examination, and initiation of treatment program for a 66-year-old chronic hemodialysis patient with fever. (Nephrology)

Hospital admission for a 40-year-old male with submaxillary cellulitis and trismus from infected lower molar. (Oral & Maxillofacial Surgery)

Initial hospital visit following admission for a 42-year-old male for observation following an uncomplicated mandible fracture. (Oral & Maxillofacial Surgery)

Initial hospital visit for a 24-year-old healthy female with benign tumor of palate. (Oral & Maxillofacial Surgery)

Initial hospital visit for a 15-year-old male with acute status asthmaticus, unresponsive to outpatient therapy. (Internal Medicine)

99223 Hospital admission of a 62-year-old smoker, established patient, with bronchitis in acute respiratory distress. (Internal Medicine/Pulmonary Medicine)

Initial hospital visit for a 45-year-old female, who has a history of rheumatic fever as a child and now has anemia, fever, and congestive heart failure. (Cardiology)

Initial hospital visit for a 50-year-old male with acute chest pain and diagnostic electrocardiographic changes of an acute anterior myocardial infarction. (Cardiology/Family Medicine/Internal Medicine)

Initial hospital visit of a 75-year-old with progressive stridor and dysphagia with history of cancer of the larynx treated by radiation therapy in the past. Exam shows a large recurrent tumor of the glottis with a mass in the neck. (Otolaryngology/Head & Neck Surgery)

Initial hospital visit for a 70-year-old male admitted with chest pain, complete heart block, and congestive heart failure. (Cardiology)

Initial hospital visit for an 82-year-old male who presents with syncope, chest pain, and ventricular arrhythmias. (Cardiology)

Initial hospital visit for a 75-year-old male with history of arteriosclerotic coronary vascular disease, who is severely dehydrated, disoriented, and confused. (Psychiatry)

Initial hospital visit for a 70-year-old male with alcohol and sedative-hypnotic dependence, admitted by family for severe withdrawal, hypertension, and diabetes mellitus. (Psychiatry)

Initial hospital visit for a persistently suicidal latency-aged child whose parents have requested admission to provide safety but are anxious about separation from her. (Psychiatry)

Initial psychiatric visit for an adolescent patient without previous psychiatric history, who was transferred from the medical ICU after an overdose. (Psychiatry)

Initial hospital visit for a 35-year-old female with severe systemic lupus erythematosus on corticosteroid and cyclophosphamide, with new onset of fever, chills, rash, and chest pain. (Rheumatology)

Initial hospital visit for a 52-year-old male with known rheumatic heart disease who presents with anasarca, hypertension, and history of alcohol abuse. (Cardiology)

Initial hospital visit for a 55-year-old female with a history of congenital heart disease; now presents with cyanosis. (Cardiology)

Initial hospital visit for a psychotic, hostile, violently combative adolescent, involuntarily committed for his and other's safety. (Psychiatry)

Initial hospital visit for a now subdued and sullen teenage male with six-month history of declining school performance, increasing self-endangerment, and resistance of parental expectations, including running away past weekend after physical fight with father. (Psychiatry)

Initial partial hospital admission for a 17-year-old female with history of borderline mental retardation who has developed auditory hallucinations. Parents are known to abuse alcohol, and Child Protective Services is investigating allegations of sexual abuse of a younger sibling. (Psychiatry)

Initial hospital visit of a 67-year-old male admitted with a large neck mass, dysphagia, and history of myocardial infarction three months before. (Otolaryngology/Head & Neck Surgery)

Initial hospital visit for a patient with suspected cerebrospinal fluid rhinorrhea that developed two weeks after head injury. (Otolaryngology/Head & Neck Surgery)

Initial hospital visit for a 25-year-old female with history of poly-substance abuse and psychiatric disorder. The patient appears to be psychotic with markedly elevated vital signs. (Psychiatry)

Initial hospital visit for a 70-year-old male with cutaneous T-cell lymphoma who has developed fever and lymphadenopathy. (Internal Medicine)

Initial hospital visit for a 62-year-old female with known coronary artery disease, for evaluation of increasing edema, dyspnea on exertion, confusion, and sudden onset of fever with productive cough. (Internal Medicine)

Initial hospital visit for a 3-year-old female with 36-hour history of sore throat and high fever; now with sudden onset of lethargy, irritability, photophobia, and nuchal rigidity. (Pediatrics)

Initial hospital visit for a 26-year-old female for evaluation of severe facial fractures (LeFort's II/III). (Plastic Surgery)

Initial hospital visit for a 55-year-old female for bilateral mandibular fractures resulting in flail mandible and airway obstruction. (Plastic Surgery)

Initial hospital visit for a 71-year-old patient with a red painful eye four days following uncomplicated cataract surgery due to endophthalmitis. (Ophthalmology)

Initial hospital visit for a 45-year-old patient involved in a motor vehicle accident who suffered a perforating corneoscleral laceration with loss of vision. (Ophthalmology)

Initial hospital visit for a 58-year-old male who has Ludwig's angina and progressive airway compromise. (Oral & Maxillofacial Surgery)

Initial hospital visit for an adult with multiple cutaneous blisters, denuded secondarily infected ulcerations, oral lesions, weight loss, and increasing weakness refactory to high-dose corticosteroid. Initiation of new immunosuppressive therapy. (Dermatology)

Initial hospital visit for an 82-year-old male who presents with syncope, chest pain, and ventricular arrhythmias. (Cardiology)

Initial hospital visit for a 62-year-old male with history of previous myocardial infarction, comes in with recurrent, sustained ventricular tachycardia. (Cardiology)

Initial hospital visit for a chronic dialysis patient with infected PTFE fistula, septicemia, and shock. (Nephrology)

Initial hospital visit for a 1-year-old male, victim of child abuse, with central nervous system depression, skull fracture, and retinal hemorrhage. (Neurology)

Initial hospital visit for a 25-year-old female with recent C4-C5 quadriplegia, admitted for rehabilitation. (Physical Medicine & Rehabilitation)

Initial hospital visit for an 18-year-old male, post-traumatic brain injury with multiple impairment. (Physical Medicine & Rehabilitation)

Initial partial hospital admission for 16-year-old male, sullen and subdued, with six-month history of declining school performance, increasing self-endangerment, and resistance to parental expectations. (Psychiatry)

Initial hospital visit for a 16-year-old primigravida at 32 weeks gestation with severe hypertension (200/110), thrombocytopenia, and headache. (Obstetrics & Gynecology)

Initial hospital visit for a 49-year-old male with cirrhosis of liver with hematemesis, hepatic encephalopathy, and fever. (Gastroenterology)

Initial hospital visit for a 55-year-old female in chronic pain who has attempted suicide. (Psychiatry)

Initial hospital visit for a 70-year-old male, with multiple organ system disease, admitted with history of being aneuric and septic for 24 hours prior to admission. (Urology)

Initial hospital visit for a 3-year-old female with 36-hour history of sore throat and high fever, now with sudden onset of lethargy, irritability, photophobia, and nuchal rigidity. (Pediatrics/Critical Care)

Initial hospital visit for a 78-year-old male, transfers from nursing home with dysuria and pyuria, increasing confusion, and high fever. (Internal Medicine)

Initial hospital visit for a 1-day-old male with cyanosis, respiratory distress, and tachypnea. (Cardiology)

Initial hospital visit for a 3-year-old female with recurrent tachycardia and syncope. (Cardiology)

Initial hospital visit for a thyrotoxic patient who presents with fever, atrial fibrillation, and delirium. (Endocrinology)

Initial hospital visit for a 50-year-old Type I diabetic who presents with diabetic ketoacidosis with fever and obtundation. (Endocrinology)

Initial hospital visit for a 40-year-old female with anatomical stage 3, ARA functional class 3 rheumatoid arthritis on methotrexate, corticosteroid, and nonsteroidal anti-inflammatory drugs. Patient presents with severe arthritis flare, new oral ulcers, abdominal pain, and leukopenia. (Rheumatology)

Initial hospital exam of a pediatric patient with high fever and proptosis. (Otolaryngology/Head & Neck Surgery)

Initial hospital visit for a 25-year-old patient admitted for the first time to the rehab unit, with recent C4-C5 quadriplegia. (Physical Medicine & Rehabilitation)

Hospital admission, examination, and initiation of treatment program for a previously unknown 58-year-old male who presents with acute chest pain. (Cardiology)

Hospital admission, examination, and initiation of induction chemotherapy for a 42-year-old patient with newly diagnosed acute myelogenous leukemia. (Hematology/Oncology)

Hospital admission following a motor vehicle accident of a 24-year-old male with fracture dislocation of C5-C6; neurologically intact. (Neurosurgery)

Hospital admission for a 78-year-old female with left lower lobe pneumonia and a history of coronary artery disease, congestive heart failure, osteoarthritis, and gout. (Family Medicine)

Hospital admission, examination, and initiation of treatment program for a 65-year-old immunosuppressed male with confusion, fever, and a headache. (Infectious Disease)

Hospital admission for a 9-year-old with vomiting, dehydration, fever, tachypnea, and an admitting diagnosis of diabetic ketoacidosis. (Pediatrics)

Initial hospital visit for a 65-year-old male who presents with acute myocardial infarction, oliguria, hypotension, and altered state of consciousness. (Cardiology)

Initial hospital visit for a 15-year-old male with acute status asthmaticus, unresponsive to outpatient therapy. (Internal Medicine/Pediatrics/Pulmonary Medicine)

Initial hospital visit for a hostile/resistant adolescent patient who is severely depressed and involved in poly-substance abuse. Patient is experiencing significant conflict in his chaotic family situation and was suspended from school following an attack on a teacher with a baseball bat. (Psychiatry)

Initial hospital visit for 89-year-old female with fulminant hepatic failure and encephalopathy. (Gastroenterology)

Initial hospital visit for a patient with congestive heart failure, type 1 diabetes mellitus, and renal failure who has developed an acute onset of fever and a generalized bullous erythematous and purpuric eruption. (Dermatology)

Hospital admission for a 50-year-old male with new-onset left hemiparesis (Neurology)

Hospital admission for an 18-year-old male admitted to the trauma service following a motor vehicle accident for treatment of a closed head injury, liver laceration, and long bone fractures. (General Surgery)

First hour of critical care of a 15-year-old with acute respiratory failure from asthma. (Pulmonary Medicine)

Hospital admission of a 62-year-old smoker, established patient, with bronchitis in acute respiratory distress. (Pulmonary Medicine/Critical Care)

Initial hospital visit for a 15-year-old male with acute status asthmaticus, unresponsive to outpatient therapy. (Cardiology/Family Practice/General Surgery/Pulmonary Medicine/Critical Care)

Initial hospital visit for a 42-year-old female with rapidly progressing scleroderma, malignant hypertension, digital infarcts, and oligurea. (Cardiology/Family Practice/General Surgery/Pulmonary Medicine/Rheumatology/Critical Care)

Subsequent Hospital Care

99231 Subsequent hospital visit for a 65-year-old female, post-open reduction and internal fixation of a fracture. (Physical Medicine & Rehabilitation)

Subsequent hospital visit for a 33-year-old patient with pelvic pain who is responding to pain medication and observation. (Obstetrics & Gynecology)

Subsequent hospital visit for a 21-year-old female with hyperemesis who has responded well to intravenous fluids. (Obstetrics & Gynecology)

Subsequent hospital visit to re-evaluate postoperative pain and titrate patient-controlled analgesia for a 27-year-old female. (Anesthesiology)

Follow-up hospital visit for a 35-year-old female, status post-epidural analgesia. (Anesthesiology/Pain Medicine)

Subsequent hospital visit for a 56-year-old male, post-gastrectomy, for maintenance of analgesia using an intravenous dilaudid infusion. (Anesthesiology)

Subsequent hospital visit for a male with improving venous stasis ulcers. (Dermatology)

Subsequent hospital visit for a 24-year-old female with otitis externa, seen two days before in consultation, now to have otic wick removal. (Otolaryngology/Head & Neck Surgery)

Subsequent hospital visit for a 62-year-old patient with resolving cellulitis of the foot. (Orthopaedic Surgery)

Subsequent hospital visit for a 25-year-old male admitted for supra-ventricular tachycardia and converted on medical therapy. (Cardiology)

Subsequent hospital visit for a 27-year-old male with nasal fracture who was intoxicated and uncooperative on admission exam. Patient confirms no difficulty breathing and no change in nasal appearance, exam normal other than mild tenderness. (Plastic Surgery)

Subsequent hospital visit for a 76-year-old male with venous stasis ulcers. (Geriatrics)

Subsequent hospital visit for a 67-year-old female admitted three days ago with bleeding gastric ulcer; now stable. (Gastroenterology)

Subsequent hospital visit for stable 33-year-old male following a motor vehicle accident who is stable with bruised ribs and improving dyspnea. (General Surgery/Gastroenterology)

Subsequent hospital visit for a 29-year-old male with effort thrombosis of left upper extremity. (General Surgery)

Subsequent hospital visit for a 14-year-old female in middle phase of residential or day treatment who is now behaviorally stable and making satisfactory progress in treatment. (Psychiatry)

Subsequent hospital visit for a 55-year-old male with rheumatoid arthritis, two days following an uncomplicated total joint replacement. (Rheumatology)

Subsequent hospital visit for a 60-year-old dialysis patient with an access infection, now afebrile on antibiotic. (Nephrology)

Subsequent hospital visit for a 23-year-old female admitted for cellulitis following dog bite to hand, redness, pain, and swelling resolving. (Plastic Surgery)

Subsequent hospital visit for a 66-year-old female with L-2 vertebral compression fracture with resolving ileus. (Orthopaedic Surgery)

Subsequent hospital visit for an 18-year-old female responding to intravenous antibiotic therapy for ear or sinus infection. (Otolaryngology/Head & Neck Surgery)

Subsequent hospital visit for a 70-year-old male admitted with congestive heart failure who has responded to therapy. (Cardiology)

Follow-up hospital visit for a 32-year-old female with left ureteral calculus; being followed in anticipation of spontaneous passage. (Urology)

Subsequent hospital visit for a 42-year-old female, admitted for acute gastroenteritis and dehydration, requiring IV hydration; now stable but refusing oral intake. (Family Medicine/Pediatrics)

Subsequent hospital visit for a 50-year-old Type II diabetic who is clinically stable and without complications requiring regulation of a single dose of insulin daily. (Endocrinology)

Subsequent hospital visit to reassesses the status of a 65-year-old patient post-open reduction and internal fixation of hip fracture, on the rehab unit. (Physical Medicine & Rehabilitation)

Subsequent hospital visit for a 78-year-old male with cholangiocarcinoma managed by biliary drainage. (Interventional Radiology)

Subsequent hospital visit for a 50-year-old male with uncomplicated myocardial infarction who is clinically stable and without chest pain. (Family Medicine/Cardiology/Internal Medicine)

Subsequent hospital visit for a stable 72-year-old lung cancer patient undergoing a five-day course of infusion chemotherapy. (Hematology/Oncology)

Subsequent hospital visit, two days post admission for a 65-year-old male with a CVA (cerebral vascular accident) and left hemiparesis, who is clinically stable. (Neurology/Physical Medicine & Rehabilitation)

Subsequent hospital visit for now stable, 33-year-old male, status post lower gastrointestinal bleeding. (General Surgery)

Subsequent hospital visit for a 3-year-old patient in traction for a congenital dislocation of the hip. (Orthopaedic Surgery)

Subsequent hospital visit for a 4-year-old female, admitted for acute gastroenteritis and dehydration, requiring IV hydration; now stable. (Family Medicine/Internal Medicine)

Subsequent hospital visit for 50-year-old female with resolving uncomplicated acute pancreatitis. (Gastroenterology)

Subsequent hospital visit for a 30-day-old male admitted for sepsis evaluation and IV antibiotics due to fever; afebrile now with cultures pending. (Family Medicine/Pediatrics)

Subsequent hospital visit for a 10-year-old male admitted for lobar pneumonia with vomiting and dehydration; is becoming afebrile and tolerating oral fluids. (Pulmonary Medicine)

Subsequent visit on third day of hospitalization for a 60-year-old female recovering from an uncomplicated lower extremity cellulitis. (Infectious Disease/Internal Medicine/Pulmonary Medicine)

Subsequent visit for a 75-year-old female, now three days after onset of left hemiparesis, awaiting placement in a rehabilitation unit. (Neurology)

99232 Subsequent visit on third day of hospitalization for a 60-year-old female recovering from an uncomplicated pneumonia. (Infectious Disease/Internal Medicine/Pulmonary Medicine)

Subsequent hospital visit for a patient with peritonsillar cellulitis, with slow response to antibiotic therapy, with consideration for additional testing and changes in treatment plan. (Otolaryngology/Head & Neck Surgery)

Subsequent hospital visit for a 27-year-old with acute vertigo, with review of laboratory and imaging studies. (Otolaryngology/Head & Neck Surgery)

Subsequent hospital visit for a patient with venous stasis ulcers who developed fever and red streaks adjacent to the ulcer. (Dermatology/Internal Medicine/Family Medicine)

Subsequent hospital visit for a 45-year-old male admitted for IV antibiotics for cellulitis post dog bite to hand. Increased redness and fluctuance found. (Plastic Surgery)

Subsequent hospital visit for a 54-year-old female admitted for myocardial infarction, but who is now having frequent premature ventricular contractions. (Internal Medicine)

Subsequent hospital visit for an 80-year-old patient with a pelvic rim fracture, inability to walk, and severe pain; now 36 hours post-injury, experiencing urinary retention. (Orthopaedic Surgery)

Subsequent hospital visit for a 17-year-old female with fever, pharyngitis, and airway obstruction, who after 48 hours develops a maculopapular rash. (Pediatrics/Family Medicine)

Follow-up visit for a 67-year-old male with congestive heart failure who has responded to antibiotics and diuretics and has now developed a monoarthropathy. (Internal Medicine)

Follow-up hospital visit for a 58-year-old male receiving continuous opioids who is experiencing severe nausea and vomiting. (Pain Medicine)

Subsequent hospital visit for a patient after an auto accident who is slow to respond to ambulation training. (Physical Medicine & Rehabilitation)

Subsequent hospital visit for a 50-year-old diabetic, hypertensive male with back pain not responding to conservative inpatient management with continued radiation of pain to the lower left extremity. (Orthopaedic Surgery)

Subsequent hospital visit for a 37-year-old female on day five of antibiotics for bacterial endocarditis, who still has low-grade fever. (Cardiology)

Subsequent hospital visit for a 54-year-old patient, post MI (myocardial infarction), who is out of the CCU (coronary care unit) but is now having frequent premature ventricular contractions on telemetry. (Cardiology/Internal Medicine)

Subsequent hospital visit for a patient with neutropenia, a fever responding to antibiotics, and continued slow gastrointestinal bleeding on platelet support. (Hematology/Oncology)

Subsequent hospital visit for a 50-year-old male admitted two days ago for sub-acute renal allograft rejection. (Nephrology)

Subsequent hospital visit for a 35-year-old drug addict, not responding to initial antibiotic therapy for pyelonephritis. (Urology)

Subsequent hospital visit for a 79-year-old male with worsening jaundice and a pancreatic mass. (General Surgery)

Subsequent hospital care for a 62-year-old female with congestive heart failure, who remains dyspneic and febrile. (Internal Medicine)

Subsequent hospital visit for a 73-year-old female with recently diagnosed lung cancer, who complains of unsteady gait. (Pulmonary Medicine)

Subsequent hospital visit for a 20-month-old male with bacterial meningitis treated one week with antibiotic therapy; has now developed a temperature of 101 degrees. (Pediatrics)

Subsequent hospital visit for 13-year-old male admitted with left lower quadrant abdominal pain and fever, not responding to therapy. (General Surgery)

Subsequent hospital visit for a 65-year-old male with hemiplegia and painful paretic shoulder. (Physical Medicine & Rehabilitation)

Subsequent hospital visit for a patient admitted for treatment of congestive heart failure, on multiple medications, whose previous pale, diffuse rash has now generalized, brightened, and is intensely pruritic. (Dermatology)

Subsequent hospital visit for a 41-year-old female whose altered mental status improved. (General Surgery)

Subsequent hospital visit for adolescent female who continues to struggle with suicidal thoughts and has multiple questions about her antidepressant medication. (Psychiatry)

Subsequent partial hospital visit for a child with depression and severe anxiety. (Psychiatry)

Subsequent hospital visit for 59-year-old male with depression, anxiety, and medication side effects. (Psychiatry)

Subsequent partial hospital visit for a 25-year-old female with body image ruminations and high anxiety about following the prescribed meal plan. (Psychiatry)

99233 Subsequent hospital visit for a 38-year-old male, quadriplegic with acute autonomic hyperreflexia, who is not responsive to initial care. (Physical Medicine & Rehabilitation)

Follow-up hospital visit for a teenage female who continues to experience severely disruptive, violent, and life-threatening symptoms in a complicated multi-system illness. Family/social circumstances also a contributing factor. (Psychiatry)

Subsequent hospital visit for a 42-year-old female with progressive systemic sclerosis (scleroderma), renal failure on dialysis, congestive heart failure, cardiac arrhythmias, and digital ulcers. (Allergy & Immunology)

Subsequent hospital visit for a 50-year-old diabetic, hypertensive male with nonresponding back pain and radiating pain to the lower left extremity, who develops chest pain, cough, and bloody sputum. (Orthopaedic Surgery)

Subsequent hospital visit for a 64-year-old female, status post-abdominal aortic aneurysm resection, with non-responsive coagulopathy, who has now developed lower GI bleeding. (Abdominal Surgery/Colon & Rectal Surgery/General Surgery)

Follow-up hospital care of a patient with pansinusitis infection complicated by a brain abscess and asthma; no response to current treatment. (Otolaryngology/Head & Neck Surgery)

Subsequent hospital visit for a patient with a laryngeal neoplasm who develops airway compromise, suspected metastasis. (Otolaryngology/Head & Neck Surgery)

Subsequent hospital visit for a 49-year-old male with significant rectal bleeding, etiology undetermined, not responding to treatment. (Abdominal Surgery/General Surgery/Colon & Rectal Surgery)

Subsequent hospital visit for a 50-year-old male, post-aortocoronary bypass surgery; now develops hypotension and oliguria. (Cardiology)

Subsequent hospital visit for an adolescent patient who is violent, unsafe, and noncompliant, with multiple expectations for participation in treatment plan and behavior on the treatment unit. (Psychiatry)

Subsequent hospital visit for an 18-year-old male being treated for presumed PCP-induced psychosis. Patient still has moderate auditory hallucinations and is insisting on signing out against medical advice. (Psychiatry)

Subsequent hospital visit for an 8-year-old female with caustic ingestion, who now has fever, dyspnea, and dropping hemoglobin. (Gastroenterology)

Subsequent hospital visit for a 44-year-old patient with electrical burns to the left arm with ascending infection. (Orthopaedic Surgery)

Subsequent hospital visit for a type 1 diabetes mellitus patient with a new onset of fever, change in mental status, and a diffuse petechial, purpuric eruption. (Internal Medicine)

Subsequent hospital visit for a 65-year-old female, status postoperative resection of abdominal aortic aneurysm, with suspected ischemic bowel. (General Surgery)

Subsequent hospital visit for a 50-year-old male, post-aortocoronary bypass surgery, now develops hypotension and oliguria. (Cardiology)

Subsequent hospital visit for a 65-year-old male, following an acute myocardial infarction, who complains of shortness of breath and new chest pain. (Cardiology)

Subsequent hospital visit for a 65-year-old female with rheumatoid arthritis (stage 3, class 3) admitted for urosepsis. On the third hospital day, chest pain, dyspnea, and fever develop. (Rheumatology)

Follow-up hospital care of a pediatric case with stridor, laryngomalacia, established tracheostomy, complicated by multiple medical problems in PICU. (Otolaryngology/Head & Neck Surgery)

Subsequent hospital visit for a 60-year-old female, four days post uncomplicated inferior myocardial infarction who has developed severe chest pain, dyspnea, diaphoresis, and nausea. (Family Medicine)

Subsequent hospital visit for a patient with AML (acute myelogenous leukemia), fever, elevated white count and uric acid undergoing induction chemotherapy. (Hematology/Oncology)

Subsequent hospital visit for a 38-year-old quadriplegic male with acute autonomic hyperreflexia, who is not responsive to initial care. (Physical Medicine & Rehabilitation)

Subsequent hospital visit for a 65-year-old female postoperative resection of abdominal aortic aneurysm, with suspected ischemic bowel. (General Surgery)

Subsequent hospital visit for a 60-year-old female with persistent leukocytosis, fever, abdominal pain, and hypotension seven days after a sigmoid colon resection for carcinoma. (Infectious Disease)

Subsequent hospital visit for a chronic renal failure patient on dialysis, who develops chest pain, shortness of breath. (Nephrology)

Subsequent hospital visit for a 65-year-old male with acute myocardial infarction who now demonstrates complete heart block and congestive heart failure. (Cardiology)

Subsequent hospital visit for a 55-year-old male with severe chronic obstructive pulmonary disease and bronchospasm; initially admitted for acute respiratory distress requiring ventilatory support in the ICU. The patient was stabilized, extubated, and transferred to the floor but has now developed acute fever, dyspnea, left lower lobe rhonchi, and laboratory evidence of carbon dioxide retention and hypoxemia. (Family Medicine/Internal Medicine)

Subsequent hospital visit for 46-year-old female, known liver cirrhosis patient, with recent upper gastrointestinal hemorrhage from varices; now with worsening ascites and encephalopathy. (Gastroenterology)

Subsequent hospital visit for 62-year-old female admitted with acute subarachnoid hemorrhage, negative cerebral arteriogram, increased lethargy, and hemiparesis with fever. (Neurosurgery)

Subsequent partial hospital visit for an adolescent female who cut herself over the weekend following an intense family argument. (Psychiatry)

Subsequent hospital visit for an adolescent patient who is actively suicidal and experiencing significant medication side effects. (Psychiatry)

Subsequent hospital visit for a 70-year-old male with depression who had a syncopal episode on the unit. (Psychiatry)

Subsequent hospital visit for a 43-year-old male with new onset foot drop after removing a cast from his leg. (Neurology)

Consultations

Office or Other Outpatient Consultations

New or Established Patient

99241 Initial office consultation for a 40-year-old female in pain from blister on lip following a cold. (Oral & Maxillofacial Surgery)

Initial office consultation for a 62-year-old construction worker with olecranon bursitis. (Orthopaedic Surgery)

Office consultation with 25-year-old postpartum female with suspected hemorrhoids. (General Surgery)

Office consultation with 58-year-old male, referred for follow-up of creatinine level and evaluation of obstructive uropathy, relieved two months ago. (Nephrology)

Office consultation for 30-year-old female tennis player with sprain or contusion of the forearm. (Orthopaedic Surgery)

Office consultation for a 45-year-old male, requested by his internist, with asymptomatic torus palatinus requiring no further treatment. (Oral & Maxillofacial Surgery)

99242 Initial office consultation for a 29-year-old soccer player with painful proximal thigh/groin injury. (Orthopaedic Surgery)

Initial office consultation for an 8-year-old female with a five-day-old second-degree scald burn of the foot. (Plastic Surgery)

Initial office consultation for a patient with a history of discoid lupus erythematosus who has developed a new erythematous nodule on a cheek. (Dermatology)

Office consultation for management of systolic hypertension in a 70-year-old male scheduled for elective prostate resection. (Geriatrics)

Office consultation with 27-year-old female, with old amputation, for evaluation of existing above-knee prosthesis. (Physical Medicine & Rehabilitation)

Office consultation with 66-year-old female with wrist and hand pain, and finger numbness, secondary to suspected carpal tunnel syndrome. (Orthopaedic Surgery)

Office consultation for 61-year-old female, recently on antibiotic therapy, now with diarrhea and leukocytosis. (Abdominal Surgery)

Office consultation for a patient with papulosquamous eruption of elbow with pitting of nails and itchy scalp. (Dermatology)

Office consultation for a 25-year-old female seen in consultation for complaints of breast pain, with no nipple discharge, mass, or family history of breast cancer. (General Surgery)

Initial office consultation for a 60-year-old female with ptosis, muscle weakness, and thymic tumor who was referred by her neurologist for possible therapeutic plasmapheresis. (Pathology)

99243 Initial office consultation for a 60-year-old male with avascular necrosis of the left femoral head with increasing pain. (Orthopaedic Surgery)

Office consultation for a 31-year-old female complaining of palpitations and chest pains. Her internist had described a mild systolic click. (Cardiology)

Office consultation for a 65-year-old female with recurrent upper extremity cellulitis following axillary lymph node dissection for breast carcinoma. (Infectious Disease)

Office consultation for a 65-year-old male with chronic low-back pain radiating to the leg. (Neurosurgery)

Office consultation for 23-year-old female with Crohn's disease not responding to therapy. (Abdominal Surgery/ Colon & Rectal Surgery)

Office consultation for 25-year-old patient with symptomatic knee pain and swelling, with torn anterior cruciate ligament and/or torn meniscus. (Orthopaedic Surgery)

Office consultation for a 67-year-old patient with osteoporosis and mandibular atrophy with regard to reconstructive alternatives. (Oral & Maxillofacial Surgery)

Office consultation for 39-year-old patient referred at a perimenopausal age for irregular menses and menopausal symptoms. (Obstetrics & Gynecology)

Office consultation for a patient with a papulosquamous eruption of the elbows, pitting of the nails, an itchy, scaly scalp, and localized joint pains. (Dermatology)

Initial office consultation for a 40-year-old female in pain from blister on lip following a cold. (Oral & Maxillofacial Surgery)

Office consultation for a 45-year-old male, requested by his internist, with asymptomatic torus palatinus requiring no further treatment. (Oral & Maxillofacial Surgery)

Office consultation for a 16-year-old male who suffered a concussion a week ago, now fully recovered, needing an evaluation to return to playing football. (Neurology)

99244 Initial office consultation for a 28-year-old male, HIV+, with a recent change in visual acuity. (Ophthalmology)

Initial office consultation for a 15-year-old male with failing grades, suspected drug abuse. (Pediatrics)

Initial office consultation for a 36-year-old factory worker, status four months post-occupational low back injury and requires management of intractable low back pain. (Pain Medicine)

Initial office consultation for a 45-year-old female with a history of chronic arthralgia of TMJ and associated myalgia and sudden progressive symptomatology over last two to three months. (Oral & Maxillofacial Surgery)

Initial office consultation for a 23-year-old female with developmental facial skeletal anomaly and subsequent abnormal relationship of jaw(s) to cranial base. (Oral & Maxillofacial Surgery)

Initial office consultation for a 45-year-old myopic patient with a one-week history of floaters and a partial retinal detachment. (Ophthalmology)

Initial office consultation for a 65-year-old female with moderate dementia, mild unsteadiness, back pain fatigue on ambulation, intermittent urinary incontinence. (Neurosurgery)

Initial office consultation for a 33-year-old female referred by endocrinologist with amenorrhea and galactorrhea, for evaluation of pituitary tumor. (Neurosurgery)

Initial office consultation for a 34-year-old male with new onset nephrotic syndrome. (Nephrology)

Initial office consultation for a patient with multiple giant tumors of jaws. (Oral & Maxillofacial Surgery)

Initial office consultation for a patient with a failed total hip replacement with loosening and pain upon walking. (Orthopaedic Surgery)

Initial office consultation for a 60-year-old female with three-year history of intermittent tic-like unilateral facial pain; now constant pain for six weeks without relief by adequate carbamazepine dosage. (Neurosurgery)

Initial office consultation for a 45-year-old male heavy construction worker with prior lumbar disk surgery two years earlier; now gradually recurring low back and unilateral leg pain for three months, unable to work for two weeks. (Neurosurgery)

Office consultation with 38-year-old female with inflammatory bowel disease, complaints of pain in the right lower quadrant, and suspected intra-abdominal abscess. (General Surgery/Colon & Rectal Surgery)

Office consultation with 72-year-old male with esophageal carcinoma, symptoms of dysphagia and reflux. (Thoracic Surgery)

Office consultation for discussion of treatment options for a 40-year-old female with a 2 cm adenocarcinoma of the breast. (Radiation Oncology)

Office consultation for 66-year-old female, history of colon resection for adenocarcinoma six years earlier, now with severe mid-back pain; X-rays showing osteoporosis and multiple vertebral compression fractures. (Neurosurgery)

Office consultation for a patient with chronic pelvic inflammatory disease who now has left lower quadrant pain with a palpable pelvic mass. (Obstetrics & Gynecology)

Office consultation for a patient with long-standing psoriasis with acute onset of erythroderma, pustular lesions, chills, and fever. Combinations of topical and systemic treatments discussed and instituted. (Dermatology)

Office consultation for a 39-year-old female with persistent migraines failing medications prescribed by her primary care provider. (Neurology)

99245 Office consultation for young patient referred by pediatrician because of patient's short attention span, easy distractibility, and hyperactivity after a failed stimulant trial. (Psychiatry)

Initial office consultation for evaluation of a 70-year-old male with multiple medical problems and recent unexplained appetite loss and diminished energy. (Psychiatry)

Initial office consultation for an elementary school-aged patient, referred by pediatrician, with multiple somatic complaints and recent onset of behavioral discontrol. (Psychiatry)

Initial office consultation of a patient who presents with a 30-year history of smoking, hypertension, chronic obstructive pulmonary disease, and a hard, fixed right neck mass. Patient on other meds for conditions. Patient presents with CT ordered by PCP. (Otolaryngology/Head & Neck Surgery)

Initial office consultation for a 35-year-old multiple-trauma male patient with complex pelvic fractures, for evaluation and formulation of management plan. (Orthopaedic Surgery)

Initial emergency room consultation for 10-year-old male in status epilepticus, recent closed head injury, information about medication not available. (Neurosurgery)

Initial emergency room consultation for a 23-year-old patient with severe abdominal pain, guarding, febrile, and unstable vital signs. (Obstetrics & Gynecology)

Office consultation for a 67-year-old female longstanding uncontrolled diabetic who presents with retinopathy, nephropathy, and a foot ulcer. (Endocrinology)

Office consultation for a 37-year-old male for initial evaluation and management of Cushing's disease. (Endocrinology)

Office consultation for a 60-year-old male who presents with thyrotoxicosis, exophthalmos, frequent premature ventricular contractions, and congestive heart failure. (Endocrinology)

Initial office consultation for a 36-year-old patient, one year status post occupational herniated cervical disk treated by laminectomy, requiring management of multiple sites of intractable pain, depression, and narcotic dependence. (Pain Medicine)

Office consultation for a 58-year-old male with a history of MI and CHF who complains of the recent onset of rest angina and shortness of breath. The patient has a systolic blood pressure of 90 mmHG and is in Class IV heart failure. (Cardiology)

Emergency room consultation for a 1-year-old with a three-day history of fever with increasing respiratory distress who is thought to have cardiac tamponade by the ER physician. (Cardiology)

Office consultation in the emergency room for a 25-year-old male with severe, acute, closed head injury. (Neurosurgery)

Office consultation for a 53-year-old female with advanced head and neck cancer. (Radiation Oncology)

Office consultation for a 27-year-old juvenile diabetic patient with severe diabetic retinopathy, gastric atony, nephrotic syndrome, and progressive renal failure, now with a serum creatinine of 2.7, and a blood pressure of 170/114. (Nephrology)

Office consultation for independent medical evaluation of a patient with a history of complicated low back and neck problems with previous multiple failed back surgeries. (Orthopaedic Surgery)

Office consultation for an adolescent referred by pediatrician PCP for recent onset of violent and self-injurious behavior. (Psychiatry)

Office consultation for a 6-year-old male for evaluation of severe muscle and joint pain and a diffuse rash. Patient well until 4-6 weeks earlier, when he developed arthralgia, myalgias, and a fever of 102 degrees for one week. (Rheumatology)

Office consultation for a 70-year-old male with COPD, congestive heart failure, and diabetes, who presents with rectal bleeding and pain, and worsening constipation. The patient has a fixed, partially obstructing rectal mass. (General Surgery)

Office consultation for a 57-year-old male with recent onset of three events of left arm weakness lasting 30 minutes each. (Neurology)

Initial office consultation of a patient who presents with a 30 year history of smoking and hard, fixed right neck mass, HTN, COPD fo which he is on other meds and/or a suspicious epiglottic lesion on indirect laryngoscopy. He brings a CT ordered by his PCP. (Otolaryngology)

Inpatient Consultations

New or Established Patient

99251 Initial hospital consultation for a 27-year-old female with fractured incisor post-intubation. (Oral & Maxillofacial Surgery)

Initial hospital consultation for an orthopaedic patient on IV antibiotics who has developed an apparent candida infection of the oral cavity. (Oral & Maxillofacial Surgery)

Initial inpatient consultation for a 30-year-old female complaining of vaginal itching, post orthopaedic surgery. (Obstetrics & Gynecology)

Initial inpatient consultation for a 36-year-old male on orthopaedic service with complaint of localized dental pain. (Oral & Maxillofacial Surgery)

Initial hospital consultation for a 20-year-old male following a motor vehicle accident who developed cellulitis around a laceration that was sutured in the emergency room. (General Surgery)

Initial inpatient consultation for a 64-year-old bedridden male with skin irritation and pain in posterior heel. (Podiatry Surgery)

99252 Initial hospital consultation for a 45-year-old male, previously abstinent alcoholic, who relapsed and was admitted for management of gastritis. The patient readily accepts the need for further treatment. (Addiction Medicine)

Inpatient consultation for a 28-year-old female with thrombocytopenia and neurologic symptoms who was referred by her hematologist for possible therapeutic plasmapheresis for thrombotic thrombocytopenic purpura. (Pathology)

Initial hospital consultation for a 35-year-old dialysis patient with episodic oral ulcerations. (Oral & Maxillofacial Surgery)

Initial inpatient preoperative consultation for a 43-year-old female with cholecystitis and well-controlled hypertension. (Cardiology)

Initial inpatient consultation for recommendation of antibiotic prophylaxis for a patient with a synthetic heart valve who will undergo urologic surgery. (Internal Medicine)

Initial inpatient consultation for possible drug induced skin eruption in 50-year-old male. (Dermatology)

Preoperative inpatient consultation for evaluation of hypertension in a 60-year-old male who will undergo a cholecystectomy. Patient had a normal annual check-up in your office four months ago. (Internal Medicine)

Initial inpatient consultation for 66-year-old patient with wrist and hand pain and finger numbness, secondary to carpal tunnel syndrome. (Orthopaedic Surgery/Plastic Surgery)

Initial inpatient consultation for a 66-year-old male smoker referred for pain management immediately status post-biliary tract surgery done via sub-costal incision. (Anesthesiology/Pain Medicine)

Initial inpatient consultation for an asymptomatic patient with an established diagnosis of allergic rhinitis, who has gone six weeks since last allergy injection and needs a dose adjustment before the next dose is given. (Allergy & Immunology)

Initial office visit for an 86-year old male with a 2 cm lipoma on back that he is concerned is infected. (General Surgery)

Initial inpatient consultation for a 70-year-old female who has had no bowel sounds for two days following an orthopedic operation. (General Surgery)

Initial hospital consultation for a 56-year-old stroke patient with ankle venous stasis ulcerations. (Podiatry Surgery)

Initial consultation for 66-year-old patient with a grade 1 sacral decubitus following a six-hour abdominal surgical procedure. (Orthopaedic Surgery/Plastic Surgery)

99253 Initial hospital consultation for a 50-year-old female with incapacitating knee pain due to generalized rheumatoid arthritis. (Orthopaedic Surgery)

Initial hospital consultation for a 60-year-old male with avascular necrosis of the left femoral heel with increasing pain. (Orthopaedic Surgery)

Initial hospital consultation for a 45-year-old female with compound mandibular fracture and concurrent head, abdominal, and/or orthopaedic injuries. (Oral & Maxillofacial Surgery)

Initial hospital consultation for a 22-year-old female, paraplegic, to evaluate wrist and hand pain. (Orthopaedic Surgery)

Initial hospital consultation for a 40-year-old male with 10-day history of incapacitating unilateral sciatica, unable to walk now, not improved by bed rest. (Neurosurgery)

Initial hospital consultation, requested by pediatrician, for treatment recommendations for a patient admitted with persistent inability to walk following soft tissue injury to ankle. (Physiatry)

Initial hospital consultation for a 27-year-old previously healthy male who vomited during IV sedation and may have aspirated gastric contents. (Anesthesiology)

Initial hospital consultation for a 33-year-old female, post-abdominal surgery, who now has a fever. (Internal Medicine)

Initial inpatient consultation for a 57-year-old male admitted for severe abdominal pain and fever two days post lower endoscopy. (General Surgery)

Initial inpatient consultation for rehabilitation of a 73-year-old female one week after surgical management of a hip fracture. (Physical Medicine & Rehabilitation)

Initial inpatient consultation for diagnosis/management of fever following abdominal surgery. (Internal Medicine)

Initial inpatient consultation for a 42-year-old non-diabetic patient, postoperative cholecystectomy, now with an acute urinary tract infection. (Nephrology)

Initial inpatient consultation for 53-year-old female with moderate uncomplicated pancreatitis. (Gastroenterology)

Initial inpatient consultation for 45-year-old patient with chronic neck pain with radicular pain of the left arm. (Orthopaedic Surgery)

Initial inpatient consultation for a 43-year-old male with new onset foot drop after removing a cast from his leg. (Neurology)

Initial hospital consultation for an orthopaedic patient on IV antibiotics who has developed an apparent candida infection of the oral cavity. (Oral & Maxillofacial Surgery)

Initial inpatient consultation for a 36-year-old male on orthopaedic service with complaint of localized dental pain. (Oral & Maxillofacial Surgery)

Initial hospital consultation for a 35-year-old dialysis patient with episodic oral ulcerations. (Oral & Maxillofacial Surgery)

Initial hospital consultation for a 55-year-old diabetic patient on dialysis with infected ingrown toenail. (Podiatry Surgery)

99254 Initial inpatient consultation for a 35-year-old female with a fever and pulmonary infiltrate following cesarean section. (Pulmonary Medicine)

Initial hospital consultation for a 15-year-old patient with painless swelling of proximal humerus with lytic lesion by X-ray. (Orthopaedic Surgery)

Initial hospital consultation for evaluation of a 29-year-old female with a diffusely positive medical review of systems and history of multiple surgeries. (Psychiatry)

Initial hospital consultation for a 70-year-old diabetic female with gangrene of the foot. (Orthopaedic Surgery)

Initial inpatient consultation for a 47-year-old female with progressive pulmonary infiltrate, hypoxemia, and diminished urine output. (Anesthesiology)

Initial hospital consultation for a patient with failed total hip replacement with loosening and pain upon walking. (Orthopaedic Surgery)

Initial hospital consultation for a 62-year-old female with metastatic breast cancer to the femoral neck and thoracic vertebra. (Orthopaedic Surgery)

Initial hospital consultation for a 39-year-old female with nephrolithiasis requiring extensive opioid analgesics, whose vital signs are now elevated. She initially denied any drug use but today gives history of multiple substance abuse, including opioids and prior treatment for a personality disorder. (Psychiatry)

Initial inpatient consultation for evaluation of a 63-year-old in the ICU with diabetes and chronic renal failure who develops acute respiratory distress syndrome 36 hours after a mitral valve replacement. (Anesthesiology)

Initial inpatient consultation for a 66-year-old female with enlarged supraclavicular lymph nodes, found on biopsy to be malignant. (Hematology/Oncology)

Initial inpatient consultation for a 43-year-old female for evaluation of sudden painful visual loss, optic neuritis, and episodic paresthesia. (Ophthalmology)

Initial inpatient consultation for evaluation of a 71-year-old male with hyponatremia (serum sodium 114) who was admitted to the hospital with pneumonia. (Nephrology)

Initial inpatient consultation for a 72-year-old male with emergency admission for possible bowel obstruction. (Internal Medicine/General Surgery)

Initial inpatient consultation for a 35-year-old female with fever, swollen joints, and rash of one-week duration. (Rheumatology)

Initial hospital consultation for a 45-year-old female with compound mandibular fracture and concurrent head, abdominal, and/or orthopaedic injuries. (Oral & Maxillofacial Surgery)

Initial hospital consultation for a 70-year-old diabetic female with gangrene of the foot. (Podiatry Surgery)

Initial hospital consultation for a 39-year-old female with myasthenia admitted for a thymectomy surgery tomorrow. (Neurology)

99255 Initial hospital consultation for a 70-year-old female without previous psychiatric history who is now experiencing nocturnal confusion and visual hallucinations following hip replacement surgery. (Psychiatry)

Initial inpatient consultation for a 76-year-old female with massive, life-threatening gastrointestinal hemorrhage and chest pain. (Gastroenterology)

Initial inpatient consultation for a 75-year-old female, admitted to intensive care with acute respiratory distress syndrome, who is hypersensitive, and has a moderate metabolic acidosis, and a rising serum creatinine. (Nephrology)

Initial hospital consultation for patient with a history of complicated low back pain and neck problems with previous multiple failed back surgeries. (Orthopaedic Surgery/Neurosurgery)

Initial hospital consultation for a 66-year-old female, two days post-abdominal aneurysm repair, with oliguria and hypertension of one-day duration. (Nephrology/Internal Medicine)

Initial hospital consultation for a patient with shotgun wound to face with massive facial trauma and airway obstruction. (Oral & Maxillofacial Surgery)

Initial hospital consultation for patient with severe pancreatitis complicated by respiratory insufficiency, acute renal failure, and abscess formation. (General Surgery/Colon & Rectal Surgery)

Initial hospital consultation for a 35-year-old multiple-trauma male patient with complex pelvic fractures to evaluate and formulate management plan. (Orthopaedic Surgery)

Initial inpatient consultation for adolescent patient with fractured femur and pelvis who pulled out IVs and disconnected traction in attempt to elope from hospital. (Psychiatry)

Initial hospital consultation for a 16-year-old primigravida at 32-weeks gestation requested by a family practitioner for evaluation of severe hypertension, thrombocytopenia, and headache. (Obstetrics & Gynecology)

Initial hospital consultation for a 58-year-old insulin-dependent diabetic with multiple antibiotic allergies, now with multiple fascial plane abscesses and airway obstruction. (Oral & Maxillofacial Surgery)

Initial inpatient consultation for a 55-year-old male with known cirrhosis and ascites, now with jaundice, encephalopathy, and massive hematemesis. (Gastroenterology)

Initial hospital consultation for a 25-year-old male, seen in emergency room with severe, closed head injury. (Neurosurgery)

Initial hospital consultation for a 2-day-old male with single ventricle physiology and subaortic obstruction. Family counseling following evaluation for multiple, staged surgical procedures. (Thoracic Surgery)

Initial hospital consultation for a 45-year-old male admitted with subarachnoid hemorrhage and intracranial aneurysm on angiogram. (Neurosurgery)

Initial inpatient consultation for myxedematous patient who is hypoventilating and obtunded. (Endocrinology)

Initial hospital consultation for a 45-year-old patient with widely metastatic lung carcinoma, intractable back pain, and a history that includes substance dependence, NSAID allergy, and two prior laminectomies with fusion for low back pain. (Pain Medicine)

Initial hospital consultation for evaluation of treatment options in a 50-year-old patient with cirrhosis, known peptic ulcer disease, hypotension, encephalopathy, and massive acute upper gastrointestinal bleeding that cannot be localized by endoscopy. (Interventional Radiology)

Initial inpatient consultation in the ICU for a 70-year-old male who experienced a cardiac arrest during surgery and was resuscitated. (Cardiology)

Initial inpatient consultation for a patient with severe pancreatitis complicated by respiratory insufficiency, acute renal failure, and abscess formation. (Gastroenterology)

Initial inpatient consultation for a 70-year-old cirrhotic male admitted with ascites, jaundice, encephalopathy, and massive hematemesis. (Gastroenterology)

Initial inpatient consultation in the ICU for a 51-year-old patient who has a fever, respiratory failure requiring mechanical ventilation, and bilateral pulmonary infiltrates on chest radiograph two weeks after a renal transplantation. (Infectious Disease)

Initial inpatient consultation for evaluation and formulation of plan for management of multiple-trauma patient with complex pelvic fracture, 35-year-old male. (General Surgery/Orthopaedic Surgery)

Initial inpatient consultation for a 50-year-old male with a history of previous myocardial infarction, now with acute pulmonary edema and hypotension. (Cardiology)

Initial inpatient consultation for 45-year-old male with recent, acute subarachnoid hemorrhage, hesitant speech, mildly confused, drowsy. High risk group for HIV+ status. (Neurosurgery)

Initial inpatient consultation for 36-year-old female referred by her internist to evaluate a patient being followed for abdominal pain and fever. The patient has developed diffuse abdominal pain, guarding, rigidity, and increased fever. (Obstetrics & Gynecology)

Initial inpatient consultation for adolescent patient with fractured femur and pelvis who expressed feeling hopeless and suicidal. (Psychiatry)

Initial inpatient consultation for a 35-year-old male with closed head injury, pulmonary contusion, liver laceration, and complex pelvic fracture. (General Surgery)

Initial hospital consultation for a 35-year-old male patient with acute partial traumatic amputation of the forefoot for evaluation and formulation of a management plan. (Podiatry Surgery)

Initial hospital consultation for a 57-year-old male with new-onset right hemiparesis and aphasia. (Neurology)

Emergency Department Services

New or Established Patient

99281   Emergency department visit for a patient for removal of sutures from a well-healed, uncomplicated laceration. (Emergency Medicine)

Emergency department visit for a patient for tetanus toxoid immunization. (Emergency Medicine)

Emergency department visit for a patient with several uncomplicated insect bites. (Pediatrics)

99282   Emergency department visit for a 20-year-old student who presents with a painful sunburn with blister formation on the back. (Emergency Medicine)

Emergency department visit for a child presenting with impetigo localized to the face. (Emergency Medicine)

Emergency department visit for a patient with a minor traumatic injury of an extremity with localized pain, swelling, and bruising. (Emergency Medicine)

Emergency department visit for an otherwise healthy patient whose chief complaint is a red, swollen cystic lesion on his/her back. (Emergency Medicine)

Emergency department visit for a patient presenting with a rash on both legs after exposure to poison ivy. (Emergency Medicine)

Emergency department visit for a child presenting with impetigo localized to the face with use of topical OTC treatment. (Pediatrics)

Emergency department visit for a patient with a minor traumatic injury of an extremity with localized pain, swelling, and bruising (no imaging done). (Pediatrics)

99283   Emergency department visit for a sexually active female complaining of vaginal discharge who is afebrile and denies experiencing abdominal or back pain. (Emergency Medicine)

Emergency department visit for a well-appearing 8-year-old who has a fever, diarrhea, and abdominal cramps; is tolerating oral fluids and is not vomiting. (Pediatrics)

Emergency department visit for a patient with an inversion ankle injury, who is unable to bear weight on the injured foot and ankle. (Emergency Medicine)

Emergency department visit for a patient who has a complaint of acute pain associated with a suspected foreign body in the painful eye. (Emergency Medicine)

Emergency department visit for a healthy, young adult patient who sustained a blunt head injury with local swelling and bruising without subsequent confusion, loss of consciousness, or memory deficit. (Emergency Medicine)

99284   Emergency department visit for a 4-year-old who fell off a bike sustaining a head injury with brief loss of consciousness. (Emergency Medicine)

Emergency department visit for a patient with flank pain and hematuria. (Emergency Medicine)

Emergency department visit for a female presenting with lower abdominal pain and a vaginal discharge. (Emergency Medicine)

99285   Emergency department visit for a patient with a complicated overdose requiring aggressive management to prevent side effects from the ingested materials. (Emergency Medicine)

Emergency department visit for a patient exhibiting active, upper gastrointestinal bleeding. (Emergency Medicine)

Emergency department visit for a previously healthy young adult patient who is injured in an automobile accident and is brought to the emergency department immobilized and has symptoms compatible with intra-abdominal injuries or multiple extremity injuries. (Emergency Medicine)

Emergency department visit for a patient with an acute onset of chest pain compatible with symptoms of cardiac ischemia and/or pulmonary embolus. (Emergency Medicine)

Emergency department visit for a patient who presents with a sudden onset of "the worst headache of her life," and complains of a stiff neck, nausea, and inability to concentrate. (Emergency Medicine)

Emergency department visit for a patient with a new onset of a cerebral vascular accident. (Emergency Medicine)

Emergency department visit for acute febrile illness in an adult, associated with shortness of breath and an altered level of alertness. (Emergency Medicine)

Critical Care Services

99291   First hour of critical care of a 65-year-old male with septic shock following relief of ureteral obstruction caused by a stone. (Cardiology/Emergency Medicine/Family Practice/General Surgery/Internal Medicine/Pulmonary Medicine)

First hour of critical care of a 15-year-old with acute respiratory failure from asthma. (Cardiology/Emergency Medicine/Family Practice/General Surgery/Internal Medicine/Pulmonary Medicine)

First hour of critical care of a 45-year-old who sustained a liver laceration, cerebral hematoma, flailed chest, and pulmonary contusion after being struck by an automobile. (Cardiology/Emergency Medicine/Family Practice/General Surgery/Internal Medicine/Pulmonary Medicine)

First hour of critical care of a 65-year-old female who, following a hysterectomy, suffered a cardiac arrest associated with a pulmonary embolus. (Cardiology/Emergency Medicine/Family Practice/General Surgery/Internal Medicine/Pulmonary Medicine)

First hour of critical care of a 6-month-old with hypovolemic shock secondary to diarrhea and dehydration. (Cardiology/Emergency Medicine/Family Practice/General Surgery/Internal Medicine/Pulmonary Medicine/Critical Care)

First hour of critical care of a 3-year-old with respiratory failure secondary to pneumocystis carinii pneumonia. (Cardiology/Emergency Medicine/Family Practice/General Surgery/Internal Medicine/Pulmonary Medicine/Critical Care)

First hour of critical care of a 13-year-old with hypovolemic shock secondary to diarrhea and dehydration. (Cardiology/Emergency Medicine/Family Practice/General Surgery/Internal Medicine/Pediatrics/Pulmonary Medicine/Critical Care)

First hour of critical care of a 13-year-old with respiratory failure secondary to pneumocystis carinii pneumonia (Pediatrics)

Subsequent hospital visit for a 55-year-old male with severe chronic obstructive pulmonary disease and bronchospasm; initially admitted for acute respiratory distress requiring ventilatory support in the ICU. The patient was stabilized, extubated, and transferred to the floor but has now developed acute fever, dyspnea, left lower lobe rhonchi, and laboratory evidence of carbon dioxide retention and hypoxemia. (Family Medicine)

Initial hospital visit for a 15-year-old male with acute status asthmaticus, unresponsive to outpatient therapy. (Pulmonary Medicine)

Initial hospital visit for a 62-year-old male with history of previous myocardial infarction, comes in with recurrent, sustained ventricular tachycardia. (Cardiology)

Prolonged Services

Prolonged Service With Direct Patient Contact

Office or Other Outpatient

99354   A 20-year-old female with history of asthma presents with acute bronchospasm and moderate respiratory distress. Initial evaluation shows respiratory rate 30, labored breathing and wheezing heard in all lung fields. Office treatment is initiated which includes intermittent bronchial dilation and subcutaneous epinephrine. Requires intermittent time with patient over a period of 2-3 hours. (Family Medicine/Internal Medicine)

99355   A 20-year-old female with history of asthma presents with acute bronchospasm and moderate respiratory distress. Initial evaluation shows respiratory rate 30, labored breathing, and wheezing heard in all lung fields. Office treatment is initiated that includes intermittent bronchial dilation and subcutaneous epinephrine. Requires intermittent time with patient over a period of 2-3 hours. (Family Medicine/Internal Medicine/Pulmonary Medicine)

Inpatient

99356 A 34-year-old primigravida female presents to hospital in early labor. Admission history and physical reveals severe preeclampsia. Physician supervises management of preeclampsia, IV magnesium initiation and maintenance, labor augmentation with pitocin, and close maternal-fetal monitoring. Involvement includes 40 minutes of continuous bedside care until the patient is stable, then is intermittent over several hours until the delivery. (Family Medicine/Internal Medicine/Obstetrics & Gynecology)

Prolonged Service Without Direct Patient Contact

99358 An 85-year-old new patient with multiple complicated medical problems has moved to the area to live closer to her daughter. She is brought to the primary care office by her daughter and has been seen and examined by the physician. The physician indicated that past medical records would be obtained from the patient's prior physicians' and that he will communicate further with the daughter upon review of them. (Family Medicine/Internal Medicine)

99359 An 85-year-old new patient with multiple complicated medical problems has moved to the area to live closer to her daughter. She is brought to the primary care office by her daughter and has been seen and examined by the physician. The physician indicated that past medical records would be obtained from the patient's prior physicians' and that he will communicate further with the daughter upon review of them. (Family Medicine/Internal Medicine)

Physician Standby Services

99360 A 24-year-old patient is admitted to OB unit attempting VBAC. Fetal monitoring shows increasing fetal distress. Patient's blood pressure is rising and labor progressing slowly. A primary care physician is requested by the OB/GYN to standby in the unit for possible cesarean delivery and neonatal resuscitation. (Family Medicine/Internal Medicine)

Care Plan Oversight Services

99375 First month of care plan oversight for terminal care of a 58-year-old female with advanced intraabdominal ovarian cancer. Care plan includes home oxygen, diuretics IV for edema and ascites control and pain control management involving IV morphine infusion when progressive ileus occurred. Physician phone contacts with nurse, family, and MSW. Discussion with MSW concerning plans to withdraw supportive measures per patient wishes. Documentation includes review and modification of care plan and certifications from nursing, MSW, pharmacy, and DME. (Family Medicine/Internal Medicine)

▶Prolonged Clinical Staff Services with Physician or Other Qualified Health Care Professional Supervision ◀

● 99415 A 52-year-old female presents with gastroenteritis and persistent vomiting. She is unable to tolerate food or liquid by mouth. She presents with signs and symptoms of clinical dehydration. Evaluation and management is performed by the physician. The decision is made to begin IV hydration in the office. A hydration IV is initiated, consisting of normal saline. Prolonged monitoring and observation for 2 hours ensues with intermittent evaluation of the patient by the physician.

Inpatient Neonatal Intensive Care Service and Pediatric and Neonatal Critical Care Services

99477 Initial hospital visit for a 1-day-old male with cyanosis, respiratory distress, and tachypnea. (Cardiology)

Appendix D

Summary of CPT Add-on Codes

This listing is a summary of CPT add-on codes for CPT 2016. The codes listed below are identified in CPT 2016 with a + symbol.

01953	15241	22208	31633	33987	43273	61642	64783
01968	15261	22216	31637	34806	43283	61651	64787
01969	15272	22226	31649	34808	43338	61781	64832
10036	15274	22328	31651	34813	43635	61782	64837
11001	15276	22512	31654	34826	44015	61783	64859
11008	15278	22515	32501	35306	44121	61797	64872
11045	15777	22527	32506	35390	44128	61799	64874
11046	15787	22534	32507	35400	44139	61800	64876
11047	15847	22552	32667	35500	44203	61864	64901
11101	16036	22585	32668	35572	44213	61868	64902
11201	17003	22614	32674	35600	44701	62148	65757
11732	17312	22632	33141	35681	44955	62160	66990
11922	17314	22634	33225	35682	47001	63035	67225
13102	17315	22840	33257	35683	47542	63043	67320
13122	19001	22841	33258	35685	47543	63044	67331
13133	19082	22842	33259	35686	47544	63048	67332
13153	19084	22843	33367	35697	47550	63057	67334
14302	19086	22844	33368	35700	48400	63066	67335
15003	19126	22845	33369	36148	49326	63076	67340
15005	19282	22846	33419	36218	49327	63078	69990
15101	19284	22847	33508	36227	49412	63082	74301
15111	19286	22848	33517	36228	49435	63086	74713
15116	19288	22851	33518	36248	49568	63088	75565
15121	19297	22858	33519	36476	49905	63091	75774
15131	20930	26125	33521	36479	50606	63103	75964
15136	20931	26861	33522	37185	50705	63295	75968
15151	20936	26863	33523	37186	50706	63308	76125
15152	20937	27358	33530	37222	51797	63621	76802
15156	20938	27692	33572	37223	52442	64462	76810
15157	20985	29826	33768	37232	56606	64480	76812
15201	22103	31627	33884	37233	57267	64484	76814
15221	22116	31632	33924	37234	58110	64491	76937
				37235	58611	64492	77001
				37237	59525	64494	77051
				37239	60512	64495	77052
				37252	61316	64634	77063
				37253	61517	64636	77293
				38102	61610	64643	78020
				38746	61611	64645	78496
				38747	61612	64727	78730
				38900	61641	64778	81266

Appendix E

Summary of CPT Codes Exempt from Modifier 51

This listing is a summary of CPT codes that are exempt from the use of modifier 51. Procedures on this list are typically performed with another procedure but may be a stand alone procedure and not always be performed with other specified procedures. For add-on codes, see Appendix D. This is not an exhaustive list of procedures that are typically exempt from multiple procedure reductions. The codes listed below are identified in CPT 2016 with a ⊘ symbol.

81416	92973	95979	0054T
81426	92974	96361	0055T
81536	92978	96366	0076T
82952	92979	96367	0095T
86826	92998	96368	0098T
87187	93320	96370	0159T
87503	93321	96371	0163T
87904	93325	96375	0164T
88155	93352	96376	0165T
88177	93462	96411	0172T
88185	93463	96415	0174T
88311	93464	96417	0189T
88314	93563	96423	0190T
88332	93564	96570	0196T
88334	93565	96571	0205T
88341	93566	96934	0214T
88350	93567	96935	0215T
88364	93568	96936	0217T
88369	93571	97546	0218T
88373	93572	97598	0222T
88388	93609	97811	0229T
90461	93613	97814	0231T
90472	93621	99100	0289T
90474	93622	99116	0290T
90785	93623	99135	0291T
90833	93655	99140	0292T
90836	93657	99145	0294T
90838	93662	99150	0300T
90840	94645	99292	0309T
90863	94729	99354	0346T
91013	94781	99355	0361T
92547	95079	99356	0363T
92608	95873	99357	0365T
92618	95874	99359	0367T
92621	95885	99415	0369T
92627	95886	99416	0374T
92921	95887	99467	0376T
92925	95940	99486	0396T
92929	95941	99489	0397T
92934	95962	99498	0399T
92938	95967	99602	
92944	95975	99607	

17004	93456	93618
20697	93503	93631
20974	93600	94610
20975	93602	95905
31500	93603	95992
36620	93610	99143
44500	93612	99144
61107	93615	
93451	93616	

Appendix F

Summary of CPT Codes Exempt from Modifier 63

The listing is a summary of CPT codes that are exempt from the use of modifier 63. The codes listed below are additionally identified in CPT 2016 with the parenthetical instruction "(Do not report modifier 63 in conjunction with…)."

30540	33949	49495
30545	36415	49496
31520	36420	49600
33401	36450	49605
33403	36460	49606
33470	36510	49610
33502	36660	49611
33503	39503	53025
33505	43313	54000
33506	43314	54150
33610	43520	54160
33611	43831	63700
33619	44055	63702
33647	44126	63704
33670	44127	63706
33690	44128	65820
33694	46070	
33730	46705	
33732	46715	
33735	46716	
33736	46730	
33750	46735	
33755	46740	
33762	46742	
33778	46744	
33786	47700	
33922	47701	
33946	49215	
33947	49491	
33948	49492	

Appendix G

Summary of CPT Codes That Include Moderate (Conscious) Sedation

The following list of procedures includes conscious sedation as an inherent part of providing the procedure. These codes are identified in the CPT code set with a symbol.

Since these services include moderate sedation, it is not appropriate for the same physician or other qualified health care professional to report both the service and the sedation codes 99143-99145. It is expected that if conscious sedation is provided to the patient as part of one of these services, it is provided by the same physician or other qualified health care professional who is providing the service.

In the unusual event when a second physician or other qualified health care professional other than the health care professional performing the diagnostic or therapeutic services provides moderate sedation in the facility setting (eg, hospital, outpatient hospital/ambulatory surgery center, skilled nursing facility) for the procedures listed in Appendix G, the second individual can report 99148-99150. However, for the circumstance in which these services are performed by the second individual in the nonfacility setting (eg, office, freestanding imaging center), codes 99148-99150 would not be reported. Moderate sedation does not include minimal sedation (anxiolysis), deep sedation, or monitored anesthesia care (00100-01999).

The inclusion of a procedure on this list does not prevent separate reporting of an associated anesthesia procedure/ service (CPT codes 00100-01999) when performed by a physician or other qualified health care professional other than the health care professional performing the diagnostic or therapeutic procedure. In such cases, the person providing anesthesia services shall be present for the purpose of continuously monitoring the patient and shall not act as a surgical assistant. When clinical conditions of the patient require such anesthesia services or in the circumstances when the patient does not require sedation, the operating physician or other qualified health care professional is not required to report the procedure as a reduced service using modifier 52.

10030	22510	22514	31615
19298	22511	22515	31622
20982	22512	22526	31623
20983	22513	22527	31624

31625	33223	36247	37216
31626	33227	36248	37218
31627	33228	36251	37220
31628	33229	36252	37221
31629	33230	36253	37222
31632	33231	36254	37223
31633	33233	36481	37224
31634	33234	36555	37225
31635	33235	36557	37226
31645	33240	36558	37227
31646	33241	36560	37228
31647	33244	36561	37229
31648	33249	36563	37230
31649	33262	36565	37231
31651	33263	36566	37232
31652	33264	36568	37233
31653	33282	36570	37234
31654	33284	36571	37235
31660	33990	36576	37236
31661	33991	36578	37237
31725	33992	36581	37238
32405	33993	36582	37239
32550	35471	36583	37241
32551	35472	36585	37242
32553	35475	36590	37243
33010	35476	36870	37244
33011	36010	37183	37252
33206	36140	37184	37253
33207	36147	37185	43200
33208	36148	37186	43201
33210	36200	37187	43202
33211	36221	37188	43204
33212	36222	37191	43205
33213	36223	37192	43206
33214	36224	37193	43211
33216	36225	37197	43212
33217	36226	37211	43213
33218	36227	37212	43214
33220	36228	37213	43215
33221	36245	37214	43216
33222	36246	37215	43217

43220	43276	45307	47534	77600	93458	94011
43226	43277	45308	47535	77605	93459	94012
43227	43278	45309	47536	77610	93460	94013
43229	43453	45315	47538	77615	93461	0200T
43231	44360	45317	47539	92920	93462	0201T
43232	44361	45320	47540	92921	93463	0282T
43233	44363	45321	47541	92924	93464	0283T
43235	44364	45327	47542	92925	93505	0284T
43236	44365	45332	47543	92928	93530	0291T
43237	44366	45333	47544	92929	93561	0292T
43238	44369	45334	49405	92933	93562	0293T
43239	44370	45335	49406	92934	93563	0294T
43240	44372	45337	49407	92937	93564	0301T
43241	44373	45338	49411	92938	93565	0302T
43242	44376	45340	49418	92941	93566	0303T
43243	44377	45341	49440	92943	93567	0304T
43244	44378	45342	49441	92944	93568	0307T
43245	44379	45346	49442	92953	93571	0308T
43246	44380	45347	49446	92960	93572	0335T
43247	44381	45349	50200	92961	93582	0340T
43248	44382	45350	50382	92973	93583	
43249	44384	45378	50384	92974	93609	
43250	44385	45379	50385	92975	93613	
43251	44386	45380	50386	92978	93615	
43252	44388	45381	50387	92979	93616	
43253	44389	45382	50430	92986	93618	
43254	44390	45384	50432	92987	93619	
43255	44391	45385	50433	93312	93620	
43257	44392	45386	50434	93313	93621	
43259	44394	45388	50592	93314	93622	
43260	44401	45389	50593	93315	93624	
43261	44402	45390	50606	93316	93640	
43262	44403	45391	50693	93317	93641	
43263	44404	45392	50694	93318	93642	
43264	44405	45393	50695	93451	93644	
43265	44406	45398	50705	93452	93650	
43266	44407	47000	50706	93453	93653	
43270	44408	47382	57155	93454	93654	
43273	44500	47383	66720	93455	93655	
43274	45303	47532	69300	93456	93656	
43275	45305	47533	77371	93457	93657	

Appendix H

Alphabetical Clinical Topics Listing (AKA – Alphabetical Listing)

The **Alphabetical Clinical Topics Listing** (formerly Appendix H) has been removed from the CPT codebook. Since this document is a dynamic and rapidly expanding source of information to link CPT Category II codes, clinical conditions, and measure abstracts, the Alphabetical Listing is now solely accessed on the AMA CPT website at www.ama-assn.org/go/cpt.

In addition, new codes for the publication cycle (ie, the **Update to the List of Category II Codes**) will continue to be located on the AMA CPT website prior to publication in the next edition of the CPT codebook (subsequent to its listing to the Web).

Appendix I

Genetic Testing Code Modifiers

The **Genetic Testing Code Modifiers** (formerly Appendix I) has been removed from the CPT code set.

The addition of more than 100 molecular pathology codes to the 2012 code set and still more codes to the 2013 CPT code set resulted in the deletion of the stacking codes (83890–83914). The genetic testing code modifiers formerly described in Appendix I applied to those stacking codes, and therefore, the Appendix and modifiers have been removed from the code set.

For the most up-to-date information on future updates for molecular pathology coding in the CPT code set, see the AMA CPT website (www.ama-assn.org/go/cpt).

Appendix J

Electrodiagnostic Medicine Listing of Sensory, Motor, and Mixed Nerves

This summary assigns each sensory, motor, and mixed nerve with its appropriate nerve conduction study code in order to enhance accurate reporting of codes 95907-95913. Each nerve constitutes one unit of service.

Motor Nerves Assigned to Codes 95900 and 95907-95913

I. Upper extremity, cervical plexus, and brachial plexus motor nerves
  A. Axillary motor nerve to the deltoid
  B. Long thoracic motor nerve to the serratus anterior
  C. Median nerve
    1. Median motor nerve to the abductor pollicis brevis
    2. Median motor nerve, anterior interosseous branch, to the flexor pollicis longus
    3. Median motor nerve, anterior interosseous branch, to the pronator quadratus
    4. Median motor nerve to the first lumbrical
    5. Median motor nerve to the second lumbrical
  D. Musculocutaneous motor nerve to the biceps brachii
  E. Radial nerve
    1. Radial motor nerve to the extensor carpi ulnaris
    2. Radial motor nerve to the extensor digitorum communis
    3. Radial motor nerve to the extensor indicis proprius
    4. Radial motor nerve to the brachioradialis
  F. Suprascapular nerve
    1. Suprascapular motor nerve to the supraspinatus
    2. Suprascapular motor nerve to the infraspinatus
  G. Thoracodorsal motor nerve to the latissimus dorsi

H. Ulnar nerve
    1. Ulnar motor nerve to the abductor digiti minimi
    2. Ulnar motor nerve to the palmar interosseous
    3. Ulnar motor nerve to the first dorsal interosseous
    4. Ulnar motor nerve to the flexor carpi ulnaris
  I. Other
II. Lower extremity motor nerves
  A. Femoral motor nerve to the quadriceps
    1. Femoral motor nerve to vastus medialis
    2. Femoral motor nerve to vastus lateralis
    3. Femoral motor nerve to vastus intermedialis
    4. Femoral motor nerve to rectus femoris
  B. Ilioinguinal motor nerve
  C. Peroneal (fibular) nerve
    1. Peroneal motor nerve to the extensor digitorum brevis
    2. Peroneal motor nerve to the peroneus brevis
    3. Peroneal motor nerve to the peroneus longus
    4. Peroneal motor nerve to the tibialis anterior
  D. Plantar motor nerve
  E. Sciatic nerve
  F. Tibial nerve
    1. Tibial motor nerve, inferior calcaneal branch, to the abductor digiti minimi
    2. Tibial motor nerve, medial plantar branch, to the abductor hallucis
    3. Tibial motor nerve, lateral plantar branch, to the flexor digiti minimi brevis
  G. Other
III. Cranial nerves and trunk
  A. Cranial nerve VII (facial motor nerve)
    1. Facial nerve to the frontalis
    2. Facial nerve to the nasalis
    3. Facial nerve to the orbicularis oculi
    4. Facial nerve to the orbicularis oris
  B. Cranial nerve XI (spinal accessory motor nerve)
  C. Cranial nerve XII (hypoglossal motor nerve)
  D. Intercostal motor nerve
  E. Phrenic motor nerve to the diaphragm
  F. Recurrent laryngeal nerve
  G. Other
IV. Nerve Roots
  A. Cervical nerve root stimulation
    1. Cervical level 5 (CT)
    2. Cervical level 6 (C6)
    3. Cervical level 7 (C7)
    4. Cervical level 8 (C8)

B. Thoracic nerve root stimulation
  1. Thoracic level 1 (T1)
  2. Thoracic level 2 (T2)
  3. Thoracic level 3 (T3)
  4. Thoracic level 4 (T4)
  5. Thoracic level 5 (T5)
  6. Thoracic level 6 (T6)
  7. Thoracic level 7 (T7)
  8. Thoracic level 8 (T8)
  9. Thoracic level 9 (T9)
  10. Thoracic level 10 (T10)
  11. Thoracic level 11 (T11)
  12. Thoracic level 12 (T12)
C. Lumbar nerve root stimulation
  1. Lumbar level 1 (L1)
  2. Lumbar level 2 (L2)
  3. Lumbar level 3 (L3)
  4. Lumbar level 4 (L4)
  5. Lumbar level 5 (L5)
D. Sacral nerve root stimulation
  1. Sacral level 1 (S1)
  2. Sacral level 2 (S2)
  3. Sacral level 3 (S3)
  4. Sacral level 4 (S4)

Sensory and Mixed Nerves Assigned to Codes 95907-95913

I. Upper extremity sensory and mixed nerves
  A. Lateral antebrachial cutaneous sensory nerve
  B. Medial antebrachial cutaneous sensory nerve
  C. Medial brachial cutaneous sensory nerve
  D. Median nerve
    1. Median sensory nerve to the first digit
    2. Median sensory nerve to the second digit
    3. Median sensory nerve to the third digit
    4. Median sensory nerve to the fourth digit
    5. Median palmar cutaneous sensory nerve
    6. Median palmar mixed nerve
  E. Posterior antebrachial cutaneous sensory nerve
  F. Radial sensory nerve
    1. Radial sensory nerve to the base of the thumb
    2. Radial sensory nerve to digit 1
  G. Ulnar nerve
    1. Ulnar dorsal cutaneous sensory nerve
    2. Ulnar sensory nerve to the fourth digit
    3. Ulnar sensory nerve to the fifth digit
    4. Ulnar palmar mixed nerve
  H. Intercostal sensory nerve
  I. Other

II. Lower extremity sensory and mixed nerves
  A. Lateral femoral cutaneous sensory nerve
  B. Medial calcaneal sensory nerve
  C. Medial femoral cutaneous sensory nerve
  D. Peroneal nerve
    1. Deep peroneal sensory nerve
    2. Superficial peroneal sensory nerve, medial dorsal cutaneous branch
    3. Superficial peroneal sensory nerve, intermediate dorsal cutaneous branch
  E. Posterior femoral cutaneous sensory nerve
  F. Saphenous nerve
    1. Saphenous sensory nerve (distal technique)
    2. Saphenous sensory nerve (proximal technique)
  G. Sural nerve
    1. Sural sensory nerve, lateral dorsal cutaneous branch
    2. Sural sensory nerve
  H. Tibial sensory nerve (digital nerve to toe 1)
  I. Tibial sensory nerve (medial plantar nerve)
  J. Tibial sensory nerve (lateral plantar nerve)
  K. Other
III. Head and trunk sensory nerves
  A. Dorsal nerve of the penis
  B. Greater auricular nerve
  C. Ophthalmic branch of the trigeminal nerve
  D. Pudendal sensory nerve
  E. Suprascapular sensory nerves
  F. Other

The following table provides a reasonable maximum number of studies performed per diagnostic category necessary for a physician to arrive at a diagnosis in 90% of patients with that final diagnosis. The numbers in each column represent the number of studies recommended. The appropriate number of studies to be performed is based upon the physician's discretion.

Type of Study/Maximum Number of Studies			
Indication	Limbs Studied by Needle EMG (95860-95864, 95867-95870, 95885-95887)	Nerve Conduction Studies (Total nerves studied, 95907-95913	Neuromuscular Junction Testing (Repetitive Stimulation, 95937)
Carpal Tunnel (Unilateral)	1	7	—
Carpal Tunnel (Bilateral)	2	10	—
Radiculopathy	2	7	—
Mononeuropathy	1	8	—
Polyneuropathy/Mononeuropathy Multiplex	3	10	—
Myopathy	2	4	2
Motor Neuronopathy (eg, ALS)	4	6	2
Plexopathy	2	12	—
Neuromuscular Junction	2	4	3
Tarsal Tunnel Syndrome (Unilateral)	1	8	—
Tarsal Tunnel Syndrome (Bilateral)	2	11	—
Weakness, Fatigue, Cramps, or Twitching (Focal)	2	7	2
Weakness, Fatigue, Cramps, or Twitching (General)	4	8	2
Pain, Numbness, or Tingling (Unilateral)	1	9	—
Pain, Numbness, or Tingling (Bilateral)	2	12	—

Appendix K

Product Pending FDA Approval

Some vaccine products have been assigned a CPT Category I code in anticipation of future approval from the Food and Drug Administration (FDA). Following is a list of the vaccine product codes pending FDA approval status that are identified in the CPT code set with the (✗) symbol. Upon revision of the approval status by the FDA, notation of this revision will be provided via the AMA CPT "Category I Vaccine Codes" website listing (www.ama-assn.org/go/cpt-vaccine) and in subsequent publications of the CPT code set.

90625

90653

90666

90667

90668

90697

90739

Appendix L

Vascular Families

Assignment of branches to first, second, and third order in this table makes the assumption that the starting point is catheterization of the aorta. This categorization would not be accurate, for instance, if a femoral or carotid artery were catheterized directly in an antegrade direction. Arteries highlighted in bold are those more commonly reported during arteriographic procedures.

First Order	Second Order Branch	Third Order Branch	Beyond Third Order Branches
Innominate	**R. common carotid**	**R. internal carotid**	R. ophthalmic / R. p. communicating / R. middle cerebral / R. a. cerebral
		R. external carotid	R. superior thyroid / R. ascending pharyngeal / R. facial / R. lingual / R. occipital / R. p. auricular / R. superficial temporal / R. internal maxillary / R. middle meningeal
	R. subclavian & axillary	**R. vertebral**	Basilar
		R. internal thoracic (internal mammary)	
		R. thyrocervical trunk	R. inferior thyroid / R. suprascapular / R. transverse cervical
		R. costocervical trunk	R. highest intercostal / R. deep cervical
		R. lateral thoracic / R. thoracoacromial / R. humeral circumflex (A/P)	
		R. subscapular	R. circumflex scapular
		R. brachial	
		R. deep brachial	R. ulnar / R. radial / R. interosseous / R. deep palmar arch / R. superficial palmar arch / R. metacarpals and digitals
L. common carotid		L. internal carotid	L. ophthalmic / L. p. communicating / L. middle cerebral / L. a. cerebral
		L. external carotid	L. superior thyroid / L. ascending pharyngeal / L. facial / L. lingual / L. occipital / L. p. auricular / L. superficial temporal
		L. internal maxillary	L. middle meningeal

R = right, L = left, A = anterior, P = posterior

First Order	Second Order Branch	Third Order Branch	Beyond Third Order Branches
	L. vertebral		
	L. internal thoracic (internal mammary)		
	L. thyrocervical trunk	L. inferior thyroid L. suprascapular L. transverse cervical	
	L. costocervical trunk	L. highest intercostal L. deep cervical	
L. subclavian & axillary	L. lateral thoracic L. thoracoacromial L. humeral circumflex (A/P) L. subscapular **L. brachial**	L. circumflex scapular	
	L. deep brachial	L. ulnar L. radial L. interosseous	L. deep palmar arch L. superficial palmar arch L. metacarpals and digitals
Intercostals			
Bronchials			
Recurrent esophageal			
Inferior phrenic	Superior suprarenal		
	L. gastric	Esophageal branch	
	Splenic	Dorsal pancreatic Great pancreatic Caudal pancreatic Gastroepiploic Short gastrics	Inferior transverse pancreatic
Celiac trunk	Common hepatic	Gastroduodenal	P. superior pancreaticoduodenal A. superior pancreaticoduodenal
		Proper Hepatic	L. hepatic R. hepatic Cystic Gastroepiploic Supraduodenal Intermediate hepatic
Middle suprarenal			
	Middle colic		
	Inferior pancreaticoduodenal	P. inferior pancreaticoduodenal A. inferior pancreaticoduodenal	
Superior mesenteric	Jejunal Ileocolic Appendicular P. cecal A. cecal Marginal R. colic		

R = right, L = left, A = anterior, P = posterior

Appendix L

First Order	Second Order Branch	Third Order Branch	Beyond Third Order Branches

Renal ——————— Inferior suprarenal

Testicular / Ovarian

Lumbar

Inferior mesenteric
{ L. colic
{ Sigmoid
{ Rectosigmoid
{ Superior rectal

Middle sacral

Common Iliac

Internal iliac
{ Iliolumbar
Lateral sacral
Superior gluteal
Umbilical
Superior vesical
Obturator
Inferior vesical
Middle rectal
Inferior rectal
Internal pudendal
Inferior gluteal

External iliac
{ Inferior epigastric
{ Cremasteric
{ Pubic

Deep circumflex iliac ——————— Ascending deep circumflex iliac

Common femoral

Profunda femoris
{ Medial descending
Perforating branches
Lateral descending
Lateral circumflex

Deep external pudendal
Superficial external
  pudendal
Ascending lateral
  circumflex femoral
Descending lateral
  circumflex femoral
Transverse lateral
  circumflex femoral

Superficial femoral
{ Geniculate
Popliteal
A. tibial
Peroneal
P. tibial

R. & L. main pulmonary arteries
(venous selective)

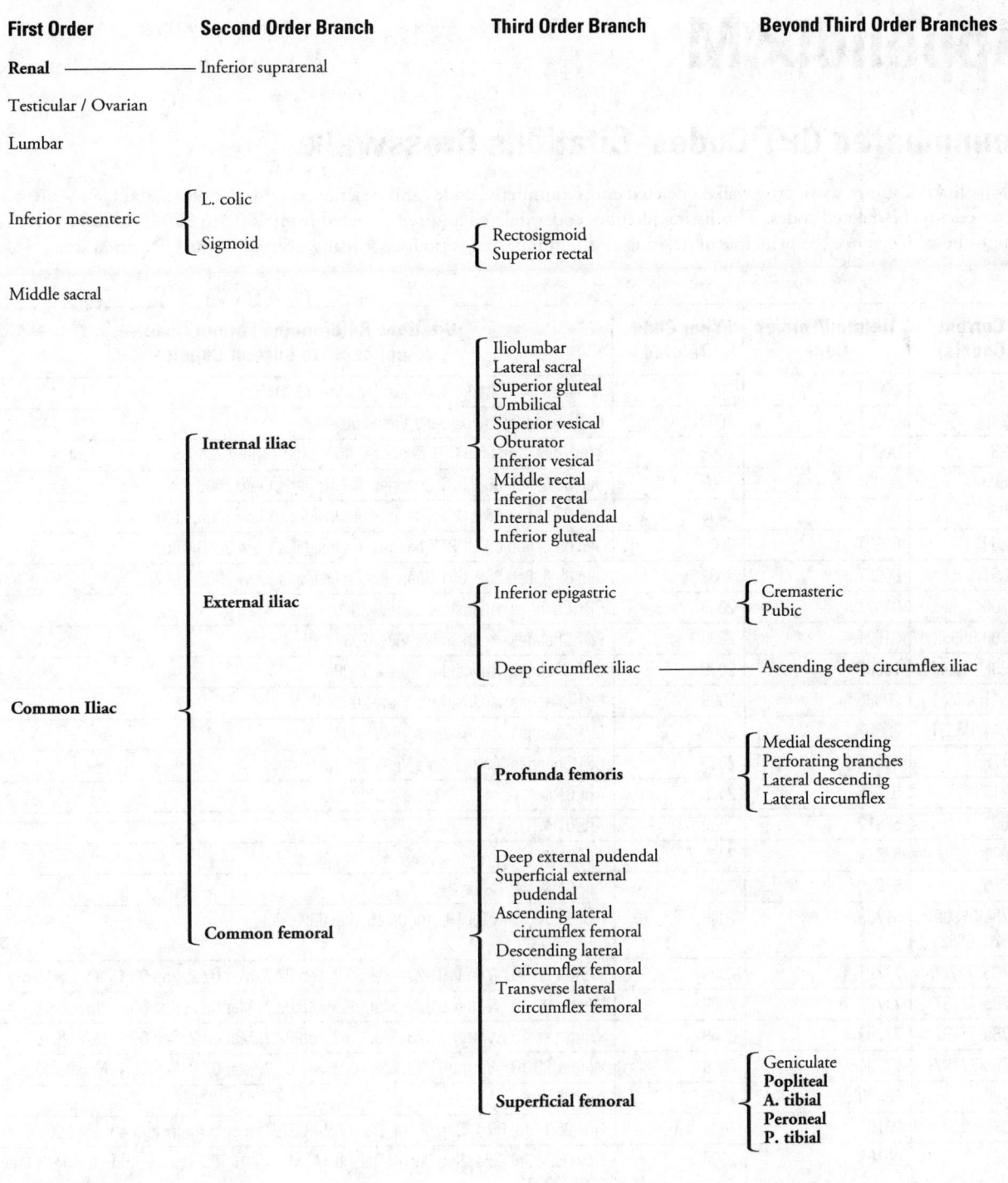

Reference: Kadir S. *Atlas of Normal and Variant Angiographic Anatomy.* Philadelphia, Pa: WB Saunders Co; 1991.
R = right, L = left, A = anterior, P = posterior

Appendix M

Renumbered CPT Codes–Citations Crosswalk

This listing is a summary of crosswalked deleted and renumbered codes and descriptors with the associated *CPT Assistant* references for the deleted codes. This listing includes codes deleted and renumbered from 2007 to 2009. Additional codes will not be added, since the principle of deleting and renumbering is no longer being utilized in the CPT code set.

Current Code(s)	Deleted/Former Code	Year Code Deleted	Citations Referencing Former Code— Applicable to Current Code(s)
89240	0058T	2009	Jun 04:8 CPT Changes: An Insider's View 2004
89240	0059T	2009	CPT Changes: An Insider's View 2004
41530	0088T	2009	May 05:7, Sep 05:9 CPT Changes: An Insider's View 2005
95803	0089T	2009	Jun 05:6, Feb 06:1 CPT Changes: An Insider's View 2006
22856	0090T	2009	Jun 05:6, Feb 06:1 CPT Changes: An Insider's View 2006, 2007
22864	0093T	2009	Jun 05:6, Feb 06:1 CPT Changes: An Insider's View 2006, 2007
22861	0096T	2009	Jun 05:6, Feb 06:1 CPT Changes: An Insider's View 2006, 2007
55706	0137T	2009	CPT Changes: An Insider's View 2006
95980-95982	0162T	2009	CPT Changes: An Insider's View 2007
1123F, 1124F	1080F	2009	CPT Changes: An Insider's View 2008
0054T, 0055T	20986	2009	CPT Changes: An Insider's View 2008
0054T, 0055T	20987	2009	CPT Changes: An Insider's View 2008
4177F	4007F	2009	CPT Changes: An Insider's View 2008
52214	52606	2009	Apr 01:4
52601	52612	2009	Apr 01:4
52601	52614	2009	Apr 01:4
52630	52620	2009	Apr 01:4
61796-61800, 63620, 63621	61793	2009	Nov 97:23, May 03:19, Apr 04:15, Jan 06:46
77785, 77786	77781	2009	Winter 90:10, Winter 91:23, Mar 99:3, Feb 02:7, Mar 02:2, Sep 05:1, Nov 05:15
77785-77787	77782	2009	Winter 90:10, Winter 91:23, Mar 99:3, Feb 02:7, Mar 02:2, Sep 05:1, Nov 05:15
77785-77787	77783	2009	Winter 90:10, Winter 91:23, Mar 99:3, Feb 02:7, Mar 02:2, Sep 05:1, Nov 05:15
77785-77787	77784	2009	Winter 90:10, Winter 91:23, Mar 99:3, Feb 02:7, Mar 02:2, Sep 05:1, Nov 05:15
88720	88400	2009	Aug 05:9
96360	90760	2009	Nov 05:1, Jul 06:4, Sep 06:14, Dec 06:14 CPT Changes: An Insider's View 2006, 2008
96361	90761	2009	Nov 05:1, Jul 06:4, Sep 06:14, Dec 06:14, Mar 07:10 CPT Changes: An Insider's View 2006, 2007
96365	90765	2009	Nov 05:1, Sep 06:14, Nov 06:22, Dec 06:14 CPT Changes: An Insider's View 2006
96366	90766	2009	Nov 05:1, Sep 06:14, Dec 06:14, Mar 07:10 CPT Changes: An Insider's View 2006, 2007
96367	90767	2009	Nov 05:1, Sep 06:14, Nov 06:22, Dec 06:14 CPT Changes: An Insider's View 2006
96368	90768	2009	Nov 05:1, Aug 06:11, Sep 06:14, Nov 06:22, Dec 06:14 CPT Changes: An Insider's View 2006
96369	90769	2009	CPT Changes: An Insider's View 2008
96370	90770	2009	CPT Changes: An Insider's View 2008
96371	90771	2009	CPT Changes: An Insider's View 2008
96372	90772	2009	Nov 05:1, Sep 06:14, Dec 06:14 CPT Changes: An Insider's View 2006
96373	90773	2009	Nov 05:1, Sep 06:14, Dec 06:14 CPT Changes: An Insider's View 2006

Current Code(s)	Deleted/Former Code	Year Code Deleted	Citations Referencing Former Code— Applicable to Current Code(s)
96374	90774	2009	Nov 05:1, Sep 06:14, Dec 06:14 CPT Changes: An Insider's View 2006
96375	90775	2009	Nov 05:1, Sep 06:14, Dec 06:14 CPT Changes: An Insider's View 2006
96376	90776	2009	CPT Changes: An Insider's View 2008
96379	90779	2009	Nov 05:1, Sep 06:14, Dec 06:14 CPT Changes: An Insider's View 2006
90951-90953, 90963, 90967	90918	2009	Fall 93:5, May 96:4, May 02:17, Jan 03:22
90954-90956, 90964, 90968	90919	2009	Fall 93:5, May 96:5, May 02:17, Jan 03:22
90957-90959, 90965, 90969	90920	2009	Fall 93:5, May 96:5, May 02:17, Jan 03:22
90960-90962, 90966, 90970	90921	2009	Fall 93:5, May 96:5, May 02:17, Jan 03:22
90951-90953, 90963, 90967	90922	2009	Fall 93:5, May 96:5, May 02:17, Jan 03:22
90954-90956, 90964, 90968	90923	2009	May 96:5, May 02:17, Jan 03:22
90957-90959, 90965, 90969	90924	2009	May 96:5, May 02:17, Jan 03:22
90960-90962, 90966, 90970	90925	2009	May 96:5, May 02:17, Jan 03:22
93285, 93291, 93298	93727	2009	Nov 99:50, Jul 00:5, CPT Changes: An Insider's View 2000
93280, 93288, 93294	93731	2009	Summer 94:23, Feb 98:11
93280, 93288, 93294	93732	2009	Summer 94:23, Feb 98:11, Mar 00:10
93293	93733	2009	Summer 94:23
93279, 93288, 93294	93734	2009	Summer 94:23, Feb 98:11
93279, 93288, 93294	93735	2009	Summer 94:23, Feb 98:11
93293	93736	2009	Summer 94:23
93282, 93289, 93292, 93295	93741	2009	Nov 99:50-51, Jul 00:5, Nov 00:9, Sep 05:8 CPT Changes: An Insider's View 2000, 2005
93282, 93289, 93292, 93295	93742	2009	Nov 99:50-51, Jul 00:5, Nov 00:9 CPT Changes: An Insider's View 2000, 2005
93283, 93289, 93295	93743	2009	Nov 99:50-51, Jul 00:5, Nov 00:9, Sep 05:8 CPT Changes: An Insider's View 2000
93283, 93289, 93295	93744	2009	Nov 99:50-51, Jul 00:5, Nov 00:9 CPT Changes: An Insider's View 2000
99466	99289	2009	May 05:1, Jul 06:4 CPT Changes: An Insider's View 2002, 2003
99467	99290	2009	CPT Changes: An Insider's View 2002
99468	99295	2009	Summer 93:1, Nov 97:4-5, Mar 98:11, Nov 99:5-6, Dec 00:14, Feb 03:15, Oct 03:1, May 05:1, Nov 05:10, CPT Changes: An Insider's View 2000, 2003, 2004, 2005
99469	99296	2009	Summer 93:1, Nov 97:4-5, Mar 98:11, Nov 99:5-6, Dec 00:14, Feb 03:15, Oct 03:1, Nov 05:10, CPT Changes: An Insider's View 2000, 2003, 2004, 2005, 2008
99471	99293	2009	Feb 03:15, Oct 03:2, Aug 04:7, 10, May 05:1, Nov 05:10, Jul 06:4, Apr 07:3 CPT Changes: An Insider's View 2003, 2004, 2005
99472	99294	2009	Feb 03:15, Oct 03:2, Aug 04:7, Nov 05:10, Jul 06:4, Apr 07:3 CPT Changes: An Insider's View 2003, 2004, 2005

Current Code(s)	Deleted/Former Code	Year Code Deleted	Citations Referencing Former Code—Applicable to Current Code(s)
99478	99298	2009	Nov 98:2-3, Nov 99: 5-6, Aug 00:4, Dec 00:15, Oct 03:2, May 05:1, Nov 05:10; CPT Changes: An Insider's View 2000, 2003
99479	99299	2009	Oct 03:2, Nov 05:10; CPT Changes: An Insider's View 2003
99480	99300	2009	CPT Changes: An Insider's View 2006
99460	99431	2009	Apr 97:10, Nov 97:9, Sep 98:5, Apr 04:14, May 05:1
99461	99432	2009	Sep 98:5, May 99:11, Apr 04:14
99462	99433	2009	Sep 98:5, Apr 03:27
99463	99435	2009	Sep 98:5, Apr 04:14
99464	99436	2009	Nov 97:9-10, Sep 98:5, Nov 99:5-6, Aug 00:3, Aug 04:9, Nov 05:15
99465	99440	2009	Summer 93:3, Mar 96:10, Nov 97:9, Sep 98:5, Nov 99:5-6, Aug 00:3, Oct 03:3, Aug 04:9, Apr 07:3
20985-20987	0054T	2008	May 04:14, Jun 04:8 CPT Changes: An Insider's View 2004
20985-20987	0055T	2008	May 04:14, Jun 04:8 CPT Changes: An Insider's View 2004, 2005
20985-20987	0056T	2008	May 04:14, Jun 04:8 CPT Changes: An Insider's View 2004
99174	0065T	2008	Mar 05:1, 3-4 CPT Changes: An Insider's View 2005
99444	0074T	2008	May 05:7, Sep 05:6 CPT Changes: An Insider's View 2005
99605-99607	0115T	2008	CPT Changes: An Insider's View 2006
99605-99607	0116T	2008	CPT Changes: An Insider's View 2006
99605-99607	0117T	2008	CPT Changes: An Insider's View 2006
50593	0135T	2008	CPT Changes: An Insider's View 2006, Clinical Examples in Radiology Winter 06:18
34806	0153T	2008	CPT Changes: An Insider's View 2007, Clinical Examples in Radiology Winter 06:19
93982	0154T	2008	CPT Changes: An Insider's View 2007, Clinical Examples in Radiology Winter 06:19
01935, 01936	01905	2008	Mar 06:15 CPT Changes: An Insider's View 2002
24357-24359	24350	2008	
24357-24359	24351	2008	
24357-24359	24352	2008	
24357-24359	24354	2008	
24357-24359	24356	2008	
3044F-3045F	3047F	2008	CPT Changes: An Insider's View 2007
3074F-3075F	3076F	2008	CPT Changes: An Insider's View 2007
32421	32000	2008	Spring 91:4, Winter 92:20
32422	32002	2008	Nov 03:14
32560	32005	2008	
32550	32019	2008	CPT Changes: An Insider's View 2005
32551	32020	2008	Fall 92:13, Nov 03:14
36591	36540	2008	Jan 02:11, Nov 02:3, Apr 03:26, Nov 05:1 CPT Changes: An Insider's View 2001, 2003
36593	36550	2008	Nov 99:20, Nov 05:1 CPT Changes: An Insider's View 2000
49203-49205, 58957, 58958	49200	2008	CPT Changes: An Insider's View 2003
49203-49205, 58957, 58958	49201	2008	
51100	51000	2008	Nov 99:32-33, Aug 00:3, Oct 03:2
51101	51005	2008	
51102	51010	2008	
60300	60001	2008	
67041, 67042, 67043	67038	2008	Aug 03:15, Sep 05:12

Current Code(s)	Deleted/Former Code	Year Code Deleted	Citations Referencing Former Code— Applicable to Current Code(s)
75557-75564	75552	2008	Fall 95:2
75557-75564	75553	2008	Fall 95:2
75557-75564	75554	2008	Fall 95:2
75557-75564	75555	2008	Fall 95:2
75557-75564	75556	2008	Fall 95:2
78610	78615	2008	CPT Changes: An Insider's View 2002
86356, 86486	86586	2008	Jul 98:11
99366-99368	99361	2008	May 05:1
99366-99368	99362	2008	
99441-99443	99371	2008	Spring 94:34, May 00:11, May 05:1, Nov 05:10
99441-99443	99372	2008	Spring 94:34, May 00:11, Nov 05:10
99441-99443	99373	2008	Spring 94:34, May 00:11, Nov 05:10
0160T, 0161T	0018T	2007	CPT Changes: An Insider's View 2002
96904	0044T	2007	CPT Changes: An Insider's View 2003, 2004
96904	0045T	2007	Jul 04:7 CPT Changes: An Insider's View 2004
77371-77373	0082T	2007	CPT Changes: An Insider's View 2005
77371-77373	0083T	2007	CPT Changes: An Insider's View 2005
22857	0091T	2007	CPT Changes: An Insider's View 2006
22865	0094T	2007	CPT Changes: An Insider's View 2006
22862	0097T	2007	CPT Changes: An Insider's View 2006
19105	0120T	2007	CPT Changes: An Insider's View 2006
15002, 15004	15000	2007	Fall 93:7, Apr 97:4, Aug 97:6, Sep 97:2, Nov 98:5, Jan 99:4, Apr 99:10, May 99:10, Nov 02:7, Aug 03:14 CPT Changes: An Insider's View 2001, 2006
15003, 15005	15001	2007	Nov 98:5-6, Jan 99:4, May 99:10, Aug 03:14
15830, 15847, 17999	15831	2007	May 01:11 CPT Changes: An Insider's View 2007
17311	17304	2007	Winter 94:19, Mar 99:11, Jun 99:10, Nov 02:7, Nov 03:15, Feb 04:11, Jul 04:2 CPT Changes: An Insider's View 2003
17312, 17314	17305	2007	Winter 94:19, Mar 99:11, Jun 99:10, Nov 02:7, Feb 04:11, Jul 04:3
17312, 17314	17306	2007	Winter 94:19, Mar 99:11, Jun 99:10, Nov 02:7, Feb 04:11, Jul 04:4
17312, 17314	17307	2007	Winter 94:19, Mar 99:11, Jun 99:10, Nov 02:7, Nov 03:15, Feb 04:11, Jul 04:4
17315	17310	2007	Winter 94:19, Mar 99:11, Jun 99:10, Nov 02:7, Feb 04:11, May 04:14, Jul 04:4 CPT Changes: An Insider's View 2003
19300	19140	2007	Feb 96:9, Apr 05:13
19301	19160	2007	Apr 05:7 CPT Changes: An Insider's View 2005
19302	19162	2007	Jun 00:11, Apr 05:7
19303	19180	2007	Apr 05:7
19304	19182	2007	Apr 05:7
19305	19200	2007	Apr 05:7
19306	19220	2007	Apr 05:7
19307	19240	2007	Apr 05:7
25606	25611	2007	Fall 93:23, Oct 99:5
25607-25609	25620	2007	
26390	26504	2007	
27325	27315	2007	
27326	27320	2007	

Current Code(s)	Deleted/Former Code	Year Code Deleted	Citations Referencing Former Code— Applicable to Current Code(s)
28055	28030	2007	
33254-33256	33253	2007	
35302-35306	35381	2007	
35506	35507	2007	
35537, 35538	35541	2007	
35539, 35540	35546	2007	
35637, 35638	35641	2007	Dec 01:7
44799	44152	2007	
44799	44153	2007	
47719	47716	2007	
48105	48005	2007	
48548	48180	2007	
49402	49085	2007	
54150	54152	2007	Sep 96:11, Dec 96:10, May 98:11, Apr 03:27 CPT Changes: An Insider's View 2007
54865	54820	2007	Oct 01:8
55875	55859	2007	Apr 04:6
56442	56720	2007	
57558	57820	2007	
67346	67350	2007	
77001	75998	2007	Dec 04:12-13 CPT Changes: An Insider's View 2004 Clinical Examples in Radiology Inaugural 04:1-2, Winter 05:9
77002	76003	2007	Fall 93:14, Jul 01:7 CPT Changes: An Insider's View 2001 Clinical Examples in Radiology Spring 05:5-6
77003	76005	2007	Nov 99:32, 34, 41, Jan 00:2, Feb 00:6, Aug 00:8, Sep 02:11, Sep 04:5 CPT Changes: An Insider's View 2000
77071	76006	2007	Nov 98:21 CPT Changes: An Insider's View 2003
72291	76012	2007	Mar 01:2 CPT Changes: An Insider's View 2001, 2006
72292	76013	2007	Mar 01:2 CPT Changes: An Insider's View 2001
77072	76020	2007	
77073	76040	2007	
77074	76061	2007	
77075	76062	2007	
77076	76065	2007	
77077	76066	2007	CPT Changes: An Insider's View 2002
77078	76070	2007	Nov 97:24 CPT Changes: An Insider's View 2002, 2003
77079	76071	2007	CPT Changes: An Insider's View 2003
77080	76075	2007	Nov 97:24, Jun 03:11 CPT Changes: An Insider's View 2005
77081	76076	2007	Nov 97:24
77082	76077	2007	CPT Changes: An Insider's View 2005
77083	76078	2007	Nov 97:24 CPT Changes: An Insider's View 2002
77051	76082	2007	CPT Changes: An Insider's View 2004
77052	76083	2007	CPT Changes: An Insider's View 2004
77053	76086	2007	
77054	76088	2007	
77055	76090	2007	Jul 96:6, Jun 99:10 CPT Changes: An Insider's View 2004
77056	76091	2007	Jul 96:6 CPT Changes: An Insider's View 2004

Current Code(s)	Deleted/Former Code	Year Code Deleted	Citations Referencing Former Code— Applicable to Current Code(s)
77057	76092	2007	Jul 96:6, Jun 99:10 CPT Changes: An Insider's View 2004
77058	76093	2007	
77059	76094	2007	
77031	76095	2007	Apr 96:9, Nov 97:24, Jan 01:9 CPT Changes: An Insider's View 2001
77032	76096	2007	Jan 01:10 CPT Changes: An Insider's View 2001
77011	76355	2007	CPT Changes: An Insider's View 2002, 2003
77012	76360	2007	Fall 93:12, Fall 94:2, Jan 01:9-10, Mar 05:2 CPT Changes: An Insider's View 2001, 2002, 2003
77013	76362	2007	Oct 02:4 CPT Changes: An Insider's View 2002, 2004
77014	76370	2007	Fall 91:12 CPT Changes: An Insider's View 2002, 2003
77021	76393	2007	Jan 01:10, Mar 05:2 CPT Changes: An Insider's View 2001, 2002
77022	76394	2007	Oct 02:4, Mar 05:5 CPT Changes: An Insider's View 2002, 2004
77084	76400	2007	
76775, 76776	76778	2007	CPT Changes: An Insider's View 2002
76998	76986	2007	CPT Changes: An Insider's View 2001
78707-78709	78704	2007	
78701-78709	78715	2007	
78761	78760	2007	
92700	92573	2007	
94002, 94004	94656	2007	Fall 92:30, Spring 95:4, Summer 95:4, Feb 96:9, Aug 00:2, Oct 03:2
94003, 94004	94657	2007	Fall 92:30, Spring 95:4, Summer 95:4, Feb 96:9, Aug 00:2, Oct 03:2

Appendix N

Summary of Resequenced CPT Codes

This is a summary of CPT codes that do not appear in numeric sequence in the listing of CPT codes. Rather than deleting and renumbering, resequencing allows existing codes to be relocated to an appropriate location for the code concept, regardless of the numeric sequence. The codes listed below are identified in CPT 2016 code set with a # symbol for location of the resequenced number within the family of related concepts. Numerically placed references (eg, **Code is out of numerical sequence. See...**) are used as navigational alerts to direct the user to the location of an out-of-sequence code.

11045	31651	37212	46946
11046	33221	37213	46947
21552	33227	37214	50430
21554	33228	38243	50431
22858	33229	43210	50432
23071	33230	43211	50433
23073	33231	43212	50434
24071	33262	43213	50435
24073	33263	43214	51797
25071	33264	43233	52356
25073	33270	43266	64461
26111	33271	43270	64462
26113	33272	43274	64463
27043	33273	43275	64633
27045	33962	43276	64634
27057	33963	43277	64635
27059	33964	43278	64636
27329	33965	44381	67810
27337	33966	44401	77085
27339	33969	45346	77086
27632	33984	45388	77295
27634	33985	45390	77385
28039	33986	45398	77386
28041	33987	45399	77387
29914	33988	46220	77424
29915	33989	46320	77425
29916	37211	46945	80081

80164	80354	88350	95938
80165	80355	88364	95939
80171	80356	88373	95940
80300	80357	88374	95941
80301	80358	88377	95943
80302	80359	90620	99177
80303	80360	90621	99224
80304	80361	90625	99225
80320	80362	90630	99226
80321	80363	90644	99415
80322	80364	90672	99416
80323	80365	90673	99485
80324	80366	92558	99486
80325	80367	92618	99490
80326	80368	92920	0253T
80327	80369	92921	0357T
80328	80370	92924	0376T
80329	80371	92925	
80330	80372	92928	
80331	80373	92929	
80332	80374	92933	
80333	80375	92934	
80334	80376	92937	
80335	80377	92938	
80336	81161	92941	
80337	81162	92943	
80338	81287	92944	
80339	81288	92973	
80340	81479	92974	
80341	82652	92975	
80342	83992	92977	
80343	86152	92978	
80344	86153	92979	
80345	87623	93260	
80346	87624	93261	
80347	87625	95782	
80348	87806	95783	
80349	87906	95800	
80350	87910	95801	
80351	87912	95885	
80352	88177	95886	
80353	88341	95887	

Appendix O

Multianalyte Assays with Algorithmic Analyses

The following list includes a set of administrative codes for Multianalyte Assays with Algorithmic Analyses (MAAA) procedures that by their nature are typically unique to a single clinical laboratory or manufacturer.

Multianalyte Assays with Algorithmic Analyses (MAAAs) are procedures that utilize multiple results derived from assays of various types, including molecular pathology assays, fluorescent in situ hybridization assays and non-nucleic acid based assays (eg, proteins, polypeptides, lipids, carbohydrates). Algorithmic analysis using the results of these assays as well as other patient information (if used) is then performed and reported typically as a numeric score(s) or as a probability. MAAAs are typically unique to a single clinical laboratory or manufacturer. The results of individual component procedure(s) that are inputs to the MAAAs may be provided on the associated laboratory report, however these assays are not reported separately using additional codes.

The list includes a proprietary name and clinical laboratory or manufacturer in the first column, an alpha-numeric code in the second column and code descriptor in the third column. The format for the code descriptor usually includes (in order):

- Disease type (eg, oncology, autoimmune, tissue rejection),

- Chemical(s) analyzed (eg, DNA, RNA, protein, antibody),

- Number of markers (eg, number of genes, number of proteins),

- Methodology(s) (eg, microarray, real-time [RT]-PCR, in situ hybridization [ISH], enzyme linked immunosorbent assays [ELISA]),

- Number of functional domains (if indicated),

- Specimen type (eg, blood, fresh tissue, formalin-fixed paraffin embedded),

- Algorithm result type (eg, prognostic, diagnostic),

- Report (eg, probability index, risk score).

MAAA procedures that have been assigned a Category I code are noted in the list below and additionally listed in the Category I MAAA section (81500-81599). The Category I MAAA section introductory language and associated parenthetical instruction(s) should be used to govern the appropriate use for Category I MAAA codes. If a specific MAAA procedure has not been assigned a Category I code, it is indicated as a four-digit number followed by the letter M.

When a specific MAAA procedure is not included in either the list below or in the Category I MAAA section, report the analysis using the Category I MAAA unlisted code (81599). The codes below are specific to the assays identified in Appendix O by proprietary name. In order to report an MAAA code, the analysis performed must fulfill the code descriptor **and**, if proprietary, must be the test represented by the proprietary name listed in Appendix O. When an analysis is performed that may potentially fall within a specific descriptor, however the proprietary name is not included in the list below, the MAAA unlisted code (81599) should be used.

Additions in this section may be released tri-annually via the AMA CPT website to expedite dissemination for reporting. The list will be published annually in the CPT codebook. Go to www.ama-assn.org/go/cpt for the most current listing.

These administrative codes encompass all analytical services required for the algorithmic analysis (eg, cell lysis, nucleic acid stabilization, extraction, digestion, amplification, hybridization and detection) in addition to the algorithmic analysis itself. Procedures that are required prior to cell lysis (eg, microdissection, codes 88380 and 88381) should be reported separately.

The codes in this list are provided as an administrative coding set to facilitate accurate reporting of MAAA services. The minimum standard for inclusion in this list is that an analysis is generally available for patient care. The AMA has not reviewed procedures in the administrative coding set for clinical utility. The list is not a complete list of all MAAA procedures.

Proprietary Name and Clinical Laboratory or Manufacturer	Alpha-Numeric Code	Code Descriptor
Administrative Codes for Multianalyte Assays with Algorithmic Analyses (MAAA)		
HCV FibroSURE™, LabCorp ►FibroTest™, Quest Diagnostics/ BioPredictive◄	▲ 0001M	Infectious disease, HCV, six biochemical assays (ALT, A2-macroglobulin, apolipoprotein A-1, total bilirubin, GGT, and haptoglobin) utilizing serum, prognostic algorithm reported as scores for fibrosis and necroinflammatory activity in liver
ASH FibroSURE™, LabCorp	0002M	Liver disease, ten biochemical assays (ALT, A2-macroglobulin, apolipoprotein A-1, total bilirubin, GGT, haptoglobin, AST, glucose, total cholesterol and triglycerides) utilizing serum, prognostic algorithm reported as quantitative scores for fibrosis, steatosis and alcoholic steatohepatitis (ASH)
NASH FibroSURE™, LabCorp	0003M	Liver disease, ten biochemical assays (ALT, A2-macroglobulin, apolipoprotein A-1, total bilirubin, GGT, haptoglobin, AST, glucose, total cholesterol and triglycerides) utilizing serum, prognostic algorithm reported as quantitative scores for fibrosis, steatosis and nonalcoholic steatohepatitis (NASH)
ScoliScore™ Transgenomic	0004M	Scoliosis, DNA analysis of 53 single nucleotide polymorphisms (SNPs), using saliva, prognostic algorithm reported as a risk score
	(0005M has been deleted, use 81507)	—
HeproDX™, GoPath Laboratories, LLC	0006M	Oncology (hepatic), mRNA expression levels of 161 genes, utilizing fresh hepatocellular carcinoma tumor tissue, with alpha-fetoprotein level, algorithm reported as a risk classifier
NETest (Wren Laboratories, LLC)	0007M	Oncology (gastrointestinal neuroendocrine tumors), real-time PCR expression analysis of 51 genes, utilizing whole peripheral blood, algorithm reported as a nomogram of tumor disease index
Prosigna Breast Cancer Assay (NanoString Technologies)	0008M	Oncology (breast), mRNA analysis of 58 genes using hybrid capture, on formalin-fixed paraffin-embedded (FFPE) tissue, prognostic algorithm reported as a risk score
VisibiliT test, Sequenom Center for Molecular Medicine, LLC	● 0009M	Fetal aneuploidy (trisomy 21, and 18) DNA sequence analysis of selected regions using maternal plasma, algorithm reported as a risk score for each trisomy
4Kscore test, OPKO Diagnostics, LLC	● 0010M	Oncology (High-Grade Prostate Cancer), biochemical assay of four proteins (Total PSA, Free PSA, Intact PSA and human kallikrein 2 [hK2]) plus patient age, digital rectal examination status, and no history of positive prostate biopsy, utilizing plasma, prognostic algorithm reported as a probability score

Category I Codes for Multianalyte Assays with Algorithmic Analyses (MAAA)		
Vectra® DA, Crescendo Bioscience, Inc.	● 81490	Autoimmune (rheumatoid arthritis), analysis of 12 biomarkers using immunoassays, utilizing serum, prognostic algorithm reported as a disease activity score (Do not report 81490 in conjunction with 86140)
Corus® CAD, CardioDx, Inc.	● 81493	Coronary artery disease, mRNA, gene expression profiling by real-time RT-PCR of 23 genes, utilizing whole peripheral blood, algorithm reported as a risk score
AlloMap®, CareDx, Inc.	● 81595	Cardiology (heart transplant), mRNA, gene expression profiling by real-time quantitative PCR of 20 genes (11 content and 9 housekeeping), utilizing subfraction of peripheral blood, algorithm reported as a rejection risk score
Risk of Ovarian Malignancy Algorithm (ROMA)™, Fujirebio Diagnostics	81500	Oncology (ovarian), biochemical assays of two proteins (CA-125 and HE4), utilizing serum, with menopausal status, algorithm reported as a risk score
OVA1™, Vermillion, Inc.	81503	Oncology (ovarian), biochemical assays of five proteins (CA-125, apoliproprotein A1, beta-2 microglobulin, transferrin, and pre-albumin), utilizing serum, algorithm reported as a risk score
Pathwork® Tissue of Origin Test, Pathwork Diagnostics	81504	Oncology (tissue of origin), microarray gene expression profiling of >2000 genes, utilizing formalin-fixed paraffin embedded tissue, algorithm reported as tissue similarity scores
PreDx Diabetes Risk Score™, Tethys Clinical Laboratory	81506	Endocrinology (type 2 diabetes), biochemical assays of seven analytes (glucose, HbA1c, insulin, hs-CRP, adiponectin, ferritin, interleukin 2-receptor alpha), utilizing serum or plasma, algorithm reporting a risk score
Harmony™ Prenatal Test, Ariosa Diagnostics	81507	Fetal aneuploidy (trisomy 21, 18, and 13) DNA sequence analysis of selected regions using maternal plasma, algorithm reported as a risk score for each trisomy

(*Continued on page 558*)

(Continued from page 557)

No proprietary name and clinical laboratory or manufacturer. Maternal serum screening procedures are well established procedures and are performed by many labs throughout the country. The concept of prenatal screens has existed and evolved for over ten years and is not exclusive to any one facility.	81508	Fetal congenital abnormalities, biochemical assays of two proteins (PAPP-A, hCG [any form]), utilizing maternal serum, algorithm reported as a risk score
	81509	Fetal congenital abnormalities, biochemical assays of three proteins (PAPP-A, hCG [any form], DIA), utilizing maternal serum, algorithm reported as a risk score
	81510	Fetal congenital abnormalities, biochemical assays of three analytes (AFP, uE3, hCG [any form]), utilizing maternal serum, algorithm reported as a risk score
	81511	Fetal congenital abnormalities, biochemical assays of four analytes (AFP, uE3, hCG [any form], DIA) utilizing maternal serum, algorithm reported as a risk score (may include additional results from previous biochemical testing)
	81512	Fetal congenital abnormalities, biochemical assays of five analytes (AFP, uE3, total hCG, hyperglycosylated hCG, DIA) utilizing maternal serum, algorithm reported as a risk score
Oncotype DX® (Genomic Health)	81519	Oncology (breast), mRNA, gene expression profiling by real-time RT-PCR of 21 genes, utilizing formalin-fixed paraffin embedded tissue, algorithm reported as recurrence score
Oncotype DX® Colon Cancer Assay, Genomic Health	● 81525	Oncology (colon), mRNA, gene expression profiling by real-time RT-PCR of 12 genes (7 content and 5 housekeeping), utilizing formalin-fixed paraffin-embedded tissue, algorithm reported as a recurrence score
Cologuard™, Exact Sciences, Inc.	● 81528	Oncology (colorectal) screening, quantitative real-time target and signal amplification of 10 DNA markers (KRAS mutations, promoter methylation of NDRG4 and BMP3) and fecal hemoglobin, utilizing stool, algorithm reported as a positive or negative result (Do not report 81528 in conjunction with 81275, 82274)
ChemoFX®, Helomics, Corp.	● 81535 ✚ ● 81536	Oncology (gynecologic), live tumor cell culture and chemotherapeutic response by DAPI stain and morphology, predictive algorithm reported as a drug response score; first single drug or drug combination each additional single drug or drug combination (List separately in addition to code for primary procedure) (Use 81536 in conjunction with 81535)
VeriStrat, Biodesix, Inc.	● 81538	Oncology (lung), mass spectrometric 8-protein signature, including amyloid A, utilizing serum, prognostic and predictive algorithm reported as good versus poor overall survival

(Continued on page 559)

(Continued from page 558)

CancerTYPE ID, bioTheranostics, Inc.	● 81540	Oncology (tumor of unknown origin), mRNA, gene expression profiling by real-time RT-PCR of 92 genes (87 content and 5 housekeeping) to classify tumor into main cancer type and subtype, utilizing formalin-fixed paraffin-embedded tissue, algorithm reported as a probability of a predicted main cancer type and subtype
Afirma® Gene Expression Classifier, Veracyte, Inc.	● 81545	Oncology (thyroid), gene expression analysis of 142 genes, utilizing fine needle aspirate, algorithm reported as a categorical result (eg, benign or suspicious)
	81599	Unlisted multianalyte assay with algorithmic analysis

Appendix O

Notes

Index

Instructions for the Use of the CPT Index

The alphabetic index is **not** a substitute for the main text of the CPT codebook. Even if only one code is present, the user must refer to the main text to ensure that the code selected accurately identifies the service(s) performed.

Main Terms

The index is organized by main terms. Each main term can stand alone, or be followed by up to three modifying terms. There are four primary classes of main entries:

1. Procedure or service.
   For example: Endoscopy; Anastomosis; Splint

2. Organ or other anatomic site.
   For example: Tibia; Colon; Salivary Gland

3. Condition.
   For example: Abscess; Entropion; Tetralogy of Fallot

4. Synonyms, Eponyms, and Abbreviations.
   For example: EEG; Bricker Operation; Clagett Procedure

The Anesthesia-section codes are indexed under the Anesthesia main entry and are not double-entered under the anatomical sites. Only specific codes within the Surgery, Medicine, Category II, and Category III sections that reference the service of anesthesia are indexed under the anatomical sites.

Modifying Terms

A main term may be followed by up to three indented terms that modify the terms they follow. For example, the main term Endoscopy is subdivided by the anatomical sites in which it is used, and within these anatomical sites, the specific purpose of the procedure is identified. In the following example, the code for an endoscopic removal of calculus from the urethra could be located:

Urethra
    Removal
        Calculus 52352

Note that in this entry, the inclusion of a subentry under "Removal" implies the reading "Removal [of]" the term that follows it. If no subheads followed "Removal," the procedure would relate to the subhead that preceded it, as in this entry for the endoscopic removal of the spleen:

Spleen
    Removal 38120

When modifying terms appear, one should review the list, as these subterms further qualify the selection of the appropriate code for the procedure.

Code Ranges

Whenever more than one code applies to a given index entry, a code range is listed. If several nonsequential codes apply, they will be separated by a comma. In the following example, three nonsequential codes apply:

Esophagus
    Reconstruction 43300, 43310, 43313

If three or more sequential codes apply, they will be separated by a hyphen. If more than one code range applies, the code ranges will be separated by a comma as in the following example:

Monitoring
    Electroencephalogram 95812-95813, 95950-95953

Conventions

As a space-saving convention, certain terms carry meaning inferred from the context. This convention is primarily used when a procedure or service is listed as a subterm. For example:

Knee
    Exploration [of] 27310, 27331

In this example, the bracketed qualifier "[of]" does not appear in the index; "of" is understood in the context of the term "Exploration." As another example:

Pelvis
    Halo [Application of] 20662

In this example, as there is no such entity as "pelvis halo," the bracketed words are inferred.

Pathology and Laboratory

The Pathology and Laboratory listing in the index presents the headings, subheadings, procedures, and analytes in the Pathology and Laboratory section of the CPT codebook. Analytes are either listed alphabetically (for example, the Chemistry analytes) or cross-referenced to the index main heads where they are alphabetically listed (for example, to reference infectious agent analytes, the entry will indicate "See Infectious Agents").

A

A Vitamin
See Vitamin, A

A-II
See Angiotensin II

Abbe-Estlander Procedure
Lip Reconstruction 40527, 40761
See Reconstruction; Repair, Cleft Lip

Abdomen
Abdominal Aorta
  Angiography. 75635
Abdominal Wall
  Debridement
    Infected. 11005, 11006
  Removal
    Mesh. 11008
    Prosthesis. 11008
  Repair
    Hernia. 49491-49496, 49501,
               49507, 49521, 49590
  Tumor
    Excision. 22900-22903
    Radical Resection. 22904, 22905
Abscess
  Incision and Drainage
    Open 49020, 49040
Anesthesia
  See Anesthesia, Abdomen
Angiography 74174, 74175, 74185, 75635
Aorta
  See Abdomen, Abdominal Aorta; Aorta,
  Abdominal
Aortic Aneurysm
  See Aorta, Abdominal, Aneurysm
Artery
  Ligation 37617
Biopsy 49000
Bypass Graft
  Excision 35907
Catheter
  Removal 49422
Celiotomy
  See Laparotomy
  for Staging 49220
CT Scan 74150, 74160, 74170,
             74174-74178, 75635
Cyst
  Destruction/Excision 49203-49205
Deliveries
  See Cesarean Delivery
Drainage
  Fluid 49082, 49083
Ectopic Pregnancy. 59130
Endometrioma
  Destruction/Excision 49203-49205
Exploration 49000, 49010
  Blood Vessel. 35840
  Staging. 58960
Hysterectomy
  See Hysterectomy, Abdominal
Incision 49000-49084
  Staging. 58960
Incision and Drainage
  Pancreatitis 48000
Infraumbilical Panniculectomy 15830

Injection
  Air. 49400
  Contrast Material. 49400
Insertion
  Catheter 49324, 49418, 49419, 49421
  Venous Shunt. 49425
Intraperitoneal
  Catheter Exit Site. 49436
  Catheter Insertion 49418-49421, 49435
  Catheter Removal 49422
  Catheter Revision. 49325
  Shunt
    Insertion 49425
    Ligation. 49428
    Removal 49429
    Revision 49426
Laparoscopy 49320-49327, 49329
Laparotomy
  Reopening 49002
  Staging. 49220, 58960
Lymphangiogram
  See Lymphangiography, Abdomen
Magnetic Resonance Imaging
(MRI) 74181-74183
Needle Biopsy (Mass). 49180
Paracentesis 49082, 49083
Radical Resection 51597
Radiation Therapy
  Placement of Guidance
    Devices. 49411, 49412
Radiographies
  See Abdomen, X-ray
Removal
  Node(s). 49220
Repair
  Blood Vessel. 35221
    with Other Graft 35281
    with Vein Graft 35251
  Hernia. 49491-49525, 49560-49587, 49590
  Suture. 49900
Revision
  Venous Shunt. 49426
Suture 49900
Tumor
  Destruction/Excision 49203-49205
Ultrasound. 76700-76705
Unlisted Services and Procedures 49999
Wall
  See Abdomen, Abdominal Wall
Wound Exploration
  Penetrating. 20102
X-ray 74000, 74010, 74020, 74022

Abdominal
See Abdomen
Aorta
  See Abdomen, Abdominal Aorta; Aorta,
  Abdominal
Aortic Aneurysm
  See Aorta, Abdominal, Aneurysm
Deliveries
  See Cesarean Delivery
Hysterectomy
  See Hysterectomy, Abdominal
Lymphangiogram
  See Lymphangiography, Abdomen
Paracentesis
  See Abdomen, Drainage
Radiographies
  See Abdomen, X-ray
Wall
  See Abdomen, Abdominal Wall

Abdominohysterectomy
See Hysterectomy, Abdominal

Abdominopelvic Amputation
See Amputation, Interpelviabdominal

Abdominoplasty
See Panniculectomy
Excision, Skin and Tissue 15830, 15847
Unlisted Procedure 17999

Ablation
Anus
  Polyp. 46615
  Tumor 46615
Bone
  Tumor
    with Adjacent Soft Tissue 20982, 20983
Colon
  Lesion. 44401, 45346, 45388
  Polyp. 44401, 45346, 45388
  Tumor 44401, 45346, 45388
Cryosurgical
  Fibroadenoma 19105
  Liver Tumor. 47381, 47383
  Renal Mass 50250
  Renal Tumor
    Percutaneous 50593
CT Scan Guidance. 77013
Endometrial. 58353, 58356, 58563
  with Ultrasound Guidance. 58356
Uterine Fibroids
  Laparoscopic 0336T
  Radiofrequency 0404T
Heart
  Arrhythmogenic Focus . . 33250, 33251, 33261,
               93653, 93654, 93655
  Atrioventricular 93650, 93653, 93654
Liver (Tumor)
  Cryosurgical 47381, 47383
  Laparoscopic 47370, 47371
  Radiofrequency 47380-47382
Lung
  Tumor
    Radiofrequency. 32998
Parenchymal Tissue
  CT Scan Guidance 77013
  Magnetic Resonance Guidance. 77022
  Ultrasound Guidance 76940
Prostate. 55873
Pulmonary Tumor 0340T, 32998
Radiofrequency
  Liver Tumor. 47382
  Lung Tumor. 32998
  Renal Tumor 50592
  Tongue Base. 41530
  Uterine Fibroid 0404T
Rectum
  Lesion. 45346
  Polyp. 45346
  Tumor 45346
Renal Cyst. 50541
Renal Mass 50542
Renal Tumor
  Cryotherapy
    Percutaneous 50593
  Radiofrequency 50592
Stereotactic
  Intracranial Lesion
    Magnetic Resonance Image
    Guided High Intensity Focused
    Ultrasound (MRgFUS). 0398T

Tongue Base
  Radiofrequency 41530
Turbinate Mucosa 30801, 30802
Uterine Tumor
  Ultrasound, Focused 0071T, 0072T
Vein
  Endovenous 36475-36479

Abortion
See Obstetrical Care
Incomplete 59812
Induced
  by Dilation and Curettage 59840
  by Dilation and Evacuation 59841
  by Saline 59850, 59851
  by Vaginal Suppositories 59855, 59856
  with Hysterotomy 59100, 59852, 59857
Missed
  First Trimester 59820
  Second Trimester 59821
Septic 59830
Spontaneous
  Complete
    See Hospital Services
  Incomplete 59812
Therapeutic
  by Saline 59850
    with Dilation and Curettage 59851
    with Hysterotomy 59852

Abrasion (Skin)
Chemical Peel 15788, 15789, 15792, 15793
Dermabrasion 15780-15783
Lesion 15786, 15787

Abscess
Bone
  Ankle
    Incision 27607
  Clavicle
    Sequestrectomy 23170
  Elbow
    Incision 23930, 23935
  Facial
    Excision 21026
  Femur
    Incision 27303
  Finger
    Incision 26034
  Foot
    Incision 28005
  Forearm
    Incision 25035
    Sequestrectomy 25145
  Humeral Head
    Incision 23174
  Humerus
    Excision 24134
    Incision and Drainage 23935
  Knee
    Incision 27303
  Leg, Lower
    Incision 27607
  Olecranon Process 24138
    Sequestrectomy 24136
  Pelvis
    Incision 26992
  Radius
    Incision, Deep 25035
    Sequestrectomy 24136
  Scapula
    Sequestrectomy 23172
  Shoulder
    Incision 23035

Thorax
  Incision 21510
Wrist
  Incision 25035
  Sequestrectomy 25145
Drainage
  with X-ray 75989
Localization
  Nuclear Medicine 78806, 78807
Tissue
  Abdomen 49040
    Incision and Drainage 49040
  Anus
    Incision and Drainage 46045-46060
  Ankle
    Incision and Drainage 27603
  Appendix
    Incision and Drainage 44900
  Arm, Lower
    Incision and Drainage 25028
  Auditory Canal, External
    Incision and Drainage 69020
  Bartholin's Gland
    Incision and Drainage 56420
  Bladder
    Incision and Drainage 51080
  Brain
    Drainage via Burr Hole 61150, 61151
    Drainage via Craniotomy 61320, 61321
    Excision 61514, 61522
  Breast
    Incision and Drainage 19020
  Ear, External
    Incision and Drainage 69000, 69005
  Elbow
    Incision and Drainage 23930, 23931
  Epididymis
    Incision and Drainage 54700
  Eyelid
    Incision and Drainage 67700
  Finger
    Incision and Drainage 26010, 26011
  Forearm
    Incision and Drainage 25028
  Gums
    Incision and Drainage 41800
  Hand
    Incision and Drainage 26034
  Hip
    Incision and Drainage 26990-26992
  Kidney
    Incision and Drainage 50020
  Knee
    Incision and Drainage 27301
  Leg, Lower
    Incision and Drainage 27603
  Liver
    Drainage
      Open 47010
      Injection 47015
      Marsupialization 47300
  Lung
    Percutaneous Drainage 32200
  Lymph Node
    Incision and Drainage 38300, 38305
  Lymphocele Drainage 49062
  Mandible
    Excision 21025
  Mouth 41015-41018
    Incision and Drainage
      Dentoalveolar 41800
      Lingual 41000
      Masticator Space 41009, 41018

Sublingual 41005, 41006, 41015
Submandibular 41008, 41017
Submental 41007, 41016
Vestibular 40800, 40801
Subfascial
  Incision and Drainage 20005
Nasal
  Incision and Drainage 30000, 30020
Neck
  Incision and Drainage 21501, 21502
Olecranon Process
  Excision 24138
Ovary
  Incision and Drainage 58820, 58822
    Abdominal Approach 58822
    Vaginal Approach 58820
Palate
  Incision and Drainage 42000
Paraurethral Gland
  Incision and Drainage 53060
Parotid Gland
  Drainage 42300, 42305
Pelvis
  Incision and Drainage . . 26990, 26991, 45000
Pericolic
Perineum
  Incision and Drainage 56405
Perirenal or Renal
  Incision and Drainage 50020
Peritoneum
  Incision and Drainage 49020
Pharynx
  Incision and Drainage 42720, 42725
Prostate
  Incision and Drainage 55720, 55725
  Transurethral Drainage 52700
Rectum
  Incision and Drainage 45005, 45020,
                                      46040, 46060
Renal
  Incision and Drainage 50020
Retroperitoneal
  Incision and Drainage 49060
Salivary Gland
  Drainage 42300-42320
Scrotum
  Incision and Drainage 54700, 55100
Shoulder
  Incision and Drainage 23030
Skene's Gland
  Incision and Drainage 53060
Skin/Superficial
  Incision and Drainage 10060, 10061
  Puncture Aspiration 10160
Spine
  Incision and Drainage 22010, 22015
Subdiaphragmatic
  Drainage 49040
Sublingual Gland
  Drainage 42310-42320
Submaxillary Gland
  Drainage 42310, 42320
Subphrenic
  Drainage 49040
Testis
  Incision and Drainage 54700
Thigh
  Incision and Drainage 27301
Thorax
  Incision and Drainage 21501, 21502
Throat
  Incision and Drainage 42700-42725

Tongue
　Incision and Drainage....... 41000-41006
Tonsil
　Incision and Drainage............ 42700
Urethra
　Incision and Drainage............ 53040
Uvula
　Incision and Drainage............ 42000
Vagina
　Incision and Drainage............ 57010
Vulva
　Incision and Drainage............ 56405
Wrist
　Incision and Drainage....... 25028, 25035
X-ray................................ 76080

Abscess, Nasal
See Nose, Abscess

Abscess, Parotid Gland
See Parotid Gland, Abscess

Absorptiometry, X-ray (DXA)
Bone Density Study
　Dual-Energy
　　Appendicular 77081
　　Axial Skeleton 77080
　　Vertebral.............. 77085, 77086
　Dual Photon 78351
　Single Photon.................... 78350
Diagnostic Screening 3095F, 3096F

Absorption Spectrophotometry, Atomic
See Atomic Absorption Spectroscopy

Accessory Nerve, Spinal
Anastomosis, Facial-Spinal 64866
Avulsion 64772
Laminectomy........................... 63191
Transection 64772
Chemodenervation, Muscles 64615

Accessory, Toe
See Polydactyly, Toe

ACE
See Angiotensin Converting Enzyme (ACE)

Acetabuloplasty 27120-27122, 29915

Acetabulum
Fracture
　Closed Treatment............. 27220-27222
　　with Manipulation 27222
　　without Manipulation.............. 27220
　Open Treatment 27226-27228
Reconstruction 27120
　with Resection, Femoral Head........ 27122
Tumor
　Excision 27076

Acetic Anhydride
Analyte 84600

Acetylcholinesterase
Blood or Urine........................ 82013

AcG (Accelerator Globulin)
See Clotting Factor

Achilles Tendon
Incision 27605, 27606
Lengthening 27612
Repair 27650-27654

Achillotomy
See Tenotomy, Achilles Tendon

Acid
Gastric................................ 82930

Acid Diethylamide, Lysergic
See Lysergic Acid Diethylamide

Acid-Fast Bacilli (AFB)
Culture............................... 87116

Acid-Fast Bacillus Culture
See Culture, Acid-Fast Bacilli

Acid-Fast Stain
Analysis.............................. 88312

Acid Perfusion Study
Esophagus.................... 91013, 91030

Acid Phosphatase ... 84060, 84061, 84066

Acid Probes, Nucleic
See Nucleic Acid Probe

Acid Reflux Test
Esophagus......... 91034, 91035, 91037, 91038
Gastroesophageal.... 91034, 91035, 91037, 91038

Acid, Adenylic
See Adenosine Monophosphate (AMP),
5-Monophosphate, Cyclic

Acid, Aminolevulinic
See Aminolevulinic Acid (ALA)

Acid, Ascorbic
See Ascorbic Acid

Acid, Deoxyribonucleic (DNA)
See Deoxyribonucleic Acid (DNA)

Acid, Folic
See Folic Acid

Acid, Glycocholic
See Cholylglycine

Acid, Lactic
See Lactic Acid

Acid, N-Acetylneuraminic
See Sialic Acid

Acid, Phenylethylbarbituric
See Phenobarbital

Acid, Uric
See Uric Acid

Acidity/Alkalinity
See Blood Gases, pH

Acids, Amino
See Amino Acids

Acids, Bile
See Bile Acids

Acids, Fatty
See Fatty Acid

Acne Surgery
Incision and Drainage
　Abscess 10060, 10061
　Comedones 10040
　Cyst 10040
　Milia, Multiple.................. 10040
　Pustules 10040

Acne Treatment
Abrasion 15786, 15787
Chemical Peel 15788-15793
Cryotherapy........................ 17340
Dermabrasion 15780-15783
Exfoliation
　Chemical 17360

Acoustic Cardiography 93799

Acoustic Evoked Brain Stem Potential
See Evoked Potential, Auditory Brainstem

Acoustic Neuroma
See Brain, Tumor, Excision; Brainstem;
Mesencephalon; Skull Base Surgery

Acoustic Recording
Heart Sounds
　with Computer Analysis............. 93799

Acoustic Respiratory Measurements
for Wheeze Rate...................... 94799

Acromioclavicular Joint
Arthrocentesis................. 20605, 20606
Arthrotomy 23044
　with Biopsy 23101
Dislocation 23540-23552
　Open Treatment 23550-23552
X-ray................................ 73050

Acromion
Excision............................. 23130

Acromionectomy
Partial............................... 23130

Acromioplasty 23415-23420
Partial............................... 23130

ACTH
See Adrenocorticotropic Hormone (ACTH)

ACTH Releasing Factor
See Corticotropic Releasing Hormone (CRH)

Actigraphy
Sleep Study.......................... 95803

Actinomyces
Antibody Detection................... 86602

Actinomycosis
Antibody Detection................... 86602

Actinomycotic Infection
See Actinomycosis

Actinotherapy.................... 96900
See Dermatology

Activated Factor X
See Stuart-Prower Factor

Activated Partial Thromboplastin Time (aPTT)
See Thromboplastin, Partial Thromboplastin Time (PTT)

Activation, Lymphocyte
See Blastogenesis

Activities of Daily Living
See Physical Medicine/Therapy/Occupational Therapy

Activity, Glomerular Procoagulant
See Thromboplastin

Acupuncture
with Electrical Stimulation 97813, 97814
without Electrical Stimulation 97810, 97811

Acute Poliomyelitis
See Polio

Acylcarnitines 82016, 82017

Adamantinoma, Pituitary
See Craniopharyngioma

Addam Operation
See Dupuytren's Contracture

Adductor Tenotomy of Hip
See Tenotomy, Hip, Adductor

Adenoidectomy
See Adenoids, Excision

Adenoids
Excision. 42830-42836
   with Tonsils 42820, 42821
Unlisted Services and Procedures 42999

Adenoma
Pancreas
   Excision 48120
Parathyroid
   Localization
      Injection Procedure. 78808
Thyroid Gland Excision 60200

Adenosine 3'5' Monophosphate
See Cyclic AMP

Adenosine Diphosphate
Blood. 82030

Adenosine Monophosphate (AMP)
5-Monophosphate, Cyclic
   Blood 82030

Adenovirus
Antibody Detection. 86603
Antigen Detection
   Immunoassay. 87301
   Immunofluorescence 87260

Adenovirus Vaccine
See Vaccines

Adenylic Acid
See Adenosine Monophosphate (AMP)

ADH
See Antidiuretic Hormone

Adhesions
Epidural. 62263, 62264
Eye
   Corneovitreal 65880
   Incision
      Anterior Segment. 65860, 65870
      Posterior Segment 65875
   Construction. 67880
      Transposition of Tarsal Plate 67882
Intestinal
   Enterolysis 44005
      Laparoscopic. 44180
Intracranial
   Dissection 62161
Intrauterine
   Lysis 58559

Labial
   Lysis 56441
Liver
   Lysis 58660
Lungs
   Pneumonolysis. 32124, 32940
Nose
   Lysis 30560
Pelvic
   Lysis 58660, 58740
Penile
   Lysis
      Post-circumcision 54162
Preputial
   Lysis 54450
Urethral
   Lysis 53500

Adipectomy
See Lipectomy

ADL
See Activities of Daily Living

Administration
Immunization
   Each Additional Vaccine/Toxoid 90472, 90474
      with Counseling 90461
   One Vaccine/Toxoid 90471, 90473
      with Counseling 90460
Occlusive Substance. 31634
Pharmacologic Agent 93463

ADP
See Adenosine Diphosphate

ADP Phosphocreatine Phosphotransferase
See CPK

Adrenal Cortex Hormone
See Corticosteroids

Adrenal Gland
Biopsy 60540-60545
Excision. 60540
   Laparoscopy. 60650
   Retroperitoneal Tumor 60545
Exploration 60540, 60545
Nuclear Medicine
   Imaging 78075

Adrenal Medulla
See Medulla

Adrenalectomy
Partial 60540, 60545, 60650
Complete. 60540, 60545, 60650
Anesthesia 00866
Laparoscopic. 50545

Adrenalin
See Catecholamines
Blood. 82383
Urine 82382, 82384

Adrenaline-Noradrenaline
Testing. 82382-82384

Adrenocorticotropic Hormone
(ACTH) 80400-80406, 80412, 80418, 82024
Blood or Urine. 82024
Stimulation Panel 80400-80406

Adrenogenital Syndrome 56805, 57335

Adult T Cell Leukemia Lymphoma Virus I
See HTLV-I

Advanced Life Support
Physician/Health Care Professional Direction 99288

Advancement
Genioglossus. 21199
Tendon
   Tibia 28238

Advancement Flap
See Skin, Adjacent Tissue Transfer

Aerosol Inhalation
See Pulmonology, Therapeutic
Pentamidine 94642

AFB
See Acid-Fast Bacilli (AFB)

Afferent Nerve
See Sensory Nerve

AFP
See Alpha-Fetoprotein (AFP)

After Hours Medical Services . . 99050

Agents, Anticoagulant
See Clotting Inhibitors

Agglutinin
Cold. 86156, 86157
Febrile. 86000

Aggregation
Platelet 85576

AHG
See Clotting Factor

AICD (Automated Implantable Cardioverter-Defibrillator)
See Implantable Defibrillator

Aid, Hearing
See Hearing Aid

AIDS Antibodies
See Antibody, Detection, Human Immunodeficiency Virus (HIV)

AIDS Virus
See HIV-1

Airway
Leak
   See Bronchoscopy
Obstruction
   Inhalation Treatment 94640

Akin Operation
See Bunion Repair

ALA
See Aminolevulinic Acid (ALA)

Alanine 2 Oxoglutarate Aminotransferase
See Transaminase, Glutamic Pyruvic

Alanine Amino Transferase (ALT) 84460

Alanine Transaminase
See Transaminase, Glutamic Pyruvic

Albumin
Ischemia modified. 82045
Serum, Plasma or Whole Blood 82040
Urine 82042-82044

Alcohol
Breath 82075
    Ethylene Glycol 82693

Alcohol Dehydrogenase
See Antidiuretic Hormone

Alcohol, Isopropyl
See Isopropyl Alcohol

Alcohol, Methyl
See Methanol

Aldolase
Blood 82085

Aldosterone
Blood 82088
Suppression Evaluation 80408
Urine 82088

Alimentary Canal
See Gastrointestinal Tract

Alkaline Phosphatase 84075,
                                         84078, 84080
Leukocyte 85540
WBC 85540

Allergen Bronchial Provocation Tests
See Allergy Tests; Bronchial Challenge Test

Allergen Challenge, Endobronchial
See Bronchial Challenge Test

Allergen Immunotherapy
Allergen
    IgE 86003, 86005
    IgG 86001
    Multiallergen Screen 86005
Allergenic Extracts
    Injection 95115, 95117
    Injection and Provision 95120-95134
        Insect Venom 95130-95134
Antigens
    Preparation and Provision 95144-95165
        Insect Venom 95145-94149
Insect, Whole Body Extract 95170
Rapid Desensitization 95180

Allergy Services/Procedures
See Allergen Immunotherapy; Office and/or Other Outpatient Services
Education and Counseling 99201-99215
Unlisted Services and Procedures 95199

Allergy Tests
Challenge Test
    Bronchial 95070, 95071
    Ingestion 95076, 95079
Eye Allergy 95060
Food Allergy 95076, 95079
Intradermal
    Allergen Extract 95024-95028
    Biologicals 95018
    Drugs 95018
    Incremental 95027
    Venoms 95017
Nasal Mucous Membrane Test 95065
Nose Allergy 95065

Patch
    Application Tests 95044
    Photo Patch 95052
Photosensitivity 95056
Skin Tests
    Allergen Extract 95004, 95024, 95027
    Biologicals 95018
    Drugs 95018
    Venoms 95017

Allogeneic Donor
Lymphocyte Infusion 38242

Allogeneic Transplantation
Hematopoietic Progenitor Cells (HPCs) 38240
See Homograft

Allograft
Aortic Valve 33406, 33413
Bone
    Elbow Joint 24370, 24371
    Shoulder Joint 23473, 23474
    Spine Surgery
        Morselized 20930
        Structural 20931
Cartilage
    Knee 27415
Cornea
    Amniotic Membrane 65780
    Endothelial 65756
    Lamellar 65710
    Penetrating 65730, 65750, 65755
    for Aphakia 65750
Skin Substitute
    Arms 15271-15274
    Digits 15275-15278
    Eyelids 15275-15278
    Face 15275-15278
    Feet 15275-15278
    Genitalia 15275-15278
    Hands 15275-15278
    Legs 15271-15274
    Mouth 15275-15278
    Orbits 15275-15278
    Scalp 15275-15278
    Trunk 15271-15274
Lung Transplant 32850

Allograft Preparation
Cornea 65757
Heart 33933, 33944
Intestines 44715-44721
Kidney 50323-50329
Liver 47143-47147
Lung 32855, 32856, 33933
Pancreas 48551, 48552
Renal 50323-50329

Allotransplantation
Intestines 44135, 44136
    Removal 44137
Renal 50360-50365
    Removal 50370

Almen Test
See Blood, Feces

Alpha-1-Antitrypsin 82103, 82104

Alpha-2 Antiplasmin 85410

Alpha-Fetoprotein (AFP)
Amniotic Fluid 82106
Serum 82105, 82107

Alpha-tocopherol 84446

ALT
See Transaminase, Glutamic-Pyruvic

Altemeier Procedure
See Procidentia, Rectum; Rectum, Prolapse, Excision

Aluminum
Blood 82108

Alveola
Fracture
    Closed Treatment 21421
    Open Treatment 21422, 21423

Alveolar Cleft
Ungrafted Bilateral 21147
Ungrafted Unilateral 21146

Alveolar Nerve
Avulsion 64738
Incision 64738
Transection 64738

Alveolar Ridge
Fracture
    Closed Treatment 21440
    Open Treatment 21445

Alveolectomy 41830

Alveoloplasty 41874

Alveolus
Excision 41830

Amide, Procaine
See Procainamide

Amikacin
Assay 80150

Amine
Vaginal Fluid 82120

Amino Acids 82127-82139

Aminolevulinic Acid (ALA)
Blood or Urine 82135

Aminotransferase
See Transaminase

Aminotransferase, Alanine
See Transaminase, Glutamic-Pyruvic

Aminotransferase, Aspartate
See Transaminase, Glutamic-Oxaloacetic

Ammonia
Blood 82140

Amniocenteses
See Amniocentesis

Amniocentesis
See Chromosome Analysis
Diagnostic 59000
Induced Abortion 59850
    with Dilation and Curettage 59851
    with Dilation and Evacuation 59851
    with Hysterotomy 59852
Therapeutic
    Amniotic Fluid Reduction 59001

Amnioinfusion
Transabdominal 59070

Amnion
Amniocentesis 59000
   with Amniotic Fluid Reduction......... 59001
Amnioinfusion
   Transabdominal 59070
Membrane Placement
   Eye 65778, 65779

Amniotic Fluid
Alpha-Fetoprotein..................... 82106
Scan 82143
Testing................. 83661, 83663, 83664

Amniotic Membrane
See Amnion

AMP
See Adenosine Monophosphate (AMP)

AMP, Cyclic
See Cyclic AMP

Amputation
See Radical Resection; Replantation
Ankle............................... 27888
Arm, Lower 25900-25905, 25915
   Revision 25907, 25909
Arm, Upper 24900-24920
   and Shoulder 23900-23921
   Cineplasty 24940
   Revision 24925-24930
   with Implant................. 24931-24935
Cervix
   Total 57530
Ear
   Partial.......................... 69110
   Total 69120
Finger 26910-26952
Foot...................... 28800-28805
Hand at Metacarpal 25927
   at Wrist 25920
     Revision 25922
   Revision 25924, 25929, 25931
Interpelviabdominal 27290
Interthoracoscapular................. 23900
Leg, Lower 27598, 27880-27882
   Revision 27884, 27886
Leg, Upper.................. 27590-27592
   at Hip 27290, 27295
   Revision 27594, 27596
Metacarpal 26910
Metatarsal 28810
Penis
   Partial.......................... 54120
   Radical 54130, 54135
   Total 54125
Thumb.................. 26910, 26951, 26952
Toe.................. 28810, 28820, 28825
Tuft of Distal Phalanx 11752
Upper Extremity 24900-24940
   Revision 24925, 24930, 24935
   with Implant.................. 24931-24935
   Cineplasty 24940

Amputation through Hand
See Hand, Amputation

Amputation, Nose
See Resection, Nose

Amylase
Blood.............................. 82150
Urine 82150

ANA
See Antinuclear Antibodies (ANA)

Anabolic Steroid
See Androstenedione

Anal Abscess
See Abscess, Tissue, Anus

Anal Bleeding
See Anus, Hemorrhage

Anal Fistula
Closure 46288
Repair 46706
Surgical Treatment ... 46270, 46275, 46280, 46285

Anal Fistulectomy
See Excision, Fistula, Anal

Anal Fistulotomy
See Fistulotomy, Anal

Anal Sphincter
Dilation 45905
Incision 46080

Anal Ulceration
See Anus, Fissure

Analgesia
See Anesthesia; Sedation

Analgesic Cutaneous Electrostimulation
See Application, Neurostimulation

Analysis
Computer Data 99090
   Cardiovascular Monitoring 93290, 93297,
                                       93299
   Device Evaluation and Programming
     Implantable Defibrillator... 93260, 93261,
                    93282-93284, 93287, 93289,
                    93295, 93296, 93640, 93641
     Leadless Pacemaker System .0388T-0391T
     Loop Recorder........... 93285, 93291,
                         93298, 93299
     Pacemaker... 93279-93281, 93293, 93294
   Electrocardiograph
     Data Analysis 0206T
   Pacemaker 93288, 93293, 93294
   Electroencephalogram
     Digital........................ 95957
   Electronic
     Drug Infusion Pump 62367-62370
   Pacing Cardioverter-Defibrillator
     Data Analysis 93289, 93295, 93296
     Initial Evaluation........... 93640, 93641
     See Pacemaker, Heart
   Neurostimulator Pulse Generator System
     with Vagus Nerve Blocking Therapy ..0317T
     Brain 95970, 95978, 95979
     Cranial Nerve 95974, 95975
     Gastric 95980-95982
     Peripheral Nerve........... 95971, 95972
     Spinal Cord............ 95971, 95972
     with Programming 95971, 95972,
                   95978-95980, 95982
     without Reprograming...... 95970, 95981
   Multianalyte Assays with Algorithmic Analysis
   (MAAA)
     Risk Score
       Endocrinology Analytes 81506
       Fetal Aneuploidy DNA Sequence..... 81507

     Fetal Congenital
       Abnormalities............. 81508-81512
       Ovarian Oncology Proteins.... 81500, 81503
     Tissue Similarity Score
       Gene Expression for Oncology 81504
       Unlisted Assay.................... 81599
Physiologic Data, Remote.............. 99091
Protein
   Tissue
     Western Blot 88372
Semen 89320-89322
   Sperm Isolation 89260, 89261
Waveform
   Central Arterial Pressure 93050

Analysis, Spectrum
See Spectrophotometry

Anaspadias
See Epispadias

Anastomosis
Arteriovenous Fistula
   Direct........................... 36821
   with Bypass Graft 35686
   with Graft............. 36825, 36830, 36832
Artery
   to Aorta 33606
   to Artery
     Cranial 61711
Bile Duct
   to Bile Duct 47800
   to Intestines................. 47760, 47780
Bile Duct to Gastrointestinal Tract .. 47780, 47785
Broncho-Bronchial.................. 32486
Caval to Mesenteric 37160
Cavopulmonary................. 33622, 33768
Colorectal 44626
Epididymis
   to Vas Deferens
     Bilateral 54901
     Unilateral 54900
Excision
   Trachea.................. 31780, 31781
Fallopian Tube..................... 58750
Gallbladder to Intestines 47720-47740
Hepatic Duct to Intestines 47765, 47802
Ileum to Anus 45113
Intestine to Intestine................ 44130
Intestines
   Colon to Anus.................. 45119
   Cystectomy.................... 51590
   Enterocystoplasty................ 51960
   Ileoanal 44157, 44158
   Resection
     Laparoscopic............ 44202-44205
Intrahepatic Portosystemic......... 37182, 37183
Jejunum 43820-43825
Microvascular
   Free Transfer
     Jejunum 43496
Nerve
   Facial to Hypoglossal.............. 64868
Oviduct 58750
Pancreas to Intestines 48520, 48540, 48548
Portocaval 37140
Pulmonary......................... 33606
Renoportal......................... 37145
Splenorenal.................. 37180, 37181
Stomach
   to Duodenum 43810, 43855
     Revision 43850
   to Jejunum....... 43820-43825, 43860-43865

Anesthesia, Local

See Injection, Anesthetic Agent

Aneurysm Repair

See Aorta; Artery

Angel Dust

See Phencyclidine

Angina Assessment

Angiocardiographies

See Angiography, specific structure or vessel

Angiography

See Aortography

Angioma

See Lesion, Skin

Angioplasties, Coronary Balloon

See Percutaneous Transluminal Angioplasty

Angioplasty

Angioscopy

Angiotensin Converting Enzyme (ACE)

Angiotensin Forming Enzyme

See Renin

Angiotensin II
Blood or Urine........................82163

Angle Deformity
Toe
    Reconstruction....................28313

Anhydride, Carbonic
See Carbon Dioxide

Anhydrides, Acetic
See Acetic Anhydrides

Animal Inoculation 87003, 87250

Ankle
See Fibula; Leg, Lower; Tibia; Tibiofibular Joint
Abscess
    Incision and Drainage 27603
Amputation....................................27888
Arthrocentesis..................... 20605, 20606
Arthrodesis 27870
Arthrography 73615
Arthroplasty 27700, 27702, 27703
Arthroscopy
    Surgical 29891, 29894-29899
Arthrotomy 27610-27612, 27620-27626
Biopsy 27613, 27614, 27620
Bursa
    Incision and Drainage 27604
Disarticulation.............................27889
Dislocation
    Closed Treatment............ 27840, 27842
    Open Treatment 27846, 27848
Exploration 27610, 27620
Fracture
    Bimalleolar............... 27808-27814
    Lateral 27786-27814
    Medial 27760-27766, 27808-27814
    Posterior......27767-27769, 27808-27814
    Trimalleolar 27816-27823
Fusion 27870
Hematoma
    Incision and Drainage 27603
Incision 27607
Injection
    Radiologic 27648
Lesion
    Excision 27630
Magnetic Resonance Imaging (MRI) 73721-73723
Manipulation.................................27860
Removal
    Foreign Body 27610, 27620
    Implant..............................27704
    Loose Body........................27620
Repair
    Achilles Tendon 27650-27654
    Ligament 27695-27698
    Tendon 27612, 27680-27687
Strapping......................................29540
Synovium
    Excision 27625, 27626
Tenotomy.......................... 27605, 27606
Tumor
    Soft Tissue
        Excision .. 27618, 27619, 27630, 27632, 27634
        Radical Resection 27615, 27616
Unlisted Services and Procedures 27899
X-ray 73600-73610
    with Contrast.....................73615

Ankylosis (Surgical)
See Arthrodesis

Annuloplasty
Intradiscal
    Percutaneous............... 22526, 22527

Anogenital Region
See Perineum

Anoplasty
Stricture 46700, 46705

Anorectal Biofeedback 90911

Anorectal Exam (Surgical) 45990

Anorectal Fistula
Repair 46706, 46707

Anorectal Myectomy
See Myomectomy, Anorectal

Anorectovaginoplasty..... 46744-46746

Anoscopy
Ablation
    Polyp................................46615
    Tumor...............................46615
Biopsy 46606
Collection of Specimen........... 46600, 46601
with Delivery of Thermal Energy 0288T
Dilation 46604
Exploration 46600
Hemorrhage 46614
High Resolution Anoscopy (HRA)
    Diagnostic 46601
    with Biopsy(ies) 46607
Injection
    Bulking Agent.......................0377T
Removal
    Foreign Body 46608
    Polyp 46610-46612
    Tumor 46610-46612

Antebrachium
See Forearm

Antecedent, Plasma Thromboplastin
See Plasma Thromboplastin, Antecedent

Antepartum Care
Cesarean Delivery.........................59510
    Previous 59610, 59618
Vaginal Delivery 59400, 59425, 59426

Anterior Chamber Fluid, Eye
See Paracentesis, Eye

Anterior Ramus of Thoracic Nerve
See Intercostal Nerve

Anthrax Vaccine
See Vaccines

Anthrogon
See Follicle Stimulating Hormone (FSH)

Anti-Australia Antigens
See Hepatitis Antigen, Detection, Immunoassay, B Surface (HBsAg)

Anti-D Immunoglobulin
See Immune Globulins, Rho(D)

Antihuman Globulin Consumption Test
See Coombs Test

Antiphospholipid Antibody
See Antibody, Detection, Anti-phosphatidylserine (Phospholipid)

Antiactivator, Plasmin
See Alpha-2 Antiplasmin

Antibiotic Administration
Injection 96372-96379
Prescribed or Dispensed 4120F, 4124F

Antibiotic Sensitivity
Susceptibility Studies....... 87181-87184, 87188
    Enzyme Detection 87185
    Minimum Inhibitory Concentration (MIC) 87186
    Minimum Lethal Concentration (MLC)... 87187

Antibodies, Thyroid-Stimulating
See Immunoglobulin, Thyroid-Stimulating

Antibodies, Viral
See Viral Antibodies

Antibody
See Antibody Identification; Microsomal Antibody Detection
Actinomyces....................86602
Adenovirus......................86603
Antinuclear.............. 86038, 86039
Anti-phosphatidylserine (Phospholipid).. 86148
Antistreptolysin O 86060, 86063
Aspergillus.....................86606
Bacterium......................86609
Bartonella......................86611
Beta-2 Glycoprotein I............86146
Blastomyces....................86612
Blood Crossmatch 86920-86923
Bordetella......................86615
Borrelia.................. 86617-86619
Brucella........................86622
Campylobacter..................86625
Candida........................86628
Cardiolipin 86147
Chlamydia 86631, 86632
Coccidioides....................86635
Coxiella Burnetii.................86638
C-Reactive Protein (CRP) 86140, 86141
Cryptococcus 86641
Cyclic Citrullinated Peptide (CCP) 86200
Cytomegalovirus (CMV)........ 86644, 86645
Cytotoxic Screen 86807, 86808
Deoxyribonuclease..............86215
Deoxyribonucleic Acid (DNA).... 86225, 86226
Diphtheria 86648
Ehrlichia 86666
Encephalitis 86651-86654
Enterovirus 86658
Epstein-Barr Virus 86663-86665
Fc Receptor 86243
Fluorescent................ 86255, 86256
Francisella Tularensis 86668
Fungus, Other...................86671
Giardia Lamblia 86674
Growth Hormone 86277
Helicobacter Pylori...............86677
Helminth.......................86682
Haemophilus Influenzae 86684
Hepatitis
    Delta Agent 86692
Hepatitis A (HAAb)......... 86708, 86709
Hepatitis B
    Core (HBcAb) 86704
    IgM 86705
    Surface(HBsAb) 86706

Antithrombin VI
See Fibrin Degradation Products

Antitoxin Assay 87230

Antiviral Antibody
See Viral Antibodies

Antrostomy
Sinus
    Maxillary 31256, 31267

Antrotomy
Sinus
    Maxillary 31020, 31030, 31032
Transmastoid........................... 69501

Antrum of Highmore
See Sinus/Sinuses, Maxillary

Antrum Puncture
Sinus
    Maxillary 31000
    Sphenoid 31002

Anus
See Hemorrhoids; Rectum
Ablation.............................. 46615
Abscess
    Incision and Drainage 46045, 46050
Anal Canal
    Delivery of Thermal Energy 0288T
Anoscopy
    See Anoscopy
Biofeedback 90911
Biopsy
    Endoscopy 46606
Crypt
    Excision 46999
Dilation
    Endoscopy 46604
Endoscopy
    Biopsy........................... 46606
    Dilation.......................... 46604
    Exploration 46600
    Hemorrhage 46614
    High Resolution Anoscopy (HRA) 46601, 46607
    Injection
        Bulking Agent.................... 0377T
    Removal
        Foreign Body..................... 46608
        Polyp...................... 46610, 46612
        Tumor 46610, 46612
Excision
    Tag 46220, 46230
Exploration
    Endoscopy 46600
    Surgical 45990
Fissure
    Destruction.................. 46940, 46942
    Excision 46200
Fistula
    Closure........................... 46288
    Excision 46270-46285
    Repair............................ 46706
Hemorrhage
    Endoscopic Control 46614
Hemorrhoids
    Clot Excision..................... 46320
    Destruction....................... 46930
    Excision 46250-46262
    Injection 46500
    Ligation 0249T, 46221, 46945, 46946
    Stapling 46947
    Suture..................... 46945, 46946

Imperforated
    Repair...................... 46715-46742
Incision
    Septum........................... 46070
    Sphincterotomy 46200
Lesion
    Destruction........... 46900-46917, 46924
    Excision 45108, 46922
Manometry 91122
Placement
    Seton 46020
Reconstruction
    Congenital Absence........... 46730-46740
    Sphincter 46750, 46751, 46760-46762
    with Graft........................ 46753
    with Implant...................... 46762
Removal
    Foreign Body 46608
    Seton 46030
    Suture........................... 46754
    Wire 46754
Repair
    Anoperineal Fistula 46715, 46716
    Cloacal Anomaly 46744, 46746, 46748
    Fistula........................... 46706
    Stricture 46700, 46705
Sphincter
    Chemodenervation................. 46505
    Electromyography 51784, 51785
    Needle 51785
    Sphincterotomy 46200
Unlisted Services and Procedures 46999

Aorta
Abdominal
    Aneurysm
        See Aneurysm Repair, Abdominal Aorta
    Angiography 75635
    Thromboendarterectomy 35331
Anastomosis
    to Pulmonary Artery 33606
Angiogram
    Radiologic Injection 93567
    See Cardiac Catheterization, Injection
Angioplasty...................... 35452, 35472
Aortography 75600, 75605, 75625, 75630
Ascending
    Graft............................ 33864
Balloon Assist Device
    Insertion............. 33967, 33970, 33973
    Removal 33968, 33971, 33974
Catheterization
    Catheter......................... 36200
    Intracatheter/Needle............... 36160
Circulation Assist Device
    Insertion............. 33967, 33970, 33973
    Removal 33968, 33971, 33974
Conduit to Heart 33404
Endograft
    Fenestrated 34839, 34841-34848
Excision
    Coarctation........... 33840, 33845, 33851
Infrarenal Abdominal
    Repair
        Endovascular 34845-34848
Insertion
    Balloon Device........ 33967, 33970, 33973
    Catheter......................... 36200
    Graft............... 33330, 33335, 33864
    Intracatheter/Needle............... 36160
Removal
    Balloon Assist Device . 33968, 33971, 33974
Repair 33320-33322, 33802, 33803
    Coarctation........... 33840, 33845, 33851

Aneurysm
    Ascending.......... 33860, 33863, 33864
    Sinus of Valsalva 33720
    Thoracic 33875, 33877
    Transverse Arch 33870
Hypoplastic or Interrupted
    Aortic Arch................ 33852, 33853
    Sinus of Valsalva ... 33702, 33710, 33720
Suspension 33800
Suture 33320-33322
Thoracic
    Catheterization................. 36221
    Repair......... 33875, 33877, 75956-75959
    Endovascular 33880, 33881, 33883,
               33884, 33886, 33889, 33891
Translocation
    Aortic Root............... 33782, 33783
Valve
    Implantation............. 33361-33369
    Incision 33415
    Repair........... 33400, 33401, 33403
    Left Ventricle 33414
    Supravalvular Stenosis........... 33417
    Replacement
        See Aortic Valve Replacement
Visceral
    Repair
        Endovascular 34839, 34841-34848
X-ray with Contrast... 75600, 75605, 75625, 75630

Aortopulmonary Transposition
See Transposition, Great Arteries

Aortic Sinus
See Sinus/Sinuses, Sinus of Valsalva

Aortic Stenosis
Repair 33415
    Nikaidoh Procedure 33782, 33783
    Supravalvular.................... 33417

Aortic Valve
Construction
    Apical-Aortic Conduit.............. 33404
Implantation
    Transcatheter................. 33361-33369
Repair
    Gusset Aortoplasty 33417
    Outflow Tract Obstruction
        Left Ventricle 33414
    Stenosis
        Idiopathic Hypertrophic 33416
        Subvalvular.................... 33415
        Supravalvular.................. 33417
    Valvuloplasty
        Open, with Cardiopulmonary Bypass.. 33400
        Open, with Inflow Occlusion 33401
        Using Transventricular Dilation 33403
Replacement
    See Aortic Valve Replacement

Aortic Valve Replacement
Ross Procedure...................... 33413
Transcatheter
    See Transcatheter Aortic Valve Replacement
    (TAVR/TAVI)
with Allograft Valve 33406
with Aortic Annulus Enlargement.... 33411, 33412
with Cardiopulmonary Bypass 33367-33369,
              33405, 33406, 33410
with Prosthesis........... 33405, 33361-33369
with Stentless Tissue Valve 33410
with Translocation, Pulmonary Valve 33413

Replantation 20802
Splint 29105
Tumor
  Soft Tissue
    Excision 24071-24076
    Radical Resection 24077-24079
  Ultrasound
    Complete 76881
    Limited 76882
  Unlisted Services and Procedures 24999
  Wound Exploration
    Penetrating 20103
X-ray
  Infant 73092

Arnold-Chiari Malformation Repair
See Decompression, Skull

Arrest, Epiphyseal
See Epiphyseal Arrest

Arrhythmogenic Focus
Heart
  Ablation 33250, 33251, 33261,
                               93653, 93654, 93656
  Catheter 93655

Arsenic
Detection 83015
Measurement 82175, 83018
Blood or Urine 82175

ART (Automated Reagin Test)
See Syphilis Test

Arterial Catheterization
See Cannulation, Arterial

Arterial Dilatation, Transluminal
See Angioplasty, Transluminal

Arterial Grafting for Coronary Artery Bypass
See Bypass Graft, Arterial, Coronary

Arterial Infusion, Thrombolysis
See Transcatheter, Therapy, Infusion, (Arterial or Venous)

Arterial Pressure
See Blood Pressure
Noninvasive Waveform Analysis 93050

Arterial Puncture
for Diagnosis 36600

Arteriography, Aorta
See Aortography

Arteriosus, Ductus
Closure
  Transcatheter Percutaneous 93582
Repair 33820-33824

Arteriosus, Truncus
Repair 33786

Arteriotomy
See Incision, Artery; Transection, Artery

Arteriovenous Anastomosis
for Increased Blood Flow 36818-36821

Arteriovenous Fistula
Cannulization
  Vein 36815
Creation 36825-36830
Hemodialysis via Fistula 4052F

Referral 4051F
Repair
  Abdomen 35182, 35189
  Head 35180, 35188
  Lower Extremity 35184, 35190
  Neck 35180, 35188
  Thorax 35182, 35189
  Upper Extremity 35184, 35190
Revision
  with Thrombectomy 36833
  without Thrombectomy 36832
Thrombectomy
  Dialysis Graft
    without Revision 36831
  Graft 36870

Arteriovenous Malformation
Carotid
  Obliteration 61613
  Occlusion 61705
Cranial
  Repair
    Carotid Artery Occlusion 61705
    Dural 61690, 61692
    Electrothrombosis 61708
    Infratentorial 61684, 61686
    Supratentorial 61680, 61682
Iliac Artery
  Repair 0254T, 34900
Spinal
  Excision 63250-63252
  Occlusion 63250-63252, 62294

Arteriovenous Shunt
Angiography 75791
Aorta to Pulmonary Artery 33755, 33762
Blalock-Taussig Shunt 33750
Dialysis Catheterization 36147, 36148
Intrahepatic Portosystemic
  Insertion 37182
  Revision 37183
Patency 78291
Peritoneal-Venous
  Evaluation 49427
  Insertion 49425
  Ligation 49428
  Removal 49429
  Revision 49426
Potts-Smith Shunt 33762
Subclavian to Pulmonary Artery 33750
Thomas Shunt 36835
Waterston Shunt 33755

Artery
Abdomen
  Angiography 75726
  Catheterization 36245-36248
  Ligation 37617
Adrenal
  Angiography 75731-75733
Anastomosis
  Cranial 61711
Angioplasty
  See Angioplasty
  Radiological Supervision 75962-75968
Aorta
  Angioplasty 35452
Aortobi-iliac
  Bypass Graft 35538, 35638
Aortobifemoral
  Bypass Graft 35540
Aortocarotid
  Bypass Graft 35526, 35626

Aortofemoral
  Bypass Graft 35539
Aortoiliac
  Bypass Graft 35537, 35637
  Embolectomy 34151-34201
  Thrombectomy 34151-34201
Aortoiliofemoral
  Thromboendarterectomy 35363
Aortoinnominate
  Bypass Graft 35526, 35626
Aortosubclavian
  Bypass Graft 35526, 35626
Arm
  Angiography 75710-75716
  Harvest 35600
Atherectomy
  Brachiocephalic 0237T
  Coronary 92924, 92925, 92933, 92934,
                         92937, 92938, 92941, 92943, 92944
  Femoral 37225, 37227
  Iliac 0238T
  Peroneal 37229, 37231
  Popliteal 37225, 37227
  Renal 0234T
  Tibial 37229, 37231
  Visceral 0235T
  Transluminal 0234T-0238T, 92924,
                         92925, 92933, 92934, 92937,
                         92938, 92941, 92943, 92944
Axillary
  Aneurysm 35011-35013
  Angioplasty 35458
  Bypass Graft 35616, 35621,
                                   35623, 35650, 35654
  Embolectomy 34101
  Thrombectomy 34101
  Thromboendarterectomy 35321
Basilar
  Aneurysm 61698, 61702
Biopsy 75970
Brachial
  Aneurysm 35011-35013
  Angiography 75658
  Bypass Graft 35510, 35512, 35522-35525
  Catheterization 36120
  Embolectomy 34101
  Exploration 24495
  Exposure 34834
  Thrombectomy 34101
  Thromboendarterectomy 35321
Brachiocephalic
  Angioplasty 35458
  Atherectomy 0237T
  Catheterization 36215-36218
Bypass Graft
  with Composite Graft 35681-35683
Cannulization
  for Extracorporeal Circulation 36823
  to Vein 36810-36815
Carotid
  Aneurysm 35001, 35002, 61697,
                         61700, 61703, 61705, 61708, 61710
  Baroreflex Activation Device
    Implantation/Replacement 0266T-0268T
    Interrogation Evaluation 0272T, 0273T
    Revision/Removal 0269T-0271T
  Bypass Graft 33891, 35501-35510,
                                 35601-35606, 35642
  Carotid Cavernous
    Fistula 61705, 61708, 61710
    Catheterization 36100, 36221-36224,
                                     36227, 36228

Aspiration Lipectomies
See Liposuction

Aspiration of Bone Marrow from Donor for Transplant
See Bone Marrow, Harvesting

Aspiration, Chest
Thoracentesis 32554, 32555
   with Imaging Guidance 32555

Aspiration, Nail
See Evacuation, Hematoma, Subungual

Aspiration, Spinal Puncture
See Spinal Tap

Assay, Tobramycin
See Tobramycin

Assay, Very Long Chain Fatty Acids
See Fatty Acid, Very Long Chain

Assisted Circulation
See Circulation Assist

AST
See Transaminase, Glutamic-Oxaloacetic

Astragalectomy
Talectomy 28130

Astragalus
See Talus

Asymmetry, Face
See Hemifacial Microsomia

Ataxia Telangiectasia
Chromosome Analysis 88248

Ataxy, Telangiectasia
See Ataxia Telangiectasia

Atherectomies, Coronary
See Artery, Coronary, Atherectomy

Atherectomy
See Revascularization, Artery
Abdominal Aorta 0236T
Brachiocephalic 0237T
Coronary 92924,
    92925, 92937, 92938, 92941, 92943, 92944
Femoral 37225, 37227
Iliac 0238T
Peroneal 37229, 37231, 37233, 37235
Popliteal 37225, 37227
Renal 0234T
Tibial 37229, 37231, 37233, 37235
Visceral 0235T

ATLV (Adult T Cell Leukemia Virus)
See HTLV-I

ATLV Antibodies
See HTLV-I, Antibody

Atomic Absorption Spectroscopy
Each Analyte 82190

ATP Creatine Phosphotransferase
See CPK

Atresia
Choanal 30540-30545
Congenital
   Auditory Canal, External 69320
   Bile Duct 47700
   Small Intestine 44126, 44127

Pulmonary Artery 33920
Tetralogy of Fallot 33697
Tricuspid 33615

Atria
Ablation
   Operative Tissue 33254-33256,
                   33265, 33266
Baffle Procedure 33774
Blalock-Hanlon Operation 33735
Cor Triatriatum
   Repair 33732
Cuff Preparation 32855, 32856
Electrogram 93615, 93616
Fibrillation
   See Fibrillation, Atrial
Endoscopy 33265, 33266
Hemodynamic Monitor System 0293T, 0294T
Left Atrial Appendage 0281T
Membrane Resection 33732
Pacemaker
   Electrode
     Removal 33229, 33236
     Repositioning 33215
     Insertion 33206, 33208
Rashkind Procedure 92992
Reconstruction 33254-33256, 33265, 33266
Septal Defect
   See Septal Defect, Atrial
Septectomy 33735, 92992, 92993
Septostomy 33735, 92992, 92993
Shunt 62190, 62220
Thrombus 33310

Atrial Electrogram
See Cardiology, Diagnostic
Esophageal Recording 93615, 93616

Atrial Fibrillation
See Fibrillation, Atrial

Atrioseptopexy
See Septal Defect, Atrial, Repair

Atrioseptoplasty
See Septal Defect, Atrial, Repair

Attachment
See Fixation

Atticotomy
Tympanic Incision 69631, 69635

Audiologic Function Tests
Acoustic Immittance 92570
Acoustic Reflex 92568, 92570
Audiometry
   Automated 0208T-0212T
   Bekesy 92560, 92561
   Comprehensive 0212T, 92557
   Conditioning Play 92582
   Groups 92559
   Pure Tone 0208T, 0209T, 92552, 92553
   Select Picture 92583
   Speech 0210T, 0211T, 92555, 92556
   Visual Reinforcement (VRA) 92579
Auditory Brainstem Implant 92640
Auditory Processing
   Treatment 92507, 92508
Central Auditory Function 92620, 92621
Ear Protector Attenuation 92596
Electrocochleography 92584
Evoked Otoacoustic Emission 92558,
                     92587, 92588
Filtered Speech 92571
Hearing Aid Evaluation 92590-92595

Loudness Balance 92562
Screening 92551
Sensorineural Acuity 92575
Short Increment Sensitivity Index (SISI) 92564
Staggered Spondaic Word Test 92572
Stenger Test 92565, 92577
Synthetic Sentence Test 92576
Tinnitus Assessment 92625
Tone Decay 92563
Tympanometry 92550, 92567, 92570

Audiometry
Bekesy 92560, 92561
Brainstem Evoked Response 92585, 92586
Comprehensive 0212T, 92557
Conditioning Play 92582
Groups 92559
Pure Tone 92552, 92553
   Automated 0208T, 0209T
Select Picture 92583
Speech 0210T, 0211T, 92555, 92556
Tympanometry 92550, 92567, 92570
Voice Prosthesis Fitting 92597

Auditory Brainstem Evoked Response
See Evoked Potential, Auditory Brainstem

Auditory Canal
Decompression 61591
External
   Abscess
     Incision and Drainage . . 69000, 69005, 69020
   Biopsy 69105
   Excision 69110, 69120
     Lesion 69140, 69145, 69150, 69155
   Hematoma 69000, 69005
   Reconstruction
     for Congenital Atresia 69320
     for Stenosis 69310
   Removal
     Cerumen 69209, 69210
     Ear Wax 69209, 69210
     Foreign Body 69200-69205
Internal
   Decompression 69960
   Exploration 69440

Auditory Canal Atresia, External
See Atresia, Congenital, Auditory Canal, External

Auditory Evoked Otoacoustic Emission
Screening 92558, 92587, 92588

Auditory Evoked Potentials
See Audiometry

Auditory Labyrinth
See Ear, Inner Ear

Auditory Meatus
X-ray 70134

Auditory Tube
See Eustachian Tube

Augmentation
Breast
   See Breast, Augmentation
Chin 21120, 21123
Cruciate Ligament 29888, 29889
Knee Ligament 27427, 27556-27558
Malar 21210, 21270
Mandibular Body 21127-21125
Facial Bones 21208

Replacement...................... 43773
Revision 43771
Port Component............. 43886-43888
Sleeve Gastrectomy 43775
Surgically Altered Stomach
　　Ultrasound Examination............. 43242

Barium..................... 83015, 83018

Barium Enema 74270-74280

Barker Operation
See Talus, Excision

Baroreflex Activation Device
Implantation/Replacement.........0266T-0268T
Interrogation Evaluation 0272T, 0273T
Revision/Removal.................0269T-0271T

Barr Bodies 88130

Barr Procedure
See Tendon, Transfer

Bartholin's Gland
Abscess
　　Incision and Drainage 56420
Cyst
　　Marsupialization 56440
Excision............................ 56740

Bartonella Detection
Antibody 86611
Nucleic Acid Probe 87470-87472

Basic Proteins, Myelin
See Myelin Basic Protein

Basilar Arteries
See Artery, Basilar

Batch-Spittler-McFaddin Operation
See Disarticulation, Knee

BCG Vaccine 90585, 90586
See Vaccines

Be Antigens, Hepatitis
See Hepatitis Antigen, Be

Bed Sores
See Pressure, Ulcer (Decubitus)

Bed Testing
See Pulmonology, Diagnostic

Bekesy Audiometry
See Audiometry, Bekesy

Belsey IV Procedure
See Fundoplasty

Bender-Gestalt Test 96101-96103

Benedict Test for Urea
See Urinalysis, Qualitative

Benign Cystic Mucinous Tumor
See Ganglion

Benign Neoplasm of Cranial Nerves
See Nerves, Neurofibroma

Bennett Fracture
Treatment 26645, 26650, 26665

Bennett Procedure
Quadricepsplasty 27430

Benzidine Test
See Blood, Feces

Benzoyl Cholinesterase
See Cholinesterase

Bernstein Test
See Acid Perfusion Study, Esophagus

Beryllium.................. 83015, 83018

Beta 2 Glycoprotein I Antibody 86146

Beta-Blocker Therapy
Performance Measures
　　Coronary Artery Disease 4008F
　　Heart Failure 4008F, 4480F, 4481F

Beta Glucosidase.............. 82963

Beta Hypophamine
See Antidiuretic Hormone

Beta Lipoproteins
See Lipoprotein, LDL

Beta Test
See Psychiatric Diagnosis

Beta-2-Microglobulin
Blood............................. 82232
Urine 82232

Beta-hydroxydehydrogenase... 80406

Bethesda System 88164-88167

Bicarbonate.................. 82374

Biceps Tendon
Reinsertion 24342
Resection 23440
Tenodesis 23430, 29828
Transplantation.................... 23440

Bichloride, Methylene
See Dichloromethane

Bicuspid Valve
See Mitral Valve

Bifrontal Craniotomy
for Craniosynostosis.................... 61557

Bilaminate Skin Substitute/ Neodermis
See Tissue, Substitute

Bile Acids 82239
Blood............................. 82240

Bile Duct
See Gallbladder
Anastomosis
　　with Intestines......... 47760, 47780-47785
Biopsy
　　Endoluminal...................... 47543
　　Endoscopy 47553
Cholangiography
　　Injection................... 47531, 47532
　　with Catheterization 47533-47537
　　with Placement of Access to
　　Small Bowel................... 47541
　　with Stent Placement 47538-47540
Cyst
　　Excision 47715
Destruction
　　Calculus (Stone)............. 43265, 47544

Dilation
　　Endoscopy 43277, 47555, 47556
　　Percutaneous..................... 47542
　　X-ray............................ 74360
Drainage
　　Catheter
　　　Change 75984
　　　Conversion of External to
　　　Internal-External.............. 47535
　　　Exchange 47536
　　　Placement............. 47533, 47534
　　　Removal 47537
Endoscopic Retrograde Cholangiopancreatography (ERCP)
　　with Optical Endomicroscopy 0397T
Endoscopy
　　Biopsy......................... 47553
　　Cannulation 43273
　　Destruction
　　　Calculus (Stone) 43265
　　Dilation............ 43277, 47555, 47556
　　Exploration..................... 47552
　　Intraoperative.................. 47550
　　Placement
　　　Stent....................... 43274
　　Removal
　　　Calculus (Stone) 43264, 47554
　　　Foreign Body................ 43275
　　Specimen Collection 43260
　　Sphincter Pressure.............. 43263
　　Sphincterotomy 43262, 43274
Exploration
　　Atresia 47700
　　Endoscopy 47552
Incision
　　Sphincter 43262, 47460
Incision and Drainage........... 47420-47425
Nuclear Medicine
　　Imaging 78226, 78227
　　Pharmacologic Intervention 78227
Placement
　　Access to Small Bowel 47541
　　Catheter
　　　Drainage............. 47533, 47534
　　　Stent................. 43274, 47801
Reconstruction
　　Anastomosis 47800
Removal
　　Calculus (Stone).. 43264, 47420, 47425, 47544
　　Foreign Body................ 43275
　　Stent...................... 43275
Repair 47701
　　Gastrointestinal Tract 47785
　　with Intestines........... 47760, 47780
Stent Placement 47538-47540, 47801
Tumor
　　Ablation 43278
　　Excision 47711, 47712
Unlisted Services and Procedures 47999
X-ray
　　Guide Dilation 74360
　　with Contrast......... 47532, 74300, 74301
　　　Calculus Removal................ 47544
　　Guide Catheter............ 74328, 74330

Bile Duct, Common, Cystic Dilatation
See Cyst, Choledochal

Bilirubin
Blood..................... 82247, 82248
Feces............................ 82252

Prostate
    Incisional 55705
    Needle or Punch. 55700, 55706
    Stereotactic 55706
    Lymph Nodes 55812, 55842, 55862
Rectum 45100, 45305, 45331
Renal Pelvis
    Endoluminal, Non-endoscopic 50606
Retroperitoneal Area 49010, 49180
Sacroiliac Joint. 27050
Salivary Gland. 42400, 42405
Shoulder 23065, 23066
Shoulder Joint. 23100, 23101, 23106, 29805
Sinus. 31237
    Sphenoid 31050
Skin Lesion 11100, 11101
Skull Base 61575, 61576
Spinal Cord
    Lesion. 63615
    Needle 62269
    Neoplasm. 63275-63290
    Transoral 61575, 61576
    Percutaneous 62269
    Stereotaxis. 63615
Stomach 43605
Tarsometatarsal Joint
    Synovium 28050
Temporomandibular Joint. 29800
Testis. 54500-54505
Thigh 27323, 27324
Thorax 21550
Throat 42800-42806
Thyroid 60100
Tongue. 41100-41105
Transcatheter 37200
Ureter 52354
    Endoluminal, Non-endoscopic 50606
    Endoscopic 50955-50957, 50974-50976
Urethra 52204, 52250, 52354, 53200
Uterus
    Endometrial 58100-58110
    Endoscopic. 58558
Uvula. 42100
Vagina 57100-57105, 57109, 57421
Vein. 37200, 75970
Vertebral Body
    Open. 20250, 20251
    Percutaneous 22510-22515
Vulva 56605, 56606, 56821
with Arthrotomy
    Acromioclavicular Joint. 23101
    Glenohumeral Joint 23100, 23105
    Sternoclavicular Joint 23101
with Cystourethroscopy 52354
Wrist 25065, 25066, 25100, 25101, 29840

Biopsy, Skin
See Skin, Biopsy

Biopsy, Vein
See Vein, Biopsy

Biostatistics
See Biometry

Biosterol
See Vitamin, A

Biotinidase 82261

Birthing Room
Newborn Care. 99460, 99463
    Attendance at Delivery 99464
    Resuscitation 99465

Bischof Procedure
See Laminectomy, with Myelotomy

Bismuth 83015

Bizzozero's Corpuscle/Cell
See Blood, Platelet

Bladder
Abscess
    Incision and Drainage 51080
Anastomosis 50780-50782, 51960
Aspiration 51100-51102
Biopsy 52204
Calculus
    Litholapaxy 52317, 52318
    Lithotripsy 51065, 52353
    Manipulation 52352
    Removal . . 51050, 51065, 52310-52315, 52352
Catheterization 51045, 51102, 51701-51703
Chemodenervation 52287
Cuff 50234, 50650
Cyst
    Urachal
        Excision 51500
Cystostomy Tube. 51705-51710
Cystourethroscopy
    See Endoscopy
Destruction
    Lesion. 51030
Dilation 52260-52265
    Ureter
        See Ureter, Dilation
Diverticulum
    Excision 51525
    Incision. 52305
    Resection 52305
Endoscopy. 52000
    Biopsy. 52204, 52224, 52250, 52354
    Dilation. 52260-52265
    Diverticulum. 52305
    Evacuation
        Clot 52001
    Excision
        Tumor 52234, 52235, 52240, 52355
    Exploration 52351
    Instillation 52005, 52010
    Fulguration 52214-52224, 52400
        Tumor 52234, 52235, 52240
    Injection, Steroid 52283
    Irrigation
        Clot 52001
    Lithotripsy 52353
    Radiotracer 52250
    Removal
        Calculus 52310-52315, 52352
        Foreign Body. 52310-52315
    Tumor
        Excision. 52234-52240, 52355
        Fulguration 52234, 52235, 52240
Excision
    Partial. 51550-51565
    Total 45126, 51570, 51580, 51590-51597
        with Nodes 51575, 51585, 51595
    Transurethral 52640
    Ureterocele 51535
Flap 50785
Fulguration 52214-52224, 52354
Incision and Drainage. 51040
Injection
    Radiologic 51600-51610
Insertion
    Stent. 51045, 52334

Instillation 51700
    Anticarcinogenic Agent 51720
Interstitial Cystitis
    Dilation. 52260-52265
Irrigation 51700
Laparoscopy 51999
Lesion
    Destruction. 51030
    Fulguration 52224
Neck
    Excision 51520
    Injection of Implant Material. 51715
    Remodel for Urinary Incontinence 53860
Nuclear Medicine
    Residual Study 78730
Pressure
    Cystometrogram (CMG) 51725-51729
    Uroflowmetry 51736-51741
    Voiding Study 51728, 51729, 51797
Radiotracer 51020, 52250
Reconstruction
    and Urethra 51800-51820
        Radiofrequency Micro-Remodeling . . . 53860
    with Intestines 51960
Removal
    Calculus . . 51050, 51065, 52310-52315, 52352
    Foreign Body 52310-52315
    Urethral Stent 52310-52315
Repair 51800-51980
    Diverticulum. 52305
    Exstrophy 51940
    Fistula. 44660, 44661,
             45800-45805, 51880-51925
    Neck. 51845
    Wound 51860-51865
Resection 52500
Tumor
    Excision 51530
    Fulguration 52234-52240
    Resection 52234-52240
Unlisted Services and Procedures 53899
Ureterocele 51535
Urethrocystography. 74450-74455
Urethrotomy 52270-52276
Urinary Incontinence Procedures
    Neck Micro-remodel 53860
    Plan of Care 0509F
    Sling Operation 51992
    Urethral Suspension 51990
X-ray 74430, 74450-74455

Bladder Voiding Pressure Studies 51728, 51729

Blalock-Hanlon Procedure 33735-33737
See Septostomy, Atrial

Blalock-Taussig Procedure
Shunt, Great Vessel 33750

Blast Cells
See Stem Cell

Blast Transformation
See Blastogenesis

Blastocyst Implantation
See Implantation, Embryo

Blastocyst Transfer
See Embryo Transfer

Blastogenesis 86353

Performance Measures
    Chronic Kidney Disease . . .0513F, 2000F, 3074F,
                                3075F, 3077F-3080F
    Coronary Artery Disease 0001F, 3074F
    Hypertension 3074F, 3075F, 3077F-3080F
Venous 93770

Blood Products
Irradiation 86945
Pooling 86965
Splitting. 86985
Volume Reduction. 86960

Blood Sample
Fetal 59030

Blood Serum
See Serum

Blood Smear
Microorganism Identification 87205-87207
Microscopic Examination 85007, 85008
Peripheral 85060
Sex Chromatin. 88140
Surgical Pathology 88312, 88313, 88319

Blood Syndrome
Chromosome Analysis 88245, 88248, 88249

Blood Tests
Coagulation
    See Blood Coagulation, Tests
Cell Count
    See Blood Cell Count
Culture, Bacteria
    See Bacteria Culture
Gas Analysis
    See Blood Gases
Iron Stores. 3160F
Kt/V. 3082F-3084F
Nuclear Medicine
    Plasma Volume. 78110, 78111
    Platelet Survival. 78190, 78191
    Red Cell Survival 78130, 78135
    Red Cell Volume. 78120, 78121
    Whole Blood Volume. 78122
Panels
    Acute Hepatitis 80074
    Electrolyte 80051
    General Health. 80050
    Hepatic Function. 80076
    Hepatitis, Acute 80074
    Lipid 80061
    Metabolic
        Basic. 80047, 80048
        Comprehensive. 80053
    Obstetric. 80055, 80081
    Renal Function 80069
Typing
    See Blood Typing, Serologic
Urea Nitrogen 84520-84525
Volume Determination 78122

Blood Transfusion, Autologous
See Autotransfusion

Blood Typing, Serologic
ABO Only. 86900
Antigen Screen 86904
Antigen Testing, Donor Blood. 86902
Compatibility. 86920-86923
Other RBC Antigens 86905
Paternity Testing 86910, 86911
Rh (D). 86901
Rh Phenotype 86906

Blood Urea Nitrogen 84520-84525

Blood Vessels
Angioscopy 35400
Endoscopy 37500, 37501
Endothelial Function Assessment
    Noninvasive 0337T
Excision
    See Arteriovenous Malformation; Bypass Graft
Exploration
    Abdomen 35840
    Carotid Artery. 35701
    Chest 35820
    Extremity 35860
    Femoral Artery 35721
    Neck. 35800
    Popliteal Artery 35741
    Vessel, Other 35761
Harvest
    See Bypass Graft, Harvest
Repair
    Aneurysm
        See Aneurysm Repair
    Aorta 33320-33322
    Fistula
        See Arteriovenous Fistula
    Direct 35201-35226
        Finger 35207
        Hand. 35207
        Intra-abdominal 35221, 35281
        Intrathoracic . . . 35211, 35216, 35271, 35276
        Lower Extremity 35226, 35286
        Neck 35201, 35231, 35261
    Great Vessel. 33320-33322
    Kidney 50100
    Upper Extremity 35236, 35266
    Malformation
        See Arteriovenous Malformation
Shunt Creation
    Direct 36818, 36821
    Thomas Shunt 36835
    with Bypass Graft 35686
    with Graft. 36825-36830
    with Transposition 36818-36820
Shunt Revision
    with Graft. 36832

Blood, Occult
See Occult Blood

Bloom Syndrome
Chromosome Analysis 88245
Gene Analysis. 81209

Blot Test, Ink
See Rorschach Test

Blotting, Western
See Western Blot

Blow-Out Fracture
Orbital Floor 21385-21395

Blue Dome Cyst
See Breast, Cyst

BMT
See Hematopoietic Progenitor Cell (HPC),
Transplantation

Boarding Home Care
Established Patient. 99334-99337
New Patient 99324-99328

Bodies
Acetone
    See Drug Assay, Drug Procedure, Definitive Drug
    Class, Alcohols
Barr
    See Barr Bodies
Carotid
    See Carotid Body
Ciliary
    See Ciliary Body
Heinz
    See Heinz Bodies
Inclusion
    See Inclusion Bodies
Ketone
    See Ketone Body

Body Cast
See Cast

Body Fluid
Abdominal
    See Paracentesis
Amniotic
    See Amniotic Fluid
Blood
    See Blood Tests
Cerebrospinal Fluid
    See Cerebrospinal Fluid
Fetal
    Procedures and Testing
        See Fetal Procedures; Fetal Testing
Pleural
    See Pleura
Semen
    See Semen Analysis
Spinal
    See Spinal Cord
Urine
    See Urinalysis

Body of Vertebra
See Vertebral Body

Boil
See Furuncle

Boil, Vulva
See Vulva, Incision and Drainage, Boil

Bone
Abscess
    See Abscess, Bone
Biopsy
    Needle 20220, 20225
    Open. 20240, 20245, 20250, 20251
    Trocar 20220, 20225
    with Vertebroplasty
        Cervicothoracic. 22510, 22512
        Lumbosacral 22511, 22512
Cast
    See Cast
Cyst
    Drainage. 20615
    Injection 20615
Debridement 11044, 11047
Density Study
    See Bone Density Study
Disease
    Evaluation and Management
    See Performance Measures, Osteoarthritis;
    Performance Measures, Osteoporosis
Excision
    See Amputation; Arthrectomy

Bronchopulmonary Lavage
See Lung, Lavage

Bronchoscopy
Ablation
    Photodynamic Therapy......... 96570, 96571
Alveolar Lavage 31624
Aspiration 31629, 31633, 31645, 31646
Balloon Occlusion 31634, 31647, 31651
Biopsy 31625-31629, 31632, 31633
Brushing/Protected Brushing 31623
Catheter Placement
    Aspiration......................... 31725
    Intracavitary Radioelement 31643
Computer-assisted Navigation 31627
Dilation 31630, 31631, 31636-31638
Exploration 31622, 31634, 31647, 31651
Fiducial Marker Placement................ 31626
Fracture Reduction 31630
Insertion of Bronchial Valve(s) 31647, 31651
Needle Biopsy..................... 31629, 31633
Removal
    Bronchial Valve 31648, 31649
    Foreign Body 31635
    Tumor 31640, 31649
Stenosis 31641
Stent Placement 31631, 31636, 31637
Stent Revision....................... 31638
with Endobronchial Ultrasound
(EBUS)...................... 31652-31654
with Airway Resizing 31647, 31648, 31649
with Assessment of Airway Leak......... 31647,
    31648, 31649
with Balloon Occlusion..... 31647, 31648, 31649
with Bronchial Thermoplasty 31660, 31661
with Insertion of Bronchial Valves 31647,
    31648, 31649

Bronchospasm Evaluation
See Pulmonology, Diagnostic, Spirometry

Bronkodyl
See Theophylline

Brow Ptosis
Repair 67900, 67909

Brucella
Antibody 86622
Antigen 86000

Bruise
See Hematoma

Brunschwig Operation
Pelvic Exenteration.................... 58240

Brush Biopsy
See Biopsy; Needle Biopsy
Bronchi 31717

Brush Border Ab
See Antibody, Detection, Heterophile

Bucca
See Cheek

Buccal Mucosa
See Mouth, Mucosa

Bulbourethral Gland
Excision............................ 53250

Bulla
Incision and Drainage
    Puncture Aspiration............... 10160

Lung
    Resection-plication 32141, 32655

BUN
See Blood Urea Nitrogen; Urea Nitrogen

Bunion Repair
by Phalanx Osteotomy 28298, 28299
Chevron Procedure 28296
Concentric Procedure 28296
Joplin Procedure...................... 28294
Keller Procedure 28292
Lapidus Procedure.................... 28297
Mayo Procedure 28292
McBride Procedure 28292
Mitchell Procedure 28296
Silver Procedure 28290
Simple Exostectomy 28290
with Implant 28293
with Metatarsal Osteotomy 28296
with Tendon Transplants................ 28294

Burgess Amputation
See Disarticulation, Ankle

Burkitt Herpesvirus
See Epstein-Barr Virus

Burns
Debridement .. 15002-15005, 16020, 16025, 16030
Dressings 16020, 16025, 16030
Escharotomy 15002-15005, 16035, 16036
First Degree, Initial Treatment 16000
Tissue Cultured Skin Grafts 15150-15152,
    15155-15157
Total Body Surface Area (TBSA) Calculation 16000

Burr Hole
for Aspiration
    Cyst 61156
    Hematoma 61156
for Biopsy
    Brain............................ 61140
    Lesion............ 61140, 61750, 61751
for Catheterization 61210
for Drainage
    Abscess 61150, 61151
    Cyst 61150, 61151
    Hematoma 61154-61156
for Exploration
    Infratentorial 61253
    Supratentorial 61250
for Implantation
    Catheter 61210
    Cerebral Monitoring Device........... 61210
    EEG Electrode.................... 61210
    Neurostimulator Array....... 61850, 61863,
        61864, 61867, 61868
    Pressure Recording Device 61210
    Reservoir 61210
    Strip Electrodes 61531
for Insertion
    Pump 61210
    Reservoir 61210
for Lesion Creation 61720
for Stereotactic Localization............. 61770
for Ventricular Puncture 61020
    with Injection, Contrast Media 61120
    with Injection, Diagnostic or Therapeutic
    Substance 61026

Burrow's Operation
See Skin, Adjacent Tissue Transfer

Bursa
Ankle
    Aspiration.................. 20605, 20606
    Incision and Drainage 27604
    Injection.................. 20605, 20606
Arm, Lower
    Aspiration.................. 20605, 20606
    Incision and Drainage 25031
    Injection.................. 20605, 20606
Arm, Upper
    Incision and Drainage 23931
Arthrocentesis
    Intermediate............... 20605, 20606
    Major 20610, 20611
    Small 20600, 20604
    with recording and reporting........ 20604,
        20606, 20611
    with ultrasound guidance 20604,
        20606, 20611
Elbow
    Aspiration.................. 20605, 20606
    Injection.................. 20605, 20606
    Excision 24105
    Incision and Drainage 23931
Femur
    Excision 27062
Finger
    Aspiration.................. 20600, 20604
    Injection.................. 20600, 20604
Foot
    Incision and Drainage 28001-28003
Hand
    Incision and Drainage 26025, 26030
Hip
    Aspiration.................. 20610, 20611
    Injection.................. 20610, 20611
    Incision and Drainage 26991
Injection 20600, 20604-20606, 20610, 20611
Ischial
    Excision 27060
Joint
    Aspiration....................... 20600,
        20604-20606, 20610, 20611
    Drainage.. 20600, 20604-20606, 20610, 20611
    Injection.. 20600, 20604-20606, 20610, 20611
Knee
    Aspiration.................. 20610, 20611
    Excision 27340
    Incision and Drainage 27301
    Injection.................. 20610, 20611
Leg, Lower........................... 27604
Leg, Upper
    Incision and Drainage 27301
Palm
    Incision and Drainage 26025, 26030
Pelvis
    Incision and Drainage 26991
Shoulder
    Aspiration.................. 20610, 20611
    Drainage....................... 23031
    Injection.................. 20610, 20611
Toe
    Aspiration.................. 20600, 20604
    Injection.................. 20600, 20604
Wrist
    Aspiration.................. 20605, 20606
    Incision and Drainage 25031
    Injection.................. 20605, 20606
    Excision 25115, 25116

Bursectomy
See Excision, Bursa

Fragmentation
Bile Duct. 43265
Bladder. 52317, 52318
Kidney 50080, 50081
Liver. 50080, 50081
Ureter. 51065, 52325, 52353
Removal
Bile Duct. 43264, 47544, 47554
Biliary Tract 47400, 47420, 47425, 47480
Bladder. 51050, 52310, 52315, 52352
Gallbladder. 47544
Kidney . . 50060, 50065, 50070, 50075, 50080,
      50081, 50130, 50561, 50580, 52352
Liver 47400
Pancreatic Duct 43264, 48020
Renal Pelvis 50075, 50080, 50081, 50130
Salivary Duct 42330, 42335, 42340
Ureter. . . 50610, 50620, 50630, 50945, 50961,
      50980, 52310, 52315, 52320, 52352

Calculus of Kidney
See Calculus, Removal, Kidney

Caldwell-Luc Procedure
See Sinus/Sinuses, Maxillary; Sinusotomy
Orbital Floor Blowout Fracture 21385

Caliper
Application/Removal 20660

Callander Knee Disarticulation
See Disarticulation, Knee

Callosum, Corpus
See Corpus Callosum

Calmette-Guerin Bacillus Vaccine
See BCG Vaccine

Caloric Vestibular Test. 92533

Calprotectin
Fecal 83993

Calycoplasty 50405

Camey Enterocystoplasty 50825

CAMP
See Cyclic AMP

Campbell Procedure 27422

Campylobacter
Antibody 86625

Campylobacter Pylori
See Helicobacter Pylori

Canal, Ear
See Auditory Canal

Canal, Semicircular
See Semicircular Canal

Canalith Repositioning. 95992

Canaloplasty 69631, 69635

Candida
Antibody 86628
Skin Test 86485

Cannulation
Arterial 36620, 36625
Arteriovenous. 36810, 36815
Common Bile Duct 43273
Fallopian Tube. 58565
Pancreatic Duct 43273

Sinus
Maxillary 31000
Ostium 31235
Sphenoid 31002
Thoracic Duct 38794
Vas Deferens. 55200
Vein to Vein. 36800
Vertebral 22513-22515
with Transcatheter Aortic Valve Replacement
(TAVR/TAVI)
Arterial and Venous 33367-33369

Cannulation, Renoportal
See Anastomosis, Renoportal

Cannulization
See Cannulation; Catheterization
Arteriovenous 36147, 36148, 36810-36815
Declotting 36593, 36860, 36861
ECMO
See Extracorporeal Membrane Oxygenation
(ECMO)
External
Declotting. 36860, 36861
Vas Deferens. 55200
Vein to Vein. 36800

Canthocystostomy
See Conjunctivorhinostomy

Canthopexy
Lateral. 21282
Medial. 21280

Canthoplasty 67950

Canthorrhaphy 67880-67882

Canthotomy. 67715

Canthus
Reconstruction 67950, 67961, 67966

Cap, Cervical
See Cervical Cap

Capsule
See Brachytherapy; Capsulectomy; Capsulodesis;
Capsulorrhaphy; Capsulotomy; Cataract
Ankle. 27612, 27630
Biopsy 44100
Elbow 24006, 24149
Eye. 66830
Finger 26160, 26520
Foot 28090, 28264, 28289
Hand 26160, 26520
Heyman 58346
Hip. 27036
Drug Delivery Implants
Contraceptive. 11976, 11981
for Clinical Brachytherapy 58346
Injection 67515
Interphalangeal Joint 26525, 28272
Knee 27347, 27405, 27435
Leg. 27630
Shoulder 23020
Tenon's 67515
Toe. 28270, 28272
Wrist 25320

Capsulectomy
Breast 19371
Elbow 24149
Foot 28090
Hand 26160, 26520
Hip. 27036

Knee 27347
Metacarpophalangeal Joint 26520

Capsulodesis
Metacarpophalangeal Joint 26516-26518
Wrist 25320

Capsulorrhaphy
Anterior. 23450, 23455, 23460, 23462
Bankart Procedure 23455
Bristow Procedure 23460
Magnuson Type 23450
Putti-Platt Procedure 23450
Glenohumeral Joint 23465, 23466
Multi-Directional Instability 23466
Posterior 23465
Shoulder 29806
Thermal 29999
Wrist. 25320
Ankle. 27630

Capsulotomy
Breast 19370
Eye. 66830
Foot 28260-28262, 28264
Hip. 27036
Interphalangeal Joint 28272
Knee 27435
Leg. 27630
Metacarpophalangeal Joint 26520
Metatarsophalangeal Joint 28270
Shoulder 23020
Toe. 28270-28272
Wrist 25085, 25320

Captopril. 80416, 80417

Car Seat Testing 94780, 94781

Carbamazepine
Assay. 80156, 80157

Carbazepin
See Carbamazepine

Carbinol
See Methanol

Carbohydrate Deficient
Transferrin. 82373

Carbon Dioxide
Blood or Urine. 82374, 82803

Carboxycathepsin
See Angiotensin II

Carboxyhemoglobin. 82375,
                                      82376, 88740

Carbuncle
Incision and Drainage. 10060, 10061

Carcinoembryonal Antigen
See Carcinoembryonic Antigen

Carcinoembryonic Antigen
Detection. 82378

Cardiac
See Coronary
Muscle
See Myocardium
Neoplasm
See Heart, Tumor
Pacemaker
See Heart, Pacemaker

Septal Defect
  See Septal Defect

Cardiac Arrhythmia, Tachycardia
See Tachycardia

Cardiac Atria
See Atria

Cardiac Catheterization
See Catheterization, Cardiac
Combined Left and Right Heart 93460, 93461
  with Left Ventriculography 93453,
                                              93460, 93461
Combined Right and Retrograde Left
  Congenital Cardiac Anomalies 93531
Combined Right and Transseptal Left
  Congenital Cardiac Anomalies . . 93532, 93533
Congenital Cardiac Anomalies 93530-93533
for Angiography
  Bypass Graft(s) . . . 93455, 93457, 93459, 93461
  Congenital Heart 93563, 93564
  Coronary 93454-93461, 93563, 93571
  Left Atrial 93565
  Left Ventricular 93565
  Pulmonary 93568
  Right Atrial 93566
  Right Ventricular 93566
for Biopsy 93505
for Congenital Prosthetic Valve
  Implantation 33477
for Dilution Studies 93561, 93562
for Flow Measurement 93571, 93572
for Measurement of O2, Cardiac Output 93451
for Opacification
  Bypass Grafts 93564
for Supravalvular Aortography 93567
Imaging 93452-93461, 93563-93568
Injection 93454-93461, 93563-93568
Insertion
  Flow Directed Catheter
    Swan-Ganz 93503
Left Heart
  by Transapical Puncture 93462
  by Transseptal Puncture through Intact
    Septum 93462
  with Ventriculography 93452,
                                            93458, 93459, 93565
Pacemaker 33210
Right Heart 93451, 93456, 93503
  Congenital Cardiac Anomalies 93530

Cardiac Electroversion
See Cardioversion

Cardiac Event Recorder
Implantation 33282
Removal 33284

Cardiac Magnetic Resonance Imaging (CMRI)
Morphology and Function 75557,
                                      75559, 75561, 75563
Stress 75559, 75563
Velocity Flow Mapping 75565

Cardiac Massage
Thoracotomy 32160

Cardiac Output
Indicator Dilution 93561, 93562

Cardiac Rehabilitation . . . 93797, 93798

Cardiac Transplantation
See Heart, Transplantation

Cardiectomy
Donor 33930, 33940

Cardioassist 92970, 92971

Cardiography
Acoustic 93799
Arterial Pressure Waveform Analysis 93050

Cardiolipin Antibody 86147

Cardiology
Diagnostic
  Acoustic Cardiography 93799
  Arrhythmia Induction 93618-93624,
                              93640, 93641, 93653-93656
  Arterial Pressure Waveform Analysis 93050
  Atrial Electrogram 93615, 93616
    Esophageal Recording 93615, 93616
  Bioimpedance-derived Analysis 93701
  Echocardiography
    See Echocardiography
  Electrocardiography
    See Electrocardiography
  Ergonovine Provocation Test 93024
  External Heart Rate Data Recording
    for Nocturnal Epilepsy
    Seizure .0381T-0386T
  Intracardiac Pacing and Mapping
    3-D Mapping 93613, 93654
    Follow-up Study 93624
    Localization 93631
    Slow Conduction Zone 93631
    Stimulation and Pacing 93623
    Tachycardia Sites 93631
  Intracardiac Pacing and Recording
    Arrhythmia Induction 93618-93624,
                              93653, 93654, 93656
    Bundle of His 93600,
                        93619, 93620, 93653, 93654, 93656
    Comprehensive 93619-93622
    Intra-Atrial 93602, 93610, 93616, 93656
    Left Ventricular 93654
    Right Ventricular 93603, 93653, 93656
    Tachycardia Sites 93609
    Ventricular 93612
  Intravascular Ultrasound 92978, 92979
  Perfusion Imaging 78451-78454
    See Nuclear Medicine
  Stress Tests
    Cardiovascular 93015-93018
    Drug Induced 93024
    Multiple Gated Acquisition (MUGA) . . 78473
    Temperature Gradient Studies 93740
    Tilt Table Evaluation 93660
    Venous Pressure Determination 93784,
                              93786, 93788, 93790
Therapeutic
  Ablation 93650, 93653-93656
  Cardioassist 92970, 92971
  Cardioversion 92960, 92961
  Intravascular Ultrasound 92978, 92979
  Pacing 92953
  Rehabilitation 93668, 93797, 93798
  Thrombolysis 92975-92977
  Thrombolysis, Coronary 92977
  Valvuloplasty 92986-92990

Cardiomyotomy
See Esophagomyotomy

Cardioplasty 43320

Cardiopulmonary Bypass
See Heart; Lung, Transplantation
  with Transcatheter Aortic Valve Replacement
  (TAVR/TAVI) 33367, 33368, 33369

Cardiopulmonary Resuscitation 92950

Cardiotomy 33310-33315

Cardiovascular Stress Test
See Exercise Stress Tests

Cardioversion 92960, 92961

Care
Custodial
  See Nursing Facility Services
Intensive
  See Intensive Care
Neonatal Intensive
  See Intensive Care, Neonatal
Self
  See Self Care

Care Plan Oversight Services
See Physician Services

Carinal Reconstruction
See Trachea, Reconstruction

Carneous Mole
See Abortion

Carnitine 82379

Carotene 82380

Caroticum, Glomus
See Carotid Body

Carotid Artery
See Artery, Carotid

Carotid Body
Tumor
  Excision 60600-60605

Carpal Bone
See Wrist
Arthroplasty
  with Implant 25443
Cyst
  Excision 25130-25136
Dislocation
  Closed Treatment 25690
  Open Treatment 25695
Excision 25210, 25215
  Partial 25145
Fracture
  Closed Treatment 25622,
                          25630, 25635, 25645
  Open Treatment 25628, 25645
    with Manipulation 25624, 25635
    without Manipulation 25630
Incision and Drainage 26034
Insertion
  Vascular Pedicle 25430
Ligament Release 29848
Osteoplasty
  Shortening 25394
Prosthetic Placement 25443
Repair
  Nonunion 25431, 25440
    with Fixation 25628
    with Styloidectomy 25440

Scaphoid (Navicular)
  Fracture 25622, 25625, 25628
    Nonunion Repair 25440
Sequestrectomy 25145
Tumor
  Excision 25130, 25135, 25136
Tunnel
  See Carpal Tunnel

Carpal Tunnel
Injection
  Therapeutic 20526
Median Nerve Neuroplasty 64721

Carpal Tunnel Syndrome
Decompression 64721

Carpals
Incision and Drainage 25035

Carpectomy 25210, 25215

Carpometacarpal Joint
Arthrodesis 25800
  Finger 26843, 26844
  Thumb 26841, 26842
Arthrotomy 26070
Biopsy 26100
Dislocation
  Closed Treatment 26670
    with Manipulation 26675, 26676
  Open Treatment 26685, 26686
Drainage 26070
Exploration 26070
Fusion
  Hand 26843, 26844
  Thumb 26841, 26842
Magnetic Resonance Imaging 73221-73225
Removal
  Foreign Body 26070
Repair 25447
Synovectomy 26130

Cartilage Graft
Costochondral 20910
Ear 21235
for Mandibular Condyle Reconstruction 21247
for Zygomatic Arch Reconstruction 21255
Harvesting 20910, 20912
Nasal Septum 20912
Rib 21230

Cartilage, Arytenoid
See Arytenoid

Cartilage, Ear
See Ear Cartilage

Cartilaginous Exostoses
See Exostosis

Case Management Services
Anticoagulant Management 99363, 99364
On-line 98969, 99444
Team Conferences 99366-99368
Telephone Calls 98966-98968, 99441-99443

Cast
See Brace; Splint
Below Knee to Toes 29405
Elbow to Finger 29075
Finger 29086
Hand and Lower Forearm 29085
Hip Spica
  1 and one-half 29325
  1 Leg 29305
  Both Legs 29325

Leg 29445, 29450
Removal 29700, 29705, 29710
Repair 29720
Shoulder Spica 29055
Shoulder to Hand 29065
Shoulder to Hip 29035
  with Head 29040
  with 1 Thigh 29044
  with Both Thighs 29046
Thigh to Ankle 29365
Thigh to Toes 29345, 29355
Type
Ambulatory 29355, 29425, 29440
  Club Foot 29450, 29750
  Cylinder 29365
  Figure-of-eight 29049
  Gauntlet 29085, 29750
  Halo
    Body Cast 29000
    Cranial 20661
    for Thin Skull Osteology 20664
    Femur 20663
    Maxillofacial 21100
    Pelvic 20662
    Removal 20665
  Long Arm 29065
  Long Leg 29358, 29450
  Minerva 29040
  Patella Tendon Bearing (PTB) 29435
  Rigid Total Contact 29445
  Risser Jacket
    Body 29010
    with Head 29015
  Short Arm 29075
  Short Leg 29405, 29450
  Spica 29055, 29305, 29720
  Velpeau 29058
  Walker 29355, 29425, 29440
Wedging 29740, 29750
Windowing 29730

Casting
Unlisted Services and Procedures 29799

Castration
See Orchiectomy

Castration, Female
See Oophorectomy

CAT Scan
See CT Scan

Cataract
Disscision 66820, 66821
Excision 66830
  Dilated Fundus Evaluation 2020F
Incision 66820, 66821
  Laser 66821
  Stab Incision 66820
Extraction/Removal
  Extracapsular 66982, 66984
  Intracapsular (ICCE) 66983
  Presurgical Measurement and
  Calculations 3073F

Catecholamines 80424, 82382-82384
Blood 82383
Panel for Pheochromocytoma 80424
Urine 82382

Cathepsin-D 82387

Catheter
See Cannulation; Catheterization; Venipuncture
Aspiration
  Nasotracheal 31720
  Tracheobronchial 31725
Balloon
  See Balloon Angioplasty
Biopsy 37200
Bladder 51701-51703
  Irrigation 51700
Blood Specimen Collection 36592, 37799
Conversion
  Biliary Drainage
    External to Internal-External 47535
    Nephrostomy to Nephroureteral 50434
Declotting 36593, 36861
Drainage
  Biliary
    Conversion 47535
    Exchange 47536
    Placement 47533, 47534
    Removal 47537
  Peritoneal 49406, 49407
  Pleural 32556, 32557
  Retroperitoneal 49406, 49407
  Spinal 62272
  Ureteral 50693
  Ventricular 62162, 62164
  Visceral 49405
Electrode Array 63650
Embolization 61624, 61626
  Peritoneal 49423
Exchange
  Nephrostomy 50435
  with Biliary Stent Placement 47538-47540
  for Cystourethroscopy 52320-52356
  for Embolectomy 34001, 34051, 34101-34111,
                           34151, 34201, 34203
  for Enteral Alimentation 44015
Flow Directed 93503
for Placement
  Radiation Source 61770
  Stent 33621, 61635
  Wireless Physiologic Sensor 34806
for Thrombectomy 34001, 34051, 34101-34111,
              34151, 34201, 34203, 34401, 34421, 34451
for Infusion
  Brachial Plexus 64416
  Femoral Nerve 64448
  Lumbar Plexus 64449
  Saline 58340
  Sciatic Nerve 64446
  Vertebral 62318, 62319
for Instillation
  Pleurodesis 32560
  Fibrinolysis 32561, 32562
Home Visit for Care 99507
Intraperitoneal, Tunneled
  Insertion
    Laparoscopic 49324
    Open 49421
    Percutaneous 49418, 49419
Obstruction Clearance 36595, 36596
Occlusion 61624, 61626
Placement
  See Catheterization
Removal
  Central Venous 36589
  Foreign Body 37197
  Peritoneal 49422
  Spinal Cord 62355
  with Biliary Stent Placement 47538-47540

Cecostomy
Laparoscopic.........................44188
Obstructive Material Removal...........49460
Skin Level............................44320
Tube
  Insertion
    Open.............................44300
    Percutaneous....................49442
    Radiologic Evaluation...........49465
    Replacement.....................49450
with Colectomy........................44141

Celiac Plexus
Destruction...........................64680
Injection
  Anesthetic........................64530
  Neurolytic........................64680

Celiac Trunk Artery
See Artery, Celiac

Celioscopy
See Endoscopy, Peritoneum

Celiotomy.........................49000
Abdomen
  for Staging.......................49220

Cell Count
B Cells...............................86355
Bacterial Colony......................87086
CD4............................86360, 86361
CD8...................................86360
CD34..................................86367
Chromosome Analysis
  See Chromosome Analysis
Body Fluid.....................86152, 86153
  Other than Blood.............89050, 89051
Natural Killer (NK)....................86357
Sperm..................89310, 89320, 89322
Stem..................................86367
T Cells.........................86359-86361

Cell, Blood
See Blood Cell

Cell, Islet
See Islet Cell

Cell, Mother
See Stem Cell

Cell-Stimulating Hormone, Interstitial
See Luteinizing Hormone (LH)

Cellobiase
See Beta Glucosidase

Cellular Inclusion
See Inclusion Bodies

Central Shunt...................33764

Central Venous Catheter Placement
Insertion
  Central
    Non-tunneled.............36555, 36556
    Tunneled without Port or
    Pump..............36557, 36558, 36565
    Tunneled with Port....36560, 36561, 36566
    Tunneled with Pump..............36563
  Peripheral
    with Port................36570, 36571
    without Port or Pump.......36568, 36569

Repair
  with Port or Pump..................36576
  without Port or Pump...............36575
Replacement
  Catheter Only.....................36578
  Complete
    Central...............36580-36583
    Peripheral............36584, 36585
Repositioning.........................36597

Central Venous Catheter Removal.....................36589

Cephalic Version
of Fetus
  Anesthesia........................01958
  External..........................59412

Cephalocele
See Encephalocele

Cephalogram, Orthodontic
See Orthodontic Cephalogram

Cerclage
Cervix................................57700
  Abdominal.........................59325
  Removal under Anesthesia..........59871
  Vaginal...........................59320
Femoral Fracture.....27244, 27245, 27506, 27507
Humeral Shaft Fracture...........24515, 24516
Tibial Shaft Fracture.............27758, 27759

Cerebellopontine Angle Tumor
See Brain, Tumor, Excision; Brainstem; Mesencephalon; Skull Base Surgery

Cerebral Cortex Decortication
See Decortication

Cerebral Death
See Brain Death

Cerebral Hernia
See Encephalocele

Cerebral Perfusion Analysis
CT Scan...............................0042T

Cerebral Ventriculographies
See Ventriculography

Cerebral Vessels
Anastomosis...........................61711
Aneurysm Surgery
  Carotid Artery Occlusion...........61705,
                    61708, 61710
  Cervical Approach.................61703
  Intracranial Approach.............61697,
             61698, 61700, 61702
Angioplasty...........................61630
Arteriovenous Malformation Surgery
  Dural......................61690, 61692
  Fistula...........................61705
  Infratentorial.............61684, 61686
  Supratentorial.............61680-61682
Dilation
  Intracranial Vasospasm.......61640-61642
Occlusion.............................61623
Placement
  Stent
    Intravascular...................61635
Thrombolysis..........................37195

Cerebrose
See Galactose

Cerebrospinal Fluid
Drainage
  Spinal Puncture...................62272
Flow Imaging
  Cisternography....................78630
  Ventriculography..................78635
  Shunt Evaluation..................78645
  Tomographic (SPECT)...............78647
  Leakage Detection and Localization....78650
Leak
  See Cerebrospinal Fluid Leak
Shunt
  See Cerebrospinal Fluid Shunt
Test
  Cell Count........................89050
  Immunoelectrophoresis.............86325
  Myelin Basic Protein..............83873
  Protein, Total....................84157

Cerebrospinal Fluid Leak
Repair
  Craniotomy........................62100
  Spinal Cord...............63707-63709
  with Skull Base Surgery.......61618, 61619
  with Nasal/Sinus Endoscopy....31290, 31291

Cerebrospinal Fluid Shunt
Creation.........62190, 62192, 62220, 62223
  Lumbar....................63740, 63741
Irrigation.................62194, 62225
Removal............62256, 62258, 63746
Replacement............62160, 62258, 63744
  Catheter.........62194, 62225, 62230
  Valve.............................62230
Reprogramming.........................62252
Torkildsen Operation..................62180
Ventriculocisternostomy....62180, 62200, 62201

Ceruloplasmin....................82390

Cerumen
Removal
  with Instrumentation..............69210
  with Irrigation/Lavage............69209

Cervical Cap.....................57170

Cervical Lymphadenectomy.........38720-38724

Cervical Mucus Penetration Test..................................89330

Cervical Plexus
Injection
  Anesthetic........................64413

Cervical Pregnancy..............59140

Cervical Puncture.........61050-61055

Cervical Smears
Cytopathology
  Automated Screen..................88174
  Hormone Evaluation................88155
  Physician Interpretation..........88141
  Partially Automated Screen....88147, 88148,
          88152, 88166, 88167, 88175
  Manual Screen..88150, 88153, 88164, 88165
Pap
  Any Reporting System........88174, 88175
  Bethesda System...........88164-88167
  Non-Bethesda.........88150, 88152-88154

Cervical Spine
See Vertebra, Cervical
Chemodenervation, Muscles.............64615

CT Scan 71250, 71260, 71270
Magnetic Resonance Angiography 71555
Magnetic Resonance Imaging
(MRI) 71550-71552
PET Imaging 78811, 78814
Ultrasound 76604
X-ray
See X-ray, Chest
Exploration
Postoperative
Hemorrhage 35820
Infection 35820
Thrombosis 35820
Penetrating Wound 20101
Exit Site, Intraperitoneal Cannula/Catheter . . 49435
Repair
Blood Vessel 35211, 35216
with Other Graft 35271-35276
with Vein Graft 35241, 35246
Tube
See Thoracostomy
Tumor
See Chest Wall

Chest Cavity
Bypass Graft 35905
Thoracoscopy
See Thoracoscopy

Chest Wall
See Pulmonology, Therapeutic
Debridement 11044, 11047
Manipulation 94667, 94668
Mechanical Oscillation 94669
Reconstruction 49904
with Lung Tumor Resection 32504
Trauma 32820
Repair 32905
Closure 32810
Fistula 32906
Lung Hernia 32800
Resection 32503
Tumor
Ablation 32998
Cryoablation 0340T
Excision 19260, 19270-19272
Unlisted Services and Procedures 32999

Chest, Funnel
See Pectus Excavatum

Chevron Procedure 28296

Chiari Osteotomy of the Pelvis
See Osteotomy, Pelvis

Chicken Pox Vaccine
Varicella Virus (VAR) 90716

Child Procedure
Pancreatectomy 48146

Chimerism 81267, 81268

Chin
Cartilage Graft 21230
Repair
Augmentation 21120
Osteotomy 21121-21123
Rhytidectomy 15828
Skin Graft 15240, 15241
Tissue Transfer
Adjacent 14040, 14041
Flap 15574, 15620
Wound Repair 13131-13133

Chinidin
See Quinidine

Chiropractic Manipulation
See Manipulation, Chiropractic

Chiropractic Treatment
Spinal
Extraspinal 98940-98943

Chlamydia
Antibody 86631, 86632
Antigen Detection
Amplified Nucleic Acid Probe . . . 87486, 87491
Direct Nucleic Acid Probe 87485, 87490
Direct Optical 87810
Immunoassay 87320
Immunofluorescence 87270
Nucleic Acid Quantification 87487, 87492
Culture 87110

Chloramphenicol 82415

Chloride
Blood 82435
Other Source 82438
Panels
Basic Metabolic 80047, 80048
Comprehensive Metabolic 80053
Electrolyte 80051
Renal Function 80069
Spinal Fluid 82438
Urine 82436

Chloride, Methylene
See Dichloromethane

Chlorinated Hydrocarbons 82441

Chlorohydrocarbon
See Chlorinated Hydrocarbons

Choanal Atresia
Repair 30540-30545

Cholangiography
Injection 47531, 47532
Intraoperative 74300, 74301
Postoperative 47531
Repair
with Bile Duct Exploration 47700
with Cholecystectomy . . . 47563, 47605, 47620
Transhepatic
Laparoscopically Guided 47579
with Conversion of Drainage Catheter 47535
with Exchange of Drainage Catheter 47536
with Placement of Access to Small Bowel . . . 47541
with Placement of Drainage
Catheter 47533, 47534
with Placement of Stent 47538-47540
with Removal of Drainage Catheter 47537

Cholangiopancreatography
See Bile Duct; Pancreatic Duct
Endoscopic Retrograde Cholangiopancreatography
(ERCP)
with Ablation
Lesion 43278
Polyp 43278
Tumor 43278
with Biopsy 43261
with Collection of Specimen(s) 43260
with Exchange
Stent 43276
with Optical Endomicroscopy 0397T
with Papillotomy 43262

with Placement
Stent 43274
with Pressure Measurement Sphincter of
Oddi 43263
with Removal
Foreign Body 43275
Stent 43275, 43276
with Removal/Destruction of
Calculus 43264, 43265
with Sphincterotomy 43262, 43274,
43276, 43277
with Transendoscopic Balloon Dilation . . 43277
Intraoperative 74300, 74301
Postoperative 47531

Cholangiostomy
See Hepaticostomy

Cholangiotomy
See Hepaticostomy

Cholecalciferol
See Vitamin, D, Blood Serum Level, 25 hydroxy

Cholecystectomy
Any Method
with Cholangiography . . . 47563, 47605, 47620
with Choledochoenterostomy 47612
with Exploration Common Duct . . 47564, 47610
Donor Liver 47143
Excision 47600-47620
Laparoscopic 47562-47564

Cholecystenterostomy
Direct 47720
with Gastroenterostomy 47721, 47741
Laparoscopic 47570
Roux-en-Y 47740, 47741

Cholecystography 47490, 74290

Cholecystostomy
Open 47480
Percutaneous 47490
with Peripancreatic Drain Placement 48000

Cholecystotomy
Open 47480
with Choledochostomy 47420
with Choledochotomy 47420

Choledochoplasty
See Bile Duct, Repair

Choledochoscopy
Biliary Endoscopy 47550

Choledochostomy
Biliary Tract 47420, 47425

Choledochotomy
Biliary Tract 47420, 47425

Choledochus, Cyst
See Cyst, Choledochal

Cholera Vaccine
Live, for Oral Use 90625

Cholesterol
Measurement
HDL 83718
LDL 83721
Panel
Lipid 80061
Serum 82465
VLDL 83719

Fracture
  Closed Treatment
    with Manipulation 23505
    without Manipulation. 23500
  Open Treatment 23515
Pinning, Wiring 23490
Prophylactic Treatment 23490
Repair
  Osteotomy 23480
  Malunion/Nonunion. 23485
Saucerization 23180
Sequestrectomy 23170
Tumor
  Excision 23140, 23145, 23146, 23200
    with Graft 23145, 23146
    Radical Resection 23200
X-ray 73000

Clavicula
See Clavicle

Claviculectomy
Arthroscopic 29824
Open
  Partial 23120
  Total 23125

Claw Finger Repair 26499

Cleft Cyst, Branchial
See Branchial Cleft, Cyst

Cleft Foot
Reconstruction 28360

Cleft Hand
Repair 26580

Cleft Lip
Repair
  Primary 40700-40702
  Secondary 40720
  with Pedicle Flap 40761
Rhinoplasty 30460-30462

Cleft Palate
Repair 42200-42225
Rhinoplasty 30460-30462

Cleft, Branchial
See Branchial Cleft

Clinical Act of Insertion
See Insertion

Clinical Chemistry Test
See Chemistry Tests, Clinical

Clinical Pathology
Consultation 80500, 80502

Clitoroplasty
Intersex State 56805

Closed [Transurethral] Biopsy of Bladder
See Biopsy, Bladder, Cystourethroscopy

Clostridial Tetanus
See Tetanus

Clostridium Botulinum Toxin
See Chemodenervation

Clostridium Difficile
Antigen Detection
  Immunoassay 87324

Immunoassay
  with Direct Optical Observation 87803
Tissue Culture 87230
Toxin Genes Detection 87493

Clostridium Tetani ab
See Antibody, Detection, Tetanus

Closure 12001-13160
See Repair, Wound
Anal Fistula 46288
Atrioventricular Valve 33600
Cystostomy 51880
Enterostomy 44227, 44620, 44625, 44626
  Laparoscopic 44227
Lacrimal Fistula 68770
Lacrimal Punctum
  Plug 68761
  Thermocauterization, Ligation or
  Laser Surgery 68760
Left Atrial Appendage
  with Implant 0281T
Rectovaginal Fistula . . 57300, 57305, 57307, 57308
Semilunar Valve 33602
Septal Defect
  Ventricular 33776, 33780, 93581
Ventricular Tunnel 33722

Closure of Esophagostomy
See Esophagostomy, Closure

Closure of Gastrostomy
See Gastrostomy, Closure

Closure, Atrial Septal Defect
See Septal Defect, Atrial, Closure

Closure, Cranial Sutures, Premature
See Craniosynostosis

Closure, Fistula, Vesicouterine
See Fistula, Closure, Vesicouterine

Closure, Meningocele Spinal
See Meningocele Repair

Closure, Vagina
See Vagina, Closure

Clot 34401-34490, 35875, 35876, 50230
See Thrombectomy; Thromboendarterectomy; Thrombolysis
Clotting
  See Blood Coagulation, Test; Clotting Factor
  Epidural Blood Patch 62273
Declotting
  Cystourethroscopic 52001
  External Cannula 36860, 36861
  Eye 65930
  Implanted Catheter 36593
  Pericardium 32658, 33020
  Vascular Access Device 36593

Clot Lysis Time
Whole Blood Dilution 85175
Euglobin Lysis 85360

Clot Retraction
Coagulation Test 85170

Clotting Disorder
See Coagulopathy

Clotting Factor
Factor I
  See Fibrinogen

Factor II (Prothrombin) 85210
Factor III (Thromboplastin)
  Inhibition 85705
  Inhibition Test 85347
  Partial Time 85730-85732
Factor IV
  See Calcium
Factor VII (Proconvertin) 85230
Factor VIII
  AHG 85240
  Related Antigen 85244
  VW factor 85245, 85246
  von Willebrand factor 85247
Factor IX (Christmas Factor 85250
Factor X (Stuart-Prower) 85260
Factor X (Thrombokinase) 85260
Factor XI (Plasma Thromboplastin, Antecedent [PTA]) 85270
Factor XII (Hageman Factor) 85280
Factor XIII (Fibrin Stabilizing) 85290, 85291

Clotting Inhibitors
Tests
  Antithrombin III 85300, 85301
  Factor Inhibitor 85335
  Mixed Screen 85611, 85732
  Protein C 85302, 85303, 85307
  Protein S 85305, 85306
  Thrombomodulin 85337
  Thromboplastin Inhibition 85705

Clotting Operation
See Excision, Nail Fold

Clotting Test
Protein C 85303, 85307
Protein S 85306
See Coagulation, Tests

Clotting Time
See Coagulation Time

Clozapine
Drug Assay 80159

Clubfoot Cast 29450
Wedging 29750

CMG
See Cystometrogram

CMRI
See Cardiac Magnetic Resonance Imaging (CMRI)

CMV
See Cytomegalovirus

CNPB
See Continuous Negative Pressure Breathing (CNPB); Pulmonology, Therapeutic

Co-Factor I, Heparin
See Antithrombin III

CO2
See Carbon Dioxide

Coagulation
Tests
  See Blood Coagulation, Tests
Unlisted Services and Procedures 85999

Coagulation Defect
See Coagulopathy

Coagulation Factor
See Clotting Factor

Congenital Cardiac Anomaly
Catheterization 93530-93533
   Injection 93563, 93564
Closure
   Interatrial Communication............ 93580
   Ventricular Septal Defect 93581
Echocardiography
   Fetal 76825, 76826
   Doppler, Fetal 76827, 76828
   for Congenital Anomalies
     Transesophageal 93315-93317
     Transthoracic 93303, 93304
Ectopy
   Ventricular
     Treatment 93654

Congenital Elevation of Scapula
See Sprengel's Deformity

Congenital Heart Septum Defect
See Congenital Cardiac Anomaly

Congenital Kidney Abnormality
Nephrolithotomy........................ 50070
Pyeloplasty 50405
Pyelotomy 50135

Congenital Laryngocele
See Laryngocele

Congenital Vascular Anomaly
See Vascular Malformation

Conisation
See Cervix, Conization

Conization
Cervix 57461, 57520, 57522

Conjoint Psychotherapy
See Psychiatric Treatment, Family

Conjunctiva
Biopsy 68100
Cyst
   Incision and Drainage 68020
Fistulization for Drainage 68745, 68750
Follicle Expression 68040
Graft 65150, 65782
   Harvesting, Living Donor 68371
Injection 68200
Insertion Stent 68750
Lesion
   Destruction........................ 68135
   Excision 68110, 68115
     with Adjacent Sclera 68130
Reconstruction 68320, 68325, 68326, 68328
   with Flap 67971, 68360, 68362
Removal
   Foreign Body 65205, 65210
Repair
   Eyelid Wound............... 67961, 67966
     Direct Closure....... 65270, 67930, 67935
     Mobilization and
     Rearrangement............ 65272, 65273
   Symblepharon
     Division 68340
     with Graft 68335
     without Graft 68330
Unlisted Services and Procedures 68399

Conjunctivo-Tarso-Muller Resection
.... 67908

Conjunctivocystorhinostomy
See Conjunctivorhinostomy

Conjunctivodacryocystostomy
See Conjunctivorhinostomy

Conjunctivoplasty 68320-68330
Reconstruction Cul-de-Sac
   with Extensive Rearrangement 68326
   with Graft........................ 68326
     Buccal Mucous Membrane 68328
Repair of Symblepharon 68330, 68335, 68340

Conjunctivorhinostomy
with Tube 68750
without Tube........................... 68745

Conscious Sedation
See Sedation

Construction
Arterial
   Conduit.................... 33920, 33608
   Tunnel.......................... 33505
Bladder from Sigmoid Colon............ 50810
Eye Adhesions......................... 67880
Finger
   Toe to Hand Transfer 26551-26556
Gastric Tube 43832
Neobladder 51596
Tracheoesophageal Fistula.............. 31611
Vagina
   with Graft........................ 57292
   without Graft 57291
Valve
   Apical-Aortic Conduit............... 33404

Consultation
Clinical Pathology 80500, 80502
Inpatient 99251-99255
   New or Established Patient..... 99251-99255
Interprofessional
   Telephone/Internet Discussion .. 99446-99449
Office and/or Other Outpatient....... 99241-99245
   New or Established Patient..... 99241-99245
Psychiatric, with Family 90887
Radiation Therapy
   Radiation Physics........... 77336, 77370
Surgical Pathology 88321, 88323, 88325
   Intraoperative......... 88329, 88331-88334
X-ray 76140

Consumption Test, Antiglobulin
See Coombs Test

Contact Lens Services
Fittings and Prescription......... 92071, 92072,
                              92310-92317
Modification 92325
Prescription...................... 92314-92317
Replacement.......................... 92326

Continuous Negative Pressure Breathing (CNPB)............ 94662

Continuous Positive Airway Pressure (CPAP) 94660

Contouring
Cranial
   Bones.......................... 21181
   Sutures......................... 61559
Forehead 21137, 21138
Frontal Sinus Wall 21139
Septoplasty 30520
Subcutaneous Injections.... 11950-11952, 11954
Tumor
   Facial Bone...................... 21029

Contraception
Cervical Cap
   Fitting.......................... 57170
Diaphragm
   Fitting.......................... 57170
Intrauterine Device (IUD)
   Insertion........................ 58300
   Removal......................... 58301

Contraceptive Capsules, Implantable
Removal 11976

Contraceptive Device, Intrauterine
See Intrauterine Device (IUD)

Contracture
Bladder Neck
   Resection........................ 52640
Elbow
   Release
     with Radical Resection of Capsule ... 24149
Finger Cast 29086
Palm
   Release 26121-26125
Scar
Shoulder
   Capsular Release.................. 23020
Thumb
   Thenar Muscle Release............. 26508
Volkmann 25315
Wrist
   Capsulotomy 25085

Contracture of Palmar Fascia
See Dupuytren's Contracture

Contralateral Ligament
Repair
   Knee............................ 27405

Contrast Aortogram
See Aortography

Contrast Bath Therapy
See Physical Medicine/Therapy/Occupational Therapy
Application of Modality 97034

Contrast Material
Injection
   Arteriovenous Dialysis Shunt 36147
   Central Venous Access Device 36598
   Colonic Tube
     for Insertion 49440-49442
     for Radiological Evaluation 49465
     for Removal of Obstruction 49460
     for Replacement 49446, 49450-49452
   Cranial
     for Ventricular Puncture 61120
   Dacryocystography................. 68850
   Peritoneal
     for Assessment of Abscess or Cyst ... 49424
     for Evaluation of Venous Shunt 49427
     for Insertion of Tunneled Catheter ... 49418
   Peritoneal Cavity 49400
   Renal Angiography........... 36251-36254
   Saline Infusion Sonohysterography
   (SIS) 58340
   Spine
     for Localization.................. 62310,
          62311, 62318, 62319, 62263
   Urethrocystography............... 51605

Correction of Lid Retraction
See Repair, Eyelid, Retraction

Correction of Malrotation of Duodenum
See Ladd Procedure

Correction of Syndactyly
See Syndactyly, Repair

Correction of Ureteropelvic Junction
Stricture 52342, 52345

Cortex Decortication, Cerebral
See Decortication

Cortical Mapping
by Electric Stimulation 95961, 95962
Initial TMS Treatment. 90867
Noninvasive 96020

Corticoids
See Corticosteroids

Corticoliberin
See Corticotropic Releasing Hormone (CRH)

Corticosteroid Binding Globulin
See Transcortin

Corticosteroid Binding Protein
See Transcortin

Corticosteroids
Blood 83491
Urine 83491

Corticosterone
Blood or Urine 82528

Corticotropic Releasing Hormone (CRH)
Stimulation Panel 80412

Cortisol 80400,
80402, 80406, 80418, 80420, 80436, 82530
Stimulation 80412
Total 82533

Cortisol Binding Globulin 84449

Costectomy
See Rib, Excision

Costen Syndrome
See Temporomandibular Joint (TMJ)

Costotransversectomy 21610

Cothromboplastin
See Proconvertin

Cotte Operation
Uterine Suspension. 58400, 58410

Cotton Procedure
Bohler Procedure. 28405

Counseling
See Preventive Medicine
Smoking and Tobacco Use
Cessation 99406, 99407

Counseling and/or Risk Factor Reduction Intervention, Preventive Medicine, Individual Counseling
See Preventive Medicine, Counseling, Risk Factor Reduction Intervention

Count
Blood Cell
  See Blood Cell Count
Blood Platelet
  See Blood, Platelet, Count
Cell
  See Cell Count
Complete Blood
  See Complete Blood Count (CBC)
Erythrocyte
  See Red Blood Cell (RBC), Count
Leukocyte
  See White Blood Cell, Count
Reticulocyte
  See Reticulocyte, Count

Counterimmunoelectrophoresis 86185

Counters, Cell
See Cell Count

Countershock, Electric
See Cardioversion

Coventry Tibial Wedge Osteotomy
See Osteotomy, Tibia

Cowper's Gland
Excision. 53250

Coxa
See Hip

Coxiella Burnetii
Antibody 86638

Coxsackie
Antibody 86658

CPAP
See Continuous Positive Airway Pressure (CPAP)

CPK
Blood. 82550-82552

CPR (Cardiopulmonary Resuscitation)
Cardiac Arrest. 92950

Cranial Bone
See Craniectomy; Craniotomy
Bone Graft
  See Bone Graft
Burr Hole
  See Burr Hole
Frontal Bone Flap 61556, 61557
Halo Application
  Thin Skull Osteology 20664
Parietal Bone Flap. 61556
Reconstruction
  Extracranial 21181-21184
Temporal Bone
  Implantation
    Cochlear Device 69930
    Hearing Device. 69710, 69711
    Osseointegrated Implant 69714, 69715
    Removal of Tumor 69970
    Resection 69535
    Unlisted Procedure. 69979
Tumor
  Excision 61563, 61564

Cranial Halo. 20661

Cranial Nerve
Avulsion 64732-64760, 64771

Cranial Nerve II
  See Optic Nerve
Cranial Nerve V
  See Trigeminal Nerve
Cranial Nerve VII
  See Facial Nerve
Cranial Nerve X
  See Vagus Nerve
Cranial Nerve XI
  See Accessory Nerve, Spinal
Cranial Nerve XII
  See Hypoglossal Nerve
Decompression 61458, 61460, 64716
Injection
  Anesthetic
    Trigeminal Nerve 64400
    Vagus Nerve 64408
    Neurolytic. 64600, 64605, 64610
Neuroplasty. 64716
Neurostimulator
  See Neurostimulators
Release 64716
Repair
  Suture, with or without Graft . . . 64864, 64865
Transection 64732-64760, 64771
Transposition. 64716

Cranial Tongs
Application/Removal 20660
Removal 20665

Craniectomy. 61501
See Craniotomy
Abscess Drainage. 61320, 61321
Anesthesia 00211
Compression 61450
Craniosynostosis
  Single Suture 61550
  Multiple Sutures 61552, 61558, 61559
Decompression 61322, 61323, 61340, 61343
  Cranial Nerves 61458
  Sensory Root of Gasserian Ganglion. . . . 61450
Drainage 61320, 61321
Evacuation of Hematoma 61312-61315
Excision
  Abscess 61514, 61522
  Bone Lesion 61500
  Fenestration of Cyst. 61516, 61524
  Meningioma. 61512, 61519
  Tumor 61500, 61510, 61518, 61520, 61521
Exploratory 61304, 61305, 61458
for Electrode
  Cortical. 61860, 61870
  Subcortical. 61863, 61864, 61867, 61868
for Osteomyelitis. 61501
Release Stenosis 61550-61552
Section 61450, 61460
Tractotomy 61480
with Craniotomy 61316, 61530
Wound Treatment 61571

Craniofacial Procedures
Unlisted Services and Procedures 21299

Craniofacial Separation
Bone Graft. 21436
Closed Treatment 21431
External Fixation. 21435
Open Treatment 21432, 21433, 21435, 21436
Wire Fixation. 21431, 21432

Craniomegalic Skull
Reduction 62115, 62117

Nose............. 17280-17284, 17286
Penis................... 54056, 54065
Skin 17000, 17003, 17004,
.... 17106-17108, 17110, 17111
Urethra........................ 52224
Vagina.................. 57061, 57065
Vulva................... 56501, 56515
Prostate................. 52214, 55873
Trichiasis...................... 67825
Tumor
Bladder......... 52234, 52235, 52240
Rectum....................... 45190
Urethra........................ 52214

Cryotherapy
Ablation
Renal Tumor.................... 50593
Acne 17340
Bronchial Stenosis 31641
Destruction
Bronchial Tumor............... 31641
Ciliary Body.................. 66720
Retinopathy.................. 67227
Lesion
Cornea 65450
Retina....................... 67208
Retinal Detachment
Prophylaxis.................. 67141
Repair..... 67101, 67107, 67108, 67113
Retinopathy
Destruction.................. 67227
Treatment
Preterm Infant............. 67229
Trichiasis...................... 67825

Cryptectomy
Unlisted Procedure, Anus............. 46999

Cryptococcus
Antibody...................... 86641
Antigen Detection
Immunoassay.................. 87327

Cryptococcus Neoformans
Antigen Detection
Immunoassay.................. 87327

Cryptorchism
See Testis, Undescended

Cryptosporidium
Antigen Detection
Immunofluorescence 87272
Immunoassay.................. 87328

Crystal Identification
Any Body Fluid 89060
Tissue 89060

CSF
See Cerebrospinal Fluid

CT Scan
3-D Rendering.............. 76376, 76377
Not Requiring Independent
Workstation................ 76376
Requiring Independent Workstation 76377
Bone
Density Study................. 77078
Brain 70450-70470
Stroke Diagnosis 3110F-3112F
Computed Tomographic Angiography
See Computed Tomographic Angiography
Drainage 75989

Follow-up Study 76380
Guidance
Localization 77011
Needle Placement.............. 77012
Parenchymal Tissue Ablation.......... 77013
Radiation Therapy 77014
Visceral Tissue Ablation 77013
Heart
Evaluation
Angiography............... 75574
for Coronary Calcium 75571
for Structure and
Morphology 75572, 75573
Optical Coherence Tomography
Axillary Lymph Node 0351T, 0352T
Breast..............0351T-0354T
Intravascular 0291T, 0292T
Parathyroid Gland 78072
Unlisted Services and Procedures 76497
with Contrast 70460
Abdomen 74160, 74177
Arm......................... 73201
Brain.............. 0042T, 70460
Cerebral Blood Flow/Volume........... 0042T
Ear 70481
Face 70487
Head........................ 70460
Leg 73701
Maxilla 70487
Neck 70491
Orbit 70481
Pelvis 72193, 74177
Sella Turcica................. 70481
Spine
Cervical.................. 72126
Lumbar 72132
Thoracic.................. 72129
Thorax 71260
without and with Contrast
Abdomen 74170,
.... 74174, 74175, 74178, 75635
Arm........................ 73202
Brain 70470, 70496
Chest 71275
Ear 70482
Face 70488
Head.............. 70470, 70496
Leg 73702-73706, 75635
Maxilla 70488
Neck 70492, 70498
Orbit 70482
Pelvis 72194, 74174, 74178
Sella Turcica................. 70482
Spine
Cervical.................. 72127
Lumbar 72133
Thoracic.................. 72130
Thorax 71270
without Contrast 70450
Abdomen 74150, 74176, 74178
Arm........................ 73200
Brain....................... 70450
Colon
Colonography 74261-74263
Ear 70480
Face 70486
Head........................ 70450
Leg 73700
Maxilla 70486
Neck 70490
Orbit 70480
Pelvis 72192, 74176, 74178

Sella Turcica.................. 70480
Spine
Cervical.................... 72125
Lumbar 72131
Thoracic................... 72128
Thorax 71250

CT Scan, Radionuclide
See Emission Computerized Tomography

Cuff, Rotator
See Rotator Cuff

Culdocentesis
See Colpocentesis

Culture
Acid Fast Bacilli 87116
Amniotic Fluid
Chromosome Analysis............. 88235
Bacteria
Aerobic........ 87040-87071, 87077
Anaerobic........... 87073-87076
Blood 87040
Other 87070-87075
Screening.................. 87081
Stool........... 87045, 87046
Urine.......... 87086, 87088
Bone Marrow
Chromosome Analysis............. 88237
Neoplastic Disorders............. 88237
Chlamydia..................... 87110
Chorionic Villus
Chromosome Analysis............. 88235
Fertilized Oocytes
for In Vitro Fertilization 89250
Co-Culture of Embryo 89251
Fungus
Blood 87103
Hair....................... 87101
Nail....................... 87101
Skin 87101
Source Other than Blood 87102
Lymphocyte
Chromosome Analysis............. 88230
HLA Typing.......... 86821, 86822
Mold 87107
Mycobacteria 87118
Mycoplasma 87109
Oocyte/Embryo 89250
Co-Culture of Oocyte/Embryo 89251
Extended Culture 89272
Pathogen
Presumptive 87081-87084
Skin
Chromosome Analysis............. 88233
Tissue
Homogenization.................. 87176
Infectious Agent Drug
Resistance 87903, 87904
Toxin/Antitoxin.............. 87230
Virus............... 87252, 87253
Tubercle Bacilli 87116
Tumor Tissue
Chromosome Analysis............. 88239
Typing 87140-87158
Unlisted Services and Procedures 87999
Yeast........................ 87106

Curettage
See Dilation and Curettage
Anal Fissure 46940
Cervix
Endocervical.......... 57454, 57456, 57505

Obstruction Clearance	36595, 36596
Imaging	75901, 75902
Removal	36590
Repair	36576
Replacement	36582, 36583, 36585
Catheter	36578

Ventricular Assist
See Ventricular Assist Device (VAD)

Device Handling
Order Expediting 99002

Device, Intrauterine
See Intrauterine Device (IUD)

Device, Orthotic
See Orthotics

Dexamethasone
Suppression Panel 80420

DHA Sulfate
See Dehydroepiandrosterone Sulfate

DHEA
See Dehydroepiandrosterone

DHEA Sulfate
See Dehydroepiandrosterone Sulfate

Diagnosis, Psychiatric
See Psychiatric Diagnosis

Diagnostic Amniocentesis
See Amniocentesis

Diagnostic Aspiration, Eye
See Paracentesis, Eye, Anterior Chamber Fluid Removal

Diagnostic Radiologic Examination
See X-ray

Diagnostic Skin and Sensitization Tests
See Allergy Tests

Diagnostic Ultrasound
See Echography

Diagnostic Ultrasound of Heart
See Echocardiography

Dialyses, Peritoneal
See Dialysis, Peritoneal

Dialysis
Anesthesia	01844
Arteriovenous Fistula	36831-36833
Arteriovenous Shunt	36147, 36148

End Stage Renal Disease
See End-Stage Renal Disease Services, Dialysis

Hemodialysis
See Hemodialysis

Hemoperfusion	90997
Hepatitis B Vaccine (HepB)	90740, 90747
Kt/V Level	3082F-3084F
Nephropathy Treatment Documented	3066F

Patient Training
Completed Course	90989
Per Session	90993
Peritoneal	90945, 90947, 4055F
Catheter Insertion	49418, 49419, 49421
Catheter Removal	49422
Home Infusion	99601, 99602
Plan of Care Documented	0507F
Unlisted Services and Procedures	90999

Dialysis, Extracorporeal
See Hemodialysis

Diaphragm
Assessment	58943, 58960
Contraception	57170

Imbrication
for Eventration	39545

Repair
Hernia	39540, 39541
Esophageal Hiatal	43280-43282, 43325
Neonatal	39503
Laceration	39501
Resection	39560, 39561
Unlisted Diaphragm Procedures	39599

Diaphragm Contraception
See Contraception, Diaphragm

Diaphysectomy
Calcaneus	28120
Clavicle	23180
Femur	27360
Fibula	27360, 27641
Humerus	23184, 24140
Metacarpal	26230
Metatarsal	28122
Olecranon Process	24147

Phalanges
Finger	26235, 26236
Toe	28124
Radius	24145, 25151
Scapula	23182
Talus	28120
Tarsal	28122
Tibia	27360, 27640
Ulna	24147, 25150

Diastase
See Amylase

Diastasis
See Separation

Diathermy
See Physical Medicine/Therapy/Occupational Therapy

Destruction
Ciliary Body	66700

Lesion
Retina	67208, 67227

Retinal Detachment
Prophylaxis	67141
Repair	67101
Treatment	97024

Diathermy, Surgical
See Electrocautery

Dibucaine Number 82638

Dichloride, Methylene
See Dichloromethane

Dichlorides, Ethylene
See Dichloroethane

Diethylamide, Lysergic Acid
See Lysergic Acid Diethylamide

Diethylether 84600

Differential Count
See White Blood Cell Count

Differentiation Reversal Factor
See Prothrombin

Diffusion Test, Gel
See Immunodiffusion

Digestive Tract
See Gastrointestinal Tract

Digit
See Finger; Toe
Destruction	64632
Injection	64455
Replantation	20816-20822

Digital Artery Sympathectomy 64820

Digital Slit-Beam Radiograph
See Scanogram

Digits
See Digit

Dihydroxyethanes
See Ethylene Glycol

Dihydroxyvitamin D 82652

Dilatation, Transluminal Arterial
See Angioplasty, Transluminal

Dilation
See Dilation and Curettage; Dilation and Evacuation

Anal
Endoscopy	46604
Sphincter	45905, 46940
Aortic Valve	33403

Bile Duct
Balloon	47542
Endoscopy	43277, 47555, 47556
Stricture	74363
with Stent Placement	47538-47540

Biliary Ampulla
Balloon	47542

Bladder
Cystourethroscopy	52260, 52265

Bronchi
Endoscopy	31630, 31636

Cerebral Vessels
Intracranial Vasospasm	61640-61642

Cervix
Canal	57800
Stump	57558

Colon
Endoscopy	45386

Colon-Sigmoid
Endoscopy	45340
Esophagus	43450, 43453
Balloon	43195, 43213, 43214, 43220, 43233, 43249
Endoscopy	43195, 43196, 43212, 43213, 43220, 43226, 43229, 43233, 43453
Gastric/Duodenal Stricture	43245
Surgical	43510
Intestines	44615
Endoscopy	44370
Stent Placement	44379, 44384, 44402
Kidney	50080, 50081, 50395
Intra-Renal Stricture	52343, 52346
Lacrimal Punctum	68801

Larynx
Endoscopy	31528, 31529

Nasolacrimal Duct
Balloon Catheter	68816

Nose
Balloon	31295-31297

Leg
   Knee............................. 27560-27562
      Closed Treatment 27550, 27552,
                               27560, 27562
      Open Treatment 27556-27558,
                               27566, 27730
      Recurrent 27420-27424
   Patella
      Closed Treatment 27560, 27562
      Open Treatment 27566
      Recurrent 27420, 27424
   Tibiofibular Joint
      Closed Treatment 27830, 27831
      Open Treatment 27832
Lunate
   Closed Treatment................. 25690
   Open Treatment 25695
   with Manipulation 25690
Metacarpophalangeal Joint
   Closed Treatment.......... 26700-26706
   Open Treatment 26715
Percutaneous 26705
Metatarsophalangeal Joint
   Closed Treatment.......... 28630, 28635
   Open Treatment 28645
   Percutaneous Fixation 28636
Patella
   Closed Treatment.......... 27560, 27562
   Open Treatment 27566
   Recurrent 27420, 27424
Pelvic Ring
   Closed Treatment.......... 27193, 27194
   Open Treatment 27217, 27218
   Percutaneous Fixation 27216
   without Manipulation 27193, 27194
Peroneal Tendons 27675, 27676
Radiocarpal
   Closed Treatment................. 25660
   Open Treatment 25670
Radioulnar
   Closed Treatment................. 25675
   Open Treatment 25676
Radioulnar Joint
   Closed Treatment................. 25520
   Galeazzi 25520, 25525, 25526
   Open Treatment 25525, 25526
Radius
   Closed Treatment................. 24640
   with Fracture
      Closed Treatment............. 24620
      Open Treatment 24635
Shoulder
   Closed Treatment with
      Manipulation 23650, 23655
   Open Treatment 23660
   with Greater Tuberosity Fracture
      Closed Treatment............. 23665
      Open Treatment 23670
   with Surgical or Anatomical Neck Fracture
      Closed Treatment............. 23675
      Open Treatment 23680
Skin
   Debridement 11010-11012
Sternoclavicular Joint
   Closed Treatment
      with Manipulation 23525
      without Manipulation........... 23520
   Open Treatment 23530, 23532
Talotarsal Joint
   Closed Treatment.......... 28570, 28575
   Open Treatment 28585
   Percutaneous Fixation 28576

Tarsal
   Closed Treatment........... 28540, 28545
   Open Treatment 28555
   Percutaneous Fixation 28546
Tarsometatarsal Joint
   Closed Treatment........... 28600, 28605
   Open Treatment 28615
   Percutaneous Fixation 28606
Temporomandibular Joint
   Closed Treatment........... 21480, 21485
   Open Treatment 21490
Thumb
   Closed Treatment........... 26641, 26645
   Open Treatment 26665
   Percutaneous Fixation 26650
   with Fracture 26645
      Open Treatment 26665
      Percutaneous Fixation 26650
   with Manipulation 26641, 26645, 26650
Tibiofibular Joint
   Closed Treatment........... 27830, 27831
   Open Treatment 27832
Toe
   Closed Treatment................. 26770,
                26775, 28630-28635
   Open Treatment 28645
   Percutaneous Fixation 26776, 28636
Trans-Scaphoperilunar
   Closed Treatment................. 25680
   Open Treatment 25685
Vertebra
   Additional Segment
      Open Treatment 22328
   Cervical
      Open Treatment 22318, 22319, 22326
   Closed Treatment
      with Manipulation, Casting
      and/or Bracing 22315
   Lumbar
      Open Treatment 22325
   Thoracic
      Open Treatment 22327
Wrist
   Closed Treatment....... 25660, 25675, 25680
   Intercarpal 25660
      Open Treatment 25670
   Open Treatment 25670, 25685
   Percutaneous Fixation 25671
   Radiocarpal 25660
      Open Treatment 25670
   Radioulnar
      Closed Treatment............. 25675
      Open Treatment 25676
      Percutaneous Fixation 25671
   with Fracture
      Closed Treatment............. 25680
      Open Treatment 25685
   with Manipulation 25660, 25675, 25680

Dislocation, Radiocarpal Joint
See Radiocarpal Joint, Dislocation

Disorder
Blood Coagulation
   See Coagulopathy
Penis
   See Penis
Retinal
   See Retina

Displacement Therapy
Nose 30210

Dissection
Axial Vessel
   for Island Pedicle 15740
Cavernous Sinus.................... 61613
Cranial Adhesions.................. 62161
Donor Organ
   Heart 33944
   Heart/Lung 33933
   Kidney 50323, 50325
   Liver 47143
   Lung 32855
   Pancreas....................... 48551
Facial Nerve 42420
for Debulking..................... 58952, 58953
Hygroma, Cystic
   Axillary/Cervical........... 38550, 38555
Infrarenal Aneurysm 34825, 34826,
            34800, 34802, 34830-34832
Lymph Nodes 38542
Mediastinal................. 60521, 60522
Neck
   See Radical Neck Dissection
Neurovascular..................... 32503
Sclera 67107
Urethra 54328, 54332, 54336, 54348, 54352

Dissection, Neck, Radical
See Radical Neck Dissection

Distention
See Dilation

Diverticula, Meckel's
See Diverticulum, Meckel's

Diverticulectomy 44800
Cervical Esophagus................. 43180
Esophagus............. 43130, 43135, 43180
Hypopharynx....................... 43180

Diverticulectomy, Meckel's
See Meckel's Diverticulum, Excision

Diverticulum
Bladder
   See Bladder, Diverticulum
Large Intestine 44604, 44605
Meckel's
   Excision 44800
   Unlisted Procedure.............. 44899
Small Intestine 44602, 44603
Urethra
   Excision 53230, 53235
   Marsupialization 53240
   Urethroplasty.............. 53400, 53405

Division
Anal Sphincter 46080
Flap 15600, 15610, 15620, 15630
Intrauterine Septum 58560
Muscle
   Foot 28250
   Neck
      Scalenus Anticus 21700, 21705
      Sternocleidomastoid 21720, 21725
Plantar Fascia
   Foot 28250
Rectal Stricture..................... 45150
Saphenous Vein 37700, 37722, 37735
Symblepharon...................... 68340

Division, Isthmus, Horseshoe Kidney
See Symphysiotomy, Horseshoe Kidney

DXA
See Dual X-ray Absorptiometry (DXA)

Dynamometry
See Osteotomy, Calcaneus
Venous Studies
  See Osteotomy, Calcaneus
with Ophthalmoscopy 92260

E

E Antigens
See Hepatitis Antigen, Be

E B Virus
See Epstein-Barr Virus

E Vitamin
See Tocopherol

E1
See Estrone

E2
See Estradiol

E3
See Estriol

Ear
Collection of Blood 36416
Drum
  See Tympanic Membrane
External Ear
  Biopsy............... 69100, 69105
  Blood Specimen Collection 36416
  Debridement
    Mastoidectomy Cavity 69220-69222
  Drainage
    Abscess 69000, 69005
    Hematoma 69000, 69005
  Excision
    Partial 69110
    Total 69120
  Exostosis Excision 69140
  Graft
    See Graft, Ear
  Lesion
    Shaving......................... 11310
    Destruction, Malignant 17280
    Excision............ 11400-11444, 11446,
             69145, 69150, 69155
    Excision, Malignant ... 11640-11644, 11646
  Mastoid
    See Mastoid
  Piercing 69090
  Reconstruction
    External Auditory Canal 69310, 69320
    Protruding Ear.................... 69300
    with Tissue Transfer......... 14060, 14061
  Prosthesis, Custom 21086
  Removal
    Foreign Body.............. 69200, 69205
    Impacted Cerumen 69209, 69210
  Repair
    Complex 13151, 13152, 13153
    Intermediate..................... 12051
    Simple.......................... 12011
    Superficial 12011

Tympanic Membrane
  See Tympanic Membrane
Unlisted Services and Procedures...... 69399
Inner Ear
  CT Scan 70480-70482
  Endolymphatic Sac........... 69805, 69806
  Labyrinth
    Excision................. 69905, 69910
    Incision for Perfusion 69801
  Insertion
    Cochlear Device 69930
  Semicircular Canal 69820, 69840
  Unlisted Services and Procedures...... 69949
  Vertigo
    See Canalith Repositioning
  Vestibular Nerve Section 69915
Meatoplasty 69310
  for Congenital Atresia 69320
Middle Ear
  CT Scan 70480-70482
  Exploration 69440
  Excision
    Polyp 69540
    Glomus Tumor........ 69550, 69552, 69554
  Facial Nerve Decompression.... 69720, 69725
  Facial Nerve Suture 69740, 69745
  Repair
    Fistula................... 69666, 69667
  Stapes
    Mobilization 69650
    Stapedectomy............... 69660-69662
    Stapedotomy 69660-69662
  Tumor
    Excision........... 69550, 69552, 69554
Temporal Bone
  Bone Conduction Hearing Device
    Implantation 69710
    Removal 69711
    Repair 69711
  Osseointegrated Implant
    Implantation 69714, 69715
    Removal 69717
    Replacement..................... 69717
  Resection 69535
  Unlisted Services and Procedures..... 69799

Ear Canal
See Auditory Canal

Ear Cartilage
Graft
  Autogenous
    Ear Cartilage to Nose or Ear......... 21235
    Rib Cartilage to Ear 21230

Ear Lobes
Pierce 69090

Ear Protector Attenuation
Measurements 92596
See Hearing Aid Services

Ear Wax
See Cerumen

Ear, Nose, and Throat
Audiologic Function Tests
  See Audiologic Function Tests
Audiometry
  See Audiometry
Binocular Microscopy 92504
Diagnostic Analysis
  Auditory Brainstem Implant.......... 92640
  Cochlear Implant 92601-92604

Evaluation
  Auditory Rehabilitation Status 92626,
             92627, 92630, 92633
  Language Comprehension and
    Expression 92523
  Laryngeal Sensory Testing...... 92614-92617
  Prescription of Communication Device
    Non-speech-generating 92605, 92618
    Speech Generating.......... 92607, 92608
  Speech Fluency 92521
  Speech Sound Production 92522
  Swallowing 92610-92613, 92616
  Voice and Resonance
    Behavioral Analysis 92524
Examination under Anesthesia........... 92502
Facial Nerve Function Study............ 92516
Laryngeal Function Study 92520
Nasal Function Study 92512
Nasopharyngoscopy 92511
Treatment
  Hearing, Language and Speech
    Disorder 92507, 92508
  Oral Function for Feeding............ 92526
  Swallowing Dysfunction 92526
  Use and Programming of Communication
    Device
    Non-speech-generating 92606
    Speech-generating................ 92609
Vestibular Function Tests
  See Vestibular Function Tests

Ebstein Anomaly Repair
Tricuspid Valve 33468

Eccrine Glands
Chemodenervation
  Axillae 64650
  Feet 64999
  Hands........................... 64999
  Other Area 64653

ECG
See Electrocardiography

Echinococcosis 86171, 86280

Echocardiography
Doppler
  See Doppler Echocardiography
Congenital Cardiac Anomaly
  Fetal 76825, 76826
  Doppler, Fetal............. 76827, 76828
  Transesophageal 93315-93317
  Transthoracic 93303, 93304
Intracardiac...................... 93662
Transesophageal.......... 93312-93318, 93355
Transthoracic....... 93306-93308, 93350-93352
  Congenital Cardiac Anomalies .. 93303, 93304
  with Stress Test 93350-93352

Echoencephalography
Intracranial...................... 76506

Echography
See Ultrasound

Echotomography
See Echography

Extracorporeal Life Support (ECLS)
See Extracorporeal Membrane Oxygenation (ECMO)

ECMO
See Extracorporeal Membrane Oxygenation (ECMO)

Microvolt T-wave Alternans 93025
Recording 0295T, 0296T
Scanning Analysis with Report . . 0295T, 0297T
Tracing 93005, 93041
Tracing and Evaluation 93040
Signal Averaged 93278
Symptom-Related Memory Loop 93268,
93270-93272

Electrocautery
Inferior Turbinates Soft Tissue 30801, 30802
Prostate Resection 52601
Ureteral Stricture 52341-52346

Electrochemistry
See Electrolysis

Electroconvulsive Therapy 90870

Electrocorticogram
Intraoperative 95829, 61536, 61538

Electrode, Depth
See Depth Electrode

Electrodesiccation 17000-17286
Lesion
Penis 54055

Electroejaculation
Reproductive 55870

Electroencephalography (EEG)
Brain Death 95824
Coma 95822
Digital Analysis 95957
Electrode Placement 95830
Intraoperative 95955
Monitoring . . . 95812, 95813, 95950-95953, 95956
with Drug Activation 95954
with Physical Activation 95954
with WADA Activation 95958
Standard 95819

Electrogastrography 91132, 91133

Electrogram, Atrial
Esophageal Recording 93615, 93616

Electrolysis 17380

Electromyographs
See Electromyography, Needle

Electromyography
Anorectal with Biofeedback 90911
Fine Wire
Dynamic 96004
Needle
Cranial Nerve Supplied Muscle . . 95867, 95868
Extremities 95860-95864
Extremity 95860, 95885, 95886
Face and Neck Muscles 95867, 95868
Guidance
for Chemodenervation 64617, 95874
Hemidiaphragm 95866
Larynx 95865
Non-extremity 95887
Ocular 92265
Other than Thoracic Paraspinal 95870
Single Fiber Electrode 95872
Thoracic Paraspinal Muscles 95869
Sphincter Muscles
Anus 51784, 51785
Needle 51785
Urethra 51784, 51785
Needle 51785

Surface
Dynamic 96002, 96004

Electron Microscopy
Diagnostic 88348

Electronic Analysis
Implantable Defibrillator
Pacing Cardioverter-Defibrillator
Device Interrogation 93287, 93289,
93295, 93296
Evaluation of Programming . . . 93292-93294
Subcutaneous Implantable Defibrillator
Device Interrogation 93261, 93289,
93295, 93296
Evaluation of Programming 93260,
93282-93284, 93287, 93640, 93642
Drug Infusion Pump 62367-62370
Pulse Generator
Field Stimulation 0285T
Gastric Neurostimulator 95980-95982
Neurostimulator
with Vagus Nerve Blocking Therapy . . 0317T
Brain 95970, 95978, 95979
Cranial Nerve 95974, 95975
Gastric 95980-95982
Peripheral Nerve 95971, 95972
Spinal Cord 95971, 95972
Loop Recorder, Implantable
Data Analysis 93291, 93298, 93299
Evaluation of Programming 93285, 93291,
93298, 93299

Electrophoresis
Counterimmuno- 86185
Hemoglobin 83020
High Resolution 83701
Immuno- 86320, 86325, 86327
Immunofixation 86334, 86335
Protein 84165, 84166
Unlisted Electrophoretic Technique 82664

Electrophysiology
Procedure 93600-93660

Electroretinogram
See Electroretinography

Electroretinography 92275

Electrostimulation, Analgesic
Cutaneous
See Application, Neurostimulation

Electrosurgery
Lesions
Anal 46924
Cutaneous Vascular
Proliferative 17106-17108
Penile 54065
Skin, Benign 17110, 17111
Skin, Malignant 17266
Arms, Legs, or Trunk 17260-17264
Face, Ears, Eyelids, Nose, Lips, Mucous
Membrane 17280-17284, 17286
Scalp, Neck, Hands, Feet, or
Genitalia 17270-17274, 17276
Skin, Premalignant 17000, 17003, 17004
Vaginal 57061, 57065
Vulva 56501, 56515
Trichiasis
Epilation 67825
Tumor
Rectal 45190

Electroversion, Cardiac
See Cardioversion

Elevation, Scapula, Congenital
See Sprengel's Deformity

Elliot Operation
See Excision, Lesion, Sclera

Eloesser Procedure
See Thoracostomy, Empyema

Eloesser Thoracoplasty
See Thoracoplasty

Embolectomy
Aortoiliac Artery 34151, 34201
Axillary Artery 34101
Brachial Artery 34101
Carotid Artery 34001
Celiac Artery 34151
Femoral 34201
Iliac 34151-34201
Innominate Artery 34001-34101
Mesentery Artery 34151
Peroneal Artery 34203
Popliteal Artery 34201, 34203
Pulmonary Artery 33910, 33915, 33916
Radial Artery 34111
Renal Artery 34151
Subclavian Artery 34001, 34101
Tibial Artery 34203
Ulnar Artery 34111

Embolization
Central Nervous System 61624
Non,àíCentral Nervous System
Head or Neck 61626
Intra-arterial
for Aneurysm 61710
for Carotid-Cavernous Fistula 61710
for Vascular Malformation 61710
Ureteral 50705
Vascular
Arterial 37242
for Hemorrhage 37244
for Infarction 37243
for Lymphatic Extravasation 37244
for Organ Ischemia 37243
for Tumors 37243
Venous 37241

Embryo
Biopsy 89290, 89291
Carcinoembryonic Antigen 82378
Cryopreservation 89258
Thawing 89352
Culture 89250
with Co-Culture Oocyte 89251, 89272
Hatching, Assisted 89253
Implantation
See Implantation, Embryo
Preparation
for Transfer 89255
Storage 89342
Transfer
See Embryo Transfer

Embryo Implantation
See Implantation, Embryo

Embryo Transfer
In Vitro Fertilization 58970, 58974, 58976
Intrafallopian 58976

Removal
　Foreign Body 62163
Bronchi
　Aspiration 31645, 31646
　Biopsy 31625-31629, 31632, 31633
　Computer-assisted Image-guided 31627
　Destruction
　　Lesion 31641, 96570, 96571
　　Tumor 31641, 96570, 96571
　Dilation 31630, 31631, 31636-31638
　Excision
　　Tumor 31640
　Exploration 31622
　Lesion
　　Destruction 31641, 96570, 96571
　Needle Biopsy 31629, 31633
　Occlusion 31634
　Placement
　　Fiducial Markers 31626
　　Radioelement Catheter 31643
　　Stent 31636, 31637
　Removal
　　Foreign Body 31635
　Revision
　　Stent 31638
　Specimen Collection 31623, 31624
　Stenosis 31641, 96570, 96571
　through Tracheostomy 31615
　Tumor
　　Destruction 31641, 96570, 96571
　with Alveolar Lavage 31624
　with Brushing 31623
　with Cell Washing 31622
　with Endobronchial Ultrasound (EBUS)
　Sampling 31652, 31653
Cervix 57452
　Biopsy 57421, 57454, 57455, 57460
　Curettage 57454, 57456
　Exploration 57452
　Loop Electrode Biopsy 57460
　Loop Electrode Conization 57461
Chest Cavity
　Diagnostic 32601, 32604, 32606
　Surgical 32650-32674
Colon
　Ablation
　　Lesion 45388
　　Polyp 45388
　　Tumor 45388
　Biopsy 44389, 45380, 45392
　Band Ligation 45350, 45398
　Decompression 45337
　Destruction
　　Lesion 44401
　　Tumor 44401
　Dilation 45386, 45388
　　Transendoscopic Balloon 45386
　Exploration 44388, 45378
　Hemorrhage Control 44391, 45382
　Injection 45381
　Mucosal Resection 45349
　Placement
　　Decompression Tube 45337
　　Stent 45389
　Removal
　　Foreign Body 44390, 45379
　　Polyp 44392, 45384, 45385
　　Tumor 44392, 45384, 45385
　Specimen Collection 45380
　Ultrasound 45391, 45392
　via Stoma 44388-44394, 44402

Colon-Sigmoid
　Ablation
　　Lesion 45346
　　Polyp 45346
　　Tumor 45346
　Band Ligation 45350
　Biopsy 45331
　Decompression 45337
　Dilation
　　Transendoscopic Balloon 45340
　Exploration 45330
　Hemorrhage 45334
　Injection 45335
　Mucosal Resection 45349
　Needle Biopsy 45342
　Placement
　　Decompression Tube 45337
　　Stent 45327, 45347
　Removal
　　Foreign Body 45332
　　Polyp 45333, 45338
　　Tumor 45333, 45338
　Specimen Collection 45330
　Ultrasound 45341, 45342
　Volvulus 45321, 45337
Duodenum
　Ultrasound Examination 43253
Endomicroscopy
　Esophageal 43206
　Gastrointestinal 43252
Esophagus
　Biopsy 43198, 43202
　Collection of Specimen 43197, 43200
　Dilation . . . 43195, 43196, 43212-43214, 43220,
　　　　　　　43226, 43229, 43233, 43248, 43249
　Exploration 43200
　Hemorrhage 43227
　Injection 43192, 43201, 43204
　Injection Varices 43243
　Insertion Stent 43212
　Needle Biopsy 43232
　Removal
　　Foreign Body 43194, 43215
　　Polyp 43216, 43217, 43229
　　Tumor 43216, 43217, 43229
　Ultrasound 43231, 43232, 43237,
　　　　　　　　　　　　43238, 43242, 43253
　Vein Ligation 43205
　with Optical Endomicroscopy 43206
Eye 66990
Foot
　Plantar Fasciotomy 29893
Gastrointestinal
　See Laparoscopy
　Ablation
　　Lesion 43270
　　Polyp 43270
　　Photodynamic Therapy 96570, 96571
　　Tumor 43270
　Capsule 91110, 91111
　Upper 3130F, 3132F, 3140F, 3141F
　　Biopsy 43239
　　Catheterization 43241
　　Dilation 43245, 43248, 43249
　　Drainage of Pseudocyst 43240
　　Exploration 43235, 43252
　　Foreign Body 43247
　　Hemorrhage 43255
　　Inject Varices 43243
　　Injection 43236, 43253
　　Needle Biopsy 43238, 43242
　　Referral 3132F
　　Removal 43247, 43250, 43251

Stent Placement 43266
Thermal Radiation 43257
Tube Placement 43246
Ultrasound 43237-43242,
　　　　　　　　　43253, 43259, 76975
Vein Ligation 43244
with Optical Endomicroscopy 43252
Heart
　Atria 33265, 33266
Ileum
　Biopsy 44382
　Stent Placement 44384
　via Stoma 44384
Intestines, Small
　Ablation
　　Polyp 44369
　　Tumor 44369
　Biopsy 44361, 44377
　Destruction
　　Lesion 44369
　　Tumor 44369
　Diagnostic 44376
　Exploration 44360
　Hemorrhage 44366, 44378
　Placement
　　Stent 44370, 44379
　　Tube 44372, 44373, 44379
　Removal
　　Foreign Body 44363
　　Lesion 44365
　　Polyp 44364, 44365
　　Tumor 44364, 44365
　Tube Placement 44372
　Tube Revision 44373
　via Stoma 44380, 44382, 44384
　Tumor 44364, 44365
Intracranial 62160-62165
Intraluminal Imaging
　Colon 0355T
　Gastrointestinal Tract 91110, 91111
Jejunum
　Ultrasound Examination 43253
Kidney 50551, 50570
　Biopsy 50555, 50557, 50574-50576, 52354
　Catheterization 50553, 50572
　Destruction 50557, 50576, 52354
　Dilation
　　Stricture 52343, 52346
　Excision
　　Tumor 50562, 52355
　Exploration 52351
　Lithotripsy 52353
　Removal
　　Calculus 50561, 50580, 52352
　　Foreign Body 50561, 50580
　via Incision 50570, 50572,
　　　　　　　　50574-50576, 50580
　via Stoma 50551, 50553,
　　　　　　　50555, 50557, 50561, 50562
Larynx
　Arytenoidectomy 31560, 31561
　Aspiration 31515
　Biopsy 31510, 31535, 31536
　Dilation 31528, 31529
　Direct 31515, 31520, 31525-31529
　　Diagnostic 31520, 31525, 31526
　　Operative . . . 31530, 31531, 31535, 31536,
　　　　　　31540, 31541, 31545, 31546, 31561
　Epiglottis Stripping 31540, 31541
　Excision
　　Tumor 31540
　Fiberoptic 31575-31579
　Indirect 31505, 31510-31513

Infusion
  for Other Than Thrombolysis . . 61650, 61651
    for Thrombolysis. 61645
  Injection 61645
  Thrombectomy 61645
Occlusion
  Arterial Balloon 61623
  Transcatheter 61624, 61626
Vascular Catheterization. 61630, 61635

Enema
Contrast. 74270, 74280
Home Visit for Fecal Impaction. 99511
Therapeutic
  for Intussusception 74283

Energies, Electromagnetic
See Irradiation

ENT
See Ear, Nose, and Throat; Otorhinolaryngology

Entamoeba Histolytica
Antigen Detection
  Immunoassay. 87336, 87337

Enterectomy
Donor. 44132, 44133
Partial 44133
Laparoscopic. 44202, 44203
Small Intestine 44120, 44121
  for Congenital Atresia 44126-44128
  with Enterostomy. 44125
Transplanted Allograft 44137

Enterocele
Repair
  Abdominal Approach 57270
  Vaginal Approach. 57268, 57556
  with Colporrhaphy 57265
  with Hysterectomy. 58263, 58270, 58280,
                                    58292, 58294

Enterocystoplasty
with Intestinal Anastomosis. 51960
Camey. 50825

Enteroenterostomy
See Anastomosis, Intestines

Enterolysis 44005
Laparoscopic. 44180

Enteropancreatostomy
See Anastomosis, Pancreas to Intestines

Enterorrhaphy 44602, 44603, 44615

Enterostomy
Closure 44227, 44620, 44625, 44626
Placement. 44300
with Enterectomy
  Intestine, Small 44125
with Enteroenterostomy 44130
with Proctectomy 45119, 45397

Enterotomy
Biopsy 44020
Decompression. 44021
Excision
  Lesion. 44110, 44111
Exploration 44020
Foreign Body Removal 44020
Intestinal Stricturoplasty 44615

Enterovirus
Antibody. 86658, 87267, 87498

Entropion
Repair 67921-67924
  Excision Tarsal Wedge. 67923
  Suture. 67921
  Thermocauterization 67922

Enucleation
Cyst
  Mandible 21040
  Maxilla. 21030
  Zygoma. 21030
Eye. 65101, 65103, 65105
Empyema
  Pleural 32540
Prostate. 52649
Tumor, Benign
  Mandible 21040
  Maxilla. 21030
  Zygoma. 21030

Enucleation, Cyst, Ovarian
See Cystectomy, Ovarian

Enucleation, Prostate
See Prostate, Enucleation

Environmental Intervention
for Psychiatric Patients 90882

Enzyme Activity
Constituents 88319
Detection. 87185
Incubation 86977
Immunoassay
  See Antigen Detection, Enzyme Immunoassay
Specific Analytes
  See Pathology and Laboratory, Enzymes
Infectious Agent 87905
Ova and Parasites. 87185

Enzyme, Angiotensin Converting
See Angiotensin Converting Enzyme (ACE)

Enzyme, Angiotensin-Forming
See Renin

EOG
See Electro-oculography

Eosinocyte
See Eosinophils

Eosinophils
Nasal Smear 89190

Epicondylitises, Lateral Humeral
See Tennis Elbow

Epicondylitis, Radiohumeral
See Tennis Elbow

Epidemic Parotitis
See Mumps

Epididymectomy
Bilateral. 54861
Unilateral 54860
with Excision of Spermatocele. 54840

Epididymis
Incision and Drainage. 54700
Anastomosis
  to Vas Deferens
    Bilateral 54901
    Unilateral 54900
Biopsy. 54800, 54865

Epididymography. 74440
Excision
  Bilateral 54861
  Unilateral 54860
Exploration
  Biopsy. 54865
Lesion
  Excision
    Local 54830
    Spermatocele 54840
Needle Biopsy. 54800
Spermatocele
  Excision 54840
Unlisted Services and Procedures 55899
X-ray with Contrast. 74440

Epididymograms 55300

Epididymography 74440

Epididymoplasty
See Repair, Epididymis

Epididymovasostomy
Bilateral. 54901
Unilateral 54900

Epidural
Administration
  Drug 62310, 62311
    Hospital Management 01996
  Device 62360-62362, 62365
    Analysis 62367
Anesthesia
  See Epidural Anesthesia
Catheterization 62350, 62351
  Removal 62355
Electrode
  Insertion 61531, 63650, 63655
  Removal 61535
Injection 62281, 62282, 62310,
                                62311, 62318, 62319
  Transforaminal . . . 64479, 64480, 64483, 64484
    Ultrasound Guidance 0228T-0231T
  Blood or Clot Patch 62273
  Neurolytic Substance. 62281, 62282
  with Disc Decompression 62287
Lysis 62263, 62264

Epidural Anesthesia
Infusion 62318, 62319
Injection 62310, 62311

Epidurography 72275

Epigastric
Hernia Repair 49570, 49572
  Laparoscopic. 49652

Epiglottidectomy. 31420

Epiglottis
Excision. 31420
Stripping 31540, 31541

Epikeratoplasty
Eye. 65767

Epilation
See Removal, Hair

Epinephrine
See Catecholamines
Blood. 82383, 82384
Urine 82384

Excision
  Diverticula 43130, 43135
  Partial 43116-43118, 43121-43124
  Total 43107, 43108, 43112, 43113, 43124
Exploration
  Endoscopy 43200
Hemorrhage 43227
Incision 43020, 43045
  Muscle 43030
Imaging Studies 91110, 91111
  Motility 78258
  Obstructions 74360
  Reflux 78262
  Removal of Foreign Body 74235
  Strictures 74360
  Swallowing Function
    Cineradiography 74230
  X-ray 74210, 74220
Injection
  Sclerosis Agent 43204
  Submucosal 43192, 43201
Insertion
  Sengstaken Tamponade 43460
  Stent 43212
  Tamponade 43460
  Tube 43510
Lengthening 43283, 43338
Lesion
  Excision 43100, 43101
Ligation 43405
Motility Study 78258, 91010, 91013
  with Perfusion 91013
  with Pressure Topography 91299
  with Stimulation 91013
Mucosal Resection 43211
Needle Biopsy
  Endoscopy 43232
Nuclear Medicine
  Imaging (Motility) 78258
  Reflux Study 78262
Reconstruction 43300, 43310, 43313
  Creation
    Stoma 43351, 43352
  Esophagostomy 43351, 43352
  Fistula 43305, 43312, 43314
  Gastrointestinal 43360, 43361
Removal
  Foreign Bodies 43020, 43045,
                  43194, 43215, 74235
  Lesion 43216
  Polyp 43216, 43217
Repair 43300, 43310, 43313
  Esophagogastroduodenoscopy . . 43235-43259
  Esophagogastric Fundoplasty 43325,
                        43327, 43328
    Esophagogastroduodenoscopic 43210
    Laparoscopic 43280
  Esophagogastrostomy 43320
  Esophagojejunostomy 43340, 43341
  Esophagomyotomy 43279
  Esophagoplasty . . 43300, 43305, 43310, 43312
  Fistula 43305, 43312, 43314, 43420, 43425
  Heller Esophagomyotomy 32665
  Muscle 43330, 43331
  Nissen Procedure 43280
  Paraesophageal Hernia
    Laparoscopic 43281, 43282
    via Laparotomy 43332, 43333
    via Thoracoabdominal
      Incision 43336, 43337
    via Thoracotomy 43334, 43335
  Pre-existing Perforation 43405
  Thal-Nissen Procedure 43325

Toupet Procedure 43280
  Varices 43401
  Wound 43410, 43415
Sphincter Augmentation
  Device Placement 0392T
  Device Removal 0393T
Suture 43405
  Wound 43410, 43415
Ultrasound
  Endoscopy 43231, 43232
Unlisted Services and Procedures . . . 43289, 43499
Vein
  Ligation 43205, 43400

Esophagus Neoplasm
See Tumor, Esophagus

Esophagus, Varix
See Esophageal Varices

Established Patient
Checkout for Orthotic/Prosthetic Use 97762
Counseling
  See Counseling
Critical Care 99291, 99292
Domiciliary or Rest Home Visit 99334-99337,
                           99339, 99340
Emergency Department Services 99281-99285
Evaluation Services
  Basic Life and/or Disability 99450
  Work-related or Medical Disability 99455
Home Services 99347-99350, 99606
Hospital Inpatient Services 99221-99223,
             99231-99236, 99238, 99239
Hospital Observation Services 99217-99220,
             99224-99226, 99235, 99236
Inpatient Consultations 99251-99255
Nursing Facility 99304-99310,
              99315, 99316, 99318
Office and/or Other Outpatient
Consultations 99241-99245
Office Visit 99211-99215
Online Medical Evaluation 98969, 99444
Ophthalmological Services 92012, 92014
Outpatient Visit 99211-99215
Preventive Medicine 99391-99397
Prolonged Services
  with Patient Contact 99354-99357
    with Physician Supervision . . . 99415, 99416
  without Patient Contact 99358, 99359
Telephone Services 98966-98968, 99441-99443

Establishment
Colostomy
  Abdominal 50810
  Perineal 50810

Estes Operation
See Ovary, Transposition

Estlander Procedure 40525

Estradiol 82670
Response 80415

Estriol
Blood or Urine 82677

Estrogen
Blood or Urine 82671, 82672
Receptor Assay 84233

Estrone
Blood or Urine 82679

Ethanediols
See Ethylene Glycol

Ethanol
Breath 82075

Ethmoid
Artery Ligation 30915
Excision
  See Ethmoidectomy
Nasoethmoid
  See Nasoethmoid Complex
Repair
  Leak, Cerebrospinal Fluid 31290
Sinus
  See Sinus/Sinuses, Ethmoid

Ethmoid, Sinus
See Sinus/Sinuses, Ethmoid

Ethmoidectomy
Anterior 31200
Partial 31254
Total 31201, 31205, 31255
Endoscopic 31254, 31255
Skull Base Surgery 61580, 61581

Ethosuccimid
See Ethosuximide

Ethosuximide
Assay 80168

Ethyl Alcohol
See Ethanol

Ethylene Dichlorides
See Dichloroethane

Ethylene Glycol 82693

Ethylmethylsuccimide
See Ethosuximide

Etiocholanalone Measurement
See Etiocholanolone

Etiocholanolone 82696

ETOH
See Drug Assay, Drug Procedure, Definitive Drug Class, Alcohols

Euglobulin Lysis 85360

European Blastomycosis
See Cryptococcus

Eustachian Tube
Inflation
  Myringotomy 69420
  Anesthesia 69421

Eutelegenesis
See Artificial Insemination

Evacuation
Clots
  Endoscopic 52001
Hematoma
  Brain 61108, 61154, 61312-61315
  Anesthesia 00211
  Subungual 11740
Hydatidiform Mole 59870
Intraspinal Lesion 63265
Meibomian Glands 0207T
Pregnancy
  See Dilation and Evacuation
  Cervical 59140
Stomach 43753

Nail Fold 11765
Nails 11750-11752
Neck
   Tumor 21552, 21554-21556
Neoplasm
   Spine 63275-63290
Nerve
   Foot 28055
   Hamstring Muscle 27325
   Neurofibroma 64788-64792
   Neurolemmoma 64788-64792
   Neuroma 64774-64786
   Popliteal 27326
   Sympathetic
      See Sympathectomy
Neurofibroma 64788-64790
Neurolemmoma 64788-64792
Neuroma 64774-64786
Nose
   Cyst 30124, 30125
   Lesion 30117, 30118
   Polyp 30110-30115
   Rhinectomy 30150, 30160
   Skin 30120
   Turbinate, Inferior 30130, 30140
Odontoid Process 22548
Olecranon Process 24147
   Cyst 24120, 24125, 24126
   Tumor 24120, 24125, 24126
Omentum 49255
Operculum 41821
Orbit
   Lesion 61333, 67412, 67420
Ovary
   Cystectomy 58925
   Oophorectomy 58940, 58943
   Salpingo-oophorectomy 58720
   Wedge Resection/Bisection 58920
Oviduct 58700, 58720
Palate 42120, 42145
   Lesion 42104, 42106, 42107
Pancreas
   See Pancreatectomy
   Ampulla of Vater 48148
   Lesion 48120
   Peripancreatic Tissue 48105
Parathyroid Gland 60500, 60502, 60505
   Tumor 42410, 42415, 42420, 42425, 42426
Parotid Gland
   Partial 42410-42415
   Total 42420-42426
Patella 27350
Pelvis
   Tumor 27043, 27045,
      27047, 27048, 27049, 27059
Penis
   Amputation 54120, 54125, 54130, 54135
   Circumcision 54150, 54160, 54161, 54163
   Frenulotomy 54164
   Lesion 54060
   Plaque 54110-54112
   Post-Circumcision Adhesion 54162
Pericardium 33030, 33031
   Cyst 32661
   Mass 32661
   Tumor 32661
Peritoneum
   Tumor 49203-49205
Petrous Temporal Apex 69530
Phalanges
   Cyst
      Finger 26210, 26215
      Toe 28108

Finger 26235, 26236
Toe 28124, 28126, 28150, 28153
Hemiphalangectomy 28160
Tumor 26210, 26215,
   26260, 26262, 28108, 28175
Pharynx 42145, 42890, 42892, 42894
   Cyst 42810, 42815
   Lesion 42808
   with Larynx 31390, 31395
Pituitary Gland 61546, 61548
   Tumor 61546, 61548, 62165
Plaque
   Penis 54110-54112
Pleura 32310-32320
   Thoracoscopic 32656
Polyp
   Nose 30110, 30115
      Endoscopic 31237
   Urethra 53260
      Caruncle 53265
Presacral
   Tumor 49215
Prostate
   See Proctectomy
Pterygium 65420, 65426
Pulmonary Artery 33910, 33915, 33916
Pubic Symphysis 27070, 27071
   Cyst 27065-27067
   Tumor 27065-27067
Radius 24130, 24145, 25151
   Cyst 24120, 24125,
      24126, 25120, 25125, 25126
   Styloid Process 25230
   Tumor 24120, 24125, 25120, 25125, 25126
Rectum
   See Proctectomy
   Lesion 45108
   Prolapse 45130, 45135
   Stricture 45150
   Tumor 45160, 45171, 45172
Redundant Skin of Eyelid
   See Blepharoplasty
Retroperineal
   Tumor 49203-49205
Ribs 21600, 21610, 21615, 21616
Sacrococcygeal
   Tumor 49215
Salivary Gland Duct
   Cyst 42408
Scalp
   Tumor 21011-21014
Scapula 23172, 23182, 23190
   Cyst 23140, 23145, 23146
   Tumor 23140, 23145, 23146
Sclera 66150, 66155, 66160, 66170
   Lesion 66130
Scrotum 55150
Semilunar Cartilage of Knee
   See Knee, Meniscectomy
Seminal Vesicle . . . . : . . . 55650
   Mullerian Duct Cyst 55680
Sesamoid Bone
   Toe 28315
   Shoulder
      Tumor 23071, 23073, 23075, 23076
Sinus
   Ethmoid 31200, 31201, 31205
   Maxilla 31225, 31230
Skene's Glands 53270
Skin
   Excess 15830, 15832-15839, 15847

Lesion, Benign 11400-11404, 11406,
   11420-11424, 11426, 11440-11444, 11446,
   11450, 11451, 11462, 11463, 11470, 11471
Lesion, Malignant 11600-11604, 11606,
   11620-11624, 11626, 11640-11644, 11646
Nose 30120
Skin Graft
   Infected
      Abdomen 35907
      Extremity 35903
      Neck 35901
      Thorax 35905
   Site Preparation 15002-15005
Skull 61501
   Lesion 61500
      Anterior 61600, 61601
      Base 61575, 61576
      Middle 61605-61608
      Posterior 61615, 61616
   Tumor 61500
Spermatic Cord
   Lesion 55520
   Variocele 55530, 55535, 55540
Spermatocele 54840
Spine
   Lesion 63300-63308
   Neoplasm 63275-63278, 63280-63283,
      63285-63287, 63290
Spinal Cord
   Lesion 61575, 61576, 63265-63268,
      63270-63273, 63300-63308
Spleen 38100-38102
Stapes 69660, 69661
Sternum 21620, 21627, 21630, 21632
Stomach
   See Gastrectomy
   Tumor 43610, 43611
Sublingual Gland 42450
   Cyst 42408
Submandibular (Submaxillary)
   Gland 42440, 42509
Sweat Glands
   Axillary 11450, 11451
   Inguinal 11462, 11463
   Perianal 11470, 11471
   Perineal 11470, 11471
   Umbilical 11470, 11471
Synovium
   See Synovectomy
Talus 28120, 28130
   Cyst 28100, 28102, 28103
   Osteochondral Defect 29891
   Tumor 28100, 28102, 28103
Tarsal 28116, 28122
   Cyst 28104, 28106, 28107
   Tumor 28104, 28106, 28107
Temporal Bone 69530, 69535
Tendon
   Finger 26180, 26390, 26415
   Forearm 25109
   Hand 26390, 26415
   Palm 26170
   Wrist 25109
Tendon Sheath
   Cyst 28092
   Finger 26145
   Foot 28086-28088
   Forearm 25115, 25116
   Bursa 25115, 25116
   Cyst 25120, 25125, 25126
   Lesion 25110
   Synovia 25115, 25116
   Tumor 25120, 25125, 25126

Leg
　Lesion 27630
　Palm 26145
　Wrist
　　Ganglion 25111, 25112
　　Lesion 25110
　　Bursa 25115, 25116
　　Synovectomy 25118, 25119
　　Synovia 25115, 25116
Testis
　See Orchiectomy
　Lesion 54512
　Tumor 54530, 54535
Thigh
　Tumor 27327, 27328, 27337, 27339
Thorax
　Tumor 21552, 21554-21556
Thrombus
　See Thrombectomy
Thromboendarterectomy
　See Thromboendarterectomy
Thymus Gland 60520-60522
Thyroglossal Duct
　Cyst 60280, 60281
Thyroid Gland
　See Thyroidectomy
　Lobectomy
　　Partial 60210, 60212
　　Total 60220, 60225
　Tumor 60200
Tibia 27360, 27640
　Cyst 27635, 27637, 27638
　Osteochondral Defect 29891
　Tumor 27635, 27637, 27638
Toe
　Lesion 28092
　Tumor 28039, 28041, 28043, 28045, 28175
Tongue
　See Glossectomy
　Lesion 41110, 41112-41114
　Lingual Frenum 41115
Tonsils 42820, 42821, 42825, 42826
　Lingual 42870
　Radical Resection 42842, 42844, 42845
　Tag 42860
Torus Mandibularis 21031
Trachea
　Stenosis and Anastomosis 31780, 31781
　Tumor 31785, 31786
Tricuspid Valve 33460
Tumor
　Abdomen 49203-49205
　Abdominal Wall 22900-22903
　Acetabulum 27076
　Ankle 27618, 27619, 27632, 27634
　Arm, Lower 25071, 25073, 25075, 25076
　Arm, Upper 24071, 24073, 24075, 24076
　Back/Flank 21930, 21933
　Bile Duct 47711, 47712
　Bladder 51530
　Brain 61510, 61518, 61520, 61521,
　　　　　　　　　　61526-61530, 61545, 62164
　Breast 19120, 19125, 19126
　　Chest Wall 19260, 19271, 19272
　Bronchi 31640
　Calcaneus 28100-28103
　Carpal 25130-25136
　Carotid Body 60600, 60605
　Cervix 58550, 58555
　Cheekbone 21030, 21034
　Clavicle 23140, 23145, 23146
　Colorectal 45126
　Cranial Bone 61563, 61564

Dentoalveolar Structures 41825-41827
Ear, Middle 69550, 69552, 69554
Elbow 24071, 24073, 24075, 24076
Face
　Bone 21029, 21030,
　　　　　　　　　21034, 21040, 21046-21049
　Soft Tissue 21011-21014
Femur 27065-27067, 27327, 27328,
　　　　　　　　　27337-27339, 27355-27358
Fibula 27635, 27637, 27638
Finger 26111-26118
Flank
　See Excision, Tumor, Back/Flank
Foot
　Soft Tissue 28039, 28041, 28043, 28045
Forearm 25071, 25073, 25075, 25076
Greater Trochanter, Femur 27065-27067
Gums 41825-41827
Hand 26111-26118
Heart 33120-33130
Hip 27043-27048, 27065-27067
Humerus 23150, 23155,
　　　　　　　　　23156, 24110, 24115, 24116
Ilium 27065-27067, 27075, 27076
Innominate 27077
Ischium
　Radical Resection Including
　　Acetabulum 27076
　Ramus
　　Radical Resection 27075
　Tuberosity
　　Radical Resection 27078
Knee 27327, 27328, 27337-27339
Lacrimal Gland 68540, 68550
Larynx 31300, 31540, 31541
Leg, Lower 27615-27619,
　　　　　　　　27632, 27634, 27645, 27646
Leg, Upper 27327-27329,
　　　　　　　　　27337-27339, 27365
Lung 32503, 32504
Mandible 21040, 21044-21047
Maxilla 21030, 21034, 21048, 21049
Mediastinum 32662
Mesentery 49203-49205
Metacarpal 26200-26205
Metatarsal 28104, 28106, 28107
Neck 21552, 21554-21556
Olecranon Process 24120, 24125, 24126
Parotid Gland 42410-42426
Pelvis 27043, 27045,
　　　　　　　　27047, 27048, 27049, 27059
Pericardium 32661
Peritoneum 49203-49205
Phalanges 26210-26215, 26260, 26262
　Toe 26215, 28108, 28175
Pituitary Gland 61546, 61548, 62165
Presacral 49215
Pubis 27065-27067, 27075, 27076
Radius . . . 24120-24125, 25120, 25125, 25126
Rectum 45160-45172
Retroperineal 49203-49205
Sacrococcygeal 49215
Scalp 21011-21016
Scapula 23140, 23145, 23146
Shoulder 23071-23078
Skull 61500
Stomach 43610, 43611
Talus 28100, 28102, 28103
Tarsal Bones 28104, 28106, 28107
Testis 54530, 54535
Thigh 27327, 27328, 27337, 27339
Thorax 21552, 21554-21556

Thyroid 60200
Tibia 27635, 27637, 27638
Toe 28039-28045, 28175
Trachea 31785, 31786
Ulna 25120, 25125, 25126
Ureter
　Radical Resection 52355
Urethra 53220
Uterus
　Fibroid 58140, 58145, 58146
　Hydatidiform Mole 59100
　Intramural Myoma 58545, 58546
　Leiomyomata 58561
Ulna
　Darrach Procedure 25240
　Tumor 25120, 25125, 25126
Ureter
Urethra
　Tumor 53220
Uterus
　Fibroid 58140, 58145, 58146
　Hydatidiform Mole 59100
　Intramural Myoma 58545, 58546
　Leiomyomata 58561
Uvula
　Lesion 42104, 42106, 42107
　Vagina 57135
　Vertebra, Cervical 22100
　Vertebra, Lumbar 22102
　Vertebra, Thoracic 22101
　Wrist 25071-25076
　Zygoma 21030, 21034
Turbinate, Inferior 30130, 30140
Tympanic Nerve 69676
Ulcer
　Pressure
　　Coccyx 15920, 15922
　　Ischium 15940, 15941, 15944-15946
　　Sacrum 15931, 15933-15937
　　Trochanter 15950-15953, 15956, 15958
　　Stomach 43610
Ulna 24147, 25150, 25240
　Darrach Procedure 25240
　Cyst 25120, 25125, 25126
Umbilicus 49250
Urachus
　Cyst 51500
Ureter
　See Ureterectomy
Ureterocele 51535
Urethra
　Bulbourethral Gland 53250
　Diverticulum 53230, 53235, 53240
　Lesion 52224
　Prolapse 53275
　Skene's Glands 53270
　Urethrectomy 53210, 53215
Uterus
　See Hysterectomy
　Myoma 58545, 58546
　Tumor . . . . 58140 , 58145, 58146
Uvula 42140, 42145
Vagina
　Cyst 57135
　Lumen 57120
　Septum 57130
　Vaginectomy
　　Complete 57110-57112, 58275, 58280
　　Partial 57106, 57107, 57109
Varicocele
　Spermatic Cord 55530, 55535, 55540
Vas Deferens 55250

Vascular Malformation
    Finger 26111, 26113, 26115, 26116
    Hand 26111, 26113, 26115, 26116
Vein
    Varicose 37765, 37766
Vertebra
    Additional Segment 22103, 22116
    Cervical 22110
      for Tumor 22100, 22110
    Lumbar 22102
      for Tumor 22114
    Thoracic 22112
      for Tumor 22101
Vertebral Body 63081-63103
    Corpectomy 63081, 63082,
           63085-63088, 63090, 63091
Vitreous
   See Vitrectomy
Vulva
   See Vulvectomy
Wrist
    Radial Styloidectomy 25230
    Tendon Sheath 25109
Zygoma
    Cyst 21030

Exclusion
Duodenum 48547
Small Intestine 44700

Exenteration
Orbit
    Removal Orbital Contents 65110
      with Muscle or Myocutaneous Flap . . . 65114
      with Therapeutic Removal of Bone . . . 65112
    Anterior Cranial Fossa
      Craniofacial 61581
      Orbitocranial 61585
      with Maxillectomy 31230
Pelvis 45126, 51597, 58240

Exercise Stress Tests
Cardiovascular 93015-93018, 93464
Pulmonary 94620, 94621

Exercise Test
See Electromyography, Needle
Ischemic Limb 95875

Exercise Therapy
See Physical Medicine/Therapy/Occupational
Therapy

Exfoliation
Chemical 17360

Exocrine, Pancreas
See Pancreas

Exomphalos
See Omphalocele

Exostectomy
Foot 28288, 28290
Silver-type Procedure 28290

Exostosis
Excision
    External Auditory Canal 69140
    Fibula 27635
    Foot 28288, 28290
    Palate 21031, 21032
    Tibia 27635

Expander, Skin, Inflatable
See Tissue, Expander

Expired Gas Analysis
See Pulmonology, Diagnostic, Expired Gas Analysis

Exploration
Abdomen 49000, 49002, 54535, 54560
    Penetrating Wound 20102
    Staging 58960
Adrenal Gland 60540, 60545, 60650
Anal
    Endoscopy 46600
Ankle 27610, 27620
Anus
    Surgical 45990
Arm, Lower 25248
Artery
    Brachial 24495
    Carotid 35701
    Femoral 35721
    Other 35761
    Popliteal 35741
Back
    Penetrating Wound 20102
Bile Duct 47420, 47425, 47480
    Atresia 47700
    Endoscopy 47552
Blood Vessel
    Abdomen 35840
    Chest 35820
    Extremity 35860
    Neck 35800
Brain
    Infratentorial 61305
    Supratentorial 61304
    via Burr Hole
      Infratentorial 61253
      Supratentorial 61250
Breast 19020
    Nipple 19110
Bronchi
    Endoscopy 31622
Bronchoscopy 31622
Cardiotomy 33310, 33315
Cauda Equina 63005, 63011, 63017
Chest 32100, 32601
    Penetrating Wound 20101
Colon
    Colotomy 44025
    Endoscopic 44388, 45378
Colon-Sigmoid
    Endoscopic 45330, 45335
Common Bile Duct
    with Cholecystectomy 47564, 47610
Duodenum 44010
Ear, Middle 69440
Elbow 24000, 24101
Epididymis 54865
Esophagus
    Endoscopy 43200
Extremity
    Penetrating Wound 20103
Finger Joint 26075-26080
Flank
    Penetrating Wound 20102
Forearm 25248
Gallbladder 47480
Gastrointestinal Tract, Upper
    Endoscopy 43235, 43252
Hand Joint 26070
Heart 33310, 33315
Hepatic Duct 47400
Hip 27033

Intestines, Small
    Endoscopy 44360
    Enterotomy 44020
Joint
   See Joint, Exploration
Kidney 50010, 50045, 50120
Lacrimal Duct 68810, 68811, 68815, 68816
    Canaliculi 68840
Larynx 31320
    Endoscopy 31505, 31510-31513,
          31520, 31525, 31526, 31575
Laparoscopic
    Surgical
      Pelvis 49321-49327
Liver 47400
    Wound 47361, 47362
Mediastinum 39000, 39010, 60505
Nasolacrimal Duct . . . 68810, 68811, 68815, 68816
Neck
    Penetrating Wound 20100
Nerves
    Cranial 61458, 61460
Nose
    Endoscopy 31231, 31233, 31235
Ocular
    for Strabismus 67340
Orbit 61332, 61333
    with/without Biopsy 67450
    without Bone Flap 67400
Parathyroid Gland 60500, 60502, 60505
Pelvis 49320
Rectum
    Injury 45562, 45563
    Surgical 45990
Retroperitoneal Area 49010
Scrotum 55110
Shoulder Joint 23040-23044, 23107
Sinus
    Frontal 31070-31075, 31255
    Maxillary 31020-31030
Spinal Cord 63001, 63003, 63005, 63011,
        63015-63017, 63040, 63042-63044
Spine Fusion 22830
Stomach 43500
Testis
    Undescended 54550, 54560
Toe Joint 28024
Ureter 50600
Vagina 57000
    Endocervical 57452
Wound
   See Wound, Exploration
Wrist 25101, 25248
    Joint 25040

Exploration, Larynx by Incision
See Laryngotomy, Diagnostic

Exploratory Laparotomy
See Abdomen, Exploration

Expression
Conjunctiva 68040

Exteriorization, Small Intestine
See Enterostomy

External Auditory Canal
See Auditory Canal

External Cephalic Version 59412

External Ear
See Ear, External Ear

Eye Allergy Test
See Allergy Tests

Eye Evisceration
See Evisceration, Ocular Contents

Eye Exam

Eye Exercises

Eye Muscles

Eye Prosthesis
See Prosthesis, Ocular; Prosthesis, Orbital

Eye Socket
See Orbit; Orbital Contents; Orbital Floor;
Periorbital Region

Eyebrow

Eyeglasses
See Spectacle Services

Factor Inhibitor Tests
See Pathology and Laboratory, Factor Inhibitor Tests

Factor, Intrinsic
See Intrinsic Factor

Factor, Rheumatoid
See Rheumatoid Factor

Factor, Sulfation
See Somatomedin

Fallopian Tube
Anastomosis 58750
Biopsy 49321
Cannulation 58565
Catheterization 58345, 74742
Destruction
　　Endoscopic 58670
Ectopic Pregnancy 59121
　　with Salpingectomy and/or
　　Oophorectomy 59120, 59151
Excision 58661, 58700, 58720, 58943, 58950,
　　　　　　　　　　　　　　　　　 58953, 58956
Ligation 58600, 58611
Lysis
　　Adhesions 58740
Occlusion 58615
　　Endoscopic 58671
Placement
　　Implant for Occlusion 58565
Repair 58752
　　Anastomosis 58750
　　Create Stoma 58673, 58770
Tumor
　　Resection . . 58950, 58952-58954, 58956-58958
Unlisted Services and Procedures 58999
X-ray
Hysterosalpingography 74740

Fallopian Tube Pregnancy
See Ectopic Pregnancy, Tubal

Fallot, Tetralogy of
See Tetralogy of Fallot

Family Adaptive Behavior
Treatment Guidance 0370T
Multiple-Family 0371T

Family Psychotherapy
See Psychotherapy, Family of Patient

Fanconi Anemia
Chromosome Analysis 81242, 88248

Farnsworth-Munsell Color Test
See Color Vision Examination

Farr Test
See Gammaglobulin, Blood

Fasanella-Servat Procedure . . . 67908

Fascia Graft 15840

Fascia Lata Graft
Harvesting 20920-20922

Fascial Defect
Leg 27656
Urostomy 50728

Fascial Graft
Cheek 15840
Fascia and Skin
　　Flap 15732, 15734, 15736, 15738
Free
　　Microvascular Anastomosis 15758
Harvest 20920, 20922
Reconstruction
　　Collateral Ligament 26541
　　Hamstring Muscle 27386
　　Infrapatellar Tendon 27381
　　Quadriceps Muscle 27386
　　Tendon Pulley 26502
Sternoclavicular Dislocation 23532

Fasciectomy
Foot 28060-28062
Palm 26121-26125

Fasciocutaneous Flaps
Muscle 15732-15738
Pharyngeal Wall 42894

Fasciotomy
Arm, Lower 24495, 25020-25025
Buttock
　　Decompression 27027
　　　with Debridement 27057
Foot 28008
Hand Decompression 26037
Hip 27025
Knee 27305, 27496-27499
Leg, Lower 27600-27602, 27892-27894
Leg, Upper 27305, 27496-27499, 27892-27894
Palm 26040-26045
Pelvis
　　Decompression 27027
　　　with Debridement 27057
Plantar
　　Endoscopic 29893
Thigh 27025
Toe 28008
Wrist 25020-25025

FAST
See Allergen Immunotherapy

Fat
Feces 82705-82715
Removal
　　Lipectomy 15876-15879

Fat Stain
Feces 89125
Respiratory Secretions 89125
Sputum 89125
Urine 89125

Fatty Acid
Blood 82725
Long-Chain Omega-3
　　Red Blood Cell (RBC) Membranes 0111T
Very Long Chain 82726

Favre-Durand Disease
See Lymphogranuloma Venereum

Fc Receptor 86243

FDP
See Fibrin Degradation Products

Fecal Microbiota Transplant . . . 44705

Feedback, Psychophysiologic
See Biofeedback; Training, Biofeedback

Female Castration
See Oophorectomy

Female Gonad
See Ovary

Femoral Arteries
See Artery, Femoral

Femoral Nerve
Injection
　　Anesthetic 64447, 64448

Femoral Stem Prosthesis
See Arthroplasty, Hip

Femoral Vein
See Vein, Femoral

Femur
See Hip; Knee; Leg, Upper
Abscess
　　Incision 27303
Amputation 27590
Bone Graft 27170, 27177, 27470
Bursa
　　Excision 27062
Craterization 27070, 27071, 27360
Cyst
　　Excision 27065-27067, 27355-27358
Diaphysectomy 27360
Drainage 27303
Excision 27070, 27071, 27360
Femoroplasty 29914
Fracture 27244
　　Closed Treatment 27501-27503,
　　　　　　　　　　　　　　　　　　　 27267, 27268
　　Distal 27508, 27510, 27514
　　Distal, Medial or Lateral Condyle 27509
　　　Open Treatment 27514
　　Epiphysis 27516-27519
　　　Open Treatment 27519
　　Intertrochanteric 27244
　　　Closed Treatment 27238
　　　Treatment with Implant 27244
　　　with Implant 27245
　　　with Manipulation 27240
　　Neck
　　　Closed Treatment 27230-27232
　　　Open Treatment 27236,
　　　　　　　　　　　　　　 27177-27179, 27181
　　　Percutaneous Fixation 27235
　　Open Treatment 27245, 27269,
　　　　　　　　　　　　　 27506, 27507, 27511-27513
　　Percutaneous Fixation 27509
　　Peritrochanteric 27244
　　　Closed Treatment 27238
　　　Open Treatment 27236, 27269
　　　Treatment with Implant 27244
　　　with Implant 27245
　　　with Manipulation 27240
　　Proximal End, Head
　　　Closed Treatment 27267, 27268
　　Shaft 27500, 27502, 27506, 27507
　　Subtrochanteric 27244
　　　Closed Treatment 27238
　　　Treatment with Implant 27244
　　　with Implant 27245
　　　with Manipulation 27240
　　Supracondylar 27501-27503, 27509,
　　　　　　　　　　　　　　　　　 27511-27513
　　　Open Treatment 27511, 27513
　　Transcondylar 27501-27503, 27509,
　　　　　　　　　　　　　　　　　 27511-27513
　　　Open Treatment 27511, 27513

Osteotomy
   Femur 27165, 27181, 27450
   Foot
      Calcaneus. 28300
      Talar 28302
      Tarsal 28304
Repair of Nonunion. 25628
   Carpal Bone 25431, 25440
   Clavicle. 23485
   Fibula 27726
without Fracture
   Interdental 21497

Fixation (Device)

See Spinal Instrumentation
Ankle
   Dislocation. 27842, 27846, 27848
   Fracture
      Bimalleolar 27814
      Malleolar 27766, 27769
      Trimalleolar. 27822, 27823
      Manipulation 27860
Bennett Fracture. 26650, 26665
Carpal Bone. 25431, 25440, 25628
Clavicle 23485, 23515
Craniofacial. 21432, 21435, 21436
Elbow 24635
External
   See External Fixation
Femur
   Condylar Fracture. 27509, 27511,
                    27513, 27514
   Curettage 27358
   Cyst Excision 27358
   Epiphyseal Separation. 27519, 27509
   Head Fracture. 27254, 27269
   Neck Fracture. 27235, 27236
   Osteotomy 27165, 27181, 27450
   Shaft Fracture 27506
   Trochanteric Fracture 27248
   Tumor Excision 27358
Fibula
   Fracture 27826, 27828, 27780, 27792
   Nonunion or Malunion. 27726
   Tibiofibular Syndesmosis. 27829, 27832
Finger
   Arthrodesis. 26843, 26850, 26860
   Dislocation. 26706, 26715
   Fracture . . 26607, 26608, 26615, 26756, 26765
   Joint Dislocation 26776, 26785
   Joint Fracture. 26746
   Nonunion 26546
   Shaft. 26727, 26735
Foot
   Dislocation
      Interphalangeal 28675
      Metatarsophalangeal. 28636, 28645
      Talotarsal. 28576, 28585
      Tarsal 28546, 28555
      Tarsometatarsal 28606, 28615
   Fracture
      Calcaneus. 28406, 28415
      Great Toe 28496, 28505
      Metatarsal 28476, 28485
      Sesamoid 28531
      Talus 28436, 28445
      Tarsus 28456, 28465
   Osteotomy
      Calcaneus. 28300
      Talar 28302
      Tarsal 28304

Hand
   Carpometacarpal 26676, 26685,
                    26706, 26715
Harrington Rod 22840, 22850
Hip
   Acetabular Fracture 27226-27228
   Dislocation. 27216-27218
Humerus 23615, 23630, 24400, 24538
   Condylar . . 24545, 24546, 24566, 24579, 24582
Interdental. 21110, 21421, 21431, 21462
   without Fracture. 21497
Knee
   Dislocation. 27556
   Fracture 27524, 27540, 29850
   Joint Manipulation 29887, 29892
   Osteochondritis Dissecans 29885, 29887
Malar. 21365
Mandibular . . . 21196, 21452-21454, 21462, 21470
Maxillofacial. 21100, 21110,
             21345, 21346, 21421, 21435
Nasal. 21330, 21339, 21340, 21345, 21346
Odontoid Process 22318
Pelvis
   Dislocation. 27216-27218
   Fracture 27216-27218
   Spinal Instrumentation 22848
Radius. 24665, 25606-25609, 25671
   Shaft. 25515, 25525, 25526, 25574, 25575
Removal 20670, 20680
Rib 21811-21813
Scapula 23585
Shoulder 23670, 23680, 23700
Sternum. 21825
Temporomandibular Dislocation. 21485
Thumb
   Arthrodesis. 26841, 26850, 26860
   Dislocation. 26650, 26665
   Fracture 26756, 26765
   Joint Dislocation 26776, 26785
   Joint Fracture. 26746
   Shaft Fracture 26727, 26735
Tibia
   Fracture 27535, 27536,
          27827, 27828, 29855, 29856
   Shaft Fracture 27756, 27758
   Tibiofibular Syndesmosis. 27829, 27832
Tongue. 41500
Ulnar Fracture. 24685, 25671
   Shaft. 25545, 25574, 25575
   Styloid 25651
Wrist
   Fracture 29847
   Arthroplasty 25332
   Caliper 20660
   Cranial Tong 20660
   Interdental 21110
   Multiplane 20692
   Stereotactic Computer
      Assisted 20696, 20697
   Pin/Wire. 20650
   Skeletal
      Humeral Epicondyle
         Percutaneous 24566
   Stereotactic Frame. 20660
   Uniplane 20690
   Vertebral with Arthroplasty 0202T
Spinal
   See Spinal Instrumentation

Fixation Test, Complement

See Complement, Fixation Test

Fixation, External

See External Fixation

Fixation, Kidney

See Nephropexy

Fixation, Rectum

See Proctopexy

Fixation, Tongue

See Tongue, Fixation

Flank

See Back/Flank

Flap

See Skin Graft and Flap

Flatfoot Correction 28735

Flea Typhus

See Murine Typhus

Fletcher Factor. 85292

Flow Cytometry 88182-88189

Diagnostic/Pretreatment 3170F

Flow-Volume Loop

See Pulmonology, Diagnostic

Flu Vaccines

See Vaccines, Influenza

Fluid Collection

Amniocentesis
   See Amniocentesis
Arterial Catheter. 37799
Catheter
   Percutaneous 10030
Image Guided 10030
   Percutaneous 49405, 49406
   Transrectal 49407
   Transvaginal 49407
Incision and Drainage
   Cerebrospinal Fluid 62272
   Hematoma 10140
   Skin 10140
Soft Tissue
   Percutaneous 10030
Sputum 89220
Sweat 89230
Tears 83861
Venipuncture 36415
Venous Access Device 36591
Venous Catheter 36592

Fluid, Amniotic

See Amniotic Fluid

Fluid, Body

See Body Fluid

Fluid, Cerebrospinal

See Cerebrospinal Fluid

Fluorescein

Angiography, Ocular 92230, 92235, 92287
Intravenous Injection
   Vascular Flow Check, Graft 15860

Fluorescein Angiography

See Angiography, Fluorescein

G

Gabapentin
Assay. 80171

Gait Training 97116

Galactogram 77053, 77054
Injection 19030

Galactokinase
Blood. 82759

Galactose
Blood. 82760
Urine 82760

Galactose-1-Phosphate
Uridyl Transferase. 82775, 82776

Galeazzi Fracture/Dislocation
Radial Shaft 25520, 25525, 25526

Gall Bladder
See Gallbladder

Gallbladder
See Bile Duct
Anastomosis
　　with Intestines 47720, 47721,
　　　　　　　　　　　　　　　　　　 47740, 47741
Biopsy 43261
Diagnostic Imaging
　　Nuclear Medicine 78226, 78227
　　X-ray with Contrast 74290
Destruction
　　Calculi (Stone) 47544
Excision
　　See Cholecystectomy
Exploration 47480
　　Endoscopic Retrograde
　　Cholangiopancreatography (ERCP) 43260
Fistulization. 47480, 47490
Incision 47480
Incision and Drainage. 47480
Pharmacologic Intervention 78227
Removal
　　Calculi (Stone) 47480, 47544
Repair
　　with Gastroenterostomy 47741
　　with Intestines . . . 47720, 47721, 47740, 47741
Stimulation 43757
Unlisted Services and Procedures 47999

Galvanocautery
See Electrocautery

Galvanoionization
See Iontophoresis

Gamete Intrafallopian Transfer
(GIFT) 58976

Gamete Transfer
In Vitro Fertilization. 58976

Gamma Camera Imaging
See Nuclear Medicine, Diagnostic

Gamma Glutamyl Transferase . . 82977

Gamma Seminoprotein
See Antigen, Prostate Specific

Gammacorten
See Dexamethasone

Gammaglobulin
Blood 82784, 82785, 82787

Gamulin Rh
See Immune Globulins, Rho(D)

Ganglia, Trigeminal
See Gasserian Ganglion

Ganglion
Cyst
　　Aspiration/Injection 20612
　　Drainage. 20612
　　Wrist
　　　Excision. 25111, 25112
Gasserian
　　See Gasserian Ganglion
Geniculate
　　Facial Nerve
　　　Decompression. 69720, 69725
　　　Suture. 69740, 69745
Injection
　　Anesthetic
　　　Sphenopalatine 64505
　　　Stellate 64510
Stellate
　　See Stellate Ganglion

Ganglion Cervicothoracicum
See Stellate Ganglion

Ganglion Pterygopalatinum
See Sphenopalatine Ganglion

Ganglion, Gasser's
See Gasserian Ganglion

Gardner Operation
See Meningocele Repair

Gardnerella Vaginalis
Detection 87510-87512

Gasser Ganglion
See Gasserian Ganglion

Gasserian Ganglion
Sensory Root
　　Compression 61450
　　Decompression 61450
　　Section. 61450
Creation of Lesion
　　Stereotactic 61790

Gastrectomy
Longitudinal 43775
Partial 43631-43635, 43845, 48150, 48152
　　with Gastrojejunostomy. 43632
Proximal 43117, 43118, 43121-43123
Sleeve 43775
Total 43620-43622
　　with Esophagoenterostomy 43620
with Gastroduodenostomy 43631

Gastric Acid
Analysis. 82930

Gastric Analysis Test
Secretory Study. 43754, 43755

Gastric Electrodes
Neurostimulator
　　Implantation
　　　Laparoscopic. 43647
　　　Open 43881

Removal
　　Laparoscopic. 43648
　　Open 43882
Replacement
　　Laparoscopic. 43647
　　Open 43881
Revision
　　Laparoscopic. 43648
　　Open 43882

Gastric Intubation
Diagnostic. 43754-43757
Therapeutic. 43753

Gastric Lavage, Therapeutic
Intubation 43753

Gastric Tests
Acid Reflux 91034, 91035, 91037, 91038
Motility. 91020

Gastric Ulcer Disease
See Stomach, Ulcer

Gastrin 82938-82941

Gastrocnemius Recession
Leg, Lower. 27687

Gastroduodenostomy
Establishment 43810
Revision. 43850, 43855
with Gastrectomy 43631

Gastroenterology, Diagnostic
B-12 Absorption Study 78270-78272
Breath Test
　　Hydrogen 91065
　　Methane. 91065
　　Urea 78267, 78268
Motility Study
　　Colon 91117
　　Esophagus 91010, 91013
　　Gastric 91020
Esophagus Tests
　　Acid Perfusion 91030
　　Acid Reflux. 91034-91038
　　Balloon Distension Study. 91040
　　　with Provocation. 91040
　　Intubation with Specimen
　　　Collection. 43754, 43755
　　Motility Study 91010, 91013
Gastric Tests
　　Emptying Imaging Study 78264
　　　with Small Bowel Transit. 78265
　　　with Small Bowel and Colon Transit . . 78266
　　Motility. 91020
Gastroesophageal Reflux Test
　　See Acid Reflux Test, Gastroesophageal
Imaging
　　Gastrointestinal Tract
　　　See Gastrointestinal Tract
Manometry 91010, 91013, 91020, 91022
Rectum
　　Sensation, Tone, and Compliance Test . . 91120
Rectum/Anus
　　Manometry. 91122
Stomach
　　Stimulation of Secretion 43755
Unlisted Services and Procedures 91299

Gastroenterostomy
for Obesity
　　Laparoscopic 43644, 43645
for Repair 47721, 47741

Gastroesophageal Reflux Test
with Electrode Placement.............. 91034,
91035, 91037, 91038

Gastrointestinal Endoscopies
See Endoscopy, Gastrointestinal

Gastrointestinal Exam
Capsule Endoscopy
  Colon............................ 0355T
  Esophagus................. 91110, 91111
CT Scan
  Colon................... 74261-74263
Endoscopic Imaging
  Intraluminal
    Colon............................ 0355T
    Esophagus................. 91110, 91111
Radiologic Imaging
  Bile Ducts....... 47531, 47532, 74300, 74301
  Colon................... 74270, 74280
  Duodenum....................... 74260
  Esophagus............... 74210, 74220
    Swallowing Function.............. 74230
  Gallbladder............... 74290, 78226
  Gastrointestinal Tract
    See Gastrointestinal Tract, Imaging,
    Esophagus
  Pharynx....................... 74210
  Protein Loss..................... 78282
  Small Intestine.............. 74249-74251
Nuclear Medicine
  Blood Loss Study............... 78278
  Esophageal Motility............... 78258
  Gastric Emptying Imaging Study....... 78264
    with Small Bowel Transit.......... 78265
    with Small Bowel and Colon Transit .. 78266
  Gastric Mucosa Imaging........... 78261
  Gastroesophageal Reflux Study....... 78262
  Hepatobiliary............... 78226, 78227
  Intestine....................... 78290
  Liver............. 78201, 78215, 78216
    SPECT....................... 78205
    with Vascular Flow......... 78202, 78206
  Peritoneal-Venous Shunt Patency...... 78291
  Protein Loss Study................. 78282
  Salivary Gland.............. 78230-78232
  Spleen....................... 78215
  Unlisted Diagnostic Nuclear Medicine
  Procedure..................... 78299
Ultrasound
  Endoscopic..................... 76975

Gastrointestinal Pathogen 87505-87507

Gastrointestinal Tract
Imaging
  CT Scan
    Colon................... 74261-74263
  Endoscopic
    Esophagus................. 91110, 91111
  Radiological.....................74340
  Colon................... 74270, 74280
  Duodenum....................... 74260
  Small Intestine....... 74245, 74249-74251
  Upper .. 74240, 74241, 74245-74247, 74249
Measurements
  Transit....................... 91112
  Pressure....................... 91112
Reconstruction.............. 43360, 43361
Upper
  Dilation................... 43249, 74360
X-ray........... 74240, 74241, 74245
  Guide Dilator................... 74360

Guide Intubation.................. 74340
  with Contrast............... 74246-74249

Gastrointestinal, Upper
Biopsy........................ 43239
Dilation
  Endoscopy 43245
  Esophagus 43249
    Passage of Dilator 43248
Endoscopy
  Ablation
    Lesion...................... 43270
    Polyp...................... 43270
    Tumor...................... 43270
  Biopsy...................... 43239
  Catheterization.................. 43241
  Collection of Specimen 43235
  Dilation............. 43245, 43248, 43249
  Drainage
    Pseudocyst 43240
  Esophageal Ultrasound .. 43237, 43238, 43253
  Examination 43235, 43252
    Ultrasound 43253
  Hemorrhage 43255
  Injection 43236, 43253
  Injection, Varices 43243
  Ligation, Varices.............. 43244
  Mucosal Resection 43254
  Needle Biopsy 43238, 43242
  Removal
    Foreign Body.................. 43247
    Lesion...................... 43251
    Polyp...................... 43251
    Tumor...................... 43251
  Stent Placement................. 43266
  Thermal Radiation 43257
  Tube Placement 43246
  Ultrasound 43237, 43238,
                43242, 43253, 43259, 76975
Exploration
  Endoscopy 43235, 43252
Hemorrhage
  Endoscopic Control 43255
Imaging
  Radiologic 74240, 74241,
                74245-74247, 74249
  Ultrasound Endoscopy 43237, 43238,
                43242, 43259, 76975
Injection
  Submucosal 43236
  Transmural 43253
  Varices...................... 43243
Lesion
  Ablation...................... 43270
Ligation of Vein.............. 43244
Needle Biopsy
  Endoscopy 43238, 43242
Reconstruction
  Esophageal.................. 43360
Removal
  Foreign Body.................. 43247
  Lesion...................... 43250
  Polyp................. 43250, 43251
  Tumor...................... 43250
Tube Placement
  Endoscopy 43246
Ultrasound
  Endoscopy 43237, 43238,
                43242, 43259, 76975

Gastrojejunostomy
Conversion from Gastrostomy Tube........ 49446
Contrast Injection..................... 49465
Removal of Obstructive Material.......... 49460

Replacement of Tube.................. 49452
Revision of Gastrojejunal
Anastomosis................... 43860, 43865
Whipple Procedure................. 48150
  with Duodenal Exclusion 48547
  with Pancreatectomy 48150
  with Partial Gastrectomy 43632
  with Vagotomy 43825
  without Vagotomy............... 43820

Gastroplasty
Collis....................... 43338
Esophageal Lengthening......... 43283, 43338
Laparoscopic........... 43279, 43280, 43283
Revision
  for Obesity 43644, 43645,
             43842, 43843, 43845-43848
Wedge....................... 43338

Gastroplasty with Esophagogastric Fundoplasty
Laparoscopic................... 43820

Gastrorrhaphy
Injury....................... 43840
Perforated Ulcer.................. 43840
Wound....................... 43840

Gastroschises
See Gastroschisis

Gastroschisis
Repair....................... 49605
with Prosthesis.................. 49605
  Removal of Prosthesis.............. 49606

Gastrostomy
Closure....................... 43870
Laparoscopic
  Temporary 43653
Temporary....................... 43830
  Laparoscopic 43653
  Neonatal 43831
Radiological Assessment............... 49465
Tube
  See Gastrostomy Tube
with Pancreatic Drain.................. 48001
with Pyloroplasty 43640
with Vagotomy 43640, 43641

Gastrostomy Tube
Change
  Percutaneous...................... 43760
  with Fluoroscopic Guidance........... 49450
Contrast Injection 49465
Conversion
  to Gastro-jejunostomy Tube.......... 49446
  to Jejunostomy Tube............ 44373
Obstructive Material Removal 49460
  Placement
    Endoscopic 43246
    Percutaneous 49440
    with Conversion to Gastro-jejunostomy
    Tube 49446
Replacement....................... 49450
Repositioning
  Feeding Tube 43761

Gastrotomy
Exploration....................... 43500
Foreign Body Removal 43500
Suture Repair
  Bleeding Ulcer 43501
  Esophagogastric Laceration........... 43502
with Esophageal Tube Insertion........... 43510

GDH
See Glutamate Dehydrogenase

Gel Diffusion
Detection 86331

Gel Diffusion Test
See Immunodiffusion

Gene Analysis
Analytes

ABCA4 (ATP-binding cassette, sub-family
A [ABC1], member 4) 81408
ABCC8 (ATP-binding cassette, sub-family
C [CFTR/MRP], member 8) 81400,
81401, 81407
ABCD1 (ATP-binding cassette, sub-family
D [ALD], member 1) 81405
ABL1 (ABL proto-oncogene 1, non-receptor
tyrosine kinase) 81170, 81401
ACADM (acyl-CoA dehydrogenase,
C-4 to C-12 straight chain) 81400, 81401
ACADS (acyl-CoA dehydrogenase,
C-2 to C-3 short chain) 81404, 81405
ACADVL (acyl-CoA dehydrogenase,
very long chain) 81406
ACE (angiotensin I converting
enzyme [peptidyl-dipeptidase A] 1) 81400
ACTA2 (actin, alpha 2, smooth muscle,
aorta) 81405
ACTC1 (actin, alpha, cardiac muscle 1) . . 81405
ACTN4 (actinin, alpha 4) 81406
ADRB2 (adrenergic, beta-2-, receptor,
surface) 81401
AFF2 (AF4/FMR2 family, member
2 [FMR2]) 81401, 81404
AFG3L2 (AFG3 ATPase family gene 3 like 2
[S. cerevisiae]) 81406
AGL (amylo-alpha-1, 6-glucosidase,
4-alpha-glucanotransferase) 81407
AHI1 (Abelson helper integration
site 1) 81407
AIRE (autoimmune regulator) 81406
ALDH7A1 (aldehyde dehydrogenase
7 family, member A1) 81406
ANG (angiogenin, ribonuclease,
RNase A family, 5) 81403
ANKRD1 (ankyrin repeat domain 1) 81405
ANO5 (anoctamin 5) 81406
APOB (apolipoprotein B) 81401
APOE (apolipoprotein E) 81401
APP (amyloid beta [A4] precursor
protein) 81406
AGTR1 (angiotensin II receptor, type 1) . . 81400
APC (adenomatous polyposis
coli) 81201, 81202
APTX (aprataxin) 81405
AQP2 (aquaporin 2 [collecting duct]) 81404
AR (androgen receptor) 81401, 81405
ARSA (arylsulfatase A) 81405
ARX (aristaless related
homeobox) 81403, 81404
ASPA (aspartoacylase) 81200
ASPM (asp [abnormal spindle] homolog,
microcephaly associated [Drosophila]) . . 81407
ASS1 (argininosuccinate synthase 1) . . . 81406
ATL1 (atlastin GTPase 1) 81406
ATM (ataxia telangiectasia mutated) . . . 81408
ATN1 (atrophin 1) 81401
ATP1A2 (ATPase, Na+/K+ transporting,
alpha 2 polypeptide) 81406
ATP7B (ATPase, Cu++ transporting,
beta polypeptide) 81406
ATXN1 (ataxin 1) 81401

ATXN2 (ataxin 2) 81401
ATXN3 (ataxin 3) 81401
ATXN7 (ataxin 7) 81401
ATXN8OS (ATXN8 opposite strand
[non-protein coding]) 81401
ATXN10 (ataxin 10) 81401
AVPR2 (arginine vasopressin
receptor 2) 81404
BBS1 (Bardet-Biedl syndrome 1) 81406
BBS2 (Bardet-Biedl syndrome 2) 81406
BBS10 (Bardet-Biedl syndrome 10) 81404
BCKDHA (branched chain keto acid
dehydrogenase E1, alpha
polypeptide) 81400, 81405
BCKDHB (branched chain keto acid
dehydrogenase E1, beta
polypeptide) 81205, 81406
BCL1/IgH, t(11;14) 81401
BCR/ABL1 (chronic myelogenous leukemia)
Translocation 81206-81208
BCS1L (BCS1-like [S. cerevisiae]) 81405
BEST1 (bestrophin 1) 81406
BLM (Bloom syndrome,
RecQ helicase-like) 81209
BMPR2 (bone morphogenetic protein
receptor, type II [serine/threonine
kinase]) 81405, 81406
BRAF (B-Raf proto-oncogene,
serine/threonine kinase) 81210, 81406
BRCA1, BRCA2
(breast cancer 1 and 2) . . 81162, 81211-81213
BRCA1 (breast cancer 1) 81214, 81215
BRCA2 (breast cancer 2) 81216, 81217
BSCL2 (Berardinelli-Seip congenital
lipodystrophy 2 [seipin]) 81406
BTD (biotinidase) 81404
BTK (Bruton agammaglobulinemia tyrosine
kinase) 81406
C10orf2 (chromosome 10 open reading
frame 2) 81404
CACNA1A (calcium channel,
voltage-dependent, P/Q type, alpha 1A
subunit) 81401, 81407
CACNB2 (calcium channel,
voltage-dependent, beta 2 subunit) 81406
CALR (calreticulin) (eg, myeloproliferative
disorders) 81219
CAPN3 (calpain 3) 81406
CASQ2 (calsequestrin 2
[cardiac muscle]) 81405
CASR (calcium-sensing receptor) 81405
CAV3 (caveolin 3) 81404
CBFB/MYH11 (inv (16)) 81401
CBS
(cystathionine-beta-synthase) . . . 81401, 81406
CD40LG (CD40 ligand) 81404
CCND1/IGH (BCL1/IgH, t(11;14)) 81401
CCR5 (chemokine C-C motif receptor 5) . . 81400
CDH1 (cadherin 1, type 1, E-cadherin
[epithelial]) 81406
CDH23 (cadherin-related 23) 81408
CDKL5 (cyclin-dependent
kinase-like 5) 81405, 81406
CDKN2A (cyclin-dependent kinase
inhibitor 2A) 81404
CEBPA (CCAAT/enhancer binding protein
[C/EBP], alpha) 81218
CEL (carboxyl ester lipase [bile salt
stimulated lipase]) 81403
CEP290 (centrosomal protein 290kDa) . . 81408
CFH/ARMS2 (complement
factor H/age-related maculopathy
susceptibility 2) 81401

CFTR (cystic fibrosis transmembrane
conductance regulator) 81220-81224
CHD7 (chromodomain helicase DNA
binding protein 7) 81407
CHRNA4 (cholinergic receptor, nicotinic,
alpha 4) 81405
CHRNB2 (cholinergic receptor, nicotinic,
beta 2 [neuronal]) 81405
Chromosome 1p-/19q- 81402
Chromosome 18q- 81402
CLCN1 (chloride channel 1,
skeletal muscle) 81406
CLCNKB (chloride channel,
voltage-sensitive Kb) 81406
CLRN1 (clarin 1) 81400, 81404
CNBP (CCHC-type zinc finger, nucleic acid
binding protein) 81401
CNTNAP2 (contactin associated
protein-like 2) 81406
COL1A1 (collagen, type I, alpha 1) 81408
COL1A1/PDGFB (t(17;22)) 81402
COL1A2 (collagen, type I, alpha 2) 81408
COL4A1 (collagen, type IV, alpha 1) 81408
COL4A3 (collagen, type IV, alpha 3
[Goodpasture antigen]) 81408
COL4A4 (collagen, type IV, alpha 4) 81407
COL4A5 (collagen, type IV,
alpha 5) 81407, 81408
COL6A1 (collagen, type VI, alpha 1) 81407
COL6A2 (collagen, type VI,
alpha 2) 81406, 81407
COL6A3 (collagen, type VI, alpha 3) 81407
COX6B1 (cytochrome c oxidase subunit
VIb polypeptide 1) 81404
COX10 (COX10 homolog, cytochrome c
oxidase assembly protein) 81405
COX15 (COX15 homolog, cytochrome c
oxidase assembly protein) 81405
CPT1A (carnitine palmitoyltransferase 1A
[liver]) 81406
CPT2 (carnitine palmitoyltransferase 2) . . 81404
CRB1 (crumbs homolog 1 [Drosophila]) . . 81406
CREBBP (CREB binding protein) . . 81406, 81407
CRX (cone-rod homeobox) 81404
CSTB (cystatin B [stefin B]) 81401, 81404
CTNNB1 (catenin [cadherin-associated
protein], beta 1, 88kDa) 81403
CYP1B1 (cytochrome P450, family 1,
subfamily B, polypeptide 1) 81404
CYP21A2 (cytochrome P450, family 21,
subfamily A, polypeptide 2) 81402, 81405
CYP2C19 (cytochrome P450, family 2,
subfamily C, polypeptide 19) 81225
CYP2C9 (cytochrome P450, family 2,
subfamily C, polypeptide 9) 81227
CYP2D6 (cytochrome P450, family 2,
subfamily D, polypeptide 6) 81226
CYP3A4 (cytochrome P450, family 3,
subfamily A, polypeptide 4) 81401
CYP3A5 (cytochrome P450, family 3,
subfamily A, polypeptide 5) 81401
CYP11B1 (cytochrome P450, family 11,
subfamily B, polypeptide 1) 81405
CYP17A1 (cytochrome P450, family 17,
subfamily A, polypeptide 1) 81405
CYP21A2 (cytochrome P450, family 21,
subfamily A, polypeptide2) 81402, 81405
Constitution 81228, 81229
Neoplasia 81406
DAZ/SRY (deleted in azoospermia and
sex determining region Y) 81403
DBT (dihydrolipoamide branched chain
transacylase E2) 81405, 81406

PDHA1 (pyruvate dehydrogenase [lipoamide] alpha 1) 81405, 81406

PDHB (pyruvate dehydrogenase [lipoamide] beta) 81405

PDHX (pyruvate dehydrogenase complex, component X) 81406

PDX1 (pancreatic and duodenal homeobox 1) 81404

PHEX (phosphate regulating endopeptidase homolog, X-linked) 81406

PHOX2B (paired-like homeobox 2b) 81403, 81404

PIK3CA (phosphatidylinositol-4,5-bisphosphate 3-kinase, catalytic subunit alpha) 81404

PINK1 (PTEN induced putative kinase 1) 81405

PKD1 (polycystic kidney disease 1 [autosomal dominant]) 81407

PKD2 (polycystic kidney disease 2 [autosomal dominant]) 81406

PKHD1 (polycystic kidney and hepatic disease 1) 81408

PKP2 (plakophilin 2) 81406

PLCE1 (phospholipase C, epsilon 1) 81407

PLN (phospholamban) 81403

PLP1 (proteolipid protein 1) 81404, 81405

PML/RARalpha, (t(15;17)) (promyelocytic leukemia/retinoic acid receptor alpha) 81315, 81316

PMP22 (peripheral myelin protein 22) 81324-81326

PMS2 (PMS2 postmeiotic segregation increased 2 [S. cerevisiae]) 81317-81319

PNKD (paroxysmal nonkinesigenic dyskinesia) 81406

POLG (polymerase [DNA directed], gamma) 81406

POMGNT1 (protein O-linked mannose beta1, 2-N-acetylglucosaminyltransferase) 81406

POMT1 (protein-O-mannosyltransferase 1) 81406

POMT2 (protein-O-mannosyltransferase 2) 81406

POU1F1 (POU class 1 homeobox 1) 81405

PPP2R2B (protein phosphatase 2, regulatory subunit B, beta) 81401

PQBP1 (polyglutamine binding protein 1) 81404, 81405

PRKAG2 (protein kinase, AMP-activated, gamma 2 non-catalytic subunit) 81406

PRKCG (protein kinase C, gamma) 81406

PRNP (prion protein) 81404

PROP1 (PROP paired-like homeobox 1) . . 81404

PRPH2 (peripherin 2 [retinal degeneration, slow]) 81404

PRSS1 (protease, serine, 1 [trypsin 1]) 81401, 81404

PRX (periaxin) 81405

PSEN1 (presenilin 1) 81405

PSEN2 (presenilin 2 [Alzheimer disease 4]) 81406

PTEN (phosphatase and tensin homolog) 81321-81323

PTPN11 (protein tyrosine phosphatase, non-receptor type 11) 81406

PYGM (phosphorylase, glycogen, muscle) 81401, 81406

RAB7A (RAB7A, member RAS oncogene family) 81405

RAF1 (v-raf-1 murine leukemia viral oncogene homolog 1) 81404, 81406

RAI1 (retinoic acid induced 1) 81405

REEP1 (receptor accessory protein 1) . . . 81405

RET (ret proto-oncogene) 81404-81406

RHD (Rh blood group, D antigen) 81403

RHO (rhodopsin) 81404

RP1 (retinitis pigmentosa 1) 81404

RPE65 (retinal pigment epithelium specific protein 65kDa) 81406

RPS19 (ribosomal protein S19) 81405

RRM2B (ribonucleotide reductase M2 B [TP53 inducible]) 81405

RUNX1/RUNX1T1(t(8;21)) 81401

RYR1 (ryanodine receptor 1, skeletal) . . 81406, 81408

RYR2 (ryanodine receptor 2 [cardiac]) . . 81408

SCN1A (sodium channel, voltage-gated, type I, alpha subunit) 81407

SCN1B (sodium channel, voltage-gated, type I, beta) 81404

SCN4A (sodium channel, voltage-gated, type IV, alpha subunit) 81406

SCN5A (sodium channel, voltage-gated, type V, alpha subunit) 81407

SCNN1A (sodium channel, nonvoltage-gated 1 alpha) 81406

SCNN1B (sodium channel, nonvoltage-gated 1, beta) 81406

SCNN1G (sodium channel, nonvoltage-gated 1, gamma) 81406

SCO1 (SCO cytochrome oxidase deficient homolog 1) 81405

SCO2 (SCO cytochrome oxidase deficient homolog 2 [SCO1L]) 81404

SDHA (succinate dehydrogenase complex, subunit A, flavoprotein [Fp]) 81406

SDHB (succinate dehydrogenase complex, subunit B, iron sulfur) 81405

SDHC (succinate dehydrogenase complex, subunit C, integral membrane protein, 15kDa) 81404, 81405

SDHD (succinate dehydrogenase complex, subunit D, integral membrane protein) . . 81404

SEPT9 (septin 9) 81401

SERPINA1 (serpin peptidase inhibitor, clade A [alpha-1 antiproteinase, antitrypsin], member 1) 81332

SERPINE1 (serpine peptidase inhibitor clade E, member 1, plasminogen activator inhibitor 1, PAI 1) 81400

SETX (senataxin) 81406

SGCA (sarcoglycan, alpha [50kDa dystrophin-associated glycoprotein]) 81405

SGCB (sarcoglycan, beta [43kDa dystrophin-associated glycoprotein]) 81405

SGCD (sarcoglycan, delta [35kDa dystrophin-associated glycoprotein]) 81405

SGCE (sarcoglycan, epsilon) 81405, 81406

SGCG (sarcoglycan, gamma [35kDa dystrophin-associated glycoprotein]) 81404, 81405

SH2D1A (SH2 domain containing 1A) 81403, 81404

SH3TC2 (SH3 domain and tetratricopeptide repeats 2) 81406

SHOC2 (soc-2 suppressor of clear homolog) 81400, 81405

SHOX (short stature homeobox) 81405

SIL1 (SIL1 homolog, endoplasmic reticulum chaperone [S. cerevisiae]) 81405

SLC9A6 (solute carrier family 9 [sodium/hydrogen exchanger], member 6) 81406

SLC2A1 (solute carrier family 2 [facilitated glucose transporter], member 1) 81405

SLC12A1 (solute carrier family 12 [sodium/potassium/chloride transporters], member 1) 81407

SLC12A3 (solute carrier family 12 [sodium/chloride transporters], member 3) . . . 81407

SLC16A2 (solute carrier family 16, member 2 [thyroid hormone transporter]) . . . 81404, 81405

SLC22A5 (solute carrier family 22 [organic cation/carnitine transporter], member 5) 81405

SLC25A4 (solute carrier family 25 [mitochondrial carrier; adenine nucleotide translocator], member 4) 81404

SLC25A20 (solute carrier family 25 [carnitine/acylcarnitine translocase], member 20) 81404, 81405

SLC26A4 (solute carrier family 26, member 4) 81406

SLC37A4 (solute carrier family 37 [glucose-6-phosphate transporter], member 4) 81406

SLCO1B1 (solute carrier organic anion transporter family, member 1B1) 81400

SMAD4 (SMAD family member 4) 81405, 81406

SMN1 (survival of motor neuron 1, telomeric) 81400, 81403, 81405

SMN1/SMN2 (survival of motor neuron 1, telomeric/survival of motor neuron 2, centromeric) 81401

SMPD1 (sphingomyelin phosphodiesterase 1, acid lysosomal) 81330

SNRPN/UBE3A (small nuclear ribonucleoprotein polypeptide N/ubiquitin protein ligase E3A) 81331

SOD1 (superoxide dismutase 1, soluble) 81404

SOS1 (son of sevenless homolog 1) 81406

SPAST (spastin) 81405, 81406

SPG7 (spastic paraplegia 7 [pure and complicated autosomal recessive]) 81405, 81406

SPG11 (spastic paraplegia 11 [autosomal recessive]) 81407

SPINK1 (serine peptidase inhibitor, Kazal type 1) 81404

SPRED1 (sprouty-related, EVH1 domain containing 1) 81405

SPTBN2 (spectrin, beta, non-erythrocytic 2) 81407

SRY (sex determining region Y) 81400

SS18/SSX1 (t(X;18)) 81401

SS18/SSX2 (t(X;18)) 81401

STAT3 (signal transducer and activator of transcription 3 [acute-phase response factor]) 81405

STK11 (serine/threonine kinase 11) 81404, 81405

STXBP1 (syntaxin binding protein 1) 81406

SURF1 (surfeit 1) 81405

TACO1 (translational activator of mitochondrial encoded cytochrome c oxidase I) 81404

TARDBP (TAR DNA binding protein) 81405

TAZ (tafazzin) 81406

TBP (TATA box binding protein) 81401

TBX5 (T-box 5) 81405

TCF4 (transcription factor 4) 81405, 81406

TGFBR1 (transforming growth factor, beta receptor 1) 81405

TGFBR2 (transforming growth factor, beta receptor 2) 81405

TH (tyrosine hydroxylase) 81406

THAP1 (THAP domain containing, apoptosis associated protein 1) 81404

THRB (thyroid hormone receptor, beta) . . 81405

TK2 (thymidine kinase 2,
mitochondrial) 81405
TMEM43 (transmembrane protein 43) . . 81406
TMEM67 (transmembrane protein 67) . . 81407
TNNC1 (troponin C type 1 [slow]) 81405
TNNI3 (troponin I, type 3 [cardiac]) 81405
TNNT2 (troponin T, type 2 [cardiac]) 81406
TOR1A (torsin family 1, member A
[torsin A]) 81400, 81404
TP53 (tumor protein 53) 81404, 81405
TPM1 (tropomyosin 1 [alpha]) 81405
TPMT (thiopurine
S-methyltransferase) 81401
TRB@ (T cell receptor beta
locus) 81340, 81341
TRD@ (T cell antigen receptor, delta)
Rearrangement 81402
TRG@ (T cell receptor gamma locus) . . . 81342
TRPC6 (transient receptor potential cation
channel, subfamily C, member 6) 81406
TSC1 (tuberous sclerosis 1) 81405, 81406
TSC2 (tuberous sclerosis 2) 81406, 81407
TTPA (tocopherol [alpha] transfer
protein) 81404
TTR (transthyretin) 81404
TWIST1 (twist homolog 1
[Drosophila]) 81403, 81404
TYMP (thymidine phosphorylase) 81405
TYMS (thymidylate synthetase) 81401
TYR (tyrosinase [oculocutaneous
albinism IA]) 81404
UBA1 (ubiquitin-like modifier activating
enzyme 1) 81403
UBE3A (ubiquitin protein ligase E3A) . . . 81406
UGT1A1 (UDP glucuronosyltransferase 1
family, polypeptide A1) 81350
UMOD (uromodulin) 81406
Uniparental disomy (UPD) 81402
USH1C (Usher syndrome 1C [autosomal
recessive, severe]) 81407
USH1G (Usher syndrome 1G [autosomal
recessive]) 81404
USH2A (Usher syndrome 2A [autosomal
recessive, mild]) 81408
VHL (von Hippel-Lindau tumor
suppressor) 81403, 81404
VKORC1 (vitamin K epoxide reductase
complex, subunit 1) 81355
VPS13B (vacuolar protein sorting
13 homolog B [yeast]) 81407, 81408
VWF (von Willebrand factor) 81401,
81403-81406, 81408
WAS (Wiskott-Aldrich syndrome
[eczema-thrombocytopenia]) 81406
WDR62 (WD repeat domain 62) 81407
WT1 (Wilms tumor 1) 81404
ZEB2 (zinc finger E-box binding
homeobox 2) 81404, 81405
ZNF41 (zinc finger protein 41) 81404
Chimerism Analysis 81267, 81268
Comparative Analysis Using Short Tandem
Repeat (STR) Markers 81265, 81266
Cytogenomic Constitutional Targeted Microarray
Analysis
Chromosome 22q13 81405
Cytogenomic Microarray Analysis,
Neoplasia 81406
HLA Class I and II Typing,
Low Resolution 81370, 81371
HLA Class I Typing, Low Resolution . . 81372-81374
HLA Class II Typing,
Low Resolution 81375-81377
HLA Class I and II Typing, High Resolution . . . 81378

HLA Class I Typing,
High Resolution 81379-81381
HLA Class II Typing, High Resolution   81382, 81383
Human Platelet Antigen Genotyping 81400
Long QT Syndrome Gene Analysis . . . 81280-81282
Microsatellite Instability Analysis 81301
Short Tandem Repeat
(STR) Analysis 81265, 81266, 81402
Translocation Analysis
BCR/ABL1 (t(9;22)) 81206-81208
CCND1/IGH (BCL1/IgH, t(11;14)) . . . 81401
COL1A1/PDGFB (t(17;22)) 81402
E2A/PBX1 (t(1;19)) 81401
EML4/ALK (inv(2)) 81401
ETV6/NTRK3 (t(12;15)) 81401
ETV6/RUNX1 (t(12;21)) 81401
EWSR1/ATF1 (t(12;22)) 81401
EWSR1/ERG (t(21;22)) 81401
EWSR1/FLI1 (t(11;22)) 81401
EWSR1/WT1 (t(11;22)) 81401
FOXO1/PAX3 (t(2;13)) 81401
FOXO1/PAX7 (t(1;13)) 81401
FUS/DDIT3 (t(12;16)) 81401
IGH@/BCL2 (t(14;18)) 81402
MLL/AFF1 (t(4;11)) 81401
MLL/MLLT3 (t(9;11)) 81401
NPM1/ALK (t(2;5)) 81401
PAX8/PPARG (t(2;3)) (q13;p25)) 81401
PML/RARalpha (t(15;17)) 81315, 81316
RUNX1/RUNX1T1 (t(8;21)) 81401
SS18/SSX1 (t(X;18)) 81401
SS18/SSX2 (t(X;18)) 81401

Gene Product
See Protein

Genioplasty
Augmentation 21120, 21123
Osteotomy 21121-21123

Genitourinary Sphincter, Artificial
See Prosthesis, Urethral Sphincter

Genomic Sequencing Procedures (GSPs) and other Molecular Multianalyte Assays
Ashkenazi Jewish Associated Disorders 81412
Aortic Dysfunction or Dilation 81410, 81411
Exome 81415-81417
Fetal Chromosomal Aneuploidy 81420
Genome 81425-81427
Hearing Loss 81430, 81431
Hereditary Breast Cancer-Related
Disorders 81432, 81433
Hereditary Colon Cancer Disorders . . 81435, 81436
Hereditary Neuroendocrine Tumor
Disorders 81437, 81438
Hereditary Retinal Disorders 81434
Noonan Spectrum Disorders 81442
Nuclear Encoded Mitochondrial Genes 81440
Targeted Genomic Sequence
Analysis Panel 81445, 81450, 81455
Whole Mitochondrial Genome 81460, 81465
X-linked Intellectual Disability
(XLID) 81470, 81471

Genotype Analysis
by Nucleic Acid
Hepatitis C Virus 87902
HIV-1 . . . . 87901, 87906
Protease/Reverse Transcriptase
Regions 87901
Vancomycin Resistance 87500
Human Platelet Antigen 81400

Gentamicin
Assay 80170

Gentamycin Level
See Gentamicin

Gentiobiase
See Beta Glucosidase

Genus: Human Cytomegalovirus Group
See Cytomegalovirus

GERD
See Gastroesophageal Reflux Test

German Measles
See Rubella

Gestational Trophoblastic Tumor
See Hydatidiform Mole

GGT
See Gamma Glutamyl Transferase

GI Tract
See Gastrointestinal Tract

Giardia
Antigen Detection
Immunoassay 87329
Immunofluorescence 87269

Giardia Lamblia
Antibody 86674

Gibbons Stent
Ureteral 52332

GIF
See Somatostatin

GIFT
See Gamete Intrafallopian Transfer (GIFT)

Gill Operation
Laminectomy 63012

Gillies Approach
Fracture
Zygomatic Arch 21356

Gingiva
See Gums

Gingiva, Abscess
Incision and Drainage 41800

Gingivectomy
Each Quadrant 41820

Gingivoplasty
Each Quadrant 41872

Girdlestone Laminectomy
See Laminectomy

Girdlestone Procedure
See Acetabulum, Reconstruction

Gla Protein (Bone)
See Osteocalcin

Gland
See Specific Gland

Gland, Adrenal
See Adrenal Gland

Gland, Bartholin's
See Bartholin's Gland

Gland, Bulbourethral
See Bulbourethral Gland

Gland, Lacrimal
See Lacrimal Gland

Gland, Mammary
See Breast

Gland, Parathyroid
See Parathyroid Gland

Gland, Parotid
See Parotid Gland

Gland, Pituitary
See Pituitary Gland

Gland, Salivary
See Salivary Glands

Gland, Sublingual
See Sublingual Gland

Gland, Sweat
See Sweat Glands

Gland, Thymus
See Thymus Gland

Gland, Thyroid
See Thyroid Gland

Glasses
See Spectacle Services

Glaucoma
Counseling 4174F
Cryotherapy. 66720
Cyclophotocoagulation 66710, 66711
Diathermy 66700
Filtration Implant
   See Aqueous Shunt
Fistulization of Sclera 66150
     Through Ciliary Body 66999
Iridectomy 66625, 66630
Plan of Care. 0517F
Provocative Test 92140

Glaucoma Drainage Implant
See Aqueous Shunt

Glenn Procedure 33766, 33767

Glenohumeral Joint
Arthrodesis 23800, 23802
Arthrotomy 23040
    with Biopsy 23100
    with Drainage 23040
    Foreign Body Removal 23040
    with Exploration. 23040, 23107
    with Synovectomy 23105
Arthroplasty 23470, 23472-23474
Capsulorrhaphy. 23465, 23466
Exploration 23040, 23107
Removal
    Foreign or Loose Body 23040, 23107

Glenoid Fossa
Allograft 23473, 23474
Arthroplasty 23473, 23474
Reconstruction 21255

Globulin
Antihuman
   Coombs Test
     Direct 86880, 86885, 86886
     Indirect 86850, 86870

Immune
  Administration 96365-96368
  Product
    Botulinum Antitoxin 90288
    Botulism 90288
    Cytomegalovirus (CMV-IgIV) 90291
    Diphtheria Antitoxin 90296
    Gammaglobulin 82784, 82785
    Hepatitis B (HBIg) 90371
    Ig. 90281
    IgIV 90283
    Rabies (RIg/Rig-HT)) 90375, 90376
    Respiratory Syncytial Virus 90378
    Rho(D) (RhIg/RhIgIV) 90384-90386
    SCIg 90284
    Tetanus (TIg) 90389
    Unlisted 90399
    Vaccinia 90393
    Varicella-zoster 90396
Sex Hormone Binding 84270

Globulin, Corticosteroid-Binding
See Transcortin

Globulin, Rh Immune
See Immune Globulins, Rho(D)

Globulin, Thyroxine-Binding
See Thyroxine Binding Globulin

Glomerular Procoagulant Activity
See Thromboplastin

Glomus Caroticum
See Carotid Body

Glossectomy
Complete. 41140, 41145
Composite 41150, 41153, 41155
Partial 41135
   Half. 41130
   Less than Half 41120

Glossopexy
See Tongue, Fixation

Glossorrhaphy
See Suture, Tongue

Glucagon
Measurement 82943
Tolerance Panel. 80422, 80424
Tolerance Test. 82946

Glucose
Blood Test 82947, 82948, 82950
   Home Test 82962
Body Fluid 82945
Interstitial Fluid
   Continuous Monitoring 95250, 95251
    Data Interpretation. 99091
Panel
   Basic Metabolic. 80047, 80048
   Comprehensive Metabolic. 80053
   Glucagon Tolerance 80422, 80424
   Growth Hormone Suppression. 80430
   Insulin Tolerance 80434, 80435
   Insulin-induced C-peptide Suppression. . 80432
   Renal Function 80069
Tolerance Test. 82951, 82952
   Intravenous Push 96374
Urinalysis 81000-81003, 81005

Glucose Phosphate Isomerase
See Phosphohexose Isomerase

Glucose Phosphate Isomerase Measurement
See Phosphohexose Isomerase

Glucose-6-Phosphate
Dehydrogenase 82955-82960

Glucosidase 82963

Glucuronide Androstanediol . . 82154

Glue
Anal Fistula Repair 46706
Bronchoscopy
    Balloon Occlusion 31634
Cornea Wound 65286
Sclera Wound 65286

Glukagon
See Glucagon

Glutamate Dehydrogenase
Blood. 82965

Glutamate Pyruvate Transaminase
See Transaminase, Glutamic Pyruvic

Glutamic Alanine Transaminase
See Transaminase, Glutamic Pyruvic

Glutamic Aspartic Transaminase
See Transaminase, Glutamic Oxaloacetic

Glutamic Dehydrogenase
See Glutamate Dehydrogenase

Glutamyltransferase, Gamma . . 82977

Glutathione 82978

Glutathione Reductase 82979

Glycanhydrolase, N-Acetylmuramide
See Lysozyme

Glycated Hemoglobins
See Glycohemoglobin

Glycated Protein 82985

Glycerol Phosphoglycerides
See Phosphatidylglycerol

Glycerol, Phosphatidyl
See Phosphatidylglycerol

Glycerophosphatase
See Alkaline Phosphatase

Glycinate, Theophylline Sodium
See Theophylline

Glycocholic Acid
See Cholylglycine

Glycohemoglobin
Glycosylated Hemoglobin 83036

Glycol, Ethylene
See Ethylene Glycol

Glycols, Ethylene
See Ethylene Glycol

Glycosaminoglycan
See Mucopolysaccharides

Goeckerman Treatment
Photochemotherapy 96910, 96912, 96913

Gol-Vernet Operation
See Pyelotomy, Exploration

Goldwaite Procedure
Knee 27422

Golfer's Elbow
See Tennis Elbow

Gonadectomy, Female
See Oophorectomy

Gonadectomy, Male
See Excision, Testis

Gonadotropin
Chorionic 84702-84704
   Stimulation Panel 80414
FSH 83001
ICSH 83002
LH 83002
Stimulation Panel 80426

Gonadotropin Panel
Stimulation 80426

Gonioscopy
Ophthalmic 92020

Goniotomy
Congenital Glaucoma 65820

Gonococcus
See Neisseria Gonorrhoeae

Goodenough Harris Drawing Test
Psychological Testing 96101-96103

GOTT
See Transaminase, Glutamic Oxaloacetic

GPUT
See Galactose-1-Phosphate, Uridyl Transferase

Graft
Anal 46753
Aorta 33840-33851, 33860-33877
Artery
   Bypass Graft
     See Bypass Graft, Arterial; Bypass Graft,
     Arterial-Venous
   Coronary 33503
Bone
See Bone Graft
Bone Marrow
   SeeHematopoietic Progenitor Cell (HPC),
   Transplantation
Bone and Skin 20969, 20970, 20972, 20973
Cartilage
   See Cartilage Graft
Conjunctiva 65782
   Harvesting 68371
Cornea
   with Lesion Excision 65426
Cornea Transplant
   See Cornea, Transplantation
Dura
   Cranial
     Craniectomy 61343
     Anterior Cranial Fossa 61601
     Middle Cranial Fossa 61606, 61608
     Posterior Cranial Fossa 61616
   Spinal Cord 63710
     Laminectomy 63180, 63182
Ear
   Dermal Autograft 15135, 15136
   Epidermal Autograft 15115, 15116

Full-thickness Graft, Free 15260, 15261
   Preparation of Recipient Site 15004, 15005
   Skin Substitute Graft 15275-15278
   Split-thickness Autograft 15120, 15121
   Tissue Cultured Skin Autograft . . 15155-15157
Eye
   Amniotic Membrane 65778-65780
   Conjunctiva 65782
   Stem Cell 65781
for Facial Nerve Paralysis
   Fascia 15840
   Muscle 15841, 15842, 15845
Fascia
   See Fascial Grafts
Fascia Lata
   Harvesting 20920, 20922
Gum Mucosa 41870
Intestine 43116, 46748
Muscle
   See Muscle Flaps; Muscle Grafts
Nail Bed
   Reconstruction 11762
Nerve
   See Nerve Graft
Oral Mucosa 40818
Organ
   See Transplantation
Pancreas
   See Pancreas, Transplantation
Patency
   Blood Flow Check 15860
   Vascular Flow Check 15860
Skin
   See Skin Graft and Flap
Skin Substitute
   See Skin Substitute Graft
Tendon
   Finger 26392, 26416, 26420, 26428, 26434
   Hand 26392, 26412, 26416
   Harvesting 20924
Tissue
   Harvesting 20926
Vein
   Bypass Graft
     See Bypass Graft, Venous
   Cross-Over 34520

Grain Alcohol
See Drug Assay, Drug Procedure, Definitive Drug
Class, Alcohols

Granulation Tissue
Cauterization, Chemical 17250

Gravis, Myasthenia
See Myasthenia Gravis

Gravities, Specific
See Specific Gravity

Great Toe
Arthrodesis
   Interphalangeal Joint 28755
     with Tendon Transfer 28760
   Metatarsophalangeal Joint 28750
Fracture
   Skeletal Fixation 28496
   Closed Treatment 28490
   Open Treatment 28505
Osteocutaneous Flap 20973
Toe-to-Hand Transfer 20973
   Wrap-around with Bone Graft 26551

Great Vessels
Graft Insertion 33330, 33335
Shunt
   Aorta to Pulmonary Artery
     Ascending 33755
     Descending 33762
   Central 33764
   Subclavian to Pulmonary Artery 33750
   Vena Cava to Pulmonary Artery . . 33766, 33767
Suture Repair 33320-33322
Translocation
   Aortic Root 33782, 33783
Transposition Repair
   Aortic Pulmonary Artery
     Reconstruction 33778-33781
   Atrial Baffle Procedure 33774-33777
   with Subpulmonary Stenosis 33770, 33771
   with Ventricular Septal Defect . . 33770, 33771
Unlisted Services and Procedures 33999

Great Vessels Transposition
See Transposition, Great Arteries

Greater Tuberosity Fracture
Humeral
   Closed Treatment 23620, 23625, 23665
   Open Treatment 23630, 23670
with Shoulder Dislocation
   Closed Treatment 23665
   Open Treatment 23670

Greater Vestibular Gland
See Bartholin's Gland

Green Operation
See Scapulopexy

Grippe, Balkan
See Q Fever

Gritti Operation
See Amputation, Leg, Upper; Radical Resection;
Replantation

Groin Area
Incision
   Femoral Artery Exposure 34812
Repair
   Hernia 49550-49557
Revision
   Femoral Arterial Bypass Graft 35883

Group Adaptive Behavior
Treatment 0366T, 0367T

Group Health Education
Genetic 98961, 98962, 99078
Physical 99078
Preventive Medicine 99411
Self-Management, Condition or
Treatment 98961, 98962

Grouping, Blood
See Blood Typing, Serologic

Growth Factors, Insulin-Like
See Somatomedin

Growth Hormone 83003
Human
   Measurement 83003
   Antibody 86277
Growth Hormone Stimulation Panel 80428
Growth Hormone Suppression Panel 80430
Insulin Tolerance Panel 80435
Pituitary Evaluation Panel 80418

Growth Hormone Release Inhibiting Factor
See Somatostatin

Growth Stimulation Expressed Gene 2 83006

GTT
See Glucose, Tolerance Test
See Hydatidiform Mole

Guaiac Test
See Blood, Feces

Guard Stain
Special Stain, Group II 88313

Gullet
See Esophagus

Gums
Abscess
    Incision and Drainage 41800
Alveolus
    Excision 41830
Cyst
    Incision and Drainage 41800
Excision
    Gingiva 41820
    Operculum 41821
Graft
    Mucosa 41870
Hematoma
    Incision and Drainage 41800
Lesion
    Destruction 41850
    Excision 41825-41827
Mucosa
    Excision 41828
    Graft 41870
Reconstruction
    Alveolus 41874
    Gingiva 41872
Removal
    Bone 41806
    Foreign Body 41805
Tuberosities
    Excision 41822, 41823
Tumor
    Excision 41825-41827
Unlisted Services and Procedures 41899

Gunning-Lieben Test
See Drug Assay, Drug Procedure, Definitive Drug Class, Alcohols

Guthrie Test
Phenylalanine (PKU) 84030

H

H Flu
See Haemophilus Influenza (H Flu)

H1N1
Immunization
    See Vaccines

HAA (Hepatitis Associated Antigen)
See Hepatitis Antigen, B Surface

HAAb
See Antibody, Detection, Hepatitis A (HAAb)

Haemoglobin F
See Fetal Hemoglobin

Haemophilus Influenza (H Flu)
Antibody 86684
Antigen Detection 87275
Immunoassay 87804
Nucleic Acid Detection
    Reverse Transcription, Amplified
    Probe 87501-87503
Vaccines
    Hib-HepB 90748
    Hib-MenCY 90644
    Hib, PRP-OMP Conjugate 90647
    Hib, PRP-T Conjugate 90648, 90748

Haemorrhage
See Hemorrhage

Haemorrhage Rectum
See Hemorrhage, Endoscopic Control, Rectum

Hageman Factor
Clotting Factor XII 85280

HAI Test
See Hemagglutination Inhibition Test

Hair
Cell
    Ear, Function Analysis 92588
Electrolysis 17380
Fungi Isolation 87101
KOH Examination 87220
Microscopic Evaluation 96902
Transplant
    Punch Graft 15775, 15776
    Strip Graft 15220, 15221

Hair Removal
See Removal, Hair

Hallux
See Great Toe

Halo
Body Cast 29000
Cranial 20661
    for Thin Skull Osteology 20664
Femur 20663
Maxillofacial 21100
Pelvic 20662
Removal 20665

Haloperidol
Assay 80173

Halstead-Reitan Neuropsychological Battery
Neuropsychological Testing 96118, 96119

Halsted Mastectomy
See Mastectomy, Radical

Halsted Repair
See Hernia, Repair, Inguinal

Ham Test
See Hemolysins

Hammertoe Repair
Correction 28285, 28286

Hamster Penetration Test
Sperm Evaluation 89329

Hand
Amputation
    at Metacarpal 25927, 26910
    at Wrist 25920
        Revision 25922
    Ray Amputation 26910
    Revision 25924, 25929, 25931
Bone
    Cyst
        Curettage 26210, 26215
        Excision 26210, 26215
        Osteotomy, Metacarpal 26565
    Incision and Drainage 26034
Casts, Splints, and Strapping 29065, 29085
    Compression System 29584
    Gauntlet Cast 29085
    Long Arm Cast 29065
    Long Arm Splint 29105
    Short Arm Cast 29075
    Short Arm Splint 29125, 29126
    Strapping 29280
Decompression 26035
Diagnostic Imaging
    Magnetic Resonance Imaging
    (MRI) 73218-73220
        Angiography 73225
    X-ray 73120, 73130
Drainage
    Bursa 26025, 26030
Fasciectomy 26121, 26123, 26125
Fasciotomy
    Decompressive 26037
    Injection, Enzyme 20527, 26341
    Open 26045
    Percutaneous 26040
Fracture
    Carpometacarpal 26645, 26650
    Interphalangeal
        See Interphalangeal Joint, Fracture
    Metacarpal
        Closed Treatment 26600, 26605, 26607
        Open Treatment 26615
        Skeletal Fixation 26608
    Metacarpophalangeal 26740-26746
    Phalangeal 26720-26735, 26750-26765
Insertion
    Tendon Graft 26392
Joint
    See Carpometacarpal Joint; Intercarpal Joint
Manipulation
    Carpometacarpal Fracture 26645, 26650
    Dupuytren's Cord 26341
    Joint Dislocation
        See Carpometacarpal Joint; Intercarpal Joint
    Metacarpal Fracture 26605, 26607
    Palmar Fascial Cord 26341
Nerve
    Graft 64890, 64891, 64895, 64896
    Neuroma, Excision 64782, 64783
    Neuroplasty 64704
    Suture
        Additional Nerve 64837
        Common Sensory 64834
        Digital 64831
Reconstruction
    Tendon Pulley 26500-26502
Removal
    Implantation 26320
    Tube/Rod 26390-26392, 26416
Repair
    Blood Vessel 35207
    Cleft Hand 26580

Palate 42280, 42281
Retina 0100T
Skull Plate 62142, 62143
Spectacle
    Fitting 92352, 92353
    Repair 92371
Speech Aid 31611
Temporomandibular Joint 21243
Voice 31611
Unlisted Maxillofacial Prosthetic
Procedure 21089
Lipectomy, Suction Assisted 15876
Nerve
    Graft 64885, 64886
Other Procedures 21299, 21499
Repair/Revision and/or Reconstruction
    See Cranioplasty; Face; Mandible
Rhytidectomy
    See Rhytidectomy
Unlisted Services and Procedures 21499

Head Rings, Stereotactic
See Stereotactic Frame

Headbrace
See Halo

Heaf Test
See TB Test

Health Behavior
See Evaluation and Management, Health Behavior

Health Risk Assessment Instrument
See Preventive Medicine, Health Risk Assessment

Hearing Aid
Device
    Attenuation Measurements 92596
    Check 92592, 92593
    Evaluation, Electroacoustic 92594, 92595
    Examination and Selection 92590, 92591
Implants
    Bone Conduction
        Implantation 69710
        Removal 69711
        Repair 69711
        Replacement 69710
    Brainstem
        Implantation 61863, 61867
        Programming 92640
    Cochlear
        Implantation 69930
        Programming 92601-92604
        Rehabilitation 92626, 92627
    Osseointegrated
        Implantation 69714, 69715
        Replacement 69717, 69718

Hearing Aid Check 92592, 92593

Hearing Aid Services
Attenuation Measurements
    Ear Protector 92596
Electroacoustic Test 92594, 92595
Examination 92590, 92591

Hearing Tests
See Audiologic Function Tests

Hearing Therapy
Evaluation 92626, 92627
for Hearing Loss
    Postlingual 92633
    Prelingual 92630

Individual 92507
Group 92508
Cochlear Implant
    Analysis and Programming 92601-92604
    Rehabilitation 92626, 92627

Heart
Ablation
    Arrythmogenic Focus . . . 33250, 33251, 33261
    Atrial Tissue 33254-33259
        Endoscopic 33265, 33266
Anomaly
    Repair 33615, 33617
Aorta
    See Aorta
Arrhythmia
    See Tachycardia
Artificial Heart
    Implantation 0051T
    Repair 0052T, 0053T
Atria
    See Atria
Balloon Device
    Insertion 33973
    Removal 33974
Biopsy 93505
    UltrasonicGuidance 76932
Blood Vessel
    Repair 33320-33322
Cardiac Output Measurements 93451,
                                      93561, 93562
Cardiac Rehabilitation 93797, 93798
Cardioassist
    Circulation 92970, 92971
Cardiopulmonary Bypass
    with Aortic Aneurysm Repair 33877
    with Ascending Aorta Graft 33860, 33863,
                                            33864
    with Atrial Septectomy/Septostomy 33736
    with Chamber Fistula Repair 33500
    with Descending Thoracic Aorta Graft . . 33875
    with Lung Transplant 32852, 32854
    with Operative Ablation 33251,
                          33256, 33259, 33261
    with Pericardiectomy 33031
    with Pulmonary Artery Repair . . 33910, 33916,
                                    33922, 33926
    with Replacement of Ventricular
    Assist Device 33983
    with Septal Defect Repair
        See Septal Defect
    with Sinus of Valsalva Repair . . . 33720, 33702
    with Transcatheter Aortic Valve
    Replacement (TAVR/TAVI) 33367-33369
    with Transverse Arch Graft 33870
    with Tumor Excision/Resection 33120
    with Valve Repair
        See Aortic Valve; Mitral Valve; Tricuspid
        Valve; Pulmonary Valve
    with Wound Repair 33305
Cardioversion 92960, 92961
Catheterization
    See Cardiac Catheterization
Cardiac Event Recorder
    Implantation 33282
    Removal 33284
Coronary Artery Bypass Graft
    See Coronary Artery Bypass Graft (CABG)
Cor Triatriatum
    Repair 33732
Cyst
    Pericardial
        Resection 33050

Diagnostic Imaging
    Acoustic Cardiography 93799
    Angiography
        See Angiography, Heart
        Blood Pool 78472, 78473,
                    78481, 78483, 78496
        SPECT 78494
    CT Scan 75571-75573
        Angiography 75574
    Magnetic Resonance
        See Cardiac Magnetic Resonance Imaging
        (CMRI)
    Myocardial Imaging
    Quantitative Assessment of
    Mechanics 0399T
        Infarct Avid 78466, 78468, 78469
        Perfusion 78451-78454
        Perfusion Study 78491, 78492
        PET Metabolic Evaluation 78459
        SPECT 0332T, 78451, 78452, 78469
        Sympathetic Innervation 0331T, 0332T
    Shunt Detection 78428
    Unlisted Cardiovascular Diagnostic
    Nuclear Medicine Procedure 78499
    Ventriculography
        See Ventriculography
Electrical Recording
    See Electrophysiology Procedure
Electrode
    Insertion 33202, 33203, 33210,
          33211, 33216, 33217, 33224, 33225
    Removal 33238
        Single/Dual Chamber 33243, 33244
Electrophysiologic Study
    See Electrophysiology Procedure
Exploration 33310-33315
External Heart Rate Data Recording
    for Nocturnal Epilepsy Seizure . . . 0381T-0386T
Foreign Body Removal 33310
Great Vessels
    See Great Vessels
Heart-Lung Bypass
    See Cardiopulmonary Bypass
Heart-Lung Transplantation
    See Transplantation, Heart-Lung
Hemodynamic Monitoring
    Noninvasive 93880, 93882,
            93922-93931, 93965-93990, 93998
    with Pharmacologic Agent 93463
    with Physiologic Exercise Study 93464
Infundibular Stenosis 33476-33478
Injection
    Radiologic
        See Cardiac Catheterization, Injection
Intracardiac Ischemia Monitoring System
    Evaluation 0305T, 0306T
    Insertion
        Complete System 0302T
        Device Only 0304T
        Electrode Only 0303T
        Interrogation Device 0306T
        Programming Device 0305T
        Removal 0307T
    Removal/Replacement
        Complete System 0302T
        Device Only 0304T
        Electrode Only 0303T
Intraoperative Pacing and Mapping 93631
Ligation
    Fistula 37607
Myocardium
    Imaging 78466-78469

Nail
    Evacuation 11740
Nasal Septum
    Incision and Drainage 30020
Neck
    Incision and Drainage 21501, 21502
Nose
    Incision and Drainage 30000, 30020
Pelvis
    Incision and Drainage 26990
Scrotum
    Incision and Drainage 54700
Shoulder
    Incision and Drainage 23030
Skin
    Incision and Drainage 10140
    Puncture Aspiration 10160
Subdural 61108
Subungual
    Evacuation 11740
Testis
    Incision and Drainage 54700
Thigh
    Incision and Drainage 27301
Thorax
    Incision and Drainage 21501
Tongue 41000, 41005, 41006, 41015
Vagina
    Incision and Drainage 57022, 57023
Wrist 25028

Hematopoietic Progenitor Cell (HPC)

Donor Search and Cell Acquisition 38204
Harvesting 38205, 38206
HPC Boost 38243
Transplant Preparation
    Cell Concentration 38215
    Cell Depletion 38210-38214
    Cryopreservation and Storage 38207
    Thawing 38208, 38209
Transplantation 38240-38242

Hematopoietic Stem Cell Transplantation

See Stem Cell, Transplantation

Hematopoietin

See Erythropoietin

Hematuria

See Blood, Urine

Hemic System

Unlisted Procedure, Hemic System 38999
Unlisted Procedure, Spleen
    Laparoscopic 38129

Hemiepiphyseal Arrest

Elbow 24470

Hemifacial Microsomia

Reconstruction
    Mandibular Condyle 21247

Hemilaminectomy 63020-63044

Hemilaryngectomy 31370-31382

Hemipelvectomies

See Amputation, Interpelviabdominal

Hemiphalangectomy

Toe 28160

Hemispherectomy

Brain
    Partial 61543

Hemocytoblast

See Stem Cell

Hemodialyses

See Hemodialysis

Hemodialysis 90935-90937

Access
    Anastomosis
        Arteriovenous 36818-36821
    Cannulation
        Arteriovenous 36810
    Closure 36815
    Revision 36815
    Vein to Vein 36800
Blood Flow Study 90940
Duplex Scan of Access 93990
Home Visit 99512
Kt/V Level 3082F-3084F
Plan of Care Documented 0505F
Procedure
    via Catheter 4054F
    via Functioning Arteriovenous Fistula . . . 4052F
        Thrombectomy 36831
    via Functioning Arteriovenous Graft 4053F
    with Evaluation 90935, 90937

Hemofiltration

Dialysis Procedure 90945, 90947

Hemoglobin

Analysis
    O_2 Affinity 82820
A1c (HbA1c) Level 3044F, 3045F
Carboxyhemoglobin 82375, 82376, 88740
Chromatography 83021
Concentration 85046
Electrophoresis 83020
Fetal 83030-83033, 85460, 85461
Fractionation and Quantitation 83020
Glycosylated (A1C) 83036, 83037
Hgb
    Transcutaneous Testing 88738
Methemoglobin 83045-83050
    Transcutaneous 88741
Non-Automated 83026
Plasma 83051
Sulfhemoglobin 83060
Thermolabile 83065-83068
Transcutaneous 88740
Urine 83069

Hemoglobin F

Fetal Hemoglobin
    Copper Sulfate 83030-83033
    Differential Lysis 85460, 85461

Hemoglobin, Glycosylated

See Glycohemoglobin

Hemogram

Complete Blood Count
    Added Indices 85025-85027
    Automated 85025-85027
    Manual 85014-85018, 85032

Hemolysins

Acid 85475
with Agglutinins 86940, 86941

Hemolytic Complement

See Complement, Total Hemolytic

Hemolytic Complement, Total

See Complement, Total Hemolytic

Hemoperfusion

Dialysis 90997

Hemophil

See Clotting Factor

Hemorrhage

Control
    Gastrointestinal 43753
    Liver 47350
    Lung 32110
    Nasal (Epistaxis)
        Complex 30903
        Initial 30905
        Simple 30901
        Subsequent 30906
    Nasopharynx 42970-42972
    Neck 35800
    Oropharynx 42960-42962
    Prostate, Transurethral Fulguration 52214
    Throat 42960-42962
    Uterus
        Postpartum 59160
    Vagina 57180
Endoscopic Control
    Anus 46614
    Chest Cavity 32654
    Colon 44391, 45382
    Colon-Sigmoid 45334
    Esophagus 43227, 43460
    Gastrointestinal, Upper 43255
    Intestines, Small 44366, 44378
    Nose 31238
    Rectum 45317
Vascular 37244

Hemorrhoidectomy

Complex 46260
    with Fissurectomy 46261, 46262
External Complete 46250
Ligation 46221, 46945, 46946
Simple 46255
    with Fissurectomy 46257, 46258

Hemorrhoidopexy

Stapling 46947

Hemorrhoids

Band Ligation
    with Colonoscopy 45398
    with Sigmoidoscopy 45350
Destruction 46930
Excision
    See Hemorrhoidectomy
Incision
    External 46083
Injection
    Sclerosing Solution 46500
Ligation 0249T, 46945, 46946
Stapling 46947
Suture 46945, 46946

Hemosiderin

Qualitative 83070

Heparin

Assay 85520
Neutralization 85525
Protamine Tolerance Test 85530

Heparin Cofactor I

See Antithrombin III

Hernia, Rectovaginal
See Rectocele

Hernia, Umbilical
See Omphalocele

Heroin Screen
See Drug Assay

Herpes Simplex
Antibody 86694-86696
Antigen Detection
　Immunofluorescence 87273, 87274
　Nucleic Acid. 87528-87530
Identification
　Smear and Stain 87207

Herpes Smear and Stain
Inclusion Bodies 87207

Herpes Virus-4 (Gamma), Human
See Epstein-Barr Virus

Herpes Virus-6
Detection. 87531, 87532
Quantification 87533

Herpetic Vesicle
Destruction
　Penis. 54050, 54055-54057, 54060, 54065
　Anus. 46900, 46910,
　　　　　　　　　　46916, 46917, 46922, 46924

Heteroantibodies
See Antibody, Detection, Heterophile

Heterophile Antibody
Screening 86308-86310

Heterotropia
See Strabismus

Hex B
See b-Hexosaminidase

Hexadecadrol
See Dexamethasone

Hexosephosphate Isomerase
See Phosphohexose Isomerase

Heyman Procedure
Femoral Neck 27179
Midtarsal. 28264

Hg Factor
See Glucagon

HGB
See Hemoglobin, Concentration

HGH
See Growth Hormone, Human

HHV-4
See Epstein-Barr Virus

HIAA
See Hydroxyindoleacetic Acid, Urine

Hib Vaccine
4 Dose Schedule
　PRP-T 90648
PRP-OMP
　3 Dose Schedule 90647

Hibb Operation 22610, 22612, 22614

Hidradenitis
See Sweat Gland
Excision. 11450-11471
Suppurative
　Incision and Drainage 10060, 10061

High Altitude Simulation Test
HAST. 94452, 94453

High Density Lipoprotein
See Lipoprotein

High Molecular Weight Kininogen
See Fitzgerald Factor

High Resolution Anoscopy (HRA)
Diagnostic. 46601
Biopsy 46607

Highly Selective Vagotomy
See Vagotomy, Highly Selective

Highmore Antrum
See Sinus/Sinuses, Maxillary

Hill Procedure
See Gastroplasty with Esophagogastric
Fundoplasty

Hinton Positive
See RPR

Hip
See Femur; Pelvis
Abscess
　Incision and Drainage 26990, 26991
Arthrocentesis. 20610, 20611
Arthrodesis 27284-27286
Arthrography. 73525
Arthroplasty 27130-27132
Arthroscopy 29860-29863, 29914-29916
Arthrotomy 27030-27033
Biopsy 27040-27045
Bone
　Drainage. 26992
Bursa
　Incision and Drainage 26990, 26991
Capsulectomy
　with Release, Flexor Muscles 27036
Cast 29305-29325
Craterization 27070
Cyst
　Excision 27065-27067
Denervation. 27035
Echography
　Infant 76885, 76886
Endoprosthesis
　See Prosthesis, Hip
Excision 27070
Exploration 27033
Fasciotomy 27025
Fusion 27284-27286
Hematoma
　Incision and Drainage 26990
Injection
　Radiologic 27093-27096
　Radiostereometric Analysis (RSA) 0350T
Reconstruction
　Total Replacement. 27130
Removal
　Cast 29710
　Foreign Body 27033, 27086, 27087
　　Arthroscopic. 29861-29863
　Loose Body
　　Arthroscopic. 29861-29863
　Prosthesis. 27090, 27091

Repair
　Muscle Transfer . . 27100-27105, 27110, 27111
　Osteotomy 27146-27156
　Tendon 27097
Replacement
　Partial. 27125
　Total 27130, 27132
Saucerization 27070
Stem Prostheses
　See Arthroplasty, Hip
Strapping. 29520
Tenotomy
　Abductor Tendon 27006
　Adductor Tendon 27000-27003
　Iliopsoas 27005
Total Replacement 27130-27132
Tumor
　Excision 27047, 27048, 27065-27067
　Radical Resection 27049, 27059
Ultrasound
　Infant 76885, 76886
X-ray
　Bilateral 73521-73523
　Unilateral 73501-73503
　with Contrast 73525

Hip Joint
Arthroplasty 27132
　Revision 27134-27138
Arthrotomy 27052, 27054
Biopsy 27052
Capsulotomy
　with Release, Flexor Muscles 27036
Dislocation 27250-27252
　Congenital 27256-27259
　Open Treatment 27253, 27254
　without Trauma 27265, 27266
Manipulation. 27275
Reconstruction
　Revision 27134-27138
Synovium
　Excision 27054
　　Arthroscopic 29860-29863
Total Replacement 27132

Hip Stem Prostheses
See Arthroplasty, Hip

Hippocampus
Excision. 61566

Histamine
Measurement 83088

Histamine Release Test
Leukocyte 86343

Histochemistry
Stain on Frozen Tissue Block 88314
Enzyme Constituents. 88319

Histocompatibility Testing
See Tissue, Typing

Histoplasma
Detection
　Immunoassay
　　Antibody 86698
　　Antigen 87385

Histoplasma capsulatum
Antigen Detection
　Immunoassay 87385

Histoplasmin Test
See Histoplasmosis, Skin Test

Hot Pack Treatment
Application 97010

House Calls
Established Patient 99347-99350
New Patient 99341-99345

HPC
See Hematopoietic Progenitor Cell (HPC)

HPL
See Lactogen, Human Placental

HTLV-I
Antibody
    Confirmatory Test 86689
    Detection 86687

HTLV-II
Antibody 86688

HTLV-III
See HIV

HTLV-III Antibodies
See Antibody, Detection, Human Immunodeficiency
Virus, HIV

HTLV-IV
See HIV-2

Hubbard Tank Therapy
Each 15 minutes 97036

Hue Test
Color Vision Exam 92283

Huggin Operation
See Orchiectomy, Simple

Huhner Test
Semen Analysis 89300, 89320

Human Chorionic Gonadotropin
See Chorionic Gonadotropin

Human Chorionic Somatomammotropin
See Lactogen, Human Placental

Human Cytomegalovirus Group
See Cytomegalovirus

Human Epididymis Protein 86305

Human Growth Hormone (HGH)
Anterior Pituitary Evaluation Panel 80418
Antibody 86277
Insulin Tolerance Panel 80435
Measurement 83003
Stimulation Panel 80428
Suppression Panel 80430

Human Herpes Virus 4
See Epstein-Barr Virus

Human Immunodeficiency Virus
See HIV

Human Immunodeficiency Virus 1
See HIV-1

Human Immunodeficiency Virus 2
See HIV-2

Human Leukocyte Antigen (HLA)
Antibody Analysis 86828-86835
Crossmatch 86825, 86826

Molecular Pathology 81370-81383
Tissue Typing 86812, 86813,
                  86816, 86817, 86821, 86822

Human Papillomavirus
Vaccine
   See Vaccines, Human Papillomavirus (HPV)

Human Papillomavirus Detection
Nucleic Acid Probe 87623-87625

Human Placental Lactogen
See Lactogen, Human Placental

Human T Cell Leukemia Virus I
See HTLV I

Human T Cell Leukemia Virus I Antibodies
See Antibody, Detection, HTLV I

Human T Cell Leukemia Virus II
See HTLV-II

Human T Cell Leukemia Virus II Antibodies
See Antibody, Detection, HTLV-II

Humeral Epicondylitises, Lateral
See Tennis Elbow

Humeral Fracture
See Fracture, Humerus

Humerus
See Arm, Upper; Shoulder
Abscess
    Incision and Drainage 23935
Craterization 23184, 24140
Cyst
    Excision 23150, 24110
      with Allograft 23156, 24116
      with Autograft 23155, 24115
Diaphysectomy 23184, 24140
Excision 23174, 23184, 23195,
                  24134, 24140, 24150
Fracture
    Closed Treatment 24500-24505
      with Manipulation 23605
      without Manipulation 23600
    Condyle
      Closed Treatment 24576, 24577
      Open Treatment 24579
      Percutaneous Fixation 24582
    Epicondyle
      Closed Treatment 24560-24565
      Open Treatment 24575
    Skeletal Fixation
      Percutaneous 24566
    Greater Tuberosity Fracture
      Closed Treatment with
      Manipulation 23625
      Closed Treatment without
      Manipulation 23620
      Open Treatment 23630
    Open Treatment 23615, 23616
    Shaft 24500-24505, 24516
      Open Treatment 24515
    Supracondylar
      Closed Treatment 24530-24535
      Open Treatment 24545, 24546
      Percutaneous Fixation 24538
    Transcondylar
      Closed Treatment 24530-24535
      Open Treatment 24545, 24546

      Percutaneous Fixation 24538
      with Dislocation 23665-23670
Osteomyelitis 24134
Pinning, Wiring 23491, 24498
Prophylactic Treatment 23491, 24498
Radical Resection 23220, 24150
    Radial Head or Neck 24152
Repair 24430
    Nonunion, Malunion 24430-24435
    Osteoplasty 24420
    Osteotomy 24400-24410
    with Graft 24435
Resection Head 23195
Saucerization 23184, 24140
Sequestrectomy 23174, 24134
Tumor
    Excision . . 23150, 23220, 24071-24076, 24110
    with Allograft 23156, 24116
    with Autograft 23155, 24115
X-ray 73060

Hummelshein Operation
See Strabismus, Repair

Humor Shunt, Aqueous
See Aqueous Shunt

HVA
See Homovanillic Acid

Hybridization Probes, DNA
See Nucleic Acid Probe

Hydatid Disease
See Echinococcosis

Hydatid Mole
See Hydatidiform Mole

Hydatidiform Mole
Evacuation and Curettage 59870
Excision 59100

Hydration
Intravenous 96360, 96361
Rehydration Oral Solution 4056F
Status 2030F, 2031F

Hydrocarbons, Chlorinated
See Chlorinated Hydrocarbons

Hydrocele
Aspiration 55000
Excision
    Bilateral
      Tunica Vaginalis 55041
    Unilateral
      Spermatic Cord 55500
      Tunica Vaginalis 55040
Repair 55060

Hydrochloric Acid, Gastric
See Acid, Gastric

Hydrochloride, Vancomycin
See Vancomycin

Hydrocodon
See Dihydrocodeinone

Hydrogen Ion Concentration
See Blood Gases, pH

Hydrolase, Acetylcholine
See Acetylcholinesterase

Hydrolase, Triacylglycerol
See Lipase

Hydrolases, Phosphoric Monoester
See Phosphatase

Hydrotherapy (Hubbard Tank)
Application 97036
See Physical Medicine/Therapy/Occupational
Therapy

Hydrotubation
See Chromotubation

Hydroxycorticosteroid 83491

Hydroxyindoleacetic Acid
Urine 83497
    Qualitative 81005

Hydroxypregnenolone
3 Beta-hydroxydehydrogenase Deficiency
Panel 80406
Quantitative 84143

Hydroxyprogesterone
ACTH Stimulation Panel 80402, 80406
Quantitative 83498, 83499

Hydroxyproline
Free 83500
Total 83505

Hydroxytyramine
See Dopamine

Hygroma
Cystic
    Axillary/Cervical
        Excision 38550-38555

Hymen
Excision 56700
Incision 56442

Hymenal Ring
Revision 56700

Hymenectomy 56700

Hymenotomy 56442

Hyoid
Bone
    Fracture
        Open Treatment 21495
Muscle
    Incision and Suspension 21685

**Hyperbaric Oxygen
Pressurization** 99183

Hypercycloidal X-ray 76101, 76102

Hyperdactylies
See Supernumerary Digit

**Hyperglycemic Glycogenolytic
Factor**
See Glucagon

Hyperhidrosis 64650-64653

Hypertelorism of Orbit
See Orbital Hypertelorism

Hyperthermia Therapy
See Thermotherapy

Hyperthermia Treatment . . 77600-77620

Hypnotherapy 90880

Hypodermis
See Subcutaneous Tissue

Hypogastric Plexus
Destruction 64681
Injection
    Anesthetic 64517
    Neurolytic 64680, 64681

Hypoglossal Nerve
Anastomosis
    Facial-Hypoglossal 64868
    Facial-Spinal 64866

Hypoglossal-Facial Anastomosis
See Hypoglossal Nerve, Anastomosis,
Facial-Hypoglossal

Hypopharynges
See Hypopharynx

Hypopharynx
Diverticulectomy 43130, 43180

Hypophysectomy 61546-61548, 62165

Hypophysis
See Pituitary Gland

Hypopyrexia
See Hypothermia

Hypospadias
Repair 54300, 54352
    Complications 54340-54348
    First Stage 54304
        Proximal Penile or Penoscrotal 54332
    One Stage
        Meatal Advancement 54322
        Perineal 54336
    Urethroplasty
        Local Skin Flaps 54324
        Local Skin Flaps and Mobilization of
        Urethra 54326
        Local Skin Flaps, Skin Graft Patch and/or
        Island Flap 54328
    Urethroplasty for Second
    Stage 54308, 54312, 54316
        Free Skin Graft 54316
    Urethroplasty for Third Stage 54318

Hypothermia
Treatment
    Neonatal
        Selective 99184
        Total 99184

Hypoxia
Breathing Response 94450
High Altitude Simulation Test 94452, 94453

Hysterectomy
Abdominal
    Radical 58210
    Resection of Ovarian Malignancy 58951,
                              58953, 58954, 58956
    Supracervical 58180
    Total 58150, 58200, 58956
        with Colpo-Urethrocystopexy 58152
        with Omentectomy 58956
        with Partial Vaginectomy 58200
Cesarean
    after Cesarean Delivery 59525
    with Closure of Vesicouterine Fistula . . . 51925
Laparoscopic 58541-58544
    Radical 58548

Total 58570-58573
Removal
    Lesion 59100
Supracervical
    Laparoscopic 58541-58544
Vaginal 58260-58270,
              58290-58294, 58550-58554
    Laparoscopic 58550, 58570-58573
    Radical 58285
    Removal Tubes/Ovaries 58262, 58263,
                              58291, 58292, 58552, 58554
    Repair of Enterocele . . . 58263, 58292, 58294
    with Colpectomy 58275-58280
    with Colpo-Urethrocystopexy . . . 58267, 58293

Hysterolysis
See Lysis, Adhesions, Uterus

Hysteroplasty 58540

Hysterorrhaphy 58520, 59350

Hysterosalpingography 74740
Catheterization 58345
Injection Procedure 58340

Hysterosalpingostomy
See Implantation, Tubouterine

Hysteroscopy
Ablation
    Endometrial 58563
Diagnostic 58555
Lysis
    Adhesions 58559
Placement
    Fallopian Tube Implants 58565
Removal
    Impacted Foreign Body 58562
    Leiomyomata 58561
Resection
    of Intrauterine Septum 58560
Surgical with Biopsy 58558
Unlisted Services and Procedures . . . 58578, 58579

Hysterosonography
See Ultrasound; Sonohysterography

Hysterotomy
See Cesarean Delivery
Abdominal 59100
with Failed Abortion 59852, 59857
with Tubal Ligation 58611

Hysterotrachelectomy
See Amputation, Cervix

I

I Antibodies, HTLV
See Antibody, Detection, HTLV-I

I, Angiotensin
See Angiotensin I

I, Coagulation Factor
See Fibrinogen

I, Heparin Co-Factor
See Antithrombin III

ICCE
See Cataract, Extraction/Removal, Intracapsular (ICCE)

Ichthyosis, Sex Linked
See Syphilis Test

ICSH
See Luteinizing Hormone (LH)

Identification
Antibody
   See Antibody Identification
Antigen
   See Antigen Detection
Axial Vessel
   for Island Pedicle 15740
Crystal, Light Microscopy 89060
Microbe
   See Infectious Agent; Bacteria Culture; Ova;
   Parasites
Oocyte
   from Follicular Fluid 89254
Sex Chromatin. 88130, 88140
Sperm
   Medicolegal. 88125
   from Aspiration 89257
   from Tissue. 89264
Urate Crystal. 89060

IDH
See Isocitric Dehydrogenase, Blood

IG
See Immune Globulins

IgA 82784

IgD 82784

IgE 82785, 86003-86005

IgG 82784, 82787, 86001

IgM 82784

II, Coagulation Factor
See Prothrombin
See Gene Analysis

II, Cranial Nerve
See Optic Nerve

Ileal Conduit
Visualization 50690

Ileoscopy
via Stoma 44380-44382, 44384

Ileostomy 45136
Continent (Kock Procedure). 44316
Ileoanal Reservoir 45136
Laparoscopic 44186, 44187
Non-Tube. 44310, 44187
Revision. 44312-44314

Iliac Arteries
See Artery, Iliac

Iliac Crest
Microvascular Anastomosis
   Bone Graft 20956
   Free Osteocutaneous Flap 20970

Iliohypogastric Nerve
Injection
   Anesthetic 64425

Ilioinguinal Nerve
Injection
   Anesthetic 64425

Ilium
Craterization 27070
Cyst
   Excision 27065-27067
Excision. 27070
Fracture
   Open Treatment 27215, 27218
Saucerization 27070
Tumor
   Excision 27065-27067, 27075, 27076

Ilizarov Procedure
Monticelli Type 20692
   See Application, Bone Fixation Device

IM Injection
See Injection, Intramuscular

Imaging
See Vascular Studies

Imaging, Gamma Camera
See Nuclear Medicine, Diagnostic

Imaging, Magnetic Resonance
See Magnetic Resonance Imaging (MRI)

Imaging, Ultrasonic
See Echography

Imbrication
Diaphragm. 39545

Immune Complex Assay 86332

Immune Globulin Administration
Intravenous Infusion . . 96365-96368, 96374, 96375
Injection 96372

Immune Globulin E
See IgE

Immune Globulins
Antitoxin
   Botulinum. 90287
   Diphtheria 90296
Botulism 90288
Cytomegalovirus 90291
Hepatitis B 90371
Human. 90281, 90283, 90284
Rabies 90375, 90376
Respiratory Syncytial Virus. 90378
Rho(D) 90384-90386
Tetanus 90389
Unlisted Immune Globulin 90399
Vaccinia. 90393
Varicella-Zoster. 90396

Immunization Administration
Each Additional Vaccine/Toxoid 90472, 90474
   with Counseling 90461
One Vaccine/Toxoid 90471, 90473
   with Counseling 90460

Immunization, Mumps
See Mumps, Immunization

Immunoassay
Amniotic Fluid Protein. 84112
Analyte 83516, 83518-83520
   Calprotectin, Fecal 83993
   Hemoglobin, Fecal 82274

Cellular Function
   Detection of Biomarker 86352
Infectious Agent
   See Infectious Agent
Other than Infectious Agent
Antibody/Antigen 83516, 83518, 83519
Tumor Antigen
   Qualitative/Semiquantitative 86294
   Quantitative
      CA-125 86304
      CA 15-3. 86300
      CA 19-9. 86301
      Other Antigen 86316
      Human Epididymis Protein 4 (HE4) 86305

Immunoblotting, Western
See Western Blot

Immunochemical, Lysozyme (Muramidase)
See Lysozyme

Immunocytochemistry
Antibody 88341, 88342, 88344

Immunodeficiency Virus Type 1, Human
See HIV 1

Immunodeficiency Virus Type 2, Human
See HIV 2

Immunodeficiency Virus, Human
See HIV

Immunodiffusion
Gel Diffusion
   Antibody or Antigen. 86331
Ouchterlony. 86331
Unspecified. 86329

Immunoelectrophoresis
Crossed/2-dimensional Assay 86320
Fluids Other Than Serum 86325
Serum 86320

Immunofixation Electrophoresis
Fluids Other Than Serum 86335
Serum 86334

Immunofluorescence Microscopy
Antibody Stain Procedure. 88346, 88350
Antiserum Culture Typing 87140
Infectious Agent Antigen Detection
   See Infectious Agent, Antigen Detection,
   Immunofluorescence

Immunogen
See Antigen

Immunoglobulin 82784-82787
Platelet Associated Antibody 86023
Thyroid Stimulating. 84445

Immunoglobulin E
See IgE

Immunoglobulin Receptor Assay 86243

Immunologic Skin Test
See Skin, Tests

Immunohistochemistry
Antibody 88341, 88342, 88344

Ankle. 27607
    Tendon 27605, 27606
Anus
    See Anus, Incision
Aortic Valve
    for Stenosis 33415
Artery
    Nose. 30915-30920
Atrial Septum 33735-33737
Bile Duct
    Sphincter 43262, 47460
Bladder
    Catheterization. 51045
    with Destruction 51020-51030
    with Radiotracer 51020
Bladder Diverticulum 52305
Brachial Artery
    Exposure. 34834
Brain
    Amygdalohippocampectomy 61566
    Subpial 61567
Breast
    Capsules. 19370
Burn Scab 16035, 16036
Buttock 27027, 27057
Cataract
    Secondary
      Laser Surgery 66821
      Stab Incision Technique 66820
Chest
    Biopsy. 32096-32098
    with Therapeutic Wedge
    Resection 32505, 32506
Colon
    Exploration. 44025
    Stoma
      Creation 44320-44322
      Revision 44340-44346
Cornea
    for Astigmatism 65772
    Laser
      for Keratoplasty 0289T, 0290T
Corpus Callosum. 61541
Cricothyroid Membrane 31605
Dentate Ligament 63180-63182
Duodenum. 44010
Ear, Inner
    Labyrinth
      Transcanal 69801
Elbow 24000
Esophagus. 43020, 43045
    Muscle 43030
Exploration
    Heart 33310-33315
    Kidney 50010
Eye
    Adhesions 65880
      Anterior Segment. 65860-65865
      Anterior Synechiae. 65870
      Corneovitreal 65880
      Posterior 65875
    Anterior Chamber. 65820
    Trabeculae 65850
Eyelid
    Canthus 67715
    Margin
      for Biopsy 67810
      Sutures 67710
Femoral Artery
    Exposure. 34812, 34813
Fibula. 27607
Finger
    Decompression 26035

Tendon 26060, 26455-26460
Tendon Sheath 26055
Foot 28005
    Capsule 28260-28264
    Fasciotomy. 28008
    for Infection 28002, 28003
    Tendon 28230, 28234
Gallbladder 47490
Hand Decompression 26035-26037
    Tendon 26450, 26460
Heart
    Exploration. 33310-33315
Hemorrhoids
    External 46083
Hepatic Ducts
    See Hepaticostomy
Hip
    Denervation 27035
    Exploration 27033
    Fasciotomy. 27025
    Joint Capsule
      for Flexor Release. 27036
    Tendon
      Abductor 27006
      Adductor 27000-27003
      Iliopsoas 27005
Hymen
    See Hymen, Incision
Hymenotomy. 56442
Hyoid
    Muscle 21685
Iliac Artery
    Exposure. 34820, 34833
Intercarpal Joint
    Dislocation 25670
Interphalangeal Joint
    Capsule 26525
Intestines (Except Rectum)
    See Enterotomy
Intestines, Small 44010
    Biopsy. 44020
    Creation
      Pouch 44316
      Stoma 44300-44310, 44314
    Decompression 44021
    Exploration 44020
    Incision. 44020
    Removal
      Foreign Body. 44020
    Revision
      Stoma 44312
Iris 66500-66505
Kidney 50010, 50045
Knee
    Capsule 27435
    Exploration. 27310
    Fasciotomy. 27305
    Removal of Foreign Body. 27310
Lacrimal Punctum 68440
Lacrimal Sac
    See Dacryocystotomy
Larynx 31300-31320
Leg, Lower
    Fasciotomy. 27600-27602
Leg, Upper
    Fasciotomy. 27305
    Tenotomy 27306, 27307, 27390-27392
Lip
    Frenum 40806
Liver
    See Hepatotomy
Lung
    Biopsy. 32096, 32097

Decortication
    Partial 32225
    Total 32220
Lymphatic Channels 38308
Mastoid
    See Mastoidotomy
Mesencephalic Tract. 61480
Metacarpophalangeal Joint
    Capsule 26520
Mitral Valve 33420-33422
Muscle
    See Myotomy
Nerve. . .64568, 64575-64580, 64595, 64702-64772
    Foot 28035
    Root 63185-63190
    Sacral 64581
    Vagus 43640, 43641
Nose
    See Rhinotomy
Orbit
    See Orbitotomy
Palm
    Fasciotomy. 26040-26045
Pancreas
    Sphincter 43262
Pelvis
    Fasciotomy. 27027, 27057
Penis
    Prepuce 54000, 54001
      Newborn. 54000
Pericardium
    with Clot Removal 33020
    with Foreign Body Removal 33020
    with Tube 33015
Pharynx
    Stoma. 42955
Pleura
    Biopsy. 32098
Pleural Cavity
    Empyema 32035, 32036
Prostate
    Exposure
      Bilateral Pelvic Lymphadenectomy . . . 55865
      Insertion Radioactive Substance 55860
      Lymph Node Biopsy 55862
      Transurethral 52450
Pterygomaxillary Fossa. 31040
Pulmonary Valve 33470, 33471, 33474
Pyloric Sphincter. 43520
Retina
    Encircling Material. 67115
Sclera
    Fistulization
      Sclerectomy with Punch or Scissors
      with Iridectomy. 66160
      Thermocauterization with
      Iridectomy. 66155
      Trabeculectomy ab Externo in Absence
      Previous Surgery. 66170
      Trephination with Iridectomy 66150
Semicircular Canal
    Fenestration 69820
    Revision 69840
Seminal Vesicle 55600-55605
    Complicated 55605
Shoulder
    Bone 23035
    Capsular Contracture Release. 23020
    Removal
      Calcareous Deposits. 23000
      Tenomyotomy. 23405, 23406
Shoulder Joint. 23040-23044

Interphalangeal Joint
    Toe 28024
Intertarsal Joint 28020
Kidney 50040, 50125
Knee 27303, 27310
Lacrimal Gland 68400
Lacrimal Sac 68420
Liver
    Abscess or Cyst 47010
Mediastinum 39000-39010
Metatarsophalangeal Joint 28022
Milia, Multiple 10040
Onychia 10060, 10061
Orbit 67405, 67440
Paronychia 10060, 10061
Pelvic
    Bone 26992
Penis 54015
Pericardium 33025
Phalanges
    Finger 26034
Pilonidal Cyst 10080, 10081
Pustules
    Skin 10040
Radius 25035
Seroma
    Skin 10140
Shoulder
    Abscess 23030
    Arthrotomy
        Acromioclavicular Joint 23044
        Sternoclavicular Joint 23044
    Bursa 23031
    Hematoma 23030
Shoulder Joint
    Arthrotomy
        Glenohumeral Joint 23040
Spine
    Abscess 22010-22015
Tarsometatarsal Joint 28020
Tendon Sheath
    Finger 26020
    Palm 26020
Thorax
    Deep 21510
Toe 28024
Ulna 25035
Ureter 50600
Vagina 57020
Wound Infection
    Skin 10180
Wrist 25028, 25040

Incisional Hernia Repair
See Hernia Repair, Incisional

Inclusion Bodies
Fluid 88106
Smear 87207, 87210

Incomplete Abortion
See Abortion, Incomplete

Indicator Dilution Studies
Cardiac Output 93562
Thermodilution 93561

Induced Abortion
See Abortion

Induced Hyperthermia
See Thermotherapy

Induced Hypothermia
See Hypothermia

Induratio Penis Plastica
See Peyronie Disease

Indwelling Catheter
Percutaneous, Lung
    See Pleural Cavity, Catheterization

Infant, Newborn, Intensive Care
See Intensive Care, Neonatal

Infantile Paralysis
See Polio

Infection
Diagnosis
    Group A Strep Test 3210F
Immunoassay 86317, 86318
Rapid Test 86403, 86406
Treatment
    Antibiotic Prescribed 4045F

Infection, Actinomyces
See Actinomycosis

Infection, Bone
See Osteomyelitis

Infection, Filarioidea
See Filariasis

Infection, Postoperative Wound
See Postoperative Wound Infection

Infection, Wound
See Wound, Infection

Infectious Agent
Antibody Detection
    Immunoassay, Multistep
        Actinomyces 86602
        Adenovirus 86603
        Aspergillus 86606
        Bacterium 86609
        Bartonella 86611
        Blastomyces 86612
        Bordetella 86615
        Borrelia 86617-86619
        Brucella 86622
        Campylobacter 86625
        Candida 86628
        Chlamydia 86631, 86632
        Coccidioides 86635
        Coxiella Burnetii 86638
        Cryptococcus 86641
        Cytomegalovirus (CMV) 86644, 86645
        Diphtheria 86648
        Ehrlichia 86666
        Encephalitis 86651-86654
        Enterovirus 86658, 87498
        Epstein-Barr Virus 86663-86665
        Francisella Tularensis 86668
        Fungus, Other 86671
        Giardia Lamblia 86674
        Helicobacter Pylori 86677
        Helminth 86682
        Haemophilus Influenzae 86684
        Hepatitis
        Delta Agent 86692
        Hepatitis A (HAAb) 86708, 86709
        Hepatitis B
            Core 86704
            IgM 86705
            Surface 86706
        Hepatitis Be 86707
        Hepatitis C 86803, 86804
        Herpes Simplex 86694-86696

Histoplasma 86698
HIV 86689, 86701-86703
HIV-1 . . . . 86701, 86703, 87389, 87806
HIV-2 . . . . 86702, 86703, 87389, 87806
HTLV-I 86687, 86689
HTLV-II 86688
Influenza Virus 86710
Legionella 86713
Leishmania 86717
Leptospira 86720
Listeria Monocytogenes 86723
Lyme Disease 86617
Lymphocytic Choriomeningitis 86727
Lymphogranuloma Venereum 86729
Malaria 86750
Mucormycosis 86732
Mumps 86735
Mycoplasma 86738
Neisseria Meningitidis 86741
Nocardia 86744
Parvovirus 86747
Plasmodium 86750
Protozoa 86753
Respiratory Syncytial Virus 86756
Rickettsia 86757
Rotavirus 86759
Rubella 86762
Rubeola 86765
Salmonella 86768
Shigella 86771
Tetanus 86774
Thyroglobulin 86800
Toxoplasma 86777, 86778
Treponema Pallidum 86780
Trichinella 86784
Tuberculosis 86580
Varicella-Zoster 86787
Virus, Other 86790
West Nile Virus 86788, 86789
Yersinia 86793
Immunoassay, Other Antibody
    Quantitative 86317
Immunoassay, Single Step
    Qualitative/Semiquantitative 86318
Antigen Detection
    Direct Fluorescence
        Bordetella 87265
        Chlamydia Trachomatis 87270
        Cryptosporidium 87272
        Cytomegalovirus 87271
        Enterovirus 87267
        Giardia 87269
        Influenza A 87276
        Legionella Pneumophila 87278
        Respiratory Syncytial Virus 87280
        Treponema Pallidum 87285
        Varicella-Zoster 87290
    Immunoassay
        Adenovirus 87301, 87809
        Aspergillus 87305
        Chlamydia Trachomatis 87320
        Clostridium Difficile 87324
        Cryptococcus Neoformans 87327
        Cryptosporidium 87328
        Cytomegalovirus 87332
        Entamoeba Histolytica Dispar Group . . 87336
        Entamoeba Histolytica Group 87337
        Escherichia coli 0157 87335
        Giardia 87329
        Helicobacter Pylori 87338, 87339
        Hepatitis B Surface Antigen (HBsAg) . . 87340
        Hepatitis B Surface Antigen (HBsAg)
        Neutralization 87341

Nebulizer............................ 94664
Home Visit........................... 99503

Inhibin A........................ 86336

Inhibition Test, Hemagglutination
See Hemagglutination Inhibition Test

Inhibition, Fertilization
See Contraception

Inhibitor, Alpha 1-Protease
See Alpha-1 Antitrypsin

Inhibitor, Alpha 2-Plasmin
See Alpha-2 Antiplasmin

Inhibitory Concentration, Minimum
See Minimum Inhibitory Concentration

Initial Inpatient Consultations
New or Established Patient........ 99251-99255

Injection
See Allergen Immunotherapy; Infusion
Abdomen
    Air............................. 49400
    Contrast Material................. 49400
Anesthetic Agent
    Paravertebral Block (PVB)...... 64461, 64462
    Sacroiliac Joint.................. 27096
    Spine
        Cervical...... 0228T, 0229T, 62310, 62318
        Lumbar....... 0230T, 0231T, 62311, 62319
        Sacral....... 0230T, 0231T, 62311, 62319
        Thoracic..... 0228T, 0229T, 62310, 62318
Angiography
    Pulmonary....................... 75746
Ankle
    Radial.......................... 27648
Antibiotic
    See Antibiotic Administration
Antigen (Allergen)................ 95115-95125
Anus
    Bulking Agent.................... 0377T
    Sclerosing Solution............... 46500
Aorta (Aortography)
    Radiologic....................... 93567
Aponeurosis......................... 20550
Arthrography
    Sacroiliac Joint.................. 27096
Bile Duct
    Cholangiography............. 47531, 47532
Bladder
    for Chemodenervation.............. 52287
    Radiologic.................. 51600-51610
Brain Canal......................... 61070
Bursa........ 20600, 20604, 20605, 20610, 20611
Cardiac Catheterization............ 93454-93464,
                              93563-93568
Carpal Tunnel
    Therapeutic...................... 20526
Chemotherapy........... 96401-96542, 96549
Cistern
    Medication or Other............... 61055
Contrast............................ 49465
    via Catheter................. 36598, 49424
Corpora Cavernosa................... 54235
Cyst
    Bone............................ 20615
    Kidney.......................... 50390
    Pelvis.......................... 50390
    Thyroid......................... 60300
Diagnostic
    Additional Sequential, Each Push.... 96376

Elbow
    Arthrography
        Radiologic...................... 24220
Epidural
    See Epidural, Injection
Esophageal Varices
    Endoscopy................... 43204, 43243
Esophagus
    Sclerosing Agent.................. 43204
    Submucosal.......... 43192, 43201, 43236
Extremity
    Pseudoaneurysm................... 36002
Eye
    Anterior Segment
        Air............................ 66020
        Medication...................... 66030
    Posterior Segment
        Intravitreal.................... 67028
Eyelid
    Subconjunctival.................. 68200
Foot
    Nerve........................... 64455
Fluid Collection
    Sclerosant....................... 49185
Ganglion
    Anesthetic.................. 64505, 64510
Ganglion Cyst....................... 20612
Gastric Secretion Stimulant............. 43755
Gastric Varices
    Endoscopy....................... 43243
Heart Vessels
    Cardiac Catheterization........ 93454-93464,
                            93563-93568
        See Catheterization, Cardiac
    Radiologic.................. 93454-93461
Hemorrhoids
    Sclerosing Solution............... 46500
Hip
    Radiologic.................. 27093-27095
Insect Venom.................... 95130-95134
Intervertebral Disc
    Chemonucleolysis Agent............. 62292
    Radiological................ 62290, 62291
Intra-amniotic...................... 59852
Intra-arterial.................. 96373, 96379
    Thrombolytic.......... 37184-37186, 61645
Intradermal
    for Tattooing................ 11920-11922
Intralesional
    Skin....................... 11900, 11901
Intramuscular....................... 96372
    Therapeutic................. 96372, 99506
Intravenous......................... 96379
    Nuclear Diagnostic Localization....... 78808
    Thrombolytic................ 37187, 37188
    Unlisted........................ 96379
    Vascular Flow Check, Graft........... 15860
Intravenous Push................. 96374-96376
Joint........ 20600, 20604-20606, 20610, 20611
Kidney
    Drugs........................... 50391
    for Nephrostogram........... 50430, 50431
Knee
    Radiologic....................... 27370
Lacrimal Gland
    Radiologic....................... 68850
Left Heart
    Radiologic....................... 93565
Lesion
    Skin....................... 11900, 11901
Ligament............................ 20550
Liver............................... 47015
Mammary Ductogram/Galactogram........ 19030

Muscle Endplate
    Facial.......................... 64612
Nerve
    Anesthetic...... 01991, 01992, 64400-64530
    Neurolytic Agent............. 64600-64640,
                           64680, 64681
Orbit
    Retrobulbar
        Alcohol........................ 67505
        Medication...................... 67500
    Tenon's Capsule.................. 67515
Pancreatography..................... 48400
Paravertebral Facet Joint/Nerve
    with Image Guidance.......... 64490-64495
    with Ultrasound Guidance...... .0213T-0218T
Penis
    for Erection..................... 54235
    Peyronie Disease................. 54200
        with Surgical Exposure of Plague.... 54205
    Radiology....................... 54230
    Vasoactive Drugs................. 54231
Peritoneal Cavity Air
    See Pneumoperitoneum
Platelet Rich Plasma................. 0232T
Prophylactic
    Additional Sequential, Each Push...... 96376
Radiologic
    Breast.......................... 19030
    Cholangiography........... 47531, 47532
Rectum
    Sclerosing Solution............... 45520
Right Heart
    See Cardiac Catheterization, Injection
    Radiologic....................... 93566
Sacroiliac Joint
    for Arthrography................. 27096
Salivary Duct....................... 42660
Salivary Gland
    Radiologic....................... 42550
Sclerosing Agent
    Esophagus....................... 43204
    Intravenous................. 36470, 36471
Sentinel Node
    Identification.............. 38792, 38900
Shoulder
    Arthrography
        Radiologic...................... 23350
Shunt
    Peritoneal
        Venous......................... 49427
Sinus Tract......................... 20500
    Diagnostic...................... 20501
Spider Veins
    Telangiectasia................... 36468
Spinal Artery....................... 62294
Spinal Cord
    Anesthetic.................. 62310-62319
    Blood........................... 62273
    Neurolytic Agent............ 62280-62282
    Other....................... 62310-62319
    Radiological..................... 62284
Steroids
    Spine
        Cervical....... 0228T, 0229T, 62310, 62318
        Lumbar....... 0230T, 0231T, 62311, 62319
        Sacral....... 0230T, 0231T, 62311, 62319
        Thoracic...... 0228T, 0229T, 62310, 62318
Urethral Stricture.................. 52283
Subcutaneous........................ 96372
    Silicone.................... 11950-11954
    Therapeutic..................... 96372
Temporomandibular Joint
    Arthrography..................... 21116

Inspiratory Positive Pressure Breathing

See Intermittent Positive Pressure Breathing (IPPB)

Instillation

Instillation, Bladder

See Bladder, Instillation

Instrumentation

See Application; Bone, Fixation; Spinal Instrumentation

Insufflation, Eustachian Tube

See Eustachian Tube, Inflation

Insulin

Insulin C-Peptide Measurement

See C-Peptide

Insulin-Like Growth Factors

See Somatomedin

Insurance

Integumentary System

Fusion...............................28755
  with Tendon Transfer..............28760
Removal of Foreign Body.................26080
Repair
  Collateral Ligament...........26540, 26545
  Volar Plate.......................26548
Synovectomy............................26140
Toe....................................28272
  Arthrotomy........................28024
  Dislocation..........28660-28665, 28675
    Percutaneous Fixation............28666
  Excision..........................28160
  Exploration.......................28024
  Removal
    Foreign Body.....................28024
    Loose Body.......................28024
  Synovial
    Biopsy...........................28054

Interprofessional Telephone Assessment and Management
............99446-99449

Interruption
Vein
  Femoral............................37650
  Iliac..............................37660
  Lower Leg..........................37735
  Saphenous Vein.....................37700

Intersex State
Clitoroplasty..........................56805
Vaginoplasty...........................57335

Intersex Surgery
Female to Male.........................55980
Male to Female.........................55970

Interspace
Arthrodesis
  Presacral
    See Arthrodesis, Vertebra, Lumbar

Interstitial Cell Stimulating Hormone
See Luteinizing Hormone (LH)

Interstitial Cystitides, Chronic
See Cystitis, Interstitial

Interstitial Cystitis
See Cystitis, Interstitial

Interstitial Fluid Pressure
Monitoring.............................20950

Interstitial Cell Stimulating Hormone
See Luteinizing Hormone (LH)

Interstitial Radiation Therapy
See Brachytherapy, Interstitial Application
Radioelement Application...............77778
  Device Placement
    Breast..................19296-19298
    Genitalia........................55920
    Head.............................41019
    Neck.............................41019
    Pelvis...........................55920
    Uterus...........................57155
    Vagina...................57155, 57156
  Heyman Capsules Insertion..........58346
  Ultrasonic Guidance................76965

Intertarsal Joint
Arthrotomy...................28020, 28050
Biopsy.................................28050
Drainage...............................28020
Exploration............................28020
Removal
  Foreign Body.......................28020
  Loose Body.........................28020
Synovectomy............................28070

Interthoracoscapular Amputation
See Amputation, Interthoracoscapular

Intertrochanteric Femur Fracture
See Femur, Fracture, Intertrochanteric

Intervertebral Chemonucleolysis
See Chemonucleolysis

Intervertebral Disc
Annuloplasty..................22526, 22527
Arthroplasty
  Artificial Disc.....0163T, 0375T, 22856-22858
    Removal......0095T, 0164T, 22864, 22865
    Revision......0098T, 0165T, 22861, 22862
Aspiration.............................62267
Biopsy.................................62267
Decompression................63075-63078
  by Needle..........................62287
Discectomy
  See Discectomy
Discography
  Cervical...........................72285
    Injection........................62291
  Lumbar....................62292, 72295
    Injection........................62290
  Thoracic...........................72285
    Injection........................62291
Herniated
  Excision
    Cervical......63020, 63035, 63040, 63043
    Lumbar...............63030, 63035,
                 63042-63044, 63056, 63057
    Thoracic......63055, 63057, 63064, 63066
Injection
  Chemonucleolysis Agent.............62292
  X-ray.....................62290, 62291
Removal
  Artificial Disc....0095T, 0164T, 22864, 22865
  by Needle..........................62287
Revision
  Artificial Disc Arthroplasty..........0098T,
                         0165T, 22861, 22862

Intestinal Anastomosis
See Anastomosis, Intestines

Intestinal Invagination
See Intussusception

Intestinal Peptide, Vasoactive
See Vasoactive Intestinal Peptide

Intestines
Alimentation...........................44015
Allotransplantation...........44135, 44136
  Removal............................44137
Anastomosis.........44130, 44625, 44626
  Camey Enterocystoplasty............50825
  Closure............................44227
  Koch Pouch.........................50825
    with Cystectomy..................51590
    with Intestinal Replacement of Ureter..50840
  Laparoscopic.......................44227

Biopsy.................................44100
Closure
  Enterostomy.........44620, 44625, 44626
    Large or Small...44227, 44625, 44626
  Fistula.............44640, 44650, 44660
    with Resection...................44661
  Stoma.....................44620-44625
Construction
  Neobladder.........................51596
  Ureter.............................50840
Enteroenterostomy......................44130
Enterolysis............................44005
  Laparoscopic.......................44180
Enterostomy
  Closure.............44620, 44625, 44626
  Laparoscopic........44227, 44625, 44626
Excision
  Donor.....................44132, 44133
Fecal Microbiota Transplantation
  Preparation of Specimen............44705
Graft.......................43116, 46748
Ladd Procedure.........................44055
Laparoscopic Resection
  with Anastomosis..........44202, 44203
Exteriorization.............44602-44605
Lesion
  Excision..................44110, 44111
Lysis
  Laparoscopic.......................44180
  of Adhesions.......................44005
  of Duodenal Bands..................44050
Malrotation
  Correction.........................44055
Mobilization..43108, 43113, 43118, 43123, 43361
Nuclear Medicine
  Imaging............................78290
Obstruction
  Stricturoplasty....................44615
Plication..............................44680
Reconstruction
  Bladder............................50820
  Colonic Reservoir..................45119
  for Obstruction....................44615
  Pouch....................43622, 43634
Resection..............................44661
  Laparoscopic.......................44227
Transplantation
  Allograft Preparation.....44715-44721
  Donor Enterectomy.........44132, 44133
  Removal of Allograft...............44137
Unlisted Services and Procedures.......44799
  Laparoscopic.......................44238
Ureteroenterostomy.....................50800
Volvulus
  Reduction..........................44050

Intestines, Large
See Anus; Colon; Rectum

Intestines, Small
Anastomosis.................43845, 44130
  Closure............................44227
Laparoscopic Resection........44202, 44203
Biopsy.................................44020
  Endoscopy..........................44361
Catheterization
  Jejunum............................44015
Decompression..........................44021
Destruction
  Lesion.............................44369
  Tumor..............................44369
Endoscopy..............................44364

J

Jaboulay Operation
See Gastroduodenostomy

Jaboulay Operation Gastroduodenostomy
See Gastroduodenostomy

Jannetta Procedure
See Decompression, Cranial Nerve; Section

Japanese Encephalitis Virus
See Vaccine

Japanese, River Fever
See Scrub Typhus

Jatene Type Procedure ... 33770-33781

Jaw Joint
See Facial Bones; Mandible; Maxilla

Jaws
Muscle Reduction 21295, 21296
Orthopantogram X-ray
    for Orthodontics 70355

Jejunostomy
Catheterization 44015
Contrast. 49465
Conversion
    from Gastrostomy Tube 44373
        Endoscopic 44373
        Percutaneous 49446
Insertion
    Catheter 44015
    Endoscopic 44372
    Percutaneous 49441
Laparoscopic 44186, 44187
Non-Tube. 44187, 44310
Obstructive Material Removal 49460
Replacement 49451
with Pancreatic Drain 48001

Jejunum
Creation
    Stoma
        See Jejunostomy
Endoscopy
    Examination 43242
    Needle Aspiration 43242
    Needle Biopsy 43242
    Ultrasound 43259
Transfer
    with Microvascular Anastomosis
        Free. 43496

Johannsen Procedure
Urethroplasty 53400

Joint
Acromioclavicular
    See Acromioclavicular Joint
Arthrocentesis
    Bursa 20600, 20604
    Intermediate Joint 20605, 20606
    Large Joint 20610, 20611
    Small Joint. 20600, 20604
Aspiration 20600, 20604,
                         20605, 20606, 20610, 20611
Dislocation
    See Dislocation

Drainage 20600, 20604,
                         20605, 20606, 20610, 20611
Exploration
    Acromioclavicular 23044
    Ankle 27610, 27620
    Carpometacarpal 26070
    Elbow 24101
    Finger 26075-26080
    Glenohumeral. 23040, 23107
    Hand 26070
    Hip 27033
    Interphalangeal
        Finger 26080
        Toe 28024
    Intertarsal. 28020
    Knee 27310, 27331
    Metacarpophalangeal 26070
    Metatarsophalangeal 28022
    Midcarpal. 25040
    Radiocarpal 25040
    Sternoclavicular. 23044
    Tarsometatarsal 28020
    Wrist 25101
Finger
    See Finger, Joint
Fixation (Surgical)
    See Arthrodesis
Foot
    See Talotarsal Joint; Tarsal Joint;
    Tarsometatarsal Joint
Hip
    See Hip Joint
Injection 0213T-0218T, 20600, 20604, 20605,
                         20610, 20611
Intertarsal
    See Intertarsal Joint
Knee
    See Knee Joint
Ligament
    See Ligament
Magnetic Resonance Imaging
    Extremity, Lower 73721
    Extremity, Upper. 73221
Metacarpophalangeal
    See Metacarpophalangeal Joint
Metatarsophalangeal
    See Metatarsophalangeal Joint
Nuclear Medicine
    Imaging 78300, 78305, 78306, 78315
    SPECT 78320
Radiology
    Stress Views 77071
    Survey Views 77077
Replacement
    Temporomandibular 21243
    Vertebral. 0202T, 20931, 20938, 22554,
             22556, 22851, 63081, 63085, 63087, 63090
Sacroiliac
    See Sacroiliac Joint
Shoulder
    See Glenohumeral Joint
Sternoclavicular
    See Sternoclavicular Joint
Survey 77077
Temporomandibular
    See Temporomandibular Joint (TMJ)
    Arthrography 70332
    Magnetic Resonance Imaging 70336
    Radiology 70328
Dislocation Temporomandibular
    See Dislocation, Temporomandibular Joint
Implant
    See Prosthesis, Temporomandibular Joint

Wrist
    See Radiocarpal Joint

Joint Syndrome, Temporomandibular
See Temporomandibular Joint (TMJ)

Jones and Cantarow Test
See Blood Urea Nitrogen; Urea Nitrogen, Clearance

Jones Procedure
Arthrodesis 28760

Joplin Procedure
Hallux Vagus Correction 28294

Jugal Bone
See Zygomatic Arch

Jugular Vein
See Vein, Jugular

K

K-Wire Fixation
Tongue. 41500

Kader Operation
See Incision, Stomach, Creation, Stoma; Incision
and Drainage

Kala Azar Smear 87207

Kallidin I /Kallidin 9
See Bradykinin

Kallikrein HK3
See Antigen, Prostate Specific

Kallikreinogen
See Fletcher Factor

Kasai Procedure 47701

Kedani Fever
See Scrub Typhus

Keel
Insertion/Removal
    Laryngoplasty. 31580

Kelikian Procedure 28280

Keller Procedure 28292

Kelly Urethral Plication 57220

Keratectomy
Partial
    for Lesion 65400

Keratomileusis 65760

Keratophakia 65765

Keratoplasty
Endothelial 65756
    Allograft Preparation 65757
Lamellar
    Anterior 65710
    Laser Preparation. 0289T, 0290T
Penetrating 65730
    in Aphakia 65750
    Laser Preparation. 0289T, 0290T
    in Pseudophakia. 65755

Keratoprosthesis 65770

Keratotomy
Radial 65771

Ketogenic Steroids 83582

Ketone Body 82009, 82010

Ketosteroids 83586, 83593

Kidner Procedure 28238

Kidney
Abscess
  Incision and Drainage 50020
    Open 50020
Anesthesia 00862
Biopsy 50200, 50205
  Endoscopic 50555, 50557, 52354
Catheterization
  Endoscopic 50572
  Nephroureteral 50387
Cyst
  Ablation 50541
  Aspiration 50390
  Excision 50280, 50290
  Injection 50390
  X-ray 74470
Destruction
  Calculus 50590
  Endoscopic 50557, 50576, 52354
Dilation 50395
Endoscopy
  Biopsy 50555, 50574-50576, 52354
  Catheterization 50553, 50572
  Destruction 50557, 50576, 52354
Dilation
  Intra-Renal Stricture 52343, 52346
  Ureter 50553
Excision
  Tumor 52355
Exploration 52351
Lithotripsy 52353
Removal
  Calculus 50060-50075
  Foreign Body 50561, 50580
  via Incision 50562, 50570,
         50572, 50574-50576, 50580
  via Stoma 50551, 50553,
         50555, 50557, 50561
Excision
  Donor 50300, 50320, 50547
  Partial 50240
    Laparoscopic 50543
  Laparoscopic 50545-50548
  Recipient 50340
  Transplantation 50370
  with Ureters 50220, 50225,
         50230, 50234, 50236
Exploration 50010, 50045, 50120
Incision 50010, 50045
Incision and Drainage 50040, 50125
Injection
  Drugs 50391
  for Nephrostogram 50430, 50431
Insertion
  Guide 50395
  Stoma 50400
Instillation
  Drugs 50391
Lithotripsy 50590
Manometry
  Pressure 50396

Mass
  Ablation 50542
    Cryosurgical 50250
    Radiofrequency 50592
Needle Biopsy 50200
Nuclear Medicine
  Function Study 78725
  Imaging 78700, 78701, 78707-78710
  Unlisted Services and Procedures 78799
Placement
  Catheter
    Nephrostomy 50432
    Nephroureteral 50433
Removal
  Calculus 50060, 50065,
         50070, 50075, 50080, 50130, 50561
  Foreign Body 50561, 50580
  Tube
    Nephrostomy 50389
Repair
  Blood Vessels 50100
  Fistula 50520, 50525, 50526
  Fixation 50400, 50405
  Horseshoe Kidney 50540
  Wound 50500
Solitary 50405
Suture
  Fistula 50520, 50525, 50526
  Horseshoe Kidney 50540
Transplantation
  Allograft Preparation 50323-50329
  Anesthesia
    Donor 00862
    Recipient 00868
  Donor 00862
  Donor Nephrectomy 50300, 50320, 50547
  Implantation of Graft 50360
  Recipient Nephrectomy 50340, 50365
  Reimplantation Kidney 50380
  Removal Transplant Renal Autograft 50370
Tumor
  Ablation
    Cryotherapy 50593
Ultrasound 76770, 76775, 76776
X-ray with Contrast
  Guide Catheter 50433

Kidney Stone
See Calculus, Removal, Kidney

Killian Operation
See Sinusotomy, Frontal Sinus

Kinase, Creatine
See CPK

Kineplasty
See Cineplasty

Kinetic Therapy 97530
See Physical Medicine/Therapy/Occupational Therapy

Kininase A
See Angiotensin Converting Enzyme (ACE)

Kininogen 85293

Kininogen, High Molecular Weight
See Fitzgerald Factor

Kleihauer-Betke Test 85460

Kloramfenikol
See Chloramphenicol

Knee
See Femur; Fibula; Patella; Tibia
Abscess 27301
Arthrocentesis 20610, 20611
Arthrodesis 27580
Arthroplasty 27440-27445, 27447
  Revision 27486, 27487
Arthroscopy
  Diagnostic 29870
  Surgical 29866-29868,
       29871, 29873-29877, 29879-29889
Arthrotomy 27310, 27330-27335, 27403
Autograft, Osteochondral, Open 27416
Biopsy 27323, 27324, 27330, 27331
  Synovium 27330
Bone
  Drainage 27303
  Graft 29885
Bone Graft 29885
Bursa 27301
  Excision 27340
Cyst
  Excision 27345-27347
Disarticulation 27598
Dislocation 27550-27552,
    27556-27558, 27560-27562, 27566
  Open Treatment 27556-27558, 27566
Drainage 27310
Excision
  Cartilage 27332, 27333
  Ganglion 27347
  Lesion 27347
  Patella 27350, 27424
  Synovium 27334, 27335
Exploration 27310, 27331
Fasciotomy 27305, 27496-27499
Fracture 27520-27524, 27538, 27540
  Arthroscopic Treatment 29850, 29851
Fusion 27580
Hematoma 27301
Incision
  Capsule 27435
Injection
  X-ray 27370
Magnetic Resonance Imaging
(MRI) 73721-73723
Manipulation 27570
Meniscectomy 27332, 27333
Patella
  See Patella
Radiostereometric Analysis (RSA) 0350T
Reconstruction 27437, 27438
  Ligament 27427-27429
  with Prosthesis 27445
Removal
  Foreign Body 27310, 27331, 27372
  Loose Body 27331
  Prosthesis 27488
Repair
  Ligament 27405-27409
    Collateral 27405
    Collateral and Cruciate 27409
    Cruciate 27407-27409
  Meniscus 27403
  Tendon 27380, 27381
Replacement 27447
  Intraoperative Use, Kinetic Balance
  Sensor 0396T
Retinacular
  Release 27425
Strapping 29530
Suture
  Tendon 27380, 27381

Laminaria
Insertion
    for Cervical Dilation................59200
    for Abortion 59855

Laminectomy
Arthrodesis.............22630, 22632-22634
for Decompression
    Cervical 0274T, 61343,
        63001, 63015, 63045, 63048
    Lumbar...............0275T, 63005, 63012,
        63017, 63047, 63048
    Sacral.......................63011
    Thoracic.. 0274T, 63003, 63016, 63046, 63048
for Excision
    Arteriovenous Malformation....63250-63252
    Intraspinal Lesion.............63300-63308
    Neoplasm.................63275-63278,
       63280-63283, 63285-63287, 63290
    Other than Neoplasm.......63265-63268,
       63270-63273
for Implantation of Electrodes.......63655
Lumbar 0202T, 22630, 63012
with Discectomy...........0274T, 0275T, 63020
with Exploration
    Cervical 63001, 63015, 63045, 63048
    Lumbar........63005, 63017, 63047, 63048
    Thoracic.......63003, 63016, 63046, 63048
    Sacral.......................63011
with Cordotomy................63194-63199
with Creation of Shunt.............63740
with Diagnostic/Therapeutic Injection......62351
with Drainage............63172, 63173
with Dural/Cerebrospinal Fluid Leak Repair.. 63709
with Facetectomy...............0202T, 0274T,
       0275T, 63045-63048
with Foraminotomy..............0202T, 0274T,
       0275T, 63045-63048
with Ligamentous Resection 0274T,
       0275T, 63180, 63182
with Myelotomy.................63170
with Nerve Resection 63191
with Rhizotomy...............63185, 63190
with Spinal Cord Release.............63200

Laminoplasty
Cervical......................63050, 63051

Lamotrigine
Drug Assay....................80175

Langerhans Islands
See Islet Cell

Language Evaluation
Language Comprehension and Expression...92523
Speech Fluency....................92521
Speech Sound Production...........92522
Voice and Resonance
    Behavioral Analysis.................92524

Language Therapy
Individual......................92507
Group........................92508

LAP
See Leucine Aminopeptidase

Laparoscopic Appendectomy
See Appendectomy, Laparoscopic

Laparoscopic Biopsy of Ovary
See Biopsy, Ovary

Laparoscopy

Abdomen
    Aspiration
      Cavity 49322
      Cyst......................49322
    Biopsy.......................49321
    Collection of Specimen 49320
    Diagnostic 49320
    Drainage
      Lymphocele.................49323
    Placement
      Interstitial Radiation Device........49327
    Unlisted Procedures................49329
Adrenal Gland
    Biopsy......................60650
    Excision 60650
Appendix
    Appendectomy 44970
Aspiration 49322
Biopsy 49321
    Lymph Nodes 38570
Bladder
    Repair
      Sling Operation.................51992
      Urethral Suspension.............51990
      Unlisted 51999
      Laparoscopic 44188
Biliary Tract
    Cholangiography 47563
      with Biopsy.................47579
    Cholecystectomy 47562-47564
    Cholecystenterostomy 47570
Colon
    Cecostomy 44188
    Colectomy
      Partial............. 44204-44208, 44213
      Total....................44210-44212
Colostomy.....................44188
Destruction
    Lesion......................58662
Ectopic Pregnancy.................59150
    with Salpingectomy and/or
    Oophorectomy 59151
Esophagus
    Lengthening 43283
    Esophagogastric Fundoplasty 43280
    Esophagomyotomy Fundoplasty 43279
    Heller Type Esophagomyotomy 43279
    Hernia Repair 43281, 43282
    Sphincter Augmentation
      Device Placement...............0392T
      Device Removal 0393T
Gastric Restrictive Procedures 43644, 43645,
43770-43775
Hernia Repair
    Epigastric
      Incarcerated or Strangulated 49653
      Reducible 49652
    Incisional
      Incarcerated or Strangulated 49655
      Reducible 49654
    Incisional Recurrent
      Incarcerated or Strangulated 49657
      Reducible 49656
    Inguinal
      Initial.....................49650
      Recurrent 49651
    Paraesophageal 43281, 43282
    Spigelian
      Incarcerated or Strangulated 49653
      Reducible 49652
    Umbilical
      Incarcerated or Strangulated 49653
      Reducible 49652

Ventral
      Incarcerated or Strangulated........49653
      Reducible 49652
    Unlisted Procedures................49659
Intestines
    Enterectomy 44202, 44203
    Enterolysis 44180
    Enterostomy
      Closure 44227
      Ileostomy 44187
      Jejunostomy............. 44186, 44187
    Reconstruction with Gastric Bypass 43645
    Resection
      with Anastomosis..........44202, 44203
Kidney
    Ablation
      Cysts.....................50541
      Lesions 50542
    Allograft Preparation 50325
    Nephrectomy 50544-50548
    Donor 50547
Liver
    Ablation
      Tumor 47370, 47371
Lymph System
    Biopsy.......................38570
    Lymphadenectomy...........38571, 38572
Lysis of Adhesions 58660
Lysis of Intestinal Adhesions 44180
Nephrectomy..........50545-50548
    Partial......................50543
Omentum
    Collection of Specimen 49320
    Diagnostic 49320
    Omentopexy 49326
    Unlisted Procedures...............49329
Ovary/Oviduct
    Ectopic Pregnancy 59150
      with Salpingectomy and/or
      Oophorectomy 59151
    Excision of Lesions................58662
    Fimbrioplasty 58672
    Fulguration
      Lesions 58662
      Oviducts 58670
    Lysis of Adhesions 58660
    Occlusion of Oviducts 58671
    Oophorectomy 58661
    Removal
      Ovary(s)...........58544, 58552, 58554
      Tube(s) 58544, 58552, 58554
    Oviduct Surgery 58670, 58671, 58679
    Salpingectomy..................58661
    Salpingostomy 58673
    Unlisted Procedure...............58679
Pelvis..........................49320
    Placement
      Interstitial Radiation Device........49327
    Pyeloplasty....................50544
Peritoneum
    Collection of Specimen 49320
    Diagnostic 49320
    Catheter Insertion 49324
    Placement
      Interstitial Radiation Device........49327
    Removal of Obstructive Material....49325
    Unlisted Procedures...............49329
Prostate
    Prostatectomy 55866
Rectum
    Proctectomy
      Complete 45395
      with Creation of Colonic Reservoir ...45397

Exploration
  Blood Vessel. 35860
Fasciotomy. 27600-27602, 27892-27894
Hematoma
  Incision and Drainage. 27603
Incision. 27607
Lesion
  Excision. 27630
Neurectomy 27325, 27326
Repair
  Blood Vessel. 35226
  Blood Vessel with Other Graft 35286
  Blood Vessel with Vein Graft 35256
  Fascia 27656
  Tendon 27612, 27650, 27652,
             27654, 27656, 27658-27692
Revascularization. 37228-37235
Splint 29515
Strapping
  Compression. 29581
  Unna Boot. 29580
Suture
  Tendon 27658-27665
  Nerve 64856, 64857, 64859
Tenotomy 27605, 27606
Tumor
  Excision. 27618, 27619, 27632, 27634
  Radical Resection. 27615, 27616
Ultrasound
  Complete 76881
  Limited 76882
Unlisted Services and Procedures. 27899
Unna Boot 29580
Vein
  Ligation. 37718, 37760, 37761
  Division. 37718
  Stripping. 37718
  X-ray. 73592
Magnetic Resonance Imaging
(MRI). 73718-73720
Neuroplasty. 64708, 64712
Nerve Graft 64892, 64897, 64898
Splint. 29505
Strapping
  Multi-layer Compression
  System 29581, 29582
Upper
  See Femur
  Abscess
    Incision and Drainage. 27301
  Amputation 27590-27592
    at Hip 27290-27295
    Revision 27594-27596
  Angiography. 73706, 75635
  Artery
    Ligation 37618, 37650
  Biopsy. 27323, 27324
  Body Cast 29044, 29046
  Bursa 27301
    Incision and Drainage. 27301
  Bypass Graft. 35903
  Cast 29345-29355, 29365, 29450
  Cast Brace 29358
  CT Scan 73700-73706, 75635
  Exploration
    Blood Vessel. 35860
  Fasciotomy. 27025, 27305,
      27496-27499, 27892-27894
  Halo Application 20663
  Hematoma 27301
    Incision and Drainage. 27301
  Lipectomy. 15832
  Neurectomy 27325, 27326

Removal
  Cast. 29705
  Foreign Body. 27372
Repair
  Blood Vessel with Other Graft 35286
  Blood Vessel with Vein Graft 35256
  Muscle 27385, 27386, 27400, 27430
  Tendon 27393-27400
Revascularization. 37224-37227
Splint 29505
Strapping
  Compression. 29582
  Unna Boot. 29580
Suture
  Muscle 27385, 27386
  Nerve 64856-64859
Tendon Transfer/Transplant. . . . 27396, 27397,
                27400
Tenotomy 27306, 27307, 27390-27392
Transplantation
  Testis to Thigh 54680
Tumor
  Excision. 27327, 27328, 27337-27339
  Resection 27329, 27364, 27365
Ultrasound
  Complete 76881
  Limited 76882
Unlisted Services and Procedures. 27599
Unna Boot 29580
X-ray. 73592
Varicose Vein
  Division 37785
  Excision 37785
  Ligation 37785
  Phlebectomy. 37765, 37766
Vein
  Ligation
    Great Saphenous 37700, 37722, 37735
    Perforator 37760, 37761
  Division 37700, 37722, 37735
  Stripping. 37722, 37735
Wound Exploration
  Penetrating. 20103

Leg Length Measurement X-ray
See Scanogram

Legionella
Antibody 86713
Antigen 87277, 87278, 87540-87542

Legionella Micdadei
Antigen Detection
  Immunofluorescence 87277

Legionella Pneumophila
Antigen Detection
  Direct Fluorescence 87278
  Amplified Probe 87541
  Direct Probe 87540
  Quantification 87542

Leiomyomata
Removal 58140, 58145, 58545, 58546, 58561

Leishmania
Antibody 86717

Lengthening, Tendon
See Tendon, Lengthening

Lens
Contact
  See Contact Lens Services
Extracapsular 66940
Incision 66821, 66825

Intracapsular. 66920
  Dislocated 66930
Intraocular
  Exchange 66986
  Reposition 66825
Laser 66821
Prosthesis
  Insertion 66983
    Manual or Mechanical
    Technique 66982, 66984
    Not Associated with Concurrent Cataract
    Removal 66985
    Ocular Telescope 0308T
  Removal
    Crystalline. 0308T
  Repositioning 66825
Removal 67108, 67113
  Cataract
    See Cataract
  Foreign Body 65235
  Lens Material
    Aspiration Technique 66840
    Extracapsular 66940
    Intracapsular. 66920-66930
    Pars Plana Approach 66852
    Phacofragmentation Technique 66850

Lens Material
Removal
  Aspiration Technique 66840
  Extracapsular 66940
  Intracapsular 66920-66930
  Pars Plana Approach 66852
  Phacofragmentation Technique 66850

Leptomeningioma
See Meningioma

Leptospira
Antibody 86720

Leriche Operation 64809
See Sympathectomy, Thoracolumbar

Lesion
See also Tumor
Ablation
  Endoscopic Retrograde
  Cholangiopancreatography (ERCP) 43278
  Stereotactic
    Magnetic Resonance Image Guided
    High Intensity Focused Ultrasound
    (MRgFUS) 0398T
Anal
  Destruction. 46900-46917, 46924
  Excision 45108, 46922
Ankle
  Tendon Sheath
    Excision. 27630
Arm, Lower
  Tendon Sheath
    Excision. 25110
Auditory Canal, External
  Excision
    Exostosis. 69140
    Radical with Neck Dissection 69155
    Radical without Neck Dissection. 69150
    Soft Tissue 69145
Bladder
  Destruction. 51030
  Fulguration. 52224, 52234, 52235, 52240
  Resection 52234, 52235, 52240
  Treatment. 52224

Brain
  Excision 61534, 61536,
                61600-61608, 61615, 61616
Brainstem
  Excision 61575, 61576
Breast
  Detection
    Mammography............77051, 77052
  Excision 19120-19126
  Localization Device Placement
    with Magnetic Resonance
      Guidance...... 19085, 19086, 19287, 19288
    with Mammographic
      Guidance.................. 19281, 19282
    with Stereotactic Guidance 19081,
                19082, 19283, 19284
    with Ultrasound Guidance 19083,
                19084, 19285, 19286
Chemotherapy..................96405, 96406
Choroid 67220, 67221, 67225
Ciliary Body
  Destruction........................ 66770
Colon
  Ablation 44401, 45388
  Excision 44110, 44111
Conjunctiva
  Destruction........................ 68135
  Excision 68110-68130
    Over 1 cm 68115
    with Adjacent Sclera 68130
Cornea
  Destruction........................ 65450
  Excision 65400
    of Pterygium............... 65420-65426
Cranium
  Radiosurgery 61796-61800
  Stereotactic Radiation Therapy........ 77432
Ear, Middle
  Excision 69540
Epididymis
  Excision 54830
Esophagus
  Ablation 43229
  Excision 43100, 43101
  Removal 43216, 43217
Eyelid
  Destruction........................ 67850
  Excision
    Multiple, Different Lids 67805
    Multiple, Same Lid................ 67801
    Single 67800
    Under Anesthesia............... 67808
    without Closure 67840
Facial
  Destruction.......17000-17004, 17280-17286
Finger
  Tendon Sheath
    Excision........................ 26160
Foot
  Excision 28080, 28090
Gums
  Destruction........................ 41850
  Excision 41825-41828
Hand Tendon Sheath................... 26160
Intestines
  Excision 44110
Intestines, Small
  Ablation 44369
  Excision 44111
Iris
  Destruction........................ 66770
Larynx
  Removal 31512, 31545, 31546, 31578

Leg, Lower
  Tendon Sheath
    Excision........................ 27630
Mesentery
  Excision 44820
Mouth
  Destruction........................ 40820
  Excision 40810-40816, 41116
  Vestibule
    Destruction.................... 40820
    Repair 40830
Nose
  Intranasal
    Excision.................. 30117, 30118
Orbit
  Excision 61333, 67412, 67420
Ovary
  Excision 58662
Palate
  Destruction........................ 42160
  Excision 42104, 42106, 42107
Pancreas
  Excision 48120
Pelvis
  Excision 58662
Penis
  Destruction
    Cryosurgery.................... 54056
    Electrodesiccation 54055
    Extensive 54065
    Laser Surgery 54057
    Simple........................ 54050-54060
    Surgical Excision 54060
  Excision 54060
    Penile Plaque 54110-54112
Peritoneum
  Excision 58662
Pharynx
  Destruction........................ 42808
  Excision 42808
Radiosurgery
  Cranial 61796-61800
Rectum
  Excision 45108
Renal Pelvis
  Biopsy...................... 52354
  Fulguration................. 52354
Retina
  Destruction
    Extensive 67227, 67228
    Localized................. 67208-67210
  Radiation by Implantation of Source.... 67218
Sclera
  Excision 66130
Skin
  Abrasion.................... 15786, 15787
  Biopsy..................... 11100, 11101
  Destruction
    Benign........... 17110, 17111, 17250
    Malignant................. 17260-17286
    Premalignant 17000-17004
  Excision
    Benign................. 11400-11471
    Malignant................. 11600-11646
  Injection.................... 11900, 11901
  Multi-spectral Analysis 0400T, 0401T
  Paring or Curettement 11055-11057
  Reflectance Confocal Microscopic
    Imaging 96931
  Shaving 11300-11313
Skin Tags
  Removal 11200, 11201

Skull
  Excision .. 61500, 61600-61608, 61615, 61616
Spermatic Cord
  Excision 55520
Spinal Cord
  Destruction................. 62280-62282
  Excision 61575, 61576,
                63265-63273, 63300-63308
Stereotactic Radiation Therapy 77432, 77435
Testis
  Excision 54512
Toe
  Excision 28092
Tongue
  Excision 41110-41114
Ureter
  Biopsy....................... 52354
  Destruction................. 52341, 52342,
                52344, 52345, 52354
  Fulguration................... 52354
Urethra
  Fulguration............. 52224, 53265
  Treatment.................... 52224
Uvula
  Destruction........................ 42160
  Excision 42104-42107
Vagina
  Destruction................. 57061-57065
Vulva
  Destruction
    Extensive 56515
    Simple........................ 56501
Wrist Tendon
  Excision 25110

Leu 2 Antigens
See CD8

Leucine Aminopeptidase 83670

**Leukemia Lymphoma Virus I
Antibodies, Human T Cell**
See Antibody, Detection, HTLV-I

**Leukemia Lymphoma Virus I, Adult
T Cell**
See HTLV I

**Leukemia Lymphoma Virus II
Antibodies, Human T Cell**
See Antibody, Detection, HTLV-II

**Leukemia Virus II, Hairy Cell
Associated, Human T Cell**
See HTLV II

Leukoagglutinins 86021

Leukocyte
See White Blood Cell
  Alkaline Phosphatase.................... 85540
  Antibody 86021
  Count.............. 85032, 85048, 89055
  Fecal Assessment..................... 89055
  Histamine Release Test 86343
  Human Leukocyte Antigen (HLA)
    See HLA
  Phagocytosis......................... 86344
  Transfusion 86950
  Urinalysis 81000

Levarterenol
See Noradrenalin

Lipophosphodiesterase I
See Tissue, Typing

Lipoprotein
(a)	83695
Apolipoprotein	82172
Blood	83695, 83700-83721
Delipidation	
HDL	0342T
HDL	83718
LDL	83700-83704, 83721
Phospholipase A2	83698
VLDL	83719

Lipoprotein, Alpha
See Lipoprotein

Lipoprotein, Pre-Beta
See Lipoprotein, Blood

Liposuction
15876-15879

Lisfranc Operation
See Amputation, Foot; Radical Resection; Replantation

Listeria Monocytogenes
Antibody 86723

Lithium
Assay 80178

Litholapaxy
52317, 52318

Lithotripsy
See Extracorporeal Shock Wave Therapy
Bile Duct Calculi (Stone)	
Endoscopy	43265
Bladder	52353
Kidney	50080, 50081, 50590, 52353
Pancreatic Duct Calculi (Stone)	
Endoscopy	43265
Ureter	52353
Urethra	52353
with Cystourethroscopy	52353
with Indwelling Ureteral Stent Insertion	52356

Lithotrity
See Litholapaxy

Liver
See Hepatic Duct
Ablation	
Tumor	47380-47383
Laparoscopic	47370, 47371
Abscess	
Aspiration	47015
Incision and Drainage	
Open	47010
Injection	47015
Aspiration	47015
Biopsy	47700
Needle	47000, 47001
Wedge	47100
with Staging Laparotomy	49220
Assist System	
Care Plan Oversight	0405T
Cyst	
Aspiration	47015
Incision and Drainage	
Open	47010
Injection	47015
Drainage	47400
Image Guided Fluid Collection	49405
Excision	
Extensive	47122

Partial	47120, 47125-47130
Donor	47140-47142
Total	
Donor	47133
Exploration	47400
Hemorrhage	47350-47362
Injection	47015
Lobectomy	47125-47130
Partial	47120
Needle Biopsy	47000, 47001
Nuclear Medicine	
Imaging	78201-78216
Vascular Flow	78206
Removal	
Calculus	47400
Repair	
Abscess	47300
Cyst	47300
Wound	47350-47362
Suture	
Wound	47350-47362
Transplantation	
Partial	47135, 47144, 47145
Whole	47135
Allograft Preparation	47143-47147
Lobe Split	47145
Trisegment Split	47144
Trisegmentectomy	47122
Ultrasound	
Elastography, Shear Wave	91200
Unlisted Services and Procedures	47379, 47399

Living Activities, Daily
See Activities of Daily Living

Lobectomy
Brain	61323, 61537-61540
Partial	61539, 61540
Temporal Lobe	61537, 61538
Contralateral Subtotal	
Thyroid Gland	60212, 60225
Liver	47120-47130
Donor	47141, 47142
Lung	32480-32482
Sleeve	32486
Thoracoscopic	32663, 32670
Parotid Gland	42410-42415
Sleeve	32486
Temporal Lobe	61537, 61538
Thoracoscopic	
Lung	32663, 32670
Thyroid Gland	
Partial	60210-60212
Total	60220-60225

Local Excision Mastectomies
See Breast, Excision, Lesion

Local Excision of Lesion or Tissue of Femur
See Tumor, Femur

Localization of Nodule
Breast	
Device Placement	
with Magnetic Resonance Guidance	19085, 19086, 19287, 19288
with Mammographic Guidance	19281, 19282
with Stereotactic Guidance	19081, 19082, 19283, 19284
with Ultrasound Guidance	19083, 19084, 19285, 19286
Soft Tissue	
Device Placement	10035, 10036

Log Hydrogen Ion Concentration
See Blood Gases, pH

Long Acting Thyroid Stimulator
See Thyrotropin Releasing Hormone (TRH)

Long-Term Care Facility Visits
See Nursing Facility Services

Longmire Operation
See Anastomosis, Hepatic Duct to Intestines

Loopogram
See Urography, Antegrade

Loose Body
Removal	
Ankle Joint	27620, 29894
Carpometacarpal Joint	26070
Elbow Joint	24101, 29834
Glenohumeral Joint	23107
Hip Joint	27033
Interphalangeal Joint	28024
Intertarsal Joint	28020
Knee Joint	27331
Metatarsophalangeal Joint	28022
Shoulder Joint	29819
Subtalar Joint	29904
Tarsometatarsal Joint	28020
Toe	28022
Wrist Joint	25101

Lord Procedure
See Anal Sphincter, Dilation

Louis Bar Syndrome
See Ataxia Telangiectasia

Low Birth Weight Intensive Care Services
99478-99480

Low Density Lipoprotein
See Lipoprotein, LDL

Low Frequency Ultrasound
97610

Low Vision Aids
See Spectacle Services
Fitting 92354, 92355

Lower Extremities
See Extremity, Lower

Lower GI Series
See Barium Enema

LRH
See Luteinizing Releasing Factor

LSD
See Lysergic Acid Diethylamide

LTH
See Prolactin

Lumbar
See Spine

Lumbar Plexus
Decompression	64714
Infusion	
Anesthetic	64449
Neuroplasty	64714
Repair/Suture	64862

Lumbar Puncture
See Spinal Tap

Lymphocytes, CD4
See CD4

Lymphocytes, CD8
See CD8

Lymphocytic Choriomeningitis
Antibody 86727

Lymphocytotoxicity 86805, 86806

Lymphogranuloma Venereum
Antibody 86729

Lymphoma Virus, Burkitt
See Epstein-Barr Virus

Lynch Procedure 31075

Lysergic Acid Diethylamide
Drug Assay
    Alkaloids, Not Otherwise Specified 80323

Lysis
Adhesions
    Epidural 62263, 62264
    Fallopian Tube 58660, 58740
    Foreskin 54450
    Intestinal 44005, 44180
    Labial 56441
    Lung 32124, 32940
    Nose 30560
    Ovary 58660, 58740
    Oviduct 58660, 58740
    Penile
        Post-Circumcision 54162
    Ureter 50715-50725
    Urethra 53500
    Uterus 58559
Clot
    Time 85175
Euglobulin 85360
Fibrosis
    Urethral 52285
Hemoglobin 85460, 85461
Intranasal Synechia 30560

Lysozyme 85549

M

Macrodactylia
Repair 26590

Macroscopic Examination
Arthropod 87168
Parasite 87169
Tissue 88387, 88388

Magnesium 83735

Magnet Operation
See Ciliary Body; Cornea; Eye, Removal, Foreign Body; Iris; Lens; Retina; Sclera; Vitreous

Magnetic Resonance Angiography (MRA)
Abdomen 74185
Arm 73225
Chest 71555
Head 70544-70546
Leg 73725

Neck 70547-70549
Pelvis 72198
Spine 72159

Magnetic Resonance Imaging (MRI)
Diagnostic
    3-D Rendering 76376, 76377
        Not Requiring Independent
        Workstation 76376
        Requiring Independent Workstation . . 76377
    Abdomen 74181-74183
    Ankle 73721-73723
    Arm 73218-73220
        Joint 73221-73223
    Bone Marrow Study 77084
    Brain 70551-70555
        Intraoperative 70557-70559
    Chest 71550-71552
    Elbow 73221
    Face 70540-70543
    Fetal 74712, 74713
    Finger Joint 73221-73223
    Foot 73718, 73719
    Foot Joints 73721-73723
    Hand 73218-73220, 73223
    Heart 75557-75565
    Joint
        Lower Extremity 73721-73723
        Upper Extremity 73221-73223
    Knee 73721-73723
    Leg 73718-73720
        Joint 73721-73723
    Obstetrical
        Maternal Pelvis 74712, 74713
    Neck 70540-70543
    Orbit 70540-70543
    Pelvis 72195-72197
    Spectroscopy 76390
    Spine
        Cervical 72141, 72142, 72156
        Lumbar 72148, 72149, 72158
        Thoracic 72146, 72147, 72157
    Temporomandibular Joint (TMJ) 70336
    Toe 73721-73723
    Wrist 73221
Guidance
    Arthrography, Enhanced
        Shoulder
            Injection 23350
    Brain
        Stereotactic Lesion Ablation
            Magnetic Resonance Image Guided High
            Intensity Focused Ultrasound
            (MRgFUS) 0398T
        Stereotactic Lesion Biopsy 61751
    Breast 77058, 77059
        Biopsy 19085, 19086
        Lesion Localization Device
        Placement 19085, 19086, 19287, 19288
        with Computer-aided Detection 0159T
    Needle Placement 77021
    Orthopedic Procedure
        Computer-assisted Navigation 0055T
    Parenchymal Tissue Ablation 77022
Unlisted Procedure 76498

Magnetic Resonance Spectroscopy
76390

Magnetic Stimulation
Transcranial 0310T, 90867-90869

Magnetoencephalography (MEG) 95965-95967

Magnuson Procedure 23450

MAGPI Operation 54322

MAGPI Procedure
See Hypospadias, Repair

Major Vestibular Gland
See Bartholin's Gland

Malar Area
Augmentation 21270
Bone Graft 21210
Fracture
    Open Treatment 21360-21366
    with Bone Graft 21366
    with Manipulation 21355
Reconstruction 21270

Malar Bone
See Cheek, Bone

Malaria Antibody 86750

Malaria Smear 87207

Malate Dehydrogenase 83775

Maldescent, Testis
See Testis, Undescended

Male Circumcision
See Circumcision

Malformation, Arteriovenous
See Arteriovenous Malformation

Malic Dehydrogenase
See Malate Dehydrogenase

Malignant Hyperthermia Susceptibility
Caffeine Halothane Contracture Test
(CHCT) 89049

Malleolus
See Ankle; Fibula; Leg, Lower; Tibia; Tibiofibular Joint

Mallet Finger Repair 26432, 26433

Maltose
Tolerance Test 82951, 82952

Malunion Repair
Clavicle 23485
Femur
    with Graft 27472
    without Graft 27470
Fibula 27726
Humerus
    with Graft 24435
    without Graft 24430
Metatarsal Bone 28322
Radius
    with Graft 25405, 25420
    without Graft 25400, 25415
Tarsal Bone 28320
Tibia
    by Synostosis with Fibula 27725
    with Graft 27722, 27724
    without Graft 27720
Ulna
    with Graft 25405, 25420
    without Graft 25400, 25415

Mammalian Oviduct
See Fallopian Tube

Mammaplasty
Augmentation 19324, 19325
Reduction 19318

Mammary Abscess
See Abscess, Tissue, Breast

Mammary Arteries
See Artery, Mammary

Mammary Duct
X-ray 77053, 77054
    Contrast Injection. 19030

Mammary Ductogram
X-ray 77053, 77054
Contrast Injection 19030

Mammary Stimulating Hormone
See Prolactin

Mammillaplasty
See Nipples, Reconstruction

Mammogram 77055-77057

Mammography 77055-77057
Localization, Lesion
    Device Placement 19281, 19282
Magnetic Resonance Imaging
(MRI) 77058, 77059
    with Computer-Aided Detection 0159T
Screening Mammography. 77057
Tomosynthesis 77061-77063
with Computer-Aided Detection. 77051, 77052

Mammoplasty
See Mammaplasty

Mammotomy
Mastotomy
    Drainage of Abscess 19020
    Exploration. 19020

Mammotropic Hormone, Pituitary
See Prolactin

Mammotropic Hormone, Placental
See Lactogen, Human Placental

Mammotropin
See Prolactin

Mandated Services
On Call Services 99026, 99027

Mandible
See Facial Bones; Maxilla; Temporomandibular
Joint (TMJ)
Abscess
    Excision 21025
Bone Graft. 21215
Condyle
    See Mandibular Condyle
Cyst
    Excision 21040, 21046, 21047
Disarticulation. 61590
Excision
    Abscess 21025
    Bone. 21025
    Cyst 21040, 21046, 21047
    Torus Mandibularis 21031
    Tumor 21040, 21044, 21045, 21046, 21047

Fracture
    Closed Treatment
        Alveolar Ridge 21440
        with Interdental Fixation 21453
        with Manipulation 21451
        without Manipulation. 21450
    Open Treatment 21454-21470
        Alveolar Ridge 21445
        Condylar Fracture 21465
        External Fixation. 21454
        with Interdental Fixation 21462
        without Interdental Fixation. 21461
    Percutaneous Treatment 21452
Osteotomy. 21198, 21199
    with Cyst Excision 21046, 21047
    with Tumor Excision 21046, 21047
Prosthesis
    Impression 21081
Rami
    See Mandibular Rami
Reconstruction
    with Implant. 21244-21246, 21248, 21249
Removal
    Foreign Body 41806
Resection
    with Glossectomy 41150, 41155
Splitting. 61576
Torus Mandibularis
    Excision 21031
Tumor
    Excision 21040-21047
X-ray 70100-70110

Mandibular Body
Augmentation
    with Bone Graft 21127
    with Prosthesis 21125

Mandibular Condyle
Fracture
    Open Treatment 21465
Reconstruction 21247

Mandibular Condylectomy
See Condylectomy

Mandibular Fracture
See Fracture, Mandible

Mandibular Rami
Reconstruction
    with Bone Graft 21194
    with Internal Rigid Fixation 21196
    without Bone Graft 21193
    without Internal Rigid Fixation 21195

**Mandibular Resection
Prosthesis** 21081

Mandibular Staple Bone Plate
Reconstruction
    Mandible 21244

Manganese 83785

Manipulation
Chest Wall 94667, 94668
Chiropractic. 98940-98943
Clubfoot Cast Application. 29450
Dislocation and/or Fracture
    Acetabulum 27222
    Acromioclavicular 23545
    Ankle 27810, 27818, 27860
    Bennett Fracture 26645, 26650
    Calcaneal 28405, 28406
    Carpal. 25635

Carpal Scaphoid. 25624
Carpometacarpal 26670-26676
    Thumb Dislocation 26641, 26645, 26650
Clavicular. 23505
Elbow 24300, 24620, 24640
Femoral . . 27232, 27268, 27503, 27510, 27517
    Peritrochanteric 27240
Femoral Shaft. 27502
Fibula 27781, 27788
Finger 26725-26727, 26742, 26755
    Joint 26340
Greater Tuberosity
    Humeral 23625
Hand. 26670-26676
Heel 28405, 28406
Hip 27257
Hip Socket 27222
Humeral 23605, 24505, 24535
    Condyle. 24577, 24582
    Epicondyle 24565, 24566
    Tuberosity 23625
Intercarpal 25660
Interphalangeal Joint. 26340, 26742,
26770-26776, 28666
Knee. 27538, 29850
Lunate 25690
Malar Area 21355
Mandibular. 21451
Metacarpal. 26605-26607
Metacarpophalangeal . . . 26700-26706, 26742
Metacarpophalangeal Joint . 26700-26706,
26340, 26742
Metatarsal 28475, 28476
Metatarsophalangeal Joint. 28636
Monteggia 24620
Navicular 25624
Orbit 21401
Pelvis 27275
Pelvic Ring 27194
Phalangeal Shaft 26727
    Distal, Finger or Thumb 26755
    Finger/Thumb 26725, 26727
Phalanges. 28495, 28496, 28510
    Finger 26742, 26755, 26770-26776
    Finger/Thumb 26727
    Great Toe 28495, 28496
    Toes 28515
Radial 24655, 25565, 25605
Radial Shaft 25505, 25565
Radiocarpal 25660
Radioulnar 25675
Scapular 23575
Shoulder. 23650-23655
    Joint 23700
    with Greater Tuberosity 23665
Sternoclavicular 23525
    with Neck Fracture 23675
Talotarsal 28576
Talus. 28435, 28436
Tarsal 28455, 28456, 28546
Tarsometatarsal Joint 28606
Thumb 26641-26650
Tibial. 27532, 27752, 27762, 27768, 27825
Trans-Scaphoperilunar. 25680
Ulnar. 24675, 25605
Ulnar Shaft 25535, 25565
Vertebral. 22315
Wrist 25259, 25624, 25635,
                    25660, 25675, 25680, 25690
Dupuytren's Cord. 26341
Slipped Epiphysis
    Femur 27178
Foreskin. 54450

Maxillectomy 31225-31230
Partial 21049
with Craniofacial Procedures 61581

Maxillofacial Fixation
See Fixation (Device), Maxillofacial

Maxillofacial Impressions
Auricular Prosthesis 21086
Facial Prosthesis 21088
Mandibular Resection Prosthesis 21081
Nasal Prosthesis 21087
Obturator Prosthesis
    Definitive 21080
    Interim 21079
    Surgical 21076
Oral Surgical Splint 21085
Orbital Prosthesis 21077
Palatal Prosthesis
    Augmentation 21082
    Lift 21083
Speech Aid Prosthesis 21084

Maxillofacial Procedures
Fixation
    See Fixation (Device), Maxillofacial
Reconstruction
    See Face, Reconstruction
Unlisted Services and Procedures 21299

Maxillofacial Prosthetics 21076-21088
Impressions
    See Maxillofacial Impressions
Unlisted Services and Procedures 21089

Maydl Operation 45563, 50810
See Colostomy

Mayo Hernia Repair 49582

Mayo Procedure 28292

Maze Procedure
Endoscopic 33265, 33266
Open 33254-33256

McBride Procedure 28292

McBurney Operation 49582

McCannel Procedure 66682

McKissock Surgery 19318

McVay Operation 49582

Measles Uncomplicated
See Rubeola

Measles Vaccine
See Vaccines

Measles, German
See Rubella

Meat Fibers
Feces 89160

Meatoplasty
External Auditory Canal 69310
Urethra 53450, 53460

Meatotomy
Cystourethroscopy 52281
Infant 53025
Prostate
    Laser Coagulation 52647
    Laser Enucleation 52649

    Laser Vaporization 52648
    with Prostatectomy 55801, 55821
    Transurethral Resection 52630
        Electrosurgical 52601
Ureter 52290
Urethral 52285, 53020
    Infant 53025

Meckel's Diverticulum
Excision 44800
Unlisted Services and Procedures 44899

Median Nerve
Decompression 64721
Neuroplasty 64721
Release 64721
Repair/Suture
    Motor Thenar 64835
Transposition 64721

Median Nerve Compression
See Carpal Tunnel Syndrome

Mediastinal Cyst
See Cyst, Mediastinal; Mediastinum, Cyst

Mediastinoscopy
Biopsy
    Mediastinal Lymph Node 39402
    Mediastinal Mass 39401

Mediastinotomy
Cervical Approach 39000
Transthoracic Approach 39010

Mediastinum
Cyst
    Excision 32662
    Resection 39200
Drainage
    Image Guided Fluid Collection 49405
Endoscopy
    Biopsy 39401, 39402
Excision
    Cyst 32662
    Mass 32662
    Lymph Node 19272, 21632, 32674, 38746
    Tumor 32662
Exploration 39000-39010, 60505
Incision and Drainage 39000-39010
Lymph Node
    Biopsy
        Medianoscopy 39402
    Lymphadenectomy 19272,
               21632, 32674, 38746
Sampling
    Endobronchial Ultrasound (EBUS)
    Guided 31652, 31653
Mass
    Biopsy
        Medianoscopy 39401
        Needle Biopsy 32405
    Excision 32662
Radical Dissection 60522
Removal
    Foreign Body 39000-39010
Resection
    Cyst 39200
    Tumor 39220
Thoracoscopy
    Biopsy 32606
    Diagnostic 32601
Excision
    Cyst 32662
    Mass 32662
    Tumor 32662

Tumor
    Excision 32662
    Resection 39220
Unlisted Procedure 39499

Medical Disability Evaluation Services 99455, 99456

Medical Genetics 96040
Genetic Counseling 96040

Medical Team Conference 99366-99368

Medical Testimony 99075

Medication Therapy Management
Pharmacist Provided 99605-99607
Psychiatric 90863

Medicine, Preventive
See Preventive Medicine

Medicine, Pulmonary
See Pulmonology

Medulla
Creation of Lesion
    Stereotactic 61791
Decompression
    Craniectomy 61343

Megacolon
Decompression
    with Colonoscopy 45393
    with Sigmoidoscopy 45337

Meibomian Cyst
See Chalazion

Membrane Oxygenation, Extracorporeal
See Extracorporeal Membrane Oxygenation (ECMO)

Membrane, Mucous
See Mucosa

Membrane, Tympanic
See Tympanic Membrane

Meninges
Excision
    Tumor 61512, 61519
Meningitis, Meningococcal
    Antibody 86741
    Vaccine . . . 90620, 90621, 90644, 90733, 90734
Repair
    Meningocele 63700, 63702
    Myelomeningocele 63704, 63706
    Pseudomeningocele 63709

Meningioma
Excision 61512, 61519

Meningitis, Lymphocytic Benign
See Lymphocytic Choriomeningitis

Meningocele Repair
Meningocele 63700, 63702
Myelomeningocele 63704, 63706
Pseudomeningocele 63709

Meningococcal
See Vaccines

Meningococcal Vaccine
See Vaccines

Meningococcus
See Neisseria Meningitidis

Meningomyelocele
See Myelomeningocele

Meniscectomy
Knee Joint.........................27332, 27333
   Arthroscopic................29880, 29881
Temporomandibular Joint................21060

Meniscus
Knee
   Excision.......................27332, 27333
      Arthroscopic...............29880, 29881
   Lesion
      Excision..........................27347
   Repair.................................27403
      Arthroscopic...............29882, 29883
   Transplantation.....................29868

Mental Nerve
Avulsion...............................64736
Incision...............................64736
Transection............................64736

Mercury
Quantitative...........................83825
Screen.................................83015

Mesencephalic Tract
Incision...............................61480
Section................................61480

Mesencephalon
Tractotomy.............................61480

Mesenteric Arteries
See Artery, Mesenteric

Mesentery
Lesion
   Excision..............................44820
Repair.................................44850
Suture.................................44850
Unlisted Services and Procedures.........44899

Mesh
for Exclusion
   Small Intestine from Pelvis...........44700
Implantation
   Hernia Repair... 43282, 43333, 43335, 43337,
        49652-49654, 49568, 49652-49657
Insertion
   Pelvic Floor..........................57267
Removal
   Abdominal, Infected..................11008

Metabisulfite Test
See Red Blood Cell (RBC), Sickling

Metabolite
Thromboxane............................84431

Metacarpal
Amputation.............................26910
Graft..................................26546
Craterization..........................26230
Cyst
   Excision....................26200, 26205
Diaphysectomy..........................26230
Excision
   Bone...............................26230
   Cyst........................26200-26205
   Tumor.......................26200-26205
Fracture
   Closed Treatment............26600, 26605

with Fixation..........................26607
Open Treatment.........................26615
Percutaneous Fixation..................26608
with Manipulation...............26605-26607
without Manipulation...................26600
Ray Amputation.........................26910
Repair
   Lengthening...........................26568
   Non-union............................26546
   Osteotomy............................26565
Resection
   Tumor................................26250
Saucerization..........................26230
Tumor
   Excision....................26200-26205
   Radical Resection....................26250

Metacarpophalangeal Joint
Arthrodesis....................26850-26852
Arthroplasty...................26530, 26531
Arthroscopy
   Diagnostic...........................29900
   Surgical.....................29901, 29902
   with Debridement.....................29901
Arthrotomy.............................26075
Biopsy
   Synovium.................26105, 29900
Capsule
   Excision.............................26520
   Fixation.....................26516-26518
   Incision.............................26520
Capsulodesis...................26516-26518
Dislocation
   Closed Treatment............26700, 26705
   Open Treatment.......................26715
   Percutaneous Fixation................26706
   with Manipulation....................26340
Drainage...............................26075
Exploration............................26075
Fracture, Articular
   Closed Treatment.....................26740
   Open Treatment.......................26746
   with Manipulation....................26742
Fusion..............26516-26518, 26850-26852
Implantation
   Prosthetic
      Joint............................26531
Reconstruction
   Collateral Ligament.........26541, 26542
Removal of Foreign Body................26075
Repair
   Collateral Ligament..................26540
Synovectomy............................26135

Metadrenaline
See Metanephrines

Metals, Heavy
See Heavy Metal

Metanephrines........................83835

Metatarsal
See Foot
Graft
   Bone.................................20957
      Osteocutaneous..................20972
   Amputation...........................28810
Condyle
   Excision.............................28288
   Craterization........................28122
Cyst
   Excision....................28104-28107
Diaphysectomy..........................28122
Excision........28110-28114, 28122, 28140

Fracture
   Closed Treatment
      with Manipulation........28475, 28476
      without Manipulation............28470
   Open Treatment.......................28485
   Percutaneous Fixation................28476
Microvascular Anastomosis
   Bone Graft...........................20957
   Free Osteocutaneous Flap.............20972
Repair
   Lengthening.................28306-28309
   Nonunion or Malunion.................28322
   Osteotomy...................28306-28309
   Shortening..................28306-28309
Saucerization..........................28122
Sequestrectomy.........................28122
Tumor
   Excision....................28104-28107
   Radical Resection....................28173

Metatarsectomy....................28140

Metatarsophalangeal Joint
Amputation.............................28820
Arthrotomy.....................28022, 28052
Biopsy.................................28052
Capsulotomy............................28270
Cheilectomy............................28289
Dislocation
   Closed Treatment............28630-28635
   Open Treatment.......................28645
   Percutaneous Fixation................28636
Drainage...............................28022
Exploration............................28022
Great Toe
   Arthrodesis..........................28750
   Fusion...............................28750
Removal
   of Foreign Body......................28022
   of Loose Body........................28022
Repair
   Hallux Rigidus.......................28289
Synovial
   Biopsy...............................28052
   Excision.............................28072

Methaemoglobin
See Methemoglobin

Methane Test.....................91065

Methbipyranone
See Metyrapone

Methemalbumin...................83857

Methemoglobin............83045-83050

Methenamine Silver Stain......88312

Methopyrapone
See Metyrapone

Methoxyhydroxymandelic Acid
See Vanillylmandelic Acid

Methyl Alcohol
See Methanol

Methylene Bichloride
See Dichloromethane

Methylfluorprednisolone
See Dexamethasone

Metroplasty
See Hysteroplasty

Metyrapone
Panel 80436

MIC
See Minimum Inhibitory Concentration

Micro-ophthalmia
Orbit Reconstruction 21256

Microalbumin
Urine 82043, 82044

Microbiology 87003-87999
See Pathology and Laboratory, Microbiology

Microbiota, Transplantation Fecal Matter 44705

Microdissection 88380, 88381

Microfluidic Analysis 83861

Microfluorometries, Flow
See Flow Cytometry

Microglobulin, Beta 2
Blood 82232
Urine 82232

Micrographic Surgery
Mohs Technique 17311-17315

Micrographic Surgery, Mohs
See Mohs Micrographic Surgery

Micropigmentation
Correction 11920-11922

Microsatellite Instability Analysis 81301

Microscope, Surgical
See Operating Microscope

Microscopic Evaluation
Blood Smear 85007, 85008
Hair 96902
Necropsy 88020, 88025,
               88027-88029, 88036, 88037
Surgical Pathology 88302, 88304, 88305,
               88307, 88309, 88399
Urinalysis 81015

Microscopies, Electron
See Electron Microscopy

Microscopy
Binocular
     Ear Exam 92504
Reflectance Confocal Microscopy (RCM)
     Skin Imaging 96931-96936
     Lesion 96932
Specular
     Endothelial Cell Analysis 92286

Microsomal Antibody 86376

Microsomia, Hemifacial
See Hemifacial Microsomia

Microsurgery
Operating Microscope 69990

Microvascular Anastomosis
Bone Graft
     Fibula 20955
     Iliac Crest 20956
     Metatarsal 20957
     Other Site 20962

Fascial Flap, Free 15758
Finger Transfer 26555
Intestinal Graft, Free 43116
Jejunum Transfer, Free 43496
Muscle Flap, Free 15756
Myocutaneous Flap
     Breast Reconstruction 19368
     Pharyngeal Wall Resection
       with Closure 42894
Omental Flap, Free 49906
Osteocutaneous Flap 20969
     Iliac Crest 20970
     Metatarsal 20972
     Great Toe with Web 20973
Skin Flap, Free 15757
Toe Joint, Free 26556
Toe-to-Hand Transfer 26551, 26553, 26554

Microvite A
See Vitamin, A

Microwave Therapy 97024
See Physical Medicine/Therapy/Occupational Therapy

Midbrain
See Brain; Brainstem; Mesencephalon; Skull Base Surgery

Midcarpal Medioccipital Joint
Arthrotomy 25040

Middle Cerebral Artery Velocimetry 76821

Middle Ear
See Ear, Middle Ear

Midface
Reconstruction
     Forehead
       Advancement 21159, 21160,
                21172, 21175, 21263
       Alteration 21175
       Entire/Majority 21179, 21180
       with Bone Graft 21145-21160, 21188
       without Bone Graft 21141-21143
       LeFort I 21141-21143,
              21145-21147, 21155, 21160
       LeFort II 21150, 21151
       LeFort III 21154, 21155, 21159, 21160

Migration Inhibitory Factor (MIF) 86378

Mile Operation
See Colectomy, Total, Laparoscopic, with Proctectomy

Milia, Multiple
Removal 10040

Miller Procedure 28737

Miller-Abbott Intubation
Introduction 44500
     with Radiologic Guidance 74340

Minerva Cast
Application 29040
Removal 29710

Minimum Inhibitory Concentration 87186

Minimum Lethal Concentration 87187

Minnesota Multiphasic Personality Inventory
See MMPI

Miscarriage
Incomplete Abortion 59812
Missed Abortion
     First Trimester 59820
     Second Trimester 59821
Septic Abortion 59830

Missed Abortion
See Abortion

Mitchell Procedure 28296

Mitogen Blastogenesis 86353

Mitral Valve
Incision 33420, 33422
Repair 33425-33427
     Transcatheter 0345T, 33418, 33419
Replacement 33430

Mitrofanoff Operation 50845

Miyagawanella
See Chlamydia

MLC
See Lymphocyte, Culture

MMPI 96101-96103
Computer-Assisted 96103

MMR Shots 90707
See Vaccines

Mobilization
Conjunctiva 65272, 65273
Cranium 61595-61597, 61590, 61591
Intestine 43108, 43113, 43118, 43123, 43361
Nerve 64874
Splenic Flexure 44139
     Laparoscopic 44213
Stapes 69650
Urethra 54300, 54326, 54344

Moderate Sedation
See Sedation

Modified Radical Mastectomy
See Mastectomy, Modified Radical

Mohs Micrographic Surgery 17311-17315

Molar Pregnancy
See Hydatidiform Mole

Mold
Cast 29450
Culture 87107

Mole, Carneous
See Abortion

Mole, Hydatid
See Hydatidiform Mole

Molecular Cytogenetics . . 88271-88275
Interpretation and Report 88291

Molecular Diagnostics
Reverse Transcription and Amplified Probe
     Enterovirus 87498
     Hepatitis C 87521
     HIV-1 87535
     HIV-2 87538

Reverse Transcription and Quantification
  Hepatitis C 87522
  HIV-1 87536
  HIV-2 87539

Molecular Oxygen Saturation
See Oxygen Saturation

Molecular Pathology 81161,
81200-81383, 81400-81408
See Gene Analysis
Unlisted Procedure 81479

Molecular Probes 88120

Molluscum Contagiosum
Destruction 17110, 17111, 46900,
46910, 46916, 46917, 54050-54065
Excision
  Anus 46922
  Penis 54060

Monilia
See Candida

Monitoring
Ablation Therapy
  Incompetent Vein 36475,
36476, 36478, 36479
  Parenchymal Tissue 76940, 77013, 77022
  Renal Mass 50250, 50542
ACE/ARB Therapy 4188F
Anticonvulsant Therapy 4191F
Atrial Hemodynamic Monitor
System 0291T, 0292T
Blood Pressure, 24 Hour 93784-93790
by Arterial Catheterization 36620
Digoxin Therapy 4189F
Diuretic Therapy 4190F
ESRD 90951-90959, 90963-90965
Evaluation and Programming
  Implantable Defibrillator
    Transvenous 93282-93284, 93287
    Wearable 93292
  Loop Recorder . . . 93285, 93291, 93298, 93299
  Pacemaker 93279-93281, 93294-93296
Electrocardiogram 93015, 93268, 93270-93272,
93318, 93351, 93660, 93798
  See Electrocardiography
Electroencephalogram 95812, 95813,
95950-95953, 95956
  with Drug Activation 95954
  with Physical Activation 95954
  with WADA Activation 95958
Fetal
  During Labor 59050, 59051, 99500
    Interpretation Only 59051
Glucose
  Home Device 82962
  Interstitial Fluid 95250, 95251
  Tolerance Test 82951, 82952
Interstitial Fluid Pressure 20950
Intracardiac Ischemia Monitoring System
  Evaluation 0305T, 0306T
  Insertion
    Complete System 0302T
    Device Only 0304T
    Electrode Only 0303T
  Interrogation Device Evaluation 0306T
  Programming Device 0305T
  Removal 0307T
  Removal and Replacement
    Complete System 0302T
    Device Only 0304T
    Electrode Only 0303T

Intraocular Pressure 0329T
Neurological
  Arterial Occlusion 61623
Neurophysiologic
  Intraoperative 95940, 95941
Pediatric Apnea 94774-94777
Retinal Disease 92228
Seizure 0381T-0386T, 61531-61533, 61760
with Contrast
  Biliary Drainage 47533-47540
  Catheter 75984, 93503

Monitoring, Sleep 95800, 95801
See Polysomnography

Monoethylene Glycol
See Ethylene Glycol

Mononuclear Cell Antigen 86356

Mononucleosis Virus, Infectious
See Epstein-Barr Virus

Monophosphate, Adenosine
See Adenosine Monophosphate (AMP)

Monophosphate, Adenosine Cyclic
See Cyclic AMP

Monospot Test
See Rapid Test for Infection

Monoxide, Carbon
Diffusing Capacity 94729

Monteggia Fracture 24620-24635

Monticelli Procedure
See Application, Bone Fixation Device

Morbilli
See Rubeola

Morphometric Analysis
Computer-Assisted 88367, 88373, 88374
Manual 88368, 88369, 88377
Nerve 88356
Skeletal Muscle 88355
Tumor 88358-88361
Urinary Tract Specimen 88120, 88121

Morton's Neuroma
Excision 28080

Mosaicplasty 27416

Mosenthal Test
See Urinalysis, Routine

Mother Cell
See Stem Cell

Motility Study
Colon 91117
Duodenal 91022
Esophagus 91010
  with Perfusion 91013
  with Stimulation 91013
  Imaging 78258
Sperm 89300

Motion Analysis
by Video and 3-D Kinematics 96000, 96004
Computer-based 96000, 96004

Motion Management Simulation
Respiratory 77293

Mouth
Abscess
  Incision and Drainage 40800, 40801,
41005-41009, 41015-41018
Biopsy 40808, 41108
Cyst
  Incision and Drainage 40800, 40801,
41005-41009, 41015-41018
Excision
  Frenum 40819
Gums
  See Gums
Hematoma
  Incision and Drainage 40800, 40801,
41005-41009, 41015-41018
Lesion
  Destruction 40820
  Excision 40810-40816, 41116
Vestibule
  Destruction 40820
Lips
  See Lip
Mucosa
  Donor Excision 40818
Lesion
  Excision 40810, 40812, 40814, 40816
Reconstruction 40840-40845
Removal
  Foreign Body 40804, 40805
Repair
  Laceration 40830, 40831, 41250, 41252
Resection
  with Glossectomy 41150, 41153, 41155
Skin Graft
  Dermal Autograft 15135, 15136
  Epidermal Autograft 15115, 15116
  Recipient Site Preparation 15004, 15005
  Skin Substitute 15275-15278
  Split-Thickness 15120, 15121
  Tissue-cultured Autograft 15155-15157
Tongue
  See Tongue
Unlisted Services and Procedures . . . 40899, 41599
Vestibule
  Biopsy 40808
  Destruction
    Lesion 40820
    Scar 40820
  Excision
    Frenum 40819
  Incision and Drainage
    Abscess 40800, 40801
    Cyst 40800, 40801
    Hematoma 40800, 40801
  Removal
    Foreign Body 40804, 40805
  Repair 40830-40845
  Unlisted Procedures 40899
Wound Repair 13131-13133

Move
See Transfer
Finger 26555
Toe Joint 26556
Toe to Hand 26551-26554

MPD Syndrome
See Temporomandibular Joint (TMJ)

MPR
See Multifetal Pregnancy Reduction

MR Spectroscopy
See Magnetic Resonance Spectroscopy

MRA
See Magnetic Resonance Angiography (MRA)

MRI
See Magnetic Resonance Imaging (MRI)
See Multiple Sleep Latency Testing (MSLT)

Mucin
Synovial Fluid 83872

Mucocele
Sinusotomy
   Frontal 31075

Mucopolysaccharides 83864

Mucormycoses
See Mucormycosis

Mucormycosis
Antibody 86732

Mucosa
Ablation
   Turbinates 30801, 30802
Advancement
   Lip 40500
   Urethra 53450
Biopsy
   Vaginal 57100-57105
   Gross and Microscopic Examination
     Oral 88305
     Nasal 88305
     Vaginal 88302
Ectopic Gastric Imaging 78290
Excision
   Alveolar, Hyperplastic 41828
   Vestibule of Mouth, Donor 40818
Fulguration
   Hypertrophic Folds
     Urethra 52400
Lesion
   Ablation
     Vestibule of Mouth 40810-40818
     Photodynamic Therapy 96567
   Periodontal Grafting 41870
Polyp
   Sinus
     Removal 31051
Stripping
   Sinus 31051
Resection
   Endoscopy 43211
   Hypertrophic Folds
     Urethra 52400
Turbinates
   Ablation 30801, 30802
Vaginal

Mucosa, Buccal
See Mouth, Mucosa

Mucous Cyst
Tendon Sheath/Joint Capsule
   Excision
     Hand or Finger 26160

Mucous Membrane
See Mouth, Mucosa
Cutaneous
   Biopsy 11100, 11101
   Excision
     Benign Lesion 11440-11446
     Malignant Lesion 11640-11646

   Layer Closure, Wounds 12051-12057
   Simple Repair, Wounds 12011-12018
Excision
   Sphenoid Sinus 31288
Graft
   Buccal 67835, 68325, 68328, 68335
Lesion
   Destruction 17000-17004, 17280-17286
   Excision
     Benign 11440-11446
     Malignant 11640-11646
     Shaving 11310-11313
Rectum
   Proctoplasty for Prolapse 45505
Repair
   Trichiasis 67835
   Wound
     Superficial 12011, 12013-12018
     Intermediate 12051-12057
Tests
   Nasal 95065
   Ophthalmic 95060
Unlisted Procedure 17999

Mucus Cyst
See Mucous Cyst

MUGA (Multiple Gated Acquisition) 78472, 78473, 78483

Muller Procedure
See Sleep Study

Multianalyte Assays with Algorithmic Analyses 81500-81599,
                      0001M-0004M
Administrative 0001M-0004M
Autoimmune
   Rheumatoid Arthritis 81490
Cardiology
   Heart Transplant 81595
Coronary Artery Disease 81493
Endocrinology 81506
Fetal
   Congenital Abnormalities 81508-81512
   Fetal Aneuploidy 81507
Oncology
   Breast 81519
   Colon 81525
   Colorectal 81528
   Gynecologic 81535, 81536
   Lung 81538
   Ovarian 81500, 81503
   Thyroid 81545
   Tissue of Origin 81504
   Tumor of Unknown Origin 81540
Unlisted Multianalyte Assay with Algorithmic
Analysis 81599

Multifetal Pregnancy Reduction 59866

Multiple Sleep Latency Testing (MSLT) 95805

Multiple Valve Procedures
See Valvuloplasty

Mumford Operation
See Claviculectomy, Open, Partial

Mumford Procedure 29824

Mumps
Antibody 86735
Immunization 90707, 90710

Vaccine
   MMR 90707
   MMRV 90710

Muramidase 85549

Murine Typhus 86000

Muscle
See specific muscle
Abdomen
   See Abdominal Wall
Biofeedback Training
   Perineal 90911
Biopsy 20200-20206
   Extraocular 67346
   Needle 20206
Chemodenervation 64612, 64615-64617,
               64642-64647, 67345
   Guidance 95873, 95874
Compartment Syndrome
   Detection 20950
Cutting
   Pyloric 43520
Debridement 11011, 11012,
          11043, 11044, 11046, 11047
   Infected 11004-11006
   Nonviable 25023, 25025,
           27057, 27497, 27499
   Leg 27892-27894
Delivery
   Thermal Energy
     Anus 0288T
     for Gastroesophageal Reflux
     Disease 43257
Division
   See Muscle Division
Excision
   Lip 40816
   Pectoral 19305-19307
Fasciotomy
   See Fasciotomy
Flaps
   Fasciocutaneous 15732,
          15734, 15736, 15738
   Muscle, Free 15842
   with Microvascular
     Anastomosis 15756, 42894
   Myocutaneous 15732, 15734,
          15736, 15738, 61619
Grafts
   Muscle, Free 15841, 25265, 25274
Heart
   See Myocardium
Imbrication
   Anus 46761
Implantation
   Eye 65105, 65140, 65155
   Nerve to Muscle 64787
Incision
   Esophagus 32665, 43130,
          43279, 43330, 43331
   Hyoid 21685
   Pharynx 43030, 43130
   Pylorus 43520
Injection 20552, 20553
Masseter, Reduction
   See Masseter Muscle/Bone
Interstitial Fluid Pressure
   Monitoring 20950
Neck
   See Neck Muscle
Neurectomy
   Hamstring 27325

N

N. Meningitidis
See Neisseria Meningitidis

Naffziger Operation
See Decompression, Orbit; Section

Nagel Test
See Color Vision Examination

Nail Bed
Reconstruction 11762
Repair 11760

Nail Fold
Excision
    Wedge 11765

Nail Plate Separation
See Nails, Avulsion

Nails
Avulsion 11730-11732
Biopsy 11755
Debridement 11720, 11721
Drainage 10060, 10061
Evacuation
    Hematoma, Subungual 11740
Excision 11750-11752
KOH Examination 87220
Reconstruction 11762
Removal 11730-11732, 11750-11752
Trimming 11719

Narcosynthesis
Diagnostic and Therapeutic 90865

Nasal Abscess
See Nose, Abscess

Nasal Area
Bone Graft. 21210

Nasal Bleeding
See Epistaxis

Nasal Bone
Bone Graft. 21210
Fracture
    Closed Treatment. 21310-21320
    Open Treatment 21325-21335
    with Manipulation 21315-21320
    without Manipulation 21310
Reconstruction
    See Rhinoplasty
X-ray 70160

Nasal Deformity
Repair 40700-40761

Nasal Function Study 92512

Nasal Polyp
See Nose, Polyp

Nasal Prosthesis
Impression. 21087

Nasal Septum
Abscess
    Incision and Drainage 30020
Fracture
    Closed Treatment. 21337
    Open Treatment 21336

Hematoma
    Incision and Drainage 30020
Insertion
    Button Prosthesis. 30220
Repair 30630
    Septoplasty 30520
Submucous Resection. 30520

Nasal Sinuses
See Sinus/Sinuses

Nasal Smear
Eosinophils 89190

Nasal Turbinate
Fracture
    Therapeutic 30930

Nasoethmoid Complex
Fracture
    Open Treatment 21338, 21339
    Percutaneous Treatment 21340
Reconstruction 21182-21184

Nasogastric Tube
Placement 43752

Nasolacrimal Duct
Dilation 68816
Exploration 68810
    with Anesthesia. 68811
Insertion
    Catheter 68816
    Stent. 68815
    Tube 68815
Repair 21340
X-ray
    with Contrast. 70170

Nasomaxillary
Fracture
    Closed Treatment. 21345
    Open Treatment 21346-21348
    with Bone Grafting. 21348

Nasopharynges
See Nasopharynx

Nasopharyngoscopy 92511

Nasopharynx
See Pharynx
Biopsy
    Lesion. 42804-42806
Hemorrhage 42970-42972
Unlisted Services and Procedures 42999

Natriuretic Peptide 83880

Natural Killer (NK) Cells
Count. 86357

Natural Ostium
Sinus
    Maxillary 31000
    Sphenoid 31002

Navicular Bone
Carpal
    Arthroplasty
        with Implant 25443
    Fracture
        Closed Treatment 25622
        Open Treatment 25628
        with Manipulation 25624
    Repair
        Nonunion 25431, 25440

Tarsal
    Arthrodesis. 28737
    Excision 28238

Navigation
Computer Assisted Procedures
Bronchoscopy 31627
    Cranial 61781, 61782
    Musculoskeletal. 20985
    Orthopedic 0054T, 0055T
    Spinal 61783

Neck
Angiography 70498, 70547-70549
Artery
    Ligation 37615
Biopsy 21550
Bypass Graft 35901
CT Scan. 70490-70492, 70498
    with PET Scan 78814
Dissection, Radical
    See Radical Neck Dissection
Exploration
    Blood Vessel. 35800
    Lymph Nodes 38542
Incision and Drainage
    Abscess 21501, 21502
    Hematoma 21501, 21502
Lipectomy, Suction Assisted. 15876
Magnetic Resonance Angiography
(MRA) 70547-70549
Magnetic Resonance Imaging
(MRI). 70540-70543
Muscle
    Chemodenervation. 64616
Nerve
    Graft 64885, 64886
Nuclear Medicine
    Thyroid Carcinoma Imaging. 78015
PET Scan 78811
    with CT Scan 78814
Repair
    Blood Vessel. 35201
        with Other Graft 35261
        with Vein Graft 35231
Rhytidectomy 15828
Skin
    Graft 15240, 15241
    Revision 15819
Tissue Transfer
    Adjacent. 14040, 14041
    Flap. 15574, 15620
Tumor
    Excision 21552-21558
    Radical Resection 21557, 21558
Ultrasound Exam. 76536
Unlisted Services and Procedures, Surgery . . 21899
Urinary Bladder
    See Bladder, Neck
Wound
    Exploration 20100
    Repair. 13131-13133
X-ray 70360

Neck Muscle
Division
    Scalenus Anticus 21700-21705
    Sternocleidomastoid 21720-21725

Necropsy
Coroner's Exam 88045
Forensic Exam. 88040
Gross and Micro Exam 88020-88029
Gross Exam 88000-88016
Organ. 88037

Nerve XI, Cranial
See Accessory Nerve, Spinal

Nerve XII, Cranial
See Hypoglossal Nerve

Nerves
Anastomosis
   Facial to Hypoglossal 64868
   Facial to Spinal Accessory 64866
Application
   Surface Neurostimulator 64550
Avulsion 64732-64772
Biopsy 64795
Cervical
   Neurostimulator Implant 0282T, 0283T
Closure
   Amputation, Ankle 27888
Decompression 64702-64727
   Cranial 61458, 61460
   Laminotomy/Laminectomy 0274T, 0275T
Denervation 27035
Destruction 64600-64681
   Laryngeal, Recurrent 31595
Excision
   See Neurectomy
Graft 64885-64907
Implantation
   Electrode Array . . . 0282T, 0283T, 64553-64581
   to Bone 64787
   to Muscle 64787
Incision 28035, 43640, 43641, 64732-64772
Injection
   Anesthetic 01991, 01992, 64400-64530
Diagnostic Agent 0213T, 64493-64495
   Neurolytic Agent 64600-64681
   Therapeutic Agent 0213T, 64490-64495
Insertion
   Electrode Array 64553-64581
Lesion
   Excision 64774-64792
Lumbar
   Neurostimulator Implant 0282T, 0283T
Neurofibroma
   Excision 64788-64792
Neurolemmoma
   Excision 64788-64792
Neurolytic
   Internal 64727
Neuroma
   Destruction 64632
   Excision 64774-64786
   Injection 64455
Neuroplasty 64702-64721
Removal
   Electrode Array 64585
Repair
   Graft 64885-64911
   Microdissection 69990
   Suture 64831-64876
Revision
   Electrode Array 64585
Spinal Accessory
   Incision 63191
   Section 63191
Suture 64831-64876
Sympathectomy
   Excision 64802-64818
Thoracic
   Neurostimulator Implant 0282T, 0283T
Transection 64732-64772
Vagus Nerve 43640, 43641
   Laparoscopic 43651, 43652

Transposition 64718-64721
Unlisted Services and Procedures 64999

Nervous System
Skull, Meninges, and Brain 61000-62258
Spine and Spinal Cord 62263-63746
Extracranial, Peripheral Nerves and Autonomic
Nervous System 64400-64999
Nuclear Medicine
   Unlisted Services and Procedures 78699

Nesidioblast
See Islet Cell

Neural Conduction
See Nerve Conduction

Neural Ganglion
See Ganglion

Neurectomy
Foot 28055
Gastrocnemius 27326
Hamstring Muscle 27325
Hip
   Obturator 27003
Leg, Lower 27326
Leg, Upper 27325
Morton 28080
Popliteal 27326
Tympanic 69676

Neuroendoscopy
Intracranial 62160-62165

Neurofibroma
Excision
   Cutaneous Nerve 64788
   Extensive 64792
   Peripheral Nerve 64790

Neurolemmoma
Excision
   Cutaneous Nerve 64788
   Extensive 64792
   Peripheral Nerve 64790

Neurologic System
See Nervous System

Neurology
Brain Cortex Magnetic Stimulation 0310T,
   90867-90869
Brain Mapping 0310T, 90867, 96020
Brain Surface Electrode
   Stimulation 95961, 95962
Central Motor
   Motor Function Mapping 0310T
   Transcranial Motor Stimulation . . 95928, 95929
Cognitive Performance 96125
Diagnostic
   Anal Sphincter 51785
   Autonomic Function Tests
     Heart Rate Response 95921, 95943
     Parasympathetic 95943
     Pseudomotor Response 95921-95924
     Sympathetic Function . . 95921-95924, 95943
     Valsalva Maneuvers 95922, 95943
   Electrocorticogram
     Intraoperative 95829
   Electroencephalogram (EEG) . . 95812-95827, 95955
     Brain Death 95824
     Electrode Placement 95830
     Intraoperative 95955
     Monitoring 95812, 95813,
     95950-95953, 95956

   Physical or Drug Activation 95954
   Sleep 95800, 95801, 95822, 95827
   Standard 95819
   WADA Activation 95958
Electroencephalography (EEG)
   Digital Analysis 95957
Electromyography
   Fine Wire
     Dynamic 96004
   Ischemic Limb Exercise Test 95875
   Needle 51785, 95860-95872
   Surface
     Dynamic 96002-96004
Evoked Potentials
   Auditory 92585, 92586
   Central Motor 95928, 95929, 95939
   Somatosensory Testing . . 95925-95927, 95938
   Visual 95930, 0333T
Higher Cerebral Function
   Aphasia Test 96105
   Cognitive Function Tests 96116
   Developmental Tests 96110, 96111
   Neurobehavioral Status 96116
   Neuropsychological Testing 96118-96120
   Neuropsychological Testing,
     Computer-Assisted 96120
Magnetoencephalography (MEG) 95965-95967
Motion Analysis
   by Video and 3-D Kinematics . . . 96000, 96004
   Computer-based 96000, 96004
Muscle Testing
   Manual 95831-95834
Nerve Conduction
   Motor and Sensory Nerve 95905-95913
Neurofunctional Testing 96020
Neuromuscular Junction Tests 95937
Neurophysiological Monitoring
   Intraoperative 95940, 95941
Neuropsychological Testing 96118-96120
   Cognitive Performance 96125
   Computer-Assisted 96120
Plantar Pressure Measurements
   Dynamic 96001, 96004
Polysomnography 95782, 95783, 95808-95811
Range of Motion 95851, 95852
Reflex
   Blink Reflex 95933
Sleep Study 95800, 95801, 95805-95811
   Actigraphy Testing 95803
Somatosensory Testing 95925-95927,
   95938, 95939
Cholinesterase Inhibitor Challenge Test 95857
Therapeutic
   Magnetic Stimulation
     Transcranial 90867-90869
Unlisted Services and Procedures 95999
Urethral Sphincter 51785

Neurolysis
Internal 64727
with Neuroplasty 64702-64721

Neuroma
Acoustic
   See Brain, Tumor, Excision
Excision
   Cutaneous Nerve 64774
   Digital Nerve 64776-64778
   Foot 28080
   Foot Nerve 64782, 64783
   Hand Nerve 64782, 64783
   Peripheral Nerve 64784
   Sciatic Nerve 64786

Injection
    Anesthetic Agent 64455
    Steroid 64455
Interdigital
    Morton
        Excision 28080

Neuromuscular Junction Tests 95937

Neuromuscular Pedicle
Reinnervation
    Larynx 31590

Neuromuscular Reeducation . . . 97112
See Physical Medicine/Therapy/Occupational Therapy

Neurophysiologic Testing
Autonomic Nervous Function
    Heart Rate Response 95921-95924
    Pseudomotor Response 95921-95924
    Sympathetic Function 95921-95924
Intraoperative 95940, 95941

Neuroplasty
Cranial Nerve 64716
Digital Nerve 64702, 64704
Peripheral Nerve 64708, 64712-64714,
               64716, 64718, 64719, 64721
    Arm 64708
    Brachial Plexus 64713
    Cranial 64716
    Leg 64708
    Lumbar Plexus 64714
    Median at Carpal Tunnel 64721
    Sciatic 64712
    Ulnar at Elbow 64718
    Ulnar at Wrist 64719

Neuropsychological Testing 96118-96120
Computer-Assisted 96120

Neurorrhaphy 64831-64876
Peripheral Nerve
    Conduit 64910, 64911
    with Graft 64885-64907

Neurostimulators
Analysis
    with Vagus Nerve Blocking Therapy 0317T
    Brain 95970, 95978, 95979
    Cranial Nerve 95974, 95975
    Gastric 95980-95982
    Peripheral Nerve 95971, 95972
    Spinal Cord 95971, 95972
Application 64550, 64566
Implantation
    Electrode Array 64553-64565
        by Burr Hole 61863, 61864
        by Craniectomy 61863,
        61864, 61867, 61868
        Vagus Nerve 0312T
        with Image Guidance 64561
    Electrodes 0282T,
        0283T, 43647, 43881, 64568
        by Burr Hole 61850
        by Craniectomy 61860
    Pulse Generator
        Vagus Nerve 0312T
Insertion
    Pulse Generator . . 61885, 61886, 64568, 64590
    Receiver 61885, 61886, 64590

Removal
    Electrode Array
        Vagus Nerve 0314T
    Electrodes 43648, 43882, 61880, 64570
    Pulse Generator 61888, 64595, 64570
        Vagus Nerve 0314T, 0315T
    Receiver 61888, 64595
Replacement 61885
    Electrode Array
        Vagus Nerve 0313T
    Pulse Generator
        Vagus Nerve 0316T
    Electrodes 43647, 43881, 64569, 64570
Revision
    Electrode Array
        Vagus Nerve 0313T
    Electrodes 61880, 64569

Neurotomy, Sympathetic
See Gasserian Ganglion, Sensory Root, Decompression

Neurovascular Pedicle Flaps . . 15750

Neutralization Test
Virus 86382

New Patient
Domiciliary or Rest Home Visit 99324-99328
Emergency Department Services 99281-99288
Home Services 99341-99345
Hospital Inpatient Services 99221-99239
Hospital Observation Services 99217-99220
Initial Office Visit 99201-99205
    See Evaluation and Management; Office and
    Other Outpatient
Inpatient Consultations 99251-99255
Office and/or Other Outpatient
Consultations 99241-99245

Newborn Care 99460-99465, 99502
Attendance at Delivery 99464
Blood Transfusion
    Exchange 36450
    Push 36440
Circumcision
    Clamp or Other Device 54150
    Surgical Excision 54160
History and Examination 99460, 99463
Home Visit 99502
Initial Care
    Birthing Room 99460, 99463
    Hospital 99460, 99463
    Other Site 99461
Laryngoscopy 31520
Normal 99460-99463
Prepuce Slitting 54000
Preventive
    Office 99461
Resuscitation 99465
Standby for Cesarean Delivery 99360
Subsequent Hospital Care 99462
Umbilical Artery Catheterization 36660

Next Generation Sequencing (NGS) and Other Molecular Multianalyte Assays
Aortic Dysfunction or Dilation 81410, 81411
Exome 81415-81417
Fetal Chromosomal Aneuploidy 81420
Genome 81425-81427
Hearing Loss 81430, 81431
Hereditary Breast Cancer-Related
Disorders 81432, 81433

Hereditary Colon Cancer Disorders . . 81435, 81436
Hereditary Neuroendocrine Tumor
Disorders 81437, 81438
Hereditary Retinal Disorders 81434
Noonan Spectrum Disorders 81442
Nuclear Encoded Mitochondrial Genes 81440
Targeted Genomic Sequence Analysis
Panel 81445, 81450, 81455
Whole Mitochondrial Genome 81460, 81465
X-linked Intellectual Disability
(XLID) 81470, 81471

Nickel 83885

Nicolas-Durand-Favre Disease
See Lymphogranuloma Venereum

Nidation
See Implantation

Nikaidoh Procedure
Aortic Root Translocation 33782, 33783

Nipples
See Breast
Exploration 19110
Inverted 19355
Lesion
    Excision 19120
Reconstruction 19350

Nissen Operation
See Fundoplasty, Esophagogastric

Nissen Procedure
See Gastroplasty with Esophagogastric Fundoplasty

Nitrate Reduction Test
See Urinalysis

Nitric Oxide
Administration 93463
Expired Gas Determination 95012

Nitroblue Tetrazolium Dye Test 86384

Nitrogen, Blood Urea
See Blood Urea Nitrogen

NMR Imaging
See Magnetic Resonance Imaging (MRI)

NMR Spectroscopies
See Magnetic Resonance Spectroscopy

No Man's Land
Tendon Repair 26356-26358

Noble Procedure
See Repair; Suture

Nocardia
Antibody 86744

Nocturnal Penile Rigidity Test 54250

Nocturnal Penile Tumescence Test 54250

Node Dissection, Lymph
See Dissection, Lymph Nodes

Node, Lymph
See Lymph Nodes

Nodes
See Lymph Nodes

Non-Invasive Vascular Imaging
See Vascular Studies

Non-Office Medical Services .. 99056
Emergency Care 99060

Non-Stress Test, Fetal 59025
with Biophysical Profile 76818

Nonunion Repair
Carpal 25431, 25440
Clavicle 23485
Femur
　with Graft. 27472
　without Graft 27470
Fibula. 27726
Humerus 24430-24435
Metacarpal 26546
Metatarsal 28322
Phalanx 26546
Radius 25400-25405, 25415-25420
Tarsal. 28320
Tibia 27720, 27722, 27724, 27725
Ulna. 25400, 25415, 25415, 25415, 25420
with Bone Graft. 23485, 25405, 25415, 26546,
　　　　　　　　　27470, 27722, 27724, 28322

Noradrenalin
Blood 82383, 82384
Urine 82384

Norepinephrine
See Catecholamines
Blood 82383, 82384
Urine 82384

Norwood
Procedure 33611, 33612, 33619
See Repair, Heart, Ventricle; Revision

Nose
Abscess
　Incision and Drainage 30000-30020
Artery
　Ligation 30915-30920
Biopsy
　Intranasal. 30100
　Endoscopic. 31237
Debridement
　Endoscopic. 31237
Dermoid Cyst
　Excision
　　Complex 30125
　　Simple. 30124
Displacement Therapy 30210
Endoscopy
　Diagnostic 31231-31235
　Surgical 31237-31294
Excision
　Rhinectomy 30150-30160
　Turbinate 30140
Fracture
　Closed Treatment. 21345
　Open Treatment 21325-21336, 21338,
　　　　　　　　　　　21339, 21346, 21347
　Percutaneous Treatment 21340
　with Fixation 21330, 21340, 21345-21347
Hematoma
　Incision and Drainage 30000-30020
Hemorrhage Control
　Cauterization 30901-30906

Packs 30901-30906
　Endoscopic 31237
Insertion
　Septal Prosthesis 30220
Lesion
　Destruction or Excision
　　External Approach 30118
　　Internal Approach. 30117
Lysis of Adhesions 30560
Polyp
　Excision
　　Endoscopic 31237
　　Extensive 30115
　　Simple. 30110
Reconstruction
　Cleft Lip/Cleft Palate 30460-30462
　Complete 30410
　Dermatoplasty 30620
　Primary 30400, 30420
　Secondary 30430-30450
　Septum. 30520
Removal
　Foreign Body 30300
　　by Lateral Rhinotomy 30320
　　with Anesthesia 30310
Repair
　Adhesions 30560
　Cleft Lip 40700-40761
　Choanal Atresia 30540, 30545
　Complex 13151-13153
　Fistula 30580-30600, 42260
　Rhinophyma 30120
　Septum 30540-30545, 30630
　Synechia. 30560
　Vestibular Stenosis 30465
Skin
　Excision 30120
　Surgical Planing 30120
Submucous Resection Turbinate
　Excision 30140
Turbinate
　Excision 30130-30140
　Fracture 30930
　Injection 30200
Turbinate Mucosa
　Cauterization 30801, 30802
Unlisted Services and Procedures 30999

Nose Bleed
Cauterization 30901-30906
Packs 30901-30906
　Endoscopic. 31237

NTD 86384
See Nitroblue Tetrazolium Dye Test

Nuclear Antigen
Antibody 86235

Nuclear Imaging
See Nuclear Medicine
Planar
　Parathyroid Gland 78070
Subtraction
　Parathyroid Gland 78070

Nuclear Magnetic Resonance Imaging
See Magnetic Resonance Imaging (MRI)

Nuclear Magnetic Resonance Spectroscopy
See Magnetic Resonance Spectroscopy

Nuclear Matrix Protein 22 86386

Nuclear Medicine
Diagnostic
　Adrenal Gland Imaging 78075
　Bile Duct
　　Imaging. 78226, 78227
　Bladder
　　Residual Study 78730
　Blood
　Bone and Joint
　　Bone Density Study 78350, 78351
　　Imaging. 78300-78320
　　SPECT 78320
　　Ultrasound 76977
　　Flow Imaging 78445
　　Plasma Volume 78110-78121
　　Platelet Survival 78190, 78191
　　Red Cell Sequestration. 78140
　　Red Cell Survival 78130-78135
　　Red Cells Volume 78120, 78121
　　Unlisted Services and Procedures. 78199
　　Whole Blood Volume 78122
　Bone Marrow
　　Imaging 78102-78104
　Brain
　　Blood Flow 78610
　　Cerebrospinal Fluid Imaging. . . 78630-78650
　　Imaging. 78600-78609
　　PET Imaging 78608, 78609
　　Vascular Flow 78601, 78606, 78610
　Endocrine System
　　Parathyroid Gland Imaging. . . . 78070-78072
　　Unlisted Services and Procedures 78099
　Esophagus
　　Imaging (Motility). 78258
　　Reflux Study 78262
　Gallbladder
　　Imaging. 78226, 78227
　Gastric
　　Emptying Imaging Study. 78264-78266
　　Mucosa Imaging. 78261
　　Urea Breath Test. 78267, 78268
　　Vitamin B-12 Absorption
　　　Study. 78270-78272
　Gastroesophageal Reflux Study 78262
　Gastrointestinal
　　Blood Loss Imaging 78278
　　Intestine Imaging 78290
　　Peritoneal-Venous Shunt Patency 78291
　　Protein Loss Study 78282
　　Unlisted Services and Procedures 78299
　Genitourinary System
　　Unlisted Services and Procedures 78799
　Heart
　　Angiography 78445
　　Blood Flow 78414
　　Blood Pool Imaging. 78472, 78473,
　　　　　　　　　　　　78481-78483
　　Blood Pool SPECT Imaging 78494-78496
　　Myocardial Imaging . . . 78459, 78466-78469
　　Myocardial PET Imaging. 78459,
　　　　　　　　　　　　78491, 78492
　　Myocardial Perfusion
　　　Imaging 78451-78454
　　Shunt Detection 78428
　　Vascular Flow Imaging 78445
　　Venography. 78445
　　Venous Thrombosis Imaging . . 78456-78458
　　Unlisted Services and Procedures. 78499
　Hepatic Duct
　　Imaging. 78226, 78227

O

O2 Saturation
See Oxygen Saturation

Ober-Yount Procedure 27025
See Fasciotomy, Hip

Obliteration
Mastoid.......................... 69670
Vagina
    Total 57110-57112
    Vault 57120

Oblongata, Medulla
See Medulla

Observation 99217-99220,
                99224-99226, 99234-99236
See Evaluation and Management; Hospital
Services

Observational Behavioral Follow-Up Assessment 0360T, 0361T

Obstetrical Care
Abortion
    Induced
        by Amniocentesis Injection ... 59850-59852
          See Abortion; Cesarean Delivery; Ectopic
          Pregnancy
        by Dilation and Curettage 59840
        by Dilation and Evaluation 59841
    Missed
        First Trimester.................. 59820
        Second Trimester 59821
    Spontaneous 59812
    Therapeutic 59840-59852
Antepartum Care.................. 59425, 59426
Cesarean Delivery................. 59618-59622
    Only 59514
    Routine......................... 59510
    with Hysterectomy................. 59525
Curettage
    Hydatidiform Mole................. 59870
Evacuation
    Hydatidiform Mole................. 59870
External Cephalic Version.............. 59412
Miscarriage
    Surgical Completion.......... 59812-59821
Placenta Delivery 59414
Postpartum Care.................. 59430, 59514
Septic Abortion..................... 59830
Total (Global)........... 59400, 59610, 59618
Unlisted Services and Procedures ... 59898, 59899
Vaginal
    after Cesarean (VBAC)......... 59610-59614
Vaginal Delivery.............. 59409, 59410
    Delivery after Cesarean........ 59610-59614

Obstruction
See Occlusion

Obstruction Clearance
Venous Access Device 36595, 36596

Obstruction Colon
See Colon, Obstruction

Obturator Nerve
Avulsion 64763-64766
Incision 64763-64766
Transection 64763-64766

Obturator Prosthesis 21076
Definitive........................ 21080
Insertion
    Larynx....................... 31527
Interim........................... 21079

Occipital Nerve, Greater
Avulsion 64744
Incision 64744
Injection
    Anesthetic 64405
Transection 64744

Occlusion
Bronchi
    Balloon............. 31634, 31647, 31651
Vascular
    Arterial, other than Hemorrhage
    or Tumor...................... 37242
    Carotid Artery............... 37606, 61705
    during Endovascular Therapy.......... 34820
    for Hemorrhage 37244
    for Infarction 37243
    for Lymphatic Extravasation 37244
    for Organ Ischemia.............. 37243
    for Tumors 37243
    Nervous System
        Cranial 61623, 61624, 61626
        Spinal .. 61624, 61626, 62294, 63250-63252
    Placement of Occlusion Device........ 34808
    Veinous, other than Hemorrhage..... 37241
    with Ligation 37606
Fallopian Tube
    Oviduct.......... 58565, 58615, 58671
Penis
    Vein 37790
Umbilical Cord..................... 59072
Ureteral.......................... 50705

Occlusive Disease of Artery
See Repair, Artery; Revision

Occult Blood 82270-82272
by Hemoglobin Immunoassay............ 82274

Occupational Therapy
Evaluation 97003, 97004

Ocular Implant
See Orbital Implant
Insertion
    Drainage Device. ..0191T, 0253T, 0376T, 66183
    in Scleral Shell................. 65130
    Muscles, Attached................ 65140
    Muscles, Not Attached 65135
Modification 65125
Reinsertion 65150
    with Foreign Material 65155
Removal 65175

Ocular Muscle
See Eye Muscles

Ocular Orbit
See Orbit

Ocular Screening.......... 99174, 99177

Ocular Prostheses
See Prosthesis, Ocular

Oculomotor Muscle
See Eye Muscles

Oddi Sphincter
See Sphincter of Oddi

Odontoid Dislocation
Open Treatment/Reduction.............. 22318
    with Grafting 22319

Odontoid Fracture
Open Treatment/Reduction.............. 22318
    with Grafting 22319

Odontoid Process
Excision.......................... 22548

Oesophageal Neoplasm
See Tumor, Esophagus

Oesophageal Varices
See Esophageal Varices

Oesophagus
See Esophagus

Oestradiol
See Estradiol

Office and/or Other Outpatient Services
Consultation
    See Consultation
Established Patient................ 99211-99215
New Patient................... 99201-99205
Normal Newborn 99461
Office Visit
    Established Patient 99211-99215
    New Patient.................. 99201-99205
Outpatient Visit
    Established Patient 99211-99215
    New Patient.................. 99201-99205
    Prolonged Services 99354,
                99355, 99415, 99416

Office Medical Services
After Hours 99050
Emergency Care 99058
Extended Hours..................... 99051

Office or Other Outpatient Consultations
See Consultation, Office and/or Other Outpatient

Olecranon
See Elbow; Humerus; Radius; Ulna
Bursa
    Arthrocentesis 20605, 20606
Cyst
    Excision 24125, 24126
Tumor
    Cyst 24120
    Excision 24125, 24126

Olecranon Process
Craterization 24147
Diaphysectomy 24147
Excision.......................... 24147
    Abscess 24138
Fracture
    See Elbow; Humerus; Radius
    Closed Treatment............. 24670-24675
    Open Treatment 24685
Osteomyelitis 24138, 24147
Saucerization 24147
Sequestrectomy 24138

Oligoclonal Immunoglobulins .. 83916

Omentectomy 49255, 58950-58958
Laparotomy........................ 58960
Oophorectomy...................... 58943
Resection Ovarian Malignancy...... 58950-58952

Sofield Procedure 24410
Ssbanejew-Frank Operation 43830-43832
Stamey Procedure. 51845
Steindler Stripping 28250
Stenger Test 92565, 92577
Stookey-Scarff Procedures 62200
Strassman Procedure 58540
Strayer Procedure 01474
Sturmdorf Procedure 57520
Swanson Procedure 28309
Swenson Procedure 45120
Syme Procedure 27888
Takeuchi Procedure. 33505
Tenago Procedure 53431
Thal-Nissen Procedure 43325
Thiersch Operation 15050
Thiersch Procedure 46753
Thompson Procedure 27430
Tompkins metroplasty 58540
Torek Procedure 00930
Torkildsen Procedure 62180
Touroff Operation 37615
Tuffier Vaginal Hysterectomy 00944, 58260
Von Kraske Proctectomy 45111
Waldius Procedure 27445
Walsh Modified Radical 00865
Waterston Procedure 33755
Watson-Jones Procedure 27695-27698
Wertheim Operation 00846
Whipple Procedure 48150
Whitman Astragalectomy. 28120, 28130
Whitman Procedure 27120
Winiwater Operation 47720-47740
Winter Procedure 54435
Witzel Operation 43500, 43520, 43830-43832

Operation Microscopes
See Operating Microscope

Operculectomy 41821

Operculum
See Gums

Ophthalmic Mucous Membrane
Test 95060
See Allergy Tests

Ophthalmology
Unlisted Services and Procedures 92499
  See Ophthalmology, Diagnostic

Ophthalmology, Diagnostic
Color Vision Exam 92283
Computerized Scanning
    Anterior 92132
    Posterior. 92133, 92134
Dark Adaptation 92284
Electro-oculography 92270
Electromyography, Needle 92265
Electroretinography. 92275
Endoscopy. 66990
Evoked Potentials
    Acuity 0333T
    Central Nervous System 95930
Eye Exam
    Established Patient 92012-92014
    New Patient. 92002-92004
    with Anesthesia. 92018, 92019
Glaucoma Provocative Test. 92140
Gonioscopy 92020
Instrument-based Screening. 99172, 99174
Ocular Photography
    External 92285
Ophthalmoscopy. 92225, 92226

with Dynamometry. 92260
with Fluorescein Angiography. 92235
with Fluorescein Angioscopy. 92230
with Fundus Photography 92250
with Indocyanine-Green Angiography. . 92240
    Remote Imaging. 92227, 92228
Refractive Determination 92015
Retinal Imaging. 0380T
Sensorimotor Exam. 92060
Tear Film Imaging 0330T
Tonometry
    Serial 92100
Ultrasound. 76511-76529
Visual Acuity Screen. 99172, 99173
Visual Field Exam 0378T, 0379T, 92081-92083
Visual Function Screen 99172, 99174, 99177

Ophthalmoscopy 92225, 92226
See Ophthalmology, Diagnostic

Optic Nerve
Decompression 67570
    with Nasal/Sinus Endoscopy. 31294
Diagnostic Imaging
    Computerized Scanning. 92133
Head Evaluation 2027F

Optical Coherence Tomography
Axillary Lymph Node. 0351T, 0352T
Breast 0351T-0354T
Intravascular 0291T, 0292T

Optical Endomicroscopy
Esophageal 43206
Gastrointestinal 43252
with Endoscopic Retrograde
Cholangiopancreatography (ERCP) 0397T

Optokinetic Nystagmus Test
See Nystagmus Tests, Optokinetic

Oral Lactose Tolerance
Test 82951, 82952
See Glucose, Tolerance Test

Oral Mucosa
See Mouth, Mucosa

Oral Surgical Splint 21085

Orbit
See Orbital Contents; Orbital Floor; Periorbital
Region
Biopsy 61332
    Exploration 67450
    Fine Needle Aspiration or Orbital
    Contents. 67415
    Orbitotomy without Bone Flap. 67400
Bone Graft. 21182-21184,
        21256, 21260, 21267, 21395, 21408
CT Scan. 70480-70482
Decompression 61330
    Bone Removal 67414, 67445
Exploration 61332, 67400, 67450
Lesion
    Excision. 61333
Fracture
    Closed Treatment
        with Manipulation 21401
        without Manipulation. 21400
    Open Treatment 21406-21408
        Blowout Fracture 21385-21395
Incision and Drainage 67405, 67440
Injection
    Retrobulbar 67500-67505
    Tenon's Capsule 67515

Insertion
    Implant. 67550
Lesion
    Excision 67412, 67420
Magnetic Resonance Imaging
(MRI) 70540-70543
Removal
    Bone 67445
    Foreign Body 67413, 67430
    Implant 67560
    Lesion. 61333
Sella Turcica 70482
Unlisted Services and Procedures 67599
X-ray 70190-70200

Orbit Area
Reconstruction
    Secondary 21275

Orbit Wall
Decompression
    with Nasal/Sinus Endoscopy. . . . 31292, 31293

Orbital Contents
Aspiration 67415

Orbital Floor
See Orbit; Periorbital Region
Fracture
    Blow Out 21385-21395

Orbital Hypertelorism
Osteotomy
    Periorbital. 21260-21263

Orbital Implant
See Ocular Implant
Insertion 67550
Removal 67560

Orbital Prosthesis 21077

Orbital Rim and Forehead
Reconstruction 21172-21180

Orbital Rims
Reconstruction 21182-21184

Orbital Transplant 67560

Orbital Walls
Reconstruction 21182-21184

Orbitocraniofacial Reconstruction
Secondary 21275

Orbitotomy
with Bone Flap
    for Exploration 67450
    Lateral Approach 67420
    with Drainage 67440
    with Removal Foreign Body. 67430
    with Removal of Bone for
    Decompression 67445
with Removal Foreign Body 67413
with Removal of Bone for Decompression. . . 67414
without Bone Flap
    for Exploration 67400
    with Drainage Only 67405
    with Removal Lesion 67412

Orchidectomies
See Excision, Testis

Orchidopexy
See Orchiopexy

Orchidoplasty
See Repair, Testis

P

Oxidoreductase, Alcohol-Nad+
See Antidiuretic Hormone

Oximetry (Noninvasive)
See Pulmonology, Diagnostic
Blood O2 Saturation Determination
    Ear or Pulse 94760-94762
    Pulse, Recording
      Car Seat/Bed Testing 94780, 94781
    with Pulmonary Stress Testing . . 94620, 94621

Oxoisomerase
See Phosphohexose Isomerase

Oxosteroids
See Ketosteroids

Oxygen Saturation 82805-82810

Oxygenation, Extracorporeal Membrane
See Extracorporeal Membrane Oxygenation (ECMO)

Oxyproline
See Hydroxyproline

Oxytocin Stress Test, Fetal 59020

P

P&P
See Proconvertin

P B Antibodies
See Antibody, Detection, Heterophile

Pacemaker, Heart
See Cardiology; Electrocardiography
Conversion
    Single to Dual Chamber 33214
Data Analysis 93288, 93293, 93294
Electronic Analysis 93288
    Antitachycardia System 93724
Evaluation and Programming
    Dual Lead 93280, 93286, 93288, 93289
    Implantable Subcutaneous
      Lead 93260, 93261
    In Person 93261, 93279-93281,
                    93286, 93288, 93289
    Multiple Lead 93281, 93286, 93288, 93289
    Remote 93293, 93294, 93296
    Single Lead 93279, 93286, 93288, 93289
Insertion 33206-33208
    Electrode 33202, 33203, 33216,
                    33217, 33224, 33225
    Pulse Generator Only 33212, 33213, 33221
    Temporary Catheter or
    Electrode 33210, 33211, 93583
Leadless System
    Device Evaluation, in Person
      Interrogation 0391T
      Peri-procedural 0390T
      Programming 0389T
    Transcatheter Insertion 0387T
    Transcatheter Removal 0388T
    Transcatheter Replacement 0387T
Placement
    Lead 33202, 33203
Relocation
    Skin pocket 33222

Removal
    Pulse Generator Only 33233
    Transvenous Electrodes 33234, 33235
    via Thoracotomy 33236, 33237
Repair
    Electrode 33218-33220
Replacement
    Catheter 33210
    Electrode 33210, 33211
    Insertion 33206-33208
    Pulse Generator 33227-33229
Repositioning
    Electrode 33215, 33226
Telephonic Analysis 93293
Upgrade 33214

Pachymetry
Cornea 76514
    with Collagen Cross-Linking 0402T

Packing
Nasal Hemorrhage 30901-30906

Pain Management
Electrical Reprocessing 0278T
Epidural/Intrathecal 62350, 62351,
             62360-62362, 99601, 99602
Intravenous Therapy . . . 96365-96368, 96374-96379

Palate
Abscess
    Incision and Drainage 42000
Biopsy 42100
Bone Graft 42210
Excision
    Lesion 42120
Fracture
    Closed Treatment 21421
    Open Treatment 21422, 21423
Lesion
    Destruction 42160
    Excision 42104-42120
Prosthesis
    Augmentation 21082
    Impression 42280
    Insertion 42281
    Lift 21083
Reconstruction
    Lengthening 42226, 42227
Repair
    Cleft Palate 42200-42225
    Laceration 42180-42182
    Vomer Flap 42235
Unlisted Services and Procedures 42299

Palate, Cleft
See Cleft Palate

Palatoplasty 42145, 42200-42225

Palatoschisis
See Cleft Palate

Palm
Arch
    Sympathectomy 64823
Bursa
    Incision and Drainage 26025-26030
Dupuytren's Contracture
    Injection 20527
    Manipulation 26341
Fascial Cord
    Enzyme Injection 20527
    Manipulation 26341
Fasciectomy 26121-26123
Fasciotomy 26040-26045

Injection, Enzyme
    Fascial Cord 20527
    Dupuytren's Contracture 20527
Tendon
    Excision 26170
    Incision 26450
    Lysis 26440, 26442
    Transfer 26485, 26489
Tendon Sheath
    Excision 26145
    Incision and Drainage 26020

Palsy, Seventh Nerve
See Facial Nerve Paralysis

Pancreas
Anastomosis
    with Intestines 48520-48540, 48548
Biopsy 48100
    Needle Biopsy 48102
Cyst
    Anastomosis 48520-48540
    Repair 48500
Debridement
    Peripancreatic Tissue 48105
Dilation
    Ampulla of Vater 47542, 43277
Endoscopy
    See Endoscopy, Pancreatic Duct
Excision
    Ampulla of Vater 48148
    Duct 48148
    Partial 48140-48146, 48150, 48154, 48160
    Peripancreatic Tissue 48105
    Total 48155-48160
Lesion
    Ablation 43278
    Excision 48120
Needle Biopsy 48102
Placement
    Drainage 48000, 48001
Polyp
    Ablation 43278
Pseudocyst
    Drainage
      Open 48510
      Percutaneous 49405
Removal
    Calculi (Stone) 43264, 48020
Removal Transplanted Allograft 48556
Repair
    Cyst 48500
Resection 48105
Suture 48545
Transplantation 48160, 48550, 48554-48556
    Allograft Preparation 48550-48552
Tumor
    Ablation 43278
Unlisted Services and Procedures 48999
X-ray 74300, 74301
    Injection Procedure 48400

Pancreas, Endocrine Only
See Islet Cell

Pancreatectomy
Donor 48550
Partial 48140-48146, 48150-48154, 48160
Total 48155-48160
with Transplantation 48160

Pancreatic DNAse
See DNAse

Index

Peans' Operation
See Amputation, Leg, Upper, at Hip; Radical Resection; Replantation

Pectoral Cavity
See Chest Cavity

Pectus Carinatum
Reconstructive Repair. 21740-21743
　　with Thoracoscopy. 21743

Pectus Excavatum
Reconstructive Repair. 21740-21742
　　with Thoracoscopy. 21743

Pediatric Critical Care 99471, 99472

Pediatric Intensive Care 99478

Pedicle Fixation
Insertion 22840, 22842-22844

Pedicle Flap
Abbe-Estlander Type. 40761
for Breast Reconstruction
　　Double 19369
　　Single. 19367
for Cerebrospinal Fluid Leak. 61619
for Eyelid Repair 67961
for Lip Repair. 40761
for Vaginal Lengthening 46748
Formation 15570-15576
Island. 15740
Neurovascular. 15750
Transfer. 15650
Vascular 15731

PEEP
See Pressure Breathing, Positive

Pelvi-Ureteroplasty
See Pyeloplasty

Pelvic Adhesions
See Adhesions, Pelvic

Pelvic Exam
Preventive 99397
under Anesthesia 57410

Pelvic Exenteration 45126,
　　　　　　　　　　　　　　　　51597, 58240

Pelvic Fixation
See Spinal Instrumentation

Pelvic Lymphadenectomy 38770,
　　　　　　　　38780, 55845, 55865, 57531,
　　　　　　　　58210, 58210, 58548, 58958

Pelvimetry 74710

Pelviolithotomy 50130

Pelvis
See Hip
Abscess
　　Incision and Drainage 26990, 45000
Angiography 72191, 74174
Biopsy. 27040, 27041
Bone
　　Drainage. 26992
Brace Application 20662
Bursa
　　Incision and Drainage 26991
CT Scan. 72191-72194, 74174, 74176-74178
Destruction
　　Lesion. 58662

Endoscopy
　　Destruction of Lesion. 58662
　　Lysis of Adhesions 58660
Exclusion
　　Small Intestine. 44700
Exenteration 45126, 51597, 58240
Fasciotomy
　　Decompression 27027
　　　　with Debridement. 27057
Halo. 20662
Hematoma
　　Incision and Drainage 26990
Lysis
　　Adhesions 58660
Magnetic Resonance Angiography. 72198
Magnetic Resonance Imaging
(MRI) 72195-72197
　　Obstetric. 74712, 74713
Removal
　　Foreign Body 27086, 27087
Repair
　　Osteotomy 27158
　　Tendon 27098
Ring Dislocation/Fracture
　　Closed Treatment. 27193, 27194
　　　　with Manipulation 27194
　　Open Treatment 27217, 27218
　　　　with Internal Fixation 27217, 27218
　　Percutaneous Skeletal Fixation 27216
Tumor
　　Excision 27043-27048
　　Radical Resection 27049, 27059
Ultrasound. 76856, 76857
Unlisted Services and Procedures for
Hips and Hip Joint 27299
X-ray 72170-72190
　　with Hip(s) 73501-73503, 73521-73523
　　Manometry. 74710

Pemberton Osteotomy of Pelvis 27158

Penectomy
See Amputation, Penis

Penetrating Keratoplasties
See Keratoplasty, Penetrating

Penile Induration
See Peyronie Disease

Penile Prosthesis
Insertion
　　Inflatable 54401-54405
　　Noninflatable. 54400
Removal
　　Inflatable 54406, 54410-54417
　　Semi-rigid. 54415-54417
Repair
　　Inflatable 54408
Replacement
　　Inflatable 54410, 54411, 54416, 54417
　　Semi-rigid. 54416, 54417

Penile Rigidity Test 54250

Penile Tumescence Test 54250

Penis
Amputation
　　Complete 54125
　　Partial. 54120
　　Radical 54130-54135
　　Replanted. 54438
Biopsy 54100-54105

Circumcision
　　Lysis of Adhesions 54162
　　Repair. 54163
　　Surgical Excision
　　　　Newborn. 54150, 54160, 54161
Destruction
　　Lesion. . . . 54050, 54055-54057, 54060, 54065
Drainage 54015
Excision
　　Partial. 54120
　　Prepuce 54150-54161, 54163
　　Total 54125-54135
Frenulotomy 54164
Incision
　　Frenulum 54164
　　Prepuce 54000, 54001
Incision and Drainage 54015
Injection
　　for Erection. 54235
　　Peyronie Disease 54200
　　　　Surgical Exposure Plaque. 54205
　　Vasoactive Drugs. 54231
　　X-ray. 54230
Insertion
　　Prosthesis
　　　　Inflatable 54401-54405
　　　　Noninflatable 54400
Irrigation
　　Priapism. 54220
Lesion
　　Destruction
　　　　Cryosurgery. 54056
　　　　Electrodesiccation 54055
　　　　Extensive 54065
　　　　Laser Surgery 54057, 54065
　　　　Simple. 54050-54060
　　　　Surgical Excision 54060
　　Excision 54060
　　　　Penile Plaque 54110-54112
Nocturnal Penile Tumescence Test. 54250
Occlusion
　　Vein 37790
Plaque
　　Excision 54110-54112
Plethysmography. 54240
Prepuce
　　Adhesions
　　　　Lysis 54450
　　Slitting 54000, 54001
　　Stretching. 54450
Removal
　　Foreign Body 54115
　　Prosthesis
　　　　Inflatable 54406, 54410-54417
　　　　Semi-rigid. 54415-54417
Repair
　　Angulation 54360
　　Chordee 54300-54304, 54328
　　Complications 54340-54348
　　Epispadias 54380-54390
　　Fistulization 54435
　　Hypospadias. 54328-54352
　　Injury 54440
　　Priapism with Shunt. 54420-54430
　　Prosthesis
　　　　Inflatable 54408
　　　　Corporeal Tear(s) 54437
Replacement
　　Prosthesis
　　　　Inflatable 54410, 54411, 54416, 54417
　　　　Semi-rigid. 54416, 54417
Replantation 54438
Revascularization 37788

Pericardiocentesis 33010, 33011
Ultrasound Guidance 76930

Pericardiostomy
Tube 33015

Pericardiotomy
Removal
    Clot 33020
    Foreign Body 33020

Pericardium
Biopsy
    Endoscopic 32604
Cyst
    Excision 32661
    Resection 33050
Diagnostic Thoracoscopy 32601
Excision 33030, 33031
    Window, for Drainage 32659, 33025
Incision
    Removal
        Clot 33020
        Foreign Body 33020
    Pericardiostomy 33015
Incision and Drainage 33025
Mass
    Excision 32661
Puncture Aspiration 33010, 33011
Removal
    Endoscopic
        Clot 32658
        Foreign Body 32658
Tumor
    Excision 32661
    Resection 33050

Peridural Anesthesia
Infusion 62318, 62319
Injection 62310, 62311

Peridural Injection
See Epidural, Injection

Perineal Prostatectomy
See Prostatectomy, Perineal

Perineoplasty 56810

Perineorrhaphy
Repair
    Rectocele 57250

Perineum
Abscess
    Incision and Drainage 56405
Biopsy
    Lesion 56605, 56606
Colostomy 50810
Anogenital Examination
    with Magnification and Image
    Recording 99170
Debridement
    Infected 11004, 11006
Removal
    Prosthesis 53442
Repair 56810
X-ray with Contrast 74775

Perionychia
See Paronychia

Periorbital Region
Reconstruction
    Osteotomy with Graft 21267, 21268
Repair, Osteotomy 21260-21263
Treatment

Orbital Floor Blowout Fracture 21386,
                                21390, 21395

**Peripheral Artery Disease (PAD)
Rehabilitation** 93668

Peripheral Nerve
Repair/Suture
    Major 64856, 64857, 64859

Periprosthetic Capsulectomy
Breast 19371

Peristaltic Pumps
See Infusion Pump

**Peritoneal
Dialysis** 90945-90947, 4055F
Catheter Insertion 49418, 49419, 49421
Catheter Removal 49422
Home Infusion 99601, 99602
Kt/V Level 3082F-3084F
Plan of Care Documented 0507F

Peritoneal Free Air
See Pneumoperitoneum

Peritoneal Lavage 49084

Peritoneoscopy
See Peritoneum, Endoscopy

Peritoneum
Abscess
    Incision and Drainage 49020
        Percutaneous 49406
Chemotherapy Administration 96446
    See Chemotherapy
Drainage
    Image Guided Fluid Collection ... 49406, 49407
    Intramedullary Cyst/Syrinx 63173
    Lymphocele 49062, 49323
Endoscopy
    Biopsy 49321
    Diagnostic 49320
    Drainage
        Lymphocele 49323
    Insertion
        Catheter 49324
    Revision
        Cannula/Catheter 49326
Exchange
    Drainage Catheter 49423
Injection
    Air 49400
    Contrast 49400
        via Catheter 49424
Insertion
    Catheter 49418, 49419
        for Dialysis 49421
    Shunt
        Peritoneal-Venous 49425
        Subarachnoid/Subdural-
        Peritoneal 62192, 63740, 63741
        Ventriculo-Peritoneal 62223
Lavage 49084
Lesion
    Excision
        Laparoscopic 58662
    Fulguration
        Laparoscopic 58662
Ligation
    Shunt 49428

Removal
    Catheter 49422
    Foreign Body 49402
    Shunt 49429
Shunt, Peritoneal-Venous
    Insertion 49425
    Ligation 49428
    Radiologic Evaluation 78291
        Injection, Contrast 49427
    Removal 49429
    Revision 49426
Tumor
    Destruction 49203-49205
    Excision 49203-49205
    Resection 58950-58958
Unlisted Services and Procedures 49999
    Laparoscopic 49329
Venous Shunt
    Injection 49427
X-ray 74190
    Injection
        Air/Contrast 49400

Persistent Truncus Arteriosus
See Truncus Arteriosus

**Persistent, Omphalomesenteric
Duct**
See Diverticulum, Meckel's

Personal Care
See Self Care

Personality Test 96101-96103
Computer-Assisted 96103

Pessary
Insertion 57160

Pesticides
Chlorinated Hydrocarbons 82441

PET
See Positron Emission Tomography (PET)

Petrous Temporal
Excision
    Apex 69530

Peyronie Disease
Excision
Penile Plaque 54110-54112
Excision with Graft 54110-54112
Injection 54200
Surgical Exposure 54205

pH
Blood Gases 82800, 82803
Exhaled Breath Condensate 83987
Gastric Acid 82930
Other Fluid 83986
Urine 81000-81003, 83986

Phacoemulsification
Removal
    Extracapsular Cataract 66982, 66984
    Secondary Membranous Cataract 66850

Phagocytosis
White Blood Cells 86344

Phalangectomy
Toe 28150
    Partial 28160

Photography
Fundus 92250
Ocular 92285
Skin
　　Monitoring 96904

Photography, Ocular 92285

Photon Beam Therapy
See Radiation Therapy, Treatment Delivery

Photopheresis
Blood 36522
See Actinotherapy; Photochemotherapy

Photoradiation Therapies
See Actinotherapy

Photosensitivity Testing 95056
See Allergy Tests

Phototherapies
See Actinotherapy

Phototherapy, Ultraviolet
See Actinotherapy

Phrenic Nerve
Anastomosis
Avulsion 64746
Incision 64746
Injection
　　Anesthetic 64410
Transection 64746

Physical Medicine/Therapy/ Occupational Therapy
See Neurology, Diagnostic
Activities of Daily Living 97535, 99509
Aquatic Therapy
　　with Exercises 97113
Athletic Training
　　Evaluation 97005
　　Re-Evaluation 97006
Check-Out
　　Orthotic/Prosthetic 97762
Cognitive Skills Development 97532
Community/Work Reintegration 97537
Evaluation
　　Athletic Training 97005, 97006
　　Occupational Therapy 97003, 97004
　　Physical Therapy 97001, 97002
Kinetic Therapy 97530
Manual Therapy 97140
Modalities
　　Contrast Baths 97034
　　Diathermy Treatment 97024
　　Electric Stimulation
　　　　Attended, Manual 97032
　　　　Unattended 97014
　　Hot or Cold Pack 97010
　　Hydrotherapy (Hubbard Tank) 97036
　　Infrared Light Treatment 97026
　　Iontophoresis 97033
　　Microwave Therapy 97024
　　Paraffin Bath 97018
　　Traction 97012
　　Ultrasound 97035
　　Ultraviolet Light 97028
　　Unlisted Modality 97039
　　Vasopneumatic Device 97016
　　Whirlpool Therapy 97022
Orthotics Training 97760
Osteopathic Manipulation 98925-98929
Procedures
　　Aquatic Therapy 97113

Direct 97032-97039
Gait Training 97116
Group Therapeutic 97150
Massage Therapy 97124
Neuromuscular Reeducation 97112
Physical Performance Test 97750
Supervised 97010-97028
Therapeutic Exercises 97110
Traction Therapy 97140
Work Hardening 97545, 97546
Prosthetic Training 97761
Self-care Training 97535
Sensory Integration 97533
Therapeutic Activities
　　One-on-one Patient Contact 97530
Unlisted Services and Procedures ... 97139, 97799
Wheelchair Management 97542
Work Reintegration 97537

Physical Therapy
See Physical Medicine/Therapy/Occupational Therapy

Physician Services
Care Plan Oversight Services 99339, 99340, 99374-99380
　　Domiciliary Facility 99339, 99340
　　Home Health Agency Care 99374, 99375
　　Home or Rest Home Care 99339, 99340
　　Hospice 99377, 99378
　　Liver Assist System Patient
　　　Oversight 0405T
　　Nursing Facility 99379, 99380
Case Management Services 99366-99368
Consultation, Interprofessional
　　Telephone/Internet Discussion .. 99446-99449
Direction, Advanced Life Support 99288
Online 99444
Prolonged
　　with Direct Patient Contact 99354-99357
　　　Inpatient 99356, 99357
　　　Outpatient/Office 99354,
　　　　　　　　　　　99355, 99415, 99416
　　without Direct Patient Contact .. 99358, 99359
Standby 99360
Supervision, Care Plan Oversight Services .. 99339, 99340, 99374-99380
Team Conference 99367
　　Telephone 99441-99443

Piercing of Ear Lobe 69090

Piles
See Hemorrhoids

Pilonidal Cyst
Excision 11770-11772
Incision and Drainage 10080, 10081

Pin
See Wire
Application, Uniplane External Fixation System
　See External Fixation
Insertion/Removal
　　Skeletal Traction 20650
Retention, Palatal Prosthesis 42281
Prophylactic Treatment
　　Femur 27187
　　Humerus 24498
　　Shoulder 23490, 23491
Removal 20670, 20680

Pinch Graft 15050

Pinna
See Ear, External Ear

Pinworms
Examination 87172

Pirogoff Procedure 27888

Pituitary Epidermoid Tumor
See Craniopharyngioma

Pituitary Gland
Excision 61546-61548
Tumor
　　Excision 61546-61548, 62165

Pituitary Growth Hormone
See Growth Hormone

Pituitary Lactogenic Hormone
See Prolactin

Pituitectomy
See Pituitary Gland, Excision

PKU
See Phenylalanine

Placement
Adjustable Gastric Restrictive Device 43770
Catheter
　　Aneurysm Sac
　　　Pressure Sensor 34806
　　　　Complete Study 93982
　　Brain
　　　for Chemotherapy 0169T
　　Breast
　　　for Interstitial Radioelement
　　　　Application 19296-19298, 20555, 41019
　　Bronchus
　　　for Intracavitary Radioelement
　　　　Application 31643
　　　　See Catheterization
　　Head
　　　Interstitial Radioelement
　　　　Application 41019
　　Kidney
　　　Nephrostomy 50432
　　　Nephroureteral 50433
　　Neck
　　　Interstitial Radioelement
　　　　Application 41019
　　Pelvic Organs
　　　Interstitial Radioelement
　　　　Application 55920
　　Prostate 55875
　　Renal Artery
　　　Selective 36251, 36252
　　　Superselective 36253, 36254
　　Ureter via Kidney 50695
Catheter, Cardiac 93503
　　See Catheterization, Cardiac
Cecostomy Tube 44300, 49442
Dosimeter
　　Prostate 55876
Drainage
　　Pancreas 48001
Duodenostomy Tube 49441
Endoscopic Access
　　Biliary Tract 47541
Endovascular Prosthesis
　　Aorta 33883-33886
Enterostomy Tube 44300
Esophageal Sphincter Augmentation
　　Device 0392T
Fiducial Markers
　　Bronchus 31626
　　Prostate 55876
Gastrostomy Tube 43246, 49440

Pleurectomy
Parietal 32310-32320
   Endoscopic 32656

Pleuritis, Purulent
See Pleural Cavity, Incision, Empyema

Pleurocentesis
See Thoracentesis

Pleurodesis
Thoracoscopic 32650
Instillation of Agent 32560

Pleurosclerosis
See Pleurodesis

Pleurosclerosis, Chemical
See Pleurodesis, Instillation of Agent

Plexectomy, Choroid
See Choroid Plexus, Excision

Plexus
Brachialis
   See Brachial Plexus
Cervicalis
   See Cervical Plexus
Choroid
   See Choroid Plexus
Coeliacus
   See Celiac Plexus
Lumbalis
   See Lumbar Plexus

PLGN
See Plasminogen

Plication, Sphincter, Urinary Bladder
See Bladder, Repair, Neck

Pneumocisternogram
See Cisternography

Pneumococcal Vaccine
See Vaccines

Pneumocystis Carinii
Antigen Detection
   Immunofluorescence 87281

Pneumogastric Nerve
See Vagus Nerve

Pneumogram
Infant 94772

Pneumolysis
See Pneumonolysis

Pneumonectomy 32440-32445
Thoracoscopic 32671
Completion 32488
Donor 32850, 33930
Sleeve 32442

Pneumonology
See Pulmonology

Pneumonolysis 32940
Intrapleural 32652
Open Intrapleural 32124

Pneumonostomy 32200

Pneumonotomy
See Incision, Lung

Pneumoperitoneum
Injection of Air 49400

Pneumothorax
Pleurodesis 32560
Pleural Scarification for Repeat 32215
Therapeutic
   Injection Intrapleural Air 32960

Polio
Antibody Detection 86658
Vaccine 90713

Poliovirus Vaccine
See Vaccines

Pollicization
Digit 26550

Polya Gastrectomy
See Gastrectomy, Partial

Polydactylism
See Polydactyly; Supernumerary Digit

Polydactyly
Finger
   Reconstruction 26587
   Repair 26587
Toe 28344

Polyp
Ablation
  Endoscopic
    Anus 46615
    Colon 44401, 45388
    Esophagus 43229
    Rectum 45320, 45346
    Small Intestine 44369
    Upper Gastrointestinal Tract . . 43270, 43278
Antrochoanal
  Removal 31032
Anus
  Ablation
    Endoscopic 46615
  Removal
    Endoscopic 46610-46612
Colon
  Ablation 44401, 45388
  Removal 44392, 44394, 45384, 45385
Esophagus
  Ablation 43229
  Removal 43216, 43217
Excision
  Ear 69540
  Nose
    Endoscopic 31237-31240
    Extensive 30115
    Simple 30110
  Urethra 53260
  Uterus 58558
Fulguration
  Urethra 53260
  Endoscopic
    Bladder 52285
    Urethra 52285
Nose
  Excision
    Endoscopic 31237-31240
    Extensive 30115
    Simple 30110
Rectum
  Ablation
    Endoscopic 45320, 45346
  Removal
    Endoscopic 45308, 45309, 45315, 45333

Removal
  Endoscopic
    Anus 46610-46612
    Colon 44392, 44394, 45384, 45385
    Esophagus 43216, 43217
    Rectum 45308, 45309, 45315, 45333
    Small Intestine 44364, 44365
    Upper Gastrointestinal Tract . 43250, 43251
Small Intestine
  Ablation
    Endoscopic 44369
  Removal
    Endoscopic 44364, 44365
Sphenoid Sinus
  Removal 31051
Urethra
  Excision 53260
  Fulguration 53260
Uterus
  Excision 58558

Polypectomy
Nose
  Endoscopic 31237-31240
  Extensive 30115
  Simple 30110
Urethra 53260
Uterus 58558

Polypeptide, Vasoactive Intestinal
See Vasoactive Intestinal Peptide

Polysomnography 95782,
              95783, 95808-95811

Pomeroy's Operation
See Tubal Ligation

Pooling
Blood Products 86965
Cardiac Blood Pool Imaging
   See Blood Pool Imaging

Popliteal Arteries
See Artery, Popliteal

Popliteal Synovial Cyst
See Baker's Cyst

Poradenitistras
See Lymphogranuloma Venereum

PORP (Partial Ossicular Replacement Prosthesis) 69633, 69637

Porphobilinogen
Urine 84106-84110

Porphyrin Precursors 82135

Porphyrins
Feces 84126
Urine 84119, 84120

Port Image(s) 77417

Portal Vein
See Vein, Hepatic Portal

Portoenterostomies, Hepatic
See Hepaticoenterostomy

Portoenterostomy 47701

Positional Nystagmus Test
See Nystagmus Tests, Positional

Placement 34806
Ulcer (Decubitus)
  Excision
    Coccygeal 15920, 15922
    Ischial 15940, 15941, 15944-15946
    Sacral 15931, 15933-15937
    Trochanteric . . . 15950-15953, 15956, 15958
    Unlisted Procedure 15999
Venous
  See Blood Pressure, Venous
Voiding
  See Voiding Pressure Studies

Pretreatment
Red Blood Cell
  Antibody Identification 86970-86972
Serum
  Antibody Identification 86975-86978

Prevention & Control
See Prophylaxis

Preventive Medicine
Behavior Change Intervention
  Individual
    Substance Abuse Other Than
      Tobacco 99408, 99409
    Tobacco Use Cessation 99406, 99407
  Group
    Diabetes Prevention 0403T
    Risk Factor Reduction 99411, 99412
Comprehensive
  Established Patient 99382-99397
  New Patient 99381-99387
Counseling
  Individual
    Behavior Change 99406-99408
    Exercise 4019F
    Risk Factor Reduction
      Intervention 99401-99404
    Self-Examination for Moles 5005F
  Group Counseling. 99411, 99412
Fluoride Varnish Application. 99188
Health Risk Assessment 99420
Immunization
  See Immunization Administration; Vaccines
Interventions
  See; Performance Measures, Preventive Care
  and Screening
Newborn Care
  See Newborn Care, Normal
Unlisted Services and Procedures 99429

Priapism
Repair
  Fistulization 54435
  with Shunt 54420-54430

Primidone
Assay. 80188

PRL
See Prolactin

Procalcitonin (PCT) 84145

Pro-Insulin C Peptide
See C-Peptide

Proalbumin
See Prealbumin

Probes, DNA
See Nucleic Acid Probe

Probes, Nucleic Acid
See Nucleic Acid Probe

Procainamide
Assay. 80190-80192

Procalcitonin (PCT) 84145

Process
Coracoid
  Transfer 23462
Coronoid
  Coronoidectomy. 21070
Odontoid
  Excision 22548
  Fracture 22318
Olecranon
  Craterization. 24147
  Diaphysectomy. 24147
  Excision, Cyst or Tumor . . 24120, 24125, 24126
  Saucerization 24147
  Sequestrectomy. 24138
Spinous
  Wiring 22841
  Insertion, Distraction Device 0171T, 0172T
Styloid
  Fracture 25650, 25652
  Styloidectomy 25230, 25440
Vertebral
  Excision 22100-22103, 22110, 22116
  Fracture 22305

Procidentia
Rectum
  Excision 45130-45135
  Reduction 45900

Procoagulant Activity, Glomerular
See Thromboplastin

Proconvertin 85230

Proctectasia
See Dilation, Rectum

Proctectomy
Partial
  Open 45113-45116, 45123
Total 45110-45112, 45119-45121
  Laparoscopic 45395-45397
  Open. 45110, 45112, 45119, 45120
with Colectomy. 44155-44158, 45121
  Laparoscopic 44211, 44212
with Colectomy/Ileostomy
  Laparoscopic 44212
  Open 44155
with Pelvic Exenteration. 45126

Proctocele
See Rectocele

Proctopexy
Laparoscopic. 45400-45402
  with Sigmoid Resection. 45402
Open 45540, 45541
  with Sigmoid Excision 45550

Proctoplasty. 45500-45505

Proctorrhaphy
See Rectum, Suture

Proctoscopies
See Anoscopy

Proctosigmoidoscopy
Ablation
  Polyp or Lesion. 45320
Biopsy. 45305
Collection of Specimen. 45300

Destruction
  Tumor. 45320
Diagnostic. 45300
Dilation 45303
Exploration 45300
Hemorrhage Control 45317
Placement
  Stent. 45327
Removal
  Foreign Body 45307
  Polyp. 45308-45315
  Tumor. 45315
Volvulus Repair. 45321

Products, Gene
See Protein

Proetz Therapy
Nose 30210

Profibrinolysin
See Plasminogen

Progenitor Cell
See Stem Cell

Progesterone. 84144

Progesterone Receptors 84234

Progestin Receptors
See Progesterone Receptors

Proinsulin 84206

Projective Test
Psychological Testing 96101-96103
Psychiatric Evaluation. 90885

Prokallikrein
See Fletcher Factor

Prokallikrein, Plasma
See Fletcher Factor

Prokinogenase
See Fletcher Factor

Prolactin. 80418, 84146

Prolapse
See Procidentia

Prolapse, Rectal
See Procidentia, Rectum

Prolastin
See Alpha-1 Antitrypsin

Prolonged Services 99354-99360
with Direct Patient Contact 99354-99357
  Inpatient. 99356, 99357
  Outpatient/Office. 99354, 99355
    Clinical Staff with Physician
    Supervision. 99415, 99416

Prophylactic Treatment
See Preventive Medicine
Antibiotic. 4042F, 4045F, 4046F-4049F
Antimicrobial
  Cefazolin or Cefuroxime. 4041F, 4043F
Clavicle
  Methylmethacrylate. 23490
  Nailing 23490
  Pinning 23490
  Plating 23490
  Wiring 23490
Deep Vein Thrombosis 4070F

Radial Head 24666
Radius, Distal 25441, 25446
Scaphoid Carpal 25443
Trapezium 25445
Ulnar 25442, 24363
Revision 24370, 24371
Wrist 25446

Knee
Arthroplasty
Insertion 27438, 27445
Intraoperative Use, Kinetic Balance
Sensor 0396T
Removal 27488

Lens
Insertion 66982-66985
Repositioning 66825
without Cataract Removal 66985

Mandible 21125
Nasal Septum
Insertion 30220

Ocular 65770, 66982-66985
Telescope Prosthesis 0308T
Temporary 92358

Orbital 21179

Orthotic
Check-Out 97762
Training 97761

Ossicle Reconstruction
Chain 69633

Palate 42280, 42281
Penis
Insertion 54400-54405
Removal 54406, 54415
Repair 54408
Replacement 54410, 54411, 54416, 54417

Perineum
Removal 53442

Retina
Placement
Pulse Generator 0100T
Receiver 0100T

Shoulder
Removal 23334, 23335

Skull Plate
Removal 62142
Replacement 62143

Spectacle
Fitting 92352, 92353
Repair 92371

Speech Aid
Insertion 31611

Spine
Insertion 22851

Synthetic 69633, 69637

Temporomandibular Joint
Arthroplasty 21243

Testis
Insertion 54520, 54660

Tissue Expander, Other than Breast
Insertion 11960
Removal without Prosthesis Insertion . . 11971
Replacement with Prosthesis 11970

Training 97761

Unlisted Maxillofacial Prosthetic
Procedure 21089

Urethral Sphincter
Insertion 53444, 53445
Removal 53446, 53447
Repair 53449
Replacement 53448

Vagina
Insertion 57267
Removal 57295, 57296, 57426

Revision 57295, 57296, 57426
Wrist
Insertion 25443-25446
Removal 25250, 25251

Prosthetic Valve, Aortic Valve Replacement
See Aortic Valve Replacement, with Prosthesis

Protease F
See Plasmin

Protein
A, Plasma (PAPP-A) 84163
Apoliproprotein A1 81503
Analysis, Tissue
Western Blot 88371
Beta-2 Microglobulin 81503
C
Activated (APC) 85307
Activator 85337
Activity 85303
Antigen 85302
Reactive 86140, 86141
Resistance Assay 85307
CA-125 . . . . 81500, 81503
Cerebrospinal Fluid 83873
DIA 81509
Electrophoresis 84165, 84166
Western Blot 84181, 84182
Other Fluids 84166
Glycated 82985
hCG 81508, 81509
HE4 81500
Human Epididymis Protein 4 86305
Myelin Basic 83873
Nuclear Matrix Protein 22 (NMP22) 86386
Osteocalcin 83937
PAPP-A 81508, 81509
Prealbumin 81503, 84134
S
Free 85306
Total 85305
Serum, Plasma or Whole Blood 84155, 84165
Total 84155-84157
by Refractometry 84160
Transferrin 81503
Urine 84156
Urine 84156
Dipstick 81000
Western Blot 84181, 84182, 88371, 88372

Protein Analysis, Tissue
Western Blot 88371

Protein Blotting
See Western Blot

Protein C Activator 85337

Protein C Antigen 85302

Protein C Assay 85303

Protein C Resistance Assay . . 85307

Protein S
Assay 85306
Total 85305

Prothrombase
See Thrombokinase

Prothrombin 85210

Prothrombin Time 85610, 85611

Prothrombinase
See Thromboplastin

Prothrombokinase 85230

Protime
See Prothrombin Time

Proton Treatment Delivery
Complex 77525
Intermediate 77523
Simple 77520-77522

Protoporphyrin 84202, 84203

Protozoa
Antibody 86753

Provitamin A
See Vitamin, A

Provocation Test
Allergy
See Allergy Tests
Bronchospasm, Evaluation 94070
Ergonovine 93024
Esophageal Balloon Distension Study 91040
for Glaucoma 92140
with Electrogastrography 91133

Prower Factor
See Stuart-Prower Factor

PSA
See Prostate Specific Antigen

Pseudocyst
Esophagus
Drainage 43240
Pancreas
Drainage 48510

Pseudophakia
See Keratoplasty

PSG
See Polysomnography

Psoriasis Treatment 96910-96922
See Dermatology; Photochemotherapy

Psychiatric Diagnosis
Assessment
Brief Emotional/Behavioral 96127
Behavior Identification 0359T-0363T
Evaluation of Records or Reports 90885
Evaluation 90791
with Medical Services 90792
Interactive Complexity 90785
Performance Measures
Dementia
See Performance Measures, Dementia
Major Depressive Disorder (MDD)
See Performance Measures, Major
Depressive Disorder
Psychological Testing 96101-96103, 96125
Computer-Assisted 96103
Suicide Risk Assessment 3085F
Unlisted Services and Procedures 90899

Psychiatric Treatment
Adaptive Behavior
Family 0370T, 0371T
Group 0366T, 0367T, 0372T
Individual 0364T, 0365T, 0373T, 0374T
Biofeedback Training 90875, 90876
Consultation with Family 90887

Removal/Revision 0284T,
61888, 64595, 64570
Systems
See Baroreflex Activation Device; Implantable
Defibrillator; Neurostimulators; Pacemaker,
Heart

Pulse Rate Increased
See Tachycardia

Pump
See Chemotherapy, Pump Services; Infusion Pump

Pump Services
Oxygenator/Heat Exchanger 99190-99192
Maintenance
Drug Delivery Pump . . 95990, 95991, 96521-96523

Pump, Infusion
See Infusion Pump

Punch Graft 15775, 15776

Puncture
Artery
Diagnosis 36600
Chest
Drainage 32554-32557
with Imaging Guidance 32555, 32557
Cisternal
See Cisternal Puncture
Cornea 65600
Follicle
Oocyte Retrieval 58970
Lumbar
See Spinal Tap
Pericardium 33010, 33011
Pleural Cavity
Drainage 32556, 32557
Sinus
for Endoscopy 31233, 31235
Skull
Drain Fluid 61000-61020
Cistern 61050
Inject Cistern 61055
Inject Ventricle 61026
Shunt
Drain Fluid 61070
Injection 61070
Spinal Cord
Diagnostic 62270
Drain Fluid 62272
Lumbar 62270
Tracheal
Aspiration and/or Injection 31612
Vein
See Venipuncture
Ventricle
See Ventricular Puncture

Puncture Aspiration
Abscess
Skin 10160
Bulla 10160
Cyst
Breast 19000, 19001
Skin 10160
Hematoma 10160
Hydrocele 55000
Pleural Cavity 32554
with Imaging Guidance 32555
Tunica Vaginalis 55000

Puncturing
See Puncture

Pupillometry 0341T

Pure-Tone Audiometry
See Audiometry, Pure Tone

Pustules
Removal 10040

Putti-Platt Procedure 23450

PUVA
See Dermatology; Photochemotherapy; Ultraviolet
Light Therapy

Pyelogram
See Urography, Intravenous; Urography, Retrograde

Pyelography 74400, 74425

Pyelolithotomy 50130
Anatrophic 50075
Coagulum 50130

Pyeloplasty 50400-50405, 50544
Foley-Y 50400
Repair
Horseshoe Kidney 50540
Secondary 50405

Pyeloscopy
with Cystourethroscopy 52351
Biopsy 52354
Destruction 52354
Lithotripsy 52353
Removal
Calculus 52352
Tumor Excision 52355

Pyelostolithotomy
Percutaneous 50080, 50081

Pyelostomy
with drainage 50125
with Pyeloplasty 50400, 50405
Change Tube 50435

Pyelotomy
Complicated 50135
Exploration 50120
with Drainage 50125
with Removal of Calculus 50130
with Renal Endoscopy 50570

Pyeloureteroplasty
See Pyeloplasty

Pyloric Sphincter
Incision 43520
Reconstruction 43800

Pyloromyotomy 43520

Pyloroplasty 43800
with Vagotomy 43640

Pyothorax
See Abscess, Bone, Thorax

Pyridoxal Phosphate 84207

Pyrophosphate, Adenosine
See Adenosine Diphosphate

Pyrophosphorylase, Udp Galactose
See Galactose-1-Phosphate, Uridyl Transferase

Pyruvate 84210-84220

Q

Q Fever 86000, 86638

Q Fever ab
See Antibody, Detection, Coxiella Burnetii

QST
See Quantitative Sensory Testing (QST)

Quadrantectomy 19301, 19302

Quadriceps Repair 27430
Suture 27385, 27386

Quantitative Sensory Testing (QST)
Cooling Stimuli 0108T
Heat-Pain Stimuli 0109T
Other Stimuli 0110T
Touch Pressure Stimuli 0106T
Vibration Stimuli 0107T

Quick Test
See Prothrombin Time

Quinidine
Assay 80194

Quinine 84228

R

Rabies Vaccine
See Vaccines

Rachicentesis
See Spinal Tap

Radial Artery
See Artery, Radial

Radial Head, Subluxation
See Nursemaid Elbow

Radial Keratotomy 65771

Radiation
See Irradiation

Radiation Physics
Consultation 77336-77370
Unlisted Services and Procedures 77399

Radiation Therapy
Consultation
Radiation Physics 77336-77370
Dose Plan 77300, 77301, 77306, 77307, 77331
Brachytherapy 0394T, 0395T, 77316-77318
Intensity Modulated Radiation Treatment
(IMRT) 77338
Multi-leaf Collimator (MLC) Device . . . 77338
Radiotherapy
3-Dimensional 77295
Teletherapy 77306, 77307, 77321
Field Set-up 77280, 77285, 77290
Guidance
CT 77014
for Localization of Target Volume 77387
Interstitial Devices, Placement . . 49411, 49412
Planning 77261-77263, 77299

Mammography
　See Mammography
Nuclear Medicine
　See Nuclear Medicine
Radiation Oncology
　Device Design/
　Construction 77332-77334, 77338
　Dosimetry
　　See Dosimetry
　Medical Physics Consultation . . . 77336, 77370
　Treatment Delivery
　　See Radiation Therapy, Treatment Delivery
　Treatment Planning 77261-77263, 77299
　　Field Setting . . . 77280, 77285, 77290, 77293
Radiation Therapy
　See Radiation Therapy
Radiologic Guidance
　Computed Tomography 77011-77014
　Fluoroscopy 77001-77003
　Magnetic Resonance 77021, 77022
X-ray
　See X-ray
Unlisted Services and Procedures
　Brachytherapy 77799
　Computed Tomography 76497
　Fluoroscopy 76496
　Magnetic Resonance 76498
　Nuclear Medicine 78099, 78199, 78299,
　　78399, 78499, 78599, 78699, 78799, 78999
　Radiation Physics 77399
　Radiographic 76499
　Radiopharmaceutical 79999
　Treatment Management 77499
　Treatment Planning 77299
　Ultrasound 76999

Radionuclide CT Scan
See Emission Computerized Tomography

Radionuclide Imaging
See Nuclear Medicine, Diagnostic

Radionuclide Therapy
See Radiopharmaceutical Therapy

Radionuclide Tomography, Single-Photon Emission-Computed
See SPECT

Radiopharmaceutical Localization
Inflammatory Process 78805-78807
Injection 78808

Radiopharmaceutical Therapy
Interstitial 79300
Intra-Arterial 79445
Intra-Articular 79440
Intracavitary 79200
Intravenous 79101, 79403
Oral 79005
Unlisted Services and Procedures 79999

Radiostereometric Analysis (RSA) 0347T-0350T

Radiosurgery
Brain
　Lesion 61796-61800
　Treatment Delivery 77371, 77372

Radiotherapeutic
See Radiation Therapy

Radiotherapies
See Irradiation

Radiotherapy, Surface
See Application, Radioelement, Surface

Radioulnar Joint
Arthrodesis
　with Resection of Ulna 25830
Arthrotomy 25107
Dislocation
　Closed Treatment 25520, 25525
　　with Manipulation 25675
　Open Treatment 25526, 25676
　Percutaneous Fixation 25671
Reconstruction 25337

Radius
See Arm, Lower; Elbow; Ulna
Amputation
　See Amputation, Arm, Lower
Arthroplasty 24365
　with Implant 24366, 25441
Craterization 24145, 25151
Cyst
　Excision 24125, 24126, 25120-25126
Diaphysectomy 24145, 25151
Dislocation
　Partial 24640
　Subluxate 24640
　with Fracture
　　Closed Treatment 24620
　　Open Treatment 24635
Excision
　Epiphyseal Bar 20150
　Head 24130
　Partial 24136, 25145, 25151
　Styloid Process 25230, 25440
Fracture
　Colles
　　Treatment 25600
　Distal 25600-25609
　　Closed Treatment 25600-25605
　　Open Treatment 25607-25609
　　Percutaneous Fixation 25606
　Head/Neck
　　Closed Treatment 24650-24655
　　Open Treatment 24665, 24666
　Shaft
　　Closed Treatment 25500-25505, 25520,
　　　25560, 25565
　　Open Treatment 25515, 25525, 25526,
　　　25574, 25575
　　Manipulation 25505, 25565
　　with Ulna 25560-25565, 25574, 25575
　Smith Type
　　Closed Treatment 25600, 25605
　　with Ulna
　　　Open Treatment 25575
Implant
　Removal 24164
Incision and Drainage 25035
Osteomyelitis 24136, 24145
Osteoplasty
　Lengthening 25391, 25393
　Shortening 25390, 25392
Osteotomy 25350, 25355, 25365, 25370, 25375
　Sofield Type 25370
Prophylactic Treatment 25490, 25492
Repair
　Defect, with Graft 25425, 25426
　Epiphyseal Arrest 25450-25455
　Epiphyseal Separation
　　Closed 25600
　　Closed with Manipulation 25605
　　Open Treatment 25607-25609

Percutaneous Fixation 25606
Malunion or Nonunion 25400,
　　25405, 25415, 25420
Osteotomy 25350-25355, 25370-25375
　and Ulna 25365
　with Graft 25405, 25420-25426
Replacement with Prosthesis
　Distal 25441, 25446
　Radial Head 24666
Replantation 20805
Saucerization 24145, 25151
Sequestrectomy 24136, 25145
Styloidectomy 25230, 25440
Tumor
　Cyst 24120
　Excision . . 24125, 24126, 25120-25126, 25170
　Radical Resection 24152, 25170

Ramstedt Operation
See Pyloromyotomy

Ramus Anterior, Nervus Thoracicus
See Intercostal Nerve

Range of Motion Test
Body, Total
　with Hands 95834
　without Hands 95833
Cholinesterase Inhibitor Challenge 95857
Extremities or Trunk
　with Hand 95852
　without Hand 95851
Eye 92018, 92019
for Myasthenia Gravis 95857
Hand 95832, 95834, 95852
Muscle 95831

Rapid Heart Rate
See Tachycardia

Rapid Plasma Reagin Test 86592, 86593

Rapid Test for Infection 86308,
　　86403-86406
Monospot Test 86308

Rapoport Test 52005

Rashkind Procedure 33735-33737

Rat Typhus
See Murine Typhus

Rathke Pouch Tumor
See Craniopharyngioma

Rays, Roentgen
See X-ray

Raz Procedure 51845
See Repair, Bladder, Neck

RBC
See Red Blood Cell (RBC)

RBC ab
See Antibody, Detection, Red Blood Cell

Reaction, Polymerase Chain
See Genomic Sequencing Procedures (GSPs) and Other Molecular Multianalyte Assays

Realignment
Femur
　Shaft 27454
Hand
　Extensor Tendon 26437

Reductase, Lactic Cytochrome
See Lactic Dehydrogenase

Reduction
Amniotic Fluid 59001
Collateral Ligament
    Ulnar 29902
Craniomegalic Skull 62115, 62117
Ear, Protruding 69300
for Dislocation
    Carpometacarpal 26686
for Fracture
    Laryngeal 31584
    Odontoid 22318, 22319
    Tracheal 31630
    Vertebral 22325-22328
Forehead 21137-21139
Internal Hernia
    Mesentery 44050
Intussusception 44050
Mammaplasty 19318
Masseter Muscle/Bone 21295, 21296
Osteoplasty
    Facial Bones 21209
Overcorrection of Ptosis 67909
Pregnancy
    Multifetal 59866
Procidentia 45900
Skull
    Craniomegalic 62115, 62117
Tissue 30801
Torsion
    Testis 54600
Tumor
    Bone
        Ablation Therapy 20982, 20983
    Breast
        Microwave Thermotherapy 0301T
    Pulmonary 32998
Volume
    Blood Products 86960
    Lung 32491
Volvulus 44050, 44055
with Reconstruction
    Hip 27147, 27156
    Radioulnar Joint 25337
    Wrist 25230

Reflex Test
Blink Reflex 95933

Reflux Study 78262
Gastroesophageal 91034-91038

Refraction
Ophthalmological 92015

Rehabilitation
Artery
    Occlusive Disease 93668
Auditory
    Post-Lingual Hearing Loss 92633
    Pre-Lingual Hearing Loss 92630
    Status Evaluation 92626, 92627
Cardiac 93797, 93798

Rehabilitation Facility
Discharge Services 1110F, 1111F

Rehabilitative
See Rehabilitation

Reimplantation
Arteries
    Aorta
        Prosthesis 35697

Carotid 35691, 35694, 35695
Coronary Ostium 33783
Subclavian 35693-35695
Vertebral 35691-35693
Visceral 35697
Kidney 50380
Pulmonary Artery 33788
Ureters 51565

Reinnervation
Larynx
    Neuromuscular Pedicle 31590

Reinsch Test 83015

Reinsertion
Drug Delivery Implant 11983
Ocular Implant 65150, 65155
Spinal Fixation Device 22849
Tendon
    Biceps 24342
    Triceps 24342

Relative Density
See Specific Gravity

Release
Capsule
    Ankle 27612
    Elbow 24149
    Foot 28260
    Knee 27435
    Metatarsophalangeal Joint 28289
    Shoulder 23020
Carpal Tunnel 64721
Choroidal Fluid 67015
Fascia
    Finger/Thumb 26123
    Heel 28119
Flexor Muscles
    Hip 27036
Knee Joint 29873
Ligament
    Coracoacromial 23130, 23415, 29826
    Knee
        Retinacular 27425
    Transverse Carpal 29848
Metacarpophalangeal Joint 26135
Muscle
    Abductor Hallucis 28240
    Hamstring 27097
    Hand 26508, 26593
    Hip 27036
    Knee 27422
Nerve 64702-64726
    Neurolytic 64727
Penis
    Chordee 54352
    from Scrotum 54318
Retina
    Encircling Material 67115
    Fluid 67015
Scar 11042, 14040, 14041
    Colostomy 44340
    Eye 67343
    Ileostomy 44312
Spinal Cord 63200
Stapes 69650
Tarsal Tunnel 28035
Tendon 24332, 25295
    Vitreous 67015

Release-Inhibiting Hormone, Somatotropin
See Somatostatin

Relocation
Skin Pocket
    Implantable Defibrillator 33223
    Pacemaker 33222

Removal
Adjustable Gastric Restrictive
    Device 43772-43774
Allograft
    Intestinal 44137
Artificial Intervertebral Disc
    Cervical Interspace 0095T, 22864
    Lumbar Interspace 0164T, 22865
Balloon
    Intra-Aortic 33974
Balloon Assist Device
    Intra-Aortic 33968, 33971
Baroreflex Activation Device 0269T-0271T
Blood Clot
    Eye 65930
Blood Component
    Apheresis 36511-36516
Breast
    See Mastectomy
Bronchial Valve 31648, 31649
Calcareous Deposits
    Subdeltoid 23000
Calculi (Stone)
    See Calculus, Removal
Capsules
    Breast 19371
Cardiac Event Recorder 33284
Cast 29700, 29705, 29710
Cataract
    See Cataract, Removal/Extraction
Catheter
    Central Venous 36589
    Peritoneum 49422
    Pleural Cavity 32552
    Spinal Cord 62355
Cerclage
    Cervix 59871
Cerumen
    Auditory Canal, External 69209, 69210
Clot
    Pericardium 33020
    Endoscopic 32658
Comedones 10040
Contraceptive Capsules 11976
Cranial Tongs 20665
Cyst 10040
Dacryolith
    Lacrimal Duct 68530
    Lacrimal Gland 68530
Drug Delivery Implant 11982, 11983
Ear Wax
    Auditory Canal, External 69209, 69210
Electrode
    Array
        Nerve 64585
    Brain 61535, 61880
    Heart 33238
    Spinal Cord 63661-63664
    Stomach 43648, 43882
Embolus
    See Embolectomy
Esophageal Sphincter Augmentation
    Device 0393T
External Fixation System 20694
Eye
    Bone 67414, 67445
    Epithelium 65435, 65436

Renal Abscess

Renal Arteries

Renal Autotransplantation

Renal Calculus

Renal Cyst

Renal Dialyses

Renal Disease Services

Renal Transplantation

Renin

Renin-Converting Enzyme

Reoperation

Repair

Thromboendarterectomy 35301-35321,
35341-35390
Tibioperoneal 37228-37235
Viscera 35450, 35471
Arytenoid Cartilage 31400
Atria
Laparoscopic 33265, 33266
Open 33254-33256
Bile Duct 47701
with Intestines 47760, 47780-47785
Wound 47900
Bladder
Exstrophy 51940
Fistula 44660, 44661, 45800-45805,
51880-51925
Neck 51845
Resection 52500
Wound 51860-51865
Blepharoptosis
Frontalis Muscle Technique with
Fascial Sling 67902
Blood Vessel
Abdomen 35221
with Other Graft 35281
with Vein Graft 35251
Chest 35211-35216
with Other Graft 35271-35276
with Vein Graft 35241-35246
Finger 35207
Graft Defect 35870
Hand 35207
Kidney 50100
Lower Extremity 35226
with Other Graft 35286
with Vein Graft 35256
Neck 35201
with Other Graft 35261
with Vein Graft 35231
Upper Extremity 35206
with Other Graft 35266
with Vein Graft 35236
Body Cast 29720
Brain
Wound 61571
Breast
Suspension 19316
Bronchi
Fistula 32815
Brow Pyrosis 67900
Bunion 28290-28299
Bypass Graft 35901-35907
Fistula 35870
Calcaneus
Osteotomy 28300
Cannula 36860, 36861
Carpal 25440
Carpal Bone 25431
Cervix
Cerclage 57700
Abdominal 59320-59325
Suture 57720
Chest Wall 32905
Closure 32810
Fistula 32906
Chin
Augmentation 21120, 21123
Osteotomy 21121-21123
Clavicle
Osteotomy 23480-23485
Cleft Hand 26580
Cleft Lip 40525-40527, 40700-40761
Nasal Deformity . . 40700, 40701, 40720-40761

Cleft Palate
See Cleft Palate, Repair
Colon
Fistula 44650-44661
Hernia 44050
Malrotation 44055
Obstruction 44050
Cornea
See Cornea, Repair
Coronary Chamber Fistula 33500, 33501
Cyst
Bartholin's Gland 56440
Liver 47300
Diaphragm
for Eventration 39545
Hernia 39503, 39540, 39541
Laceration 39501
Ductus Arteriosus 33820-33824, 93582
Ear, Middle
Oval Window Fistula 69666
Round Window Fistula 69667
Elbow
Hemiepiphyseal Arrest 24470
Ligament 24343-24346
Muscle 24341
Muscle Transfer 24301
Tendon 24340-24342
Each 24341
Tendon Lengthening 24305
Tendon Transfer 24301
Tennis Elbow 24357-24359
Encephalocele 62121
Endovascular
See Endovascular Repair
Enterocele
Hysterectomy 58270, 58294
Epididymis 54900, 54901
Epiphysis
Femur 27177-27181, 27475,
27479, 27485, 27742, 27516-27519
Fibula 27477, 27479, 27485,
27732, 27734, 27740, 27742
Tibia 27477-27485, 27730-27742
Epispadias 54380-54390
Esophagus 43300, 43310, 43313
Esophagogastrostomy 43320
Esophagojejunostomy 43340, 43341
Fistula . . . 43305, 43312, 43314, 43420-43425
Fundoplasty 43210, 43325
Laparotomy 43327
Thoracotomy 43328
Lengthening 43283, 43338
Muscle 43330, 43331
Pre-Existing Perforation 43405
Varices 43401
Wound 43410-43415
Eye
Ciliary Body 66680
Suture 66682
Conjunctiva 65270-65273
Wound 65270-65273
Cornea 65275
with Amniotic Membrane 65778-65780
Astigmatism 65772-65775
with Glue 65286
Wound 65275-65285
Fistula
Lacrimal Gland 68770
Iris
Suture 66682
with Ciliary Body 66680
Lacrimal Duct
Canaliculi 68700

Lacrimal Punctum 68705
Retina
Detachment 67101, 67105,
67107, 67108, 67110, 67113
Sclera
Reinforcement 67250-67255
Staphyloma 66220-66225
with Glue 65286
with Graft 66225
Wound 65286, 66250
Strabismus
Chemodenervation 67345
Symblepharon
Division 68340
with Graft 68335
without Graft 68330
Trabeculae 65855
Eye Muscles
Strabismus
Adjustable Sutures 67335
One Horizontal Muscle 67311
One Vertical Muscle 67314
Posterior Fixation Suture
Technique 67334, 67335
Previous Surgery, Not Involving Extraocular
Muscles 67331
Release Extensive Scar Tissue 67343
Superior Oblique Muscle 67318
Two Horizontal Muscles 67312
Two or More Vertical Muscles 67316
Wound
Extraocular Muscle 65290
Eyebrow
Ptosis 67900
Eyelashes
Epilation
by Forceps 67820
by Other than Forceps 67825
Incision of Lid Margin 67830
with Free Mucous Membrane Graft . . . 67835
Eyelid 21280-21282
Ectropion 67916, 67917
Suture 67914
Thermocauterization 67915
Entropion 67924
Excision Tarsal Wedge 67923
Suture 67921-67924
Thermocauterization 67922
Excisional 67961-67966
Lagophthalmos 67912
Ptosis
Conjunctivo-Tarso-Muller's Muscle-Levator
Resection 67908
Frontalis Muscle Technique . . . 67901, 67902
Levator Resection 67903, 67904
Reduction of Overcorrection 67909
Superior Rectus Technique 67906
Retraction 67911
Wound
Suture 67930-67935
Facial Bones 21208, 21209
Facial Nerve
Paralysis 15840-15845
Suture
Intratemporal, Lateral to Geniculate
Ganglion 69740
Intratemporal, Medial to Geniculate
Ganglion 69745
Fallopian Tube 58752
Anastomosis 58750
Create Stoma 58770
Fascial Defect 50728
Femur 27470-27472

Respiratory Syncytial Virus Immune Globulin
See Immune Globulins
Antigen Detection
　See Immune Globulins, Respiratory Syncytial Virus

Response, Auditory Evoked
See Auditory Evoked Potentials

Rest Home Visit
See Domiciliary Services

Resuscitation
Cardiac
　See Cardiac Massage
Cardiopulmonary 92950
Newborn 99465

Reticulocyte
Count 85044-85046

Retina
Diagnostic Imaging
　Computerized Scanning 92134
　Electroretinography 92275
　Fluorescein Angiography 92235
　Ophthalmoscopy 92225, 92226
　Remote 92227, 92228
Incision
　Encircling Material 67115
Lesion
　Destruction
　　Extensive 67227, 67228
　　Localized 67208-67218
Macular/Fundus Exam, Dilated 2019F-2021F
　Findings Communicated for Diabetes Management 5010F
Monitoring
　Time Series Images
　　Computer Aided Animation, Analysis 0380T
Prophylaxis
　Retinal Detachment 67141, 67145
Prosthesis 0100T
Release
　Encircling Material 67115
Removal
　Implanted Material 67120
Repair
　Detachment 67113
　by Scleral Buckling 67107, 67108, 67113
　Cryotherapy . . . 67101, 67107, 67108, 67113
　Diathermy 67101
　Encircling 67107
　Imbrication 67107
　Injection of Air 67110
　Photocoagulation 67105, 67107, 67108
　Scleral Dissection 67107
　Tamponade 67108, 67113
　with Drainage of Subretinal Fluid . . . 67101, 67105, 67107, 67108, 67113
　with Removal of Lens 67113
　with Vitrectomy 67108, 67113
　Prophylaxis
　　Detachment 67141-67145
Retinopathy
　Detection 92225-92228
　Destruction
　　Cryotherapy, Diathermy 67227
　Treatment
　　Cryotherapy 67229
　　Photocoagulation 67228, 67229
　　Preterm Infant 67229

Macular Degeneration
　Dilated Macular Exam 2019F
Time Series Images
　Computer Aided Animation, Analysis . . . 0380T

Retinacular
Knee
　Release 27425

Retinopathy
Detection 92225-92228
Destruction
　Cryotherapy, Diathermy 67227
Treatment
　Cryotherapy 67229
　Photocoagulation 67228, 67229
　Preterm Infant 67229
Macular Degeneration
　Dilated Macular Exam 2019F

Retraction, Clot
See Clot Retraction

Retrieval
Cranial Bone Graft 62148
Filter
　Vena Cava 37193
Foreign Body
　Intracranial 62163
　Intravascular 37197
Oocyte 58970
Suture
　from Iris 66682

Retrocaval Ureter
Ureterolysis 50725

Retrograde Cholangiopancreatographies, Endoscopic
See Cholangiopancreatography

Retrograde Cystourethrogram
See Urethrocystography, Retrograde

Retrograde Pyelogram
See Urography, Retrograde

Retroperitoneal Area
Abscess
　Incision and Drainage
　　Open 49060
　　Percutaneous 49406
Biopsy 49010
Cyst
　Destruction/Excision 49203-49205
Endometriomas
　Destruction/Excision 49203-49205
Exploration 49010
Needle Biopsy
　Mass 49180
Tumor
　Destruction/Excision 49203-49205

Retroperitoneal Fibrosis
Ureterolysis 50715

Retropubic Prostatectomies
See Prostatectomy, Retropubic

Revascularization
Artery
　Coronary . . 92937, 92938, 92941, 92943, 92944
　Femoral/Popliteal 37224-37227
　Iliac 37220-37223
　Tibial/Peroneal 37228-37235

Coronary Artery Bypass Graft 92937, 92938, 92941, 92943, 92944
Distal Revascularization and Interval Ligation (DRIL) 36838
Distal Upper Extremity
　with Interval Ligation 36838
Interval Ligation
　Distal Revascularization and Interval Ligation (DRIL) 36838
Penis 37788
Transmyocardial 33140, 33141

Reversal, Vasectomy
See Vasovasorrhaphy

Reverse T3
See Triiodothyronine, Reverse

Reverse Triiodothyronine
See Triiodothyronine, Reverse

Revision
See Reconstruction
Abdomen
　Intraperitoneal Catheter 49325
Adjustable Gastric Restrictive Device . . . 43771
Aorta 33404
Baroreflex Activation Device 0269T-0271T
Blepharoplasty 15820-15823
Bronchial Stent 31638
Bronchus 32501
Bypass Graft
　Vein Patch 35685
Cervicoplasty 15819
Colostomy
　See Colostomy, Revision
Cornea
　Prosthesis 65770
　Reshaping
　　Epikeratoplasty 65767
　　Keratomileusis 65760
　　Keratophakia 65765
Ear, Middle 69662
External Fixation System 20693
Eye
　Aqueous Shunt 66184, 66185
Gastric Restrictive Procedure
　Other than Adjustable Gastric Restrictive Device 43848
Gastrostomy Tube 44373
Hip Replacement
　See Replacement, Hip, Revision
Hymenal Ring 56700
Ileostomy
　See Ileostomy, Revision
Infusion Pump
　Intraarterial 36261
　Intravenous 36576-36578, 36582, 36583
Iris
　Iridoplasty 66762
　Iridotomy 66761
Jejunostomy Tube 44373
Lower Extremity Arterial Bypass 35879-35881
Pulse Generator 0284T
Rhytidectomy 15824-15829
Semicircular Canal
　Fenestration 69840
Shoulder
　See Arthroplasty, Shoulder Joint
Shunt
　Intrahepatic Portosystemic 37183
Sling 53442
Stapedectomy
　See Stapedectomy, Revision

Stomach
for Obesity 43848
Subcutaneous Port
for Gastric Restrictive Procedure 43886
Tracheostomy
Scar 31830
Urinary-Cutaneous Anastomosis 50727, 50728
Vagina
Prosthetic Graft 57295, 57296, 57426
Sling
Stress Incontinence 57287
Venous Access Device 36576-36578,
36582, 36583, 36585
Ventricle
Ventriculomyectomy 33416
Ventriculomyotomy 33416

Rh (D)
See Blood Typing, Serologic

Rh Immune Globulin
See Immune Globulins, Rho (D)

Rheumatoid Factor 86430, 86431

Rhinectomy
Partial 30150
Total 30160

Rhinomanometry 92512

Rhinopharynx
See Nasopharynx

Rhinophyma
Repair 30120

Rhinoplasty
Cleft Lip/Cleft Palate 30460-30462
Primary 30400-30420
Secondary 30430-30450

Rhinoscopy
See Endoscopy, Nose

Rhinotomy
Lateral 30118, 30320

Rhizotomy 63185-63190

Rho Variant Du 86905

Rhomboid Flap 14000-14302

Rhytidectomy 15824-15829

Rhytidoplasties
See Face Lift

Rib
Excision 21600-21616, 32900
Fracture
External Fixation 21899
Open Treatment
with Internal Fixation 21811-21813
Graft
to Face 21230
Resection 19260-19272, 32900
X-ray 71100-71111

Riboflavin 84252

**Richardson Operation
Hysterectomy**
See Hysterectomy, Abdominal, Total

Richardson Procedure 53460

Rickettsia
Antibody 86757

Ridell Operation
See Sinusotomy, Frontal Sinus

Ridge, Alveolar
See Alveolar Ridge

Right Atrioventricular Valve
See Tricuspid Valve

Right Heart Cardiac Catheterization
See Cardiac Catheterization, Right Heart

Ripstein Operation 45540, 45541
See Proctopexy

Risk Factor Reduction Intervention
Group 99411, 99412
Diabetes Prevention 0403T
Individual 99401-99404

Risser Jacket
Application 29010-29015
Removal 29710

**Rocky Mountain Spotted
Fever** 86000

Roentgen Rays
See X-ray

Roentgenographic
See X-ray

Roentgenography
See X-ray

Ropes Test 83872

Rorschach Test 96101

**Ross Information Processing
Assessment** 96125

Ross Procedure 33413

Rotation Flap
See Skin, Adjacent Tissue Transfer

Rotator Cuff
Repair 23410-23420

Rotavirus
Antibody 86759
Antigen Detection
Immunoassay 87425

Rotavirus Vaccine
3 Dose 90680
2 Dose 90681

Round Window
Repair Fistula 69667

Round Window Fistula
Repair 69667

Roux-En-Y Procedure 43621,
43633, 43634, 43644, 43846,
47740, 47741, 47780-47785, 48540

RPR
See Syphilis Test

RSV
See Immune Globulins; Respiratory Syncytial Virus

RT3
See Triiodothyronine, Reverse

Rubbing Alcohol
See Isopropyl Alcohol

Rubella
Antibody 86762
Vaccine 90707, 90710

Rubella HI Test
See Hemagglutination Inhibition Test

Rubella/Mumps
See Vaccines

Rubeola
Antibody 86765
Antigen Detection
Immunofluorescence 87283

Rubeolla
See Rubeola

**Russell Viper Venom
Time** 85612, 85613

S

Sac, Endolymphatic
See Endolymphatic Sac

Saccomanno Technique 88108

Sacral Nerve
Implantation
Electrode Array 64561, 64581

Sacral, Pre-
Arthrodesis
See Arthrodesis, Vertebra, Lumbar

Sacroiliac Joint
Arthrodesis
Open 27280
Percutaneous 27279
Arthrotomy 27050
Biopsy 27050
Dislocation
Open Treatment 27218
Fusion 27280
Injection for Arthrography 27096
X-ray 72200-72202

Sacrum
Augmentation
Percutaneous 0200T, 0201T
Bone Biopsy 0200T, 0201T
Sacroplasty
Percutaneous 0200T, 0201T
Tumor
Excision 49215
X-ray 72220

Sahli Test
See Gastroenterology, Diagnostic, Stomach

Salicylate
Assay 80329-80331

Saline-Solution Abortion
See Abortion, Induced, by Saline

Salivary Duct
Catheterization 42660
Dilation 42650-42660

Diversion 42507-42510
Ligation 42665, 42510
Repair 42500-42505
   Fistula. 42600

Salivary Gland Virus
See Cytomegalovirus

Salivary Glands
Abscess
   Incision and Drainage
      Parotid 42300-42305
      Sublingual. 42310
      Submaxillary. 42310-42320
Biopsy 42405
Calculi (Stone)
   Excision 42330-42340
Chemodenervation 64611
Cyst
   Marsupialization 42409
   Excision 42408
Duct
   See Salivary Duct
Excision
   Parotid Gland 42410, 42415,
            42420, 42425, 42426
   Sublingual Gland 42450
   Submandibular Gland 42440, 42509
Injection
   X-ray. 42550
Needle Biopsy. 42400
Nuclear Medicine
   Function Study 78232
   Imaging 78230, 78231
Tumor
   Parotid
      Excision. 42410, 42415,
            42420, 42425, 42426
Unlisted Services and Procedures 42699
X-ray 70380-70390
   with Contrast 70390

Salmonella
Antibody 86768

Salpingectomy
Complete or Partial 58700
   Laparoscopic 58661
for Ectopic Pregnancy 59120
   Laparoscopic 59151
with Vaginal Hysterectomy 58262,
          58263, 58291, 58292
   Laparoscopic 58552, 58554
with Oophorectomy. 58943

Salpingo-Oophorectomy 58720
Resection Ovarian Malignancy. 58950-58958
Resection Peritoneal Malignancy. . . . 58950-58958
Resection Tubal Malignancy. 58950-58958

Salpingohysterostomy
See Implantation, Tubouterine

Salpingolysis 58740
Laparoscopic. 58660

Salpingoneostomy 58673, 58770

Salpingoplasty
See Fallopian Tube, Repair

Salpingostomy 58673, 58770
Laparoscopic. 58673

Salter Osteotomy of the Pelvis
See Osteotomy, Pelvis

Sampling
See also Biopsy; Brush Biopsy; Needle Biopsy
Blood
   Arterial 36620
   Fetal Scalp 59030
   Ocular. 0198T
   Organ 36500
   Plasma 78110, 78111
   Red Cell 78120, 78121
   Venous 75893
Chorionic Villus 59015, 76945
Endometrium. 58100, 58558
Lymph Node
   Endobronchial Ultrasound (EBUS) Guided
      Hilar 31652, 31653
      Mediastinal 31652, 31653
   Para-Aortic 57109, 57112, 57531,
            58200, 58210, 58548
   Pelvic 58200
   Periaortic 38572
   Retroperitoneal 38570
Stereotactic Template Guided 55706

Sang-Park Procedure 33735-33737

Sao Paulo Typhus
See Rocky Mountain Spotted Fever

Saucerization
Calcaneus 28120
Clavicle 23180
Femur 27070, 27360
Fibula. 27360, 27641
Hip. 27070
Humerus 23184, 24140
Ileum 27070
Metacarpal 26230
Metatarsal 28122
Olecranon Process 24147
Phalanges
   Finger 26235, 26236
   Toe 28124
Pubis 27070
Radius 24145, 25151
Scapula 23182
Symphysis Pubis 27070, 27071
Talus 28120
Tarsal. 28122
Tibia. 27360, 27640
Ulna. 25150

Saundby Test
See Blood, Feces

Scabies
See Tissue, Examination for Ectoparasites

Scalenotomy
See Muscle Division, Scalenus Anticus

Scalenus Anticus
Division 21700-21705

Scaling
See Exfoliation

Scalp
Skin Graft
   Dermal Autograft 15135, 15136
   Epidermal Autograft 15115, 15116
   Flap. 15610
   Pedicle Formation 15572
   Recipient Site Preparation. 15004, 15005
   Skin Substitute. 15275-15278
   Split-Thickness. 15120, 15121
   Tissue-cultured Autograft 15155-15157

Lesion
   Destruction. 17270-17274, 17276
   Excision
      Benign. 11420-11424, 11426
      Malignant. 11620-11624, 11626
      Shaving 11305-11308
Tissue Transfer
   Adjacent. 14020, 14021
Tumor
   Excision 21011-21014
   Radical Resection 21015, 21016
Venipuncture
   Child. 36405
Wound
   Repair. 12001, 12002, 12004-12007,
      12031, 12032, 12034-12037, 13120-13122

Scalp Blood Sampling
Fetal 59030

Scan
See Nuclear Medicine, Diagnostic
Abdomen
   See Abdomen, CT Scan
CT
   See CT Scan
MRI
   See Magnetic Resonance Imaging (MRI)
PET
   See Positron Emission Tomography (PET)
Radionuclide
   See Emission Computerized Tomography
SPECT
   See SPECT

Scanning, Radioisotope
See Nuclear Medicine, Diagnostic

Scanogram 77073

Scaphoid
Fracture
   Closed Treatment. 25622
   Open Treatment 25628
   with Manipulation 25624
Nonunion
   Repair. 25440
Replacement 25443

Scapula Bone
Craterization 23182
Cyst
   Excision 23140
      with Allograft 23146
      with Autograft 23145
Diaphysectomy 23182
Excision
   Partial. 23172, 23182, 23190
Fracture
   Closed Treatment
      with Manipulation 23575
      without Manipulation. 23570
   Open Treatment 23585
Ostectomy. 23190
Repair
   Fixation. 23400
   Scapulopexy. 23400
Saucerization 23182
Sequestrectomy 23172
Tumor
   Excision 23140, 23210
      with Allograft 23146
      with Autograft 23145
      Radical Resection 23210
X-ray 73010

Scapulopexy 23400

Scarification
Pleural 32215

Scarification of Pleura
See Pleurodesis

Schanz Operation
See Femur, Osteotomy

Schauta Operation
See Hysterectomy, Vaginal, Radical

Schede Procedure 32905, 32906

Scheie Procedure 66155

Schilling Test 78270
See Vitamin B-12 Absorption Study

**Schlatter Operation Total
Gastrectomy** 43620-43622

Schlicter Test 87197
See Bactericidal Titer, Serum

Schuchard Procedure
Osteotomy
　Maxilla 21206

Schwannoma, Acoustic
See Brain, Tumor, Excision

Sciatic Nerve
Decompression 64712
Administration, Anesthetic
　Infusion 64446
　Injection 64445, 64446
Neuroma
　Excision 64786
Neuroplasty 64712
Release 64712
Repair/Suture 64858

Scintigraphy
See Nuclear Medicine, Diagnostic
Computed Tomographic
　See Emission Computerized Tomography

Scissoring
Skin Tags 11200, 11201

Sclera
Aqueous Drainage Device
　to Extraocular Reservoir 66179, 66180
　without Extraocular Reservoir ... 0376T, 66183
Excision
　Sclerectomy with Punch or Scissors 66160
Fistulization
　for Glaucoma
　　Through Ciliary Body 66999
　Sclerectomy with Punch or Scissors with
　　Iridectomy 66160
　Thermocauterization with Iridectomy ... 66155
　Trabeculectomy ab Externo 66170, 66172
　Trephination with Iridectomy 66150
Lesion
　Excision 66130
Repair
　Reinforcement
　　with Graft 67255
　　without Graft 67250
　Staphyloma
　　with Graft 66225
　　without Graft 66220
　with Glue 65286
　Wound

Operative 66250
Tissue Glue 65286

Scleral Buckling Operation
See Retina, Repair, Detachment

Scleral Ectasia
See Staphyloma, Sclera

Sclerectomy 66160

Sclerotherapy
Esophageal Varices 43204, 43243
Fluid Collection 49185
Gastric Varices 43243
Hemorrhoids 46500
Perirectal 45520
Venous 36468-36471

Sclerotomy
See Incision, Sclera

Screening, Drug
See Drug Screen
Alcohol and/or Substance Abuse 99408, 99409

Scribner Cannulization 36810

Scrotal Varices
See Varicocele

Scrotoplasty 55175-55180

Scrotum
Abscess
　Incision and Drainage 54700, 55100
Exploration 55110
Hematoma
　Incision and Drainage 54700
Removal
　Foreign Body 55120
Repair 55175-55180
Resection 55150
Ultrasound 76870
Unlisted Services and Procedures 55899

Scrub Typhus 86000

Second Look Surgery
See Reoperation

Section
See Decompression
Cesarean
　See Cesarean Delivery
Cranial Nerve 61460
　Spinal Access 63191
Dentate Ligament 63180-63182
Gasserian Ganglion
　Sensory Root 61450
Mesencephalic Tract 61480
Nerve Root 63185-63190
Spinal Accessory Nerve 63191
Spinal Cord Tract 63194-63199
Vestibular Nerve
　Transcranial Approach 69950
　Translabyrinthine Approach 69915

Sedation
Moderate 99143-99150
　with Independent Observation .. 99143-99145

Seddon-Brookes Procedure 24320

Sedimentation Rate
Blood Cell
　Automated 85652
　Manual 85651

Segmentectomy
Breast 19301, 19302
Lung 32484
　Thoracoscopic 32669

Seidlitz Powder Test
See X-ray, with Contrast

Selective Catheterization
Arterial
　First Order
　　Abdominal 36245
　　Brachiocephalic Branch 36215
　　Lower Extremity 36245
　　Pelvic 36245
　　Renal 36251, 36252
　　Thoracic Branch 36215
　Second Order
　　Abdominal 36246
　　Brachiocephalic Branch 36216
　　Lower Extremity 36246
　　Pelvic 36246
　　Thoracic Branch 36216
　Superselective
　　Abdominal 36247, 36248
　　Brachiocephalic Branch 36217, 36218
　　Lower Extremity 36247, 36248
　　Pelvic 36247, 36248
　　Renal 36253, 36254
　　Thoracic Branch 36217, 36218
　Pulmonary 36014, 36015
Venous
　First Order Branch 36011
　Second Order Branch 36012
with Angiography
　Carotid Arch 36223, 36224
　Carotid Artery 36222-36224, 36227, 36228
　Cervicocerebral Arch 36222-36226
　Innominate Artery 36222, 36223, 36225
　Subclavian Artery 36225
　Vertebral Vessels 36225, 36226, 36228

**Selective Cellular Enhancement
Technique** 88112

Selenium 84255

Self Care
See Physical Medicine/Therapy/Occupational
Therapy
Training 97535, 98960-98962, 99509

Sella Turcica
CT Scan 70480-70482
X-ray 70240

Semen
See Sperm

Semen Analysis 89300-89322
Sperm Analysis 89331
　Antibodies 89325
with Sperm Isolation 89260, 89261

Semenogelase
See Antigen, Prostate Specific

Semicircular Canal
Fenestration 69820
　Revised 69840

Semilunar
Bone
　See Lunate
Ganglion
　See Gasserian Ganglion

Biopsy
  Deep.............................23066
  Soft Tissue......................23065
Blade
  See Scapula Bone
Bone
  Excision
    Acromion......................23130
    Clavicle...................23120-23125
    Incision......................23035
  Tumor
    Excision....................23140-23146
Bursa
  Aspiration...............20610, 20611
  Drainage.......................23031
  Injection.................20610, 20611
Capsular Contracture Release...........23020
Cast/Splint
  Figure Eight....................29049
  Long Arm Cast...................29065
  Long Arm Splint.................29105
  Removal.........................29710
  Shoulder to Hips................29035
  Spica...........................29055
  Velpeau.........................29058
Clavicle
  See Clavicle
Disarticulation..................23920, 23921
Dislocation
  Closed Treatment
    with Manipulation....23650-23655, 23665,
    23675
  Open Treatment........23660, 23670, 23680
Exploration...........................23107
Hematoma
  Drainage........................23030
Joint
  See Acromioclavicular Joint, Glenohumeral
  Joint; Sternoclavicular Joint
Manipulation
  Application of Fixation Apparatus......23700
Prophylactic Treatment............23490, 23491
Removal
  Calcareous Deposits...............23000
  Cast............................29710
  Foreign Body
    Intramuscular...................23333
    Subcutaneous....................23330
    Subfascial......................23333
  Foreign or Loose Body.............23107
Repair
  Capsule..................23450-23466
  Ligament Release.................23415
  Muscle Transfer............23395-23397
  Rotator Cuff...............23410-23420
  Seddon-Brookes Procedure.........24320
  Tendon.......23410-23412, 23430-23440
  Tenomyotomy..............23405, 23406
Replacement...........................23472
  Revision..................23473, 23474
Scapula
  See Scapula Bone
Strapping.............................29240
Surgery
  Unlisted Services and Procedures......23929
Tumor
  Soft Tissue
    Excision.................23071-23076
    Radical Resection........23077, 23078
Unlisted Services and Procedures.........23929
X-ray.........................73020-73030
X-ray with Contrast....................73040
    Injection......................23350

Shoulder Joint
See Glenohumeral Joint
Arthroplasty
  with Implant..........23470, 23472-23474
Arthrotomy
  with Biopsy...............23100, 23101
  with Synovectomy..........23105, 23106
Dislocation
  Open Treatment..................23660
  with Greater Tuberosity Fracture
    Closed Treatment..............23665
    Open Treatment................23670
  with Surgical or Anatomical Neck Fracture
    Closed Treatment with Manipulation 23675
    Open Treatment................23680
Excision
  Torn Cartilage..................23101
Exploration...............23040-23044
Incision and Drainage..........23040-23044
Removal
  Foreign Body............23040-23044
X-ray.............................73050

Shunt(s)
Aqueous
  to Extraocular Reservoir.......66179, 66180
    Revision.................66184, 66185
  without Extraocular Reservoir...0376T, 66183
Arteriovenous
  See Arteriovenous Shunt
Brain
  Creation................62180-62223
  Removal.................62256-62258
  Replacement.............62160, 62194,
                    62225-62230, 62258
  Reprogramming...................62252
Cerebrospinal Fluid
  See Cerebrospinal Fluid Shunt
Creation
  Arteriovenous
    Direct........................36821
    ECMO
      See Extracorporeal Membrane
      Oxygenation (ECMO)
    Thomas Shunt..................36835
    Transposition..........36818-36820
    with Bypass Graft.............35686
    with Graft.............36825-36830
  Cerebrospinal Fluid.............62200
Fetal.................................59076
Great Vessel
  Aorta...........................33321
  Pulmonary.......................33924
  Aorta to Pulmonary Artery
    Ascending.....................33755
    Descending....................33762
  Central.........................33764
  Subclavian to Pulmonary Artery......33750
  Vena Cava to Pulmonary Artery..33766-33768
Intra-Atrial................33735-33737
LeVeen
  See LeVeen Shunt
Nonvascular
  X-ray...........................75809
Peritoneal
  Venous
    Injection.....................49427
    Ligation......................49428
    Removal.......................49429
    X-ray.........................75809
Pulmonary Artery
  See Pulmonary Artery, Shunt

Revision
  Arteriovenous...................36832
Spinal Cord
  Creation..................63740, 63741
  Irrigation......................63744
  Removal.........................63746
  Replacement.....................63744
Superior Mesenteric-Caval
  See Anastomosis, Caval to Mesenteric
Thomas Shunt.........................36835
Ureter to Colon......................50815
Ventriculocisternal with Valve
  See Ventriculocisternostomy

Shuntogram.....................75809

Sialic Acid....................84275

Sialodochoplasty......42500-42505

Sialogram
See Sialography

Sialography....................70390

Sickling
Electrophoresis.....................83020

Siderocytes....................85536

Siderophilin
See Transferrin

Sigmoid
See Colon, Sigmoid

Sigmoid Bladder
Creation............................50810
Cystectomy..........................51590

Sigmoidoscopy
Ablation
  Lesion..........................45346
  Polyp...........................45346
  Tumor...........................45346
Band Ligation.......................45350
Biopsy..............................45331
Collection
  Specimen........................45330
Decompression.......................45337
Diagnostic..........................45330
Dilation, balloon...................45340
Exploration.................45330, 45335
Hemorrhage Control..................45334
Hemorrhoid Ligation.................45350
Injection
  Submucosal......................45335
Mucosal Resection...................45349
Needle Biopsy.......................45342
Placement
  Decompression Tube...............45337
  Stent...........................45347
Removal
  Foreign Body....................45332
  Polyp...................45333, 45338
  Tumor...................45333, 45338
Repair
  Volvulus........................45337
Resection...........................45349
Ultrasound...............45341, 45342

**Signal-Averaged
Electrocardiography**
See Electrocardiography, Signal Averaged

Silica..........................84285

Silicon Dioxide
See Silica

Silicone
Contouring Injections 11950-11954

Silver Operation
See Keller Procedure

Silver Procedure 28290

Simple Mastectomies
See Mastectomy

Single Photon Absorptiometry
See Absorptiometry, X-ray, Single Photon

Single Photon Emission Computed Tomography
See SPECT

Sinus, Sphenoid
See Sinus/Sinuses, Sphenoid

Sinus/Sinuses
Carotid
   Baroreflex Activation Device
     See Baroreflex Activation Device
   Injection 64508
Cranial
   Decompression 61595
   Excision of Lesion 61607
   Ligation 61598
   Resection 61591
Dilation 31295-31297
Endoscopy
   Diagnostic 31231, 31233, 31235
   Surgical 31237-31240, 31254-31256,
     31267, 31276, 31287, 31288, 31290-31297
   Biopsy 31237
   Debridement 31237
   Decompression 31292-31294
   Dilation 31295-31297
   Exploration 31276
   Hemorrhage Control 31238
   Polypectomy 31237
Ethmoid
   Excision 31200-31205
   with Nasal/Sinus Endoscopy . . 31254, 31255
   Drug-Eluting Implant
     Placement 0406T, 0407T
   Repair of Cerebrospinal Leak 31290
Ethmoidectomy
   Excision 31254, 31255
Excision
   See Excision, Sinus
Frontal
   Destruction 31080-31085
   Dilation 31296
   Exploration 31070-31075
   with Nasal/Sinus Endoscopy 31276
   Fracture
     Open Treatment 21343, 21344
   Incision 31070-31087
Injection 20500
   Diagnostic 20501
Maxillary
   Antrostomy 31256-31267
   Caldwell-Luc Operation 21385
   Dilation 31295
   Excision 31225-31230
   Exploration 31020-31032
   with Nasal/Sinus Endoscopy 31233
   Incision 31020-31032, 31256-31267
   Irrigation 31000

Skull Base 61581
   Surgery 61581
Multiple
   Incision 31090
   Paranasal
     Incision 31090
Pilonidal
   See Cyst, Pilonidal
Pyriform
   Resection 42892
Sinus of Valsalva
   Repair 33702-33722
Sinus Venosus
   Repair 33645
Sphenoid
   Biopsy 31050, 31051
   Dilation 31295
   Exploration 31050, 31051
     with Nasal/Sinus Endoscopy 31235
   Incision 31050, 31051
     with Nasal/Sinus Endoscopy . . 31287, 31288
   Irrigation 31002
   Repair of Cerebrospinal Leak 31291
   Sinusotomy 31050, 31051
   Skull Base Surgery 61580, 61581
Unlisted Services and Procedures 31299
X-ray 70210-70220

Sinusectomy, Ethmoid
See Sinus/Sinuses, Ethmoidectomy

Sinusoidal Rotational Testing
See Ear, Nose, and Throat

Sinusoscopy
Sinus
   Maxillary 31233
   Sphenoid 31235

Sinusotomy
Combined 31090
Frontal Sinus
   Exploratory 31070-31075
   Nonobliterative 31086, 31087
   Obliterative 31080-31085
Maxillary 31020-31032
   Caldwell-Luc Operation 21385
Multiple
   Paranasal 31090
Sphenoid Sinus 31050, 31051

Sirolimus
Drug Assay 80195

SISI Test 92564

Sistrunk Operation
See Cyst, Thyroid Gland, Excision

Six Minute Walk Test 94620

Size Reduction, Breast
See Breast, Reduction

Skeletal Fixation
Ankle Dislocation 27842, 27846
Bennett Fracture 26650
Calcaneal Fracture 28406
Carpometacarpal Fracture
Dislocation 26650, 26676
Femoral Fracture 27235, 27509
Humeral Fracture 24538, 24566, 24582
Interphalangeal Joint Dislocation . . 26776, 28666
Metacarpal Fracture 26608
Metacarpophalangeal Dislocation 26706
Metatarsal Fracture 28476

Metatarsophalangeal Dislocation 28636
Pelvic Bone Fracture/Dislocation 27216
Phalangeal Fracture 26727, 26756, 28496
Radial Fracture 25525, 25606
Radioulnar Dislocation 25671
Sternal Fracture 21825
Talar Fracture 28436
Talotarsal Joint Dislocation 28576
Tarsal Dislocation 28546
Tarsal Fracture 28456
Tarsometatarsal Joint Dislocation 28606
Tibial Fracture 27756
Ulnar Fracture 25651

Skeletal Traction
Insertion/Removal
   Pin/Wire 20650
Acetabulum Fracture 27220
Femoral Fracture 27232, 27240,
                 27502, 27503, 27517
Hip Socket 27220
Humerus Fracture 23605, 24505, 24535
Phalangeal Fracture 26725
Scapula Fracture 23575
Tibia Fracture 27532, 27752, 27762, 27825

Skene's Gland
Abscess
   Incision and Drainage 53060
Destruction 53270
Excision 53270

Skilled Nursing Facilities (SNFs)
See Nursing Facility Services

Skin
Abrasion 15786, 15787
   Chemical Peel 15788-15793
   Dermabrasion 15780-15783
Abscess
   See Abscess, Tissue, Skin/Superficial
Adjacent Tissue Transfer 14000-14350
Allografts
   See Allograft, Skin Substitute
Biopsy 11100, 11101
Chemical Exfoliation 17360
Complete Physical Examination 2029F
Cyst
   See Cyst, Skin
Debridement 11000-11006,
          11010-11012, 11042-11047
   Eczematous 11000, 11001
   Infected 11000-11006
   Subcutaneous Tissue 11042-11047
     Infected 11004-11006
   with Open Fracture and/or
     Dislocation 11010-11012
Decubitus Ulcer(s)
   See Pressure Ulcer (Decubitus)
Desquamation
   See Exfoliation
Destruction
   Benign Lesions
     One to Fourteen 17110
     Fifteen or More 17111
   Flat Warts 17111
   Lesions 17106-17108
   Malignant Lesions 17260-17286
     by Photodynamic Therapy 96567
   Premalignant Lesions
     by Photodynamic Therapy 96567
     Fifteen or More Lesions 17004
     First Lesion 17000
     Two to Fourteen Lesions 17003

Index

Index

Extraocular Muscles 67340
One Horizontal Muscle 67311
One Vertical Muscle 67314
Posterior Fixation Suture
Technique 67334, 67335
Previous Surgery, Not Involving
Extraocular Muscles 67331
Release Extensive Scar Tissue 67343
Superior Oblique Muscle............ 67318
Transposition 67320
Two Horizontal Muscles 67312
Two or More Vertical Muscles........ 67316

Strapping
See Cast; Splint
Ankle.................................. 29540
    Compression 29581, 29582
Arm
    Compression 29583, 29584
Chest................................. 29200
Elbow................................. 29260
Finger................................ 29280
    Compression 29584
Foot.................................. 29540
    Compression 29581, 29582
Hand 29280
    Compression 29584
Hip................................... 29520
Knee 29530
Leg
    Compression 29581, 29582
Shoulder 29240
Thorax................................ 29200
Toes.................................. 29550
Unlisted Services and Procedures 29799
Unna Boot............................. 29580
Wrist................................. 29260

Strassman Procedure 58540

Strayer Procedure
Leg, Lower.............................. 27687

Streptococcus pneumoniae Vaccine
See Vaccines

Streptococcus, Group A
Antigen Detection
    Immunoassay...................... 87430
    Nucleic Acid............... 87650-87652
Direct Optical Observation 87880

Streptococcus, Group B
by Immunoassay
    with Direct Optical Observation 87802

Streptokinase, Antibody 86590

Stress Tests
Cardiovascular 93015-93024
Multiple Gated Acquisition (MUGA). 78472, 78473
Myocardial Perfusion Imaging 78451-78454
Pulmonary 94620, 94621
    See Pulmonology, Diagnostic

Stricture
Dilation
    Gastric/Duodenal.................. 43245
    Ureteral
        Balloon 50706
        Endoscopy.......... 50553, 50572,
                 50575, 50953, 50972
        with Cystourethroscopy 52341-52343
        with Ureteroscopy 52344-52346

Repair
    Urethra..................... 53400-53405
Urethra
    See Urethral Stenosis

Stricturoplasty
Intestines 44615

Stroboscopy
Larynx 31579

STS 86592, 86593
See Syphilis Test

Stuart-Power Factor........... 85260

Study, Color Vision
See Color Vision Examination

Sturmdorf Procedure 57520

Styloid Process
Radial
    Excision 25230

Styloidectomy
Radial 25230

Stypven Time
See Russell Viper Venom Time

Subacromial Bursa
Arthrocentesis.................. 20610, 20611

Subclavian Arteries
See Artery, Subclavian

Subcutaneous Infusion
See Infusion, Subcutaneous

Subcutaneous Injection
See Injection, Subcutaneous

Subcutaneous Mastectomies
See Mastectomy, Subcutaneous

Subcutaneous Tissue
Excision................. 15830-15839, 15847

Subdiaphragmatic Abscess
See Abscess, Tissue, Subdiaphragmatic

Subdural Electrode
Insertion 61531-61533
Removal 61535

Subdural Hematonia
See Hematoma, Subdural

Subdural Puncture 61105-61108

Subdural Tap............... 61000, 61001

Sublingual Gland
Abscess
    Incision and Drainage 42310-42320
Calculi (Stone)
    Excision 42330
Cyst
    Drainage....................... 42409
    Excision 42408
Excision............................. 42450

Subluxation
Elbow 24640

Submandibular Gland
Calculi (Stone)
    Excision 42330-42335
Excision............................. 42440

Submaxillary Gland
Abscess
    Incision and Drainage 42310-42320

Submucous Resection of Nasal Septum
See Nasal Septum, Submucous Resection

Subperiosteal Implant
Reconstruction
    Mandible 21245, 21246
    Maxilla.................... 21245, 21246

Subphrenic Abscess
See Abscess, Tissue, Subphrenic

Subtrochanteric Fracture
See Femur, Fracture, Subtrochanteric

Sucrose Hemolysis Test
See Red Blood Cell (RBC), Fragility, Osmotic

Suction Lipectomies
See Liposuction

Sudoriferous Gland
See Sweat Glands

Sugar Water Test
See Red Blood Cell (RBC), Fragility, Osmotic

Sugars 84375-84379

Sugiura Procedure
See Esophagus, Repair, Varices

Sulfate
Chondroitin
    See Chondroitin Sulfate
DHA
    See Dehydroepiandrosterone Sulfate
Urine................................. 84392

Sulfation Factor
See Somatomedin

Sulphates
See Sulfate

Sumatran Mite Fever
See Scrub Typhus

Superficial Musculoaponeurotic System (SMAS) Flap
Rhytidectomy 15829

Supernumerary Digit
Reconstruction 26587
Repair............................... 26587

Supply
See Chemotherapy
Educational Materials.................. 99071
Low Vision Aids
    See Spectacle Services
Materials............................. 99070
Prosthesis
    Breast......................... 19396

Suppositories, Vaginal
See Pessary

Suppression................. 80400-80408

Suppression/Testing
See Evocative/Suppression Test

Suppressor T Lymphocyte Marker
See CD8

Sweat Test 82435
See Chloride, Blood

Swenson Procedure 45120

Syme Procedure 27888

Sympathectomy
Artery
    Digital 64820
    Radial 64821
    Superficial Palmar Arch 64823
    Ulnar 64822
Cervical 64802
Cervicothoracic 64804
Digital Artery
    with Magnification 64820
Lumbar 64818
Presacral 58410
Thoracic 32664
Thoracolumbar 64809
with Rib Excision 21616

Sympathetic Nerve
Excision 64802-64818
Injection
    Anesthetic 64508, 64520-64530

Sympathins
See Catecholamines

Symphysiotomy
Horseshoe Kidney 50540

Symphysis, Pubic
See Pubic Symphysis

Syncytial Virus, Respiratory
See Respiratory Syncytial Virus

Syndactylism, Toes
See Webbed, Toe

Syndactyly
Repair 26560-26562

Syndesmotomy
See Ligament, Release

Syndrome
Adrenogenital
    See Adrenogenital Syndrome
Ataxia-Telangiectasia
    See Ataxia Telangiectasia
Bloom
    See Bloom Syndrome
Carpal Tunnel
    See Carpal Tunnel Syndrome
Costen's
    See Temporomandibular Joint (TMJ)
Erb-Goldflam
    See Myasthenia Gravis
Ovarian Vein
    See Ovarian Vein Syndrome
Synechiae, Intrauterine
    See Adhesions, Intrauterine
Treacher Collins
    See Treacher-Collins Syndrome
Urethral
    See Urethral Syndrome

Syngesterone
See Progesterone

Synostosis (Cranial)
See Craniosynostosis

Synovectomy
Ankle 27625, 27626
    Partial 29895
Elbow 24102, 29836
    Partial 29835
    with Prosthesis Removal
        Humeral and Ulnar Components 24160
        Radial Head 24164
Carpometacarpal Joint 26130
Finger
    Joint 26135-26140
    Tendon Sheath 26145
Foot
    Tendon Sheath 28086, 28088, 28090
Glenohumeral Joint 23105
Hip Joint 27054, 29863
Interphalangeal Joint 26140
Intertarsal Joint 28070
Knee Joint 27334, 27335
    Partial 27441, 27443, 29875, 29876
Metacarpophalangeal Joint 26135
Metatarsophalangeal Joint 28072
Palm
    Tendon Sheath 26145
Shoulder
    with Prosthesis Removal 23334, 23335
Shoulder Joint 29821
    Partial 29820
Sternoclavicular Joint 23106
Subtalar Joint 29905
Tarsometatarsal Joint 28070
Wrist
    Joint 25105, 29845
    Partial 29844
    Radical 25115, 25116
    Tendon Sheath 25118, 25119

Synovial
Bursa
    See Bursa
Cyst
    See Ganglion
Membrane
    See Synovium
Popliteal Space
    See Baker's Cyst

Synovium
Biopsy
    Carpometacarpal Joint 26100
    Interphalangeal Joint 26110
    Knee Joint 27330
    Metacarpophalangeal Joint
        with Synovial Biopsy 26105
Excision
    Carpometacarpal Joint 26130
    Finger Joint 26135-26140
    Hip Joint 27054
    Interphalangeal Joint 26140
    Knee Joint 27334, 27335

Syphilis ab
See Antibody, Detection, Treponema Pallidum

Syphilis Test 86592, 86593

Syrinx
Spinal Cord
    Aspiration 62268

System
Endocrine
    See Endocrine System

Hemic
    See Hemic System
Lymphatic
    See Lymphatic System
Musculoskeletal
    See Musculoskeletal System
Nervous
    See Nervous System

T

T Cell Leukemia Virus I Antibodies, Adult
See Antibody, Detection, HTLV-I

T Cell Leukemia Virus I, Human
See HTLV I

T Cell Leukemia Virus II Antibodies, Human
See Antibody, Detection, HTLV-II

T Cell Leukemia Virus II, Human
See HTLV II

T Cells
CD4
    Absolute 86361
Count 86359
Gene Rearrangement 81340-81342
Ratio 86360

T Lymphotropic Virus Type III Antibodies, Human
See Antibody, Detection, HIV

T-3
See Triiodothyronine

T3 Free
See Triiodothyronine, Free

T-4 .... 84436-84439, 86360

T4 Molecule
See CD4

T4 Total
See Thyroxine, Total

T-7 Index
See Thyroxine, Total

T-8
See CD8; T-Cells, Ratio

T-Cell T8 Antigens
See CD8

T-Phyl
See Theophylline

Taarnhoj Procedure
See Decompression, Gasserian Ganglion, Sensory Root; Section

Tachycardia
Mapping of Sites 93609, 93654
Treatment
    Ventricular 93653, 93654

Tacrolimus
Drug Assay 80197

Tag, Skin
See Skin, Tags

Tail Bone
Excision 27080
Fracture 27200-27202

Takeuchi Procedure 33505

Talectomy
See Astragalectomy

Talotarsal Joint
Dislocation 28570-28575, 28585
   Percutaneous Fixation 28576

Talus
Arthrodesis
   Pantalar 28705
   Subtalar 28725
   Triple 28715
Arthroscopy
   Surgical 29891, 29892
      Subtalar 29904-29907, 29915, 29916
Autograft, Osteochondral 28446
Craterization 28120
Cyst
   Excision 28100-28103
Diaphysectomy 28120
Excision 28120, 28130
Fracture
   Open Treatment 28445
   Percutaneous Fixation 28436
   with Manipulation 28435, 28436
   without Manipulation 28430
Repair
   Osteochondritis Dissecans 29892
   Osteotomy 28302
Saucerization 28120
Subtalar Joint
   Implant for Stabilization 0335T
Tumor
   Excision 28100-28103
   Radical Resection 27647

TAP (Transversus Abdominis Plane) Block
Cisternal
   See Cisternal Puncture
Lumbar Diagnostic
   See Spinal Tap
Somatic Nerves 64486-64489

Tarsal
Fracture
   Percutaneous Fixation 28456

Tarsal Bone
See Repair, Tarsal

Tarsal Joint
See Foot
Arthrodesis 28730-28735, 28740
   with Advancement 28737
   with Lengthening 28737
Craterization 28122
Cyst
   Excision 28104-28107
Diaphysectomy 28122
Dislocation 28540-28545, 28555
   Percutaneous Fixation 28545, 28546
Excision 28116, 28122
Fracture
   Open Treatment 28465
   with Manipulation 28455, 28456
   without Manipulation 28450

Fusion 28730-28735, 28740
   with Advancement 28737
   with Lengthening 28737
Repair
   Nonunion or Malunion 28320
   Osteotomy 28304, 28305
Saucerization 28122
Tumor
   Excision 28104-28107
   Radical Resection 28171

Tarsal Strip Procedure 67917-67924

Tarsal Tunnel Release 28035

Tarsal Wedge Procedure 67916, 67923

Tarsometatarsal Joint
Arthrodesis 28730-28735, 28740
Arthrotomy 28020, 28050
Dislocation 28600-28605, 28615
   Percutaneous Fixation 28606
Exploration 28020
Fusion 28730-28735, 28740
Removal
   Foreign Body 28020
   Loose Body 28020
Synovial
   Biopsy 28050
   Excision 28070

Tarsorrhaphy 67875
Median 67880
Severing 67710
   with Transposition of Tarsal Plate 67882

Tattoo
Cornea 65600
Skin 11920-11922

TAVR/TAVI
See Transcatheter Aortic Valve Replacement (TAVR/TAVI)

TB Test
Antigen Response 86480, 86481
Skin Test 86580

TBG
See Thyroxine Binding Globulin

TBS
See Bethesda System

TCT
See Thrombin Time

Td Shots
See Tetanus

Team Conference
Case Management Services 99366-99368

Tear Duct
See Lacrimal Duct

Tear Film Imaging 0330T

Tear Gland
See Lacrimal Gland

Technique
Pericardial Window
   See Pericardiostomy
Projective
   See Projective Test

Teeth
X-ray 70300-70320

Telangiectasia
Chromosome Analysis 88248
Injection 36468

Telangiectasia, Cerebello-Oculocutaneous
See Ataxia Telangiectasia

Telephone
Consultation 99446-99449
Evaluation and Management
   Nonphysician 98966-98968
   Physician 99441-99443
Pacemaker Analysis 93293

Teletherapy
Dose Plan 77306, 77307

Temperature Gradient Studies 93740

Temporal Arteries
See Artery, Temporal

Temporal Bone
Electromagnetic Bone Conduction Hearing Device
   Implantation/Replacement 69710
   Removal/Repair 69711
Excision 69535
Resection 69535
Tumor
   Removal 69970
Unlisted Services and Procedures 69979

Temporal, Petrous
Excision
   Apex 69530

Temporomandibular Joint (TMJ)
Arthrocentesis 20605, 20606
Arthrography 70328-70332
   Injection 21116
Arthroplasty 21240-21243
Arthroscopy
   Diagnostic 29800
   Surgical 29804
Arthrotomy 21010
Cartilage
   Excision 21060
Condylectomy 21050
Coronoidectomy 21070
Dislocation
   Closed Treatment 21480-21485
   Open Treatment 21490
Injection
   Radiologic 21116
Magnetic Resonance Imaging (MRI) 70336
Manipulation 21073
Meniscectomy 21060
Prostheses
   See Prosthesis, Temporomandibular Joint
Reconstruction
   See Reconstruction, Temporomandibular Joint
X-ray with Contrast 70328-70332

Tenago Procedure 53431

Tendinosuture
See Suture, Tendon

Tendon
Achilles
   See Achilles Tendon

Thermocoagulation
See Electrocautery

Thermotherapy
Microwave
    Breast Tumor 0301T
    Prostate Tissue. 53850
Radiofrequency. 53852
    Prostate Tissue. 53852

Thiamine 84425

Thiersch Operation 15050
See Pinch Graft

Thiersch Procedure 46753

Thigh
Fasciotomy 27025
    See Femur; Leg, Upper

Thin Layer Chromatographies
See Chromatography, Thin-Layer

Thiocyanate 84430

Third Disease
See Rubella

Thompson Procedure 27430

Thoracectomy
See Thoracoplasty

Thoracentesis 32554, 32555
with Imaging Guidance. 32555

Thoracic
Anterior Ramus
    See Intercostal Nerve
Aorta
    See Aorta, Thoracic
Arteries
    See Artery, Thoracic
Cavity
    See Chest Cavity
Duct
    See Lymphatics
    Cannulation 38794
    Ligation 38380
        Abdominal Approach 38382
        Thoracic Approach 38381
    Suture
        Abdominal Approach 38382
        Cervical Approach 38380
        Thoracic Approach 38381
Empyema
    See Pleural Cavity, Incision, Empyema
Surgery
    Video-Assisted
        See Thoracoscopy
Vertebra
    See Vertebra, Thoracic
Wall
    See Chest Wall

Thoracocentesis
See Thoracentesis

Thoracoplasty 32905
with Closure Bronchopleural Fistula. 32906

Thoracoscopy
Diagnostic
    with Biopsy 32604, 32606, 32607-32609
    without Biopsy. 32601
Surgical. 32650-32674
    with Control Traumatic Hemorrhage 32654

with Creation Pericardial Window 32659
with Diagnostic Wedge Resection 32668
with Esophagomyotomy. 32665
with Excision Mediastinal Cyst, Tumor
    and/or Mass. 32662
with Excision Pericardial Cyst, Tumor
    and/or Mass. 32661
with Lobectomy 32663
with Mediastinal Lymphadenectomy 32674
with Open Treatment of Rib Fracture
    Internal Fixation Placement . . . 21811-21813
with Parietal Pleurectomy 32656
with Partial Pulmonary Decortication . . 32651
with Pleurodesis 32650
with Regional Lymphadenectomy 32674
with Removal Intrapleural Foreign Body 32653
with Removal of Clot/Foreign Body. 32658
with Resection of Thymus 32673
with Resection-Plication of Bullae 32655
with Sternum Reconstruction 21743
with Therapeutic Wedge
    Resection 32666, 32667
with Thoracic Sympathectomy 32664
with Total Pulmonary Decortication . . . 32652

Thoracostomy
Drainage 32551
Empyema. 32035, 32036
Hemothorax. 32551
Tube. 32551

Thoracotomy
Cardiac Massage 32160
Lymphadenectomy
    Thoracic 38746
for Post-Op Complications 32120
Hemorrhage 32110
Removal
    Bullae. 32141
    Cyst 32140
    Defibrillator 33243
    Electrodes 33238
    Foreign Body
        Intrapleural. 32150
        Intrapulmonary 32151
    Pacemaker 33236, 33237
Repair
    Paraesophageal Hiatal Hernia. . . 43334, 43335
Resection
    Diagnostic Wedge 32507
    Therapeutic Wedge 32505, 32506
Transmyocardial Laser
Revascularization 33140, 33141
with Biopsy. 32096, 32097
with Lung Repair. 32110
with Open Intrapleural Pneumolysis. 32124
with Resection-Plication of Bullae 32141

Thorax
See Chest; Chest Cavity; Mediastinum
Angiography 71275
Biopsy. 21550
CT Scan. 71250-71275
Incision
    Empyema 32035, 32036
Incision and Drainage
    Abscess 21501, 21502
    Deep. 21510
    Hematoma 21501, 21502
Stereotactic Body Radiation Therapy
    Target Delineation 32701
Strapping. 29200
Tube Thoracostomy. 32551

Tumor
    Excision 21552-21558
    Excision/Resection. 21557, 21558
Unlisted Services and Procedures, Surgery . . 21899

Three Glass Test
See Urinalysis, Glass Test

Three-Day Measles
See Rubella

Throat
See Pharynx
Abscess
    Incision and Drainage 42700-42725
Biopsy 42800-42806
Hemorrhage 42960-42962
Reconstruction 42950
Removal
    Foreign Body 42809
Repair
    Pharyngoesophageal 42953
    Wound 42900
Suture
    Wound 42900
Unlisted Services and Procedures 42999

Thrombectomy
See Thromboendarterectomy
Aortoiliac Artery 34151-34201
Arteriovenous Fistula
    Graft. 36870
Axillary Artery. 34101
Axillary Vein 34490
Brachial Artery 34101
Bypass Graft
    Other than Hemodialysis Graft
    or Fistula 35875, 35876
Carotid Artery 34001
Celiac Artery 34151
Dialysis Graft 36831, 36833
Femoral. 34201
Femoropopliteal Vein 34421-34451
Iliac 34151-34201
Iliac Vein 34401-34451
Innominate Artery. 34001-34101
Mesentery Artery 34151
Percutaneous
    Coronary Artery 92973
    Intracranial Artery 61645
    Noncoronary Artery 37184-37186
    Fluoroscopic Guidance. 37184-37188
    Mechanical Arterial. 37184-37186
    Mechanical Venous 37187, 37188
Peroneal Artery. 34203
Popliteal Artery 34201-34203
Radial Artery. 34111
Renal Artery 34151
Subclavian Artery 34001-34101
Subclavian Vein 34471-34490
Tibial Artery. 34203
Ulnar Artery. 34111
Vena Cava 34401-34451
Vena Caval 50230

Thrombin Inhibitor I
See Antithrombin III

Thrombin Time 85670-85675

Thrombocyte (Platelet)
See Blood, Platelet

Thrombocyte ab
See Antibody, Detection, Platelet

without Manipulation 27824
Incision 27607, 27455-27457,
27705, 27709-27712
Manipulation. . 27532, 27752, 27762, 27768, 27825
Neurostimulation
Posterior 64566
Osteoplasty
Lengthening 27715
Prophylactic Treatment 27745
Reconstruction 27418
at Knee 27440-27443, 27446
Repair 27720-27725
Epiphysis 27477-27485, 27730-27742
Malunion/Nonunion. 27720,
27722, 27724, 27725
Osteochondritis Dissecans
Arthroscopy 29892
Osteotomy 27455-27457,
27705, 27709-27712
Pseudoarthrosis 27727
Realignment 27712
Skeletal Traction
See Skeletal Traction, Tibia Fracture
Tubercleplasty 27418
Revascularization 37228-37235
Saucerization 27360, 27640
Tibiofibular Joint
Arthrodesis. 27871
Dislocation 27830-27832
Disruption. 27829
Tumor
Excision 27635-27638
Radical Resection 27645
X-ray 73590

Tibial
Arteries
See Artery, Tibial
Nerve
Repair/Suture
Posterior 64840

Tibiofibular Joint
Arthrodesis 27871
Dislocation 27830-27832
Disruption
Open Treatment 27829
Fusion 27871

TIG
See Immune Globulins, Tetanus

Time
Bleeding
See Bleeding Time
Prothrombin
See Prothrombin Time
Reptilase
See Thrombin Time

Tinnitus
Assessment. 92625

Tissue
Crystal Identification. 89060
Culture
Chromosome Analysis 88230-88239
Homogenization 87176
Non-neoplastic Disorder 88230, 88237
Skin Grafts 15100, 15101, 15120, 15121
Harvesting 15040
Solid Tumor 88239
Toxin/Antitoxin. 87230
Virus 87252, 87253
Dissection, Macroscopic 88387, 88388

Examination, Macroscopic 88387, 88388
Enzyme Activity. 82657
Examination for Ectoparasites 87220
Examination for Fungi 87220
Expander
Breast Reconstruction with 19357
Insertion
Skin. 11960
Removal
Skin. 11971
Replacement
Skin. 11970
Grafts
Harvesting 20926
Granulation
See Granulation Tissue
Homogenization 87176
Hybridization In Situ 88364-88366
Morphometric Analysis
Computer-Assisted. . . . 88367, 88373, 88374
Manual 88368, 88369, 88377
Implant
Biological 15777
Mucosal
See Mucosa
Preparation
Macroscopic. 88387, 88388
Previously Diagnosed/Archived
Retrieved/Selected for Examination 88363
Skin Harvest for Culture 15040
Soft
Abscess 20005
Drainage. 10030
Fluid Collection 10030
Tumor
See Tumor, Excision
See Tumor, Radical Resection
Substitute 15271-15278
Transfer
Adjacent
Eyelids 67961
Skin. 14000-14350
Facial Muscles 15845
Finger Flap 14350
Toe Flap 14350
Typing
Culture 87140-87158
Human Leukocyte Antigen (HLA)
Antibodies 86812-86817
Crossmatch. 86825, 86826
Lymphocyte Culture 86821, 86822

Tissue Culture
from Skin Harvest 15040
Skin Grafts 15150-15157

Tissue Factor
See Thromboplastin

TLC
See Chromatography, Thin-Layer
Screen. 84375

TMJ
See Temporomandibular Joint (TMJ)
Manipulation, Therapeutic
See Manipulation, Temporomandibular Joint(s)
(TMJ)
Prostheses
See Prosthesis, Temporomandibular Joint

TMS
See Psychiatric Treatment, Transcranial Magnetic
Stimulation (TMS)

Tobacco
See Performance Measures

TMVR
See Transcatheter, Mitral Valve Repair

Tobramycin
Assay. 80200

Tocolysis 59412

Tocopherol 84446

Toe
Amputation 28810-28825
Arthrocentesis. 20600, 20604
Bone
Condyle
Excision. 28126
Craterization. 28124
Cyst
Excision. 28108
Diaphysectomy. 28124
Excision 28150, 28810, 28820
Joint 28160, 28825
Partial 28124
Proximal End. 28160
Fracture
Closed Treatment 28510, 28515
Open Treatment 28525
with Manipulation 28515
without Manipulation 28510
Repair
Osteotomy 28310-28312
Resection
Base 28126
Condyle. 28153
with Macrodactyly Reconstruction . . 28341
Saucerization 28124
Transfer
Joint 26556
Toe-to-Hand 26553, 26554
Tumor
Excision. 28108
Radical Resection. 28175
Capsulotomy 28270-28272
Dislocation
See Dislocation, Toe
Fasciotomy 28008
Graft
Bone 26551
Flap. 14350, 20973
Tendon 20974
Lesion
Excision 28092
Reconstruction
Angle Deformity. 28313
Extra Toes. 28344
Hammertoe 28285, 28286
Macrodactyly 28340, 28341
Polydactyly 28344
Syndactylization. 28280
Syndactyly 28345
Webbed Toe 28345
Repair
Bunion 28290-28299
Cock-up Fifth 28286
Muscle 28240
Tendon 28232-28234, 28240
Webbed 28280
Webbed Toe 28345
Strapping. 29550
Tendon
Graft 20924
Incision 28010, 28011, 28232-28234

Unlisted Services and Procedures
  Bronchi.........................31899
Wound
  Suture
    Cervical.......................31800
    Intrathoracic...................31805

Tracheal
Stent
  Placement.......................31631
Tubes
  See Endotracheal Tube

Trachelectomy...................57530
Radical............................57531

Tracheloplasty
See Cervicoplasty

Trachelorrhaphy...............57720

Tracheo-Esophageal Fistula
Repair...................43305, 43312, 43314

Tracheobronchoscopy
through Tracheostomy...................31615

Tracheoplasty
Cervical...........................31750
Intrathoracic......................31760
Tracheopharyngeal Fistulization..........31755

Tracheostoma
Revision......................31613, 31614

Tracheostomy
Emergency................31603-31605
Planned....................31600, 31601
Revision
  Scar..........................31830
Surgical Closure
  with Plastic Repair.................31825
  without Plastic Repair...............31820
Tracheobronchoscopy through.............31615
with Flaps............................31610

Tracheotomy
Tube Change......................31502

Tracking Tests (Ocular)........92545
See Ear, Nose, and Throat

Tract, Urinary
See Urinary Tract

Traction Therapy
See Physical Medicine/Therapy/Occupational
Therapy
Manual.............................97140
Mechanical.........................97012

Tractotomy
Mesencephalon......................61480

Training
Activities of Daily Living...........97535, 99509
Biofeedback............90875, 90901-90911
Cognitive Skills......................97532
Community/Work Reintegration...........97537
Compensatory.................97532, 97535
Home Management...........97535, 99509
Orthoptic/Pleoptic...................92065
Orthotics............................97760
Prosthetics.........................97761
Self Care.........97535, 98960-98962, 99509
Sensory Integration...................97533
Walking (Physical Therapy)............97116
Wheelchair Management................97542

TRAM Flap
Breast Reconstruction............19367-19369

Trans-Scaphoperilunar
Fracture/Dislocation
  Closed Treatment..................25680
  Open Treatment....................25685

Transaminase
Glutamic-Oxaloacetic..................84450
Glutamic-Pyruvic.....................84460

Transanal Endoscopic Microsurgery (TEMS)
See Rectum, Tumor, Excision, Transanal Endoscopic

Transcatheter
Aortic Valve Replacement (TAVR/TAVI)
  Open Axillary Artery Approach........33363
  Open Femoral Artery Approach........33362
  Open Iliac Artery Approach..........33364
  Percutaneous Femoral Artery
  Approach..........................33361
  Transaortic Approach...............33365
  Transapical Approach...............33366
  with Cardiopulmonary Bypass
  Support...............33367, 33368, 33369
Biopsy............................37200
Closure
  Percutaneous
    Ductus Arteriosus................93582
    Heart.......................93580-93582
  Transmyocardial
    Cranial.....................61624-61626
Denervation
  Renal Sympathetic...........0338T, 0339T
Embolization
  Cranial......................61624-61626
  Vascular.....................37241-37244
Insertion
  Leadless Pacemaker System...........0387T
Mitral Valve Repair.......33418, 33419, 0345T
Occlusion
  Cranial......................61624-61626
  Vascular.....................37241-37244
Placement
  Intravascular Stent...........0075T, 0076T,
                    37215-37218, 37236-37239, 92928, 92929
  Sensor, Aneurysmal Sac............34806
Removal
  Leadless Pacemaker System..........0388T
Replacement
  Leadless Pacemaker System..........0387T
Retrieval
  Foreign Body (Fractured Catheter)......37197
Therapy
  Embolization...............75894, 75898
  Infusion (Arterial or Venous)....37211-37214,
                    61650, 61651
    Radiological Supervision..........75898
  Perfusion
    Cranial.....................61624-61626
  Septal Reduction...................93583

Transcatheter Aortic Valve Replacement (TAVR/TAVI)
Axillary Artery Approach...............33363
Femoral Artery Approach.........33361, 33362
Iliac Artery Approach.................33364
Transaortic Approach..................33365
Transapical Exposure..................33366

with Cardiopulmonary Bypass
Support......................33367-33369
with Arterial/Venous Cannulation...33367-33369

Transcatheter Foreign Body
Retrieval...........................37197

Transcortin.......................84449

Transcranial
Doppler Study (TCP)..............93886-93893
Stimulation, Magnetic............90867-90869
Stimulation, Motor.............95928, 95929

Transcutaneous Testing
Bilirubin............................88720
Carboxyhemoglobin...................88740
Hemoglobin (Hgb)....................88738
Unlisted In Vivo Procedure.............88749
Methemoglobin.......................88741

Transcutaneous Electric Nerve Stimulation
See Application, Neurostimulation

Transdermal Electrostimulation
See Application, Neurostimulation

Transcutaneous Electrical Modulation Pain Reprocessing...................0278T

Transection
Artery
  Carotid......................61610-61612
Blood Vessel
  Kidney..........................50100
Brain
  Subpial..........................61567
Nerve........................64732-64772
  Vagus......................43640, 43641
Pulmonary Artery.....................33922

Transesophageal
Doppler Echocardiography...93312-93318, 93355
  during Heart Procedure..............93355

Transfer
Blastocyst
  See Embryo Transfer
Gamete Intrafallopian
  See GIFT
Jejunum
  with Microvascular Anastomosis
    Free............................43496
Preparation
  Embryo..........................89255
    Cryopreserved..................89352
Surgical
  See Transposition
Tendon
  See Tendon, Transfer
Finger.............................26555
Toe Joint...........................26556
Toe to Hand...................26551-26556

Transferase
Alanine Amino.......................84460
Aspartate Amino.....................84450
Glutamic Oxaloacetic.................84450

Transferrin......................84466

Transformation
Lymphocyte.........................86353

Scapula
  Excision 23140, 23210
    with Allograft 23146
    with Autograft 23145
Shoulder
  Soft Tissue
    Excision 23071-23076
    Radical Resection 23077, 23078
Skin
  Mohs Micrographic Surgery 17311-17315
Skull
  Excision 61500
Spinal Cord
  Excision 63275-63290
Stomach
  Excision 43610, 43611
Talus
  Excision 28100-28103
  Radical Resection 27647
Tarsal
  Excision 28104-28107
  Radical Resection 28171
Temporal Bone
  Removal 69970
Testis
  Excision 54530-54535
Thigh
  Excision 27327, 27328, 27337, 27339
  Radical Resection 27329, 27364, 27365
Thorax
  Excision 21552-21558
  Radical Resection 21557, 21558
Thyroid
  Excision 60200
Tibia 27365, 27635-27638
  Radical Resection 27645
Toe
  Excision 28039-28045
  Radical Resection 28046, 28047
Torus Mandibularis 21031
Trachea
  Excision
    Cervical 31785
    Thoracic 31786
Ulna 25120-25126, 25170
  Excision 24120
  with Allograft
    Excision 24126
  with Autograft
    Excision 24125
Ureter
  Excision 52355
Urethra
  Excision 53220, 52355
  Fulguration 52234-52240
Uterus
  Excision 58140-58146
  Resection 58950-58958
Vagina
  Excision 57135
Vertebra
  Additional Segment
    Excision 22116
  Cervical
    Excision 22100
  Lumbar 22102
  Thoracic
    Excision 22101
Wrist
  Bone
    Curettage 25130, 25135, 25136
    Excision 25130, 25135, 25136
    Radical Resection 25077, 25078

Subcutaneous
  Excision 25071, 25075
Subfascial
  Excision 25073, 25076

Tunica Vaginalis
Hydrocele
  Aspiration 55000
  Excision 55040, 55041
  Repair 55060

Turbinate
Excision 30130-30140
Fracture
  Therapeutic 30930
Injection 30200
Submucous Resection
  Nose Excision 30140

Turbinate Mucosa
Cauterization 30801, 30802

Turcica, Sella
See Sella Turcica

TURP
See Prostatectomy, Transurethral

Tylectomy
See Breast, Excision, Lesion

Tympanic Membrane
Create Stoma 69433, 69436
  Myringoplasty 69620
  Myringotomy 69421
  Neurectomy 69676
  Repair 69610
  Tympanolysis 69450
  Tympanoplasty
    See Tympanoplasty
  Tympanostomy 69433, 69436
    Removal of Tube 69424

Tympanic Nerve
Excision 69676

Tympanolysis 69450

Tympanomastoidectomy
See Tympanoplasty

Tympanometry 92550, 92567, 92570
See Audiologic Function Tests

Tympanoplasty
See Myringoplasty
  with Ossicular Chain Reconstruction 69646
with Antrotomy or Mastoidotomy 69635
  with Ossicular Chain Reconstruction . . . 69636
  and Synthetic Prosthesis 69637
with Mastoidectomy 69641
  Radical or Complete 69645
  with Intact or Reconstructed Wall 69643
  and Ossicular Chain Reconstruction . 69644
  with Ossicular Chain Reconstruction . . . 69642
without Mastoidectomy 69631
  with Ossicular Chain Reconstruction . . 69632
  and Synthetic Prosthesis 69633

Tympanostomy
Local Anesthetic 69433
General Anesthesia 69436
Removal of Tube 69424

Tympanotomy
See Myringotomy

Typhoid Vaccine
Oral 90690
Intramuscular 90691

Typhus
Endemic
  See Murine Typhus
Mite-Borne
  See Scrub Typhus
Sao Paulo
  See Rocky Mountain Spotted Fever
Tropical
  See Scrub Typhus

Typing, Blood
See Blood Typing, Serologic

Typing, HLA
See Human Leukocyte Antigen (HLA), TissueTyping

Typing, Tissue
See Tissue, Typing

Tyrosine 84510

Tzank Smear 88160, 88161

U

UDP Galactose Pyrophosphorylase
See Galactose-1-Phosphate, Uridyl Transferase

UFR
See Uroflowmetry

Ulcer
Anal
  See Anus, Fissure
Decubitus
  Excision
    Coccygeal 15920, 15922
    Ischial 15940, 15941, 15944-15946
    Sacral 15931, 15933-15937
    Trochanteric . . . 15950-15953, 15956, 15958
    Unlisted Procedure 15999
Pinch Graft 15050
Pressure 15920-15999
Stomach
  Excision 43610

Ulcerative, Cystitis
See Cystitis, Interstitial

Ulna
See Arm, Lower; Elbow; Humerus; Radius
Arthrodesis
  Radioulnar Joint
    with Bone Graft 25830
    with Resection 25830
Arthroplasty
  with Implant 25442
Bone Graft 25830
Centralization or Wrist 25335
Craterization 24147, 25150, 25151
Cyst
  Excision 24125, 24126, 25120-25126
Diaphysectomy 24147, 25150, 25151
Excision 24138
  Abscess 24138
  Complete 25240
  Epiphyseal Bar 20150

Unilateral Simple Mastectomy
See Mastectomy

Unlisted Services and Procedures 99499, 99600
Abdomen............... 22999, 49329, 49999
Allergy/Immunology..................... 95199
Anal............................... 46999
Anesthesia.......................... 01999
Arm................................ 25999
Arthroscopy......................... 29999
Autopsy............................ 88099
Bile Duct........................... 47999
Bladder............................ 51999
Brachytherapy....................... 77799
Breast............................. 19499
Bronchi............................ 31899
Cardiac............................ 33999
Cardiovascular Studies................. 93799
Casting............................ 29799
Cervix............................. 58999
Chemistry Procedure.................. 84999
Chemotherapy....................... 96549
Chest.............................. 32999
Coagulation......................... 85999
Colon.............................. 45399
Conjunctiva Surgery.................. 68399
Craniofacial........................ 21299
CT Scan............................ 76497
Cytogenetic Study.................... 88299
Cytopathology....................... 88199
Dermatology........................ 96999
Dialysis............................ 90999
Diaphragm.......................... 39599
Ear
    External........................ 69399
    Inner.......................... 69949
    Middle......................... 69799
Endocrine System.................... 60699
Epididymis.......................... 55899
Esophagus.................... 43289, 43499
Evaluation and Management Services...... 99499
Eye
    Extraocular Muscle................ 67399
Eye Surgery
    Anterior Segment................. 66999
    Posterior Segment................ 67299
Eyelid............................. 67999
Fluoroscopy......................... 76496
Forearm............................ 25999
Gallbladder......................... 47999
Gastroenterology Test................. 91299
Gum............................... 41899
Hand.............................. 26989
Hemic System....................... 38999
Hepatic Duct........................ 47999
Hip Joint........................... 27299
Home Services....................... 99600
Hysteroscopy........................ 58579
Immunization........................ 90749
Immunology......................... 86849
Infusion............................ 96379
Injection........................... 96379
Injection of Medication................ 96379
Intestine
    Laparoscopic.................... 44238
    Small.......................... 44799
Kidney............................. 53899
Lacrimal System...................... 68899
Laparoscopy........ 38129, 38589, 43289, 43659,
44238, 44979, 47379, 47579, 49329, 49659, 50549,
50949, 54699, 55559, 58578, 58679, 59898, 60659
Larynx............................. 31599

Lip................................ 40799
Liver.......................... 47379, 47399
Lungs.............................. 32999
Lymphatic System.................... 38999
Magnetic Resonance.................. 76498
Maxillofacial........................ 21299
Maxillofacial Prosthetics.............. 21089
Meckel's Diverticulum................. 44899
Mediastinum........................ 39499
Mesentery Surgery................... 44899
Microbiology........................ 87999
Mouth......................... 40899, 41599
Musculoskeletal................ 25999, 26989
Musculoskeletal Surgery
    Abdominal Wall.................. 22999
    Neck........................... 21899
    Spine.......................... 22899
    Thorax......................... 21899
Musculoskeletal System............... 20999
    Ankle.......................... 27899
    Arm, Upper...................... 24999
    Elbow.......................... 24999
    Head........................... 21499
    Knee........................... 27599
    Leg, Lower...................... 27899
    Leg, Upper...................... 27599
Necropsy........................... 88099
Nervous System Surgery............... 64999
Neurology/Neuromuscular Testing........ 95999
Noninvasive Vascular Study............. 93998
Nose.............................. 30999
Nuclear Medicine..................... 78999
    Blood.......................... 78199
    Bone........................... 78399
    Endocrine System................. 78099
    Genitourinary System.............. 78799
    Heart.......................... 78499
    Hematopoietic System.............. 78199
    Lymphatic System................. 78199
    Musculoskeletal System............ 78399
    Nervous System.................. 78699
    Therapeutic..................... 79999
Obstetrical Care.................. 59898, 59899
Omentum...................... 49329, 49999
Ophthalmology...................... 92499
Orbit.............................. 67599
Otorhinolaryngology.................. 92700
Ovary......................... 58679, 58999
Oviduct........................ 58679, 58999
Palate............................. 42299
Pancreas Surgery.................... 48999
Pathology.......................... 89240
Pelvis............................. 27299
Penis.............................. 55899
Peritoneum..................... 49329, 49999
Pharynx............................ 42999
Physical Therapy.......... 97039, 97139, 97799
Pleura............................. 32999
Pressure Ulcer....................... 15999
Preventive Medicine.................. 99429
Prostate............................ 55899
Psychiatric.......................... 90899
Pulmonology........................ 94799
Radiation Physics.................... 77399
Radiation Therapy.................... 77499
    Planning....................... 77299
Radiology, Diagnostic................. 76499
Radionuclide Therapy................. 79999
Radiopharmaceutical Therapy........... 79999
Rectum........................ 45499, 45999
Reproductive Medicine
    Laboratory Procedure.............. 89398
Salivary Gland....................... 42699

Scrotum............................ 55899
Seminal Vesicle...................... 55899
Shoulder Surgery.................... 23929
Sinuses............................ 31299
Skin............................... 17999
Special Services and Reports............ 99199
Spine.............................. 22899
Stomach........................ 43659, 43999
Strapping........................... 29799
Surgical Pathology................... 88399
Temporal Bone...................... 69979
Testis......................... 54699, 55899
Throat............................. 42999
Tongue............................. 41599
Tonsil/Adenoid...................... 42999
Toxoid............................. 90749
Trachea............................ 31899
Transfusion......................... 86999
Ultrasound.......................... 76999
Ureter............................. 50949
Urinary System...................... 53899
Uterus................ 58578, 58579, 58999
Uvula.............................. 42299
Vaccine............................ 90749
Vagina............................. 58999
Vas Deferens........................ 55899
Vascular............................ 37799
Vascular Endoscopy.................. 37501
Vascular Injection.................... 36299
Vascular Studies................. 93799, 93998
Wrist.............................. 25999

Unna Paste Boot 29580
Removal............................ 29700

UPP
See Urethra Pressure Profile

Upper
Digestive System Endoscopy
    See Endoscopy, Gastrointestinal, Upper
Extremity
    See Arm, Upper; Elbow; Humerus
Gastrointestinal Bleeding
    See Gastrointestinal, Upper, Hemorrhage
Gastrointestinal Endoscopy, Biopsy
    See Biopsy
    Planning
        See Biopsy, Gastrointestinal, Upper
        Endoscopy; Endoscopy, Gastrointestinal
GI Tract
    See Gastrointestinal Tract, Upper

Urachal Cyst
See Cyst, Urachal

Urea Breath Test 78267, 78268, 83014

Urea Nitrogen
Blood.......................... 84520-84525
Clearance.......................... 84545
Quantitative........................ 84520
Semiquantitative..................... 84525
Urine.............................. 84540

Urea Nitrogen, Blood
See Blood Urea Nitrogen

Urecholine Supersensitivity Test
See Cystometrogram

Ureter
Anastomosis
    to Bladder.................. 50780-50785
    to Colon.................... 50810-50815

Index

Index

Index

X

X, Coagulation Factor
See Stuart-Prower Factor

X, Cranial Nerve
See Vagus Nerve

X-Linked Ichthyoses
See Syphilis Test

X-ray

Index

X-ray Tomography, Computed
See CT Scan

Xa, Coagulation Factor
See Thrombokinase

Xenoantibodies
See Antibody, Detection, Heterophile

Xenografts, Skin
See Allograft, Skin Substitute

Xenotransplantation
See Allograft

XI, Coagulation Factor
See Plasma Thromboplastin, Antecedent

XI, Cranial Nerve
See Accessory Nerve, Spinal

XII, Coagulation Factor
See Hageman Factor

XII, Cranial Nerve
See Hypoglossal Nerve

XIII, Coagulation Factor
See Fibrin Stabilizing Factor

Xylose Absorption Test
Blood 84620
Urine 84620

Y

Yacoub Procedure
See Heart, Cardiopulmonary Bypass, with
Ascending Aorta Graft

Yeast
Culture 87106

Yellow Fever Vaccine 90717

Yersinia
Antibody 86793

**YHrium-Aluminum-Garnet
(YAG) Laser**
See Eye, Incision

Z

Ziegler Procedure
Discission Secondary Membranous
Cataract 66820

Zinc 84630

**Zinc Manganese Leucine
Aminopeptidase**
See Leucine Aminopeptidase

Zonisamide
Drug Assay 80203

Zygoma
See Zygomatic Arch

Zygomatic Arch
Fracture
    Open Treatment 21356-21366
    with Manipulation 21355
Reconstruction 21255

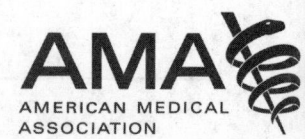